RADIOLOGY OF THE HEART AND GREAT VESSELS

Third Edition

VOLUMES OF
GOLDEN'S DIAGNOSTIC RADIOLOGY SERIES

RADIOLOGY OF THE HEART AND GREAT VESSELS
Third Edition

Robert N. Cooley, M.D.
Professor of Radiology
University of Texas Medical Branch
Galveston, Texas

and

Melvyn H. Schreiber, M.D.
Professor and Chairman
Department of Radiology
University of Texas Medical Branch
Galveston, Texas

with a section on

Coronary Arteriography
by

Luis B. Morettin, M.D.
Associate Professor of Radiology
University of Texas Medical Branch
Galveston, Texas

The Williams & Wilkins Company   Baltimore

GOLDEN'S DIAGNOSTIC RADIOLOGY
Laurence L. Robbins, M.D., Editor

Made in the United States of America

Library of Congress Cataloging in Publication Data
Cooley, Robert N.
    Radiology of the heart and great vessels.

    (Golden's diagnostic radiology; section 4)
    Bibliography: p.
    Includes index.
    1. Cardiovascular system—Radiography. I. Schreiber, Melvyn H., joint author. II. Morettin, Luis B. III. Title. [DNLM: 1. Angiocardiography. WG141 C774r]
RC78.G6   sect. 4   [RC683.5.R3]   616.07'572'08s   77-20171
ISBN 0-683-02103-6   [616.1'2'07572]

Composed and printed at the
Waverly Press, Inc.
Mt. Royal and Guilford Aves.
Baltimore, Md. 21202, U.S.A.

DEDICATION

To our wives, Grace and Tina

Preface to the Third Edition

In attempting a second revision the authors realize that they could not aspire to produce a work that would cover in a detailed manner all aspects of cardiac radiology as practiced in a large medical center. The personal experience of three authors is limited to certain specific areas of practice. The literature is enormous and to a degree unmanageable. Also, the practice of cardiac radiology is rapidly changing. Consequently, certain compromises were accepted. The section on abdominal aortography found in previous editions was eliminated. The relatively new radiologic modalities of echocardiography and nuclear imaging are mentioned frequently where in the authors' experience they have been helpful. Useful references are provided, but no attempt is made to provide interpretations or describe technical details of these procedures. This we believe is best done by those intimately engaged in the performance of the procedures.

As was the case in earlier editions this book is directed to the resident in training and the general practitioner of diagnostic radiology. For this reason, we have included much basic material and hopefully have presented it in a straightforward manner. We make no apologies for many older references. Most are quite valid, and much of the new literature is not concerned with basic radiologic procedures that have been in use for many years.

For the resident in training cardiac radiology often has a low priority because many of the special studies are often provided by other disciplines or the training is relegated to a fourth year to be spent entirely in the subspeciality. In order to participate in combined teaching sessions and the activities of cardiac catheterization laboratories, certain basic physiologic and clinical knowledge is required. We hope that we have provided a minimum but sufficient amount of information in these areas to enable the resident

in radiology of participate in these activities with understanding and profit.

The general diagnostic radiologist, using conventional chest films, is often influential in the initial disposition of patients with cardiac disease and their subsequent follow-up. Also, if the patient is referred to a cardiac center for surgical or medical treatment, an understanding of the procedures and treatment employed is necessary for adequate management and follow-up. We hope that the emphasis on conventional film interpretation will be useful in this regard.

The literature is too vast to permit a complete review for each entity. We are fearful that either through poor judgment or lack of time we have not used references of outstanding value and merit. For this we apologize.

Many of the active contributors to the literature and our friends have graciously allowed us to use their illustrations and other material. These are acknowledged in the legends and in the text. We express our sincere thanks to them.

We freely acknowledge our debt to a number of standard reference works in closely allied fields. Two most helpful books have been *Heart Disease in Infancy and Childhood,* 2nd edition, 1967, by J. D. Keith, R. P. Rowe, and P. Vlad; and *Heart Disease in Infants, Children and Adolescents,* edited by A. J. Moss and F. P. Adams. We have also freely consulted *Heart Disease* by P. D. White, *Congenital Malformations of the Heart* by H. B. Taussig, and *The Diagnosis of Congenital Heart Disease* by S. R. Kjellberg, E. Mannheimer, U. Rudhe, and B. Jonsson.

We express our thanks to Ms. Ruby Richardson of The Williams & Wilkins Company for her cooperation and encouragement and for her toleration of the many delays in preparing the manuscript.

The reproductions were provided by the painstaking efforts of Mr. Milan Autengruber and Mr. Lester Murray of our photographic department. We express our appreciation for their cooperation and tolerance of our many intrusions into their routine duties.

Words cannot express our appreciation of the efforts and cooperation of our secretaries, Mrs. Teresa Vargas and Ms. Tina Gourley, who gathered references, typed and retyped the manuscript, and kept our offices operating smoothly for the last several years.

ROBERT N. COOLEY, M.D.
MELVYN H. SCHREIBER, M.D.

Preface to the Second Edition

In the medical field the addition of new knowledge over a period of a very few years is ample justification for a revision of a previous work. When the revision is attempted the authors naturally aspire to remedy and eliminate the shortcomings of their first efforts. However, the burgeoning field of cardiovascular radiology presents special problems to those who attempt even a revision of a work on this subject. Because of the great mass of accumulated knowledge and the limitations of human capacity, two authors cannot hope to cover the entire subject in a detailed and exhaustive manner. An indication of this problem is the recent trend toward composite works with multiple authors, each limiting himself to a relatively narrow area in the field of cardiovascular radiology, which may be treated in an exhaustive manner. With a number of such works now available and the large space devoted to this subject in current radiologic literature, the question might well be asked: "Why a compendium of cardiovascular radiology?"

We have been active in residency training and in the teaching of medical students for some time. The usual habit of both of these groups is to gravitate to a number of standard reference works which they can keep at hand and which although not exhaustive are sufficiently inclusive to give some basic information on nearly all aspects of the subjects with which they deal. Likewise, the general radiologist, who frequently must deal with problems in cardiovascular radiology, prefers to begin his reading by referring to simple and rather straightforward descriptions of the conditions or entities in which he is interested. It is primarily to this group that this work is directed. We readily admit that for the specialists in cardiovascular radiology the present work brings little that is new or of special interest, though we hope that they will agree with our approach to many problems with which they are already familiar.

We have not by any means relied entirely on our own material. We have used contemporary literature freely, but even here we may not have reviewed all available sources. Indeed, we are fearful that either through poor judgment or limited time we may have omitted references to papers of outstanding value and merit. For this we apologize.

Many of the active contributors to the literature and many of our own friends have graciously allowed us to use their illustrations and other material. These are acknowledged in the legends of the illustrations and in the text. We express our sincere thanks to them.

We are indebted to Dr. Leonard C. Harris of the Department of Pediatric Cardiology who read the section on congenital anomalies and offered many valuable suggestions.

We freely acknowledge our debt to a number of standard reference works in closely allied fields. A most helpful book has been *Heart Disease in Infancy and Childhood* by J. D. Keith, R. P. Rowe, and P. Vlad. We have also freely consulted *Heart Disease* by P. D. White, *Congenital Malformations of the Heart* by H. B. Taussig, and *The Diagnosis of Congenital Heart Disease* by S. R. Kjellberg, E. Mannheimer, U. Rudhe, and B. Jonsson.

We appreciate the kindly way in which our editor, Dr. Laurence L. Robbins, has nursed us along in our efforts in preparing this work. We have taken advantage of his editorial comments with great profit. Also, Mr. Francis F. Old, Jr., of The Williams & Wilkins Company has been ever ready to place the entire resources and experience of his firm at our disposal. We express our thanks to both of these gentlemen.

Words can hardly express our admiration of

and appreciation for the efforts of our secretaries and particularly the work of Mrs. Teresa Vargas who personally typed all of the final manuscript and checked the numerous references.

ROBERT N. COOLEY, M.D.
MELVYN H. SCHREIBER, M.D.

Galveston, Texas
May 1, 1966

Contents

Key to Abbreviations

AO	— Aorta		MI	— Mitral Insufficiency
AI	— Aortic Insufficiency		MS	— Mitral Stenosis
AS	— Aortic Stenosis		MV	— Mitral Valve
ASD	— Atrial Septal Defect			
			PA	— Pulmonary Artery (Pulmonary Trunk)
CAS	— Congenital Aortic Stenosis		PAPVC	— Partial Anomalous Pulmonary Venous Connection
CPA	— Coarctation of Pulmonary Artery		PDA	— Patent Ductus Arteriosus
CTA	— Coarctation of Thoracic Aorta		PTA	— Persistent Truncus Arteriosus
			PTE	— Pulmonary Thromboembolism
IHSS	— Idiopathic Hypertrophic Subaortic Stenosis		RA	— Right Atrium
IIVC	— Interruption of Inferior Vena Cava		RAA	— Right Atrial Appendage
IVC	— Inferior Vena Cava		RAO	— Right Anterior Oblique (Left Posterior Oblique)
			RPA	— Right Pulmonary Artery
JAA	— Juxtaposition of Atrial Appendages		RSVC	— Right Superior Vena Cava
			RV	— Right Ventricle
LA	— Left Atrium			
LAA	— Left Atrial Appendage		SVC	— Superior Vena Cava
LAO	— Left Anterior Oblique (Right Posterior Oblique)		TAPVC	— Total Anomalous Pulmonary Venous Connection
LPA	— Left Pulmonary Artery			
LSVC	— Left Superior Vena Cava		VSD	— Ventricular Septal Defect
LV	— Left Ventricle			

1

Procedures

FLUOROSCOPY

Recent emphasis on the risks of radiation exposure has greatly curtailed the use of fluoroscopy in the examination of the heart and great vessels. When one considers that a good chest film can be obtained with less radiation than is applied during 0.5 sec of fluoroscopy, it is evident that fluoroscopy is an inefficient means of using radiation. Also, most patients with cardiovascular disease may be followed for significant periods of time with repeated and special examinations requiring the continued application of radiation. Particularly in children where the gonadal dose is high and where life expectancy and the reproductive period are longer, it is mandatory that radiation be used as efficiently as possible. For these reasons, fluoroscopy is no longer a routine procedure even in patients who are suspected of having a definite cardiac abnormality. Instead, it is occasionally used but only after viewing an adequate set of radiographs and with a certain definite objective in mind. The use of image amplification systems has reduced the amount of radiation necessary for fluoroscopy from ½ to ⅕ of that necessary for conventional apparatus; but even then, when compared with filming, the amount of radiation is abundant.

The advantages of fluoroscopy are that it is relatively inexpensive, can be performed quickly and with minimum discomfort to the patient, and, with an experienced observer, provides more information than any other simple procedure. Also, one much neglected advantage is the manner in which it brings the radiologist into intimate contact with the patient. Here the opportunity is given to question and examine firsthand and to assess the patient's problems. Although each patient comes with a satisfactory written history, a short period of questioning improves understanding and helps to cement a good doctor-patient relationship. Also, pertinent and obvious physical findings may be checked. Deform-

ities of the thorax which may alter the cardiac contour are easily appraised; familiarity with murmurs and thrills may be improved; the general appearance, habitus, and occupational and social status may be quickly noted and serve the experienced radiologist in his evaluation of the patient.

Adequate cardiac fluoroscopy should be carried out in 2–3 min of fluoroscopic time, but this requires considerable skill and experience. The question might well be raised that if fluoroscopy is to become infrequent, how will younger radiologists become trained in this field? This can be partially overcome by having a collection of film strips of fluoroscopy for teaching purposes. These film strips can be obtained by the experienced fluoroscopist on older persons and then reviewed with the entire resident staff at leisure, or better yet, a tape or disc system can record the entire procedure without a need for additional radiation.

Our opinion is that cardiac fluoroscopy will not become an extinct procedure and that radiologists should still be trained to perform it adequately and rapidly. It is the opinion of some clinicians that the radiologist should reach his conclusions only from objective findings and that he should make no attempt to obtain clinical information which might affect his opinion, or at least the clinical findings should be not be known until all the objective radiologic changes have been elicited. Although there may be considerable merit in this position and while such a routine may be helpful in the training period of students, it may hamper the well qualified radiologist who has accustomed himself to differentiate between demonstrated facts and less reliable opinion. Objective findings are much more plentiful when they are looked for; therefore, the patient's problems should be clearly in mind before the fluoroscopic examination is approached. The routine use of fluoroscopy in all cardiac patients, either at the initial visit or as a check-up procedure, is condemned.

Equipment

In the United States, image amplification is now widely available, and our discussion is limited to this modality. The apparatus must meet the minimum specifications for fluoroscopes as set forth in Handbook #60 of the National Bureau of Standards. The prescribed maximum output of 10 r/min as measured at the tabletop is much too high, and most equipment will provide satisfactory images at outputs of 2–3 r/min, and these should be measured directly. For infants and children, the output may be reduced to as little as 0.5 r/min depending on the size of the patient. For adults, our routine settings are 1.8 ma, 101 pkv, 3 mm aluminum filtration, and focal spot tabletop distance of 18 inches. In infants and children, the ma may be reduced to as low as 0.5, but we rarely use less than 90 pkv since lower pkv's are less efficient in image production.

For conventional fluoroscopy, a tilt table is useful because the recumbent position is occasionally necessary and helpful. A spot film device may occasionally provide an addition to routine radiography, particularly if the film is of high quality. For cardiac catheterization, coronary arteriography, and other procedures, the apparatus should be more specifically designed for their special use. Horizontal tables with mobile tabletops and supplemented by revolving cradles are necessary for coronary arteriography and cardiac catheterization, and this equipment will be further discussed under the individual procedures.

The fluoroscopic image is viewed either on a mirror or on a television monitor. To produce an image on a mirror, an optical system must gather the light and focus and bend it through an angle of 180°. Also, the image must be focused so that the cone of the light that is reflected from the mirror has a sharply limited cross-sectional area. This means that the observer's eyes must be within this cone of light before he can obtain binocular vision. This cone is not large and is variable with systems of different manufacturers. This strict limitation on the position of the eyes is a minor handicap in conventional fluoroscopy of the heart, and, in cardiac catheterization, it is a severe handicap.

Television viewing requires optical coupling of a Vidicon or Plumbicon camera to the output phosphor of the image amplifier, and this adds somewhat to the expense and bulk of the apparatus. On the other hand, the image on the television monitor is brighter than that of the mirror and can be viewed from any angle. Experience with both systems has shown that mirror viewing is certainly more awkward than the older ordinary fluoroscopy but can be mastered for conventional cardiac fluoroscopy. For cardiac catheterization, television monitor viewing is essential.

The use of caesium iodide phosphors and other developments has increased the gain of image intensifier tubes from 10,000–14,000 times. Despite this seemingly large gain, there has been relatively little corresponding reduction in radiation necessary for good image quality and particularly for the needs of cinefluorography. Contrast is due in part to the statistical fluctuation of the number of photons striking the input phosphor of the image tube over the integration time of the eye. This in turn is a function of the total number of photons that strike the input phosphor, and this, unfortunately, has an irreducible minimum. In order to obtain satisfactory contrast, a minimum of 10 mr/min at the input phosphor of the image tube is necessary for fluoroscopy. Radiation at the input phosphor is 0.5–1% of entrance exposure rate, depending on the size of the patient. Consequently, even with the higher gain tubes the radiation hazard must still be considered. These newer tubes do produce a brighter image and, of course, permit cone vision which in itself permits better perception of detail. It has been our experience that tube gain as stated by the manufacturer cannot always be confirmed, and it should be remembered that the gain is not constant over the entire operating range of the instrument.

Conventional cardiac fluoroscopy can be performed quite satisfactorily with most of the available instruments, although the 22- and 25-cm diameter circular tubes are more convenient for the adult heart. The smaller 12- and 15-cm tubes provide increased resolution and are thus desirable for special uses, such as coronary arteriography using cinefluorography. Dual and triple mode tubes (15- and 22-cm and 10-, 15-, and 22-cm diameter) may be a useful compromise for all kinds of fluoroscopy where the volume of patients is insufficient for separate instruments.

Technique of Fluoroscopy

The patient is first viewed in the posteroanterior projection in the erect position. The abdomen is scanned quickly to exclude the presence of gross abnormalities, or displacement or inversion of the abdominal viscera. The right side of the diaphragm is observed for motion while the patient takes a deep breath and then exhales. The costophrenic sinus is examined carefully. The right lung field is then scanned slowly while one looks for abnormal opacities, and the prominence of the vascular shadows is evaluated at this time. The upper mediastinum is viewed briefly, including aortic knob. The width and position of the knob and the amplitude of pulsations are noted. The left lung is then covered in the same manner from apex to base, and then the motion of the left diaphragm is studied in a similar manner to that used on the opposite side. The entire diaphragm is then viewed by providing a long horizontal field so that the motion of each side of the diaphragm can be compared. The patient is then asked to sniff vigorously to further accentuate the diaphragmatic motion.

The observer then turns his attention to the heart. Momentarily the shutters are opened sufficiently to encompass the heart and aorta, and these are observed during deep inspiration and expiration. The remainder of the examination is done using a field of about 100 cm². The right border of the heart is studied in detail. The amplitude of pulsations of the right atrium and right hilus are evaluated for any rhythmic variations in contour and amplitude of pulsations. The lateral border of the ascending aorta is identified and studied. The left border of the heart is covered in the same manner, the field often being reduced to a narrow vertical slit to study pulsa-

tions. The patient is then requested to cross his arms and to rest them on his head (Fig. 1) and is then turned into a slight degree of right anterior obliquity. As this obliquity is gradually increased, the anterior surface of the right ventricle and the pulmonary artery are brought into view. The patient is turned in short intervals until he reaches the straight lateral projection and the retrocardiac space is seen in its maximum width. Posterior projections of the left atrium or left ventricle may be visualized to a degree without barium in the esophagus. Also, an anterior extension of the heart into the retrosternal space may be evaluated. The patient is then rotated in a reverse direction back to the posteroanterior and then slowly into the left oblique projection (Fig. 1B). Again the contours are studied as the obliquity increases. In this view, the posterior wall of the left ventricle can be viewed to best advantage, and some estimate of its size can often be made. Also, the anterior surface of the ascending aorta is best studied in this projection. The pulmonary window may be visible, and the anterior surface of the right ventricle is brought into contour. Rotation is continued into the left lateral position where the appearance noted in the right lateral position can be confirmed. The patient is then given a mouthful of barium paste, and, after being turned into the posteroanterior

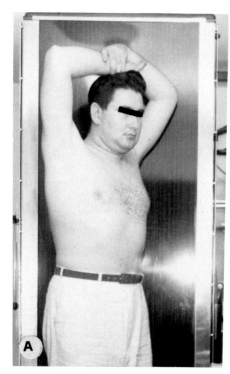 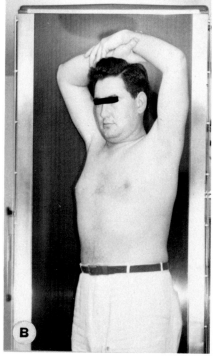

FIG. 1. POSITION OF PATIENT FOR FLUOROSCOPY IN (A) THE RIGHT ANTERIOR OBLIQUE AND (B) THE LEFT ANTERIOR OBLIQUE PROJECTIONS

projection, he is told to swallow. As the barium slowly traverses the length of the esophagus, the course and contours of this organ are determined in all projections, both in inspiration and expiration. This can be done rapidly by rotating the patient from one obliquity to the other. Finally, under certain circumstances, the patient is placed in a recumbent position, and the previous maneuvers are repeated partially or completely. Worthwhile observations concerning the presence of fluid in the pericardium or pleura may be made, although changes in the contour of the normal heart in the recumbent position must be kept in mind. Occasionally, the patient may be too sick to stand, and the entire examination must be conducted in the recumbent position; under such circumstances the procedure is less satisfactory than in the erect position. After this procedure, which lasts no longer than 5 min and requires no longer than 3 min of fluoroscopic time, the patient should be allowed to sit or lie down while the observer records his findings immediately. He should also write instructions for the technician who will take any further films that may be necessary. As an example, after the fluoroscopy of a case of mitral valvular disease with calcification, the directions would read as follows:

1. PA chest—conventional.
2. Right anterior oblique—50° rotation, 36-inch distance, extension cone, $\frac{1}{60}$-sec exposure; center to mark on anterior and posterior chest.
3. PA chest Bucky with barium.
4. Both obliques with 55° rotation with barium.

Limitations of Fluoroscopy

The surface of the heart contains a variable amount of fat which surrounds and obscures the vessels and sulci which serve to demarcate the heart chambers. The pericardium is a smooth sac which further serves to obscure the smaller surface landmarks. Consequently, only relatively gross changes in the cardiac contour can be detected by this method. In addition, in patients with heart disease there may be a number of overlying or surrounding densities which obscure the cardiac contours, such as large breasts, high diaphragm or elevation of one side of the diaphragm, areas of infiltration in the lungs, pleural fluid and excessive adipose tissue outside of the pericardium. Image amplification systems have greatly improved the information obtainable at cardiac fluoroscopy. Because of increased contrast and brightness, the subpericardial fat is frequently identified as a radiolucent stripe that permits an assessment of pericardial thickness. Also, smaller calcific densities in the coronary

arteries and heart valves are seen with ease and regularity. The size and activity of the vascular structures in the lung hilus are also more easily appraised.

The magnification inherent in the fluoroscopic image may mislead the beginner, but with the experience obtained by repeated comparisons with teleoroentgenograms, it can be adequately evaluated. The study of pulsations is enhanced by the magnification since their apparent amplitude is increased.

Fluoroscopy can ordinarily be relied upon to determine the following:

1. Presence of calcification in (a) heart valves, (b) pericardium, (c) coronary arteries, (d) atrial walls including mural thrombi, and (e) ventricular walls including cardiac aneurysm. Fluoroscopy is probably the most sensitive means of detecting these calcifications and is the best means of determining their anatomical location.

2. (a) Gross enlargement of the heart and (b) normal sized heart. Borderline heart size cannot be appraised quite as well by fluoroscopy as by roentgenography, and both procedures leave something to be desired (see Chapter 7, "Measurement of the Heart and Great Vessels").

3. Gross deviations in contour associated with definite vessel or chamber enlargement or dilatation. The pulmonary artery and aortic size can be estimated with only a fair degree of reliability. Of the cardiac chambers, the size of the left atrium is easiest to evaluate, the right ventricle is the most difficult, and the left ventricle and right atrium occupy an intermediate position.

4. (a) Amplitude of pulsation of all contours. Chamber dilatation may thus occasionally be differentiated from hypertrophy, but these two factors are so often combined as to make the differentiation unreliable. (b) Timing of pulsations. This is possible only in a gross way and is much inferior to electrokymography or roentgenkymography.

5. Gross irregularities in rhythm.

6. Abnormal vascular shadows in lung and their degree of pulsations.

7. Displacement of the heart as in kyphosis.

8. Fixation of the heart as in adhesive mediastinitis or abnormal mobility as is seen in unilateral pneumothorax or foreign body in a bronchus.

Image amplification may at times show a collection of pericardial fluid since the pericardial fat line can often be demonstrated and the distance between the epicardial fat and exterior of the heart can be seen. Normally, this is 1–2 mm in thickness, but where a larger space is visible, a diagnosis of fluid is suggested (see Fig. 477, pg. 578).

RADIOGRAPHY (CHEST FILMS)

Radiography is the most widely used method for determining the size, contour, and position of the heart and great vessels. It complements fluoroscopy in that it provides a permanent record which can be inspected whenever necessary, and in many cases it is the only roentgen procedure performed.

To reduce the magnification of the heart, the target-to-film distance is increased considerably over that usually employed in radiography, and the object-to-film distance is reduced to a minimum. These two conditions are satisfied by placing the x-ray tube at a distance of 6–7 feet (180–210 cm) from the film (teleoroentgenography) and by placing the patient in the posteroanterior position with the sternum as close to the film as possible. The distance between the anterior chest wall and the film may vary between 0.5 and 2.0 cm due to (1) the thickness of the front of the casette (0.5 cm) and (2) the covering of the cassette holder which may be 1.5 cm thick. Under these circumstances, in the average individual who can stand erect in proper position, the plane of the largest cardiac dimensions will lie about one-third of the anteroposterior diameter from the anterior chest wall or between 6 and 13 cm from the film (anteroposterior diameters of the adult chest range between 16 and 30 cm). Reference to Table 1 shows that the percentage magnification in the average examination would thus be between 4 and 6%. Also, it can be seen that increasing the target-film distance from 6 to 7 feet (180–210 cm) would decrease the magnification by the order of only 1%, but this would require an increase in the amount of x-ray energy of 36%. Table 1 also permits a rough comparison of the percentage magnification in fluoroscopy and teleoroentgenography under usual conditions. It may be seen that when the transverse diameter of the heart on the teleo-

roentgenogram is 13 cm, the actual diameter would be between 12.2 and 12.4 cm.

Short exposure times are essential if a sharp image of the heart and great vessels is to be obtained. Roesler (1946) stated that critical examination of a series of consecutive films exposed at $\frac{1}{10}$, $\frac{1}{15}$, or $\frac{1}{20}$ sec on the same individual at random periods during the cardiac cycle will show varying degrees of unsharpness due to motion. This unsharpness varies, of course, with the phase of the cardiac cycle during which the exposure happens to occur; e.g., in diastole there may be a period of as much as $\frac{2}{10}$ sec during which the heart contour scarcely changes. At $\frac{1}{20}$ sec the number of unsharp films will be minimal, but $\frac{1}{40}$-sec exposures are necessary to produce uniform films of a high degree of sharpness. On the other hand, exposure times greater than $\frac{1}{10}$ sec uniformly produce films showing some motion. Practically, this may lead to occasional difficulty in differentiating small areas of infiltration in the lung from normal vascular structures. In general, choice of exposure time depends on the degree of precision that one desires to obtain. Clear demonstration of valvular calcifications may require exposures of $\frac{1}{60}$ sec. The use of modern three-phase equipment for generation of x-rays permits still shorter exposure times with less heat load to the tube. The ripple effect found in conventional single-phase valve-tube rectified circuits is much reduced with three-phase generators, and exposure times of 8–10 msec can be obtained in chest radiography of persons of ordinary size. Condenser discharge x-ray units provide a constant potential power supply for the x-ray tube and can result in still shorter exposure times (for example, 1.8 msec for a chest film on a person whose chest measures 22 cm from front to back). The condenser discharge units require a special x-ray tube filter, but their installation is altogether somewhat less expensive by comparison with conventional units.

Scatter is reduced by the use of a collimator that limits the beam to the thoracic area.

Respiratory motion is eliminated by having the patient stop breathing during the exposure. The exact phase of respiration at which breathing should be arrested is important since the position of the diaphragm determines to a degree the contours and size of the heart and great vessels (Figs. 18 and 19). In many departments, chest films are exposed after the patient has inspired fully and is holding his breath. Thus, the diaphragm is lower, the transverse diameter of the heart is decreased, and the longitudinal

TABLE 1

PERCENTAGE MAGNIFICATION DUE TO GEOMETRIC FACTORS

AP Diameter of Chest	Target-Film Distances			
	150 cm	180 cm (6 feet)	210 cm	Fluoroscopy[a]
cm				
12	3.1	2.6	2.2	5.6
15	3.8	3.1	2.3	7.1
20	5.0	4.1	3.5	9.8
25	6.2	5.2	4.4	12.4
30	7.5	6.2	5.3	15.4

[a] 30-inch target-screen distance; numbers are approximate.

diameter is increased as compared with those seen during normal basal respiration. Occasionally, these changes may be increased further since many patients maintain inspiration by closing the glottis which in turn increases the intrathoracic pressure and decreases the venous return. This decreases the amplitude of the cardiac pulsations and the size of the heart contour. The advantage of full inspiration is that it can be obtained easily with little practice and is usually easily reproducible. Where large numbers of individuals are to be examined, this leads to savings in time and effort.

Ideally, respiration should be halted midway between normal inspiration and expiration so that the heart and great vessels would present a more normal contour. Certainly where precise and accurate evaluation of the cardiac contour is desired, exposure at the end of normal inspiration is desirable and has been used by most investigators. Of great importance, however, is the reproducibility of any chosen respiration position since comparison of films made over a period of time in different phases of respiration may lead to considerable error.

Since in infants and young children respiration is difficult to control, the position of the diaphragm may vary from full inspiration to full expiration. This makes evaluation of the cardiac contours more difficult and comparison of a series of films may be quite deceptive. Attempts have been made to overcome this difficulty by using an air-filled circular rubber bag placed around the lower thorax. Expansion of the thorax during inspiration could thus initiate an exposure. Obviously, such a device is too cumbersome for routine use. A careful technician may obtain a satisfactory inspiratory film by watching the respiratory movements of the exposed chest and thereby time the exposure for the end of inspiration. Some departments of radiology routinely expose two frontal chest films on infants in an effort to obtain one satisfactory film in inspiration.

Changes in the cardiac contour and frontal area of the heart due to cardiac phase are generally disregarded. The transverse diameter of the heart in normal persons may vary as much as 3–6% between maximal systole and diastole depending upon the position and contour (longitudinal or transverse heart). Variations in frontal area are probably somewhat less when computed by the method of Hodges and Eyster (1926) and in particular are not so greatly affected by the position of the heart since pulsations along the broad diameter tend to compensate somewhat for the lack of pulsations along

the long diameter and vice versa. Hodges (1946) recommends using the larger contour of a stereoscopic pair, however, as more nearly approaching the diastolic size of the heart. The variation in frontal area is considerable in different persons and even in the same person at different times. In general, the larger the heart, the less the amplitude of the pulsations. On the other hand, the slower the pulse, the greater the amplitude of pulsations, provided the cardiac output remains constant. This phase variation in frontal area, cardiac contour, and transverse diameter have been accepted by many investigators as part of the inherent error in the use of teleoroentgenography. Estimations of heart volume using a combination of posteroanterior and lateral teleoroentgenograms theoretically may show a variation in estimated cardiac volume between systole and diastole of 125–150 ml, or approximately 20% of the estimated systolic volume. For practical purposes, however, Kjellberg et al. (1951) believe that the effect of the cardiac cycle on the cardiac volume is inappreciable, and our studies tend to strengthen that impression.

Several devices are available which permit x-ray exposures to be made at any predetermined phase of the cardiac cycle (Fig. 2). Most are integrated parts of automatic pressure injection or monitoring devices. The exposure is timed to occur synchronous with or at a definite prese-

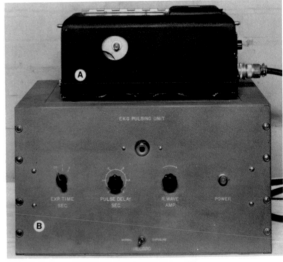

FIG. 2. ECG PULSING UNIT

Unit for obtaining exposures at any preselected phase of the cardiac cycle. An impulse is initiated by the maximum deflection of the ECG (usually the R wave in lead II). The transmission of the impulse can then be delayed for varying intervals up to 1.0 sec. The recording instrument (A) is above. (Courtesy of Dr. R. H. Morgan.)

lected time following a chosen event on the electrocardiogram, usually the R wave. For example, the exposure may be programmed to occur in maximal diastole (synchronous with the R wave) or maximal systole (simultaneous with the upstroke of the T wave). With most modern automatic injectors, both the radiographic exposure and the injection of contrast material may be timed to any desired phase of the cardiac cycle.

Tube-film distances may be reduced for oblique and lateral projections where magnification is less important, but it is inadvisable to reduce the distance to less than 4 feet (120 cm). A considerable reduction in the amount of radiation necessary to produce the exposure may thereby be accomplished. Positioning for oblique films is best determined by previous fluoroscopic control, and a protractor mounted on the cassette holder is valuable in reproducing the desired degree of obliquity. Where there has been no fluoroscopic control, the right anterior oblique is customarily made at 45° and the left anterior oblique at 60°. Routinely, right anterior oblique and lateral films are exposed with barium paste in the esophagus.

Where the cardiac contour is the center of interest, some degree of overexposure is desirable. Films exposed correctly for revealing minor lung densities may not give good contrast along the cardiac borders, particularly in the hilar and immediate supradiaphragmatic areas. Also, it is advantageous to view the barium-filled esophagus through the heart. A satisfactory plan is to expose one posteroanterior film with conventional technique and another using a high speed Potter-Bucky diaphragm, with an increase of 15–20 kv and barium in the esophagus.

Radiography is advantageous over fluoroscopy in that (1) it does not expose the patient or operator to significant amounts of radiation, (2) it conserves the physician's time, (3) it provides a permanent record, and (4) the images of the cardiovascular and pulmonary structures are much clearer and sharper on well exposed films than can be achieved with fluoroscopy. Consequently, in most departments radiography is the only routine method of examination; fluoroscopy, angiography, etc., are reserved for those cases where more detailed information is necessary. Radiography can be relied upon to demonstrate the following:

1. (a) Gross cardiac enlargement and (b) normal-sized heart. Borderline heart size is difficult to evaluate, and, even when precise radiographic studies are applied to a single doubtful case, they are probably of little value in determining whether the heart is enlarged or not.

2. Cardiac calcifications. Radiography is inferior to fluoroscopy and cinefluorography as a rule, and special techniques are necessary to demonstrate calcified valves (correct degree of obliquity, heavy exposure, and short exposure times).

3. Gross deviations in cardiac contour associated with definite chamber or vessel enlargement or dilatation. The information is about equal to that obtained from fluoroscopy, but the two procedures can be combined.

4. Displacement or fixation of the heart and mediastinum. Exposures in inspiration and expiration and lateral decubitus views in inspiration and expiration are necessary.

A classification of significant cardiovascular abnormalities that may be detected from fluoroscopy and conventional films of the chest is given in Table 2.

TABLE 2
CARDIOVASCULAR ABNORMALITIES DETECTED BY FLUOROSCOPY AND RADIOGRAPHY

I. Calcification
    A. Mitral valve—diagnostic of rheumatic mitral valvular disease.
    B. Aortic valve—diagnostic of aortic stenosis, often rheumatic but may be congenital or idiopathic.
    C. Mitral annulus fibrosus—may be the cause of a murmur but of little clinical significance. Calcification in the aortic annulus is usually an extension from valvular calcification and thus is commonly associated with aortic stenosis.
    D. Left atrial wall—suspect mural thrombus and mitral stenosis
    E. Right atrial wall—suspect mural thrombus (apparently quite rare).
    F. Myocardium—suspect:
        1. Infarction.
        2. Infarction with aneurysm.
        3. Tumor (rare).
        4. Echinococcus cyst.
    G. Right ventricle—opposite interventricular septal defect (rare).
    H. Aorta.
        1. Ascending aorta—suggestive of syphilitic aortitis but may be due to atherosclerosis or other etiologic agent.
        2. Arch—diagnostic of atherosclerosis but of minimal clinical significance.
        3. Para-aortic mass—calcium curvilinear in contour—suggestive of aneurysm although it may be a teratoma or other tumor or rarely a calcified lymph node.

TABLE 2—*continued*

I. Pericardium—suggestive of constrictive pericarditis (50–55% have calcification).

J. Coronary arteries—means coronary arteriosclerosis, but correlation between calcification and ischemic heart disease is relatively poor.

II. Cardiac Enlargement

    A. Symmetrical—suggests:

        1. Diffuse inflammation or infiltration of myocardium.

        2. Pericardial effusion (lungs often clear).

    B. Asymmetrical, including specific chamber enlargement:

        1. Left ventricle—suggests systemic hypertension or aortic valvular disease (aortic insufficiency is more common and produces more pronounced enlargement than stenosis).

        2. Combined left atrial and ventricular enlargement suggests some degree of left ventricular failure secondary to "1" above or when left atrial dilatation is relatively more pronounced, suggests predominant mitral insufficiency. Patent ductus arteriosus and interventricular septal defect may cause left atrial and left ventricular enlargement.

        3. Enlargement of all chambers with predominance of left ventricle suggests hypertension or left-sided valvular lesion with heart failure, particularly when accompanied by chronic passive congestion of lungs (exception may be Bernheim's syndrome (see text)). If lungs are clear, suggests combined valvular lesions of both sides of heart.

        4. Left atrial enlargement only is highly suggestive of predominant mitral stenosis.

        5. Left atrial and right ventricular enlargement accompanied by chronic lung stasis suggests predominant mitral stenosis of considerable duration.

        6. Left atrial, right ventricular, and right atrial enlargement with relatively clear lungs suggests right-sided heart failure secondary to mitral valvular disease; combined tricuspid and mitral valvular disease may present the same pattern.

        7. Right ventricular enlargement with (a) clear avascular lungs suggests pulmonic stenosis; (b) engorged lungs suggests congenital left-to-right shunt such as interatrial septal defect, anomalous pulmonary venous return or the Lutembacher syndrome; (c) emphysema of lungs, fibrosis or extensive infiltration suggests cor pulmonale.

        8. Right atrial and right ventricular enlargement suggests some degree of right ventricular dilatation or failure secondary to conditions listed under "7" above; structural tricuspid insufficiency may be present but this is a rare lesion.

        9. Right atrial enlargement suggests Ebstein's anomaly or tumor of right atrium.

III. Changes in Aortic Shadow

    A. Elongation—suggests atherosclerosis and is often accompanied by some degree of hypertension.

        1. Tortuosity is due to pronounced elongation—causes deviation of esophagus—may be difficult at times to differentiate from aneurysm or mediastinal mass.

    B. Dilatation—when definite is highly suggestive of aortitis—most common in ascending portion. Minor degree of dilatation may be seen with hypertension alone (dynamic dilatation). Aorta may be large in certain congenital anomalies such as truncus arteriosus and extreme tetralogy of Fallot.

        1. Localized dilatation and irregularity of contour are highly suggestive of aortitis and/or aneurysm.

        2. Diffuse dilatation suggests aneurysm.

    C. Calcification (see above under "I").

    D. Abnormal position—suggests anomaly as right aortic arch, aortic ring, etc. May cause abnormal indentation or constriction of esophagus and/or trachea.

IV. Lung Changes which Suggest Cardiac Abnormality

    A. Diffuse pulmonary fibrosis, emphysema, cystic disease or extensive bronchiectasis—suspect cor pulmonale.

    B. Increased prominence of pulmonary vascular structures (pulmonary engorgement)—suspect left-to-right shunt such as interatrial or interventricular septal defect, patent ductus arteriosus, the Lutembacher syndrome, anomalous venous return, and rupture of aortic aneurysm into right atrium or pulmonary artery. There may be increased pulmonary vascular markings in transposition of the great vessels and some cases of truncus arteriosus. (See also increased pulsations, under "V" below.)

    C. Diminished pulmonary vascularity suggests pulmonic stenosis or atresia, usually congenital in origin. If there is an associated unusual contour of the hilar shadows, suspect collateral circulation with pulmonic stenosis.

    D. Diminished pulmonary vascularity localized to one lung or a portion of one lung—suspect embolism and/or thrombosis of a major pulmonary artery.

    E. Chronic passive congestion—suspect left ventricular failure or mitral valvular disease.

    F. Chronic lung stasis (see text)—suggests mitral valvular disease.

    G. Pulmonary edema suggests left ventricular failure or mitral valvular disease. May be due a number of other causes (see text).

    H. Diffuse distribution of miliary densities suggests hemosiderosis with mitral valvular disease.

TABLE 2—*continued*

I. Localized irregular-shaped lesions which appear to have a connection with hilar structures suggest pulmonary arteriovenous fistula; if lesion diminishes definitely in size with Valsalva maneuver, this is added evidence of such a lesion.

J. Multiple small to medium-sized flame or triangular-shaped opacities scattered through both lungs suggest bacterial endocarditis such as might occur with patent ductus arteriosus.

V. Abnormal Pulsations which Suggest Cardiac Disease

    A. Increased amplitude of pulsation of:

        1. Left ventricle suggests aortic insufficiency, patent ductus arteriosus, mitral insufficiency, thyrotoxicosis, and occasionally systemic hypertension.

        2. Right ventricle (amplitude is difficult to evaluate) suggests interatrial septal defect or anomalous pulmonary venous return.

        3. Entire heart suggests hyperthyroidism and some cases of beriberi. Excursions may be quite large in some cases of bradycardia and heart block; may also be seen in pneumopericardium.

        4. Pulmonary artery and hilar shadows—usually indicates increased pulmonary blood flow. In an exaggerated form it is known as "hilar dance" and may be associated with some degree of pulmonary insufficiency. Most frequently seen in Lutembacher syndrome and interatrial septal defect; also in patent ductus arteriosus, partial anomalous pulmonary venous return, and transposition of the great vessels.

        5. Superior vena cava (this structure normally does not pulsate) suggests tricuspid insufficiency.

        6. Aorta suggests aortic insufficiency, aortitis, hypertension, hyperthyroidism, and patent ductus arteriosus.

    B. Decreased pulsations:

        1. Entire heart suggests diffuse myocarditis, pericardial effusion, or constrictive pericarditis.

        2. When localized to a single chamber is usually associated with pronounced dilatation and failure of that chamber. Diminished pulsations may be localized in constrictive pericarditis.

    C. Paradoxical pulsations are almost always limited to the left ventricle and are due to a cardiac aneurysm.

    D. Expansible pulsations of left atrium with left ventricular systole may be indicative of mitral insufficiency, but this evidence is often unreliable because of a considerable range of pulsation of the normal left atrium.

    E. Pulsations of lungs, trachea, or ribs synchronous with heart suggest adhesive pericarditis.

BODY SECTION RADIOGRAPHY

Body section radiography is a conventional or routine procedure in most diagnostic departments and therefore does not merit any special description. In connection with the cardiovascular system, it is carried out in a routine manner. It is occasionally helpful in the following conditions: (1) arteriovenous fistulas of the lungs, (2) cardiac calcifications, and, (3) rarely, in coarctation of the aorta. It has been supplanted, for the most part, by other routine and special procedures.

CARDIAC CATHETERIZATION

Cardiac catheterization refers to the procedure by which a radiopaque catheter is introduced into a cardiac chamber under fluoroscopic control. For right heart catheterization the catheter is introduced into a peripheral systemic vein; with appropriate manipulation the catheter tip can often be made to pass successively from the right atrium to the right ventricle, then into the pulmonary trunk, and finally into either the right or left pulmonary artery.

The left cardiac chambers may be catheterized in several ways: (1) direct needle puncture of the left atrium from a posterior approach, (2) percutaneous needle puncture of the left ventricle from an anterior approach, (3) transbronchial puncture of the left atrium, (4) trans-septal introduction of needle and catheter into the left from the right atrium, and (5) retrograde aortic catheterization of the left ventricle. Only the latter two routes are in common use.

Information obtained from the procedure is predominantly physiologic (oxygen content of aspirated blood samples, pressure tracings, etc.) but is also partially anatomical (position, contour, and activity of the catheter). The location of the catheter tip in relation to the various cardiac chambers and surrounding vessels is of fundamental importance and should be determined as precisely as possible during each step of the procedure. This is done by a combination of (1) fluoroscopy, (2) obtaining immediate pressure tracings which are characteristic of a particular chamber or vessel, and (3) visual and color-imetric estimations of the oxygen content of the aspirated blood. Spot films are useful as permanent records which can be reviewed at leisure when all other pertinent information has been collected. Needless to say, a great deal of cooperation and team work between the fluoroscopist, the operator, and other members of the catheterization team are necessary for the proper execution of the procedure. Ideally the functions of the radiologist should include the following: (1) to assist in the selection or even the design of the radiographic and fluoroscopic equipment to be used (the radiologist is in an excellent position to recommend the apparatus adequate to the procedures to be performed and can perform a significant service in rejecting substandard devices); (2) to prevent unnecessary and injurious amounts of radiation from reaching the patient or the operating personnel (selection of shielding and collimating devices and placement of oscilloscopes, viewing screens, oximeters, cables, and the like, such that they may be used by the personnel of the catheterization team without undue radiation exposure are properly the responsibility of the radiologist); (3) to assist the operator in determining the relative location of the catheter by the proper use of the fluoroscope; and (4) to participate in the decision to perform selective angiocardiography at the time of catheterization where indicated and oversee the injection of contrast material and subsequent filming.

Historical Background

Forssman (1929), using himself as a subject, was the first to introduce a catheter into the right atrium. Conte and Costa (1933), using catheters whose tips had been placed in the right atrium, rapidly injected contrast material and were able to obtain good opacification of the pulmonary arterial system. Cournand and Ranges (1941) were the first in this country to report on the use of the procedure for physiologic investigations. Attention was given first to heart failure, cardiorespiratory disease, and shock; later, to congenital heart disease. Brannon et al. (1945) used the procedure extensively in the study of atrial septal defects. Dexter et al. (1947) in Boston and Bing et al. (1947) in Baltimore used the procedure predominantly in congenital heart disease and particularly in the selection of patients for surgical treatment. More recently, as technical proficiency in the performance of cardiac catheterization has been attained, the procedure is being used for the investigation of all but the most routine and clear-cut cardiac abnormalities, for pre- and postoperative evaluation of cardiovascular dynamics, as a means of obtaining dye and gas dilution curves, and as a preliminary to selective angiocardiography.

Equipment and Material

If cardiac catheterization is to be performed safely while the maximum of information is obtained, adequate facilities and sophisticated equipment are required. The room should be large enough to comfortably accommodate the recording, injecting, and monitoring devices as well as the many essential and interested persons involved in the operation. Image-amplified fluoroscopy should be employed, and wall-mounted or portable television screen monitors provide ideal viewing conditions, permitting both radiologists and operator as well as other personnel to simultaneously observe the progress and position of the catheter. The ability to view the image in a dimly lit rather than a darkened room greatly facilitates the handling of instruments and catheters and may help prevent otherwise unnoticed blood loss.

A high capacity x-ray generator is ideal, and 1,000-ma capacity at 150 kv is recommended. It will provide for spot filming and will also permit angiocardiography should that be required. The equipment should include one or more provisions for recording cardiac action during catheterization and angiocardiography. A movie camera attached to the image amplifier can provide quite satisfactory cineangiographic studies (60 frames/sec required), or one may prefer to employ serial filming devices either with cut film or roll film. This equipment should be capable of providing at least 5 exposures/sec. Many modern catheterization laboratories employ video tape for recording catheter positions and for angiocardiography. Such units have the advantage of instant replay, and study of the images can permit the responsible physicians to more adequately plan the further progress of the catheterization study.

Lead aprons should be worn by all persons involved in the procedure.

The intracardiac catheters are the responsibility of the individual who is to use them, whether he is an internist, a pediatrician, a surgeon, or a radiologist. Those in common use are radiopaque, and most are sufficiently flexible that they can be easily bent into a loop of 5–6 cm in diameter. They are sufficiently rigid to prevent rotation, and considerable control of the catheter tip can be achieved by manipulating that portion of the catheter which lies outside of the patient. The catheters are usually 60–125 cm long, and the commonly used sizes vary from 6–10 French outside diameter. The lumen opens in the extreme tip in some catheters, whereas others have side openings only. Various curvatures of the tip may be shaped in advance as indicated if the catheters are homemade, but a large variety of preformed tips and catheters is commercially available. All of the catheters have Luer Lok attachments on the proximal end, and most may be cleaned, sterilized, and reused. Some inexpensive catheters are designed to be used once and discarded.

Surgical instruments, sterile supplies, fluids, syringes, manometers, strain gauges, monitoring apparatus, and other similar devices are the responsibility of the operator, but the radiologist should be familiar with their function and operation.

A detailed set of standards for cardiac catheterization laboratories has been produced in brochure form by Abrams *et al.* (1971) and more recently by a committee report by Judkins *et al.* (1976). Both of these are excellent guides for institutions sponsoring cardiac catheterization laboratories and discuss in detail personnel, equipment, electrical safety, radiation protection, and procedures and case load.

Right Heart Catheterization

The meal preceding the examination is omitted. In adults, usually no premedication is required, whereas in children morphine, barbiturates, and scopolamine may be given in preoperative amounts. In infants under the age of three months, a nipple containing a whiskey-soaked cotton ball may be quite effective. In our institution a "cardiac cocktail" is commonly employed in children. It consists of meperidine, 25 mg, chlorpromazine, 6 mg, promethazine HCl, 6 mg, in 1 ml. A dose of 1 ml/20 pounds of body weight is employed, with a maximal dose of 2 ml.

The catheter may be inserted through the external saphenous, femoral, external jugular, or one of the arm veins. In general, the arm veins are preferable except in small children or infants in whom they may be too small. When the heart and great veins are in their usual position, the left median basilic vein is preferable since it permits easier entrance into and manipulation of the catheter in the right side of the heart.

When an arm vein is used, fluoroscopy begins when the tip of the catheter approaches the axilla. The tip may enter one of the cervical veins and this should be readily corrected by withdrawing the catheter slightly and changing the direction of the tip. At the apex of the axilla there may be an apparent obstruction, but this can often be overcome by moving the arm outward and upward to varying degrees. Once the catheter enters the left innominate vein it usually passes easily into the superior vena cava and right atrium. Rarely it may enter the azygos vein and arch posteriorly, and this is best appreciated in an oblique or lateral view. Also rarely, aberrant pulmonary veins enter the superior vena cava, and the catheter will enter one of these and continue for some distance into the lung field. The color of the aspirated blood may give a clue to this possibility, and this can be confirmed by oxygen saturation measurements.

When the catheter reaches the right atrium, in many cases it is advisable to continue on into the right ventricle and pulmonary artery; however, the tip may enter either (1) the coronary sinus, (2) the inferior vena cava, (3) an interatrial septal defect or patent foramen ovale, or (4) an aberrant pulmonary vein (Jorgens *et al.*, 1952).

When the catheter enters the coronary sinus, it may at first appear to be in the right ventricle. If the patient is rotated into the lateral projection, it can be seen that the catheter is posterior (Fig. 3); also, when introduced for some distance, the catheter will emerge along the left heart border in the region below the left atrial appendage, and then it may take a slightly downward direction. Tracings may show a very low pressure, but it should be noted that pressures in the coronary sinus are quite variable and often resemble closely those obtained from the right ventricle. By slowly withdrawing the catheter, it can be seen that the point of angulation is fixed, and this does not occur if the catheter is in the right ventricle.

Rotation of the patient during cardiac catheterization to obtain far oblique and lateral views is a cumbersome procedure and is apt to lead to contamination of the operator's sterile field and may cause the catheter to change its position. Slight rotation of the patient is all that is usually necessary to locate the catheter, and where there is any question as to position, fluoroscopic observations should be supported by pressure tracings, oxygen saturation data, and small volume injections of contrast material.

When the catheter enters the inferior vena cava, the tip is usually clearly outside of the heart and its position correctly appreciated. If it should enter a hepatic vein on the left side, however, it may still appear to be within the right ventricle. The patient should be asked to

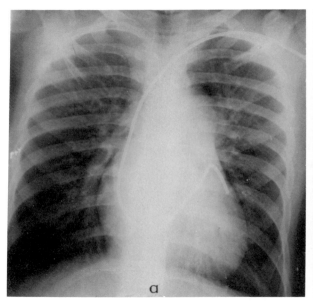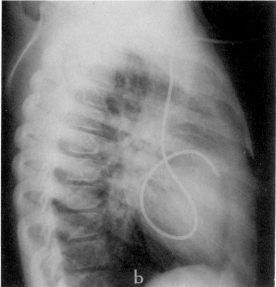

FIG. 3. APPEARANCE OF CATHETER IN CORONARY SINUS (a) AP VIEW; (b) LATERAL VIEW. TIP OF CATHETER LIES IN GREAT
CARDIAC VEIN

(Courtesy of Drs. Jorgens, La Bree, Adams, and Rigler, *American Journal of Roentgenology, Radium Therapy and Nuclear Medicine, 68:* 613, 1952.)

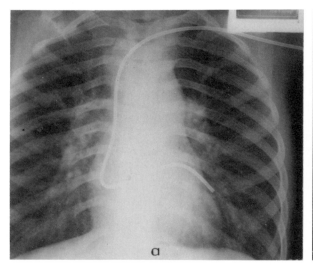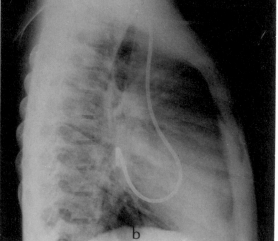

FIG. 4. CATHETER HAS ENTERED LEFT ATRIUM FROM RIGHT ATRIUM THROUGH AN INTERATRIAL SEPTAL DEFECT AND TIP
LIES IN PULMONARY VEIN

The posterior position of the catheter shows that it is not in the right ventricle. (Courtesy of Drs. Jorgens, La Bree, Adams, and Rigler, *American Journal of Roentgenology, Radium Therapy and Nuclear Medicine, 68:* 614, 1952.)

take a deep breath when, following descent of the diaphragm, it can be seen that the catheter is outside of the heart.

When the catheter enters the left atrium through an interatrial defect (Fig. 4), the appearance is similar to that seen when the catheter is in the coronary sinus. The catheter bends to the left and the tip may present near the lateral heart border. A blood sample from the left atrium is usually bright red, whereas a sample from the coronary sinus is dark, and this can be confirmed by an oximeter. The catheter tip is also more active when it is in the coronary sinus. The catheter may continue on into a pulmonary vein, and this is good evidence of an interatrial defect. Occasionally one is misled because the catheter can enter an aberrant pulmonary vein from the right atrium.

When the catheter tip is directed downward, medially, and forward, it usually enters the right ventricle without much difficulty unless there is an organic obstruction. When the catheter tip enters the ventricle, its motion increases considerably. Occasionally a loop may form which roughly outlines the size of the ventricular cavity. It is usually desirable to unwind the loop before passing the tip into the pulmonary artery. The curve of the catheter seems to favor an entrance into the right pulmonary artery, although it can often be induced to enter the left side. In the larger arteries, the catheter continues to show a waving motion and the pressure tracings may be characteristic. When the catheter tip is nearer the periphery, it may lose all motion, and the tracings are much lower and reflect the pressure changes which occur in the pulmonary capillaries. The catheter is then wedged in a smaller artery, and aspirated blood will represent reflux from the capillaries. Occasionally in congenital cyanotic heart disease (*e.g.,* tetralogy of Fallot) the catheter will enter the aorta instead of the pulmonary artery. Of course, if the catheter is extended far enough it will enter one of the brachiocephalic vessels which positively identifies its position. Usually the position of the catheter is somewhat more medial than when it is in the pulmonary artery (Fig. 5). Oxygen satura-

tions may or may not be helpful when one is dealing with congenital cyanotic heart disease.

Pressure tracings are made as the catheter is slowly withdrawn from the pulmonary artery into the right ventricle. This is the most reliable means available for determining the presence or absence of pulmonary stenosis. Where there is not an abrupt increase in pressure while the tip is being withdrawn, but rather a gradual increase while the tip is moving through a distance of 2–3 cm, one may strongly suspect that there is an infundibular chamber (infundibular pulmonary stenosis). Ranges of normal values for pressures and other important measurements at cardiac catheterization are shown in Table 3.

Blood samples for oxygen saturation determinations should be taken routinely from the pulmonary artery, right ventricle, right atrium, and superior vena cava, as the catheter is slowly withdrawn. In cases of suspected interatrial septal defect, it is well to have a sample from the inferior vena cava because this may furnish an explanation for an increase in oxygen saturation between the superior vena cava and right atrium. Oxygen saturation in the right chambers is normally 65–70%; in the left heart, oxygen saturation approaches 94–98%.

Oxygen consumption may be measured during the course of catheterization while blood samples are being collected from the pulmonary artery, if possible, or the right ventricle and a peripheral

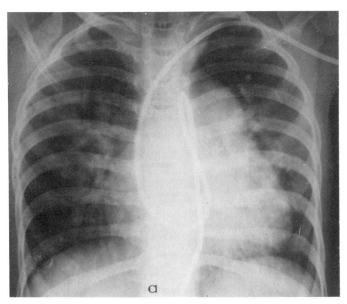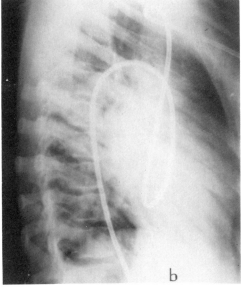

FIG. 5. CATHETER HAS PASSED FROM RIGHT VENTRICLE INTO AN OVERRIDING, DEXTROPOSED AORTA IN PATIENT WITH EISENMENGER'S COMPLEX

(A) posteroanterior view; (B) lateral view. (Courtesy of Drs. Jorgens, La Bree, Adams, and Rigler, *American Journal of Roentgenology, Radium Therapy and Nuclear Medicine, 68:* 615, 1952)

TABLE 3
TABLE OF NORMAL VALUES

Pressures in the Heart and Great Vessels (mm Hg)

	Range	Average
Right atrium		
mean	1–5	2.8
Right ventricle		
peak systolic	17–32	25
end-diastolic	1–7	4
Pulmonary artery		
mean	9–19	15
peak systolic	17–32	25
end-diastolic	4–13	9
Pulmonary artery wedge		
mean	4.5–13	9
Left atrium		
mean	2–12	7.9
Left ventricle		
peak systolic	90–140	130
end-diastolic	5–12	8.7
Brachial artery		
mean	70–105	85
peak systolic	90–140	130
end-diastolic	60–90	70

Cardiac Output and Related Measurements		± SD
O_2 uptake	143 ml/min/m^2	14.3
Arteriovenous O_2 difference	4.1 vol %	0.6
Cardiac index	3.5 L/min/m^2	0.7
Stroke index	46 ml/beat/m^2	8.1

Vascular Resistance		
Total systemic resistance	1130 dynes sec cm^{-5}	178
Total pulmonary resistance	205 dynes sec cm^{-5}	51
Pulmonary arteriolar resistance	67 dynes sec cm^{-5}	23

Ventricular Volumes	
End diastolic volume	70 ml/m^2 BSA ± 20
End systolic volume	24 ml/m^2 BSA ± 10
Stroke volume	45 ml/m^2 BSA ± 13
Ejection fraction	0.67 ± 0.08

(From Barratt-Boyes and Wood, 1958; Kennedy *et al.*, 1966; and Yang *et al.*, 1972.)

FIG. 6. NORMAL POSITIONS OF INTRACARDIAC CATHETERS

(A) The catheter traverses the right atrium and right ventricle. Its tip lies in the pulmonary trunk (AP projection). (B) The catheter entered the heart through the superior vena cava, passed through the right atrium, right ventricle and pulmonary trunk, and came to lie in the left descending pulmonary artery (lateral projection). (C) The tip of the catheter on the left lies in the left atrium where it was placed following puncture of the interatrial septum from the right atrium. The catheter on the right was introduced into the femoral artery and advanced into the thoracic aorta in retrograde fashion. Its tip was pushed past the aortic valve and is seen to lie in the left ventricle (AP projection). (D) The tip of catheter number 1 lies in the pulmonary trunk, having passed through the superior vena cava, right atrium and right ventricle. The tip of catheter number 2 lies in the left ventricle, having passed through the inferior vena cava, right atrium, left atrium (puncture of interatrial septum), and mitral valve. Contrast material injected through catheter number 2 opacifies the left ventricle and ascending aorta and, by regurgitation, the left atrium. The tip of catheter number 3 is in the ascending aorta, having passed in a retrograde manner through the abdominal and thoracic aorta. (Courtesy of Cardiopulmonary Laboratory, University of Texas Medical Branch, Galveston, Texas.)

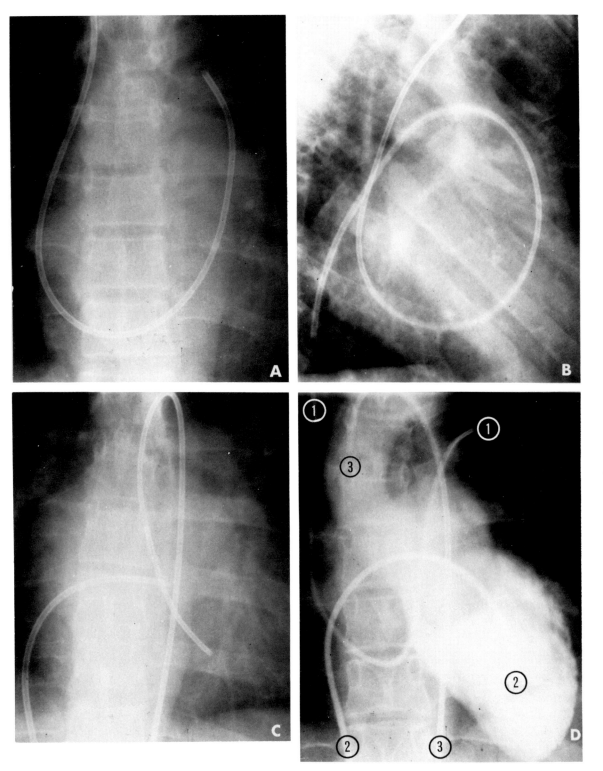

Fig. 6.

artery for oxygen saturation. Cardiac output (CO) in liters per minute may be determined by

$$CO = \frac{\text{oxygen consumption (ml/min)}}{\text{arteriovenous difference (ml/L)}}$$

Quantitative application of indicator dye dilution curves and radioactive isotopes may also be used to determine cardiac output during catheterization.

The recording of dilution curves following the introduction of an indicator dye at a specific point in the circulation has assumed great importance in the diagnosis of intracardiac shunts. At the time of catheterization a known amount of an indicator dye may be introduced into the circulation, and at some point distal to this a sensing device records the concentration of the indicator as it appears after traversing a part of the cardiovascular circuit. Thus, a dilution curve is a profile of transit times from injection site to sampling site.

In a normal subject, injection of the indicator into the pulmonary artery with sampling at the brachial artery will produce a curve similar to that shown in Figure 7A. The appearance time is the interval between the time of injection and the first detection of indicator dye at the sampling site. The build-up time is the time during which concentration increases rapidly to a maximum; this is followed by a decline toward zero concentration, after which a second peak occurs due to the indicator making a second appearance at the sampling site following circulation through the systemic capillaries and recirculation through the lungs.

The indicator dilution curve obtained in the presence of a left-to-right shunt after injection of dye into the systemic side of the cardiac circulation shows a normal appearance and build-up time, a reduced peak deflection, a prolonged disappearance phase ("wash-out" curve), and frequently the absence of an identifiable peak of dye concentration due to systemically recirculated indicator (Fig. 7B). This reflects the recirculation through the lungs of that part of the

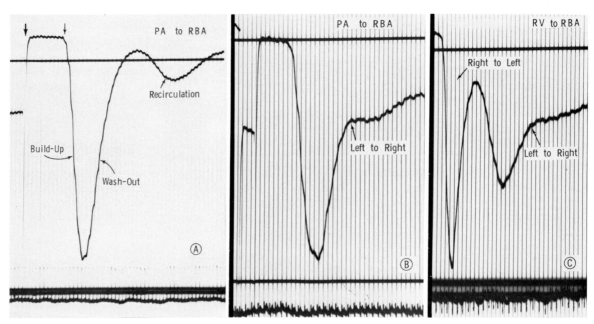

FIG. 7. INDICATOR DYE DILUTION CURVES

(A) Normal. Injection was made into the pulmonary artery with sampling at the right brachial artery. The appearance time (represented by the space between the arrows in the upper left corner) is the interval between the time of injection and the first detection of dye at the sampling site. Concentration increases rapidly to a maximum (buildup), followed by a decline toward zero concentration (washout). When the indicator makes a second appearance at the sample site following circulation through the systemic capillaries and recirculation through the lungs, a second peak of concentration is recorded (recirculation). (B) Left-to-right shunt. Injection into pulmonary artery with sampling at right brachial artery. Appearance time and buildup are normal, the peak deflection is slightly reduced, and the disappearance phase (washout curve) is prolonged. (C) Right-to-left and left-to-right shunts. Injection into the right ventricle with sampling at right brachial artery. The appearance time is very short, and there is a break in the buildup portion of the curve due to the passage of part of the indicator dye through the lungs and part directly into the systemic circulation without traversing the lungs (right-to-left shunt at or distal to the right ventricle). A left-to-right shunt is also present as evidenced by the break in the washout curve.

indicator passing from left to right through an abnormal communication.

The diagnosis of right-to-left shunt is based on an abnormally short transit time for some of the indicator from the point of injection to the point of detection. This appears as a break in the build-up portion of the curve and is due to the passage of a portion of the indicator dye directly into the systemic circulation without traversing the lungs. Such a curve is shown in Figure 7C. Injection was made into the right ventricle with detection at the brachial artery and represents a right-to-left shunt at the ventricular level. The break in the "wash-out" curve indicates that a left-to-right shunt is also present.

Substances used as indicator include (1) radio-active indicator such as iodinated human serum albumin; and (2) dyes with a high spectral absorption in the infrared region of the spectrum, such as cardiogreen. Swan (1959) believed the latter to be the ideal indicator material for the diagnostic application of dilution curves, and it is the only one in general use.

Diagnosis of left to right shunts may also be accomplished by early detection of nitrous oxide or radioactive gasses (xenon-133, krypton-85, and I^{131} methyl iodide) in the right side of the circulation after introduction of these materials into the left side via the respiratory tract. Case *et al.* (1959) found this to be a rapid, simple and accurate method of ruling out left to right shunts and detecting small shunts in which the results might be equivocal by oxygen studies.

All of the techniques utilizing indicators provide indirect evidence of the direction and magnitude of shunts. As contrast studies become incorporated into the catheterization procedure, increasing reliance is placed on them to demonstrate the structural abnormality present.

It should be emphasized that the conduct and sequence of the examination depends to a great extent upon the nature of the condition which is being investigated. In congenital heart disease, the procedure appears to be most fruitful when it is used to provide information about certain specific details, *e.g.,* the presence or absence of pulmonic stenosis, or the increase in oxygen saturation between the right ventricle and pulmonary artery, etc. The examination may be disappointing when it is conducted without any clear-cut concept of what conditions may be encountered.

Left Heart Catheterization

One of two routes to the left side of the heart may be used depending on the nature of the problem to be investigated. The transvenous route through the interatrial septum using the technique described by Ross (1959) and used by Brockenbrough and Braunwald (1960) is useful for the investigation of mitral stenosis and any condition in which direct measurements of left atrial and left ventricular pressures and blood saturations are needed. It is also desirable for any condition in which catheterization of the left and right sides of the heart is indicated. The transaortic route described by Prioton (1957) and Dotter (1960) is useful in investigations of the aortic valve and left ventricular function and is most helpful in the diagnosis and evaluation of mitral insufficiency.

In the procedure described by Brockenbrough and Braunwald (1960) the Seldinger technique is used to insert a catheter into the right femoral vein, and this is passed into the right heart for the usual purposes of right heart catheterization if necessary. This catheter is then replaced by a special polyethylene catheter 70 cm in length and with an appropriate curve. This is inserted over a guide wire, and the guide wire is then replaced by a stylet which straightens the curve in the catheter and allows it to be inserted into the right atrium. With the catheter in the right atrium the stylet is removed, and a needle measuring 71 cm is inserted into the catheter. Under fluoroscopic vision the needle is directed upward and medial and punctures the interatrial septum as is evidenced by the return of red oxygenated blood. The catheter is then passed over the needle as a guide and into the left atrium. In most cases, provided there is not a severe obstruction at the mitral valve, the catheter can be immediately inserted into the left ventricle. Blood samples may be collected, pressures recorded, and indicator dilution studies may be performed. The catheter is also suitable for the performance of selective angiography with injection into the left atrium or left ventricle. The catheter can then be withdrawn across the mitral valve and the gradient determined. It is obvious that the catheter can interfere with mitral valve function, and therefore this method is not optimum for the study of mitral insufficiency. After appropriate samples and pressures are taken from the right atrium, the catheter is then withdrawn through the atrial septum and removed. Experience and experiments in dogs show that the opening in the interatrial septum will close in about 2 weeks.

Using the transaortic route described by Dotter (1960) to the left ventricle, a suitable catheter is placed in the femoral, or less often, in the axillary or radial artery using the Seldinger technique. We prefer a radiopaque polyethylene catheter with the tip in the form of a loop or pigtail and an internal diameter of 2–2.5 mm. The catheter is inserted over a guide wire with a 1.5-cm flexible tip. The catheter is advanced into the ascending aorta under fluoroscopic control and usually, unless there is severe stenosis, will pass into the left ventricle during systole. The guide wire is then removed, and the appropriate studies can be carried out including selective left ventricular angiography if necessary. The catheter can then be withdrawn across the aortic valve detecting a gradient if it is present. A supravalvular aortic injection for aortography or evaluation of valve function can be performed.

In patients with marked atherosclerosis of the brachiocephalic and femoral vessels, it has occasionally been necessary to do a direct puncture of the left ventricle.

Reactions to Cardiac Catheterization

Minor untoward reactions are rather common, but they are rarely sufficient to disturb the patient greatly or to cause the examination to be suspended. Familiarity with these reactions, care, patience, and experience are necessary, however, if the procedure is to be carried out safely. When the catheter tip impinges on the tricuspid valve and/or the upper medial wall of the interventricular septum, arrhythmias are common and may occur in runs of three to four beats or more. These usually subside promptly after the catheter passes into the outflow tract of the right ventricle or pulmonary artery. Occasionally, they persist and become so frequent that the catheter must be entirely withdrawn from the heart. Fatal arrhythmias due to catheterization have been reported (Venables and Hiller, 1963).

Venospasm may prevent the passage of the catheter or make the manipulation quite painful to the patient. This can be greatly reduced or prevented by (1) a liberal use of local anesthetic at the site of the incision into the vein, (2) a quiet, calm, gentle approach to the patient, and (3) preoperative medication where the patient is unusually apprehensive. Where there is marked initial venospasm, it is probably wise to suspend the examination and wait for another day.

In congenital cyanotic heart disease, the entrance of air into a vein may produce cerebral air embolism. Consequently, great care must be taken in changing syringes and in taking pressure tracings, etc., that air does not enter the catheter.

Chills and fever occasionally occur several hours after the procedure and are due to pyrogenic material entering the blood stream. This can be prevented by carefully cleaning the catheters after they are used and rinsing them thoroughly with normal saline before reusing. All solutions, tubing, etc., must be free of pyrogenic substances.

Angulations and loops in the catheter which cannot be reduced are rarely seen (Skinner and Burroughs, 1961). They can be entirely avoided by careful manipulation of the catheter.

Serious complications of cardiac catheterization were summarized in detail in the report of a cooperative study on cardiac catheterization sponsored by the American Heart Association (Braunwald and Swan, 1968). Major complications included serious arrhythmia, profound hypotension, arterial thrombosis, arterial perforation and false aneurysm, perforation of the heart, serious infections, serious allergic reactions, pulmonary embolism and infarction, pneumothorax, hemothorax, systemic arterial embolism and hemorrhage. A total of 55 deaths occurred during the two years of the cooperative study, representing an overall mortality rate of 0.44% of the total of 12,367 studies carried out. The mortality was relatively higher during the first two months of life (29 deaths in 480 procedures, or 6.0%). There was an extremely low mortality rate in patients between the ages of 2 and 59 years (14 deaths in 10,004 procedures, or 0.14%).

Radiation Hazards

Before the use of image amplification, radiation exposure to the patient and operator were considerable (Hills and Stanford, 1950). With television screen monitoring of the fluoroscopic images, the time required for the procedure may be cut to a minimum and radiation exposure much reduced. The presence of a timer which automatically shuts off the exposure at the end of a 10-min period is a good reminder to the operator of fluoroscopic time elapsed. Prolonged fluoroscopy should be avoided, and the shutters should be used to keep the exposure field as small as possible. The use of a protective lead shield between the patient and operator is difficult, particularly in children, but lead aprons and other protective devices should be used whenever possible. The operator using ordinary prudence, properly operating equipment and lead protective apron and other devices should be quite safe in performing one examination daily five days a week.

Indications

Cardiac catheterization has contributed much fundamental information concerning cardiac dynamics and function in heart failure, mitral valvular disease, cardiopulmonary disease, constrictive pericarditis, and congenital heart disease. It has been of great value in congenital heart disease, and, although it should not be used indiscriminately in all cases, it has become increasingly popular as an investigative procedure in all but the simplest and most clear-cut abnormalities. It seems to be a more innocuous procedure than angiocardiography when used in the diagnosis of congenital cyanotic heart disease, but its usefulness in patients with acyanotic lesions, as in most intra- and extracardiac shunts with flow from left to right, is better established.

Cardiac catheterization is indicated in most patients in whom operation is anticipated for correction of a cardiac defect or abnormality. It is indicated for the purpose of establishing or confirming a diagnosis when appropriate therapy or prognostication depends upon accurate delineation of the nature of the cardiac defect. Cardiac catheterization may be an important diagnostic modality in those patients with heart disease whose clinical course is unfavorable and in whom watchful waiting is not sensible.

In the cooperative study on cardiac catheterization (Braunwald and Swan, 1968), the following etiologies were established in the 12,367 patients who were catheterized: no organic heart disease, 9.3%; congenital heart disease, 41.7%; rheumatic heart disease, 32.7%; arteriosclerotic heart disease, 14.5%; other forms of acquired heart disease, 4.1%; mixed or indeterminate group, 7.7%.

The most common congenital anomaly encountered was ventricular septal defect (9.2% of the total number catheterized). The second commonest anomaly was atrial septal defect which was found in 8.2% of all patients. Ventricular septal defect with obstruction to right ventricular outflow was found in 6.9% and was the third commonest anomaly. Pulmonic stenosis with intact ventricular septum was present in 6% of all patients studied.

Some of the details concerning cardiac catheterization findings in these and other conditions will be discussed under the appropriate headings.

2

Angiocardiography

Angiocardiography is a procedure in which contrast substance is injected into a systemic vein, a cardiac chamber, or the pulmonary artery so that its passage through a part or all of the heart and great vessels can be followed by serially exposed films. In classic or venous angiocardiography (Castellanos *et al.*, 1937; Robb and Stein- berg, 1939) the contrast substance is injected into an arm or leg vein. When the injection is made through a catheter or needle whose tip lies in one of the heart chambers, the procedure is known as "selective angiocardiography." Injections into the aorta are properly designated as "aortography."

HISTORY OF PROCEDURE

Forssman (1929) succeeded in threading a ureteral catheter into an elbow vein and by appropriate manipulation passed the tip into the right atrium. Shortly thereafter (1931) the same investigator, using dogs, found that if 50% Uroselectan was injected rapidly into the catheter and a single x-ray film was exposed at the end of the injection, the right heart chambers and the pulmonary artery and its branches could be visualized; also, the dogs suffered no ill effects. Encouraged by these experiments, Forssman tried the procedure on himself, but twice failed to demonstrate the right heart or pulomary artery. The amount of contrast substance was too little and the lumen of the catheter was too small to permit a significant concentration to reach the right atrium.

The Portuguese workers, Moniz *et al.* (1931), used essentially the same technique as Forssman, except that a concentrated solution of sodium iodide was substituted for Uroselectan, and obtained satisfactory visualization of the right heart chambers and pulmonary arterial system first in animals and later in man. Thus, they were able to study the arterial patterns in both normal and abnormal lungs, and probably the greatest contribution of the procedure was to demonstrate the relationships of the pulmonary artery to complex hilar shadows. Later, it was found that equally good results could be obtained by injecting the sodium iodide into a peripheral vein, and the procedure was called *l'angiopneumographie*.

A short time later, Conte and Costa (1933) attempted to shorten the injection time by placing two catheters in the right atrium (a catheter was inserted into the vein of each arm). Using 6 ml of 120% sodium iodide, they obtained good visualization of the right heart and pulmonary artery but could see nothing of the left side of the heart. Untoward effects, such as violent muscle spasm and tetany, were often observed and were attributed to the concentrated sodium iodide. These authors therefore suggested that some less toxic substance must be found before this type of examination could be successful.

In 1937, Castellanos *et al.* published an account of their use in children and infants of a procedure which they called *la angiocardiografia radio-opaca*. Their technical contributions were (1) the use of large bore trocars for the more rapid introduction of the contrast substance into the veins, (2) the use of first 35 and then 50% Perabrodil (Diodrast), and (3) the adaptation of the procedure for use in infants and children where good radiographic contrast was more easily obtained. This procedure was used on a number of patients with congenital heart disease and frequently demonstrated interatrial and interventricular defects. The left heart chambers and the aorta were still not visualized reliably, however, except in those instances in which the contrast substance passed from the right to the left side through a septal defect.

Four-chamber angiocardiography arrived in

1939 following a description by Robb and Steinberg of a technique which produced visualization of all the heart chambers, as well as the great vessels, in a higher percentage of examinations. After considerable study, these workers decided that 70% Diodrast was the most satisfactory contrast substance available at that time and that it was well tolerated in doses up to 1 ml/kg of body weight. They also developed a large bore cannula which, when used with a special syringe tip of equal diameter, permitted the injection of 50 ml of Diodrast within 2 sec or less. Their other refinements consisted of (1) stratifying blood above the contrast substance in the syringe so as to flush out the recipient vein and cause all of the contrast substance to reach the heart in the shortest possible time, (2) having the patient inspire slowly during injection so as to decrease the pressure within the thorax, (3) elevation of the arm during injection, and (4) the precise determination of arm-to-lung and arm-to-tongue circulation times. Their patients were examined in erect or sitting positions before a stereoscopic cassette changer which permitted the exposure of only two films. Their basic technique, however, was so well conceived that it has remained practically unmodified to the present time. Most of the improvements that have appeared have been in the production of more rapid serial x-ray exposures and the adaptation of the procedure for use in children in the recumbent position. More recently, Steinberg (1962) has taken advantage of the more innocuous contrast substances and has used the veins of both arms for simultaneous injection. This allows the use of up to 90 ml of highly concentrated contrast substance for a single examination.

Chavez et al. (1947) returned to the use of a catheter as a means of introducing the contrast substance into the right side of the heart. Catheter sizes of 10 French are desirable if an adequate concentration of the contrast material is to be obtained in an adult. A further refinement of this procedure introduced by A Jönsson et al. (1949) is the use of a manual pump which greatly increases the injection rate.

Manual pumps have now been replaced by power-driven, and in many instances sophisticated semi-automatic injectors which will be described below. Injectors with developing pressures of up to 1,000 psi permitted the introduction through a small bore catheter of a sufficient amount of contrast substance to produce good selective visualization of the cardiac chambers and the aorta. The introduction of catheters into the right side of the heart and aorta for physiologic and hemodynamic investigations was popularized by Cournand and Ranges (1941), and it was a rather easy step to follow this procedure by selective injection of contrast substance. It was soon found that it was necessary to substitute other types of catheters for the Cournand catheter in order to produce safe and satisfactory selective visualization of the right ventricle and pulmonary artery (Rodriguez-Alvarez and Rodriguez, 1957). The approach to the left side of the heart and the aorta underwent a considerably longer evolutionary development.

Rousthoi (1933) inserted catheters into the right carotid arteries of rabbits and threaded them into the ascending aorta and left ventricle. Following the injection of Thorotrast, he obtained visualization of the left ventricle, the thoracic aorta, and particularly the coronary arteries. Nuvoli (1936) was the first to perform aortography and left ventriculography successfully in man by inserting a strong, large bore needle directly through the sternum into the ascending aorta or the left ventricle. Radner (1945) revived this technique as applied to the aorta but apparently used it only a few times because of complications (mediastinal emphysema; extravasation of the contrast substance into the pericardium). Hoyos and Del Camp (1948) modified this procedure by inserting a needle through the left second anterior interspace into the aortic arch. In 1 of 4 cases, they found a small pneumothorax following the procedure. Ponsdomenech and Nunez (1951) employed a similar route by inserting a long needle through the chest wall from a paraxyphoid position usually into the left ventricle and injecting the contrast substance directly into this chamber. They thus were able to obtain left ventriculograms and aortograms in 30 patients. The same type of approach was explored by Lehman et al. (1957) and, although successful, was attended by a sizeable number of cardiac arrhythmias and one case of total and persistent heart block. Following the development of techniques for retrograde insertion of catheters into the aorta and left ventricle, the transternal or transthoracic approach has been largely abandoned.

Castellanos and Pereiras (1942) injected contrast substance in a retrograde direction into the brachial artery. The direction of blood flow was temporarily reversed so that a sufficiently high concentration of the contrast substance entered the aorta so as to permit quite satisfactory visualization. All of these subjects, however, were children, and more extended experience with this technique demonstrated that it was not satisfactory in adults.

Radner (1948), dissatisfied with direct puncture of the aorta, experimented with the insertion of a ureteral type catheter into the right or left radial artery and guiding the tip into the ascending aorta under fluoroscopic control. He injected 20–30 ml of 70% contrast substance as rapidly as possible using a hand syringe, but this gave only a faint visualization of the aorta. Broden et al. (1949) continued further with the technique and were able to decrease greatly the number of cases in which the procedure had to be abandoned because of arterial spasm or inability to position properly the catheter in the ascending aorta. Also, by using the pressure pump developed by Jönsson (1949) a much greater flow rate of contrast substance could be obtained, and the resultant aortograms were quite satisfactory. Numbers of workers had experience with nonopaque conventional polyethylene catheters in aortography (Helmsworth et al., 1950; Pierce, 1951). Seldinger (1953) described a most useful improvement whereby a catheter larger than the puncture needle could be inserted into either an artery or a vein. After puncture of the selected vessel, a spring guide was passed through the needle into the vessel and the needle removed. Then, a suitable catheter could be inserted around the guide and into the artery. Upon withdrawal of the catheter, the puncture wound with local compression closed spontaneously and with a minimum of complications. This procedure eliminated the need for arterial repair and cutdown procedures in most cases and stimulated the use of retrograde aortography and the approach to the left ventricle by the transaortic route. Prioton et al. (1957) described a more extensive experience in left ventriculography and aortography using the transaortic route, and this method was used more extensively in the United States by Amplatz et al. (1959) and Dotter (1960). Desilets and Hoffman (1965) have described a technique by which closed end catheters could be inserted percutaneously.

Another approach to the left side of the heart and particularly the left atrium was described by Ross (1959) and Brockenbrough and Braunwald (1960). It consists of passage of a suitable catheter over a special needle, the tip of which lies in the left atrium. After puncture of the interatrial septum, the catheter is passed over the needle into the left atrium and the needle is withdrawn. It is then possible to pass the catheter into the left ventricle, and selective left atrial and left ventricular angiography can be performed.

Image amplification and television monitor viewing became more widely available in the early fifties, and this stimulated and greatly facilitated the selective catheterization of the heart and great vessels by the procedures mentioned above. Also, image amplification, by reducing radiation exposure to acceptable levels, opened up the development of cinefluorography as a practical recording vehicle. Tape, and later disc recorders were easily adapted to the television systems and served as supplementary recording methods. Concurrently over the past 20 years, large film changers have steadily improved so that at the present time we have a wide range of available recording devices. Thus, it is seen that the present eminent status of cardioangiography is due to a convergence of several lines of advance occurring over a period of approximately 40 years. This brief sketch fails to mention many important contributions by dozens of pioneers in this field.

PATIENT PREPARATION

The vast majority of cardioangiographic procedures is carried out under local anesthesia with a conscious and, it is hoped, a cooperative patient. Only on rare occasions, usually in small children or disturbed adults, is a general anesthetic necessary. It is customary to withhold food and fluids for at least several hours preceding the examination in order to prevent aspiration of gastric contents. On the other hand, dehydration must be avoided as it distinctly increases the chances of complications from the use of contrast substance.

Premedication is generally desirable for all types of angiography. A tranquilizer, such as Valium in 5- to 10-mg doses, is desirable. This is supplemented by demerol and scopolamine or a barbiturate. In children, we prefer a mixture known as a "cardiac cocktail" containing 25 mg of demerol, 6.25 mg of phenergan, and chlorpromazine, 6.25 mg/ml. The standard dose is 1 ml for each 20 pounds of body weight.

It is customary in most hospitals to have the patient duly sign an authorization or permission form for each specific procedure. A simple signing of this form is of little medicolegal consequence unless it is accompanied by a valid and medically complete explanation of the possible hazards and consequences of the examination. This should be done in the presence of a witness if at all possible. A valid consent under these circumstances should be obtained from all patients or guardians. One or more followup visits are mandatory following completion of this procedure, and the radiologist has not discharged his responsibility until the patient has passed the critical periods of complication, usually 24–48 hr following the completion of the procedure. The radiologist must take the primary responsibility for the detection and the diagnosis of complications and the institution of proper treatment.

Test Dose for Sensitivity

We prefer to administer this procedure routinely, but only because of tradition and possible medicolegal considerations. In our experience, the test dose has not been helpful in predicting untoward or even fatal reactions. In 4 fatal reactions which we have personally observed, the test dose in no way foretold the severe reaction leading to death. On the other hand, we have seen patients become nauseated and vomit following the initial test dose and yet the regular dose was given without untoward effects. The test dose that we administer is composed of 1 ml of contrast substance which is diluted to 10 ml with normal saline for adults. For children, half of this amount is used. This is injected intravenously slowly over a period of about 1 min.

VENOUS ANGIOCARDIOGRAPHY

Experienced angiographers rarely use this procedure today. When the technique is mastered, it is a simple procedure. It suffices for a number of problems, particularly those associated with visualization of the right side of the heart and the vena cavae. In many circumstances, it may give adequate but often minimal visualization of the left side of the heart and aorta. It is particularly useful in the superior vena caval syndrome and the diagnosis of suspected pericardial effusion. It can be performed very rapidly and does not require the supporting personnel necessary for selective angiography. It is thus better adapted to the small hospital and makes useful angiography widely available. Although it is a relatively simple procedure, a rigid adherence to detail and timing is necessary to produce a satisfactory examination. For a detailed description of the fine points of this technique, the reader is referred to the classical paper of Robb and Steinberg (1939). The circulation time is determined in all patients despite the availability of as many as 30 films. Every effort should be made to reduce the number of films used consistent with proper delineation of both sides of the heart and the pulmonary circulation. The rapid injection of the contrast substance in 2 sec or less in adults is essential. To facilitate this, the cannula must be unobstructed and injection must be made during inspiration, if possible. Four sizes of Robb-Steinberg cannulas are available (#10, 0.105 inch; #12, 0.085 inch; #13, 0.074 inch; and #15, 0.054 inch). The largest cannula that can be inserted should be used.

SELECTIVE ANGIOCARDIOGRAPHY

These examinations are often done in connection with and as a part of a cardiac catheterization procedure. The injection of contrast substance may be delayed until most or all of the hemodynamic data have been collected. Again, it may be done in order to better identify a particular chamber or vessel and its relationship and as a guide to further catheterization procedures. Again, it may be performed as an isolated procedure with the object of elucidating a particular defect or disorder.

Right Atrium

Either a side- or an end-hole catheter is placed in the midportion of the right atrium. The catheter may be inserted either through the arm vein or through the femoral vein. Frequently a second injection into the pulmonary artery is anticipated as in cases of suspected pulmonary thromboembolism, and in such instances a side-hole catheter is essential. The amount of contrast substance is 40–50 ml in 1.5–2 sec. Frontal and lateral projections are commonly used.

Right Ventricle

An end-hole catheter is a hazard and should not be used because of the possibility of an intramyocardial injection. The catheter irritates the conduction system, and extra systoles are frequent. Injections of 40–45 ml of contrast substance over a period of 3–4 sec are satisfactory. Standard positions to show the outflow tract are the frontal and lateral views and occasionally 15–20° of right anterior obliquity. Other projections rarely add anything to that which can be seen in these views. Following the right ventricular injection, the catheter is immediately withdrawn into the right atrium. Right ventriculography is performed most often in the study of pulmonary stenosis, either valvular or in the tetralogy of Fallot, and also in the evaluation of tricuspid insufficiency.

Pulmonary Artery

A catheter with side holes is essential. The tip of the catheter should be placed near or at the bifurcation of the pulmonary artery. This is the preferable position for the pulmonary angiogram, and at times it can be used for visualization of the left side of the heart. Care should be taken not to insert the catheter too far into either the right or left artery since this may cause a one-sided injection. Also, the insertion should be far enough to prevent recoil into the right ventricle. Inadvertent recoil into the right ventricle may obscure the left lower lobe pulmonary arteries. The usual dose of contrast substance is 40–45 ml injected in 1.5–2 sec. The frontal projection is routine, and a lateral projection is of little help when both pulmonary arteries are injected. On the other hand, selective injections into either the right or left arteries may at times be necessary, such as in a search for small pulmonary emboli. In these instances, an oblique or lateral view may be helpful. For selective injections, the dose of contrast substance must be reduced and may vary from 5 ml injected by hand, to 20 ml by a power injector. Care should be taken not to wedge the catheter into a pulmonary artery. Injections in such circumstances may produce localized but rather profound pulmonary edema.

Left Atrium

Entrance into the left atrium is gained either through an interatrial defect or the use of the Brockenbrough catheter inserted transeptally. In the adult, 40–45 ml of contrast substance in 3–4 sec are adequate. The procedure is most often performed in children with congenital heart disease.

Left Ventricle

Entrance into the left ventricle may be obtained either transeptally via the left atrium and mitral valve, or retrograde from the aorta. The aortic valves offer a considerable obstruction to the passage of a straight catheter, and a soft molded catheter inserted over a soft tip guide-wire usually may be inserted with little difficulty. The molded catheter with side holes then assumes a ring shape when it enters the left ventricle, and the guidewire is withdrawn. The ring-shaped tip on the curved catheter is less likely to wedge itself between the columna carneae and bring on a myocardial injection. Care should be taken not to position the catheter so close to the mitral valve as to affect its activity. In an adult, 40–45 ml injected slowly over a period of 4–5 sec is recommended. A slow injection tends to reduce the incidence of extrasystoles and thus provides a more reliable study of valvular function. The right and left oblique projections are most commonly used. The right anterior oblique usually projects the largest profile of the left ventricle and is most useful in studying the ventricular dynamics. It also shows the plane of the mitral valve to the best advantage. The left anterior oblique brings the interventricular septum into good profile and is useful in the study of inter-ventricular septal defects and aneurysms of the ventricular septum. In this projection, the mitral valve is viewed en face. The frontal projection is also helpful in studying the outflow tract of the left ventricle and the location of ventricular septal defects.

THORACIC AORTOGRAPHY

Both in the performance of left ventriculography and thoracic aortography, the selection of the route for the insertion of the catheter depends on the age and condition of the patient. Also, in the case of aortography attention must be given to the particular problem and specific portion of the aorta under investigation. All segments of the aorta and its major branches, including the coronary arteries, can be reached through the femoral artery if care and the proper type of catheter are used. The technique of coronary arteriography will be described in the section devoted to that procedure. The femoral artery, because of its size and accessibility, is the most desirable route, particularly when the percutaneous technique is used. It seems less susceptible to complications than the brachial route. In an older person (over 50 years of age), the high incidence of atherosclerosis of the lower abdominal aorta and its branches makes the route more hazardous and less certain. The brachial arteries are less subject to atherosclerosis and are a very satisfactory alternate route. The artery is customarily punctured just above the antecubital fossa. Percutaneous puncture of the brachial artery may not always be satisfactory, and a cutdown and incision into the artery may be necessary in order to insert a proper catheter.

Consequently, the experienced angiographer should be familiar with the repair of small arteries. All segments of the aorta cannot be reached by a catheter from the left brachial artery under every circumstance. With advancing age and particularly in association with hypertension, the aorta elongates, and the relative position of the left subclavian orifice is shifted toward the apex of the arch. This makes entry of the catheter into the ascending aorta easy. In young persons and with relatively normal aortas, a straight catheter almost invariably passes into the descending aorta (Bosniak, 1964) when entering the aorta from the left subclavian artery. Experience in molding the catheter tip and in manipulation is of great help in these circumstances. The right brachial artery provides the most reliable and easiest route to the ascending aorta and is certainly the route of choice in selective coronary arteriography. Atherosclerosis with elongation, narrowing, and tortuosity of the subclavian and innominate arteries is a frequent occurrence in older patients and may make this route difficult or impossible.

The axillary artery on either side is readily accessible to percutaneous puncture and can be considered as a less desirable alternative route by those who are accustomed to and thoroughly familiar with its use. It is a slightly larger artery than the brachial and permits the use of a shorter catheter. The control of hematoma formation after removal of the catheter requires more attention than is the case in the femoral or brachial area.

Equipment

The equipment is the same as that found in angiographic special procedure rooms and is described in that section.

Catheters

A wide variety of catheters is available, either homemade out of stock materials or ready-made. The choice of catheters depends on the operator's preference, experience, and the specific structures under investigation. A program of inventory control should be established in order that the catheters do not become old, brittle, and otherwise outdated. If there is any question about the quality of the catheter, it should be discarded.

Hazards and Complications

These may be considered as minor, major, and fatal. The minor complications, for the most part, are associated with the insertion of a catheter into a peripheral artery and are not peculiar to thoracic aortography. Lang (1963) found the incidence of minor complications to be about 3%, but this is variable, depending on the criteria for reporting complications. The most common complication is temporary arterial spasm. Its incidence is affected by the duration of the procedure and the extent of the catheter manipulation and, of course, the skill of the operator. Dampening of the pulse distal to the arterial puncture with a mild degree of pallor is not unusual. This is more common with the brachial than the femoral artery and is more common in females, perhaps associated with the generally smaller size of their artery. It is ordinarily treated expectantly with frequent observation and perhaps the administration of papaverine. It is now realized that in many cases a small thrombus has lodged near the site of insertion of the catheter, and this may be followed by further thrombosis and a serious impairment of the circulation. This then becomes a major complication and will be considered below. If a previously strong pulse is totally suppressed for 1 hr after removal of the catheter, the possibility of a thrombosis must be strongly considered.

Local hematoma formation is common but when it exceeds an estimated 30 ml it is considered to be a minor complication. Significant hematomas can be largely prevented by proper pressure applied at the right spot after withdrawal of the catheter. Where blood continues to collect, an attempt should be made to diffuse it by massage. Halpern (1964) believes that a persistent hematoma in proximity to the artery predisposes to false aneurysm formation.

When the bleeding exceeds 500 ml and is sufficient to disturb the patient's blood pressure and pulse rate, it is a major complication and may require immediate treatment. Predisposing factors are: (1) Heparinization established during the aortographic procedure. The effect of the heparin should be promptly neutralized by appropriate injection of protamine sulfate with monitoring of the clotting time. (2) Improper site for arterial puncture. The proper site for femoral puncture is about 2–4 cm below the inguinal ligament. If the puncture is higher, the needle may enter the artery in the retroperitoneal space. The tissue in this region does not retain the hematoma. Also, the puncture site is less susceptible to external pressure. A large hematoma may form in the retroperitoneal tissues without being readily detected externally. Direct surgical intervention may be necessary in these cases to stop the hemorrhage. (3) Early ambulation may be a cause of delayed bleeding. The patient should be kept immobile for at least 6 hr.

The most common major complications are those due to thromboembolism and thrombosis at the puncture site. The incidence of these complications is about 2% (Cramer *et al.*, 1973). Siegelman *et al.* (1968) found that fresh clot was stripped from the exterior of the catheter at or near the puncture site as the catheter was being removed from the artery. The clot is usually deposited on the exterior of the catheter near the tip. This clot may partially or completely occlude the artery and form a nidus for further thrombus formation. Ovitt *et al.* (1974) demonstrated clot formation on guidewires left in place only a few minutes during the exchange of catheters. Following the insertion of the second catheter, the clot is stripped off, and this may act as an embolus. Such a clot, if dislodged in the ascending aorta, might embolize either the coronary or cerebral arteries. A significant decrease in the clot formation on catheters and guidewires can be obtained by proper heparinization during the aortographic procedure (Wallace *et al.*, 1972); Freed *et al.*, 1974). In addition, Cramer *et al.* (1973), Ovitt *et al.* (1974), and Hawkins and Kelley (1973) have advocated the coating of catheters and guidewires with benzalkonium-heparin complex. Controlled heparinization is recommended except in those cases in which there is a contraindication, such as intestinal or intracranial hemorrhage.

Thrombosis is more common in infants and young children (Cramer *et al.*, 1973; Freed *et al.*, 1974) and in women, probably associated with the smaller size of their arteries. Other factors which affect the incidence of local thrombosis and embolism are congestive heart failure, advanced age, localized atherosclerosis, and arterial spasm.

The question of the need for surgical intervention for removal of a thrombus or embolus requires considerable judgment and experience. Continuous observation by the radiologist is essential until the pulse returns to its normal volume or a decision is made for surgical intervention. Expectant treatment consists of the administration of papaverine and heparin. Most cases can be treated expectantly for periods of up to 4 hr, and some authors suggest periods of up to 48 hr, particularly if there is any observable pulse. Cramer *et al.* (1973) suggest that prompt surgical intervention is preferred if the pulse has not returned to good volume within a few hours. Even though the thrombus is not totally occlusive, it may sufficiently narrow the artery so that when the patient resumes normal activity arterial insufficiency and claudication may occur.

Another major complication is that of damage to the thoracic spinal cord. All of the commonly used contrast substances are neurotoxic and dangerous, methylglucamine or iodothalamate perhaps being the least neurotoxic (DiChiro, 1974). The true incidence of this complication is uncertain since a number of catastrophies have probably not been reported. The greatest danger occurs with the injection of the intercostal arteries, and Kardjiev *et al.* (1974) suggest that injections into the right fifth intercostal artery is particularly prone to be followed by temporary and at times permanent damage. Midstream injections have been followed by nerve damage since the contrast substance tends to stratify posteriorly and enter the intercostal arteries in high concentration. In most instances, there has been a selective injection with associated momentary occlusion of the segmental arteries. Careful monitoring is always necessary to see that the catheter tip has not inadvertently entered a segmental artery (Brodey *et al.*, 1974).

The number of admitted instances where the catheter has been thrust through the wall of an artery or has created a false passage in the artery without detectable untoward sequelae is amazing. We have seen either a guidewire or catheter clearly outside the aorta several times, and have succeeded in their withdrawal without any untoward reaction, but this is not always the case. Surgical intervention is occasionally necessary to arrest hemorrhage from a perforated aorta. Lang (1963) found 22 instances in which a major vessel had been perforated without sequelae.

Contrast substance may be injected subintimally or submurally without detectable permanent injury. Lang (1963) reported this in 136 instances in his review. Neither the perforation of a major vessel or a subintimal or intramural injection should be viewed with equanimity since in 1 case the subintimal injection ruptured the aorta and resulted in sudden death. Cooley *et al.* (1972) and Wellons and Singh (1974) report cases of dissecting aneurysm secondary to retrograde brachial approach to the ascending aorta. The tortuous innominate artery may be easily damaged and may develop a false passage that leads to a dissecting aneurysm.

False aneurysms at the puncture site and arteriovenous fistulas between the saphenous vein and the femoral artery have been reported (Pierce and Ramey, 1953).

A preventable complication is that of breakage of the guidewire. The guidewire may be faulty, and this should be detected before insertion. Wires with small kinks or angulations should be viewed with suspicion, since these are very susceptible to shearing when they are passed through the cannula.

In a survey, Abrams (1957) found 29 deaths attributed to thoracic aortography among 1,706 examinations, or a mortality of 1.7%. This included aortography performed by all means and routes and included a considerable number of countercurrent cases performed in infants. Evidence of severe brain damage was present in at least 19 of these fatalities and was strongly suspected in 3 others. Heart, renal, and respiratory failure were listed as other causes of death, in that order. Hemiplegia was noted in 13 other patients who survived, and 6 patients had convulsions during or immediately following the examination. In at least 3 instances, the catheter was placed in or near the mouth of either the carotid or innominate arteries. Brain damage must be attributed to direct action of the contrast substance on the blood brain barrier. In the more recent survey of all types of aortographies, including thoracic aortography, by Lang (1963) and Halpern (1964) there is no mention of brain damage due to contrast substance. This marked decrease is undoubtedly due to more careful monitoring of catheter placement and perhaps to the use of more innocuous diatrizoate contrast substances. The mortality from all types of percutaneous aortography in Lang's survey (1963) was only 0.06%.

In summary, most of the minor and major complications of thoracic aortography are associated with thromboembolism and with the insertion, proper placement, and withdrawal of the catheter. The incidence of thrombosis and thromboembolism has been substantially reduced by proper heparinization and treatment of the catheters. Prompt treatment of thrombosis by surgery will greatly diminish the morbidity of this complication.

Indications

Thoracic aortography is indicated in any suspected abnormality of the aorta or its major branches in which an exact diagnosis is necessary before surgical treatment can be attempted and in which simpler procedures will not suffice. Following is a list of some of the conditions in which aortography may be used to advantage.

Congenital Anomalies

1. Complicated or atypical patent ductus arteriosus. This is most likely to be present in infancy or in young children with large hearts and some degree of heart failure.
2. Aortic pulmonary window. Precise diagnosis may be of great advantage in determining the surgical approach.
3. Coarctation of the aorta.
4. Ruptured aortic sinus aneurysm.
5. Anomalies of the aortic arch.
6. Aortic valvular and supravalvular stenosis.
7. Truncus arteriosus.
8. Sequestration of the lung.

Acquired Diseases

1. Aortic aneurysm.
2. Aortic insufficiency.
3. Aortic stenosis.
4. Buckling of the aorta or buckling of the brachiocephalic arteries, particularly the innominate artery.
5. Aortic arch syndrome. This condition is often associated with so-called pulseless disease, and aortography may demonstrate the site of the obstruction to the carotid and innominate arteries.
6. Dissecting hematoma.
7. Traumatic laceration.

3

Contrast Substances

The development of better contrast substances over the past 40 years has contributed greatly to the present status of diagnostic angiographic procedures. Modern contrast substances are relatively innocuous and rarely constitute an absolute contraindication or severe hazard in the performance of angiographic procedures. Nevertheless, the ideal contrast substance has not as yet appeared, and now there is some apprehension that the untoward effects of the commonly used substances may not be receiving the attention that they deserve.

Diodrast, Neo-Iopax, and Thorotrast are mainly of historical interest. Thorotrast is a 25% colloidal suspension of thorium dioxide and is a tempting medium because of its high opacity and nonirritating effects on the endothelium of blood vessels and other organ tissue, such as that of the myocardium and kidney. Unfortunately, thorium particles are fixed by the reticuloendothelial cells, particularly of the liver and spleen, where prolonged radioactivity has been followed by extensive fibrosis and sarcoma. Also, extravasations into subcutaneous tissue around the injection sites have produced extensive and, at times, incapacitating sheets of fibrous tissue. Consequently, the risks of the use of Thorotrast outweigh its advantages. It has been withdrawn from the market and is not approved by the Federal Drug Administration.

Sodium acetrizoate (Urokon[1]) is also mentioned because of its historical interest and its close chemical resemblance to the diatrizoates in common use today. Urokon appeared in 1950 and was soon widely used. For equivalent iodine content, it had the lowest viscosity of any available contrast substance. Initially, its toxicity appeared less than its predecessors, namely Neo-Iopax and Diodrast, but more extended use and animal experiments showed a dangerously low threshold of neurotoxicity (brain and spinal cord) and nephrotoxicity. Urokon has consequently been withdrawn from the market.

In wide use today are the meglumine Na, Ca, and Mg salts of diatrizoic, iothalamic, and metrizoic acid. Diagram 1 shows the chemical formulas of some of the substances and the trade names under which they are marketed. Actually, most of these products are mixtures of two or more salts, thus Renografin[2] 60 and 76%, Hypaque[3] 75 and 90%, and Cardio-Conray[1] contain both sodium and meglumine salts. Certain of the Isopaque[3] compounds may have mixtures of three or more salts which are thought to reduce their toxicity. The descriptive leaflets that accompany each product should be consulted regarding their composition, and even more exact and definitive information can be obtained by corresponding with the manufacturer.

TOXICITY

Contrast substances are injected for the purpose of visualization of the cardiovascular system and ideally should not provoke hemodynamic or pharmacologic changes in the patient. Nevertheless, all of the presently used substances, particularly when injected rapidly and in relatively large volume as is usual in angiography, produce pharmacologic and hemodynamic effects, most of which are undesirable. Some of these effects are easily reproducible and clearly demonstrated; others are more obscure and speculative, and still others are under investigation. Of particular importance are the synergistic reactions that contrast substances may have in combination

[1] Mallinckrodt Chemical Company, St. Louis, Missouri.
[2] Squibb Pharmaceutical Company.
[3] Winthrop Drug Company.

DIAGRAM 1

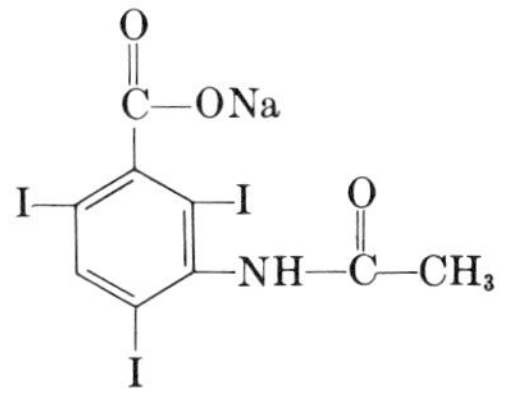

Urokon (Mallinckrodt): Sodium acetrizoate

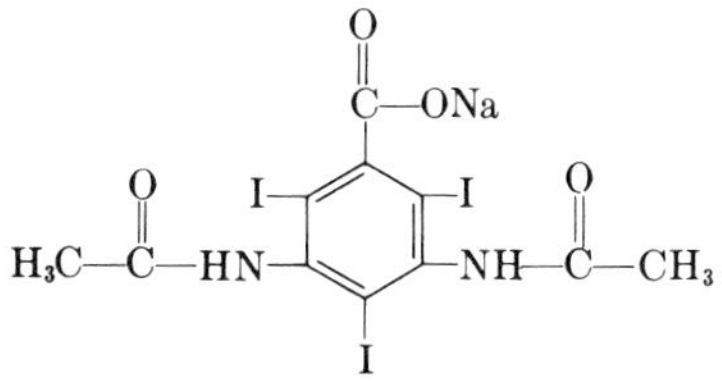

Hypaque (Winthrop): Sodium diatrizoate

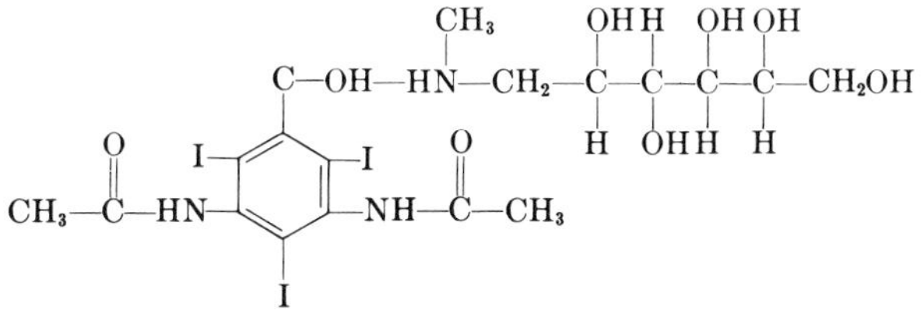

Renografin-76 (Cardiografin) (Squibb):
Methylglucamine diatrizoate

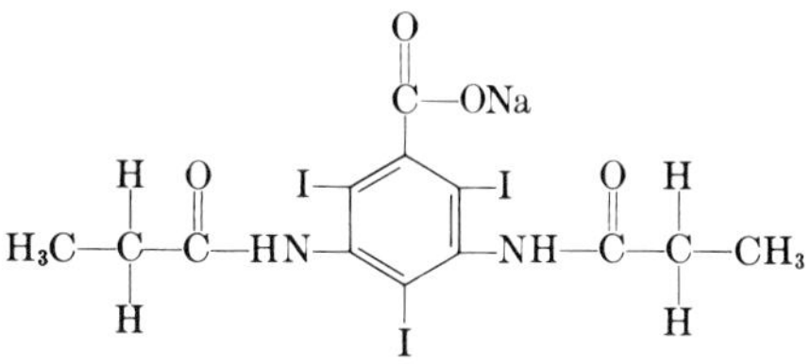

Miokon (Mallinckrodt): Sodium diprotrizoate

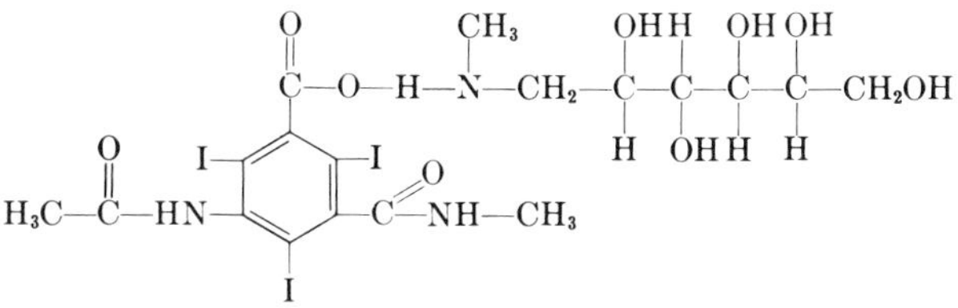

Conray (Mallinckrodt): N-Methylglucamine salt of iothalamic
acid

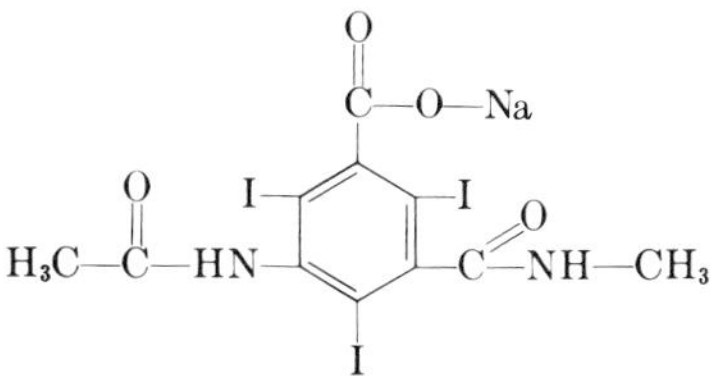

Angio-Conray (Mallinckrodt):
Sodium salt of iothalamic acid

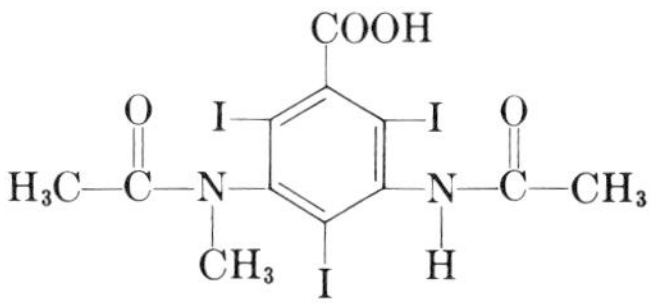

Metrizoic Acid Isopaque 440 (Winthrop): sodium, calcium and
magnesium salt of metrizoic acid

with the underlying disease processes that create the need for angiography. Also, the relationships to the therapeutic drugs that are used in the treatment of these conditions must be considered. These latter considerations perhaps have not received the attention they deserve and must always be weighed, even though our knowledge is incomplete.

All of these substances are moderately complex organic crystalline chemicals in which the iodine is firmly bound to the remainder of the molecule. They are excreted predominantly by the kidney but also by the liver, and to a much lesser degree, by the intestinal mucosa. In watery solution, they are hypertonic. Because of this hypertonicity (osmolarity 5–10 times that of blood), these substances produce an immediate dilution of the plasma with a transient reduction

in the hematocrit (Friesinger et al., 1965; Read et al., 1960). Part of the fluid is drawn from the red cells which then appear shrunken and crenated. Although hemolysis of significant degree usually does not occur, exceptions have been noted, particularly in patients with polycythemia (Cohen et al., 1969). Fluid may also enter the blood from the perivascular fluid space. The hematocrit returns to normal in 10–15 min. This reaction is not specific for contrast substance but can be produced in variable degree by a number of other hypertonic solutions, such as sodium chloride, urea, and glucose (Hilal, 1966).

Vasodilatation of peripheral vessels occurs immediately and is obviously most pronounced in the vascular bed nearest the site of injection. In peripheral angiography, the affected limb may show the effect strikingly, and this is accompanied by increased local blood flow and a decrease in peripheral resistance (Lasser, 1968). Similarly, injections into the coronary arteries in experimental animals, after a very transient decrease during immediate perfusion, are followed by an increase in the blood flow of as much as 60% (Fisher *et al.*, 1968; Friesinger *et al.*, 1965). The vasodilating effect appears to take place at the smooth muscle cell in the vessel wall, but here the mechanism is not entirely clear (Lindgren, 1970).

Intracardiac Injections

Following injections into the left side of the heart and aorta, the systemic blood pressure, after an initial transient rise, falls. The diastolic pressure falls more than the systolic, giving an increased pulse pressure. This is accompanied by an increase in heart rate, stroke volume, and cardiac output. Thus, the decrease in systemic blood pressure appears to be due to predominance of a vasodilating effect and decreased systemic resistance (Fisher, 1968). Injections into the right side of the heart or pulmonary artery are followed by somewhat different hemodynamic effects. These injections produce pulmonary hypertension, systemic hypotension and decreased cardiac output, bradycardia for varying periods of time, and diminished cardiac contractile force (Lindgren, 1970). The bradycardia and systemic hypotension are attributed to direct depressive effects of the contrast substance on the myocardium, decrease in peripheral resistance, and possibly reflex mechanisms associated with the carotid vascular system.

Some of the most disconcerting and mysterious effects of contrast substances are those that clinically resemble hypersensitivity or allergic reactions. Minor reactions, such as sneezing, urticaria, rhinorrhea, cough, headache, and laryngeal edema, are fairly common. A considerable proportion of the fatal reactions during urography appear to have been anaphylactoid in nature. These types of reactions are said to be more common in persons with allergic backgrounds or histories of allergic reactions. On the other hand, they are no more common in those who have had previous contact with contrast substances than in those who have had no contact (Lasser, 1968). None of the usual sensitivity tests permits a prediction as to the probability of these types of reaction. Attempts to produce antibodies to contrast substance in animals, for the most part, have been unsuccessful. Also, the chemical structures of the contrast substances are such that on theoretical grounds no antigen-antibody reaction is to be expected. A possible cause for allergic

reactions was suggested by Mann (1961). He postulated that certain sensitive tissues in allergic individuals might react to contrast substance by releasing histamine and the histamine in turn could produce many of the signs and symptoms of hypersensitivity. This possibility has been under active investigation (Rockoff *et al.*, 1970, 1972; Lasser *et al.*, 1971). A number of the sodium salts of contrast materials will cause an increased release of histamine from mast cells incubated in vitro. To date, the presence of increased amounts of histamine in patients showing allergic reactions to contrast substances has not been conclusively documented (Rockoff *et al.*, 1972; Lasser *et al.*, 1971).

Another fundamental mechanism associated with the effects of contrast substance is that of binding to the plasma proteins. Lasser (1968) found that the capacity to bind with plasma proteins correlated closely with the LD^{50} of the particular contrast substance (lethal dose for 50% of animals subjected to risk). The LD^{50} was lowest for those compounds with the greatest capacity to bind with the plasma proteins. Lasser's hypothesis, now supported by a considerable amount of experimental evidence, indicates that the contrast-protein combinations have an inhibiting effect on enzymes, such as acetyl cholinesterase and glucose-6-phosphate dehydrogenase, among others. This in turn might well have an effect on smooth muscle in the blood vessel walls and red blood cell permeability. In addition, evidence has accumulated suggesting that protein-bound contrast substances may alter blood coagulation mechanisms either by antifibrin or fibrinolytic activity. Also, the possibility that they may have an effect on the allergic reactions has not been excluded. All of these mechanisms are under continued investigation.

Reaction of Specific Organ Systems

Brain

The classic investigations of Broman and Olsson (1949) demonstrated that the blood brain barrier was damaged by the intracarotid injection of both Diodrast and Urokon. The extent of the damage depended on both the amount and concentration of the contrast substance, and a succession of small injections, each of which alone was well tolerated, had a cumulative damaging effect. Also, pre-existing injury or damage to the cerebral tissues enhanced the unfavorable effects of the contrast substance. Bloor *et al.* (1951) and Whiteleather and DeSaussure (1956) found Urokon to be more damaging to the brain than Diodrast and Hypaque, respectively.

Fischer and Eckstein (1961) measured systemic blood pressure and electrocardiographic responses and found that Renografin produced the least deviation from the normal of the substances then available. The brain appeared to have a very good tolerance for this substance.

Hilal (1966) found that injections into the internal carotid artery did not produce dilatation of the cerebral blood vessels. Injections into the common carotid artery produced a vasodilatation in the external carotid system with a shunting of blood from the internal to the external system. Intracarotid injections also produced systemic hypotension mediated by two distinct mechanisms: (1) stimulation of the pressure receptors in the cerebral vessels and (2) effects on the vasomotor centers of the brain. Meglumine iothalamate produced less change in the measured parameters in the dog than the other present day substances, namely Hypaque and Renografin. It is obvious that the reaction of the brain to contrast substances is of concern, not only in cerebral angiography but also in thoracic aortography where sizeable amounts of the contrast substance enter the carotid and vertebral arteries. Many of the earlier deaths associated with thoracic aortography were due to brain injury (Abrams, 1957).

Heart

The effects of injections into the cardiac chambers have been described above in connection with the general reactions to contrast substances. Part of the observed effects, particularly those having to do with contractility of the heart, may be due to perfusion of the coronary system by the contrast substance. It is likely (Friesinger *et al.*, 1965) that the perfusion of the coronary arteries is not an important factor in the changes and activity of the myocardium following left ventricular injections.

The intramyocardial injection of contrast substances occurs rarely during coronary arteriography and more frequently during right and left ventriculography. It may cause changes in the electrocardiogram but is usually well tolerated, and the contrast substance is absorbed in 10–15 min. On the other hand, arrhythmias and fatal ventricular fibrillation have occurred (Lehman *et al.*, 1959; Bookstein and Sigmann, 1963).

Coronary Vascular System

Some of the effects of the injection of contrast substances into the coronary arteries have been referred to above, such as increased blood flow, decreased myocardial contractility, and elevation of end-diastolic pressure in the left ventricle. The experiments of Gensini and DiGiorgi (1964) indicated that the sodium salts of diatrizoate caused more severe changes in the myocardial conductivity and a higher frequency of ventricular fibrillation than did the corresponding methylglucamine salts. Experience has tended to confirm these observation, and methylglucamine salts are now preferred for coronary arteriography, although the addition of a small amount of the sodium salt to the methyl glucamine seems to be an advantage. See Chapter 14, "Coronary Arteriography."

Spinal Cord

Margolis *et al.* (1958) found that injections of as little as 1 ml of 70% Urokon into the lower abdominal aorta of dogs were followed by convulsions of the lower limbs and residual paralysis. A number of instances of transverse myelitis in patients following abdominal aortography were reported (McAfee, 1957), confirming the toxicity of contrast substances to the spinal cord. Following the widespread use of the diatrizoates and iothalamates, and also greater care to avoid direct injections into the upper lumbar segmental arteries, these complications have become much rarer, although they remain a threat.

Kidney

McAfee (1957) found 39 serious reactions with 12 deaths associated with evidence of severe damage to the kidneys following lumbar aortography. In most of these cases, Urokon or Neo-Iopax had been the offending agent.

Experiments on the rabbit kidney (Idbohrn and Berg, 1954) using Diodrast, Miokon, and Urokon showed that the damage was due to a direct action on the glomeruli and tubules. Later investigations (Berg *et al.*, 1958) showed that the newer agents, namely Hypaque and Renografin, were much less toxic, and very little damage followed the use of 76% Renografin and 90% Hypaque.

Direct injections of contrast substance into the renal artery of the canine kidney produce an initial but quite transient vasodilatation that can be shown angiographically. This is apparently followed by a prolonged vasoconstriction. The activation of the renin-angiotensin system has been implicated as a cause of this phenomenon (Caldicott *et al.*, 1970).

Visceral Arterial System

Robinson (1956) reported acute pancreatitis following inadvertent injection of 20 ml of 70% Urokon into the celiac axis during lumbar aortography. On the other hand, the present authors

(Cooley *et al.*, 1964) have injected up to 4 ml/kg into the celiac axes of 5 dogs without immediate visible change in the viscera or permanent change as determined by postmortem examination 4 weeks later

Grayson *et al.* (1961) found a high incidence of patchy muscle and/or mucosal necrosis after the injection of contrast substances into the arcuate branches of the mesenteric artery. Radiographs often showed extravasation of the contrast material into the bowel wall. Doses of as little as 2 ml of 50% Miokon occasionally caused similar damage. Reaction was much less frequent with Hypaque, and in 12 experiments using up to 16 ml of 60% Renografin, no severe or permanent injury was found.

Cooley *et al.* (1964), using doses of up to 7 ml of 76% Renografin injected by catheter into the superior mesenteric artery of dogs, found no permanent damage at postmortem examination. The tolerance of the mesenteric and celiac arterial bed for Renografin seems quite ample, and this is supported by experience with celiac and mesenteric arteriography.

Possible Exaggerated and Harmful Effects of Contrast Substances on Existing Disease Processes

Several possible situations come to mind. The hypotension and decreased cardiac contractility that follow intracardiac injection of contrast substances may decrease blood flow to vital organs such as the brain, coronary circulation, and kidneys. This may occur for several minutes following the injection. A decrease in blood flow to the brain or to the heart may be critical in a patient with advanced coronary or cerebral atherosclerosis. Injections into the right ventricle or pulmonary artery produce clumping and agglutination of red cells with some resulting capillary obstruction and pulmonary hypertension. This may stimulate pulmonary edema. The sudden increase in plasma volume following the injection of contrast substance into any part of the vascular system may act as an additional load on a partially decompensated heart. This in turn could contribute to pulmonary edema and, of course, a decrease in perfusion of vital organs. Extensive hemolysis which has been noted in a few cases (Cohen *et al.*, 1969) could lead to renal tubular damage. The indication for adequate hydration during angiocardiography in such cases is quite clear. While none of these mechanisms have been documented as an important cause of morbidity or mortality, they certainly remain threats within the framework of our knowledge of the action of the contrast substance.

Other Effects of Contrast Substances

The reaction to the injection of the newer contrast substances as observed clinically varies somewhat in intensity from patient to patient. In the majority of patients, the reaction is mild and not particularly objectionable; at times, however, it is distinctly unpleasant. Five to ten seconds after the injection, depending on the circulation time, the reaction begins with a feeling of flushing and heat in the face and scalp which spreads rapidly over the entire body. Headache often localized to the occiput is occasionally seen. A metallic, irritating taste appears in the mouth and throat, and there is a tendency to cough, and in some instances, the cough may be explosive and severe. If the patient is erect, he may become dizzy. In the recumbent position this is infrequent. Some degree of nausea is not unusual, but retching is uncommon; if it persists, it often precedes some degree of circulatory reaction which may be severe. The sensation of heat may localize in the perineum or around the genitals and linger there for some minutes. In the vast majority of instances, all signs and symptoms will disappear in 10 min.

Allergic manifestations of a minor nature are rather frequent, but they are rarely alarming or severe. A small percentage of patients show several skin wheals or typical urticaria after the first injection. Occasionally, this may be widespread and produce considerable discomfort. We have frequently given a second injection after the appearance of the urticaria, and it has usually been well tolerated. If symptoms of burning and itching become severe, 3 ml (30 mg) of Benadryl are given intravenously.

FACTORS GOVERNING INJECTION

Failure to obtain an adequate concentration of iodine at a particular point of interest is a common cause of unsatisfactory angiograms. Experiments with plastic containers and phantoms show that a concentration of about 1.5–2.5% iodine produces a readily recognizable increase in density of the blood in a vessel the size of the aorta and should provide a distinct contrast between the blood and the surrounding cardiac muscle and other mediastinal contents. This var-

Contrast Substance	Iodine Content	Total Amount	Flow Rate Iodine	Flow Rate Contrast Substance
	gm/ml	ml	gm/sec	ml/sec
Renografin 76%	0.37	58	10.5	29
Renografin 60%	0.288	73	10.5	37
Hypaque 75%	0.385	55	10.5	27
Cardiografin 85%	0.40	53	10.5	26
Isopaque 440	0.44	50	10.5	25
Hypaque-M 90%	0.462	46	10.5	23
Angio-Conray 80%	0.48	46	10.5	23
Urokon 70%	0.461	47	10.5	23

[a] Comparative amounts of different contrast substances necessary to produce approximately equal and satisfactory visualization of the heart and great vessels in an adult.

iation is due to a number of factors such as thickness of the patient, amount of surrounding air-containing lung, and radiographic factors such as collimation, kilovoltage, grids, and single or biplane exposures. Table 4 shows the comparable amounts and flow rates of commonly used contrast substances necessary to obtain approximately equal and satisfactory visualization of the heart and great vessels. Where aortography or selective angiocardiography are used, the total amount and injection rate depend on a number of factors including the anatomy of the structure under investigation. Table 4 was devised to enable the radiologist to make a quick estimate as to whether a given set of circumstances with regard to catheter size will permit a minimum visualization of the desired cardiovascular structure. If such is not possible, then the examination should not be carried out because it subjects the patient to most of the risks without the possibility of obtaining useful information.

Tables and graphs (Kjellberg *et al.*, 1958; Rodriguez-Alvarez, 1957; Lehman and Debbas, 1961; Cooley and Beentjes, 1963; Cooley, 1957) showing flow rates of various contrast substances through different sizes and types of catheters and cannulas at different pressures are available, but these give only a rough approximation when applied to a particular situation due to differences in injectors, differences in temperature, and perhaps other factors. Consequently, it is advisable for the radiologist to make a number of test injections with his own equipment under actual operating conditions.

INJECTORS

For selective angiography, pressure injectors capable of generating pressures of 800–1,000 psi are necessary. In practice, most injections are made at less than 800 psi, and some catheters will not withstand pressures in excess of this level. The earlier, hand-powered, lever device units were cheap and troublefree but extremely cumbersome and were soon replaced by gas-driven devices, such as the Amplatz portable apparatus and the more massive Gidlund injector. The Amplatz apparatus still offers the advantages of lower initial cost, simplicity of operation, and portability, but it lacks many of the safety features, reproducibility, and automation of the newer generation of injectors. For the angiographer who performs often and under a variety of circumstances, the extra cost of the newer and more sophisticated injectors is worthwhile.

The three commonly used injectors are the Cordis injector (Cordis Corporation, P.O. Box 428, Miami, Florida), the Viamonte-Hobbs injector (Barber-Colman Electro-mechanical Products, Rockford, Illinois), and the Medrad injector (Allison Park, Pennsylvania). All of these injectors are driven by electric motors, and injection speeds are regulated by moderately sophisticated electronic circuits. All of these instruments are mounted on tripods or mobile stands. The Medrad has the additional advantage of a demountable syringe which considerably increases its flexibility. All of these devices have eliminated the use of tables and charts for determining flow rates applicable to individual catheters and contrast substances. In the Cordis instrument, the dials are set to produce the desired flow rate after the data on catheter size and contrast substance have been programmed into the instrument. The other two instruments automatically deliver the required or desired flow rate provided the necessary pressures are within their capabilities. This has greatly simplified the delivery of the proper amount of contrast substance. Both the Medrad and Viamonte-Hobbs injectors can be coordinated with the electrocardiogram to produce injections at the desired part of the cardiac cycle. They have sensing devices to detect increased voltages in the apparatus and thus prevent harmful currents passing down the catheter to the heart. They have positive mechanical locks that permit the injection to be terminated at a precise point and also fail-safe devices to prevent an inadvertent injection at the wrong time. All of these devices are a great advance

and have done much to take the guesswork out of the injection of contrast substance, making it more reliable and safe.

DOSAGE

Dosage is determined by the minimum amount of contrast substance necessary to produce a satisfactory angiogram and the threshold of toxicity of the contrast substance. Table 4 can be used to determine minimum dosages on a volume per weight basis (300 mg of iodine per kg total), but in individuals with large hearts larger dosages are necessary. Lethal doses for single injections of the commonly used contrast substances into the superior vena cava of dogs are of the order of 4–7 ml/kg (4–10 ml/kg, Foster *et al.*, 1962; Lehman and Debbas, 1961). In humans, doses of 1 ml/kg are commonplace and are often repeated within 30 min. Even slightly higher doses seem to be well tolerated by infants and children.

Our opinion is that higher dosages, either single or total, should be used where they can be justified by the possibility of obtaining crucial diagnostic information. The figures in Table 4 can be reduced by as much as 10% for aortography and 10–15% for selective right and left ventriculography.

No firm statement as to the total dose administered during a single procedure is possible. Total doses as high as 300 ml have been adminis-

TABLE 5

RELATIVE ORDER OF CONTRAST SUBSTANCES IN THEIR CAPACITY TO DELIVER IODINE UNDER CONDITIONS OF SELECTIVE ANGIOGRAPHY USING PRESSURES >500 psi AND CATHETER SIZES OF 7F OR LARGER ID

Contrast Substance	Specific Gravity	Viscosity Centipoise	
		25°C	37.5°C
	gm/ml		
Urokon	1.452	6.56	4.31
Angio-Conray 80%	1.505	14.4	8.4
Isopaque 440	1.470		7.1
Hypaque 90%[a]	1.450	39.0	21.0
Ditriokon	1.413	8.4	5.5
Hypaque 75%	1.425	13.4	8.35
Renovist	1.405	9.1	6.12
Renografin 60%	1.318	5.60	3.92
Renografin 76%	1.408	13.9	9.1

[a] Turbulent flow using Hypaque 90% is unobtainable under most circumstances of selective angiography.

tered over a period of 1–1½ hr without significant injury. Increasing dosages carry increasing risks. On the other hand, the need to demonstrate or elucidate a particular defect or abnormality may completely justify the increased risk.

REACTIONS

Morbidity and Mortality after Angiocardiography

Minor observed effects after angiocardiography are (1) localized infection or cellulitis at the site of cutdown or venous puncture, (2) nausea and vomiting which may persist for several hours, and (3) urticaria. Experience indicates that, if the patient survives the procedure without complications, no permanent disability will occur. Our main concern is with the immediate severe or fatal reaction.

Dotter and Jackson (1949) in a survey, found 26 deaths following a total of 6,824 angiocardiographic studies, giving a mortality of 0.38%. Since 1950, no precise information is available concerning mortality. The impression given by the literature and that obtained from personal contacts and personal experience is that the mor-

tality from venous angiocardiography, including venous abdominal aortography and placetography, is much less than 0.38%. Despite the widespread use of much larger doses of the newer contrast agents, the incidence of severe reactions has decreased to the point where it does not pose a significant problem. In approximately 750 such examinations performed at the University of Texas Medical Branch during an 8-year period there has been no mortality and only a rare severe reaction. Mortality, of course, depends on the type of patient subjected to the procedure and will be higher in patients with congenital cyanotic heart disease. Today, many of these patients have selective rather than venous angiocardiograms. The mortality from selective angiocardiography should be considered according to the chamber injected and the technique employed. The present authors are unaware of any precise evaluation in this regard. We think, however, that left ventriculography is more hazardous by any technique than is right ventricular injection. Right ventricular and right atrial injections do not appear to be significantly more hazardous than venous angiography but do require more attention and care to avoid complications.

Prevention of Severe Reactions

The intravenous sensitivity test has been unreliable in predicting a fatal reaction (Dotter and Jackson, 1949; Pendergrass et al., 1955). We have very little information about the incidence of positive reactions to the intravenous sensitivity test or the number of times angiocardiography has been abandoned because of a positive reaction. The sensitivity test itself may constitute a very minor hazard, and there is a report of a fatality following this test (Pendergrass et al., 1958). In our experience, the intravenous sensitivity test with 1 ml of contrast substance diluted in 10 ml of saline and injected over a 30-sec interval, and followed by observation of about 5 min, has been rarely positive. Only once in over 1,200 tests was the angiographic procedure abandoned because of a reaction. The test is used routinely in all patients with an allergic background or a history of previous reactions to contrast substance, but is of doubtful value.

Fischer and Doust in a recent review (1972) reported the results of a survey of 10 years of teaching hospital experience covering 3.8 million excretory urograms. The overall death rate was 19 per million. A comparison of death rates between pretested patients and those who were not pretested revealed no statistically significant differences. They concluded that there seems to be no valid reason to depend upon intravenous pretesting in the hope of avoiding serious reactions.

The routine use of antihistaminics has been recommended (Olsson, 1951), but opinion regarding their efficacy is divided (Finby et al., 1958). We do not use these substances as preliminary medication because their action is not always predictable. They may produce undue drowsiness, particularly in combination with other medications. We frequently use Benadryl, 20–50 mg intravenously, for urticaria and other minor allergic manifestations.

Preliminary treatment with corticosteroids for patients with known sensitivity to contrast substance or with an allergic history has been suggested (Abrams, 1961; Youker, 1965). Obviously this should not be a routine procedure, and we have used cortisone only with medical consulta-

tion. We have carried out angiography after preliminary treatment with cortisone without significant reaction in 8 patients who had severe reactions following contrast injection.

Treatment of Severe Reactions

If treatment is to be effective, it must be prompt, organized, and administered with coolness and equanimity (Barnhard and Barnhard, 1965). A tray is kept nearby that contains the following drugs:
Adrenalin: 1:1,000, 1-ml vial
Aramine: 1:100, 1-ml vial
Atropine sulfate: 0.4 mg/ml
Isosorbide dinitrate: 5-mg sublingual tablets
Levophed bitartrate: 2 mg/ml, 4-ml vial
Nalline hydrochloride: 0.5 mg/ml, 1-ml ampule
Sodium bicarbonate: 50-ml ampule
Sodium nembutal: 50 mg/ml, 20-ml vial
Solu-Cortef: 2-ml vial containing 100 mg

The following equipment is kept on a cart or in the room where the examination is conducted:
Blood pressure manometer and cuff
Intravenous set with dextrose and saline
Endotracheal airways of several sizes
Laryngoscope
Ambu resuscitation bag
Two or three sizes of masks
External defibrillator
Stethoscope
Ample supply of needles and syringes

Electrocardiographic monitoring with oscilloscopic viewing is a routine procedure in all children, the aged, and in many other cases. The physician should remain by the patient's side for at least 15 min after the injection of contrast substance.

Most severe reactions involve either the respiratory or circulatory system. Some of these reactions can be anticipated. Prolonged nausea, retching, pallor, and a change in heart rate should alert the physician to an impending reaction. If the blood pressure falls significantly, emergency measures should be instituted immediately. Aramine, 3 mg (0.2–0.3 ml) should be given intravenously. This should be followed by an intravenous infusion containing Aramine. The question of giving adrenalin in dosages of 0.5–1 ml often arises, and there is no unanimity of opinion regarding this. The possibility of producing ventricular fibrillation seems to be a very significant one, and unless there is an allergic manifestation, such as asthma or laryngeal edema, we prefer not to use adrenalin. In many cases the decline in blood pressure is related to reflex vagal stimulation. When this occurs, 0.5 mg of atropine sulfate is administered intravenously, slowly, usually with prompt return of blood pressure to normal. If necessary the dose may be repeated once after a 15- to 20-min delay.

Electrocardiographic monitoring is very helpful in anticipating or preventing cardiac arrest. If ventricular fibrillation appears, external chest massage is instituted immediately. This, combined with an adequate respiratory exchange, permits appraisal of the next procedure which is usually an attempt at defibrillation with an external defibrillator. The external defibrillator should be used only when the electrocardiographic tracing shows ventricular fibrillation. For cardiac arrest, closed chest massage may be continued for some time with the hope of stimulating myocardial activity.

Inadequate respiratory exchange and respiratory arrest are treated by inserting an S-shaped airway over the tongue into the hypopharynx. We do not attempt to insert an intratracheal tube but await the assistance of the anesthesiologist. The airway over the tongue serves to hold the tongue forward, and this usually suffices at least for a short time. Artificial respiration is carried out with the Ambu bag. Three sizes of masks enable a good fit over the nose and mouth. Regular rhythmic inflation of the lungs at about 12 times/min is then carried out. Oxygen can be effectively administered in high concentration by attaching a tube from the tank to the intake of the Ambu bag.

Medical consultation should be sought as soon as possible. In older patients, the possibility of myocardial ischemia and infarction, either as a cause or a result of the untoward reaction, must be considered. Also, abnormalities in rhythm and congestive heart failure are best managed by an experienced cardiologist.

Severe asthmatic attacks which acutely threaten life are immediately treated by 0.5-1 ml of adrenalin 1:1000 given intravenously. This is followed by 100 mg of Solu-Cortef intravenously or in a rapidly running saline infusion.

Mechanism of Death after Use of Contrast Substances in Angiography

When anesthesized dogs are given large doses (5–7 ml/kg) of the presently available contrast substances under circumstances similar to those used in venous angiocardiography, they become quite restless, whine, and thrash about for about 1 min. They then become quiet, defecate, salivate, retch, and vomit. Respiration becomes irregular and slow, and the heart rate becomes slower and slower and stops in 5–10 min. Convulsions occasionally occur and are of short duration; they rarely occur after the first 4 or 5 min.

In patients, the underlying disease from which the patient suffers often complicates the reaction to contrast substance. Furthermore, some of the deaths have been associated with subdural hematomas, probably secondary to extensive retching, and some to the aspiration of stomach contents. The majority of fatalities, however, appear to have been due directly to the contrast substance, but in most cases the exact mechanism or cause of death remains obscure. In 4 fatal reactions observed many years ago by one of the authors, the sequence of events seemed to have been quite similar to that seen in overdosage in dogs. Ventricular fibrillation did not appear to be present since the heart continued to beat very slowly for some minutes. Respiration was also quite slow and appeared to stop before the heart. One mechanism, however, that is clearly understood is that of ventricular fibrillation. This is most apt to occur after supravalvular or intracoronary injections of contrast substance. This type of reaction, of course, has a specific treatment, namely, external cardiac massage and defibrillation.

4

*Equipment**

CINEFLUOROGRAPHIC EQUIPMENT

A variety of equipment is available and cannot be described in detail. An attempt will be made to point out the crucial functional advantages and disadvantages of the several systems. The reader is referred to Judkins *et al.*: Report of Intersociety Commission for Heart Disease Resources. Optimal Resources for Examination of the Chest and Cardiovascular System. Circulation *53:* A1-A37, 1976. Since all systems are expensive, the radiologist should acquire that system best adapted to his needs. In many instances, it is necessary to use the equipment for examinations other than those of the cardiovascular system. Also, in order to obtain the best results from his equipment, the radiologist should be familiar with the basic physical principles governing the production of cinefluorographic images and other types of film recording systems. For this he is referred to several standard works (Christensen *et al.*, 1972; Ter Per Gossian, 1969).

For satisfactory angiocardiography, image detail is a dominant consideration. Image detail in a cinefluorographic system is a function of the performance of several components. These are: the input phosphor (size, absorptive characteristics), electrical characteristics of the image tube, degree of minification of the output phosphor, the lens system, the size of the recording surface (film size 16- or 35-mm), and film speed and development characteristics. One overriding consideration is the amount of radiation necessary for the correct exposure of a single frame. Thirty-five millimeter systems require approximately 4 times the radiation per frame as compared with 16-mm systems. Using modern high gain tubes, the reduction in photons associated with the 16-mm system may produce consider-

able undesirable quantum mottle; whereas in the similar 35-mm system, the increased radiation may eliminate this as a factor. Consequently, most 35-mm systems have appreciably better detail than the corresponding 16-mm systems using the same image tube.

Another important factor in image production and also patient exposure is the synchronization system. This system pulses the tube current so that radiation is produced only during the interval when the film is stationary. There are three commonly used systems, all of which use the electrical signals produced by a commutator and brush system in the synchronous motor that drives the camera. The grid control tube type or secondary switched capacitors deliver a controlled square wave voltage curve that can be precisely timed and produces superior results.

The brightness control system regulates the radiation rate to suit the thickness and density of the body part being examined. Movement during fluoroscopy and filming without significant change in image or film density is possible. In order to be effective, such systems must respond quite rapidly, and in all there is some lag which can be noted when continuous filming is undertaken. Most systems depend on rapid adjustments of the kilovoltage and milliamperage of the tube current. The kilovoltage should be kept within a predetermined range, particularly when using iodinated contrast substances, in order to produce maximum contrast (70–85 pkv). The operator should remember that the phototubes in these devices scan only approximately the central one-third of the output phosphor. The systems work best where the shutters are used to reduce the radiation to an area slightly smaller than the input screen of the image tube. The brightness regulator must be adjusted empirically to suit the particular film and the other

---

* Fluoroscopic equipment has been described in the section "Fluoroscopy" in Chapter 1.

factors of the examination. The system should be checked frequently for proper response if optimal results are expected.

The lens system must be properly designed, in order to avoid vignetting, and correctly focused. Some degree of overframing is routine, particularly in cardiovascular work. It is obvious that one should strive to use all of the available surface in recording the image. The available surface, however, is rectangular rather than square or round, and consequently, if one diameter is of the same size as the film area, the other diameter is either larger or smaller. Generally, equal area framing is used in which the longest diameter of the film is exposed with only a slight cutoff of the short diameter.

The Tage Arno projector is quite satisfactory for small groups but is insufficient for large audiences. Thirty-five millimeter projectors of other design are considerably more expensive

and usually more noisy than their 16-mm counterparts. Consequently, it is often necessary to reduce the 35-mm film to 16-mm for teaching large groups or for wide use as lecture material. Reduction is available commercially but gives little opportunity for editing or improving on film density and is also an extra expense. If the production of 35-mm film is extensive, it may be desirable to set up one's own reducing apparatus.

The two major drawbacks in the use of cinefluorography in comparison with large film recording for cardiac examinations are the abundant amount of radiation involved (28–64 r/min) and the rather poor detail. Its advantages are the rapidity of filming, and the integrated motion, which gives a better appreciation of all the events than does the viewing of a series of still films. Cinefluorography complements large film angiography, and both are desirable under certain circumstances.

FILM CHANGERS

A film changer is basic equipment for all angiographic procedures. The complexity and capabilities of the equipment may vary according to the type of angiographic procedure that one wishes to perform. For cardiac angiography, and particularly in children with congenital heart disease, a film-changing rate of at least 6 frames/sec is necessary. For all-around needs such as pulmonary angiography, film size of 14 × 14 inches is desirable. For peripheral angiography, as mentioned below, even larger film may be useful. When the radiologist, for economic reasons, is faced with the choice between large film recording and cinefluorography, we recommend the large film-changing systems. Their advantages are (1) increased detail of the recorded images, (2) adaptability to magnification techniques, (3) decreased radiation, (4) ease of viewing and demonstration without accessory apparatus, and (5) all-around adaptability to such procedures as cerebral and pulmonary angiography. As indicated earlier under "Cinefluorography", the two systems really are not entirely competitive but are complementary, and both can be used to advantage.

Film changers have three basic systems of film transport based on the use of cassettes, cut film, or roll film. Cassettes must have rigidity and durability and thus a modest weight which in turn brings on the problems of inertia and of providing rapid acceleration and deceleration. This puts a limit on film-changing speed, and none of the cassette devices have a film-changing

rate greater than 4/sec. However, the small mass and inertia of the cut film and roll film make the higher speeds of 6–12/sec more easily obtainable. On the other hand, the screen-film contact with cassettes can be made much more positive and even than with the rapidly opening and closing screens used in the cut and roll film devices. Air trapping and unevenness of apposition of the rapidly closing intensifying screens, despite a number of improvements in design, still remain minor problems. No attempt will be made to describe each unit in detail, but we give our appraisals of several, citing their advantages and disadvantages based on considerable experience with them.

Sanchez-Perez Film Changer

This unit has a low initial cost, is moderately rugged, and can be adapted to cerebral angiography and pulmonary angiography. It is thus a useful all-around instrument. The filming rate of 2/sec makes it unacceptable for cardiac angiography, particularly in children. It is susceptible to vibration, and also the exposure to radiation of a stacked film system produces a minor difference in density between the first and subsequent films. It can be mounted in pairs for biplane work.

Picker Amplatz Sealed Cassette Changer

The vacuum-sealed cassettes provide excellent screen contact and superior detail and resolution. The film rate of 4/sec is barely adequate for most cardiac angiography. It is not satisfactory for children with congenital heart disease. Because of its detail and resolution, it is readily adapted to magnification techniques in the lateral view. It does require a vacuumatic sealing unit, and there is an expense associated with the sealing envelopes. The units can be mounted in biplane pairs, and vibration has not been a problem.

Schonander Cut Film Changer

This unit uses conventional cut film and produces a satisfactory speed of up to 6 exposures/sec, which is adequate for most cardiac angiography. The units can be mounted in pairs for biplane examinations. It has a capacity of 30 films. Film size of 14 × 14 inches, although oversized in children, is advantageous where a considerable number of adults are examined. This film size is necessary for good pulmonary angiography. These units are expensive. They have a tendency to malfunction and must be kept in good adjustment. Care must be taken in loading the films, and constant, favorable, ambient temperature and humidity are desirable in order to maintain constant film pliability. For maximum performance, this unit should be under the surveillance of a trained service engineer, and preventative maintenance should be instituted at regular intervals of 1–2 months.

Biplane filming simultaneously significantly increases scatter and thus decreases contrast and detail, most noticeable in the frontal film. Careful collimation is essential in order to keep this within acceptable bounds. In the Schonander cut film unit, this defect can be largely overcome by placing the two changers out of phase by 180° by using an additional coupling device. Where maximum detail is essential, such as in coronary arteriography, single plane exposures should be used.

Elema Schonander Roll Film Changer

Because of the positive drive of the roll film, a speed of 12/sec is obtainable. The unit uses 100-foot rolls of film, 12 inches wide. Consequently, the horizontal film exposure is 12 × 14 inches, and the vertical is 12 × 12 inches. The two units are permanently locked and so must be used exclusively as a biplane unit. The drive mechanism is rather simple and relatively troublefree. Some of the relative disadvantages of the unit are the fact that it must be loaded in the darkroom, and there is no footage indicator. Consequently, in order to be sure that sufficient film is available one is inclined to discard short residual amounts of film.

Franklin Roll Film Changer

This changer has received rather wide acceptance. It can be used either as a single or biplane unit. The roll film is 14 inches wide, and this permits an exposure of 11 × 14 inches in each plane. The drive mechanism is very positive in operation and relatively troublefree. The magazine can be loaded and unloaded in daylight. The unit operates at a maximum speed of 6 frames/sec, which is adequate for most every type of examination. One minor disadvantage is the relatively short exposure time permitted by the drive apparatus. Consequently, the unit must be used with high capacity generators.

Amplatz See-Through Changer

This was first described by Amplatz (1968). This changer has the advantages of (1) radiolucency of the changer permitting fluoroscopy and filming without moving the patient and also monitoring of the image during filming, (2) improved screen film contact due to improved air compression system, (3) filming rates of up to 6/sec, (4) rotating Bucky diaphragm with consequent reduction in vibration, and (5) daylight loading of roll film. This changer would appear to offer many advantages, but we have had no experience with its use.

Disc and tape recorders provide an immediate playback capability that is desirable during the progress of an examination.

5

Embryology of Heart and Great Vessels

Beneath the anterior, pericardial portion of the coelom, small endothelial masses arise in the mesenchyme in the late presomite stage (about 1.5 mm). With the forward growth of the head, this cardiogenic area comes to lie above the pericardial coelom and ventral to the foregut. Fusion of isolated groups of these endothelial cells into the right and left endocardial heart tubes ensues, and each is connected cephalically with an endothelial tube representing the first aortic arch and caudally with a tube representing fused vitelline and umbilical veins. The primitive aortic arches connect with paired dorsal aortae, and these are connected by vitelline and umbilical arteries through the yolk sac to corresponding vitelline and umbilical veins. Thus, a bilaterally symmetrical circulatory system is formed and persists as such for several days (Fig. 8A).

Fusion of the endothelial tubes progresses to produce a single cardiac tube or primitive heart, continuous cephalically with the aortic arches and caudally with the dilated terminations of the vitelline and umbilical veins, the right and left sinus venosus (Fig. 8B). Each sinus venosus later receives the termination of the common cardinal veins, formed by the union of the corresponding anterior and posterior cardinal veins which drain the embryonic body wall (Fig. 8C).

The two endocardial tubes fuse when the embryo is about 2.5 mm long, at which time primitive muscle cells differentiate and surround the endothelial heart. This myocardial primordium is fused to a layer of visceral mesothelium (epicardium) to form a myoepicardial mantle about the heart (Fig. 9A). This mantle develops into myocardium and visceral pericardium, while the endothelial tube becomes the endocardium.

The single cardiac tube now develops several areas of dilatation, marked externally by grooves or sulci. From the caudal to the cranial end these are the right and left sinus venosus, the atrium (separated from the sinuses by a pair of valves), the ventricle (separated from the atrium by the atrioventricular canal produced by the ingrowth of swollen dorsal and ventral endocardial cushions), and the bulbus cordis, continuous into short ventral aortae (Fig. 9B).

Resorption of a transitory dorsal mesocardium frees the cardiac tube except at the venous entrance (caudal end) and the arterial outlet (cranial end) where the epicardium is continuous with the parietal pericardium. The primitive heart subsequently grows more rapidly than the pericardial cavity, becoming bent thereby into a U-shaped loop convex ventrally and to the right. This loop later assumes an S-shaped curve, and as it involves mainly the ventricle and bulbus, is called the bulboventricular loop (Fig. 9C). The atrium has now come to lie in the pericardial cavity dorsal to and slightly to the left of the bulboventricular loop; the right and left sinus venosus, situated on the posterior aspect of the atrium, partially fuse and open by a single sinuatrial orifice into the atrial cavity (5–6 mm stage). The left sinus horn becomes greatly reduced in size, and most of the venous blood is then shunted to the right sinus horn (owing to a rearrangement of vessels entering the sinus which produces a new venous channel, the ductus venosus in the liver). The right sinus horn enlarges, and the sinuatrial orifice is shifted to the right side of the atrium. The margins of this orifice project into the atrium as the right and left sinus valves (Fig. 10).

Increase in size and rearrangement in position produce changes in the atrium, ventricle and bulbus. The atrium increases in size transversely and develops ventral-lateral extensions, the auricular appendages, which project on either side of the bulbus (Fig. 9D). The proximal part of the bulbus is absorbed into the ventricle which is now located anteriorly and to the left. External grooves mark the internal position of a well developed atrioventricular canal.

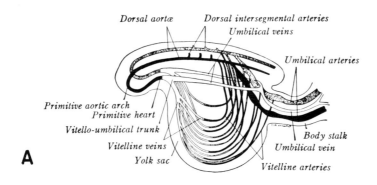

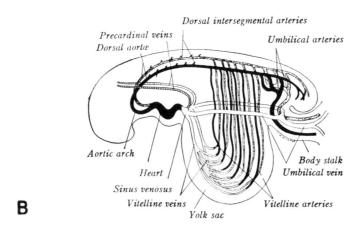

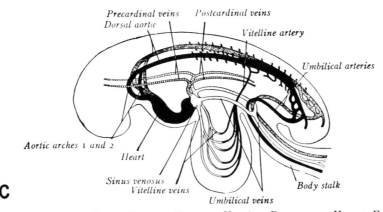

FIG. 8. ARRANGEMENT OF BLOOD VESSELS (LATERAL VIEW) IN DEVELOPING HUMAN EMBRYO

(A) For a short time a bilaterally symmetrical circulatory system is present. (B) Fusion of the endothelial heart tubes ensues, producing a single primitive heart. (C) With continued development each sinus venosus receives the terminations of the respective common cardinal, umbilical and vitelline veins. (From L. B. Arey, *Developmental Anatomy,* 5th Edition, W. B. Saunders Co., Philadelphia, 1950.)

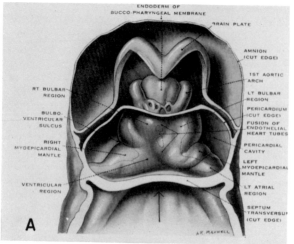

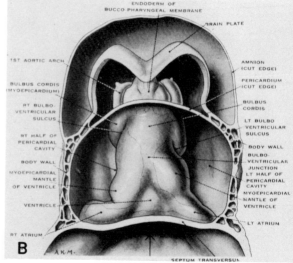

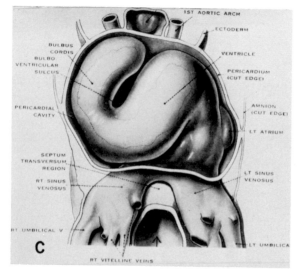

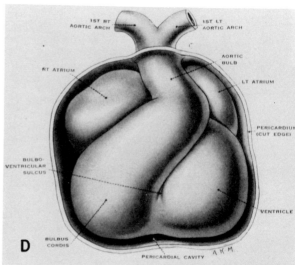

FIG. 9. VENTRAL VIEW OF RECONSTRUCTION OF HEART REGION IN 2.5-mm HUMAN EMBRYO

(A) The endothelial heart tube is indicated by interrupted lines. The arrow points into the anterior intestinal portal leading to the foregut. The myoepicardial mantle surrounds the developing cardiac chamber and consists of primitive myocardium surrounded by a layer of visceral mesothelium (epicardium). (B) The single cardiac tube becomes divided into primitive chambers. (C) With continued growth and formation of the bulboventricular loop, the atrium comes to lie dorsal and slightly to the left of the ventricle. (D) By the 5-mm stage, auricular appendages form and project on either side of the bulbus, the proximal part of which is absorbed into the ventricle. (From W. J. Hamilton, J. D. Boyd, and H. W. Mossman, *Human Embryology,* 2nd Edition, W. Heffer & Sons Ltd., Cambridge, 1957.)

INTERIOR OF HEART

At the 5-7.5 mm stage of development, septation of the heart commences.

From the midline of the atrial roof a sagittal fold, the septum primum, appears between the left valve of the sinus venosus and the single pulmonary vein (Fig. 10B). This septum extends caudally along the anterior and posterior atrial walls to join the superior and inferior (also called anterior and posterior) atrioventricular endocardial cushions which have appeared in the walls of the atrioventricular canal. This septum divides the atrium into right and left portions except inferiorly where a small foramen primum persists for a short time (Fig. 11, A and B). As it becomes obliterated by union of the septum primum with the fusing atrioventricular endocardial cushions, degeneration of the cephalic portion of the septum results in the formation of a foramen secundum which again brings the two atrial chambers into communication (Fig. 11B).

At the 18-mm stage a second septum, the septum secundum, develops from the right atrial wall between the left sinus valve and the septum primum (Fig. 11, B and C). As this partition grows anteriorly and posteriorly it develops a lower free concave edge which eventually overlaps the upper edge of the foramen secundum of the septum primum (Fig. 11, C and D). Thus, the opening between the two atrial cavities is an obliquely elongated slit bounded by the upper edge of the septum primum and the lower edge of the septum secundum. This is the foramen ovale, and the part of the septum primum which overlaps the free edge of the septum secundum is called the valve of the foramen ovale. Oxygenated blood from the inferior vena cava passes through the foramen ovale into the left atrium during fetal life; after birth the upper edge of the valve of the foramen ovale is pressed firmly against the septum secundum, fusion occurs, and eventually the two atria are completely separated from one another. Abnormalities in this developmental sequence may lead to a variety of defects in the interatrial septum.

As the interatrial septum is developing, the sinus venosus becomes absorbed into the right atrium and the single common pulmonary vein is absorbed into the left atrium. This is accompanied, on the right, by regression of the left sinus valve and division of the right sinus valve into several parts, two of which become the valve of the inferior vena cava and the valve of the coronary sinus (Thebesian valve). On the left, absorption of the common pulmonary vein leaves four separate pulmonary venous openings in the left atrium.

The superior and inferior (also sometimes called anterior and posterior) atrioventricular (A-V) endocardial cushions, arising in the wall of the transversely widened A-V canal, meet and fuse at the 11-mm stage, dividing this canal into right and left A-V canals (Fig. 12). This fusion occurs at about the time the free edge of the septum primum meets and fuses with the upper surface of the cushions.

Shortly after the appearance of the septum primum, at about the 7-mm stage, a muscular ridge appears in the floor of the ventricular cavity (Fig. 11A). This area is marked by an anteroposteriorly directed sulcus on the surface of the heart. As this interventricular septum grows, its posterior part reaches the inferior A-V cushion near its right extremity, just to the left of the right A-V orifice (Fig. 13A). The anterior part of the septum grows to reach the superior A-V cushion just to the right of the left A-V orifice (Fig. 13A). The free edge of the interventricular septum and the endocardial cushions bound the

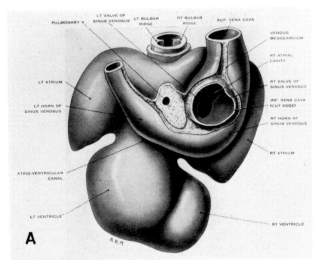
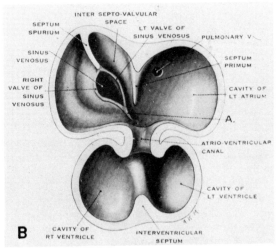

FIG. 10. HUMAN EMBRYO HEART

(A) Dorsal aspect of a reconstruction of the heart of a 10-mm human embryo. The right and left sinus venosus have partially fused and open by a single orifice into the atrial cavity. The left sinus horn is greatly reduced in size, and most of the venous blood is shunted to the larger right horn. (B) Transverse section through a reconstruction of the heart of a 7.5-mm human embryo (seen from above). A—caudal fusion of the venous valves. The atrial septum primum and the early interventricular septum grow toward the atrioventricular canal. (From W. J. Hamilton, J. D. Boyd, and H. W. Mossman, *Human Embryology*, 2nd Edition, W. Heffner & Sons Ltd., Cambridge, 1957.)

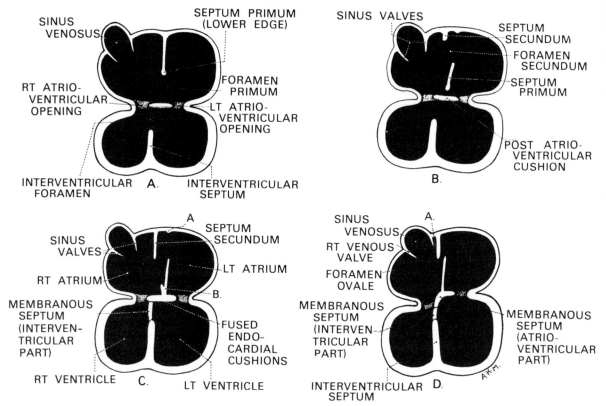

Fig. 11. Development of Interatrial and Interventricular Septums. (Schematic Transverse Sections of Heart. Atria Are Dorsal to Ventricles)

(A) The septum primum is incomplete inferiorly, forming the foramen primum. The interventricular septum extends upward from the base of the ventricle, partly dividing it into two chambers. (B) The septum primum extends ventrally to unite with the fusing endocardial cushions. Degeneration of the cephalic portion produces the foramen secundum. The septum secundum has begun to form between the septum primum and the left sinus valve. (C) The septum primum has fused with the endocardial cushions at B. (A indicates the cranial remnant of the septum primum.) The lower edge of the septum secundum now overlaps the upper edge of the septum primum, producing the foramen ovale. The membranous portion of the interventricular septum has formed and separates the two ventricles. (D) The space between the septum secundum and the left sinus valve (A) is obliterated. Since the atrial and ventricular septa are not formed opposite one another, a portion of the fused endocardial cushions comes to lie between the right atrium and the left ventricle. (From W. J. Hamilton, J. D. Boyd, and H. W. Mossman, *Human Embryology,* 2nd Edition, W. Heffer & Sons Ltd., Cambridge, 1957.)

interventricular foramen through which the bulbus cordis and both ventricular chambers communicate. The interventricular septum is oriented somewhat obliquely, especially in its upper part.

Spiral subendocardial thickenings, the bulbar ridges, arise in the distal part of the bulbus cordis at about the 5-mm stage (Fig. 14A). These ridges are attached to the lateral walls of the distal part of the bulbus (or truncus arteriosus), to the anterior and posterior walls of the intermediate part of the bulbus, and somewhat obliquely in the proximal or juxtaventricular part of the bulbus. Proximally these ridges are so situated that one projects just above the right A-V canal and one lies adjacent to the anterior part of the

interventricular septum (Fig. 13A and B). Growth and fusion of the ridges produce a spiral aorticopulmonary or conotruncal septum which divides the bulbus cordis into the aorta and the pulmonary artery at about the 20-mm stage (Figs. 13 C and 14 B).

Closure of the interventricular foramen is accomplished by the proliferation of tissue from the proximal parts of the right and left bulbar ridges and from the fused endocardial cushions. The right bulbar ridge grows downward and fuses with the posterior edge of the interventricular septum. Tissue from the left bulbar ridge fuses with the anterior edge of the interventricular septum (Fig. 13B). The right and left bulbar extensions then meet and fuse, obliterating the upper part of the interventricular foramen (Fig. 13B and C). The remainder of the interventricular foramen is closed by growth of tissue from the endocardial cushions along the free upper edge of the interventricular septum, uniting the septum with the lower margin of the fused extensions of the bulbar ridges (Fig. 13C). This sequence of events, terminating at about the 17-mm stage, separates the ventricular cavities from one another and ensures connection between the right ventricle and the anterior or pulmonary portion of the bulbus and between the left ventricle and the posterior or aortic portion of the bulbus. The right atrioventricular opening now connects the right atrium and ventricle, and the left atrioventricular orifice connects the left atrium and ventricle. Failure of fusion of the bulbar ridges and interventricular septum lead to the several varieties of high interventricular septal defect, and abnormalities of the truncoconal division may result in persistent truncus arteriosus, transposition of the great vessels, and anomalies of the origin of the aorta and pulmonary artery.

The upper portion of the interventricular septum remains as fibrous tissue throughout life. It is located partly between the right and left ventricles and partly between the right atrium and left ventricle. Proliferation of the endocardial cushions closes the lower portion of the interventricular foramen and forms that part of the of the membranous septum located between the ventricles. The part of the membranous septum between the right atrium and the left ventricle arises as a consequence of the fact that the septum primum and the interventricular septum are not attached to the endocardial cushions directly opposite one another (Fig. 11C). Consequently, that part of the fused endocardial cushions between the attachment of the two septa lies between the right atrium and the left ventricle (Fig. 11D). A cushion defect at this point may result in a septal defect between these two chambers.

After the formation of the aorticopulmonary septum, small accessory ridges appear in the proximal part of the bulbus (Fig. 14A). These ridges alternate with the main right and left bulbar ridges. Swelling of the subendothelial tissue produces three bulges which guard the orifices of the aorta and the pulmonary trunk. These swellings consist of loose connective tissue with an endothelial lining. Excavation of these ridges on their distal aspect forms the three cusps of the semilunar aortic and pulmonary valves, whose adult relations are established by their embryonic positions. Congenital valvular stenosis or insufficiency may result from abnormal development.

The atrioventricular valves arise by growth of subendocardial connective tissue in the A-V canals. These proliferations undergo excavation on their ventricular sides to form valve cusps. The cusp margins maintain connection with the ventricular wall by strands of tissue which form chordae tendineae and papillary muscles. Anomalous development may lead to congenital mitral or tricuspid atresia, stenosis, or insufficiency.

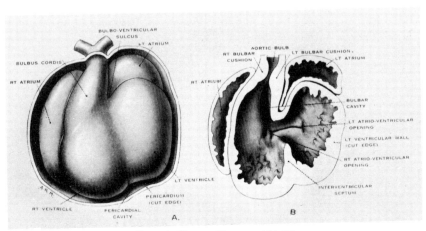

FIG. 12. HUMAN EMBRYO HEART

(A) Ventral aspect of the heart of a 10-mm human embryo. (B) Coronal section through A. The dorsal half of the model is seen from the ventral aspect. The anterior and posterior endocardial cushions (originating respectively from the cephalic and caudal aspects of the common atrioventricular canal) have not yet fused and are located between the right and left A-V openings. (From W. J. Hamilton, and J. D. Boyd, and H. W. Mossman, *Human Embryology,* 2nd Edition, W. Heffer & Sons Ltd., Cambridge, 1957.)

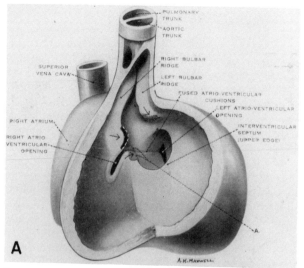

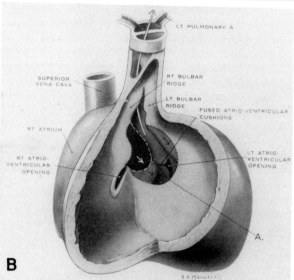

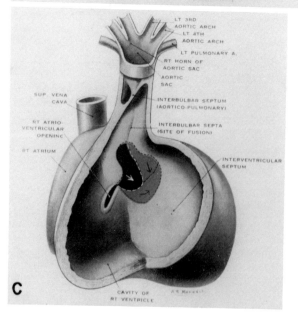

FIG. 13. DEVELOPMENT OF INTERVENTRICULAR SEPTUM
AND BULBAR RIDGES

The proliferations which eventually result in obliteration of the interventricular foramen are shaded. Proliferation from the endocardial cushions is designated by the letter A, the arrow indicating the direction of growth. The other two arrows show the directions of growth of proliferations from the right and left bulbar ridges.

(A) 12-mm human embryo. (B) 14.5-mm human embryo. Tissue from the left bulbar ridge has fused with the anterior part of the interventricular septum, and the right bulbar ridge has grown downward to fuse with the posterior part of the interventricular septum. The long white arrow indicates the course of the blood from the left ventricle to the aorta. (C) Growth of tissue from the endocardial cushions along the free upper edge of the interventricular septum finally unites the septum with the lower margin of the fused extensions of the bulbar ridges. (From W. J. Hamilton, J. D. Boyd, and H. W. Mossman, *Human Embryology*, 2nd Edition, W. Heffer & Sons Ltd., Cambridge, 1957.)

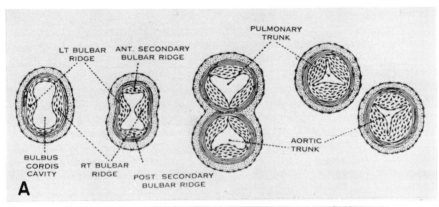

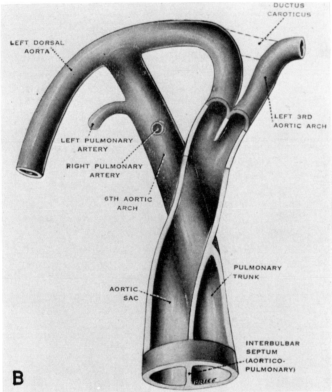

FIG. 14. HUMAN EMBRYO HEART

(A) Schematic sections showing successive stages in the subdivision of the bulbus cordis and the subsequent development of the cusps of the aortic and pulmonary semilunar valves. (B) Dissected model showing the division of the bulbus cordis by the aorticopulmonary septum. The model is seen from its right side. (From W. J. Hamilton, J. D. Boyd, and H. W. Mossman, *Human Embryology,* 2nd Edition, W. Heffer & Sons Ltd., Cambridge, 1957.)

BLOOD VESSELS

The development and fate of the branchial arch arteries and their derivatives are detailed in the section on anomalies of the aortic arch. The development of the venous system will be briefly discussed.

The right and left vitelline (omphalomesenteric) veins enter the corresponding primitive sinus venosus anterior to the liver. The left channel is transitory and regresses. The right channel ultimately forms the termination of the inferior vena cava.

The attachment of the umbilical veins to the sinus venosi persists for a short time, but by the 5-mm stage all of the blood in the umbilical veins passes into the liver. At the 6-7 mm stage the right umbilical vein atrophies, and subsequently all blood from the placenta enters the hepatic sinusoids through the left umbilical vein. As the right sinus venosus becomes dominant, a venous enlargement occurs between the left umbilical vein and the persistent part of the right vitelline vein (juxtacardiac part of inferior vena cava). This venous channel is the ductus venosus and affords a passageway for blood from the umbilical system to reach the right atrium. After birth, obliteration of the umbilical vein produces the ligamentum teres, and the ductus venosus persists as the ligamentum venosum.

Right and left anterior and posterior cardinal veins join to form the common cardinal veins (ducts of Cuvier) which empty, respectively, into the right and left sinus venosus. At the 22-mm stage a transverse connection develops between the two anterior cardinal veins (the innominate vein), and blood is thenceforth directed from the left to the lower part of the right anterior cardinal vein. This is accompanied by partial obliteration of the left duct of Cuvier (a portion persists as the lateral part of the coronary sinus). Blood from the head, neck, and upper extremities now reaches the heart via the terminal portion of the right anterior cardinal vein and the right duct of Cuvier which together become the superior vena cava.

The inferior vena cava is a complex structure which is derived from several primitive venous structures by enlargement of some vessels, anastomoses between others, and regression and disappearance of still others. These primitive vessels include the posterior cardinal veins, the right vitelline vein, the subcardinal veins, and the supracardinal veins. The result is the shifting of the pathways of venous return to the right side of the body, with the development of several alternative pathways to the right atrium: through the liver to the inferior vena cava, directly through the inferior vena cava, and via the hemiazygous and azygous systems to the superior vena cava.

Abnormalities in development of the veins may result in paired superior or inferior vena cavae, unpaired left superior or inferior vena cava, azygos vein serving as the main pathway of venous return, anomalous return of venous blood to the coronary sinus, and others.

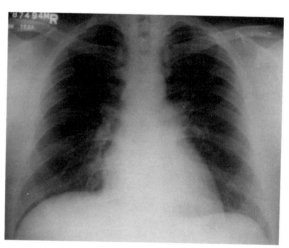

FIG. 15. TRANSVERSE HEART IN NORMAL, STOCKY
26-YEAR-OLD MAN

6

Roentgenologic Appearance of Normal Heart and Great Vessels

Our knowledge of the roentgen anatomy of the normal heart and great vessels has been obtained by correlating information gathered from the following sources:

1. Conventional roentgenography and roentgenoscopy in multiple projections. Since the heart and its contents are of homogeneous density, only contours or borders are demonstrated, and these are adequately seen only where the heart is surrounded by air-containing lung. Correlation with findings obtained from the other methods of examination listed below, however, has improved our understanding of the significance of these contours. Consequently, roentgenography and roentgenoscopy provide the greater part of the information that can be obtained from the roentgen examination of the heart.

2. Roentgenkymography and electrokymography. These provide more refined observations of amplitude and timing of pulsations of the cardiac contours. They are rarely employed in modern practice.

3. Angiocardiography and aortography which permit visualization of both exterior and interior contours of the cardiac chambers and their relations to each other and to the great vessels.

4. Cardiac catheterization when a radiopaque catheter is inserted into a particular vessel or structure (*e.g.,* coronary sinus).

5. Application of a metallic foreign body to a particular structure or border (*e.g.,* patent ductus) at operation followed by roentgenography.

6. Observation of the heart *in situ* at operation and autopsy.

7. Injection studies of the heart chambers and great vessels at autopsy followed by roentgenography (Laubry *et al.,* 1939; Wright *et al.,* 1964).

The following descriptions draw freely on all of these sources without specifically acknowledging each one.

CONTOURS AND TOPOGRAPHY OF NORMAL HEART

The normal cardiovascular contours have a considerable range of variation from (1) the transverse heart at one extreme (Fig. 15, see facing page) to (2) the long narrow heart at the other with (3) the globular heart occupying an intermediate position (Fig. 16B). This variation is due to (1) body build or habitus, (2) respiratory phase, and (3) age.

The transverse heart is common in persons of stocky, muscular, pyknic build, and in the obese. Usually, there is a wide transverse thoracic diameter and a small angle of inclination of the ribs with the horizontal accompanied by a relatively high diaphragm. The left border extends farther to the left than that of the long narrow heart and is rounded and moderately convex; the waist of the heart on the left is short but well marked, and the aortic knob is often prominent.

At the other extreme are those individuals with a long thorax, a larger angle of inclination of the ribs with the horizontal and a low diaphragm associated with a long narrow heart. The lower left border of the heart is steep and relatively straight; the waist is long and rather flat, and the aortic knob is often inconspicuous unless the aorta is elongated or dilated (Fig. 17A). All gradations of heart position between these two extremes occur, and an intermediate position produces the oblique or globular heart.

In the transverse heart a considerably greater area is in contact with the diaphragm than in the long, narrow heart, and the relative height of the

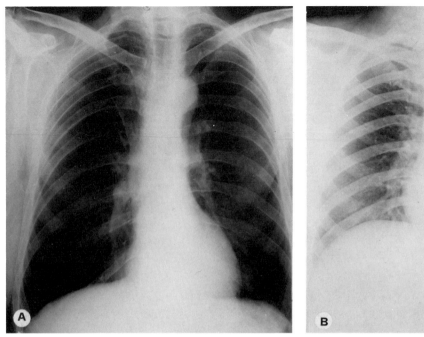

FIG. 16. NORMAL HEART
(A) A long normal heart in a healthy 70-year-old man; (B) a normal globular heart in a healthy 32-year-old man.

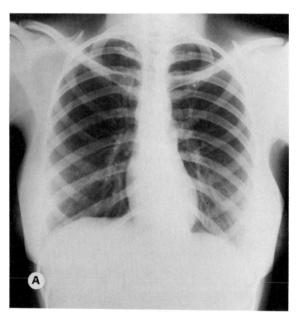
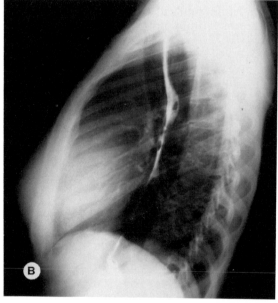

FIG. 17. NORMAL HEART
Apparently normal heart in a small, 20-year-old woman: weight, 94 lb.; height, 63 inches.

diaphragm exerts a considerable influence on the heart contour (Fig. 18, A and B). In expiration a long heart may resemble to a degree a transverse heart.

Forced inspiration causes the heart to elongate and decrease in width; forced expiration causes the heart to decrease in length and increase in width (Fig. 18, A and B). The Valsalva maneuver consists of attempting expiration against a closed glottis after forced inspiration. The intrathoracic pressure is thus increased, causing a decrease in blood flow into the heart and a decrease in size.

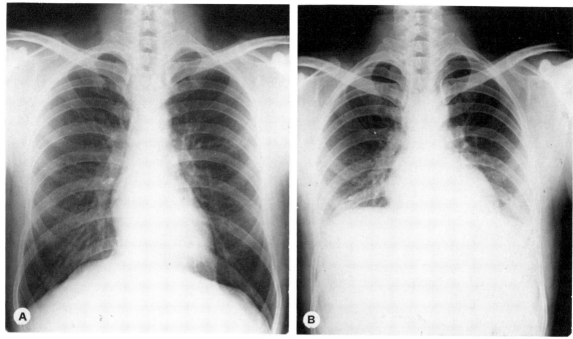

FIG. 18. LONG HEART SHOWING CHANGES IN CONTOUR IN (A) DEEP INSPIRATION AND (B) EXPIRATION

In the Müller maneuver, inspiration is attempted at the end of expiration against a closed glottis. As a result, the intrathoracic pressure drops, and there is an increased blood flow to the heart and a corresponding increase in cardiac size. During inspiration sinus arrhythmia may develop in many individuals, during which time the diastolic phase is prolonged, giving an appearance of a slight increase in cardiac size. It may be seen that the apparent cardiac size at any moment, as estimated from the frontal silhouette of the heart, depends on a variety of difficult-to-control variables, including intrathoracic pressure, venous return, phase of cardiac cycle, and perhaps even predominance of diaphragmatic or intercostal respiration (Fig. 20, A and B).

Positional Changes

Positional changes of the heart are produced by both respiration and general body position. With deep inspiration, the heart is displaced anteriorly, and there is a slight displacement toward the right; *i.e.,* both borders move toward the right. The reverse occurs during expiration. Consequently, with respiration there is a slight pendulum motion of the heart. This motion is in addition to the positional changes which occur during different phases of the cardiac cycle.

In the recumbent lateral position, the cardiovascular shadow sinks toward the dependent side during expiration with a resultant change in contour, and with deep inspiration, the shadow moves against gravity towards the midline.

In movement from the erect to the recumbent position, the heart decreases in length and increases in width, and the vascular shadows at the base of the heart widen.

During the latter months of pregnancy the heart consistently appears somewhat larger than the usual size for the individual (Fig. 21, A and B). The increased frontal surface area is due only in part to the effect of elevation of the diaphragm. Probably more important is the increased plasma volume (25–40%) in the third trimester of pregnancy. The cardiac output is usually increased, and some dilatation of the heart occurs in order to increase the stroke volume. The right atrium may be particularly prominent in such patients (Keats and Martt, 1964).

In infants, the heart is uniformly of the transverse or globular type (Fig. 22). The transverse diameter varies greatly with respiration (larger in expiration, smaller in inspiration). In addition, the thymus which reaches its greatest size in the second year, may form part of the base contour, making evaluation quite difficult. As the child grows older, the thoracic cage elongates relative to the heart so that at puberty there is a tendency to cardiac elongation. The left border may then become straight or slightly convex, simulating at times enlargement of the pulmonary trunk. Prominence of the main pulmonary artery in

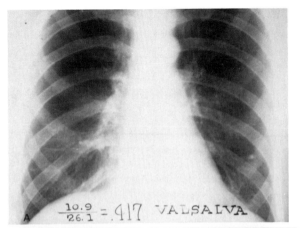

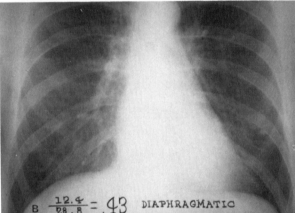

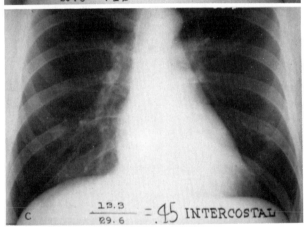

FIG. 19. NORMAL HEART

Factors affecting the transverse diameter of the heart and thorax. Fractions refer to the cardiothoracic ratio. All films are of a healthy 32-year-old man and were made within a few minutes of each other in the same degree of inspiration. (A) Film exposed at the end of 8 sec of Valsalva maneuver after a moderate inspiration. (B) Inspiration was accomplished by attempting to depress the diaphragm only. (C) The subject made a conscious effort to inspire using only his intercostal muscles.

teenaged children, especially girls, is a common normal finding. At about the 20th year, the heart reaches its definitive position and contour and thereafter remains stationary for many years. Some degree of atrophy with a consequent decrease in size occasionally occurs in old age. Elongation of the aorta with increased prominence of the aortic knob is commonly associated with aging but is due in most instances to arteriosclerosis and therefore cannot be properly considered as a normal variation.

Posteroanterior Projection

The right cardiovascular contour in the posteroanterior projection is composed of two segments: (1) a smoothly curved shadow of moderate lateral convexity extending upward from the diaphragm; and (2) an upper straight or slightly convex shadow which can be followed to the level of the clavicle (Fig. 23). These two segments converge at a usually well defined point which at times may amount to an indentation. The lower contour is due to the lateral wall of the right atrium, although in long, narrow hearts a small segment of the right ventricle may reach this lateral border. In the longer hearts in deep inspiration, a triangular shadow may appear in the right cardiophrenic angle. Sometimes it is seen mainly through the right atrial shadow and is due to the inferior vena cava with its pleural investment.

The upper slightly convex or straight right contour is due to (1) the superior vena cava and right innominate vein, and (2) occasionally, the ascending aorta. These two structures overlie each other in the area just above the heart. Higher in the thorax, the aorta bends medialward and crosses the spine so that the upper portion of the paramediastinal shadow is due entirely to the vena cava and right innominate vein. In association with some transverse hearts the aorta may extend for a short distance beyond the lateral border of the superior vena cava, but this is infrequent. The usually well defined point where the right atrial contour meets the superior vena cava contour is the cardiovascular junction and is one focus of the long diameter of the heart (Fig. 23, A and B).

The left cardiovascular contour presents three separate segments; two of these, the upper and lower, show a variable degree of lateral convexity. The midsegment, on the other hand, although frequently convex laterally, may be straight or even slightly concave, depending upon

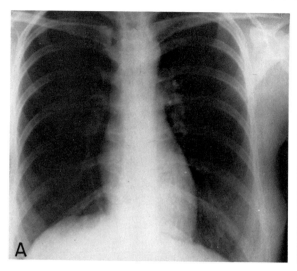 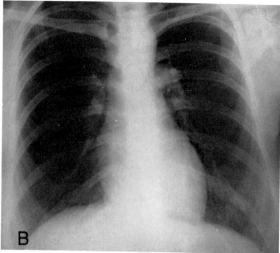

FIG. 20. NORMAL HEART

Changes in size and shape of the heart and thorax on serial films are illustrated by these two posteroanterior radiographs of the chest of a healthy 20-year-old woman. In A the transverse diameter of the heart is 10.5 cm; in B, 11.8 cm. In A the internal transverse diameter of the thorax at the level of the right hemidiaphragm is 26 cm; in B, 28 cm. Both films were exposed in the same degree of inspiration and within minutes of each other. Possible explanations for the size disparity include phase of cardiac cycle, influence of the Valsalva maneuver unconsciously performed, and effect of intercostal versus diaphragmatic respirations.

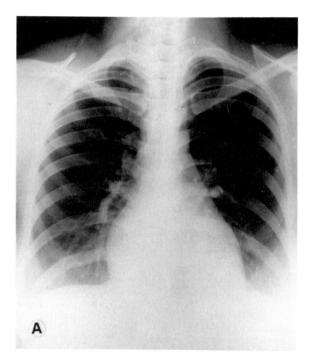 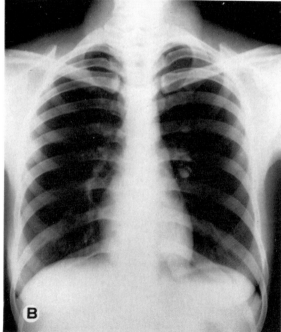

FIG. 21. CHANGE IN SIZE AND CONTOUR OF HEART DUE TO PREGNANCY

Both films were exposed in deep inspiration (A) During 28th week of pregnancy; (B) 6 months after delivery.

whether the heart is long, oblique or transverse in position.

The uppermost segment is due to the lateral wall of the greatly foreshortened aortic arch and usually a short portion of the descending aorta. The entire shadow is referred to as the aortic knob and is variable in prominence depending upon the position of the heart, the height of the

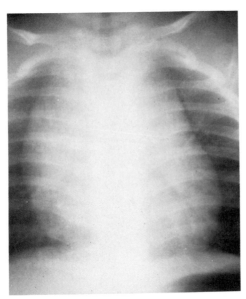

FIG. 22. NORMAL INFANT'S CHEST

Posteroanterior chest film of a normal 2-month-old male. The heart has a globular contour. The widening of the superior mediastinal shadow to the right and to the left is due to the thymus gland.

diaphragm, and the general shape of the thorax. As a part of the aging process, the knob may become more prominent, but this should not be considered a normal variation. The descending aorta, at times, occupies a paravertebral position, and it can then be identified all the way to the diaphragm. More frequently it is gradually lost in the overlying density of the spine and heart.

The middle segment is due to the lateral wall of the pulmonary trunk, and at times this blends with the contours of the descending branch of the left pulmonary artery. The pulmonary conus or infundibulum does not normally participate in this contour as has been shown repeatedly by angiocardiographic studies. In long hearts the pulmonary trunk ascends in a more vertical direction and thus may cast a longer shadow than in the transverse heart. The niche between the pulmonary trunk and the lower cardiac or left ventricular segment is filled ordinarily by the tip of the left atrial appendage. Since this is a small structure and the overlying pericardium tends to smooth out minor contour deviations, this small segment blends imperceptibly with the adjacent contours. A careful fluoroscopic study, however, may demonstrate this inactive area intervening between the actively pulsating pulmonary artery and left ventricle. In some hearts of the transverse type, the atrial appendage may not reach the left heart contour (Kerley, 1951).

The lower left cardiac segment is due entirely to the left ventricle and extends from the pulmonary trunk and atrial appendage above to the diaphragm below. The contour and convexity of this segment vary considerably. In the long heart, it is rather steep with a slight degree of lateral curve, whereas in the transverse heart the contour is more convex, rounded, and less steep. The apex of the heart on the roentgenogram is represented by that point on the left lower heart border farthest from the right cardiovascular junction (the junction of the superior vena cava with the right atrium). A shadow more translucent than the normal heart often fills in the angle between the cardiac apex and the diaphragm and is due to a fat pad. This shadow is variable in size in different patients and can be easily identified on the chest film by its contrast in density with the heart.

The area of the heart in contact with the diaphragm varies somewhat with respiratory phase and is greatest during expiration. The greater part of this area is the undersurface of the right ventricle. In deep inspiration, where some of the interior surface of the heart comes away from the diaphragm, the inferior cardiac contour may be followed for a short distance. On the left side, the stomach bubble may provide a variable amount of contrast so that a considerable segment of the cardiac contour is visible. This segment is due mainly to the undersurface of the left ventricle.

It should be noted that except for a usually negligible contribution of the left atrial appendage to the margin of the left heart border, the left atrium and right ventricle are "buried" within the cardiovascular silhouette and are not borderforming in the posteroanterior view.

Right Anterior Oblique Projection (RAO)

In 10–15° of right anterior obliquity, there is a long anterior slightly convex segment extending upward from the diaphragm to a juncture with a short, slightly convex pulmonary artery segment. The major portion of this long lower segment is due to the anterior wall of the left ventricle and a smaller upper part is due to the anterior wall of the right ventricle. Above the short pulmonary artery segment is a straight contour due to the anterior surface of the ascending aorta. Posteriorly the lower contour is formed by the right atrium but is often not well seen because of the overlying spine.

With rotation of 50–55° into the right anterior oblique (Fig. 24, A and B) the posterior surface of the heart clears the spine leaving an area of radiolucent lung posteriorly. Beginning at the diaphragm, a vertical or slightly oblique straight contour extends upward from the posterior aspect of the heart contour for a distance of 1–2 cm; this represents the inferior vena cava and its associated pleural fold. It is much better seen in the lateral view and either may fill in the posterior cardiophrenic angle or be superimposed on the cardiac contour. Just above the inferior vena caval shadow, a short segment of the right atrium participates in the posterior contour and fuses imperceptibly with a longer segment due to the posterolateral wall of the left atrium. This border begins to fade out or become indistinct about 2–3 cm before it reaches the carina. Several poorly defined densities are seen in the region of the carina and represent superimposed branches of the pulmonary arteries and veins. The descending aorta is partially projected through the carina and adds to the density of these shadows. In films of good contrast, the left main bronchus can be followed for a considerable distance into

the cardiovascular shadow, and just above and anterior to the bronchus there is an irregular rounded structure of increased density. This is the left pulmonary artery seen almost end-on. Just above the left pulmonary artery and anterior to the left main bronchus and trachea is the ascending aorta, and the aortic arch is also seen almost end-on. The distal part of the arch and the descending aorta may impinge upon the tracheal air column but usually are indistinct. Frequently, a shadow of increased density is superimposed on the posterior part of the tracheal air column and represents the anterior surface of the superior vena cava. The superior contour of the aorta is poorly outlined because of the overlying manubrium and superimposed great veins. Consequently, the major arterial branches in this projection are rarely seen.

Anteriorly in the right oblique projection there are three segments. The upper is rather straight and of moderate length and is due to the anterior

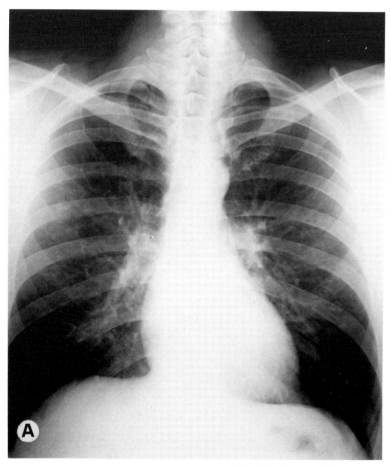

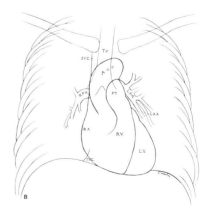

FIG. 23. NORMAL HEART

(A) Normal heart in a young man. Posteroanterior projection. (B) Sketch of A. Aor., aorta; R.P.A., right pulmonary artery; R.A., right atrium; R.V., right ventricle; I.V.C., inferior vena cava; S.V.C., superior vena cava; L.V., left ventricle; Tr., trachea.

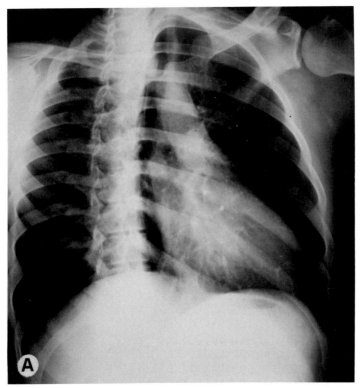

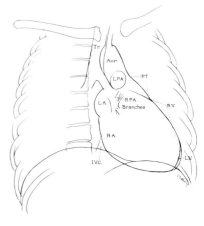

FIG. 24. NORMAL HEART

(A) Right anterior oblique projection (RAO) of a normal heart in a young man; about 50° rotation. (B) Sketch of A. Aor., aorta; I.V.C., inferior vena cava; L.A., left atrium; L.P.A., left pulmonary artery; L.V., left ventricle; P.T., pulmonary trunk; R.A., right atrium; R.V., right ventricle; Tr., trachea.

surface of the ascending aorta. This segment merges at a wide angle with the second or middle segment which is slightly convex anteriorly and is due partly to the pulmonary artery and partly to the infundibulum. The lower segment is due to the anterior surface of the right ventricle and presents a rather long, moderately convex contour. The diaphragmatic contour is indistinct but is formed for the most part by the undersurface of the right ventricle.

In the standard RAO projection the left ventricle forms little or none of the border of the heart.

Left Anterior Oblique Projection (LAO)

At 55° rotation (Fig. 25, A and B) into the left anterior oblique position, the shadow of most normal hearts will clear the spine posteriorly. Beginning just above the diaphragm anteriorly, one sees the slightly rounded anterior curve of the right ventricle which merges almost imperceptibly above with the right atrial contour. The length of this segment due to the right atrium varies considerably with the degree of obliquity

and the general shape of the heart. Usually at 55° only the atrial appendage is contour-forming. At fluoroscopy the appendage can be identified as a quiet area between the more actively pulsating right ventricle below and the surface of the ascending aorta above. Above the aortic contour there is a straight, not so dense shadow which represents the superior vena cava.

In the left oblique projection, the aortic arch is seen at approximately its maximal length, and in films of good contrast it can be followed across the tracheal air column and on into the descending portion. Underneath the arch there is a clear radiolucent area of variable size which is the aortic window. It is most clearly seen in deep inspiration and is bounded below by the left pulmonary artery; consequently the larger the artery, the smaller the area of the window. A portion of the air column of the trachea and left main bronchus are superimposed on the window and the left pulmonary artery. Below the left main bronchus posteriorly, there is a poorly defined contour which becomes much sharper as it continues downward. In its upper portion it represents the posterior lateral wall of the left atrium; in its lower portion it is due to the posterior wall of the left ventricle.

The diaphragmatic contour of the heart in this projection is best seen in long, narrow hearts in deep inspiration. Occasionally enough of this contour may be visible to permit visualization at fluoroscopy of an indentation near the midpoint in ventricular systole. This represents the inferior termination of the interventricular septum and thus serves as a dividing point between the two ventricles. In the left anterior oblique projection, the interventricular septum is almost exactly parallel to the x-ray beam. This projection is chosen for the angiographic demonstration of an interventricular septal defect.

The main pulmonary artery is not ordinarily seen in the LAO projection but is superimposed upon the density of the heart.

Lateral Projection

In the lateral projection (Fig. 26, A and B) beginning at the diaphragm anteriorly, the heart is in close relationship to the posterior surface of the sternum for a variable distance. This contour corresponds to the anterior surface of the right ventricle; with enlargement of this chamber, the length of the segment in contact with the sternum increases so that the heart impinges upon the retrosternal space above. Measurements of a series of lateral chests of normal adults of both sexes show that the length of this segment may vary from 0–10 cm, depending upon (1) the shape of the thorax (in flat-chested individuals the seg-

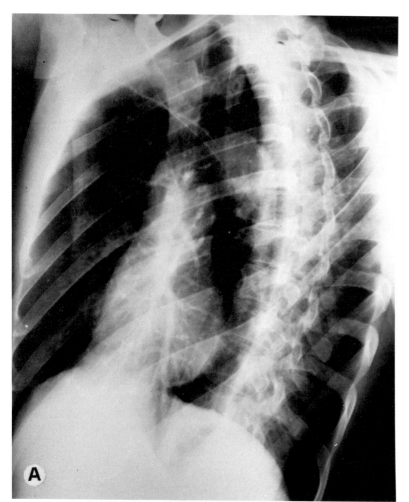

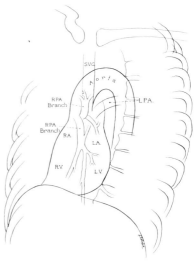

FIG. 25. NORMAL HEART

(A) Left anterior oblique projection of a normal heart in a young man; about 55° of rotation. (B) Sketch of A. L. A., left atrium; L.V., left ventricle; L.P.A., left pulmonary artery; R.A., right atrium; R.V., right ventricle; R.P.A., branch, right pulmonary artery; S.V.C., superior vena cava.

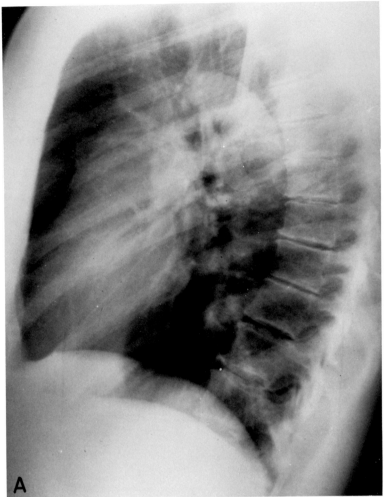

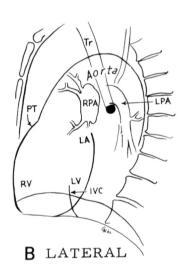

B LATERAL

FIG. 26. NORMAL HEART

(A) Right lateral projection of a normal heart in a young woman. (B) Sketch of A. Tr, trachea; R.P.A., right pulmonary artery; L.P.A., left pulmonary artery; P.T., pulmonary trunk; L.A., left atrium; L.V., left ventricle; R.V., right ventricle; I.V.C., inferior vena cava.

ment is longer), (2) the degree of cardiac mobility with respiration and diaphragmmatic height (there is forward displacement of the heart in deep inspiration), and (3) the degree of obesity (amount of pericardiac fat). Consequently, it is probable that the range of normal variation overlaps the abnormal sufficiently to make any measurement worthless (Fig. 28). Frequently, the right ventricle below and the pulmonary artery and conus above form two separate anterior convexities, the upper of which ends sharply where the pulmonary artery crosses the anterior aortic contour.

In films of high contrast, almost the entire course of the thoracic aorta is visible. The contour begins just above that of the pulmonary trunk anteriorly and extends upward for a short distance before arching posteriorly. Near the beginning of the arch anteriorly, there is a straight contour extending upward which is due to the superior vena cava. The origin of the innominate artery is rarely seen except in films of unusual contrast because its density is lost in that of the great veins. The transverse diameter of the aorta in the region of the arch is best seen where the aorta crosses the tracheal air column. The aortic arch is often shown to better advantage in the lateral than in the left anterior oblique view. The descending aorta is straight and, for the most part, anterior to the spine, although the two structures may overlap to a variable degree.

The left pulmonary artery forms a secondary arch below the aorta, although in its distal portion it overlaps the descending aorta. The pulmonary window may be visible as a roughly triangular area of radiolucency just above the arching left pulmonary artery and beneath the aortic arch. The right pulmonary artery forms a rounded, superimposed shadow, just anterior to the carina, and extends into an elongated shadow which represents the descending branch of this artery. In the lateral projection the left pulmonary artery is seen in profile as it arches over the left main bronchus while the right pulmonary artery is seen on end. The right and left pulmonary arteries form almost a right angle to one another.

Continuing from the carina downward, the posterior cardiovascular contour above is due usually to the descending branch of the right pulmonary artery and often is not sharply seen. Farther toward the diaphragm, the contour is due to the left atrium above and the left ventricle below. Together they form a smooth, slightly convex posterior segment which ends at the diaphragm. Differentiation of the left atrial and ventricular components is possible at fluoroscopy where there is a difference in amplitude of pulsation of these two chambers. The straight shadow just above the diaphragm is due to the inferior vena cava; it may be contour-forming or be superimposed on the heart contour.

The right atrium normally forms no part of the contour of the heart in the lateral projection.

Hilar and Vascular Shadows of Lung

Most of the composite hilar shadows on each side are due to the respective pulmonary arteries and their branches. The pulmonary veins probably contribute a small amount of density to the lower portion of each hilus. The shadows on each side are slightly different and will therefore be described separately.

In the left hilus associated with a long heart, a short segment of the left pulmonary artery is usually visible forming a gentle arch with convexity upwards. The artery quickly bifurcates into the major upper and lower lobe branches; the lower lobe branch is the longer and more prominent of the two and can be readily identified in most chest films as it descends in close proximity to the left heart border. The shorter upper lobe branch is further shortened by the posteroanterior projection so that a separate segment is not always seen. It ends in a bifurcation giving rise to an apical and basilar branch which may be identified with some degree of regularity. With a globular heart, the pulmonary trunk may obscure the left hilus so that only the smaller branches of the pulmonary artery are visible.

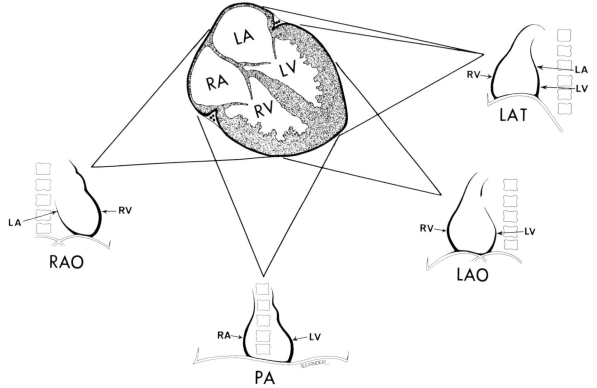

FIG. 27. SCHEMA FOR HEART CHAMBER LOCALIZATION

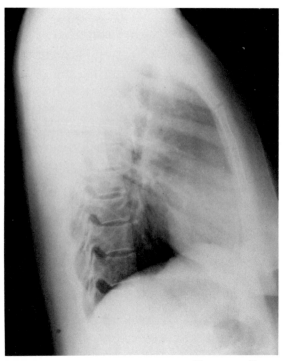

FIG. 28. LATERAL VIEW OF NORMAL HEART IN YOUNG
WOMAN

The anterior surface of the heart extends into the retrosternal space for an unusual distance. This is a normal
variation, and part of the opacity may be due to precardial
fat.

The right pulmonary artery divides into upper
and lower lobe branches before it reaches the
right cardiovascular border. Of the two major
branches, the lower is the longer and larger and
can be identified regularly coursing downward in
a direction roughly parallel to the right heart
border. It gives off a middle lobe branch and an
apical lower lobe branch and terminates in four
branches to the lower lobe, but these cannot be
identified precisely without angiocardiography.
The upper lobe branch is short and gives rise to
three divisions, namely (1) apical anterior, (2)
apical posterior, and (3) basilar. The apical
branch can be identified with some degree of
regularity.

The pulmonary veins are sizeable structures,
although they are not as large as the major
branches of the pulmonary artery. The two major veins from each lung are short and are largely
obscured by the superimposed heart shadow. It
is remarkable that vascular structures of such
size are so seldom recognized on conventional
chest films. Actually, one or two veins from the
right lower lung can frequently be identified running a straight course toward the right heart
border and crossing the pulmonary artery
branches at a moderate angle (Fig. 29B and C).
The pulmonary veins, at their point of union
with the left atrium, are located several centimeters inferior (caudal) to the right and left
pulmonary arteries.

On the lateral view, superimposition of the
inferior pulmonary veins seen on end as they
enter the left atrium may simulate a nodular
pulmonary lesion posterior to and touching the
heart (Schreiber, 1965). Knowledge of the location of the entrance of the confluence of the
pulmonary veins will largely obviate this potential difficulty.

The left hilar structures are normally located
slightly superior (cephalic) to the right hilus. A
line connecting the hilar structures may form an
angle of approximately 5° with the horizontal.

PULSATIONS OF NORMAL HEART AND GREAT VESSELS (FLUOROSCOPY AND CINEFLUOROGRAPHY)

Fluoroscopy

Posteroanterior View (PA)

The left cardiac border in the posteroanterior
projection is more active than the right. The
aortic knob consistently shows moderate pulsations, expansile and equal in all directions and
opposite in time to the left ventricular segment.
The pulmonary artery segment below the aortic
knob shows less conspicuous pulsations with the
same timing as those of the aorta. Below the
pulmonary artery is a short quiet area due to the
tip of the left atrial appendage. The left ventricular contour shows the largest amplitude of pulsations of any of the heart borders, and this is of
the order of 0.2–1.0 cm. Usually, the inward
motion of systole begins near the base and progresses as a superficial wave down the left border.
In the long narrow heart, the area of maximal
pulsation is near the apex and is relatively large;
in the transverse heart it is nearer the base and
somewhat smaller. Excursions of the heart border are not always along a horizontal axis. In the
apical region of a long heart they may be oblique
or almost vertical. The quiet left atrial tip with
the active pulsations of the left ventricle below
and opposite pulsations of the aorta and pulmonary artery above is the focus of the seesaw
activity of the left heart border. Fluoroscopy of
the apex is helpful in determining the extent of

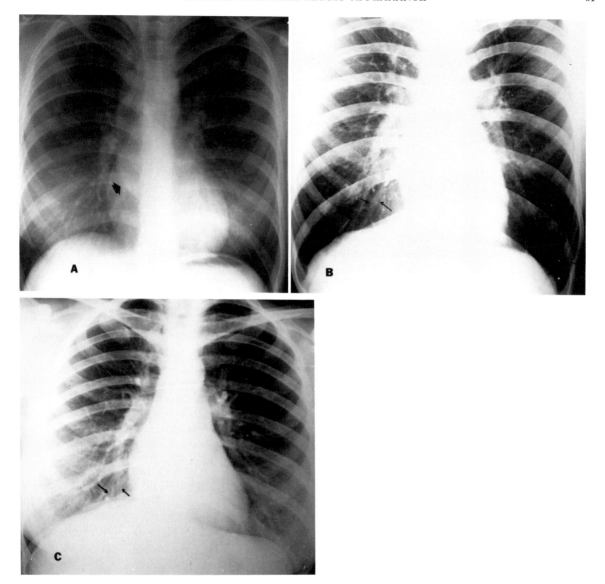

FIG. 29
(A) Normal heart in a 6-year-old boy. The normal left atrium is visible at the base of the heart and to the right of the midline (arrow). (B and C) Chest films from two different persons showing the right lower lobe pulmonary vein (arrows).

the pericardial fat pad which can be differentiated because of its lack of movement and decreased density.

Movements of the right heart border are due to a summation of both right atrial and transmitted right ventricular pulsations; the ventricular pulsations often predominate, and in an active heart their amplitude may be 0.2–0.3 cm. The timing of the pulsations is variable; the border may move laterally or medially during ventricular systole; there may be a short medial movement followed by a more pronounced lateral motion. Some of this movement is undoubtedly positional in nature.

The supracardiac shadow on the right does not show significant pulsations except in older individuals and those with a transverse heart in which case the ascending aorta may be border-forming. The superior vena cava normally does not pulsate.

Right Anterior Oblique Projection (RAO)

In about 10° rotation the anterior surface of the heart shows moderate sized movements due to the left ventricle. As the rotation is increased to 30–45°, small pulsations of the anterior surface of the right ventricle appear anteriorly below, and slightly more pronounced pulsations above are due to the pulmonary conus and artery. Posteriorly, pulsations are quite small since they arise in the right atrium below and the left above. Above 70° of obliquity, the left ventricle enters the posterior contour so that a marked increase in pulsations is noticed.

Left Anterior Oblique Projection (LAO)

In 10–15° of obliquity the anterior contour (to the observer's left) below shows small movements due mainly to the right atrium and its appendage. At 20–30° the right ventricle forms a considerable segment of the anterior contour and may show pulsations of moderate amplitude which permit differentiation from the quiet right atrial region above. Above the atrium the ascending aortic movements are visible and are best seen at about 45° rotation. At 45–60° only a small tip of the atrial appendage may be identified between the ventricle below and the ascending aorta above. Posteriorly the left ventricle is contour-forming, and consequently pulsations are of good height. At 45–60° there is a longer left ventricular segment below and a shorter left atrial segment above. Differences in timing and amplitude of movements of these two segments are usually apparent and aid in localizing the chamber borders. At this degree of obliquity (45–60°) in long hearts in deep inspiration, a considerable segment of the diaphragmatic surface is visible and pulsations are obliquely directed along the long axis of the heart. Near the central portion of this segment there is often an immobile area which marks the lower end of the interventricular septum. The exact position of the septum within the cardiac shadow, however, cannot be determined without angiocardiography.

Lateral Projection

In the lateral projection there are relatively good pulsations posteriorly over the left ventricular contour and somewhat smaller pulsations anteriorly over the right ventricle. Keats and Martt (1962) have pointed out a transient apparently paradoxical pulsation of the superior aspect of the posterior contour of the left ventricle. They suggest that the outward bulge of this portion of the ventricle during early ventricular systole is a reflection of the earliest phase of contraction of this chamber while its volume is still constant. Above the left ventricle is the contour of the left atrium which shows very feeble motion. Above the right ventricular contour is a short segment of pulmonary artery with a very small motion, and above this is the ascending aorta which usually shows well marked pulsations.

Cinefluorography

Cardiac pulsations can be permanently recorded on movie film for viewing at a later time. Such recording permits the slowing down of cardiac action for more careful study and even allows frame-by-frame analysis if needed. Either 16- or 35-mm film may be used to satisfactorily display cardiovascular pulsations. Care should be taken to open the shutters sufficiently wide that a sizeable area of the heart can be recorded. This permits comparisons to be made of the timing, amplitude, and character of cardiac pulsations in one area relative to those in another area.

RELATION OF ESOPHAGUS TO CARDIOVASCULAR CONTOURS

Beginning in the upper mediastinum the esophagus is in contact with the aortic arch and is posterior and medial to it. Continuing downward, it is posterior and in close relation to the left main bronchus and farther downward it follows closely the posterior curve of the left atrium. Just above the diaphragm it swings toward the left and crosses anterior to the descending aorta. These relationships are best demonstrated by following the passage of a bolus of barium paste through the esophagus at fluoroscopy. The aortic impression is at about the level of the aortic knob and is best seen in the posteroanterior and right oblique projections. The impression is curved or crescent-shaped and is of variable depth depending somewhat upon minor variations in the course of the aorta and degree of rotation of the heart. The indentation is on the left anterolateral aspect of the esophagus, and the convexity of the impression is therefore to the right and posterior. Continuing downward in the right anterior oblique projection, there is often a second short rounded impression due to the left main bronchus. Continuing toward the diaphragm, there may be a gentle posterior deviation of the esophagus in the area where it is in close relationship to the left atrium. This is common in children and adults with a transverse type of heart and is best seen in the far right oblique or lateral views. It is accentuated by expiration and may disappear during inspiration. In tall, slender persons with long hearts, the course of the esophagus is usually straight. The factors of body build, respiration and of heart type must therefore be evaluated before an observer can be sure that a posterior deviation of the esophagus indicates left atrial enlargement. Where the esophagus crosses the descending aorta just above the diaphragm, there is a shallow indentation with a concavity to the left. In older individuals with a tortuous aorta the indentation may be much more pronounced and result in a deviation of the entire esophagus anteriorly and to the left.

The course of the esophagus in older persons is often unreliable as an indicator of left atrial enlargement. The esophagus has no serosa and is closely applied to the aorta. As the aorta elongates, the course of the esophagus is altered accordingly, and the tortuous esophagus is an indicator only of the tortuosity of the aorta.

NORMAL ANGIOCARDIOGRAM

Contrast substance passes through the normal heart in 6–10 sec. During this time, the cardiac chambers and the great vessels are outlined in various phases of systole and diastole. Apparatus permitting regulation of exposures so as to obtain films at some preselected phase of the cardiac cycle is available. The present authors have used the Cordis heart programmer for this purpose. The apparatus allows preinjection programming of the time of the injection and of the first x-ray exposure. When using this or a similar apparatus it should be borne in mind that only the beginning of the injection and the first x-ray exposure in a series of films may be accurately timed to a portion of the cardiac cycle. If the injection lasts more than a fraction of a second, then part of the injected bolus will be entering the cardiovascular system at a phase in the cardiac cycle different from that initially programmed. Moreover, if the injection of contrast material provokes even a momentary cardiac arrhythmia, timing of the film exposures to various phases in the cardiac cycle will be disturbed. A record of exposures on a simultaneously recorded electrocardiogram permits the accurate correlation of each film of the angiocardiogram with cardiac phase. Unless this correlation is obtained, an accurate and precise description of the appearance of normal ventricular chambers as seen at angiocardiography is not possible. Usually approximately complete systole and diastole can be recognized; the intermediate phases may lead to errors.

Angiocardiography has the advantage of revealing the structure and something of the hemodynamics of the intact, functioning heart. At postmortem, the left side of the heart is almost bloodless, and the blood pressure is zero; the diaphragm is immobile, and the lungs are partially collapsed. Even after the most carefully prepared injection studies, one cannot assume that the chamber contours and relationships are precisely the same as they are during life. Thus, the anatomical information obtained from angiocardiography, although lacking somewhat in precision and depending to a degree on subjective film interpretation, is probably more valid than that obtained from other sources.

The following is a composite description and represents a theoretical average angiocardiogram. There are a number of minor variations from case to case. The descriptions are limited to the anteroposterior and lateral projections, since these have been standard with the authors for a number of years, although the right posterior oblique position has been occasionally used. For a description of the other projections, the reader is referred to the excellent work on angiocardiography by Dotter and Steinberg (1951).

Anteroposterior Projection

The superior vena cava is usually distended somewhat by the force of the injected contrast substance and in an adult is 6–8 cm in length and about 1.5–2 cm in diameter. It is formed by the junction of the right and left innominate veins and is seen as a bandlike shadow extending in a straight or slightly curved, almost vertical direction, in the right upper mediastinum. It continues inside the border of the right atrium a short distance before terminating, and in its lower portion is superimposed on the atrial appendage. The right atrium, when fully distended, is shaped like a hockey stick or golf club with the superior vena cava as the handle (Fig. 30A). The atrial appendage is not always well seen, and the medial atrial border above is usually due to the main atrial chamber. This border is vertical in its upper portion, but continuing downward it rapidly curves medially and becomes horizontal and continuous with the upper contour of the right ventricle. When the right ventricle is in partial systole or diastole (Fig. 31, A and B) the medial border of the superior vena cava, the medial and upper borders of the right atrium, the superior border of the right ventricle and the medial border of the pulmonary conus and artery form a U-shaped contour. In complete diastole the upper right ventricular contour moves lateralward and upwards and this U-shaped relationship is thus disturbed (Fig. 32, A and B). Laterally, the entire heart border is usually due

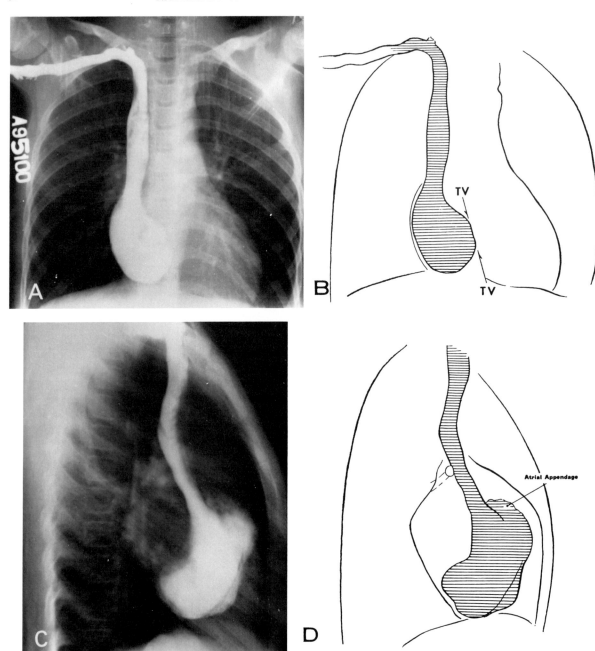

FIG. 30. SIMULTANEOUSLY EXPOSED ANTEROPOSTERIOR AND LATERAL ANGIOCARDIOGRAMS OF SUPERIOR VENA CAVA AND RIGHT ATRIUM

TV, approximate region of the tricuspid valve.

to the right atrium, and a small area of the atrium may contact the diaphragm. The atrial myocardium is 2–3 mm in thickness and is seen as a thin rim around the dense contrast substance inside the chamber. The right atrium terminates medially at the tricuspid valve. Valve leaflets are occasionally recognized, but the location of the valve is usually determined by the abrupt change

in the smooth regular contour of the atrium into the irregular and sometimes poorly defined ventricular contour. The tricuspid valve is near the midline and lies in an almost vertical plane (Fig. 30, A and B).

Regurgitation of contrast substance from the right atrium into the inferior vena cava and hepatic veins is occasionally seen in varying degree. Our experience does not permit an exact statement, but regurgitation appears to be less common in normal adults than in children, particularly those with congenital cyanotic heart disease. It is probably a function of the injection speed and right atrial volume and pressure. The inferior vena cava is seen for only a short distance and is a bandlike shadow superimposed upon the liver density. It is often obscured by the branching hepatic radicles into which the contrast substance may regurgitate for a distance of several centimeters. Those veins act as a sort of reservoir for the contrast substance as it slowly feeds back

into the right atrium; it thus may produce an appearance of reopacification which is confusing.

The right ventricle in diastole (Fig. 34A) extends about one-half to two-thirds of the way to the left heart border, and the conus or infundibulum is not borderforming. In diastole the ventricle resembles somewhat a flask with the infundibulum as the neck; in partial systole it resembles a curved powder horn. The interventricular septum is slightly curved with the convexity towards the right. During ventricular diastole the pulmonary valve sinuses are dilated frequently, permitting a precise localization of the valve and

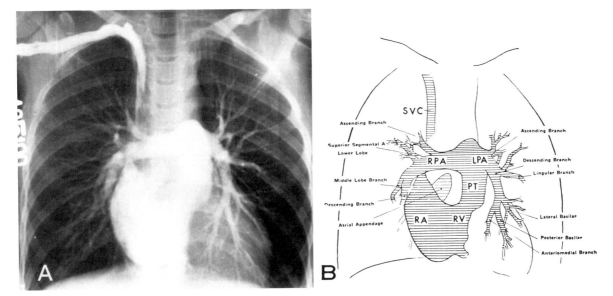

FIG. 31. NORMAL RIGHT ATRIUM, RIGHT VENTRICLE, AMD PULMONARY ARTERIAL SYSTEM
The right ventricle is in partial systole. RA, right atrium; RV, right ventricle; PT, pulmonary trunk; LPA, left pulmonary artery; RPA, right pulmonary artery; SVC, superior vena cava.

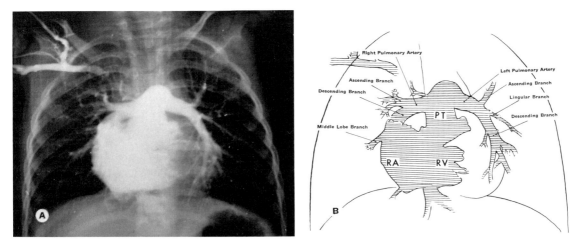

FIG. 32. NORMAL RIGHT ATRIUM, VENTRICLE, AND PULMONARY ARTERIAL SYSTEM IN 2½-YEAR-OLD CHILD
The right ventricle is in partial systole. RA, right atrium; RV, right ventricle; PT, pulmonary trunk.

a differentiation between the conus and the pulmonary trunk. The pulmonic valve is to the left of the midline and above the aortic valve.

The tubular or conical right ventricular infundibulum (pulmonary outflow tract) is confined by the septal band of the crista supraventricularis on the right and the parietal band on the left.

The pulmonary trunk runs upward and slightly toward the midline; its lateral border clearly forms the left middle cardiac segment. Its projected length is variable depending somewhat upon the cardiac type. In the transverse heart it is short and runs obliquely upward and backward; in the long heart its course is more vertical and its shadow is therefore longer. The pulmonary trunk bifurcates just to the left of the midline and in front of the left main bronchus.

The left pulmonary artery continues upward, somewhat lateralward and posterior, forming an arch, the crest of which is distinctly higher than the right pulmonary artery. After continuing laterally for a short distance, the left artery bifurcates into ascending and descending branches.

In good films, the small branches of the pulmonary arteries can be identified with regularity. Their distribution and nomenclature are similar to that of the segmental bronchi, and the terminology used by Dotter and Steinberg (1951). Boyden (1949) and Dotter (1971) will be employed in the following description. For a more detailed consideration of the variations of these segmental arteries the reader is referred to the papers by the above authors.

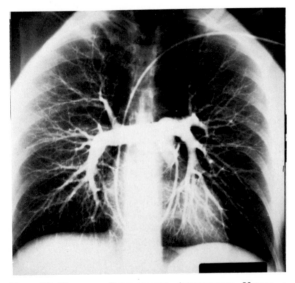

FIG. 33. NORMAL PULMONARY ANGIOGRAM USING A WEDGE FILTER IN ORDER TO BETTER PENETRATE THE MEDIASTINUM

The left ascending branch runs a short course laterally and posteriorly, and typically ends abruptly in (1) an apical posterior branch and (2) an anterior segmental branch. The apical posterior branch runs a very short, almost vertical course and divides into (a) anterior and (b) posterior apical rami. The anterior ramus runs almost vertically, is rather straight and can often be followed to the level of the clavicle. The posterior ramus in the anteroposterior projection forms a Y-shaped division with the anterior ramus and runs a more lateral, oblique course, giving off several smaller arteries as it nears the periphery.

The anterior segmental branch of the upper lobe artery runs a short, lateral and downward course, and divides into (a) an anterior and (b) a posterior ramus. The anterior ramus is foreshortened by projection and terminates in several small arterial branches. The posterior ramus continues somewhat lateralward and gives rise often to three branches which extend to the lung periphery.

The left descending artery arches posteriorly and lateralward and finally extends downward in a direction almost parallel to the left heart border. The pulmonary arch is best seen in the lateral view and is considerably foreshortened in the anteroposterior projection. Frequently in transverse or globular hearts the descending artery fuses with the lateral border of the pulmonary trunk forming a segment of the lateral cardiac border.

In contrast to the bronchial segmental arrangement, the lingular artery branch (Dotter and Steinberg, 1951) takes origin from the upper portion of the descending artery. The lingular artery is short and runs anteriorly and sharply downward and divides into (1) a superior and (2) an inferior branch. Both of these branches are superimposed to an extent on the main descending artery, and the inferior ramus usually appears between the main descending artery and the cardiac contour.

At approximately the same level as the origin of the lingular artery there is a posterior short branch, the superior or apical segmental artery of the lower lobe. This branch is quite short, runs downward and posteriorly and divides into three branches which extend roughly upward, lateralward, and downward, respectively. This particular segmental artery is best seen in the lateral projection.

The lower lobe branch terminates in a trifurcation. The three branches are (1) anteromedial, (2) lateral, and (3) posterior. The posterior branch appears as a continuation of the main lower lobe artery. It is superimposed upon the cardiac shadow in its lower portion. The antero-medial branch is the most medial and runs in a vertical direction and is also superimposed on the cardiac contour. The lateral branch is easily identified and is seen near the cardiac border and runs a straight course in an oblique lateral direction.

The right pulmonary artery is slightly lower than the left and runs in an almost horizontal direction across the vertebral column and is therefore projected in its maximum length. It divides into a smaller ascending branch just to the right of the midline (often hidden in the mediastinal opacity on plain films) and a larger descending branch just at or beyond the right heart border.

The upper or ascending branch runs obliquely upward and lateralward for a short distance and divides into (1) apical, (2) posterior, and (3) anterior branches. The apical branch in turn divides into (a) apical and (b) posterior rami. The apical ramus runs vertically upward and is lost in the extreme apex of the lung. The posterior ramus runs obliquely lateralward and upward and terminates by giving off two or three smaller branches. The posterior artery is often difficult to identify; it may be anomalous and arise from the apical branch. It runs obliquely laterally and upward and gives off two branches at its termination: (a) posterior and (b) lateral.

The anterior ramus extends lateralward for a short distance and divides into (a) anterior and (b) lateral branches. The anterior branch runs forward and slightly downward and in the anteroposterior projection is a short, almost vertical shadow. The lateral segment runs horizontally toward the lung periphery.

The right descending branch runs downward and lateralward in a graceful arch and is roughly parallel to the right heart border. It divides into the following branches in approximately the following order: (1) middle lobe, (2) superior segmental artery of the right lower lobe, (3) medial basal, (4) anterior basal, (5) posterior basal, and (6) lateral basal. The middle lobe branch extends lateralward and downward and divides into (a) superior and (b) inferior rami. These are best seen in the lateral view and may be obscured or difficult to identify in the anteroposterior projection. The superior segmental artery to the lower lobe originates at about the same level as the middle lobe branch but extends posteriorly and slightly downward and usually terminates in three branches. The medial basal artery occupies a paravertebral position and runs downward in an almost vertical direction and arises just below the origin of the superior segmental artery. The anterior basal artery is likewise superimposed on the cardiac shadow or is near the lateral cardiac contour but is difficult to positively identify. The posterior basal appears as a continuation of the

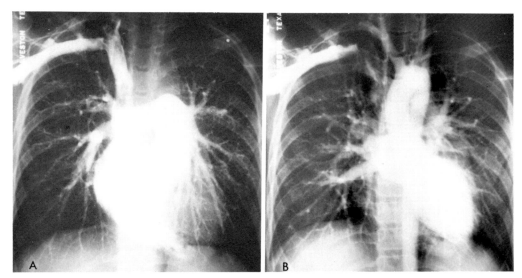

FIG. 34. NORMAL INTRAVENOUS ANGIOCARDIOGRAM IN 9-YEAR-OLD GIRL

(A) This selected early film from the serial examination shows contrast filling of the right atrium and ventricle, including the outflow tract of the right ventricle. The main pulmonary artery, its right and left branches, and its intrapulmonary ramifications are well seen. The right atrial appendage can be seen as a small opaque knob projecting just to the left of the distal most part of the superior vena cava. (B) This reproduction of a film from late in the angiocardiographic series shows pulmonary veins emptying into the left atrium and contrast filling of the left ventricle (late ventricular diastole), as well as opacification of the entire thoracic aorta and the arterial trunks originating from the arch.

main descending artery and runs posteriorly downward and is probably best seen in the lateral view. The lateral basal is best identified in the anteroposterior projection as its course runs obliquely downward and lateralward toward the base of the lung.

The pulmonary veins are often incompletely demonstrated, usually, for two reasons. In most angiocardiographic studies emphasis is placed on demonstrating either the right or left side of the heart. Consequently, intermediate phases when the pulmonary veins are most likely to be visible are neglected. Also, the somewhat more prominent pulmonary arteries tend to obscure the veins so that they are optimally demonstrated only during a short time period.

Pulmonary veins are often anomalous (Brantigan, 1947), but usually there are two veins entering the left atrium from each lung although on the right side there are frequently three (Figs. 34B; 35, A and B; and 36, A and B). On the right side the uppermost vein is usually the largest and is formed by the confluence of three sizeable branches. It is short and rather thick and runs medialward to enter the right upper aspect of the left atrium. A somewhat smaller vein appears to originate in the general region of the middle lobe and runs a short distance in a horizontal direction and either may join the larger upper vein or enter the left atrium through an independent opening. The most frequently demonstrated vein which originates in the region of the lower lobe is formed by a confluence of at least two and probably three smaller branches and runs obliquely upward where it appears to join the large upper branch before entering the left atrium; actually, they remain separate as a rule.

The uppermost vein on the left is usually straight or slightly curved and runs a relatively long course obliquely downward to join the upper lateral aspect of the left atrium. It appears to be formed by a confluence of two or three smaller branches, and before reaching the atrium it is joined by a smaller branch which probably corresponds to the middle lobe branch on the right side. The lower lobe branches largely are seen through the heart shadow. For the most part, they run upward and anterior and thus appear foreshortened. Usually two or three branches can be seen forming the main lower lobe branch which ascends to enter the atrium at its lateral inferior border.

The left atrium in the anteroposterior projection is roughly triangular in shape; the right border is narrow and represents the apex, and the left border is longer, representing the base of the triangle. It empties into the left ventricle near its inferior and lateral margin although the exact site of the mitral valve cannot often be determined at angiocardiography. The appearance of the atrium varies somewhat with cardiac phase and the chamber is largest near the end of ventricular systole (Fig. 36, A and B). The left atrial appendage is occasionally identified on the normal angiocardiogram (Fig. 35, A and B); the frequency with which it is seen, of course, depends on the concentration of contrast substance in the left atrium, the quality of the films and, most of all, the number of films exposed during left atrial filling. It is the only part of the left atrium which is borderforming in the anteroposterior projection. The left atrium is the highest or most cephalad of all of the cardiac chambers and is superimposed mainly on the structures at the base of the heart, namely the pulmonary artery and conus, and the first part of the as-

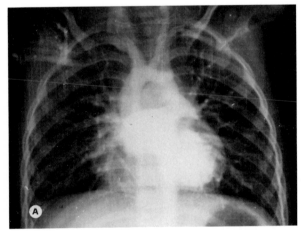
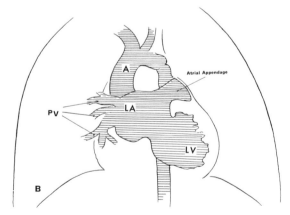

FIG. 35. NORMAL LEFT ATRIUM AND VENTRICLE IN CHILD WITH SLIGHT DEGREE OF COARCTATION OF AORTA
A, aorta; LA, left atrium; LV, left ventricle; PV, pulmonary veins.

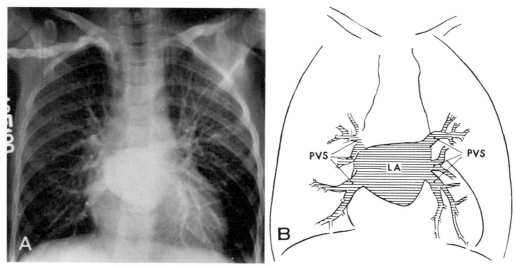

FIG. 36. LEFT ATRIUM AND PULMONARY VEINS IN NORMAL ADULT
PVS, pulmonary veins; LA, left atrium.

cending aorta. The left superior surface is in close relationship to the left main bronchus.

The left ventricular cavity contour and wall thickness vary markedly with cardiac phase. Consequently, estimates of chamber size and wall thickness are not valid unless the exposure is known to be in diastole. In diastole the cavity is projected as a somewhat asymmetrical but roughly oval or ellipsoidal shadow with a longer rounded, more convex, superolateral border and a shorter, almost straight or slightly convex inferomedial border (Figs. 34B and 35, A and B). The inferomedial border runs at an angle of about 45° with the horizontal and roughly represents the contour of the interventricular septum. In the apical region the two borders converge at a fairly sharp angle, thus forming a pointed contour. Also, at the base the margins converge to meet the outline of the ascending aorta. In complete ventricular systole a faint streak of contrast substance is usually identified, lying in an oblique plane. This, of course, represents the small ventricular space filled with residual blood.

The aortic valve, sinuses of Valsalva, and first portion of the ascending aorta are obscured somewhat by the vertebral column and at times by residual contrast substance in the left atrium. Consequently, these structures are only rarely demonstrated in the anteroposterior projection. The greater part of the ascending aorta, however, is clearly seen. The ascending aorta forms a variable lateral convexity as it sweeps toward the right. Its origin is well to the left of the midline, and occasionally it does not extend beyond the

right lateral vertebral border. As it begins to arch, it returns to the midline at about the fifth or sixth dorsal vertebra. Just to the left of the midline, the large innominate artery originates and crosses the trachea in an oblique upward direction and soon bifurcates just below the sternoclavicular joint. The first portions of the carotid and subclavian arteries may be obscured for a short distance by the bony structures of the shoulder; in their more distal portions they are easily seen. The axillary arteries bilaterally are easily seen and may be visible when there is doubt as to whether the ascending aorta contains contrast substance or not. The first parts of both the left carotid and left subclavian arteries originate just beyond the crest of the arch and are often superimposed and may appear as a single trunk.

The greatly foreshortened arch ends at the descending aorta which is somewhat variable in its distance from the midline. It always overlies the vertebral column to a slight degree and is inclined medially as it descends, so at the level of the diaphragm it is almost entirely superimposed upon the vertebral column.

Lateral Projection

The superior vena cava runs downward in a straight vertical or slightly oblique anterior course which on the average is about one-third to one-half of the anteroposterior diameter of the chest from the anterior chest wall (Figs. 37A and 38, A and B). The azygos vein is often normally filled by reflux and enters the vena cava on the upper one-third to one-half of its length. The right atrium is variable in contour due in part to the degree of distention and cardiac phase. When distended, posteriorly, it presents a straight contour which is continuous above with the superior vena cava and below with the inferior vena cava. Frequently reflux into the inferior vena cava will show that it runs obliquely forward from the diaphragm or that it has a slight posterior offset from the posterior atrial contour (Fig. 39, A–C).

Anteriorly and superiorly, the atrial appendage is frequently seen; it has a slightly rounded superior surface and ends in a pointed projection anteriorly. It is often obscured by the overlying contrast-containing pulmonary artery.

The right ventricular cavity in diastole presents a smooth, rounded, anteriorly convex contour which continues into the ventral cardiophrenic angle where it meets the diaphragmatic contour at a well defined point. Columnae carneae are often seen anteriorly as droplike or somewhat elongated areas of radiolucency within

the contrast substance. The inferior contour is straight or slightly concave downward and tends somewhat to follow the diaphragmatic contour. The posterior border of the right ventricle is often obscured by the overlying right atrium; however, it is formed for the most part by the interventricular septum which has a slight anterior curvature. Toward the base of the heart, the right ventricle narrows into a somewhat tubular or mildly funnel-shaped structure which is the conus or infundibulum. The posterior border of the outflow tract of the right ventricle is smooth and arcuate, an appearance produced by the margin of the crista supraventricularis.

The pulmonary trunk is differentiated from the conus by the frequent demonstration of the outpouching of the valve sinuses (Fig. 40) and also the less frequently seen thin, slightly curved, radiolucent shadows of the valve cusps. The pulmonary trunk is seen in almost its greatest length as it runs obliquely upward and backward. The

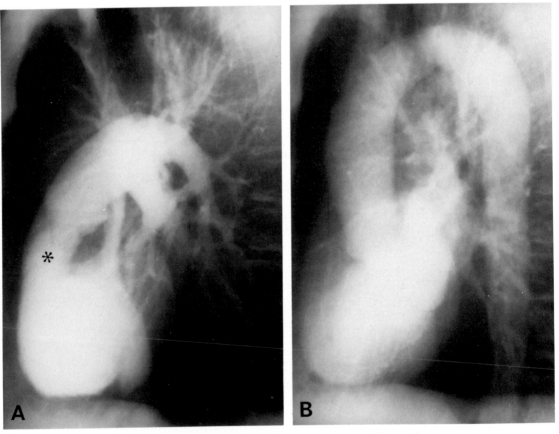

FIG. 37. NORMAL INTRAVENOUS ANGIOCARDIOGRAM IN YOUNG ADULT

(A) An early film from the lateral series shows some residual contrast material in the superior vena cava. Slight reflux into the inferior vena cava is also noted. The right atrium and ventricle are indistinguishable from one another on this film. The outflow tract of the right ventricle is located anteriorly (asterisk), and the main pulmonary artery with its right and left branches are well opacified. (B) A late film from the lateral series shows pulmonary veins converging upon the left atrium posteriorly and superiorly. The left ventricle contains a small amount of contrast material, and the entire thoracic aorta is well opacified. Observe the posterior location of the origin of the aorta relative to the origin of the pulmonary artery.

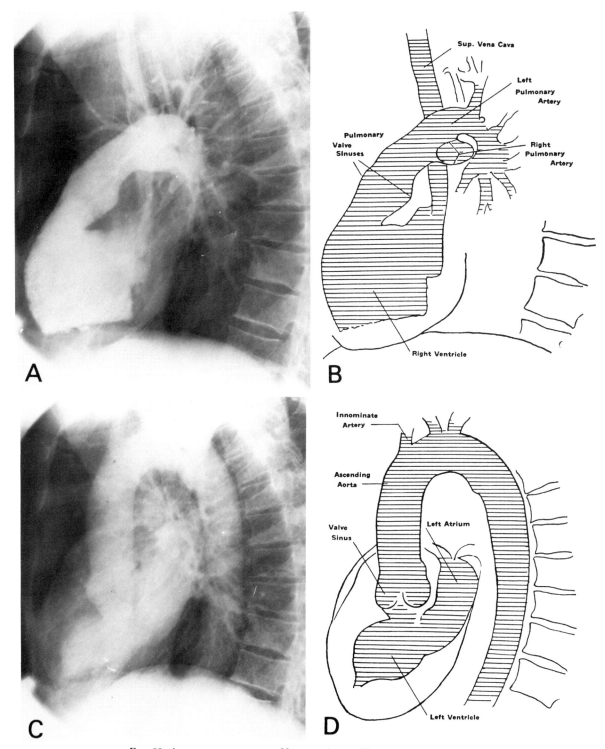

FIG. 38. ANGIOCARDIOGRAM OF NORMAL ADULT HEART, LATERAL VIEW
A and B, right heart chambers and pulmonary artery; C and D, left heart chambers and aorta.

degree of obliquity varies with the position and shape of the heart and is greater in transverse and less in long vertical hearts.

The left pulmonary artery is slightly shortened by projection and appears as a continuation of the arch of the pulmonary trunk. The ascending branch is short and arises near the apex of the arch; it is identified with some difficulty on the

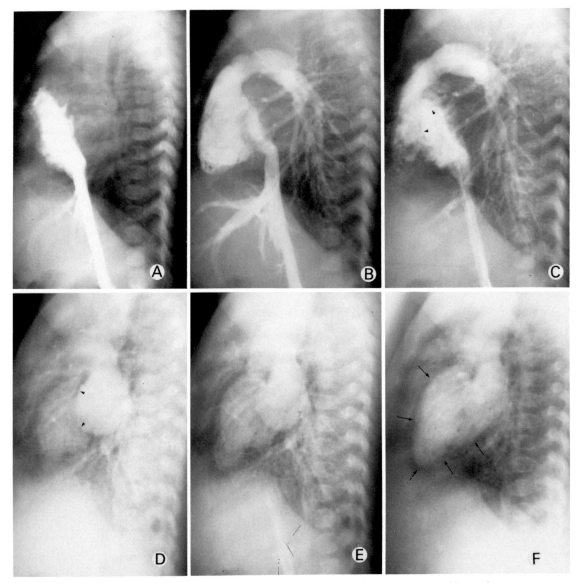

FIG. 39. NORMAL INTRAVENOUS ANGIOCARDIGRAM IN LATERAL PROJECTION IN YOUNG INFANT

(A) Contrast material opacifies the inferior vena cava, and reflux is seen into some of the hepatic veins. There is early filling of the right atrium. (B) A slightly later film shows marked reflux into the hepatic veins. The right atrium is contracted, and the right ventricle is relaxed and filled with contrast material (ventricular diastole). The right ventricular outflow tract, the main pulmonary artery and its right and left branches are well opacified. (C) A very slightly later film shows the appearance during mid ventricular systole. Arrows point to the location of the tricuspid valve. (D) A later film shows opacification of the left atrium in atrial diastole. Arrows point to the locations of the anterior and posterior mitral valve leaflets. (E) A later film shows early filling of the left ventricle. (F) A late film from the series shows the appearance in end ventricular diastole. Arrows point to the opacified relaxed left ventricle. The thoracic aorta is faintly seen.

lateral film because of its shortness and the overlapping of other structures. The descending branch of the left pulmonary artery continues obliquely posterior and downward and appears as a continuation of the pulmonary arch. Of the segmental branches the lingular and the superior segments are usually the easiest to identify. The lingular originates as the first anterior branch and runs obliquely forward and downward for a short distance before dividing into superior and inferior rami. The superior segment arises at the same level but runs posteriorly and downward. The posterior basilar artery appears as a continuation of the descending artery, is usually the largest and descends farther toward the lung base than the other segmental arteries. The other

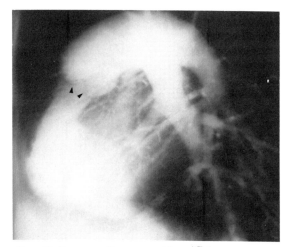

FIG. 40. LATERAL FILM FROM NORMAL INTRAVENOUS
ANGIOCARDIOGRAM

The film was exposed in ventricular diastole. Arrow heads point to fine curved radiolucent lines representing the delicate valve leaflets of the pulmonary valve. The valve is closed, and the main pulmonary artery and its right and left branches are distended.

basilar branches are easily confused with those of the opposite lung.

The right pulmonary artery in the lateral and far anterior oblique views is greatly foreshortened and appears as a rounded or oval shaped contour anterior to the trachea. The ascending branch is short and not easily identified due to overlapping. The descending branch runs obliquely posterior and downward. As on the left side, the middle lobe and superior segmental branch to the lower lobe are the easiest to recognize.

Pulmonary veins are quite distinct on the lateral angiocardiograms. At least five or six branches may be identified on a single film as they converge on the left atrium. The confluence of the inferior pulmonary veins may present a nodular appearance on the posterior wall of the left atrium at angiocardiography. A soft tissue density seen in this area on plain chest films exposed in the lateral projection may be mistaken for a pulmonary lesion (Schreiber, 1965).

The left atrium is rounded or oval in shape on the lateral view. Although its wall is somewhat thicker than that of the right atrium, it is not usually clearly seen because of a lack of contrast with surrounding structures. The curving inferior border of the atrium is usually well demarcated from the left ventricle and indicates the region of the atrioventricular annulus although the mitral leaflets are not usually demonstrated. Posteriorly at the junction of the atrial contour with the left ventricle, there is an indentation which

represents the atrioventricular groove on the exterior of the heart. The left atrium varies considerably in size and slightly in shape with changes in cardiac phase; the change in size between maximum systole and diastole is striking (Fig. 39, D–F).

The left ventricular cavity in diastole is roughly oval or triangular in shape with the apex or narrowest point anteriorly and inferiorly and

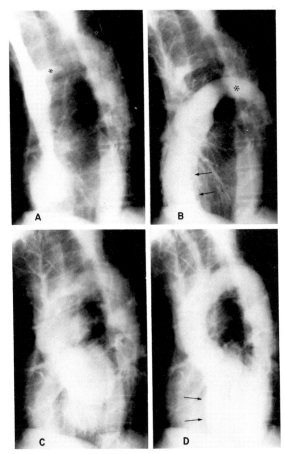

FIG. 41. NORMAL INTRAVENOUS ANGIOCARDIOGRAM IN LEFT ANTERIOR (RIGHT POSTERIOR) OBLIQUE PROJECTION

(A) An early film shows filling of the right innominate vein, the superior vena cava and the right atrium. A small amount of contrast material has refluxed into the azygos vein (asterisk). (B) A film made a few moments later shows contrast filling of the right ventricle, the main pulmonary artery and its right and left branches. Arrows point to the anterior aspect of the interventricular septum. The left pulmonary artery is particularly well seen in this view as it arches over the left main bronchus (asterisk). (C) A slightly later film shows pulmonary veins converging upon the left atrium seen here in ventricular systole (atrial diastole). (D) A late film from the series shows filling of the left ventricle (in diastole), with opacification of the entire thoracic aorta including the great vessels originating from the arch. Arrows point to the posterior aspect of the interventricular septum. The septum is seen end on in this projection.

the widest point near the base. The ventricular cavity narrows appreciably in its upper portion, however, where it joins the ascending aorta. The anterior contour of the chamber does not enter into the anterior cardiac contour in this projection but approaches it closely. The interventricular septum is not visible in the lateral projection. In about 45° of left anterior obliquity it outlines the anterior border of the left ventricular cavity (Fig. 41, B and D). In maximum systole in both anteroposterior and lateral projections, the ventricular cavity almost disappears. A small, somewhat linear collection of contrast substance can be identified, however, near the aortic opening and represents residual left ventricular blood.

The sinuses of Valsalva are best seen in the lateral (Fig. 38, C and D) or far left anterior oblique projection and during ventricular diastole when they are considerably distended. The semilunar valve cusps cast thin, slightly curved negative shadows within the surrounding contrast substance. These are best seen when the left ventricle is almost empty of the opaque material so that there is a distinct difference in the density between the aortic and left ventricular blood. The valves are seen only occasionally, however, with conventional techniques of 1–2 films/sec.

Both the right and left coronary arteries may occasionally be visualized during angiocardiography. They are commonly seen during selective left ventriculography and may be regularly visualized following the rapid injection of contrast material into the aortic root. Coronary arteriography is discussed in the section devoted to that subject.

The ascending aorta as seen in the lateral view is straight or slightly curved with an anterior convexity (Fig. 37B). It ascends in a vertical or slightly oblique posterior direction and is often parallel to the long axis of the sternum for a considerable distance. Its anterior surface is roughly about one-third of the anteroposterior diameter of the chest from the sternum. When this relative distance is decreased in congenital heart disease, it justifies a suspicion of overriding or transposition of the aorta.

Just below the origin of the innominate artery, the aorta begins to arch posteriorly. In good films, all of the major branches (innominate, left carotid, and subclavian) of the arch are visible. The left carotid and subclavian arteries may appear to arise from a single trunk. This is usually due to slight variation in their points of origin and the degree of foreshortening of the aortic arch projection.

The descending aorta is visibly smaller than the ascending portion and arch. It is parallel, or almost so, to the greater part of the lower thoracic spine and is usually superimposed upon the vertebral bodies although it may be slightly anterior, particularly in young individuals.

CARDIAC CATHETERIZATION

The course of a cardiac catheter inside the heart permits a rough appraisal of the anatomical limits of the chambers. It is much inferior in this respect to angiocardiography. The operator performing a heart catheterization relies to a considerable extent, however, on (1) the position of the catheter tip and (2) the contour of the distal portions of the catheter. The superior vena cava and right atrium usually offer little difficulty. The relatively thin wall of the atrium is seen to guide the catheter tip, and there is good contrast between the atrial borders and the surrounding lung. The catheter may be introduced into the coronary sinus in which case in the posteroanterior projection it runs toward the left and slightly upward and thus resembles the contour sometimes seen when the catheter is in the right ventricle. If the catheter is pushed far enough into the sinus, the tip may approach the lateral contour of the heart just below the left atrial tip and thus reveal its true position. It is not desirable, however, to insert the catheter to this extent. It is better to turn the patient into a left posterior oblique view and determine whether the catheter tip is anterior or posterior. Since the coronary sinus runs in the atrioventricular groove on the posterior heart surface, a posterior position of the catheter indicates that it is in the coronary sinus (Fig. 3, A and B). A more anterior position would indicate a position in the right ventricle.

From the right atrium the catheter may go into the inferior vena cava, a hepatic vein or the right ventricle. To enter the right ventricle the catheter must run medially and thus is obviously different from the position of the vena cava, etc. Also, movements of the catheter tip indicate that it is within the heart. Differentiation between the infundibulum and the pulmonary artery at or just beyond the valve is not reliable by fluoroscopy, and pressure tracings are more helpful.

NORMAL RIGHT VENTRICULOGRAM

The technique for this procedure has been described on page 23. The most frequently used projections are the frontal and lateral in 15–20° of right anterior obliquity. The contour of the right ventricle and the pulmonary artery, of course, is the same as described under the normal angiocardiogram, but detail is usually considerably better. Specifically, the septal and parietal bands, the tricuspid valve ring and the pulmonary valve leaflets are demonstrated in greater detail and more regularly than with venous angiocardiography.

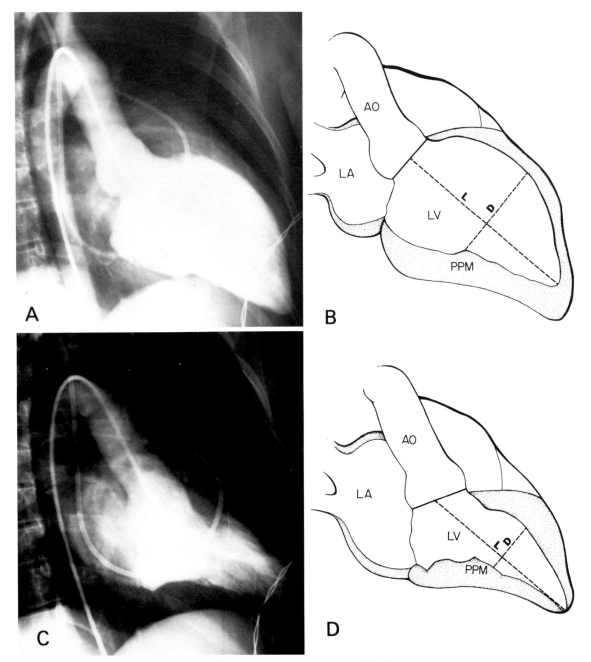

FIG. 42. NORMAL LEFT VENTRICULOGRAM IN 35° RAO PROJECTION

(A) Diastole. (B) Diagram of A. (C) Systole. (D) Diagram of C. Contrast substance in left atrium is residual from previous premature ventricular contraction. LA, left atrium, AO, aorta, LV, left ventricle, PPM, posterior papillary muscle, L, long diameter, D, short diameter (see text).

NORMAL LEFT VENTRICULOGRAM

The technique for this examination has been described on page 24. The most frequently used projections are the frontal, lateral, RAO in 25–30°, and the LAO in 55–60° of rotation.

The dynamics of the left ventricle are best studied in the right oblique projection in about 30° of rotation from the sagittal plane. Although large films exposed at rates of 4–6/sec give good detail, 35-mm cinefluorography is a better recording method for dynamic studies.

Calculations of Ventricular and Stroke Volume

In diastole the left ventricular cavity resembles somewhat an ellipse with one end, namely that at the base of the heart, truncated. The truncated base is formed mainly by the mitral and aortic valve rings. In the RAO projection the long axis of the left ventricle is approximately perpendicular to the x-ray beam, so this projection more nearly represents the true dimensions of the left ventricular cavity as seen in a single plane. Consequently, this projection is frequently used in determining ventricular volumes from a single projection (Greene *et al.*, 1967; Snow *et al.*, 1969; Green and Bunnell, 1974). The axes used in these determinations are shown in Figure 42, B and D. Actually, Greene *et al.* (1967) used as the upper locus of the long axis (L) the anterolateral margin of the opacified left ventricle, and Snow *et al.* (1969) used the midpoint of the projection of the mitral valve. The distal locus near the apex of the heart represents the greatest distance from the upper locus. Differences in selecting a point

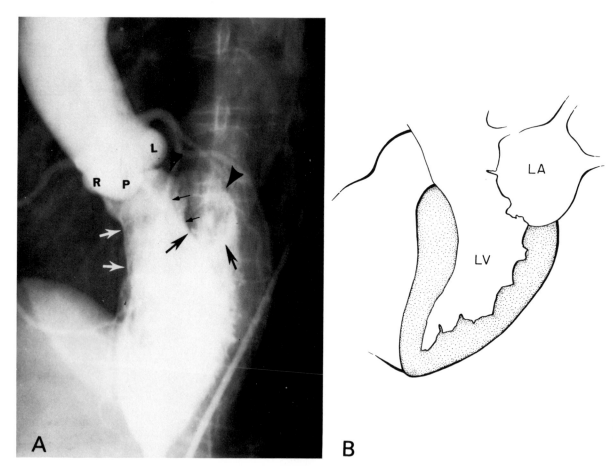

A   B

FIG. 43. LEFT VENTRICULOGRAM AND SCHEMATIC
(A) Left ventriculogram in about 60° LAO and early systole. The mitral valve is closed, and contrast substance is caught underneath the cusps and outlines the valve ring (large arrows and arrowheads). The small arrows indicate the anterior leaflet of the mitral valve. The white arrows indicate the upper portion of the ventricular septum. R; right sinus of Valsalva, P; posterior sinus of Valsalva; L; left sinus of Valsalva. (B) Diagram of A.

for the upper locus are inconsequential as a rule. D, the minor axis, is perpendicular to the major axis at its mid point. The other minor axis is at right angle to D and is assumed to be equal to D. The length of the axes must be adjusted for magnification which can be accomplished by projecting a grid pattern of 1 cm² placed at approximately the level of the heart above the film surface. The volume of the left ventricle (V) is:

$$V = \frac{4\pi}{3} \times \left(\frac{D}{2}\right)^2 \times \frac{L}{2}.$$

When this is corrected for magnification, it reduces to:

$$V = \frac{\pi}{6} \times D^2 \times L \times \frac{1}{f^3}$$
$$\times K \text{ (Green and Bunnell, 1974)}$$

where f is the ratio of the length of the projected image of the object to its actual length, and K = 0.848, a constant obtained by experiments comparing actual volumes with calculated volumes. The formula can be further simplified to:

$$V = LD^2C$$

where

$$C = \frac{\pi K}{6f^3}.$$

The determination of left ventricular volumes in systole (ESV) and diastole (EDV) permits a determination of stroke volume (SV) as:

$$SV = EDV - ESV$$

and that is equal to ml/beat. Stroke volume (SV) times heart rate (HR) equals cardiac output (CO) in ml/min as:

$$CO = SV \times HR.$$

Ejection fraction (EF) is the fraction of left ventricular volume that is expelled during systole and is determined as

$$EF = \frac{SV}{EDV}$$

Ejection fraction and cardiac output are important paramaters in the evaluation of myocardial function.

Cardiac output determined by the dye dilution or the Fick methods from a peripheral artery (CO^{per}) when subtracted from cardiac output determined by ventriculography (COv) provides an estimate of regurgitant volume as

$$V_{reg} = COv - CO^{per}.$$

This determination permits at least a rough estimate of the severity of aortic or mitral insufficiency.

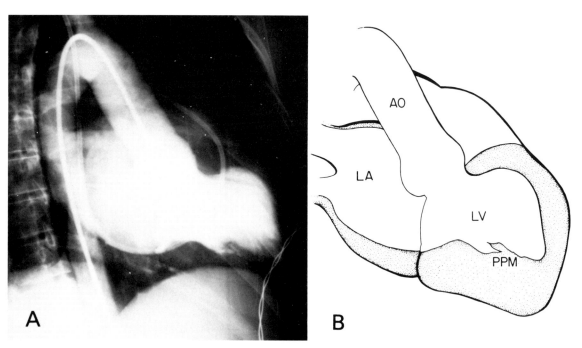

FIG. 44. LEFT VENTRICULAR EXTRASYSTOLE
Same patient as presented in Fig. 42. Moderate mitral regurgitation is usual and does not indicate abnormality of the mitral valve.

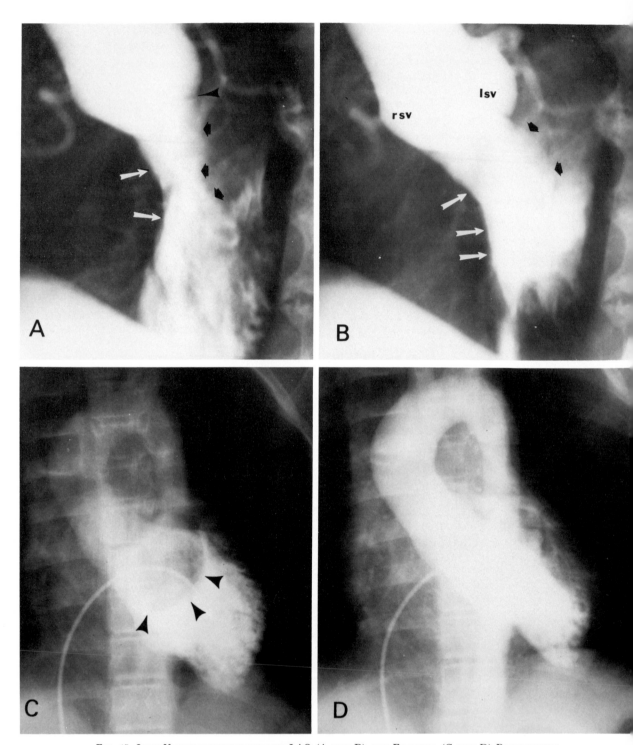

FIG. 45. LEFT VENTRICULOGRAM IN THE LAO (A AND B) AND FRONTAL (C AND D) PROJECTIONS
(A) Early systole. (B) Late systole. White arrows indicate septum. Black arrowheads indicate anterior leaflet of mitral valve. Long arrowhead indicates aortic valve ring. The septum is concave in early systole and straightens in late systole. Frontal view of left ventriculogram. (C) Beginning systole. The mitral valve has just closed and is outlined by contrast substance underneath the posterior valve cusp (arrowheads). (D) Systole. The outflow tract and aortic valve ring are obscured by the thoracic spine.

In satisfactory left ventriculography, the contrast substance outlines the entire cavity. The trabecular structure is smaller and finer than that of the right ventricle. The posterior papillary muscle (Fig. 42, A–D) is seen during diastole in at le⌐ ͻc half of the examinations. The anterior papillary muscle which protrudes from the anterior surface of the left ventricle is much less

constant during diastole. During systole both muscles become more prominent and can be identified in nearly every examination. The mitral annulus sharply defines the base of the ventricle in systole. If the aorta remains filled from the previous systole, the ring can be seen to extend to overlap the posterior sinus of Valsalva. In systole the valve cusps are immobile in the

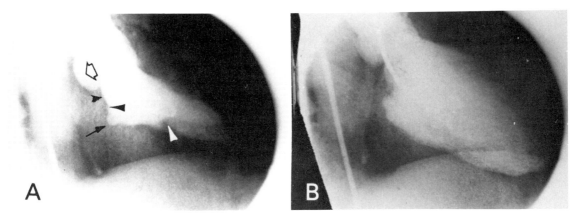

FIG. 46. CINEFLUOROGRAM, SYSTOLE AND DIASTOLE

(A) Cinefluorogram of normal mitral valve in systole in RAO projection. ➤, commisure; →, posterior cusp; ▶, anterior cusp; ⬦, posterior sinus of Valsalva; White ➤, posterior papillary muscle. (B) Diastole.

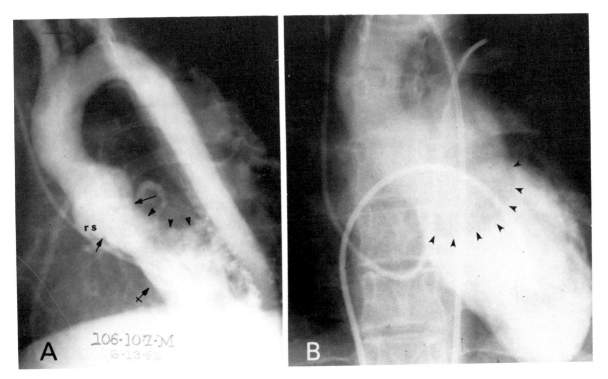

FIG. 47. LEFT VENTRICULOGRAM

(A) Normal left ventriculogram in LAO position in beginning systole and aortogram ↔, interventricular septum; ⇢, aortic valve ring; ▶, mitral valve ring; rs, right sinus of Valsalva. (B) Frontal view of left ventriculogram in early systole. Contrast substance is caught underneath the mitral valve leaflets (arrowheads) and outlines the valve ring.

approximate plane of the valve ring. In diastole the cusps cannot be identified on any single frame, although in good angiograms one can frequently obtain an estimate of their motility.

In beginning normal systole, all segments of the ventricle do not contract equally and simultaneously. The initial activity usually occurs near the apex which narrows and begins to move toward the base of the ventricle. At about the same time, and very early in systole, the base of the ventricle (the mitral and aortic rings) begins to move downward, and this occurs shortly after the short period of isometric contraction and

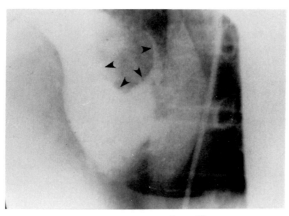

FIG. 48. CINEFLUOROGRAM OF LEFT VENTRICLE
LAO projection in beginning systole. ➤, mitral valve ring.

about the time the mitral valve is beginning to close. Intermediate segments of the ventricle may move outward at this time and should not be confused with akinesia or dyskinesia. These segments are (1) the segment just beneath the posterior leaflet of the mitral valve, and (2) the superoanterior surface of the ventricle. The segment adjacent to the posterior leaflet of the mitral valve is probably the same as that referred to by Keats and Martt (1962) as showing paradoxical pulsations in a normal heart. As systole progresses the ventricular cavity near the apex is almost completely obliterated. The papillary muscles near the midportion of the ventricle increase in size. The aortic valve is wide open, and the residual volume is concentrated near the base of the heart in the region of the mitral and under the aortic valve. The residual volume at maximum systole is usually about 30–45% of the diastolic volume given an ejection fraction of 55–70%. At maximum systole, the mitral leaflets bulge with a slight convexity toward the left atrium. At times, small separate convexities may represent scallops which are common in the posterior cusps (Ranganathan *et al.*, 1970). Any significant convexity, however, is suggestive of redundancy of the valve cusp and may bring up the question of prolapse. The normal valve is completely competent during regular systole but may be mildly incompetent during a premature

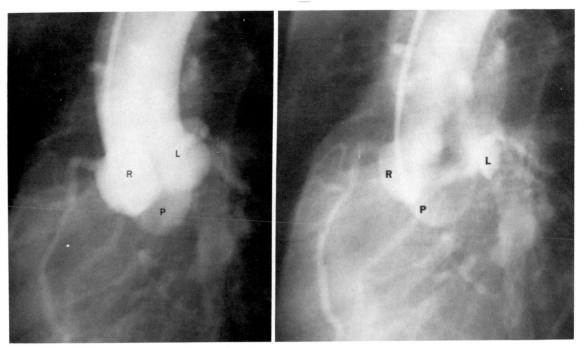

FIG. 49. AORTIC ROOT IN DIASTOLE AND SYSTOLE
Normal aortic root in diastole (A), LAO projection. R, right sinus of Valsalva; L, left sinus of Valsalva; P, posterior sinus of Valsalva. (B) In early systole.

contraction. Also, at times during the period of injection and when the catheter tip is near the orifice of the valve, contrast substance may reflux during diastole associated undoubtedly with the speed of the injection and the position of the catheter. This must not be confused with mitral insufficiency.

Premature systoles are common during ventriculography despite a slow rate of injection. Viewed serially, the premature beats can be easily recognized. The onset and development of the contraction are distinctly different from the normal systole, and the residual shape is likewise different. The initial contraction often begins near the midpoint of the ventricle and may be most pronounced along the inferior border (Fig. 44). The cavity thus assumes a narrow waist and is often accompanied by imperfect mitral closure with a jet of contrast substance penetrating the left atrium.

In the LAO projection with 60° of rotation, the ventricular septum is projected in contour, and the mitral valve is seen en face (Fig. 43). In diastole the cavity has somewhat the shape of a triangle with the base at the aortic and mitral valves. Nonopaque blood from the left atrium outlines the mitral orifice as a radiolucent disc impinging upon the left upper posterior contour of the ventricle. As systole begins, contrast substance collects momentarily underneath the valve cusps, and at times these may be separately identified. The right border of the ventricular cavity is formed by the ventricular septum, and this is normally convex toward the right. In films of good quality, the lower portion of the septum and the left lateral wall show a minor wavy pattern due to the trabeculae carnae. The upper portion of the septum is smooth. At the onset of systole, the septum momentarily increases its convexity toward the right and then straightens.

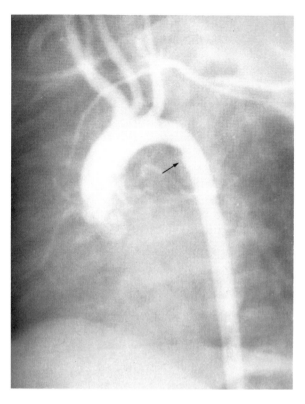

FIG. 51. NORMAL THORACIC AORTOGRAM IN YOUNG INFANT

The film was made in the right posterior oblique projection after injection of contrast material in a retrograde manner into the left brachial artery. The entire thoracic aorta is well visualized, and the right and left coronaries are faintly seen. The gentle backward arch of the thoracic aorta is well shown as well as the origin of the great vessels to the head and neck from the arch. In this patient the left carotid artery appears to originate from the innominate artery, a common variation. The arrow points to a slight out-pouching in the proximal descending thoracic aorta at the level of presumed attachment of an obliterated ductus arteriosus ("ductus diverticulum"). The aorta is smooth throughout its length.

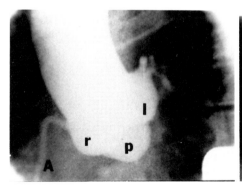
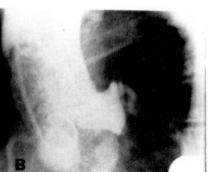

FIG. 50. AORTIC ROOT IN DIASTOLE AND SYSTOLE

Aortic root in (A) diastole in the LAO projection. (B) Early systole. r, right sinus of Valsalva; p, posterior sinus of Valsalva; l, left sinus of Valsalva.

At the height of systole, most of the contour of the muscular septum is lost due to emptying of the ventricle. A smooth segment representing the membranous septum remains distinct, and this projection is optimum for studying ventricular defects in this area. In complete systole, the apex of the ventricular cavity normally is almost completely obliterated, and the residual volume is almost entirely in the basilar portion underneath the aortic orifice and the closed mitral valve.

In the frontal projection in diastole, the ventricular cavity is shaped much like a pear; the greatest width is in the upper one-third with tapering to a rounded apex. The base is formed by the aortic valve and ring. The long axis from the middle of the valve ring to the apex forms an angle of about 40–45° with the vertical, but this is variable according to the habitus of the patient. During systole, the angle of the long axis with the vertical increases. The apex loses its rounded shape and becomes sharper and more pointed, and the upper border is decreased in convexity.

The right border of the ventricle often has a mild sigmoid-like curve. Its upper portion is formed by the ventricular septum which is typically smooth and is mildly convex to the right. The aortic valve is frequently superimposed on the thoracic spine. A single plane frontal projection may be used for the determination of cardiac volume (Dodge *et al.*, 1966).

In the lateral projection the ventricular cavity is moderately foreshortened as compared with the RAO projection. The shape is roughly triangular with the base being formed by the mitral valve and ring. The mitral valve and ring are often shown to very good advantage, and this projection is useful in studying various types of prolapse of the mitral valve. Intruding on the upper margin of the mitral ring is the aortic orifice with the left coronary sinus and valve cusp superimposed on the upper segment of the mitral ring. In this view, the aortic valve is often shown to good advantage, and the posterior cusp is usually distinctly visible and is the most dependent of the three cusps.

7

Measurement of the Heart and Great Vessels

GENERAL CONSIDERATIONS

Enlargement of a single cardiac chamber increases the heart volume and may be measured by roentgen means as generalized cardiac enlargement. The precise contribution of the enlarged chamber to the total heart volume, however, cannot be determined using current methods since only one contour of such a chamber is usually visible. Individual chamber enlargement can be recognized with a variable degree of accuracy when it produces a visible change in the cardiac contour and this is best determined by fluoroscopy and filming in various projections and will be discussed in a following section. The recognition of single chamber enlargement is of great importance because (1) it often precedes a general increase in heart size and thus represents an earlier stage of the disease and (2) it may give an important clue as to the nature and location of the underlying disease. Occasionally, however, the roentgenologist is confronted by a large cardiac contour which gives little evidence of a predominant increase in size of a single chamber.

Cardiac enlargement varies somewhat in significance depending upon (1) degree, (2) rapidity of development and duration, and (3) fundamental cause of the enlargement. Where the enlargement is persistent for weeks or months and particularly where it is progressive, it indicates a serious abnormality and is therefore of considerable diagnostic and prognostic weight. Also, changes in heart size are a reliable indicator of the effects of certain therapeutic procedures such as bed rest, surgery, and administration of drugs.

From the roentgen viewpoint, cardiac enlargement refers to an increase in cardiac volume since precise differentiation between hypertrophy and dilatation is not always possible. This is not a serious drawback since either dilatation or hypertrophy is indicative of abnormality. It does mean, however, that comparison of roentgen measurements with routine data obtained at autopsy is not entirely valid. The autopsied heart can be weighed with exactness, but to be comparable with roentgen measurements its intact volume should be determined. This requires that the heart be carefully distended with fixing solution or paraffin and its volume determined by submerging in water. Such volumetric determinations were made on the hearts of 32 children by Lind (1950) and agreed closely with premortem volumes determined by a refined roentgenographic technique. Friedman (1949) reported good agreement between postmortem determinations of heart volume by roentgenographic means and cardiac volume determined by the water displacement method. Although this indicates the ultimate accuracy of roentgenographic methods, both the pathologic and roentgenographic procedures are too laborious for routine use. Routinely the pathologist recognizes cardiac dilatation in evaluating abnormality, but cardiac weight remains as the chief criterion of heart size. The upper range of the normal heart weights accepted by the pathologist (men, 350 gm; women, 300 gm) allows for some increase in heart size or weight in many instances without definitely indicating cardiac enlargement. Furthermore, the experienced pathologist prefers to evaluate the heart size not only on the basis of weight, but also on the general development, musculature, and weight of the body and also a variety of other findings such as other evidence of cardiac disease and changes observed upon microscopic examination of the myocardium. In short, the pathologist has considerable latitude in judging heart size and prefers in the final analysis to draw upon his experience and general knowledge in determining the presence and degree of cardiac enlargement.

The object of the roentgenologist likewise is

not to determine absolute heart size but rather to ascertain whether in any given patient the heart is abnormally large. The crucial aspect of the problem is the determination of the significance of borderline measurements which unfortunately are frequent occurrences. This is due to (1) a rather wide range of variation of the volume of the normal heart and (2) certain inherent inaccuracies in routine roentgen techniques. The problem would be greatly simplified if all patients brought with them a series of teleoroentgenograms made over a preceding period of years presumably representing a period of good health. Then even a small increase in cardiac size would suggest abnormality. Since such a situation rarely obtains, the next best approach has been to obtain a series of measurements of the heart from a relatively large and representative sample of healthy individuals who are free of heart disease. Such samples included persons of both sexes and a wide range of body height, weight, and age. The cardiac measurements and data on height, weight, etc., thus obtained were tabulated and treated statistically.

These measurements, either single diameters, frontal areas, or heart volumes, are found to be distributed around an average or mean value in a symmetrical fashion known as a "standard distribution" which can be treated by relatively simple statistical methods. Although a majority of the individual measurements show only a moderate deviation from the average, there are a considerable number in which the variation is large and the range is 25–30% plus or minus the average value. To reduce this rather wide range, the cardiac measurements have been correlated with height, weight, age, etc. In general, the best correlations of the various measurements were obtained with body weight, although addition of the height factor sometimes improved the correlation to a slight degree.

This relationship or correlation between a series of factors is given a value known as a coefficient of correlation (r). A value of $r = +1$ means that a variation in one factor is accompanied by a direct proportional variation in the other; $r = -1$ means that relationship is an inverse one but still directly proportional; $r = 0$ indicates a complete lack of relationship. The value of r is such that it must be of the order of 0.6 before there is a significant (20%) reduction in the dispersion or scatter around a regression line. In other words, $r = 0.6$ will reduce a 25% deviation from the mean to 20%; r varies somewhat with the various cardiac measurements and height, weight, age, etc., and is therefore influential in determining which measurement or which criteria of correlation will produce the most accurate evaluation of heart size.

Such statistical treatment as has just been described is the basis for the tables and nomograms which have appeared in the literature. Some of these are as follows:

I. Transverse diameter
    A. related to height and weight
        1. Ungerleider and Gubner (1942)
        2. Hodges and Eyster (1924)
II. Frontal area
    A. related to height and weight
        1. Ungerleider and Gubner (1942)
        2. Hodges and Eyster (1924)
        3. Hodges (1946)
    B. related to transverse diameter of chest
        1. Hilbish and Morgan (1952)
III. Heart volume
    A. related to body surface area
        1. in children: Lind (1950)
        2. in adults: Liliestrand et al. (1939)
    B. related to body weight
        1. in children: Nghiem et al. (1967)
    C. related to body weight, surface area, and hemoglobin
        1. in men, women, and children: Kjellberg et al. (1949)

The use of these tables or nomograms permits only the following statement:

"If the cardiac diameters or frontal area exceed the average by ____ percent, the chances of a normal sized heart being present are one in ____." It might be assumed that if the heart is not normal that it is enlarged and, therefore, the nomograms permit an evaluation of the chances of enlargement. Rigid statistical considerations, however, will not permit such a statement since there are no data referable to the distribution of enlarged hearts, and the degree of overlap of the normal and abnormal ranges of heart size has not been determined. The range of normal heart measurements is surprisingly large (frontal area ± 32% of the average (Hilbish and Morgan, 1952) and ± 27% of the average (Hodges and Eyster, 1924)), and, therefore, it would seem that the probability of overlap of the normal and abnormal ranges of heart size would be considerable (a high coefficient of correlation with height, weight, body area, etc., would reduce this range somewhat). Because of this consideration, however, there is considerable skepticism regarding the value of these nomograms particularly when applied to measurements obtained from a single teleoroentgenogram because they will not permit a definite statement in borderline cases as to whether the heart is enlarged or not; they permit only a statement of the probability of normality. It should be remembered that there are very few medical tests which, from a single application, permit a uniformly positive or negative answer. Statistically, the range of normal roentgen cardiac mensuration is no greater than that of systolic blood pressures obtained from a series of normal individuals. It is also probable that a single roentgen measurement of cardiac size is of the same order of reliability in determining cardiac enlargement as a single blood pressure reading is in determining the presence of hypertension.

Measurements have their greatest value in comparing the size of the heart on one occasion to its size at another time. In this way improvement or deterioration in cardiac status may be determined. Such estimations of the size of the heart are of particular value in following the effects of therapy and are reliable indicators of the course or natural history of cardiac illness.

POSITIONING AND TECHNIQUE

Measurements are customarily obtained with the patient in the erect position in the postero-anterior projection alone or combined with the lateral projection (volumetric determinations). The recumbent position has been used by Lind (1950) in measuring heart volume in children and is advocated by Larrson and Kjellberg (1948) in adults. It has the advantage that the heart size changes less with pulse rate and the effect of stagnation of blood in the viscera is eliminated. Also, frontal and lateral films can be easily exposed without changing the patient's position, and obtaining a perfectly positioned lateral film is simplified. The standard error of a single determination in an examination in the prone position is relatively slight, presumably less than that in the upright position. While such a position requires some special apparatus and is therefore not suited for routine use, it has real advantages in volumetric determinations. For practical purposes, the erect position is employed with a target-to-film distance of 6 feet (180 cm) and the film(s) are exposed in moderate inspiration. Under these circumstances, magnification of the heart is of the order of 3–6% in adults.

Although the long and broad diameters and the frontal area of the heart may undergo considerable alterations due to the phase of respiration in which filming occurs, a study by Kjellberg et al. (1951) afforded no support to the assumption that exposure during inspiration produced a significant alteration of the cardiac volume. Kjellberg et al. (1951) found no statistically significant difference between the cardiac volume during systole and diastole, and indicate that, with the possible exception of persons with a slow pulse rate, the effect of the cardiac cycle on the cardiac volume is inappreciable and that exposure during diastole is not essential. Our experience with 20 cases in which cardiac volumes in diastole and in random phase of cardiac cycle were compared confirms this observation. Hilbish and Morgan (1952) found the difference in frontal areas of the heart obtained from random exposures and those made in diastole to average about 1%. Hodges (1946) prefers to use the larger silhouette obtained from a stereoscopic pair.

COMMONLY USED CARDIAC MEASUREMENTS

Diameters

Transverse Diameter (T) (Fig. 52)

This is the maximal transverse dimension of the heart as seen in the posteroanterior projection. It is obtained by adding the maximal distances of the right and left heart borders from the midsternal line. Its normal range is greater (Hilbish and Morgan, 1952) than that of any of the other diameters since it unduly reflects cardiac position (e.g., unduly long in the transverse heart and unduly short in the long, narrow heart). The upper limit of the normal range in adults has been placed at 50% of the internal thoracic diameter (Th) at the level of the dome of the diaphragm. Actual measurements suggest a somewhat greater variation as Clagett (1941) found 37% of 198 normal adults had a T/Th (cardio-thoracic) ratio greater than 50%, and Hilbish and Morgan (1952) found the correlation coefficient (transverse diameter of the heart versus transverse diameter of the thorax) to be only 0.56. This criterion therefore has little significance, and its main claim to consideration is that it can be quickly and easily determined by the busy roentgenologist. It may serve for a rough initial approximation but has no place where precision is required. In the first year of life the normal cardiothoracic ratio may reach as high as 60–64%.

T correlates poorly with body height and somewhat better with weight. Correlation with both height and weight is better than with either alone and is the basis of the Ungerleider and Gubner (1942) nomograms. The r used in preparing these nomograms is not stated but is probably not larger than 0.58, which is the r

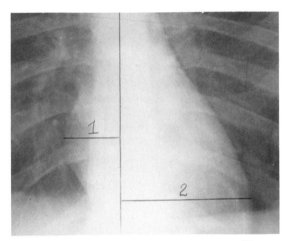

FIG. 52. DETERMINATION OF CARDIOTHORACIC RATIO

The numerator of the cardiothoracic ratio is determined by erecting perpendicular lines from a line through the midportion of the thoracic spine to the farthest point on the right (1) and left (2) heart borders. The numerator is the sum of the lengths of these two lines. The denominator is the transverse diameter of the thoracic, measured from the insides of the ribs, at the level of the right hemidiaphragm.

obtained by Hodges and Eyster (1924) using frontal plane area (A) in addition to height and weight. Because of a large normal range and only a moderate correlation coefficient with other common body measurements, T is inferior to frontal plane area in estimating heart volume (Hilbish and Morgan, 1952).

Long Diameter (L)

This is the distance from the cardiovascular junction (Fig. 53A) on the right heart border to the most distant point of the left lower pole. The point on the contour of the left lower pole is occasionally obscured by the diaphragm, but with experience this can be approximated satisfactorily. L has a large normal range and correlates with the transverse thoracic diameter only slightly better than T ($r = 0.60$). Its main use is in determining the frontal area of the heart.

Broad Diameter or Width (W)

This is the sum of two perpendicular distances. One of these is drawn from the right cardiophrenic angle to the long diameter; the other is drawn from the left upper border at the junction of the left ventricular contour with the pulmonary trunk to the long diameter. W reflects somewhat enlargement of the right ventricle. It has a slightly smaller normal range than T or L but is not superior to either of these in correlation with height and weight.

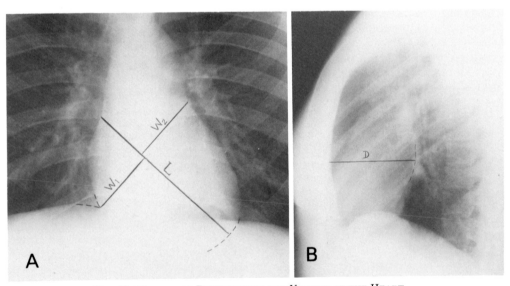

FIG. 53. METHOD OF DETERMINING THE VOLUME OF THE HEART

The length (L) is the distance from the right cardiovascular junction to the farthest point along the left heart border. The width (W_1 plus W_2) is the sum of the measurements at right angles to the length line and from that line to the cardiophrenic angle on the right and to the cardiovascular junction on the left. The depth (D) is the distance from the posterior aspect of the heart to the posterior aspect of the sternum, parallel to the horizon. The cardiac volume is determined by the formula L × W × D × 0.44. It is expressed in milliliters.

Depth Diameter

Several ways of determining the depth of the heart (D) on a lateral film have been described by Roesler (1946). The most useful measurement is the distance from the most posterior point of the cardiac contour to the posterior surface of the sternum (Fig. 53B). This dimension is, in general, perpendicular to the thoracic spine and parallel to the horizon. It is easier to determine if the esophagus is opacified with barium paste. The depth diameter is used in calculating heart volume.

Frontal Plane Area

The frontal plane area (A) can be determined by a planimeter after the upper (mediastinal) and lower (diaphragmatic) contours are drawn in. A satisfactory approximation ($r = 0.9958$) is obtained by $A = L \times W \times 0.735$ (Schwartz, 1946), and this eliminates the need for drawing in the invisible contours of the teleoroentgenogram.

Frontal plane areas of normal persons have a somewhat smaller relative range than any of the single diameters and a somewhat better correlation with height and weight. Consequently, its determination has more significance than single dimensions, and yet it is simple enough to be used routinely. Its significance can be stated as follows: using the Hodges (1946) nomograms in which A is correlated with height and weight, a heart having a frontal area 10% greater than that predicted by the formula has about 1 chance in 6 of being in the normal range; if 15% greater, the odds are about 1 chance in 11 of being in the normal range.

The work of Bardeen (1918) indicates a close relationship between the frontal plane area and heart volume (V). Roesler (1946) and Stecher (1939) in general do not support this observation. Certainly where posteroanterior and lateral films are routine a number are seen in which the heart is grossly enlarged in one projection and normal or slightly enlarged in the other. Consequently, frontal plane area is less accurate in determining true heart volume in a wide range of subjects than a method which includes the depth of the heart.

Volumetric Determinations

Rohrer in 1916 and Kahlstorf in 1932 devised formulas for radiographic determination of the cardiac volume using the frontal area (orthodiagraphically determined), the greatest depth of the heart, and a factor of 0.63, midway between the factors of 0.59 (used in determining the volume of a paraboloid) and 0.67 (used in determining the volume of a sphere). Provided that correction is made for magnification, accurate volume determinations can be made using either of two formulas:

$$\text{Volume} = A \times D \times 0.63 \quad (1)$$

$$\text{Volume} = L \times W \times D \times 0.45 \quad (2)$$

In the first formula, A is determined planimetrically. If it is determined by $A = L \times W \times 0.735$, then the two formulas agree closely.

A simplified method of cardiac volume determination may be adequate for clinical use (Schreiber, 1964). On the posteroanterior and lateral films of the chest exposed in the erect position, in moderate inspiration, and at a 72-inch target-to-film distance, cardiac volume may be accurately approximated by measuring heart length (L), width (W), and depth (D) and applying these values, uncorrected for magnification, to the following formula:

$$\text{Volume} = L \times W \times D \times 0.44 \quad (3)$$

While cardiac volume determinations are slightly more cumbersome to make, they may permit a more accurate determination of the patient's cardiac status than other roentgenographic methods utilizing uni- or bidimensional methods in selected cases. The results obtained in normal children by Lind are impressive and would indicate this method is superior to simpler determination. In his group the standard deviation of the heart volumes was ± 31.5% of the mean value; however, by correlating the heart volumes with body area, he established a regression equation which reduced this to about ± 10%. Nghiem *et al.* (1967) also established the values for normal heart volume in children with a margin of error of about 10%. Their figures allow use of a simple nomogram for determination of cardiac volume (Table 6), and normal values are related to body weight as follows: the upper limit of normal for boys equals 6.8 times weight in pounds. For girls, the normal upper limit of heart volume equals 6.3 times weight in pounds.

Keats and Enge (1965) concluded that the cardiac volume method provides the most accurate index of overall cardiac size and permits comparison with normal standards without regard to body habitus or configuration. The following values, derived from the work of Amundsen (1959), represent the upper limits of normal:

Females: 450–490 ml/m^2
Males: 500–540 ml/m^2.

TABLE 6

NOMOGRAPH FOR HEART VOLUME

(Reproduced by permission, from Nghiem, Schreiber, Harris: Circulation *35:* 509, 1967.)

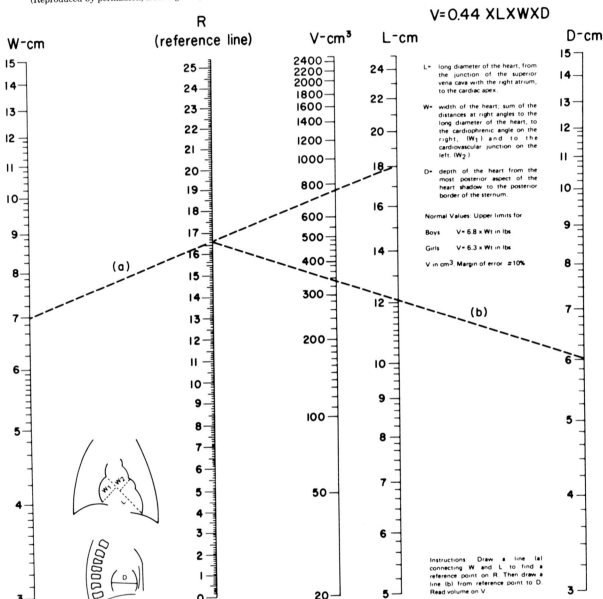

Methods for determination of left ventricular volume depend upon opacification of that chamber with contrast material. Several methods have been proposed; the chief ones are those of Arvidsson (1961) and Dodge *et al.* (1966). Biplane angiocardiography, determining left ventricular volume by the application of formulas to measurements taken from frontal and lateral films, is the classical technique. Procedures have also been described by which left ventricular chamber volume may be determined from angiocardiograms taken in the anteroposterior projection only (Sandler and Dodge, 1968), using biplane quantitative cinefluorography (Chapman *et al.,* 1966), using biplane cineangiography (Freeman *et al.,* 1970), and one plane cineangiography (Greene *et al.,* 1967; Kasser and Kennedy, 1968). Automatic computer systems have been developed and programmed to scan raw, unaltered left ventricular cineangiocardiograms and calculate the volume from each frame by an integration method (Desilets and Beckenbach, 1971). Left heart volumes have been employed in the study of congenital mitral insufficiency (Miller *et al.,* 1964), endocardial fibroelastosis (Miller *et al.,* 1965), pulsus alternans (Harris *et al.,* 1966), congenital and acquired aortic disease (Castellanos and Hernandez, 1967; Lewis *et al.,* 1971), constrictive pericarditis (Albers *et al.,* 1967) and other abnormalities.

Because of its symmetry, the left atrium lends itself well to volume determinations. The formula for the volume of a sphere is ordinarily employed, and measurements and calculations depend upon opacification of the chamber. Bjork and Lodin (1965) and Murray (1968) have studied left atrial volume in normal children and adults. Hawley *et al.* (1966) have applied the results of left atrial volume determinations to the study of cardiomyopathy, aortic valve disease, mitral valve disease, and combined aortic and mitral disease.

Right ventricular volume determinations present an especially difficult problem because of the irregular shape of the right ventricle. Goerke and Carlsson (1967) describe a method for the digital computer calculation of intracardiac ventricular volumes from biplane x-ray images, a technique applicable to both right and left ventricles. Using this method, Carlsson *et al.* (1971) compared right and left ventricular stroke volumes in 17 patients. Carlsson (1972) has recently reviewed the subject of quantitative cardiovascular data obtained from radiological images.

In routine practice we prefer to give an opinion as to whether the heart is (1) normal in size, (2) borderline, or (3) enlarged, from a simple inspection of the posteroanterior and lateral films. If a more precise evaluation is needed, the cardiothoracic ratio may be determined, but a single abnormal determination should not be considered reliable evidence of abnormality in a borderline case. The cardiothoracic ratio may have considerable value in comparing films of the same patient at different times, provided that the films are exposed in the same way. Should still more precise estimation be needed, cardiac volume is determined from frontal and lateral films and compared with the normal range of values given by Liljestrand *et al.* (1939), Kjellberg *et al.* (1949), Amundsen (1959), and Nghiem *et al.* (1967).

An area in which precise measurements of cardiac size, either frontal area or volume, is of considerable value is in the preoperative evaluation of heart cases, such as those with mitral stenosis and patent ductus arteriosus, since such a baseline is useful in evaluating objectively the effect of the operative procedure. The severity of mitral insufficiency in children may also be graded by this technique, and valuable information regarding prognosis and the most opportune time for operative treatment may be obtained (Nghiem *et al.,* 1967).

MEASUREMENTS OF GREAT VESSELS

Where the arch of the aorta crosses the barium-filled esophagus, a meniscus-like identation is produced. If the curvature of the meniscus is extended to the adjacent aortic knob, a circle is formed which approximates an anatomic cross-section (Kreuzfuchs, 1936). The diameter of this circle is larger than the actual aortic lumen because it includes (1) the thickness of the esophageal wall, (2) twice the thickness of the aortic wall, and (3) the surrounding mediastinal pleura and connective tissue. This averages about 0.3 cm and should be subtracted from the observed diameter.

The normal range is from 2.8–3.2 cm, depending upon the size and age of the patient. In films of high contrast, measurements may be made between the left border of the trachea and the lateral wall of the aortic knob. This measurement is of very little practical use and may be in considerable error if the aorta is not projected in an axial direction.

A transverse diameter of the aortic arch has been described by Ungerleider and Gubner (1942) and is the sum of maximum distances to the right and left borders of the vascular pedicle from the midsternal line. They have published a nomogram relating this diameter to height, weight, and age. This places a rough quantitative value on aortic abnormality but is probably not superior to inspection by an experienced observer.

Angiocardiography provides good visualization of the entire thoracic aorta as well as the pulmonary artery and its branches providing the optimal projections are used. The visualization is such that rather precise measurements are possible. The diameters of these vessels, however, vary considerably with cardiac phase and with the particular area which is selected for measurement.

Dotter and Steinberg (1949) have published values for the diameters of the aorta and the pulmonary artery and its branches which were obtained by direct measurements of angiograms of normal persons varying in age from 5–65 years. Cardiac phase was unknown and there was no correction for distortion. Consequently, there is a wide range of normal values. One could assume from their data that a diameter in excess of 3.8 cm in the ascending portion and 3.5 cm in the arch of the aorta is probably abnormal. The aortic and pulmonary artery walls vary between 1.5 and 2.5 mm in thickness.

8

General Symmetrical and Asymmetrical Cardiac Enlargement—Change in Size of Specific Chambers—Abnormal Pulsations

In routine practice, the roentgenologist frequently sees enlarged hearts with a symmetrical or globular contour. Although the heart is enlarged, the borders maintain their relative length and convexity and are smooth and give no clue as to increase in size of a particular chamber. Usually this type of symmetrical enlargement is associated with some diffuse disturbance of function or structure of the myocardium with subsequent enlargement of all of the cardiac chambers and is called general cardiac enlargement (Fig. 54).

In addition to general cardiac enlargement, from the roentgen viewpoint there are two other

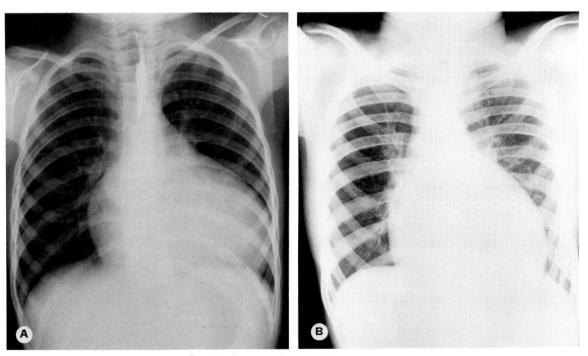

FIG. 54. GENERAL CARDIAC ENLARGEMENT
(A) Fiedler's myocarditis in a 5-year-old girl who had had symptoms for 3 months. (B) Heart in a boy 14 years of age with pseudohypertrophic muscular dystrophy.

91

common types of cardiac enlargement: (1) asymmetrical general cardiac enlargement in which all chambers are enlarged to a degree but one chamber is predominantly enlarged and (2) specific chamber enlargement where only one or at the most two chambers are enlarged. This division is determined by the cardiac contour as seen at fluoroscopy and in conventional chest films exposed in various projections.

GENERAL CARDIAC ENLARGEMENT

General cardiac enlargement of any type is due to hypertrophy or dilatation or more commonly to both and indicates myocardial strain. This strain is due to (1) an increased load on the myocardium, (2) involvement of the myocardium by inflammation, or other disease of the muscle, or (3) a combination of these factors. Hypertrophy is in part a physiologic response to an increase in work and allows the heart to carry on frequently for long periods of time. Dilatation, likewise, in the earlier stages is a response to an increase in work; in the latter stages it indicates a failing myocardium. Pulsations of a hypertrophied heart are at least normal in amplitude and are frequently exaggerated; with moderate dilatation the pulsations may still be within a normal range; with marked dilatation they are diminished or absent.

Diffuse myocarditis is a frequent cause of symmetrical generalized cardiac enlargement. It is most commonly due to rheumatic fever but occasionally occurs with acute infections such as diphtheria, influenza, pneumonia, or scarlet fever; it may be of unknown etiology, *e.g.,* Fiedler's myocarditis.

Other generalized conditions reduce the capacity of the myocardium to perform work, such as chronic anemia, myxedema, and beriberi. The myocardium may be infiltrated with amyloid (amyloidosis), glycogen (Von Gierke's disease), or hemosiderin (hemosiderosis), thus producing enlargement and probably some dilatation.

Certain poisons, such as chloroform, arsenic, and lead, destroy the cardiac musculature and severely weaken the myocardium leading to dilatation and probably some hypertrophy of the remaining muscle.

General enlargement may occur with endocrine diseases, such as hyperthyroidism and acromegaly, which increase the cardiac work. Other

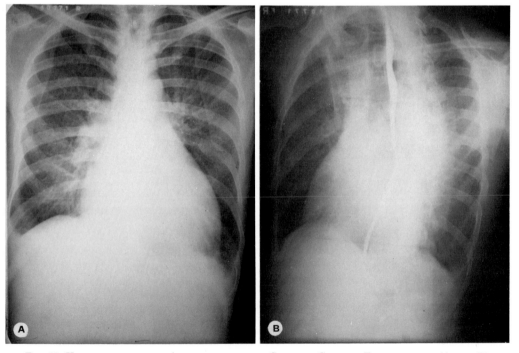

FIG. 55. HYPERTENSION WITH ASYMMETRICAL BUT GENERAL CARDIAC ENLARGEMENT (A AND B)

All of the chambers are somewhat dilated, but the left ventricle is predominantly enlarged. There are congestive changes in each lung and a small amount of fluid in the right costophrenic angle. BP, 210/120.

causes of cardiac enlargement due to myocardial abnormalities are discussed in the section on primary myocardial disease.

When the work load is evenly distributed between the two sides of the heart or where the myocardium is diffusely weakened, there is no initial specific chamber enlargement and rarely any back pressure in the pulmonary blood vessels. Consequently, even though the heart is enlarged, the lung vascular structures have a normal appearance. This helps distinguish symmetrical general cardiac enlargement due to myocardial disease from cardiac enlargement secondary to left sided heart failure in which the pulmonary vessels are apt to present a congested appearance, sometimes associated with pulmonary edema.

GENERALIZED ASYMMETRICAL CARDIAC ENLARGEMENT

Generalized asymmetrical cardiac enlargement (Fig. 55) is commonly seen in the later stages of essential hypertension, mitral regurgitation, and aortic valvular disease. Thus, it is due to an increased work load and is preceded by left ventricular enlargement. The sequence of events in essential hypertension or aortic valvular disease may be summarized as follows. The left ventricle hypertrophies in order to maintain the circulating blood volume against the increased peripheral resistance or to overcome the lack of efficiency of the aortic valve. Although it may compensate for a considerable period of time, the chamber eventually dilates and the mitral valve ring widens, producing functional mitral insufficiency. Because of the regurgitation of blood from the left ventricle, the left atrium dilates; there is an increase in pressure in the pulmonary veins and arteries and eventually in the right ventricle. The lungs become congested; the right ventricle hypertrophies and finally dilates, leading to a degree of tricuspid insufficiency and right atrial dilatation. Carried one step further, there is a persistent increase in systemic venous pressure with widening of the superior vena caval shadow and chronic passive congestion of the viscera.

Essentially the same train of events occurs in mitral valvular disease except that the left ventricle is usually not the first chamber to show signs of failure. In predominant mitral insufficiency the work of the left ventricle is increased, and it hypertrophies and dilates to a degree; with predominant stenosis it may be normal in size or small.

It should be appreciated that generalized asymmetrical enlargement is often associated with some roentgen evidence of vascular congestion of the lungs.

Other causes of asymmetrical cardiac enlargement are adhesive mediastinitis, systemic arteriovenous fistulas, cardiac tumors, and an array of congenital malformations such as complete transposition of the great vessels, patent ductus arteriosus (PDA), and anomalous origin of the left coronary artery from the pulmonary artery.

In a small minority of cases the cause of the cardiac enlargement is unknown. At times, an abnormal rhythm or tachycardia is present. Atrial fibrillation associated with mitral valvular disease, however, may exist for years without significant enlargement. Complete heart block with a slow ventricular rate may show a minor degree of enlargement. This is due (1) to prolonged diastole and (2) to the increased dilation necessary to enlarge the stroke volume which must compensate for the slower rate if the circulating blood volume is to be maintained.

General enlargement, either symmetrical or asymmetrical, is variable in onset; it may take place gradually over a period of months or years or rather rapidly. The rate of enlargement is of considerable prognostic value, indicating the severity of the underlying process. Occasionally the increase in size occurs within a few hours. A previously damaged myocardium is more susceptible to rapid dilatation. A sudden increase in heart size is always suggestive of pericardial effusion; differentiation of such an effusion from general enlargement, particularly that due to myocarditis, is very difficult except by angiocardiography or ultrasonography.

SPECIFIC CHAMBER ENLARGEMENT

Specific chamber enlargement indicates an earlier stage of disease than general cardiac enlargement. Furthermore, it suggests the site and nature of underlying structural changes. A pattern of enlargement is usually established, *i.e.*, if the left ventricle is enlarged, the aorta is often elongated, slightly dilated, and has increased pulsations; if the left atrium is dilated, there is usually enlargement of the pulmonary artery and right ventricle.

Left Ventricle

An early sign of left ventricular enlargement is an increase in length of the left heart border as measured from the lower margin of the pulmonary artery segment (point of opposite pulsations) to the apex (Fig. 56). This lengthening is due to a downward extension of the heart so that the apex often lies below the diaphragmatic curve. In addition, there may be an increased convexity or rounding out of the upper ventricular border so that it actually extends somewhat farther to the left than would be normal for the particular type of heart involved. This corresponds to enlargement of the anatomical outflow tract (area of the left ventricle extending from the apex to the semilunar valves). With further enlargement, the distance from the diaphragm to the point of opposite pulsations of the heart may actually be increased and the pulmonary artery segment relatively decreased in length. The enlarged left ventricle extends posteriorly where the contour becomes increasingly convex; consequently, in the left anterior oblique projection, a greater degree of obliquity is necessary to sep-

arate the cardiac contour from the spine and the anteroposterior diameter of the heart is thus increased (Fig. 57B). According to Hoffman and Rigler (1965), when, on a true lateral film in deep inspiration, the left ventricle extends more than 1.8 cm posterior to the posterior border of the inferior vena cava at a level 2 cm cephalad to their crossing, left ventricular enlargement can be postulated with considerable confidence. These latter changes represent enlargement of the inflow tract (area of left ventricle extending from the mitral valve to the apex). When the enlargement is due mainly to hypertrophy, the left border is well rounded and tends to approach the horizontal in its upper portion so that the waist of the heart is concave and well marked. When dilatation predominates, the left border is longer, straighter, and somewhat steeper, and the length of the ventricular segment in contact with the diaphragm is increased. Left ventricular enlargement causes some clockwise (as viewed from above) rotation of the heart so that an increased proportion of the left border is due to the left ventricle. In general, left ventricular enlargement takes place downward, posteriorly, and somewhat to the left.

The most common cause of isolated left ven-

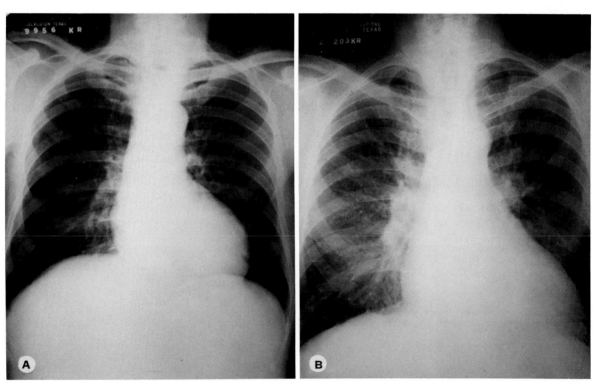

FIG. 56. ENLARGEMENT OF LEFT VENTRICLE

(A) A 67-year-old white man; BP, 200/100 for at least a year. No cardiac symptoms. (B) Asymmetrical general enlargement. Shortness of breath. BP, 200/100. There are congestive changes in the lungs. At autopsy there was coronary sclerosis with myocardial fibrosis and left ventricular dilatation and hypertrophy.

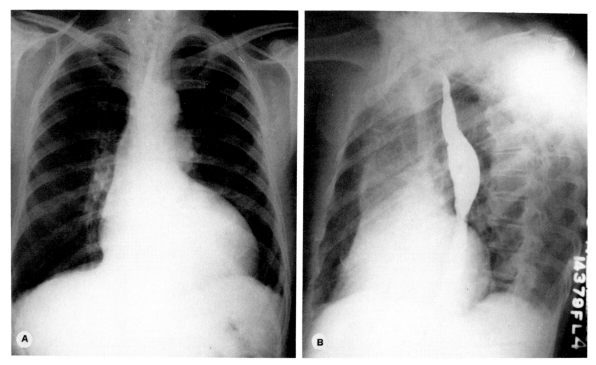

FIG. 57. LEFT VENTRICULAR ENLARGEMENT (A AND B)
The predominant lesion was aortic regurgitation of luetic origin. BP, 250/100—170/60.

tricular enlargement is essential hypertension where the heart is fully compensated. The enlargement is predominantly due to hypertrophy. Other causes include the following: chronic nephritis, coarctation of the aorta, unilateral renal disease, or any condition in which there is a persistent increase in the diastolic blood pressure.

Aortic stenosis is usually followed by predominant hypertrophy. Aortic and mitral insufficiency are accompanied by both hypertrophy and dilatation. With predominant mitral stenosis, the left ventricle may be normal in size or atrophic. Minor degrees of atrophy are difficult to recognize; the right ventricle may appear to be relatively enlarged, and the usual left ventricular contours are less convex than normal.

Dilatation is common with acute myocardial infarction and rheumatic myocarditis. Coronary arteriosclerosis causes very little change in the cardiac size unless actual infarction occurs. With the onset of failure dilatation is common.

The amplitude of pulsations of the left ventricle does not correlate with the degree of enlargement. With marked dilatation pulsations are minimal; with hypertrophy they may be normal or increased. The greatest amplitude is seen with aortic insufficiency; with hypertension the amplitude is often normal or slightly increased; with coronary arteriosclerosis with infarction, the pulsations are typically diminished and may be abnormal in contour and timing.

Left Atrium

Hypertrophy of the left atrium occurs frequently and permits the chamber to compensate for an increased intraluminal pressure for varying periods of time. There is no roentgen sign of simple hypertrophy. With a moderate degree of dilatation some posterior bulging of the left atrial contour can be seen in lateral films of good contrast. A change in contour of the barium-filled esophagus as it courses along the posterior surface of the atrium, however, is a much more sensitive and reliable indicator of dilatation. This is best studied in the right anterior oblique and lateral projections. The deviation of the esophagus begins just below the bronchial impression and consists of a backward deviation and slight flattening or an indentation in the anterior surface; the indentation is smoothly curved and actually represents the posterior surface of the atrium (Fig. 58). In normal persons there is variable redundancy of the esophagus with expiration and straightening with inspiration. Redundancy is greater in infancy and in obese or stocky individuals, and also in the recumbent position. Consequently, abnormal deviations are best evaluated in the erect position and in moderately

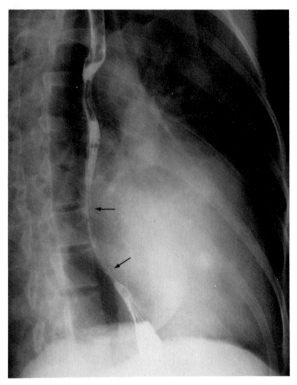

Fig. 58. Rheumatic Mitral Valvular Disease with
Predominant Insufficiency in 42-Year-Old
White Woman

This right anterior oblique view shows posterior deviation
of the opacified esophagus by an enlarged left atrium (arrows). The calcification superimposed upon the heart was in
the left lung and was thought to represent a healed granu-
loma.

deep inspiration. Some experience and a careful
technique are required in borderline cases.

Actually, the esophagus is deviated both posteriorly and to the right by the dilated atrium;
the lateral deviation is usually less pronounced
than the posterior one and is best seen in the
posteroanterior projection. In older individuals
with tortuous and slightly dilated aortas, the
esophagus deviates to follow the aorta to a degree
and is often displaced somewhat toward the left
(Fig. 488, page 000). In such cases even marked
left atrial enlargement will not necessarily cause
a displacement toward the right, and evaluation
of posterior displacement in the right anterior
oblique or lateral projections is unreliable.

In the posteroanterior projection the density
of the left atrium is superimposed upon that of
the base of the heart and is occasionally visible
as such in optimally exposed films. When the
atrium dilates, this rounded, superimposed density is easily apparent either at fluoroscopy or on
films and is a valuable sign of enlargement. The

density is frequently entirely within the cardiovascular silhouette (Figs. 88 and 89, p. 145). It is
most distinct to the right of the vertebral column
and fades away toward the left. Its lateral border
is rounded. With mitral valvular disease and
right ventricular enlargement there is usually
counterclockwise rotation of the heart (as seen
from above). This, combined with further left
atrial dilatation, may cause the right lateral contour of the left atrium to clear the cardiovascular
silhouette and form part of the right heart border. A doubly convex contour on the right is then
seen; the left atrium is above and the right is
below. With marked dilatation, the left atrium
may form the entire right heart border; in some
instances, it may reach the right lateral chest
wall. Such cases have been described as "aneurysms of the left atrium"; they may cause
compression atelectasis of the right lung and
elevation and narrowing of the right main bronchus.

The left atrium normally lies in close relation
to the tracheal carina. With moderate enlargement, it impinges mainly on the left main bronchus, and this structure is displaced upward; it
may also be slightly narrowed. Normally, the
angle between the two major bronchi at the
carina is 65–75°. When this is increased to 90°
and particularly when there is slight narrowing
of the bronchus, enlargement of the left atrium
is likely. With atrial enlargement the left recurrent laryngeal nerve may be squeezed between
the left main bronchus and the aortic arch, producing hoarseness.

Although a short segment of the left atrial
appendage, as shown by angiography, forms a
portion of the left midheart border it is smooth
and cannot be identified in the conventional
chest film of a normal heart. With minor degrees
of left atrial enlargement it may become convex
and recognizable and is considered to be a sensitive sign of left atrial enlargement, particularly
in rheumatic heart disease (Jacobson and Weidner, 1962). With moderate enlargement the left
atrial appendage uniformly forms a convexity on
the left midheart border just below the pulmonary artery. Exceptions may be due to amputation at a previous surgical procedure or extensive
inflammation and fibrosis.

Left atrial enlargement is common secondary
to a failing left ventricle and as part of a generalized cardiac enlargement; in such cases, it is
not markedly enlarged and its significance is
submerged by other aspects of the cardiac status.
Isolated or predominant dilatation, however, is
of considerable significance since it is usually
secondary to mitral valvular disease. It may be

accompanied by left ventricular enlargement and thus indicate predominant regurgitation; with predominant stenosis it may be the only enlarged chamber. This differentiation is not always easy. Other causes of left atrial enlargement are myxomas which intermittently obstruct the mitral orifice, patent ductus arteriosus, interventricular septal defects, and hyperthyroidism.

Right Ventricle

The right ventricle enlarges by extending mainly toward the left and anteriorly. There is also rotation of the heart in a counterclockwise direction (as seen from above). The left heart contour in the posteroanterior projection is somewhat altered.

Normally, the right ventricle accounts for two-thirds to three-fourths of the anterior surface area of the heart. As the chamber enlarges, the proportion of the area due to the right ventricle increases. This is due to lengthening of the anterior wall of the ventricle and the infundibulum. (The infundibulum is the portion of the right ventricle that lies above the crista supraventricularis and below the pulmonary valve.) The lengthening occurs in an oblique upward direction along the axis of the outflow tract. The outflow tract extends from the apex of the right ventricle to the pulmonary valve and is bounded anteriorly by the anterior wall of the right ventricle and posteriorly by the interventricular septum. When the increase in length is such that the infundibulum forms a part of the left midheart border as seen in the posteroanterior projection, this border straightens or becomes convex. This straightening or increased convexity takes place just below the pulmonary artery segment although the two borders fuse imperceptibly. The left ventricular border below may appear to be comparatively short. Associated counterclockwise rotation of the heart carries the left ventricle posteriorly and increases the length of the segment due to the right ventricle. This rotation also decreases the prominence of the aortic knob. With right ventricular enlargement, the aorta is frequently small (mitral stenosis, etc.) and it may be almost invisible. Thus, these factors bring about a long, straight, or slightly convex left upper border and a shorter, less convex left ventricular curve. The convex portion of the middle segment is usually due to the pulmonary artery. With more marked enlargement, the right ventricle may form the entire left heart border. The left ventricle is displaced posteriorly, and differentiation between right and left ventricular enlargement is then difficult.

One of the earliest signs of right ventricular enlargement is seen in the right anterior oblique projection. There is an increased convexity or bulge of the conus region and pulmonary artery anteriorly, and this appears before the conus becomes border-forming on the left. With more

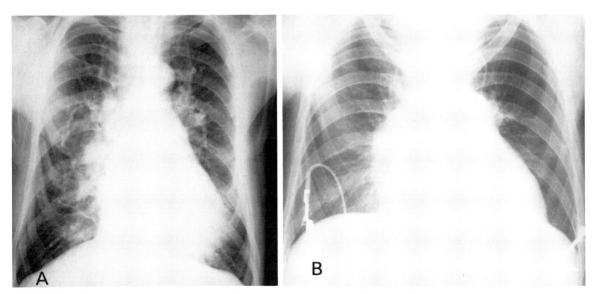

FIG. 59. COR PULMONALE AS SEEN IN PA CHEST FILM

(A) There is extensive pulmonary fibrosis and emphysema. At autopsy there was dilatation of the right atrium and dilatation and hypertrophy of the right ventricle and dilatation of the pulmonary artery. The distinctive changes in contour are some elevation of the apex of the heart and slight convexity of the pulmonary artery segment. (B) Cor pulmonale in a 25-year-old male secondary to the lateral ventricle-right atrial shunt for chronic hydrocephalus (autopsy case). The left ventricle was small, and the greater portion of the enlargement was due to the dilated right atrium and ventricle.

marked enlargement the entire anterior cardiac surface is lengthened and more convex. It may encroach to a variable degree on the clear retrosternal space, although this is difficult to evaluate. Fluoroscopy in this projection is helpful in differentiating right from left ventricular enlargement. If the left ventricle is large, the anterior border below the infundibulum will bulge; if the right ventricle is large, the conus convexity will be increased.

In the left anterior oblique projection, the anterior cardiac contour is elongated and convex. This anterior surface represents the inflow tract of the right ventricle. (The inflow tract extends from the tricuspid valve to the apex of the ventricle; it is bounded posteriorly by the lower portion of the interventricular septum and anteriorly and inferiorly by the anterior and inferior ventricular wall.)

Encroachment on the retrosternal space is best demonstrated on the lateral view. The extent of this space is so variable normally that a reduction in size is difficult to evaluate (Fig. 28). In addition, the right atrial appendage when dilated may extend into this area.

A slight to moderate degree of right ventricular enlargement cannot be objectively demonstrated by roentgen methods. This is particularly true where hypertrophy predominates. Frequently an increase in size is inferred because the pulmonary artery segment is convex and enlarged or there is fullness of the right heart border indicating a dilated right atrium. In well compensated cases of cor pulmonale, changes in the cardiac contour are often minimal and right ventricular hypertrophy may be easily overlooked (Fig. 67B, p. 115). In such cases electrocardiography may give more reliable evidence of right ventricular enlargement than roentgen studies.

Some degree of right ventricular enlargement is common following left ventricular failure due to hypertension, myocardial infarction, or aortic valvular disease. It is then a part of a generalized asymmetrical cardiac enlargement; the left ventricle remains predominantly larger than the other chambers. Mitral valvular disease sufficient to cause clinical symptoms is almost always associated with some degree of right ventricular hypertrophy. The "mitralized heart" has a steep left border which is straight in its midportion or slightly convex in the region of the pulmonary artery segment. The aortic knob is small or absent. This contour is not always due to mitral valvular disease. Other causes of right ventricular enlargement are cor pulmonale, secondary to extensive pulmonary fibrosis or emphysema, or disease of the pulmonary arteries, interatrial and high interventricular septal defects, the tetralogy of Fallot, isolated valvular pulmonic stenosis, and primary pulmonary hypertension.

Right Atrium

Isolated enlargement of the right atrium is rare; it is usually accompanied or preceded by some degree of right ventricular enlargement which tends to obscure the details of atrial enlargement.

According to Schwedel (1946), the anterior or trabeculated portion of the right atrium is the first to dilate; this includes the atrial appendage. Consequently, early enlargement is best detected in the left anterior oblique projection where the right atrial appendage is brought into contour. Normally, the atrial segment can be identified best by fluoroscopy because of a difference in pulsation between the anterior surface of the right ventricle below and the characteristic pulsations of the aorta above. The atrial segment has low but fairly typical wavelike pulsations. When there is a normal rhythm with early enlargement, this segment is elongated and, of course, is best seen at fluoroscopy. Schwedel (1946) places the upper normal length of this segment at 3 cm at 25–40° of obliquity. It may bulge anteriorly to a slight degree and can then be identified on films. With further enlargement, this segment is lengthened and elevated; in its upper portion it may approach a horizontal position.

In the posteroanterior projection, there is an increased fullness or bulging of the right lower cardiac contour, due to dilatation of the right atrium. This sign is not too reliable since displacement of the atrium due to an enlarged right ventricle or generalized cardiac enlargement will produce the same appearance. When there is a definite increase in length of this lateral segment, however, atrial enlargement is likely. A dilated vena cava may be considered as evidence of atrial dilatation. This is recognized by an increase in width of the straight bordered density adjacent to the right upper mediastinum. Rarely, a dilated inferior vena cava is detected superimposed on the right lower cardiac contour or filling in the right cardiophrenic angle.

Marked dilatation of the right atrium is seen in the right anterior oblique position. Here, the body of the atrium extends posteriorly and downward and fills in the posterior and posterolateral and cardiophrenic space. The contour of the atrium is rounded and somewhat convex posteriorly; it may rarely deviate the barium-filled esophagus.

A degree of right atrial enlargement is common

with general cardiac enlargement. Dilatation is most commonly associated with some degree of right ventricular dilatation and relative tricuspid insufficiency. Structural tricuspid insufficiency due to rheumatic fever will cause the same appearance but is rare. Tricuspid stenosis due to the same cause is also rare; it can produce isolated or predominant right atrial enlargement. In congenital tricuspid stenosis or atresia enlargement depends to a considerable degree on the size of the accompanying interatrial septal defect. In uncomplicated interatrial defect and the Lutembacher's syndrome, dilatation is common, but it may be associated with some degree of tricuspid insufficiency or right ventricular failure. Ebstein's anomaly of the tricuspid valve may produce a right atrium of very large size.

Pulmonary Artery

From the roentgen viewpoint the pulmonary arterial system may be divided into the pulmonary trunk, hilar, and intrapulmonary branches.

Enlargement of this system is due almost entirely to dilatation since thickening of the arterial walls adds very little to the total diameter. Theoretically, it would appear that dilatation would follow either an increase in intraluminal pressure or flow or a weakening of the arterial wall due to disease or a combination of these factors. In the majority of cases, the arterial wall remains intact and elastic; enlargement is then more or less reversible and represents a response to pressure and volume changes in the pulmonary circulation. Healey et al. (1949) and Campbell (1951) have studied the hemodynamic factors involved. Pulmonary artery pressures and flows were determined by right heart catheterization and were compared with the size and activity of the pulmonary trunk and the hilar and intrapulmonary branches as determined by fluoroscopy and roentgenography. Enlargement of these vessels occurs in response to (1) an increased blood flow, (2) an increased intraluminal pressure, (3) an increase in turbulent flow, or (4) a combination of these factors. Healy et al. (1949) were unable to differentiate between these factors from the roentgen appearance alone; Campbell (1951) found, however, that the pulsations in the pulmonary trunk and hilar branches were more vigorous where the flow was great (e.g., interatrial septal defect) and the pressure within normal limits. Why the pulmonary arterial system should dilate in response to an increase in flow alone is not clear; presumably there must be a minor increase in tension which is not clearly shown by present techniques.

In the posteroanterior projection, enlargement of the pulmonary trunk produces a straightening or an increase in convexity of the left midcardiac segment. If the enlargement is pronounced, the pulmonary trunk is lengthened so that the entire border between the aortic knob above and the left ventricular curve below is straight or convex. This effect is heightened if the right ventricle is enlarged sufficiently to participate in the left midborder. The aortic knob is relatively less prominent and is often actually diminished in size due to (1) a decrease in aortic caliber and (2) counterclockwise rotation of the heart as seen from above. The left ventricular segment may also appear shorter and steeper, particularly if the left ventricle is not enlarged. These changes account for the so-called "mitralized heart contour" although it is by no means always associated with mitral valvular disease. Occasionally in the posteroanterior projection, the pulmonary trunk and the arch of the left pulmonary artery may be mistaken for the aorta.

In the left anterior oblique view, the left pulmonary artery arches above the left main bronchus and below the aortic arch. With enlargement it impinges upon the radiolucent aortic window and reduces or obliterates it. This is best seen at fluoroscopy with deep inspiration. Where the obliquity is 55° or more, the right pulmonary artery appears as an oval or elongated dense opacity which suggests enlargement.

In the right oblique projection there may be an increased convexity high on the anterior surface of the heart due to the enlarged pulmonary trunk.

The portions of the pulmonary arterial system that are ordinarily known as the hilar branches in the posteroanterior projection are (1) right and left pulmonary arteries; (2) their ascending and descending branches; (3) the apical posterior, anterior segmental, and lingular branches on the left; and (4) the apical, posterior and anterior and the middle lobe branches on the right. Not all of these branches are visible in every case. With a globular or transverse heart or some enlargement, the left pulmonary artery as well as a part of the ascending and descending branches lie within the heart shadow. The right pulmonary artery is rarely identified since it is superimposed upon the other mediastinal structures and bifurcates before emerging from the lateral margin of the superior vena caval shadow. The most frequently visible major branch is the right descending. It is particularly clear-cut where it courses lateral to and parallel with the lower lobe bronchus. In its upper portion near the hilus on teleoroentgenograms, Schwedel (1946) gives the range of normal size as 9–14 mm. Chang (1962) found the upper limit of normal in width of the right descending pulmonary artery to be 15 mm in women and 16 mm in men, based on measurements of 1,085 subjects. Dotter and Steinberg (1949) gave the normal range of the right main pulmonary artery as determined by angiocardiography as 17–30 mm. Changes in size of the hilar branches, however, are generally determined by experience and on the basis of familiarity with their normal appearance.

The smaller branches of the pulmonary artery run an irregular, slightly angular but generally radiating course through the lung parenchyma. They fade out toward the outer one-third to one-fourth of the lung fields. Again recognition of dilatation or a diminution in size depends upon experience with the normal.

The pulmonary trunk may be dilated, normal, or decreased in size distal to pulmonic stenosis. In valvular pulmonic stenosis dilatation is limited to that portion of the trunk just beyond the pulmonary valve and often to the proximal part of the left pulmonary artery; the other hilar and intrapulmonary branches are usually diminished in size, although occasionally they are normal. In four such cases studied by Healey *et al.* (1949), the pulmonary blood flow was normal, the dilatation was limited entirely to the pulmonary trunk, and the hilar and intrapulmonary arteries were normal in size. The cause of such dilatation is not clear; it is presumably the result of turbulent flow in the pulmonary trunk distal to the obstruction.

In the tetralogy of Fallot with infundibular pulmonary stenosis, the blood flow through the pulmonary trunk is invariably decreased, and the pulmonary arterial system is frequently reduced in size; however, occasionally the pulmonary trunk may be normal in diameter or slightly dilated.

In cases where an increased vessel size occurs without an increase in either flow or pressure, a congenital defect in the vessel wall should be suspected.

In pulmonary emphysema, fibrosis, and primary pulmonary hypertension, the pulmonary trunk and its right and left branches are dilated; the smaller vessels in the lungs are diminished in size. Marked disparity between the size of enlarged hilar pulmonary arteries and abruptly smaller peripheral divisions is a sign of pulmonary arterial hypertension of whatever cause.

In mitral and aortic valvular disease, essential hypertension with left ventricular failure and other lesions on the left side of the heart which produce an increase in pulmonary venous pressure by obstruction, all parts of the pulmonary arterial system (trunk, hilar, and intrapulmonary branches) may be dilated. This is often accompanied by transudation of fluid into the alveoli and pleural space, thickening of the interlobular septa of the lung, and small hemorrhages into the pulmonary parenchyma, all of which produce a roentgen picture of chronic passive congestion of the lung. This will be discussed in more detail in the following section.

Dilatation of the entire arterial system which may become quite pronounced accompanies an increased pulmonary blood flow. Healey *et al.* (1949) thought that a flow in excess of 7 L/min/m^2 through the pulmonary trunk would usually produce some degree of dilatation. An increase in flow occurs typically in interatrial (IASD) and interventricular (IVSD) septal defects, persistent patency of the ductus arteriosus (PDA), and anomalous return of the pulmonary veins to the right side of the heart. There may also be an increase in pulmonary artery pressure in these conditions.

In Eisenmenger's complex, particularly in the older cases, and transposition of the great vessels, there is an increase in pressure with very slight if any increase in flow. In transposition the pulmonary arterial wall is often thickened.

A decrease in size of the pulmonary trunk is recognized in the posteroanterior projection by a concavity of the left midheart border. The heart bay is deepened. The aortic knob above and ventricular curve below may appear relatively more convex. The main branches in each hilus are usually visibly decreased in diameter, and the lungs have a clear radiolucent appearance. The pulmonary trunk is usually diminished in size distal to an infundibular stenosis such as is seen in Fallot's tetralogy; this is accompanied by a decrease in size of the hilar and intrapulmonary arteries. A small pulmonary trunk is also seen in tricuspid atresia and Ebstein's anomaly of the tricuspid valve.

The normal pulmonary artery and its proximal hilar branches show definite but minimal pulsations; with enlargement, pulsations may be increased, unchanged, or decreased. The amplitude of the pulsations depends upon (1) the hemodynamics of blood flow and (2) the condition of the arterial wall. In the majority of cases the arterial wall remains elastic and responds quickly to changes in intraluminal pressure. In mitral valvular disease and chronic passive congestion of the lungs due to other causes, pulsations are diminished or absent. In such conditions the pressure is increased and the flow is diminished. In interatrial and interventricular septal defects, patent ductus arteriosus and anomalous return of the pulmonary veins, pulsations are increased; this is best observed at fluoroscopy. "Hilar dance" is a term applied to pronounced pulsations of the hilar vessels; when viewed at fluoroscopy the entire hilus appears to expand and contract with each heart beat. Also, there is an easily appreciable change in density of the vessels which is most noticeable near the periphery of the hilus. At times, the pulsations can be seen far out in the smaller vessels in the lung. Schwedel (1946) believes that a "hilar dance" is diagnostic of pulmonary insufficiency usually on a functional basis secondary to a dilatation of the pulmonary valve ring. Essentially it represents an exaggerated degree of hilar pulsation. It is most frequent in association with interatrial septal defects or Lutembacher's syndrome (50% of the cases in Campbell's (1951) series) and is somewhat less common in patent ductus arteriosus (33% in series reported by Donovan *et al.* (1943)). In these conditions the pulmonary flow is increased; the pressure may or may not be increased. Usually the pulmonary pulse pressure is increased, and there may be some degree of functional pulmonary regurgitation.

Other conditions in which there may be an increase in pulmonary artery pulsations are hyperthyroidism, anemia, and idiopathic congenital dilatation of the pulmonary artery (Greene *et al.*, 1949). There may be a slight increase in the pulsations of the trunk and the right and left branches in pulmonary emphysema and diffuse pulmonary fibrosis.

Pulsations distal to a valvular pulmonic stenosis are described as diminished or absent (Engle and Taussig, 1950) and undoubtedly this is usual. Occasionally the pulsations are normal (Dow *et al.*, 1950) or slightly increased, and this can be confirmed by the present authors. There are many grades of severity of pulmonic stenosis. In many cases the pulmonary flow remains within normal limits and in such cases pulsations may be normal.

Aorta

The aorta may dilate (increase in diameter) or elongate (increase in length). It is rare for one of these changes to occur without the other although one type of change may predominate. Elongation produces tortuosity because a greater length of aorta must be accommodated to two or three relatively fixed points.

Dilatation and/or elongation are due to (1) disease of the aortic wall, (2) changes in pressure or blood flow through the aorta, or (3) a combination of these factors. Disease of the aortic wall is common, *e.g.*, arteriosclerosis, syphilis, rheumatic fever, and congenital defects. Changes in blood flow and pressure are also common, *e.g.*, hypertension due to any cause, aortic valvular disease, and certain congenital malformations such as truncus arteriosus, the tetralogy of Fallot, and patent ductus arteriosus. Consequently, changes in the contour of the aorta are commonly seen in the roentgen examination of the cardiovascular system.

Dilatation may be localized or diffuse. Where it is secondary to disease of the aortic wall, dilatation is often irregular and may be localized to a particular segment. An example of this is often seen in syphilitic aortitis and aneurysms of the thoracic aorta. On the other hand, dilatation secondary to systemic hypertension is more diffuse and usually involves the entire thoracic aorta. Elongation is ordinarily secondary to a diffuse process such as arteriosclerosis. A considerable length of the aorta must be involved in order to produce significant elongation.

For descriptive purposes the thoracic aorta may be divided into (1) ascending, (2) arch, and (3) descending portions.

In the posteroanterior projection, with conventional roentgenography, the first 2 or 3 cm of the ascending aorta are invisible within the cardiac contour. Beyond that point the right lateral border is superimposed upon the vena caval shadow or is borderforming in certain cases. With dilatation, a considerable length of the lateral aortic wall forms the right cardiovascular contour. This is more impressive at fluoroscopy where there is some magnification and pulsations demonstrate the maximum lateral excursion of the aortic wall. The lateral border of this segment of the ascending aorta is mildly convex. When there is localized dilatation or irregularity with bulging of this segment, syphilitic aortitis may be suspected although similar changes may accompany arachnodactyly (Goyette and Palmer, 1953).

Dilatation of the arch is indicated by an increase in size of the aortic knob. Not only is there an increase in lateral extension but the impression on the barium-filled esophagus medially is longer, indicating a larger diameter. No other portion of the aortic arch is visible unless the wall contains significant amounts of calcium.

The descending aorta is frequently visible through the cardiac silhouette just to the left of the vertebral column; with aortic dilatation this shadow increases in width and extends farther toward the left. A paravertebral position of the aorta, however, is commonly due to elongation rather than dilatation.

With 55–60° rotation into the left anterior oblique position the entire thoracic aorta may be visible, providing (1) contrast is optimum, (2) the aorta is increased in density due to small deposits of calcium and some thickening of the wall such as occurs in arteriosclerosis, or (3) the lungs are emphysematous thus providing better contrast. Even under the most favorable circumstances, the aortic borders are hazy and precise measurement is difficult. If mensuration is attempted, the upper limits of normal are as follows: ascending portion, 38 mm; arch, 35 mm; descending portion, 28 mm (Steinberg et al., 1949). Under less favorable conditions, the aortic arch may be visible only in its posterior portion and particularly where it crosses the tracheal air column. Here it should not exceed 32–35 mm in diameter.

Angiocardiography in the posteroanterior and left anterior oblique projections gives good visualization of the entire aorta, although for measurement purposes filming should be correlated with cardiac phase. Steinberg et al. (1949) found an aortic diameter in excess of 38 mm in the area just above the sinuses of Valsalva in the absence of hypertension or rheumatic aortic insufficiency was presumptive evidence of luetic aortitis. Furthermore, irregularities in the lumen and local areas of dilatation were present in 95% of their cases of luetic aortitis.

Kerley (1951) undoubtedly refers to similar changes in what he calls "a lack of parallelism" of the aortic walls in which they have an irregular ragged or jagged appearance. This is accompanied by localized areas of dilatation. Unfortunately, such changes are not always visible using conventional radiography.

Careful fluoroscopy may demonstrate local areas of minor aortic weakness and dilatation. The most important finding is the contrast in character and amplitude of the pulsations of the local dilated segment and the adjacent relatively normal aorta. The area of transition from the normal to the dilated segment is clear-cut, and the movement is exaggerated in the dilated segment. Such a finding is excellent evidence of luetic aortitis.

Elongation brings about tortuosity of the aorta and unfolding of the arch; it is often accompanied by minor degrees of dilatation. In the posteroanterior projection, the ascending aorta because of its increased length extends further to the right of the midline and forms the right upper vascular border much as it does in aortic dilatation. The aortic knob is not enlarged or dilated but is quite distinct and may be elevated so that it is at the level of the anterior end of the first rib or just below the sternoclavicular joint. The lateral border of the descending aorta as seen through the cardiac silhouette is tortuous or undulating and

lies more toward the left than normal; a paravertebral rather than a prevertebral position is common. In more advanced cases, the descending aorta wanders lateralward for a considerable distance so that it may give the appearance of a mediastinal mass. The esophagus is often carried toward the left with a tortuous aorta due to periesophageal and aortic adhesions so that its course is deviated over a considerable area (Fig. 498, page 604). In such cases, it is no longer a reliable guide to left atrial enlargement. Plaque-like areas of calcification in the arch and descending aorta are common since elongation is most often associated with arteriosclerosis.

In the far left anterior oblique and lateral projections, curvature of the aortic arch is seen to be slightly reduced. The straight line distance between the ascending and descending aorta is increased; the greater portion of the descending aortic shadow is superimposed on the vertebral bodies indicating the paravertebral position. In its lower portion, the descending aorta curves forward to pass through the diaphragm. The anterior deviation plus the unfolding of the arch above gives the entire thoracic aorta in the lateral view the appearance of a question mark.

The amplitude of pulsations of the aorta depends on (1) the elasticity of the aortic wall and (2) changes in intraluminal pressure (pulse pressure) which occur with each heart beat. Pulsations are most pronounced in the ascending portion and arch and for that reason they are best studied at fluoroscopy in the posteroanterior and left anterior oblique positions.

Hypertension, either essential or due to other causes, produces moderate diffuse dilatation of the aorta and some elongation. The dilatation is described as dynamic since in the earlier stages there are no structural changes in the aorta. There is an associated increase in pulsations in the ascending portion and arch of the aorta.

Arteriosclerosis is followed by considerable elongation and tortuosity of the aorta with minimal dilatation. In the posteroanterior projection, the appearance may be similar to that seen with hypertension. The knob may be smaller and higher, however, and in the left anterior oblique view unfolding of the aorta is seen. Calcium is commonly deposited in the arch and descending aorta in arteriosclerosis. Hypertension and arteriosclerosis frequently occur together, and precise differentiation between the radiographic manifestations of each process of little practical importance.

Syphilitic aortitis produces predominantly dilatation of the aorta; it is rarely elongated unless there is associated arteriosclerosis. Pulsations are increased in amplitude due to either changes in the aortic wall or the frequent association of aortic insufficiency.

Aortic insufficiency *per se* produces dilatation of the ascending aorta and a marked increase in pulsations. This may happen in rheumatic valvular disease where the aortic wall is uninvolved. It is typically most pronounced with syphilitic aortic valvular disease.

Dilatation of the ascending aorta is common in aortic stenosis. It is said to be due to impingement of the jet of blood coming from the stenotic valve upon the lateral aortic wall. In congenital aortic and subaortic stenosis, the dilatation may be due to an inherent structural defect in the aortic wall. Pulsations in the dilated aorta may be normal but are usually diminished.

The aorta is enlarged in the tetralogy of Fallot, patent ductus arteriosus, truncus arteriosus, and most cases of tricuspid atresia.

There is a relative decrease in aortic size in predominant mitral stenosis and in many cases of cor pulmonale and primary pulmonary hypertension; also in interatrial and interventricular septal defects, anomalous venous return of the pulmonary veins to the right atrium, and Lutembacher's syndrome. Evidence of a small aorta may be listed as follows: the aortic knob is inconspicuous or absent; the esophageal impression is small or absent; the aorta does not extend beyond the vertebral column on the right; and, in extreme cases, none of the aortic contours can be distinctly brought into profile. Then only by angiocardiography can the aorta be demonstrated.

9

Diseases of the Pulmonary Vascular System

ANATOMY AND PHYSIOLOGY

The primary functions of the pulmonary vascular system are: (1) to carry blood from the right to the left side of the heart; (2) to provide a channel to facilitate the proper exchange of gases between the blood and the air in the pulmonary alveoli; (3) to nourish the pulmonary tissues; and (4) to act as a reservoir in adapting the circulatory system to stress.

Anatomically, the pulmonary vascular system may be divided as follows: pulmonary trunk, right and left pulmonary arteries and their major branches, small muscular intrapulmonary arteries, arterioles, capillaries, venules, and pulmonary veins. In addition, there is a systemic or bronchial circulation composed of small arteries, arterioles, capillaries, venules, and veins. Numerous communications undoubtedly exist between the bronchial and pulmonary systems before their respective capillary beds are reached (Vanderhoeft, 1964). According to Marshall (1959), the bronchial arteries normally carry less than 1% of the blood to the lungs; the bronchial veins return blood to the azygos vein. The bronchial circulation is of considerable importance in maintaining the nutrition of the bronchi and pulmonary parenchyma. When a branch of the pulmonary artery is occluded, the bronchial circulation may be sufficient to maintain the involved lung segment so that infarction does not occur unless there is some degree of preceding pulmonary stasis. Similarly, the lung does not become necrotic when the bronchial arteries are interrupted. Both circulations undoubtedly contribute to the nutrition of the parenchyma of the lung.

Rarely is the bronchial circulation demonstrated roentgenographically without special techniques; the exceptions are those congenital malformations (*e.g.,* truncus arteriosus and tetralogy of Fallot) in which there is marked pul-

monic stenosis so that the bronchial circulation enlarges and carries the greater portion or all of the blood which reaches the lungs. Taussig (1960) and Campbell and Gardner (1950) have given excellent descriptions of the roentgen appearance of this collateral circulation, a considerable portion of which is due to enlarged bronchial arteries. The main branches of the pulmonary trunk (*i.e.,* the right and left pulmonary arteries) cannot be identified in the lung hilus, and the normal curve of the descending branches is missing. Instead one sees several irregular nodular shadows which tend to become confluent. They appear to be completely separate from the heart. The vascular pedicle and upper paramediastinal structures are wider than normal, are continuous with these nodular hilar densities, and are due to enlarged arteries rising from the aortic arch and extending downward toward each hilus. In the left oblique view the rather clear pulmonary window is crossed by several shadows representing these enlarged arteries. The lung parenchyma has a clear radiolucent appearance. Angiocardiography demonstrates the collateral arteries and shows their origin to be unusually high in the mediastinum; they fill only after the aorta fills, and contrast substance is slow to reach the pulmonary parenchyma.

In recent years techniques have been developed to selectively opacify the bronchial arteries (Viamonte, 1964; Newton and Preger, 1965; Noonan *et al.,* 1965). In most cases the bronchial arteries are selectively catheterized from a femoral artery approach, and most effort has been directed toward the study of inflammatory and neoplastic pulmonary lesions (Fig. 60). The demonstration of enlarged bronchial collaterals in cases of congenital or acquired heart disease may also be accomplished.

The pulmonary vascular system has a large

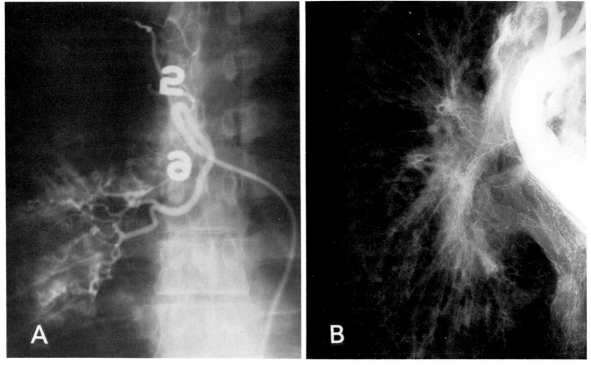

FIG. 60. BRONCHIAL ARTERIOGRAMS

(A) The film reproduced on the left is from a selective right bronchial arteriogram in the case of an inoperable bronchogenic carcinoma of the right hilum. The opacified bronchial artery is enlarged, and there is an increase in the bronchial artery supply to the hilus on the right. Some of the more peripheral bronchial arteries show an irregular contour, and an early tumor blush is noted inferiorly. (Courtesy of Thomas H. Newton, M.D.)

(B) The film reproduced on the right is a postmortem bronchial arteriogram of an intact lung and mediastinum showing the bronchial artery supply to the lung and adjacent area. The opacified aorta and its branches are seen to the right of the illustration. The myriad tiny branches to the lung parenchyma are well displayed. (Courtesy of Charles D. Noonan, M.D.)

reserve capacity for the transportation of blood. Holman and Beck (1926) and Gibbon *et al.* (1932) found that in experimental animals the cross-sectional area of the pulmonary trunk could be reduced by 61–85% without causing a drop in the systemic blood pressure. The pulmonary blood volume is said to increase by about 30% on changing from the standing to the supine position; changes in pulmonary (capillary) pressure accompanying these changes in pulmonary blood volume are relatively small, indicating relative distensibility of the pulmonary vascular bed. It is a common observation that pneumonectomy is well tolerated in human beings (Wiederanders *et al.*, 1964), and in the case of a right pneumonectomy something more than one-half of the total pulmonary vascular bed is removed. Dexter *et al.* (1950) found that pulmonary flows up to 10 L/min/m^2 of body surface, or about 3 times the normal adult pulmonary flow, were not accompanied by an increase in pressure. Friedberg (1959) states that in the normal adult lung the pulmonary vascular bed may be distended by about 3 times the normal blood flow without a

notable rise in pressure. It is obvious, therefore, in view of this large reserve that a pathologic process must obliterate large areas of the pulmonary vascular bed to produce significant obstruction. There are, however, two anatomical components of the vascular system which are more susceptible to obstruction than the others. These are (1) the pulmonary veins and (2) the arterioles. The pulmonary veins are relatively quite narrow as compared to systemic veins; consequently, obstructive processes involving these veins quite readily produce hemodynamic changes in the remainder of the pulmonary circulation and the right side of the heart.

The colloid osmotic pressure of the blood is about 25–30 mm Hg. Thus, in an otherwise normal pulmonary capillary, when the pressure exceeds 25–30 mm Hg, there will be an outflow of fluid, producing pulmonary edema. Such an elevation of intracapillary pressure (normal mean intracapillary pressure is about 9 mm Hg) is a common cause of pulmonary edema, although the same roentgenographic appearance may be due to increased capillary permeability or to a decrease in colloid osmotic pressure of the blood. Pulmonary edema does not occur, however, in many instances where the pulmonary arterial pressure is significantly or even greatly elevated. Instead, there is a marked drop in pressure between the artery and the capillaries, and this presumably takes place in the arterioles. The capillaries are thus "protected" against high pressures which might otherwise produce fatal pulmonary edema. A pressure gradient of this sort was found by Dexter *et al.* (1950) in three cases of the Eisenmenger complex and in several cases of mitral stenosis in which there was pulmonary hypertension. The mechanism of this increased resistance is not entirely clear; some of the theories of causation include (1) reactive pulmonary arteriolar vasoconstriction; (2) persistence of fetal type arterioles; (3) independent coincidental congenital disease of the pulmonary circulation; (4) degenerative or thrombo-obstructive pulmonary vascular disease (possibly secondary to high flow or pressure); (5) transmission of high left ventricular or left atrial pressure to pulmonary circulation, sometimes with associated disproportionate reactive arteriolar vasoconstriction (*e.g.,* mitral stenosis); and (6) "primary" arteriolar disease with diminution of the vascular caliber because of intimal or medial changes (Evans *et al.,* 1957; Farrar *et al.,* 1961). The extent of these changes remains controversial, however. Edwards (1957) has discussed the functional pathology of the pulmonary vascular tree in detail with particular reference to changes in congenital heart disease.

Diseases of the pulmonary vascular system most often produce their effects by (1) obstruction, (2) dilatation, or (3) a change in vascular permeability with transudation or hemorrhage into the surrounding lung. Conditions which produce obstructions are the most common.

OBSTRUCTIONS

When the vascular obstruction is distal to the pulmonary capillaries, an increase in pulmonary capillary pressure and a tendency to pulmonary edema are found (postcapillary pulmonary hypertension); if the elevated pressure persists over a period of time, pulmonary stasis and chronic passive congestion appear. In addition, there is a variable degree of dilatation of the remainder of the pulmonary vascular system and often some enlargement of the right ventricle. When the obstruction is proximal to the capillaries, edema and chronic lung stasis do not occur. Since pulmonary edema and congestion can be recognized radiologically, obstructions can be classified as to whether they are proximal or distal to the pulmonary capillaries (Goodwin, 1958).

Obstructions Distal to Pulmonary Capillaries (Conditions that Produce Postcapillary Pulmonary Hypertension)

1. Left ventricular failure secondary to essential hypertension, aortic valvular disease or myocardial infarction (Fig. 62)
2. Mitral valvular disease (Fig. 64)
3. Compression or invasion of the pulmonary veins secondary to mediastinal tumor or chronic infection (Fig. 61)
4. Left atrial tumors (myxomas)
5. Constrictive pericarditis involving the left side of the heart
6. Pulmonary veno-obstructive disease

Pulmonary Congestion

Chronic passive congestion of the lungs is almost always associated with some degree of pulmonary edema and in many cases is a prelude to the development of alveolar and interstitial transudation. The pulmonary parenchymal structure as seen on the chest film is hazy and poorly defined and in advanced cases may have an almost homogeneous structureless appearance. These changes are most pronounced in the lung bases; the apices may remain relatively normal in appearance. The major changes, however, are in the lung hilus. The pulmonary trunk, the main branches, and the intrapulmonary vessels are all dilated. The hilar shadows are enlarged, and the individual vessels in the lung parenchyma may stand out as oval-shaped areas with a considerable increase in density although their outlines are apt to be fuzzy and indistinct. The dilated smaller vessels can be followed all the way to the periphery. Fluid often collects bilaterally in the pleural spaces; it may be considerable, and there is usually more fluid on the right than on the left. In chronic passive congestion of long duration some degree of pulmonary fibrosis occurs along with pleural thickening; the interlobar fissures often appear widened and thickened. Differentiation of this appearance from small interlobar pleural effusions may be impossible.

The diaphragmatic movements are shallow, and the expansion of the lungs is poor. Chronic passive congestion is often seen in patients with mitral valvular disease but is most common following left ventricular failure in hypertension, myocardial infarction, and aortic valvular disease. Therefore, there is usually associated asymmetrical generalized cardiac enlargement.

One of the earliest findings on chest films of patients with incipient or "preclinical" left ventricular failure is produced by redistribution of pulmonary blood flow, with selective distention of upper lobe vessels in the lungs (Chait *et al.*, 1972). The cause is not clear, though patients with chronic lung stasis due to mitral valve disease may also show this finding. In both instances

it may be due to reflex spasm of lower lobe vessels related to elevation of pulmonary venous pressure, resulting in shunting of blood to the upper lobes. Indeed, McHugh *et al.* (1972) found good correlation between pulmonary capillary wedge pressure and radiologic criteria of left ventricular failure, especially redistribution of blood flow, loss of the sharp marginal contour of

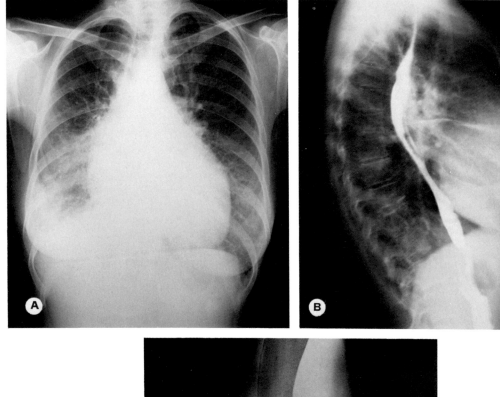

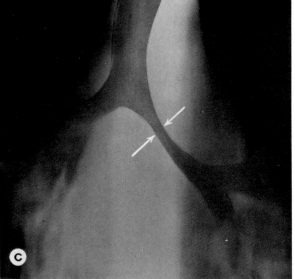

FIG. 61. CHRONIC LUNG STASIS AFTER COMPRESSION OF PULMONARY VEINS DUE TO CHRONIC MEDIASTINAL FIBROSIS (AUTOPSY CASE)

(A and B) There was a marked hypertrophy and dilatation of the right ventricle, and cardiac catheterization showed a considerable degree of pulmonary hypertension. The roentgen evidence of lung stasis resembles that seen in long-standing mitral valvular disease or other obstruction in the left side of the heart. The left atrium was not dilated, and the posterior deviation of the esophagus is due to mediastinal fibrosis. (C) Reproduction of a laminogram (retouched) showing narrowing of left main stem bronchus due to surrounding inflammation and fibrosis.

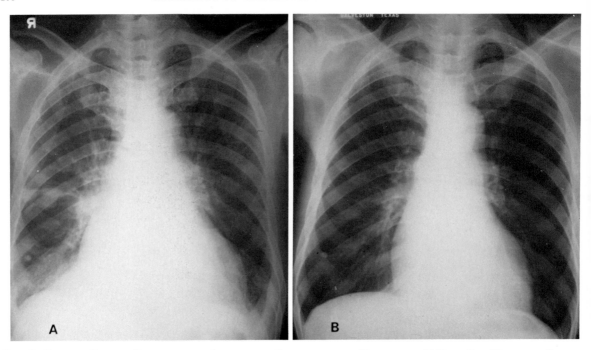

FIG. 62. CHRONIC PASSIVE CONGESTION OF LUNGS WITH CLEARING AFTER THERAPY IN 57-YEAR-OLD MAN WITH CONGES-
TIVE HEART FAILURE SECONDARY TO ARTERIOSCLEROTIC AND LUETIC CARDIOVASCULAR DISEASE
(A) The heart is enlarged, and the hilar vascular structures are increased in size and decreased in clarity. The intrapulmonary
vessels are dilated and indistinct. Pleural effusion obscures both costophrenic angles, and a small effusion is loculated in the
minor interlobar fissure. (B) The patient responded to digitalis, diuretics, bed rest, and a low salt diet. The follow-up film shows
decrease in size of the heart and pulmonary vessels, increase in definition of the hilar structures, and resorption of the pleural
effusions.

the pulmonary vessels and development of the
perihilar haze. Turner *et al.* (1972) described a
method for estimation of pulmonary arterial and
venous pressures from routine chest films; they
were able to relate the mean left atrial pressure
to the intensity of the redistribution pattern.

Angiocardiography is not required for demonstration of the upper lobe distention in early
cardiac failure, but such studies may at times
give dramatic demonstration of the redistribution of blood flow (Fig. 65).

Chronic passive congestion often improves
after adequate treatment of the underlying
cause. This may consist of digitalis, diuretics, bed
rest, etc. In some instances where the changes
appear rapidly after myocardial infarction, they
are due predominantly to edema and will clear
rapidly if the patient improves. Frequently
within a week after medical treatment the lung
haziness disappears, the peripheral vessels decrease in size and prominence, and fluid disappears from the pleural space. This may be accompanied by a decrease in heart size. Serial films
thus give objective evidence of improvement of
the condition of the pulmonary circulation, and
this parallels the clinical course of the patient
(Fig. 62). Chait *et al.* (1972) studied 94 patients

admitted to a coronary care unit and concluded
that no useful information was obtained by daily
exposure of chest films on patients clinically in
cardiac failure. Because of the precarious condition of many of these patients, there is a natural
tendency to want to obtain frequent evidences of
their improvement or lack of it, but it is likely
that films made at intervals of several days will
suffice.

Engorgement of the lungs indicates an abnormal increase in the blood volume within the
dilated vascular structures. It may follow either
an obstruction to the outflow from the lungs or
an increased inflow such as occurs in patent
ductus arteriosus or interatrial septal defect.
There is considerable similarity in the roentgen
appearance of pulmonary engorgement associated with the increased flow of the left to right
shunts and that of chronic passive congestion. In
both conditions there is enlargement of the pulmonary trunk, hilar, and intrapulmonary arteries, and the heart is usually enlarged. With increased blood flow, however, there is no haziness
of the lung due to edema, no thickening and
fibrosis of the pleura, and no pleural fluid. Although the intrapulmonary and hilar vessels are
enlarged in both conditions, their outlines are

apt to be sharp and distinct in engorgement due to increased flow but indistinct and poorly defined in congestion due to obstruction distal to the pulmonary capillaries. Furthermore, pulsations of the hilar vessels are usually increased

with increased flow (*e.g.,* patent ductus arteriosus, interatrial septal defect); they are normal or decreased in chronic passive congestion.

Chronic Lung Stasis.

Chronic lung stasis appears roentgenographically different from chronic passive congestion of the lungs and therefore merits a separate description. It accompanies a chronic increase in pulmonary capillary pressure which is probably part of the same process which gives rise to chronic passive congestion; however, some of the elements of chronic passive congestion are lacking. Chronic lung stasis most often accompanies mitral valvular disease, particularly mitral stenosis. The pulmonary trunk and right and left branches are slightly enlarged; the smaller hilar vessels are likewise increased in size so that the hilar shadows are enlarged and there is a lengthening and increased convexity of the left mid-cardiac segment. The lung parenchyma has a distinctive appearance. There are numerous fine linear areas of increased density distributed more or less evenly throughout the lung fields; they are often best seen in the lung bases and near the costophrenic angles. These linear densities intersect forming a network throughout the lung. Their intersections may be angular or rounded; when they are rounded, the appearance of lung cysts is suggested and the possibility of cystic disease of the lung was considered in several of the present authors' cases. The lung structure is sharp and well defined and there is no evidence of pulmonary edema. There is rarely any significant

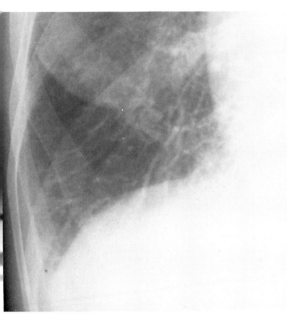

FIG. 63. COSTOPHRENIC SEPTAL LINES (KERLEY'S LINES)

Adult patient was seen with chronic elevation of the pulmonary venous pressure due to rheumatic mitral valvular disease. Seen in the right costophrenic angle are numerous roughly parallel and mostly horizontal lines thought to represent a combination of interlobular septal edema and distended lymphatics.

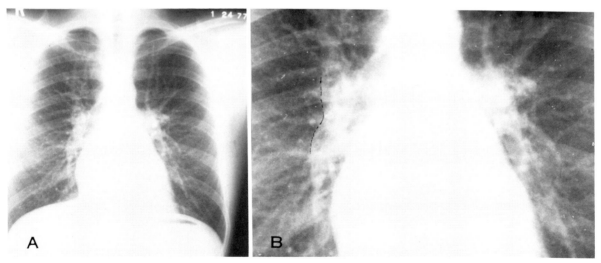

FIG. 64. PULMONARY BLOOD FLOW

(A) Redistribution of pulmonary blood flow in a case of mitral stenosis. The upper lobe arteries and veins are dilated, and the lower lobe vessels are diminished in size. (B) Enlarged view of dilated vessels in both hila. The hilar angle (angle between upper and lower lobe vessels) on the right is increased.

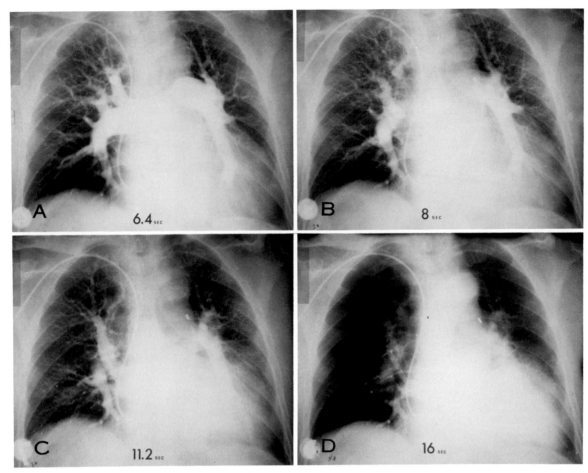

FIG. 65. REDISTRIBUTION OF FLOW IN HEART FAILURE

Pulmonary angiogram in a patient with some pulmonary congestion and chronic left ventricular failure. The arteries to the upper lobes are larger and more plentiful than in the lower lobes. In C (11.2 sec) the upper lobe veins are filled while the contrast substance is still in the arteries to the lower lobes.

amount of pleural fluid; the pleural fissures are occasionally slightly thickened.

The distinctive nature of multiple, parallel, sharply defined horizontal linear opacities in the costophrenic angles was first pointed out by Kerley (1933), who ascribed their presence to distended lymphatics secondary to passive hyperemia of the lung. More recent work by Grainger (1958), using microscopic sections and paper-mounted whole lung sections, and by Grainger and Hearn (1955) indicates that these lines are caused by thickening of pulmonary interlobular septa, usually of composite septal plates, due to extra-alveolar edema, associated with enlargement of lymphatic channels contained therein. Gough (1955) and Rossall and Gunning (1956) commenting on the radiographic changes in the lungs in mitral stenosis, affirmed the view that the anatomical basis of the lines is an increase in the bulk of the interlobular septa. Costophrenic

septal lines are probably best seen on a posteroanterior view of the chest, but occasionally oblique or lateral views will show them to advantage. They run perpendicular to the pleural surface. As a rule a single line will be of the same thickness throughout. The lines vary in number from 2 or 3–10 or 15, and they extend from 2–4 inches upward from the costophrenic angle and vary in thickness from a hairline to 2 mm in diameter (Fig. 63).

The presence of costophrenic septal lines (Kerley's lines) correlates well with pulmonary venous pressure. Carmichael *et al.* (1954) found that when these lines were present the pulmonary capillary pressure was almost invariably above 30 mm Hg. Rossall and Gunning (1956), analyzing 100 patients with mitral disease, observed that septal lines were invariably present at mean left atrial pressures exceeding 24 mm Hg, and none were found when the pressure was less than 10 mm Hg. All cases of mitral stenosis with well-marked septal lines reviewed by McMyn in 1960 had pulmonary venous pressures of greater than 20 mm Hg. No close relationship between septal lines and pulmonary arterial pressure was found. After a successful mitral valvulotomy these densities may almost entirely disappear and the lung parenchyma return to normal (Fig. 122), and this suggests that fibrosis does not play a prominent part in many patients. Not all such septal lines are due to edema, however, for some persist following operation (Harley, 1961), and in these cases fibrosis or the deposition of hemosiderin along the interlobular septa may play a role in their formation.

While Kerley's costophrenic septal lines are generally indicative of pulmonary venous hypertension in the presence of heart disease, chronic lung stasis is not the only cause. Depending upon the clinical presentation and radiographic appearance, the differential diagnosis of costophrenic septal lines should include the following entities:

Acute:
1. pulmonary edema
2. pulmonary hemorrhage
3. interstitial pneumonia

Chronic:
1. lymphangitic metastases
2. pneumoconiosis
3. mitral stenosis
4. alveolar cell carcinoma
5. sarcoidosis
6. alveolar lymphoma
7. obstruction of pulmonary veins
8. obstruction of thoracic duct
9. pulmonary lymphangiectasia
10. hyaline membrane disease
11. lipid pneumonia

Pulmonary Edema

Pulmonary edema means an excess of fluid within the lung and represents the additional feature of transudation of fluid into the alveoli, bronchi, or interstitial tissues, frequently engrafted upon existent pulmonary congestion. Actually, pulmonary edema is detected roentgenographically in a variety of conditions. Gould and Torrance (1955) found that in 64% of 100 cases the edema was unquestionably cardiac in origin, and therefore it may be presumed there was an obstructive condition or failure of the left side of the heart. In another 12 percent in which there was uremia, a cardiac factor could not be excluded. Therefore, only about three-fourths of all cases of pulmonary edema are likely to be due to obstructions of the pulmonary circulation. Other causes of pulmonary edema are (1) increase in capillary permeability and (2) decrease in colloid osmotic pressure of the blood (Barden, 1964). In uremia it is postulated that there is an increase in capillary permeability due to injury from circulating toxins (Hopps and Wisler, 1955). The colloid osmotic pressure of the blood may be reduced by excess administration of intravenous fluids or by any condition which decreases blood proteins. Capillary permeability or capillary blood pressure may be under nervous control to a degree and thus affected by central nervous system lesions. Gould and Torrance (1955) list other causes of pulmonary edema as pure uremic, 13%; anemia, 4%; central nervous system lesions, 3%; pulmonary infections, 2%; pheochromocytoma, 1%; and transfusion reactions, 1%. Inhalation of irritating gases, shock, and excessive administration of intravenous fluids are other occasional causes. The roentgenographic findings in pulmonary hemosiderosis and in Goodpasture's syndrome (hemorrhagic pulmonary-renal disease) may on occasion simulate the appearance of pulmonary edema (Sybers et al., 1965). The roentgenographic appearance of pulmonary edema does not correlate with its etiology and is rather nonspecific. For this reason it is considered in connection with its most common cause, namely pulmonary obstruction distal to the capillaries.

Pulmonary edema can occur only when the right ventricle remains adequate and continues to pump blood into the pulmonary vascular system in the face of an obstruction beyond the pulmonary capillaries. When the right ventricle fails, edema may recede. Chronic lung stasis and passive congestion will also tend to improve following right ventricular failure.

Acute pulmonary edema is characterized by the rapid onset of dyspnea, orthopnea, cyanosis, and coughing with the raising of frothy, pinkish sputum. The patient is apprehensive and restless and has a feeling of suffocation. Rhonchi and bubbling sounds originating in the bronchi are usually audible. Indeed, the appearance of the patient is so typical and the need for treatment so urgent that filming of the chest is usually not carried out; portable films are occasionally obtained under such circumstances. The attack may subside within an hour and rarely lasts longer than a few hours; however, it may end fatally. Such a clinical picture is often part of the syndrome of "paroxysmal dyspnea" and is frequently seen with a failing left ventricle or mitral valvular disease.

The roentgenographic signs of acute pulmonary edema rarely persist longer than from a few hours to days, particularly if the patient recovers. They may be present for several days before death; typically, they change rapidly. The characteristic picture consists of a diffuse increase in density around the hilar portions of both lungs; these densities are homogeneous and fade out toward the periphery. Although the opacities are commonly somewhat asymmetrical and slightly more extensive in one lung than the other, the descriptive terms "butterfly wings" and "bat wings" are reasonably good and apply to many cases. The apices and bases usually remain clear, although in severe persistent cases they may be ultimately involved (Fig. 66).

While the anatomical basis for the frequently encountered "central" distribution of pulmonary edema remains obscure, Oderr et al. (1958), from a study of emphysema by microradiologic methods, found a tendency for the central zone of the lung to be served by small twiglike branches coming off from the major trunks at near right angles and commented that the distance of capillary travel for a red cell coursing through the central zone would be long by comparison with the capillary travel distance in the periphery where the arteries and venules closely approximate each other. Herrnheiser and Hinson (1954) suggest that the formation of "butterfly" shadows depends essentially upon the disproportionate division of small prelobular and lobular vessels in the medulla or inner aspect of the lung as opposed to the prevalence of proportionate divisions in the cortex or outer aspect. Thus, any condition producing increased capillary permeability or pressure may result in selective leakage of fluid into the medullary zone of the lung if there are many more capillaries in the medullary portion than in the cortical portion (Barden, 1960).

Occasionally the opacities are blotchy and not entirely confined to the perihilar and central areas of the lung; these blotchy areas tend to become confluent. In light films the hilar vessels may appear enlarged, but this is not always so unless there is underlying chronic lung stasis or other cause for enlargement. A network of air-containing bronchi may be seen coursing through the density, and the lung vascular markings may show a slightly streaked appearance. Rarely is there any fluid in the pleural space unless there is pre-existing pulmonary congestion.

In contrast to acute pulmonary edema, symptoms and classical signs may be minimal or absent in subacute or chronic pulmonary edema. Its presence is frequently detected from the x-ray film. In addition to the central and perihilar opacities mentioned above there may be focal edema (Gould and Torrance, 1955) which is unilateral, homogeneous and frequently lobar in distribution or there may be a single rounded lesion in one lung (pseudosarcoma). However, the perihilar confluent shadows are by far the most common.

In uremia, bilateral massive opacities are often seen; these may be more dense than those seen with congestive failure due to cardiac causes and more sharply defined. In addition, there is less dilatation of the hilar blood vessels. In general, however, a precise differentiation is not possible.

Unilateral pulmonary edema, particularly when it is persistent, suggests obstruction to the pulmonary veins on one side. A single lobe only may be involved or there may be obstruction to all of the veins producing chronic edema or bilateral lung stasis. This may occur with mediastinal tumors or infections (Bindelglass and Trubowitz, 1958). Pulmonary edema due to cardiac failure may also appear to be predominantly unilateral if the patient spends any considerable time lying on one side.

Pulmonary veno-obstructive disease is a recently described entity of unknown etiology characterized by venous thrombosis and pulmonary hypertension (Liebow et al., 1973). Kerley's B lines are commonly seen as are episodes of pulmonary edema. The left atrium is not enlarged, but right ventricular hypertrophy is present. The pulmonary arteries are prominent, and the hilar vascular structures are fuzzy in outline. Pulmonary arteriography shows no evidence of arterial thromboembolism or of rapid tapering characteristic of pulmonary arterial hypertension. Stasis is seen in the arteries with varying transit times of the contrast material through the lung vasculature (indicating diffuse but spotty obstructive vascular disease). This uncommon entity is another cause of postcapillary pulmonary hypertension.

Obstructions Proximal to Pulmonary Capillaries (Conditions that Produce Precapillary Hypertension)

1. Pulmonary parenchymal abnormalities which produce vascular obstruction and cor pulmonale.

   a. Chronic obstructive emphysema.
   b. Diffuse pulmonary fibrosis secondary to (1) pneumoconiosis, (2) tuberculosis, (3) bronchiectasis, (4) collagen diseases, especially scleroderma, and (5) idiopathic.
   c. Diffuse tumor metastases (lymphohematogenous spread)

These conditions produce their effects by narrowing or obliterating large areas of the pulmo-

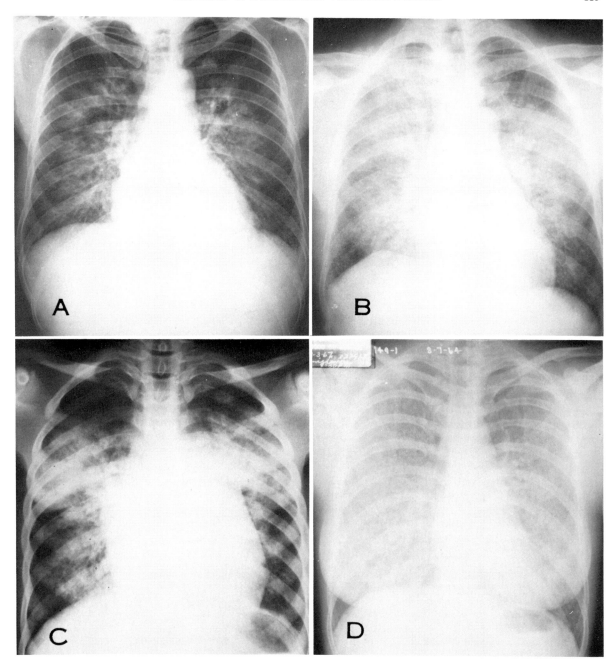

FIG. 66. PULMONARY EDEMA DUE TO VARIOUS CAUSES

(A) Uremic pulmonary edema. Fluffy infiltrations are present in the perihilar areas, sparing the apices, bases and lateral aspects of the lung. The heart is slightly enlarged because of systemic hypertension. (B) Congestive heart failure secondary to systemic hypertension. The apices and bases are spared, but alveolar infiltrations occupy the remainder of the lung fields. The cardiac apex is depressed and displaced laterally because of left ventricular enlargement. (C) Pulmonary edema due to rheumatic mitral stenosis. Because of selective shunting of blood to the upper lungs, the pulmonary edema is most marked in these areas. The enlarged heart has a "mitral" configuration. (D) Pulmonary edema secondary to near-drowning. The heart is not enlarged or deformed. The lungs are uniformly infiltrated with edema fluid.

nary vascular tree. As indicated above, it may well be that the arterioles are most vulnerable to this obliterative process, and when their number has been sufficiently reduced, there is an increase in the peripheral resistance and resultant pulmonary arterial hypertension.

Another factor which may tend to bring on or aggravate pulmonary hypertension in some cases is anoxia. Motley *et al.* (1947) found that in human beings breathing air containing 10% oxygen there was a definite increase in both systolic and diastolic pulmonary artery pressures. This was not due to an increased cardiac output but rather to an increased peripheral resistance. Consequently, it is quite possible that the low oxygen content of the alveolar air in chronic emphysema may be a further factor in increasing the vascular resistance in the lungs.

Chronic upper airway obstruction due to enlarged tonsils and adenoids may result in alveolar hypoventilation with resultant hypoxia, hypercapnia, precapillary pulmonary arterial hypertension and cor pulmonale (Levy, 1967; Gerald and Dungan, 1968). The pulmonary hypertension is reversible following tonsillectomy and adenoidectomy, but some cardiac enlargement may persist.

After an increase in vascular resistance, if the right ventricle is capable of responding, pulmonary hypertension ensues. This is followed by dilatation of the pulmonary trunk and its main branches. The smaller intrapulmonary branches remain normal or somewhat decreased in size, and it is this striking apparent attenuation in size of the pulmonary arteries as they course through the lungs toward the periphery which allows one to predict roentgenographically that pulmonary arterial hypertension is present. In emphysema, the pulmonary vessels, particularly those in and adjacent to the hilus, are sharply defined due to the exceptional contrast provided by the surrounding radiolucent lung. Although the pulmonary trunk and its branches are enlarged, they do not reach the size that is seen in interatrial septal defect and patent ductus arteriosus, and, unless there is relative pulmonic insufficiency, pulsations are minimal or absent in the pulmonary trunk and hilar vessels, whereas, in interatrial septal defect and patent ductus arteriosus, pulsations are increased in amplitude.

Fifty-nine of 62 patients with pulmonary emphysema studied by Lopez-Majano *et al.* (1966) showed well-defined areas of decreased pulmonary arterial blood flow (lung scanning with I-131 serum albumin). In the majority of cases the chest roentgenogram was inadequate for demonstrating these localized changes. The vascular damage in pulmonary emphysema, manifested as reduction in the peripheral pulmonary vascular bed, may also be shown by pulmonary angiography (Jacobson *et al.,* 1967), and its assessment may be of great importance in estimating the improvement which may be expected from therapeutic measures (Fig. 68).

The respiratory motion of the lung is undoubtedly a factor (Brenner, 1935) in propelling both the blood and lymph through the lung parenchyma although the effect of this motion on the circulation has not been precisely appraised. Certainly, respiratory changes in intrathoracic pressure are influential in causing the right heart to fill, and in emphysema where the intrathoracic pressure is permanently increased, there may be a definite impediment to filling of the right side of the heart. Overdistention of the emphysematous lungs might exert undue pressure on the exterior of the heart and thus also hamper proper filling.

Cor pulmonale

Cor pulmonale is defined as heart disease secondary to disease of the lungs or their blood vessels. In the earlier stages of cor pulmonale secondary to chronic obstructive pulmonary disease and other causes of vascular obstruction, the heart is characteristically not enlarged. Right ventricular hypertrophy is present as evidenced by thickening of the myocardium and electrocardiographic changes, but this is difficult to detect radiologically (Fig. 67B). The pulmonary artery segment on the left heart border may be increased in convexity, but this is rarely striking; it may be more noticeable in the long narrow heart than in the transverse heart and in the right anterior oblique projection than in the posteroanterior view. Likewise the descending branches of the right and left pulmonary arteries may be slightly enlarged; in emphysema these branches often stand out quite clearly. Accompanying disease in the lung parenchyma is usually evident on the chest film. Where it is extensive, one should always suspect cor pulmonale. Emphysema, however, is a clinical rather than a roentgen diagnosis, although its presence can be suspected from the chest film and particularly from fluoroscopy. Although one may find the lungs to be increased in radiolucency, the intercostal spaces to be increased in width, and the diaphragm to be flattened and irregular, these radiologic findings show only gross correlation with the patient's symptoms.

A moderate degree of cor pulmonale is present much more often than it is diagnosed; it is often unsuspected until right heart failure appears. Electrocardiography may be more helpful and reliable than the roentgen examination in indicating right ventricular hypertrophy. Right heart catheterization will often show a moderate increase in systolic and diastolic pressure with a normal or decreased flow. In the absence of

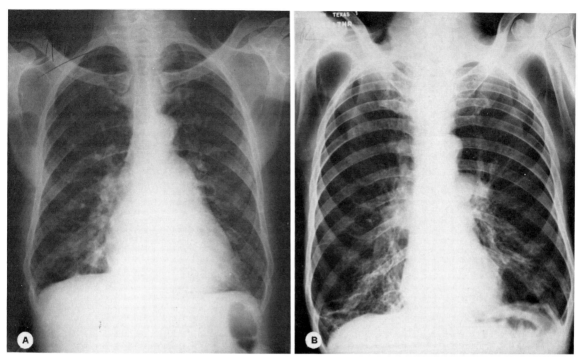

FIG. 67. ENLARGEMENT OF RIGHT SIDE OF HEART AS SEEN IN PA VIEW (COR PULMONALE)
(A) There is extensive pulmonary emphysema. At autopsy there was dilatation of the right atrium, dilatation and hypertrophy of the right ventricle, and dilatation of the pulmonary artery. The distinctive roentgen findings are a convexity of the pulmonary artery segment and a rather steep left border. (B) Patient was emaciated (84 lb) and heart weighed 250 gm. Nevertheless, at autopsy there was dilatation and hypertrophy of the right ventricle and dilatation of the pulmonary artery. There was extensive pulmonary emphysema.

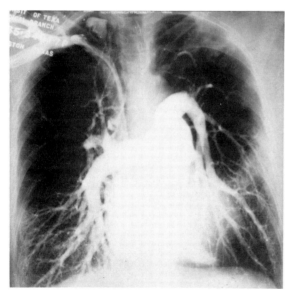

FIG. 68. ANGIOCARDIOGRAPHY IN PULMONARY EMPHYSEMA
The upper lungs are overinflated on both sides, resulting in shunting of blood into the unaffected or less affected portions of the lungs, namely the bases. The angiocardiogram shows most of the pulmonary vascular volume to reside in the lung bases.

roentgen evidence of pulmonary edema or chronic lung stasis, the inference can be drawn that there is an obstruction proximal to the pulmonary capillaries.

In advanced cor pulmonale the right ventricle extends anteriorly and to the left and encroaches upon the restrosternal space. The heart is rotated in a counterclockwise direction as seen from above; the aortic knob is decreased in prominence or invisible; the left midcardiac segment becomes longer and more convex; the left lower border may become moderately steep and straight. The right atrium eventually dilates and the transverse diameter of the heart is increased. The right ventricle may enlarge until it forms a considerable segment of the left heart border and displaces the left ventricle posteriorly. Thus, in the postero-anterior projection the heart has a pearshaped or globular appearance with little evidence of change in the aortic knob (Fig. 69). The superior vena caval shadow is often widened, and, if there is relative tricuspid insufficiency, it may pulsate with atrial systole.

Clinically at this stage there is usually cyanosis, peripheral edema, ascites, enlarged liver,

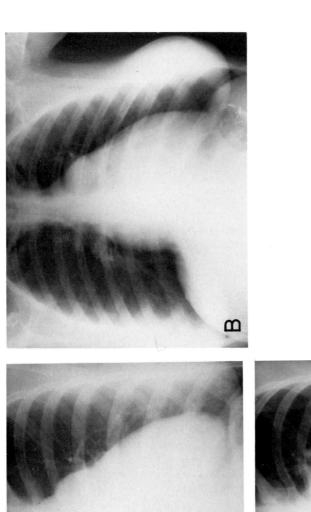

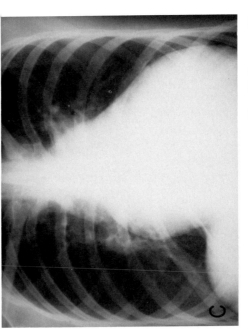

FIG. 69. PRIMARY PULMONARY HYPERTENSION

(A) Twenty-one-year-old white woman. Catheterization pressures as follows: pulmonary artery, 107/58; right ventricle, 106/ 0–9; brachial artery, 99/61. A small right-to-left shunt through the foramen ovale was present. (B) Nineteen-year-old white woman. Catheterization pressures as follows: pulmonary artery, 102/50; right ventricle, 102/14; brachial artery, 112/70. No intracardiac shunts were demonstrated. (C) Twenty-four-year-old white woman. Catheterization pressures as follows: pulmonary artery, 137/60; right ventricle, 130/0; brachial artery, 132/95. A sizeable right-to-left shunt through the foramen ovale was present.

and often clubbing of the fingers and toes. The prognosis is poor, and death may occur in a few weeks or months.

2. Pulmonary vascular abnormalities which produce obstruction and cor pulmonale.
   a. primary pulmonary hypertension
   b. pulmonary arterial hypertension associated with known cardiovascular abnormalities
      (1) rheumatic mitral valve disease
      (2) congenital heart disease
   c. pulmonary thromboembolism
   d. infections of the pulmonary vascular system
      (1) syphilis
      (2) schistosomiasis

Primary Pulmonary Hypertension

Primary or solitary pulmonary hypertension is defined as a persistent elevation of pulmonary arterial pressure sufficient to produce enlargement and ultimately failure of the right ventricle, where the cause is confined to obstruction in the lesser pulmonary arteries of intrinsic origin (Evans et al., 1957). It is about 3 times as common in women as in men and occurs predominantly between the ages of 20 and 40, although cases of both sexes and a wide age range have been reported (Farrar et al., 1961). The dominant symptom is rapidly increasing dyspnea on exertion. The electrocardiogram shows a pattern of right ventricular hypertrophy, and cardiac catheterization will exclude an intracardiac shunt and demonstrate considerable elevation of pulmonary arterial and right ventricular pressures. The clinical course is apt to be inexorably downhill, the average duration of life from the onset of cardiac symptoms being 2 1/2 years.

While considerable uncertainty with regard to the etiology of primary pulmonary hypertension exists, several hypotheses have been advanced. Civins and Edwards (1951) have described the thick muscular wall with relatively narrow lumen seen in the pulmonary arteries and arterioles of the fetus. During fetal life this serves to maintain a high resistance to blood flow through the pulmonary capillaries thus serving to shunt blood through the patent ductus into the aorta. If the fetal type of pulmonary arteriole persists after birth, primary pulmonary hypertension occurs. Van Epps (1957) has suggested that primary pulmonary hypertension in its earliest phases may be due to increased vascular tone or resistance in the precapillary vascular bed and not to any structural change in the vessels. Studies using Priscoline and hexamethonium in which the pulmonary arterial hypertension was tem-

porarily relieved or reduced after administration of the drugs would confirm this and implicate the autonomic nervous system, at least in the earlier stages. Diffuse pulmonary embolization from peripheral venous thrombosis and allergic arteritis affecting only lung vessels with subsequent thrombosis and organization have also been suggested as possible causes (Farrar et al., 1961). Rosenberg (1964), in a clinical and postmortem study of 9 patients with the diagnosis of primary pulmonary hypertension, found pulmonary emboli and thrombi to be responsible in 6. Evans et al. (1957) emphasized the frequency and importance of focal medial hypoplasia or aplasia in solitary pulmonary hypertension, supporting the view that these medial defects cause an intimal reaction to normal fluctuations in pulmonary arterial pressure and in this way initiate hypertension.

Whatever the cause, the pathologic changes in the lungs are uniform and consist of marked proliferation of the intima of the arterioles with thickening and fibrosis of the muscular wall associated with extensive thrombosis and organization and obliteration of the lumen of the arterioles over large areas of the lung. The pulmonary artery and its major divisions in the lung are moderately to greatly dilated and may be the site of arteriosclerotic plaques. Uniform musculoelastic hypertrophy in the larger arteries and a comparable increase in muscle tissue in the smaller branches may be found. Short (1956) by postmortem pulmonary arteriography, has shown widespread loss of normal peripheral arborization in primary pulmonary hypertension in contrast to the regularity of the arterial branching and the progressive decrease in caliber extending down to the finest arterioles in the normal, emphasizing the extensive and abrupt diminution in arterial and arteriolar caliber resulting from occlusive changes in the smaller vessels. Right ventricular enlargement is a consequent finding.

Radiographically the heart is seen to be slightly to moderately enlarged, and this enlargement is predominantly due to increase in the size of the right ventricle. With the development of relative tricuspid insufficiency, the right atrium may also dilate. The main pulmonary artery and its right and left branches may be considerably enlarged, but this enlargement is rapidly terminated lateral to the hilus, and the peripheral lung fields are ischemic (Fig. 69). It may be impossible radiologically to distinguish between primary pulmonary hypertension and pulmonary arterial hypertension associated with left to right intracardiac shunts or certain cases of mitral stenosis, and cardiac catheterization with employment of indicator dye dilution curves or similar maneuvers may be required to establish the diagnosis.

Pulmonary Arterial Hypertension Associated with Known Cardiovascular Abnormalities

In mitral stenosis an increase in the pulmonary arterial pressure is inevitable if the circulation is to be maintained in the face of obstruction at the mitral orifice. This natural rise in pressure is augmented in a number of patients by disproportionate pulmonary arterial hypertension producing increased pulmonary vascular resistance and forming a second barrier to the circulation in the pulmonary vessels in addition to the primary barrier at the mitral valve. While opinion on the nature of the abnormal pulmonary arterial resistance in mitral stenosis is divided, it is probably true to say that the majority of workers in this field believe that it arises from pulmonary vasoconstriction (Evans and Short, 1957). Relief from this increase in peripheral arteriolar resistance may be obtained following mitral valvulotomy, provided that severe organic changes have not developed. Eventually, organic narrowing of the peripheral arterial and arteriolar structures supervenes, and these changes consist of increase in thickness of the medial wall of the arteries associated with focal constrictions due to atheromas (Harrison, 1958). While reversal of organic changes in the pulmonary vessels probably does not occur after mitral valvulotomy, a fall in pulmonary artery pressure may none the less be obtained in many cases following operation and is probably due to the removal of vasoconstrictive stimuli produced by an abnormally high left atrial pressure (Heath and Whitaker, 1955). An occasionally striking finding in pulmonary arterial hypertension due to mitral stenosis is dilatation of the segmental arteries to the upper lobe with usually marked contraction of the vessels to the middle and lower lobes (Short, 1956). Reflex vasoconstriction secondary to increased pressure in the pulmonary venous circuit is the probable cause. Steiner (1971) speculates that blood flow in the dependent parts of the lung, just above the diaphragm, may be reduced due to the narrowing of the extra-alveolar vessels by an increased interstitial pressure (distention of the interstitial space by edema fluid) as well as by reduced expansion of the lung parenchyma in the dependent zones.

Radiographically, the main pulmonary artery and its proximal divisions are apt to be considerably enlarged, and it may be possible to appreciate differential lower zone constriction of the pulmonary arterial tree distal to the main divisions, while the upper lobe branches are normal or increased in size. The peripheral lung fields are apt to appear oligemic. Evaluation of the size of the right descending pulmonary artery on a posteroanterior teleoroentgenogram may permit fairly accurate prediction of pulmonary hypertension in mitral stenosis. Schwedel et al. (1957) and Johnson et al. (1961) have studied the width of the right descending pulmonary artery in 105 and 48 reported patients, respectively, with predominant mitral stenosis. They suggest that right descending pulmonary artery width of 15 mm or more is definitely associated with significant pulmonary arterial hypertension, although a linear correlation was not found. More recently, Chang (1962) has reported on the normal roentgenographic measurement of this vessel in 1,085 cases and states that pulmonary arterial hypertension is most likely present if the right descending pulmonary artery measures 17 mm or more in males and 16 mm or more in females. A significant increase in pulmonary artery pressure is unlikely to be present if the right descending pulmonary artery width is 14 mm or less. It is probable that within fairly broad limits the presence of pulmonary arterial hypertension in mitral stenosis can be appraised and graded, but several criteria should be used. Reliance upon a single or a few diagnostic features and their numerical expression is probably less accurate than the qualitative evaluation of several features. Viamonte et al. (1962) list 10 diagnostic criteria in mitral stenosis and found a good correlation between these radiographic signs and pulmonary artery pressure and wedge pressure, as measured at catheterization by grading the pulmonary hypertension minimal, moderate, and severe.

The relationship of pulmonary arterial hypertension to certain forms of congenital heart disease is incompletely understood, although several theories of causation have been advanced. In some cases it appears that equalization of pulmonary and systemic resistance exerts an important protective function by preventing an unequal distribution of blood (e.g., single ventricle and large ventricular septal defect); in other cases pulmonary arterial hypertension is found in association with congenital syndromes causing a left to right shunt which ordinarily show normal pulmonary artery pressures. In the first type a causal relationship between the cardiac malformation and the persistence of high pulmonary resistance appears probable, whereas in the second type pulmonary hypertension may be a coincidental complication as it appears to be unrelated to the magnitude of the shunt and to the large pulmonary blood flow (Selzer, 1954). Evans and Short (1958), examining histologic sections and postmortem arteriograms from cases of interatrial septal defect, interventricular septal defect, patent ductus arteriosus, and aortic-pulmonary window, concluded that the development of pulmonary hypertension does not appear to be related to the size of the shunt or the age of the patient but possibly to some inherent predisposition. Wood (1952) states that the high pulmonary vascular resistance in most cases of patent ductus arteriosus and interventricular septal defect is established at birth or in infancy, but does not develop until adult life in most interatrial septal defects. Pulmonary arterial hypertension is the natural condition of the fetal lung and may be caused in part by atelectasis and in part be due to the structure of the pulmonary vessels. An element of vasoconstriction cannot be excluded. Persistence of a fetal type of pulmonary arteriole with a relatively narrow lumen and thick wall into adult life may be responsible for the pulmonary hypertension seen in some congenital anomalies with left to right intracardiac shunts (Edwards, 1957). A possible relationship between narrowing of the pulmonary arterioles in congenital heart disease with left to right shunt and torrential pulmonary blood flow has been considered (Doyle et al., 1957), but there is evidence which suggests that anatomical changes in the blood vessels of the lungs do not follow directly from an increased pulmonary blood flow (Heath and Whitaker, 1957). Whatever the underlying causal factors, pulmonary arterial hypertension in congenital heart disease is associated with widespread occlusion of small arteries and arterioles with patchy intimal thickening in vessels not completely occluded. The elastic pulmonary arteries show atheromatous changes, and the media of the small muscular pulmonary arteries is hypertrophied, with intimal proliferation of fibroelastic tissue leading to partial occlusion of these small vessels. The pathologic changes differ in no important respect from those observed in solitary pulmonary hypertension or in hypertension associated with mitral stenosis.

While proportionate enlargement of the pulmonary arteries and their terminal divisions is characteristic of congenital cardiac anomalies with increased pulmonary blood flow, abrupt decrease in caliber of these vessels lateral to the hilus on either side characterizes the appearance in pulmonary arterial hypertension. The occasionally marked disparity in size between the main pulmonary artery and its proximal divisions and the clear and radiolucent peripheral lung fields is a striking finding. The importance of

radiographic identification of these changes is emphasized by the physiologic implications of the development of pulmonary hypertension, particularly in cases of left to right shunt. Cyanosis, polycythemia, and clubbing of the fingers and toes may develop, and hemoptysis from pulmonary infarction may ensue. In such cases it may be anticipated that pressure in the main pulmonary artery will not be reduced after closure of the defect, and in fact such operative treatment may cause worsening of the patient's condition and precipitate right heart failure.

It is probably safe to say that oligemia of the peripheral lung fields in congenital heart disease with intracardiac shunts usually indicates severe pulmonary arterial hypertension and actual or impending reversal of the shunt.

Pulmonary Thromboembolism

Pulmonary thromboembolism (PTE) continues to be a common cause of mortality and morbidity and is estimated by Coon et al. (1959) to be the cause of approximately 48,000 deaths a year in the United States. In recent years, a number of new diagnostic and therapeutic procedures have been developed and are being used on an increasing scale. We suspect that they will have some impact on the control of this condition, but as yet there are no concrete data that show a significant decrease in mortality or morbidity from PTE.

The literature and personal experience attest to the difficulties in diagnosis. The triad of dyspnea, tachycardia, and hemoptysis which are typically associated with acute embolism are quite nonspecific and easily masked by other causes for the same clinical signs. Hemoptysis is relatively infrequent and usually depends on the occurrence of infarction which in itself occurs in a minority of cases. The newer and more definitive diagnostic procedures, such as radioisotopic scans and pulmonary angiograms, are still not widely available or their employment is often delayed beyond the time when they can participate in the crucial decisions necessary for effective therapy.

Anticoagulant therapy has been available for at least 30 years and has been used on an increasing scale for the past 15–20 years. Heparin may have some beneficial effect in acute pulmonary thromboembolism, but anticoagulation therapy in general is only a preventative measure. Although it has been widely used and undoubtedly has had beneficial results, there are still no extensive data that show a material reduction in the overall morbidity or mortality of PTE. Furthermore, anticoagulation therapy carries certain risks and therefore should not be employed without a positive diagnosis in which case it is the lesser of two risks.

Pulmonary embolectomy for massive pulmonary thromboembolism was first advocated by Trendelenburg and used occasionally and usually without effect and as a last resort for a period of 50 years (Donaldson *et al.*, 1963). With the increased availability of hypothermia and particularly of cardiopulmonary bypass, the number of successful cases has increased (Cooley *et al.*, 1962; Cross and Mowlem, 1967). However, these sophisticated surgical procedures are not widely available, and even where they are available, they frequently cannot be mobilized in sufficient time to be effective. The combined mortality from surgical embolectomy continues to be forbiddingly high, although there must be a place for this procedure in those patients in extremis who cannot be stabilized and in whom no other therapy could possibly be effective.

Recently, fibrinolytic agents, such as Urokinase (The Urokinase Pulmonary Embolism Trial—A National Cooperative Study, *Circulation,* Supplement II, April, 1973) have been proven to increase the rate of lysis of fresh emboli. When used promptly or within a few days, they have decreased the size of large central emboli and appear to have improved the clinical course of the patient. There remains a possibility that such agents as Urokinase and perhaps Streptokinase may be useful in the massive emboli in which the condition of the patient remains unstable. In any event, any of these therapeutic measures must be used immediately, and this necessitates a prompt diagnosis.

Vena caval ligation, plication, or the insertion of sieves transvenously are maneuvers to prevent further embolization. They carry some risk in themselves and are not considered until the initial attack of PTE. Vena caval ligation particularly carries considerable undesirable risks of permanent edema of the legs and possible incapacity. Also, possibly as many as 20% of emboli originate in the right side of the heart or at sites other than in the lower extremities or pelvis.

Although massive embolization occurring as a single episode is an important aspect of PTE, it is probably not the most frequent. PTE tends to occur as a complication of left ventricular failure, rheumatic valvular disease, myocarditis, and terminal cancer. Also, obesity and fractures with immobilization and the use of oral contraceptives may be associated either with acute or chronic recurring pulmonary embolization. Smaller but chronically recurring emboli may cause few dramatic symptoms and thus be completely over-looked for a long time. The capability of fibrinolytic lysing qualities of the pulmonary blood vessels is diminished by pulmonary stasis (Paraskus *et al.*, 1973; Chait *et al.*, 1967; Dalen *et al.*, 1969). Recurrent embolization and inability of the lung to lyse repeated embolization may eventually reduce the cross-sectional area of the pulmonary vascular system to less than one-half of the normal. At this point, pulmonary hypertension appears and may be progressive producing cor pulmonale. The reduction in the cross-sectional area of the pulmonary circulation is due to organizing emboli and thrombi, plaques and atherosclerotic thickening of the intima and media, and also sizeable fibrous webs and valves which extend along the lumen of the medium-sized arteries (Korn *et al.*, 1962). Also, scars due to previous infarctions may obliterate parts of the pulmonary vascular system. All of these may lead to irreversible and usually progressive changes producing right-sided heart failure and death. The onset of chronic recurring pulmonary thromboembolism may be obscure and apparently lasts over a period of several years. It is only when the signs of pulmonary hypertension appear that the condition is suspected.

In summary, PTE may be acute or chronic. It is a quite common condition but, if the patient survives, may not recur and may leave an otherwise unimpaired pulmonary circulation. On the other hand, there is some tendency to recurrence (Barker *et al.*, 1941), and this may continue until permanent and irreversible damage is produced in the pulmonary circulation. All methods of treatment carry some risk, and this particularly applies to surgical embolectomy. Consequently, there is great emphasis on diagnosis, and the most definitive diagnostic methods are radiologic.

Radiologic Diagnosis. Radiologic diagnosis uses three modalities, namely conventional chest radiographs, radioisotopic scans, and pulmonary angiography. These procedures generally complement each other and are often used in sequence. Chest radiographs are the most widely available and are generally the first procedure in suspected PTE. Unfortunately, they are often performed with portable apparatus and are thus less than perfect technically. The incidence of abnormal findings in radiographs of the chest in patients with PTE is estimated to be 70–80% (Stein *et al.*, 1959). The present authors feel that this estimate is too high, and certainly the incidence of highly suggestive or specific findings is much lower.

CHANGES IN THE CHEST FILM DUE TO PTE. (1) Infarction. (2) Incomplete or abortive infarcts.

(3) Plate-like atelectasis. (4) Elevation of diaphragm on involved side. (5) Pleural effusion—usually minimal. (6) Diminution in size, distortion, pruning, or amputation of the midzone pulmonary arteries. (7) Enlargement and/or distortion of hilar vascular structures. (8) Enlargement of descending branches of the pulmonary artery—at least in the major portion of the course. (9) Avascular areas in the peripheral lung (Westermark sign) (1938). (10) Changes in cardiac contour.

Infarction. Infarction is a well-understood pathologic entity. Following arterial occlusion, there is gross hemorrhage into the lung, and initially this hemorrhagic area is surrounded by considerable edema and exudate, some of which contain red cells. As the infarct matures, there is some resorption of the edema, and the boundaries of the infarct become sharper and more definitive. Fibrous tissue proliferates and forms a capsule-like structure around the infarct. Heitzman *et al.* (1972) have proposed that the basic anatomic unit involved in infarction is the secondary pulmonary lobule. The fibrous tissue septa of the lobule tend to prevent entrance of collateral blood flow into this unit of the lung. Not all of the lobule needs to be involved in the infarction, however, and, of course, more than one lobule can be affected. The infarct heals by

fibrosis, and this requires several weeks to two months and usually results in a scar which may be linear or more irregular (Hampton and Castleman, 1940; Fleischner *et al.,* 1941). Most infarcts involve the pleural surface but not all (Heitzman *et al.,* 1972). The conglomerate structure consisting of several involved pulmonary lobules often has a proximal rounded appearance producing a hump-like shadow in the roentgenogram known as the Hampton hump. This is particularly noticeable when the infarct involves the lappet of the lung near the costophrenic angle (Fig. 71).

The initial shadow produced on the roentgenogram is poorly defined and has a density approximating that of a pneumonia or of other water density shadows in the lung. It is often described as "blotched". Over the ensuing two or three days, it becomes more sharply defined. It may be roughly oval or spindle-shaped and is rarely triangular as has been described in earlier literature. It usually abuts on a pleural surface that can be demonstrated by a suitable projection, but this is not always so (Heitzman *et al.,* 1972). A mature infarct may have a nodular appearance suggesting the presence of a cancer (Fig. 73). When it reaches a well-defined contour and persists for several days and particularly if it is in association with chronic heart failure or

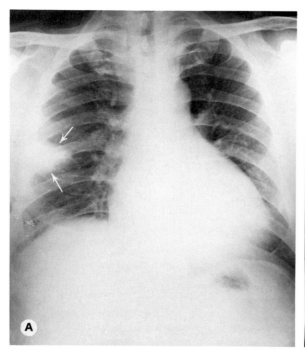
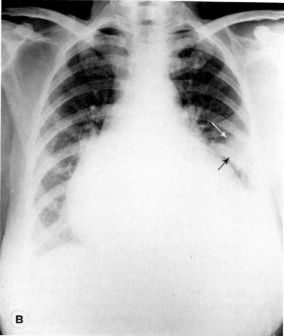

FIG. 70. TWO SEPARATE CASES OF PULMONARY INFARCTION

(A) A 51-year-old man with hypertensive and arteriosclerotic heart disease. (B) Hypertensive heart disease. There was only slight pain in the left chest.

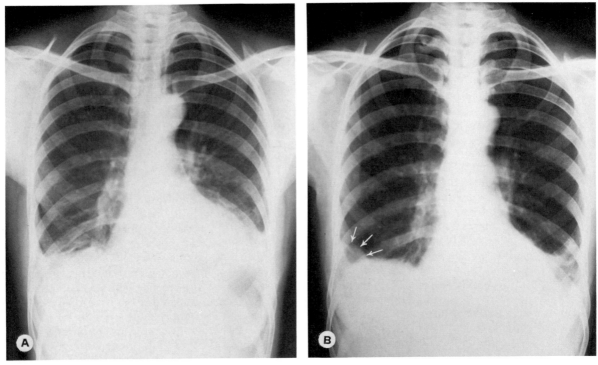

FIG. 71. PULMONARY INFARCTION

(A) Film exposed on 12th postoperative day and a few hours after onset of pain in right chest, slight fever, and tachycardia. (B) Film exposed 2 days later. There is a shadow typical of infarction in the right costophrenic angle (arrows). The shadow in the left lower lung and costophrenic angle may represent an additional infarct.

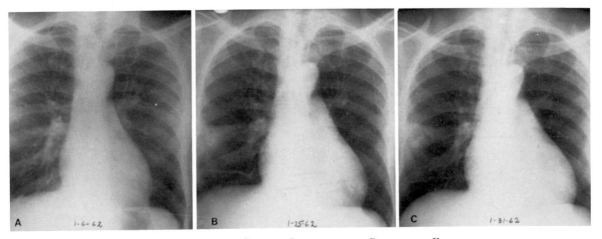

FIG. 72. PULMONARY AND CARDIAC CHANGES AFTER PULMONARY EMBOLISM

(A) Posteroanterior chest film of a 48-year-old man exposed on January 6, 1962, at which time the patient complained of shortness of breath and nonproductive cough of 3 days duration. (B) Posteroanterior chest film exposed on January 25, 1962, at which time the patient complained of sharp pain in the right lateral chest, intensified by deep breathing, along with shortness of breath and hemoptysis. The film shows the development of a wedgeshaped opacity in the lateral segment of the middle lobe on the right suggesting pulmonary infarction. In addition, the heart had enlarged moderately, and the pulmonary artery segment had become longer and more prominent. (C) The patient was treated with bed rest, antibiotics, and general supportive measures, and he improved somewhat. A posteroanterior chest film on January 31, 1962, showed little change in the area of pulmonary consolidation but slight continued enlargement of the heart. He died suddenly on February 3, 1962. At autopsy massive embolic occlusion of both pulmonary arteries was found, and the site of origin was considered to be the veins of the lower extremities. An organizing infarct was found in the right middle lobe.

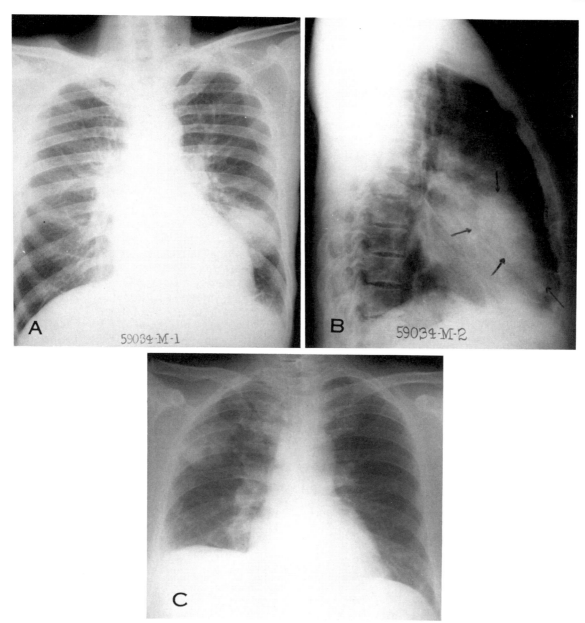

FIG. 73. INFARCTS THAT WERE RESECTED BECAUSE OF A PREOPERATIVE DIAGNOSIS OF CARCINOMA OF LUNG
(A and B) 58-year-old male with a history of hemoptysis. Infarct is in lingula. (C) 60-year-old male with hemoptysis. Large infarct is in posterior segment of right upper lobe.

some other predisposing condition, its diagnosis is easy (Fig. 70). Hampton and Castleman (1940) found that infarction was present in 58–90% of their cases of PTE examined at autopsy, the latter figure (90%) applying to cardiac patients. This is very much higher than that reported by other investigators who found that the incidence of infarction varied between 10 and 15% (Freiman et al., 1965; Smith et al., 1964). Certainly, infarction is a rare finding in massive PTE and

occurs in less than half and probably less than one-quarter of all other cases. Consequently, failure to recognize a pulmonary infarct has little value in excluding the presence of PTE.

Incomplete or Abortive Infarcts. Experimental embolism in dogs, radiologic observations in patients, and postmortem studies have shown conclusively that embolism may produce some hemorrhage and outpouring of fluid in the segment of lung supplied by the obstructed vessel. This reaction frequently stops short of infarction and tissue death and is reversible. Such changes will clear within a few days to a week and will leave no residua. Most infarcts are surrounded by such a zone of edema and hemorrhage which partially resolve leaving the final sharply defined true infarct (Hampton, 1941; Fleischner, 1962, 1966). Serial chest films and experimental studies in dogs suggest that this is a more common reaction than that of infarction and that it is the cause of the often observed pulmonary shadows seen in patients with the clinical profile of embolism. These shadows, usually of moderate size with poorly defined boundaries and water density, change in contour from day to day and frequently resolve within a few days to a week. There is reason to believe that many instances of abortive infarction have been confused with postoperative pneumonia because of the rapid resolution (Fleischner, 1966). Observations of serial chest films confirm that incomplete infarction is a more common phenomenon than frank infarction and furthermore that most frank infarcts are surrounded by an area of incomplete infarction that resolves over a period of a few days leaving the sharper outlines of the frank infarct. Both processes appear to be more common with smaller or segmental emboli and are rather uncommon in massive central embolization unless, of course, there has been preceding small vessel obstruction.

Plate-Like Atelectasis. In experimental unilateral pulmonary artery occlusion in dogs, an increased airway resistance is a common observation (Maddison *et al.,* 1967; Jaffe and Figley, 1967). Wheezing is occasionally observed in patients with confirmed pulmonary embolism (Gorham, 1961). Jaffe and Figley (1967) attempted to demonstrate bronchial spasm following experimental embolization in dogs. They outlined the bronchi by means of bronchography. They could not find convincing evidence of bronchial spasm in bronchi at the just visible level of 1.0 mm. However, the work of Nadel *et al.* (1964) suggests that spasm of the alveolar ducts does occur following microemboli. They propose that this reaction is due to the release of histamine or serotonin from the platelets trapped in the regional thromboembolus. The serotonin may have some effect upon the lung surfactant so that in association with airway obstruction the alveolus collapses and its walls tend to adhere to each other. It is a clinical observation that heparin tends to relieve patients suffering from pulmonary embolism with airway obstruction and therefore has some direct effect on this mechanism in the production of atelectasis. Whatever the cause the appearance of plate-like atelectasis is seen with some frequency in patients with pulmonary thromboembolism (Fleischner, 1966). These plate-like areas of atelectasis are more frequent in the lower lung zones. They tend to be long and reach the pleura at some point. Fleischner (1966) suggests that they can be differentiated from scars because of their length and the fact that they usually do reach the pleura. Also, they resolve and disappear, indicating conclusively that they are not scars.

Air trapping in the region of a peripheral embolus has been occasionally observed by the present authors (Fig. 74, A and B). It usually disappears in a few days and is also suggestive evidence for the presence of bronchospasm.

Elevation of Diaphragm on Involved Side. Some elevation of the diaphragm on the involved side is a common finding (Torrance, 1959; Stein, 1959). It is often associated with pleural fluid or some other radiographic finding.

Pleural Effusion. Pleural effusion is a nonspecific finding and sometimes difficult to evaluate, particularly in portable films and films made in the AP or recumbent projection. In many instances, it is simply an indication of pleural irritation. A pleural effusion in association with some other finding, such as a pulmonary infiltrate, is a common (about 50%) sign of pulmonary thromboembolism (Figley *et al.,* 1967). It is usually small in amount. As an isolated finding it is much less frequent and does not necessarily mean that infarction has occurred. When found in an appropriate clinical setting it is of considerable diagnostic significance. It may or may not be bloody.

Diminution in Size, Distortion, Pruning, or Amputation of the Midzone Pulmonary Arteries. These signs, of course, are more valid when they can be shown to be of recent origin. Comparison with previous chest films is therefore helpful. Occasionally they can be quite distinctive and are particularly distinctive when associated with avascular areas in the peripheral lung zones (Westermark sign—see below). In the present authors' experience, they are more common with chronic and recurrent embolization than they are with fresh embolization (Fig. 77). Rarely one of the major arteries may show an eccentric segmental narrowing beyond which the artery widens appreciably to almost its usual caliber. The appearance suggests an organized thromboembolus with contraction of one side of the artery. Other rarer changes are branching cylindrical calcifications representing calcified thrombus material within the pulmonary artery (McAlister and Blatt, 1962).

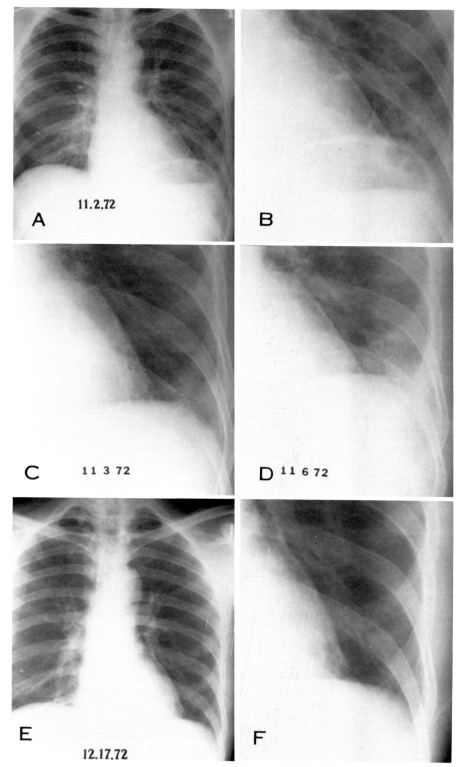

FIG. 74. ABORTIVE INFARCTION IN A 40-YEAR-OLD MALE

(A) Chest film on 11/2/72, three days after sudden onset of chest pain and hemoptysis. Ill-defined opacity in the left base and costophrenic angle. (B) Close-up of left costophrenic angle showing ill-defined density and air trapping. (C and D) One and four days later, respectively. Air trapping has disappeared. Opacity is still poorly defined—patient on anticoagulants. (E and F) Six weeks later. Chest is normal.

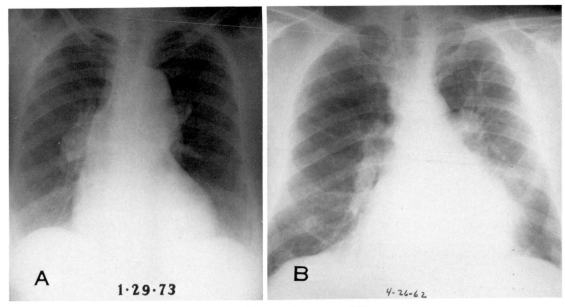

FIG. 75. MASSIVE BILATERAL PTE

(A) and (B) are chest films of two different patients with massive bilateral PTE. In (A) note the large tumor-like mass representing the right hilus that is due to the dilated right pulmonary artery filled with thrombus. The left hilus is bizarre in contour. Both patients died within a few days with right-sided heart failure.

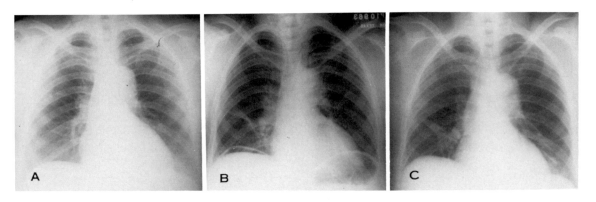

FIG. 76. PLATE-LIKE ATELECTASIS WITH POSTOPERATIVE PTE

(A) Preoperative. (B) Fourth postoperative day and after sudden onset of dyspnea. (C) Seventh postoperative day. Area of atelectasis has increased in size, and there are linear shadows in the left lung indicating probable bilateral PTE.

Enlargement and/or Distortion of Hilar Vascular Structures. This change is more common with massive and particularly recurrent embolization. The cause of the enlargement and particularly of some of the degrees of distortion is usually due to increased pulmonary artery pressure associated with extensive embolization. The enlargement of the hilar arteries may become quite striking (Fig. 75), and the shadows are often plump and rounded when seen in one projection and thus may resemble a tumor or hilar adenopathy. This finding is particularly suggestive when it is associated with amputation of the mid zone pulmonary arteries and avascularity of an adjacent segment of the lung.

Enlargement of Descending Branches of the Pulmonary Artery. Fleischner (1965), Davis (1964), and Teplick *et al.* (1964) describe enlargement of the descending branch of the pulmonary artery as strong evidence of a peripheral embolus on the same side. On the right side the descending artery is easily seen, and its diameter just distal to the hilus normally does not exceed 15 mm in the adult. Any increase of this diameter in the appropriate clinical setting is suggestive of embolization.

Avascular Areas in the Peripheral Lung. The lodgement of a thromboembolus in a segmental or larger artery greatly decreases the blood flow to the adjacent segment of lung. This increases the radiolucency of this segment, particularly when compared with adjacent portions of the same lung or comparative areas of the other lung. Westermark (1938) described such segments as seen in the chest film, and in many of these cases the radiolucent area was triangular in shape suggesting its vascular origin. An extension of this finding is seen where there is massive unilateral or predominantly unilateral embolism with diversion of most of the pulmonary blood flow to the opposite lung. Then the difference in radiolucency and prominence of the vascular structures between the two lungs becomes striking. As an isolated finding a radiolucent area in one lung and particularly a triangular-shaped one has been a most infrequent finding in the authors' experience, and this is supported by the opinion of others (Stein *et al.,* 1959). However, when it is associated with changes in the adjacent hilus or amputation and pruning of the mid zone arteries and in the appropriate clinical setting it is a helpful but sometimes misleading sign. It is most useful where there is a previous recent film for comparison. Occasionally, both lungs may be quite avascular, and the appearance of the chest film may suggest diffuse emphysema (Fig. 78).

Changes in Cardiac Contour. With extensive persistent obstruction involving more than one-half of the cross-sectional area of the pulmonary vascular bed, right ventricular pressure increases producing cor pulmonale. The main pulmonary artery enlarges producing straightening of the left cardiac border. If this condition persists, the right ventricle dilates and the cardiac silhouette enlarges, predominantly towards the left, with straightening of the upper left heart border. Such a change, even though minimal, suggests extensive bilateral embolization and is a serious prognostic sign.

Pulmonary edema does occur with thromboembolism (Fleischner, 1965) but in the authors' experience is not common. In a number of cases with massive central embolization there is some increased density in the lungs that is compatible with edema but could be attributed to simply poor aeration. Also, left heart failure could be a contributing factor. Pulmonary edema has not been an important radiographic sign of embolism.

Cavitation within sterile infarcts has received little attention and is thought to be unusual (Fig. 77). Septic infarcts typically cavitate. In our experience, sterile infarcts are occasionally associated with some degree of air trapping or bulla formation which can be confused with cavitation. Some degree of air trapping is occasionally seen adjacent to abortive infarcts (Fig. 74, A and B) and is further evidence of bronchial spasm. These areas of air trapping tend to clear rapidly, and this confirms their identity.

Despite the numerous changes that can be identified in chest films as compatible with PTE, there are still a sizeable proportion of cases in which the chest films are entirely negative or in which the findings are nonspecific. The chest film is most often normal in central massive embolization, a condition in which immediate appropriate therapy is necessary. For these reasons, the presence of a normal chest film should in no way discourage and is an indication for the use of the more definitive radiologic procedures, namely the lung scan and the pulmonary arteriogram.

The reader is referred to the papers of Wagner *et al.* (1964) and Wagner and Tow (1967) and also to standard works concerning the technique of performing the lung scan. This procedure measures the distribution of blood flow in the lungs and indicates those volumes of the lung that are under or non-perfused. Decrease or nonperfusion is reflected by an area of decreased or absent radiodensity as seen on the scan. Three basic patterns are produced by PTE as seen on the lung scan. These are the crescent-shaped peripheral defect, the lobar or large segmental defect, and the peripheral rind-like defect (Eaton *et al.,* 1969). The crescentic or triangular-shaped peripheral defect is attributed to occlusion of a small or medium-sized artery near the periphery. It may be associated with an infarct. The lobar defect is due to a larger central embolus with partial or near occlusion of a lobar artery and even more extensive central obstruction. These scans may correlate well with pulmonary angiograms. The peripheral rind type defects have been investigated and explained by Eaton *et al.* (1969). Multiple microemboli occlude many small peripheral vessels. This in turn leaves an avascular peripheral volume of lung that is underperfused. This appears as a diminution in size of the lobes. This peripheral rind may be uneven and easily recognized, but at times it is difficult to detect, particularly if more than one lobe is involved. The most striking change appears in the region of the interlobar fissures where the lobes abut on each other, and the peripheral rind of underperfused lung produces a broad stripe of decreased density that follows the course of the fissure. These stripes are best seen on the lateral scans, and consequently these should be routine

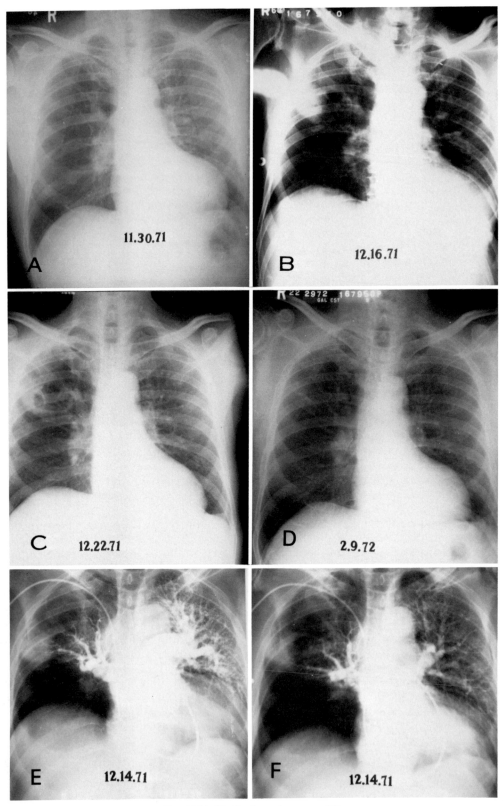

FIG. 77(A–F). See legend on page 129.

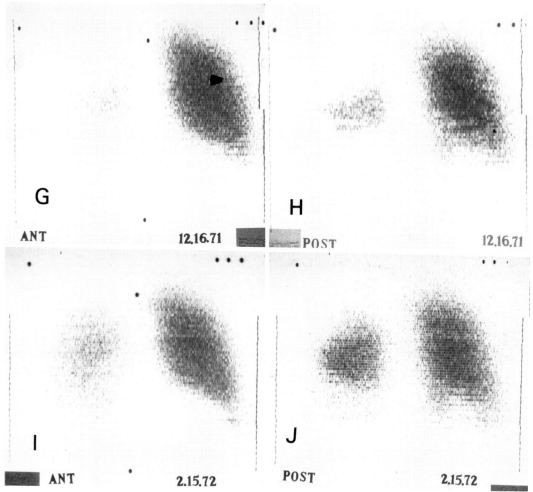

FIG. 77. RECURRENT MASSIVE PULMONARY THROMBOEMBOLISM IN A PATIENT WITH ANGINA AND A HISTORY OF MYOCARDIAL INFARCTION

(A) Chest film on admission shows a mass in the lower portion of right hilus, and entire right lung is more radiolucent than the left. (B) Chest film exposed 3 days after recurrent pain in chest and dyspnea. Peripheral opacity in right upper lung is suggestive of infarction. (C) Six days later cavitation has occurred, and the thin-walled cavity has air trapped within it. (D) Healing of infarct with residual linear scar and mass in right hilus is unchanged. (E) Pulmonary angiogram early phase shows amputation of right lower lobe artery and marked attenuation of upper lobe arteries with tortuosity and also amputation of left lower lobe artery and tortuosity of smaller upper lobe branches. (F) Late phase. Left upper lobe pulmonary veins have filled but contrast substance remains in arteries to the right lung. (G and H) Anterior and posterior scans 2 days later after angiogram. Right lung shows almost no perfusion but left lung shows that peripheral area of lung is underperfused (microemboli) and definite cutoff at left base. (I and J) Two months later some recovery of perfusion of midportion of right lung. No significant improvement in left lung.

along with the AP and PA projections. The rind or peripheral stripe sign is not specific and can be mimicked by pleural and particularly interlobar effusions (James *et al.,* 1971). Consequently, scanning with the patient in several positions is desirable in an effort to produce shifting of the pleural fluid and thus differentiate from microembolization.

Although the appearance of the lung scan may be quite suggestive of PTE, it is rarely if ever specific. Many lesions other than PTE cause underperfusion of segments or entire lobes of the lung or multiple bilateral areas of underperfusion. These are emphysematous bulla, large scars of pulmonary fibrosis, pneumonia, atelectasis and carcinoma. The conventional chest film may demonstrate an obvious cause for the underperfusion other than PTE. Consequently, all lung scans should be interpreted in comparison with a contemporary chest film. Infarcts may be rec-

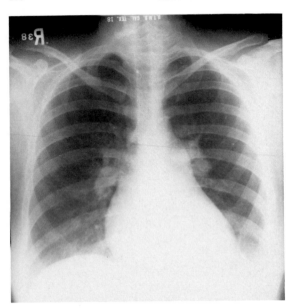

FIG. 78. CHRONIC PTE WITH ENLARGED NODULAR HILAR SHADOWS, A LARGE PULMONARY TRUNK, ENLARGEMENT OF THE RIGHT HEART AND AVASCULAR LUNGS

ognized and confirmed by the lung scan, although the area of underperfusion is typically larger than the shadow of the infarct. The combination of a positive scan with a negative chest film is highly suggestive of PTE. This is particularly likely in association with large central emboli. On the other hand, a series of technically adequate negative scans excludes PTE almost without exception. A small peripheral embolus can be missed (Fred *et al.,* 1966), particularly if both anterior and posterior and lateral scans are not of high quality. Also, there is some evidence that the scan may underestimate the extent of a large centrally placed embolus that does not completely interrupt the blood flow. The lung scan is a most valuable screening procedure. It can eliminate the possibility of PTE with a high degree of reliability, and if positive, suggests the need for pulmonary angiography for a more definitive diagnosis. The procedure has little risk, although there are reports of deaths (Dworkin *et al.,* 1966) apparently due to additional embolization imposed upon an already severely comprised pulmonary vasculature. This risk must be quite minimal since the embolization due to the microaggregated albumin could not obstruct more than 1/1,000 of the total pulmonary capillaries. The procedure does require even under good circumstances approximately one hour to perform. It is therefore difficult in an acutely ill patient. Also, performance as an emergency procedure in many hospital settings is still sometimes difficult.

Serial scans exposed several days to a week apart are useful in determining the progress and resolution or organization of PTE and associated improvement in perfusion of the lung. The natural history and fate of PTE of varying sizes are variable and to a degree unpredictable as to rate and degree of resolution and the extent if any of permanent change in the pulmonary vascular system. The embolus may be lysed by natural occurring fibrinolytic agents or it may fragment, break up, and thus be distributed into the smaller peripheral arteries or it may remain fixed and be organized leaving some scar and narrowing of the artery with obstruction to pulmonary blood flow. Pulmonary angiography is most helpful in assessing the resolution or disappearance of large central emboli, and it will provide some anatomical evidence of the state of the smaller peripheral microemboli. It is, however, not as reliable in assessing the degree of perfusion of the lung as is the scan. Tow and Wagner (1967) using serial scans found that small volumes of underperfused lung secondary to PTE returned to normal in 2–3 weeks and usually completely. Larger volumes comprising up to 50% of the total lung volume improved more slowly. In more than one-half of the cases, there were at 6 months supposedly permanent residual areas of underperfusion indicating permanent structural changes in the blood vessels. Permanent change is much more common where there is pulmonary stasis, such as congestive heart failure or the "mitral lung." In these conditions, it is so gross that it can be documented by angiography (Fred *et al.,* 1965; Chait *et al.,* 1967). From the accumulated evidence of lung scanning and angiography, most small and medium-sized PTE's in otherwise healthy lungs resolve predominantly by lysis in a few days to 2 weeks and leave no permanent impairment of perfusion. Larger impairments of flow due to PTE, particularly in association with circulatory stasis, improve very slowly over a period of months, and usually there are residual local areas of underperfusion.

PULMONARY ANGIOGRAPHY. Technique (see also section on technique). Pulmonary angiography for PTE is routinely performed in the frontal projection, and this may be supplemented when necessary by oblique projections, usually the right posterior oblique, to show the arch of the left pulmonary artery. Other selective injections into a single pulmonary artery or even localized segmental injections may be used. Magnification angiography has been used by Greenspan (1969) and is recommended for the detection of smaller peripheral emboli. A radiographic tube with 0.3 mm effective focal spot is needed, and the authors have had no experience with this procedure.

Peripheral venous injections of contrast substance can produce useful angiograms, and the exposure of a single film at the optimal time is capable of showing large central emboli. This procedure therefore could be performed in almost any radiologic department in an emergency. However, intravenous injections may be quite inadequate if there is poor action of the heart. Also, the partially opaque superior vena cava may obscure a crucial segment of the right pulmonary artery. A selective right atrial injection may be a satisfactory initial procedure, particularly since a significant proportion of emboli originate in the right atrium. Opacification of the right atrium will obscure the right lower lobe arteries, and consequently the right atrial examination must be followed by a selective injection into the pulmonary trunk. A side hold catheter is essential, and considerable care must be taken in placement so as to prevent either a right ventricular or unilateral arterial injection. Exposure factors should be such as to adequately penetrate the mediastinum and central hilar segments of the pulmonary artery or a contour filter can be used to advantage. Filming rates of 2–3/sec are quite adequate and should continue until the contrast substance reaches the aorta.

ANGIOGRAPHIC SIGNS OF PTE. The angiographic signs of PTE are:

(1) A radiolucent shadow within the contrast substance in the pulmonary artery or any of its branches. This may be and usually is accompanied by delayed, diminished or absent flow to the involved part of the lung. The embolus may have a distinct tail. This is particularly common when the embolus straddles a point of bifurcation with each end entering a separate division of the artery. This is often seen where the right artery divides into the upper and intermediate arteries. The embolus may be eccentrically placed or it may be cylindrical or tube-shaped and present in the central portion of the artery. The contrast substance may pass on each side outlining the band-like or tube-like appearance for a distance of several centimeters. In the smaller interlobar arteries, the negative shadow may be hump-shaped with segmental narrowing or droplet-shaped. Occasionally, the shadow may be plaque-like with a somewhat flattened indentation or impression on the arterial lumen. The contour and distribution of the negative filling defect seen inside the contrast-filled artery is usually so typical that it is pathognomonic of thromboembolus.

(2) Amputation of a major branch of the right or left pulmonary artery or one or more of the major interlobar branches. When the amputation involves a lobar artery, it is easily identified, but absence of filling of a smaller interlobar branch may be overlooked, especially if it occurs precisely at a point of division. The segment of the lung distal to the obstruction shows little if any perfusion and thus helps in identifying the obstruction. The amputation of a major or sizeable artery, although highly suggestive, is not pathognomonic of a thromboembolus. It can be due to invasion from adjacent neoplasm, fibrosis

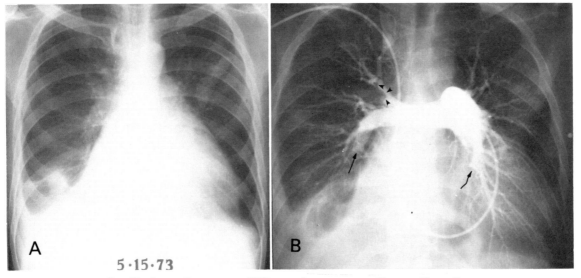

5·15·73

FIG. 79. ACUTE SUBMASSIVE PTE WITH INFARCTION AT BASE OF RIGHT LUNG

(A) Large infarct at right base with some pleural fluid. (B) Selective pulmonary angiogram shows amputation of both lower lobe arteries (arrows) and smaller clots in the right upper lobe artery (arrowheads).

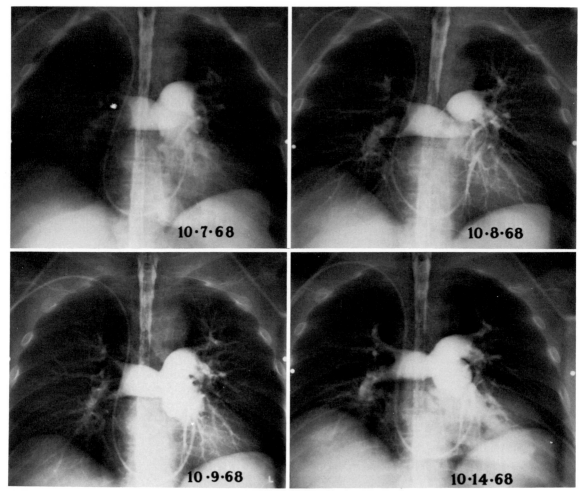

FIG. 80. SERIES OF PULMONARY ANGIOGRAMS

These angiograms were exposed over a period of 1 week to follow progress of massive central PTE. Patient was treated with heparin. Some resolution of the emboli has occurred in 7 days either by fragmentation or resolution. A large saddle embolus has lodged at the bifurcation of the right pulmonary artery with almost complete obstruction. After 2 days (10/9/68) the left lower lobe arteries are seen but are much attenuated and mildly tortuous. The patient recovered.

due to any cause, and probably from compression or displacement due to emphysematous bullae. Under the appropriate circumstances, it is a highly suggestive finding and is particularly valid if there are filling defects in other parts of the pulmonary vascular system that are diagnostic of thromboembolism. A subsequent angiogram often shows the re-establishment of flow through the amputated artery indicating either lysis and/or fragmentation of the obstructing thromboembolus.

(3) Delay or stagnation of regional or segmental blood flow. This is a secondary sign and is often seen with proximal partially occluding thromboembolism. As an isolated finding, it is most frequently seen in the basilar segments of the lung. The involved segment shows a distinct

delay in filling of the blood vessels with the contrast substance. This is noted in comparison with the other parts of the lung. The arterial segments may be filled while the veins from the other parts of the lung are opacified (Fig. 77F). It is a nonspecific sign. It could, of course, be associated with peripheral microemboli in the involved segment. It is most often due to an underlying disturbance of the circulatory dynamics of the lung. The most common cause is left ventricular failure or valvular obstructions in the left side of the heart such as mitral stenosis (Fleischner, 1966).

(4) Irregular narrowing and pruning of the mid zone and peripheral pulmonary arteries. This is a secondary and nonspecific sign. Presumably it could be associated with chronic or re-

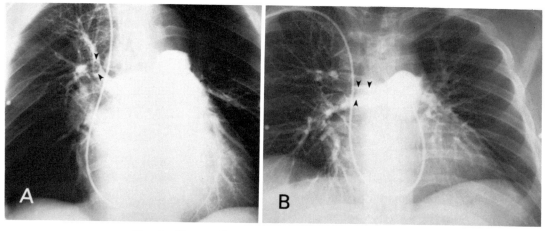

FIG. 81. MASSIVE BILATERAL PTE. TWO SEPARATE CASES

(A) Oval lozenge-shaped embolus partially occludes right upper lobe branch (arrowheads). Right lower lobe and left upper lobe branches are amputated. (B) Long tubular embolus lies in right pulmonary artery and extends into and occludes upper lobe branch and partially occludes lower and middle lobe branches. Numerous smaller emboli give numerous nodular or drop-like negative shadows that obstruct the left pulmonary artery.

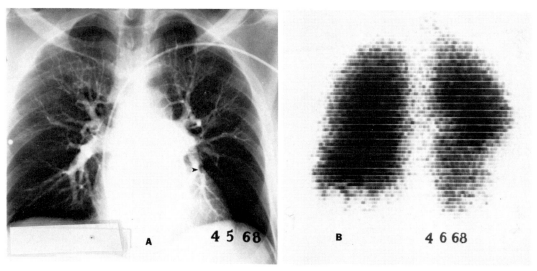

FIG. 82. SUBLOBAR PTE

Sublobar PTE lodged at origin of anteromedial and lateral basilar branches of lower lobe artery on left (A). There may be amputation of several small arteries in the right lower and middle lobes, and the accompanying scan shows a small corresponding indentation (B). Absence of perfusion at the left base is clearly shown by scan.

peated thromboemboli or conceivably could be due to spasm. As an isolated finding, it is non-specific.

(5) Tortuosity of the smaller peripheral branches of the pulmonary artery. This has been noted repeatedly (Ferris *et al.,* 1967) in patients with known PTE (Fig. 77E). It may occur distal to an obvious partial obstruction or it may occur without other evidence of PTE. In this latter situation, it must be regarded as a very secondary and unreliable sign. The cause of the tortuosity is unexplained but could be attributed to arterial

spasm. It could be also associated with regional extensive microembolism.

(6) Dilatation of the pulmonary trunk and proximal pulmonary arteries. Pulmonary angiography adds very little to that which can be seen on the conventional chest film. As an isolated finding, it is, of course, nonspecific.

In summary, the only specific angiographic sign of pulmonary thromboembolism is the visualization of the embolus as a negative shadow within the contrast substance of the partially filled pulmonary artery. Contrast substance must partially surround the embolus at some point to produce the recognizable contour. Amputation or complete obstruction is highly suggestive, particularly if the contrast substance at the point of complete interruption has a tail-like appearance or even a convex (toward the hilus) appearance. In large central embolization, these findings occur with almost 100% certainty. The detection of smaller peripheral emboli is much less certain. This may require selective injections, films of superior technical quality, and magnification techniques, if available.

The detection of small and perhaps inconsequential thromboemboli is of considerable importance because of the tendency of continued embolization. In a statistical study, Barker et al. (1941) found that there was a distinct tendency of recurrence of pulmonary thromboembolism. Poe et al. (1969) found suggestive evidence that even massive embolization may be preceded by minor emboli. Certainly, some cases of pulmonary hypertension appear to be triggered by recurring emboli (Fowler et al., 1966; Goodwin et al., 1963). The question of long-term anticoagulation therapy arises along with the possibility of surgical treatment of the inferior vena cava.

In massive embolization, angiography is indispensable to diagnosis even if it is of very primitive type. Intravenous angiogram may be sufficient to demonstrate large central emboli and confirm the cause of the patient's severe distress. In this connection, it now appears that Urokinase and Streptokinase (1970) as fibrinolytic agents have much to offer but are expensive and carry some risk. Also, the conventional type anticoagulation therapy and supportive measures are better managed following a correct diagnosis.

Repeated and often serial angiograms have been used in the study of the effect of fibrinolytic agents (Urokinase Study, 1970; Dickie et al., 1967) and also in observations on the natural course of large emboli (Fred et al., 1965; Sautter et al., 1964). Generally, the progress and fate of the thromboembolism can be documented satisfactorily from serial scans, and angiography is not recommended for this purpose routinely. The contrast substance may have some untoward effects on the coagulability of the blood (Lasser, 1968).

There has been some reluctance to use pulmonary angiography in patients in actual or threatened shock even where there is suspicion of thromboembolism (Torrance, 1959). In patients in shock with low and unstable blood pressure, the addition of the vasodilating effects of the contrast substance can present an additional hazard. However, a wide experience indicates that pulmonary angiography is well tolerated (Greenspan, 1969; Urokinase Pulmonary Thromboembolism Trials, 1973; Dickie et al., 1967). The risk of the procedure can be lessened by proper supportive therapy and familiarity with resuscitation techniques. Certainly, when compared with the possible benefits, the risks of pulmonary angiography are amply justified.

Infections of Pulmonary Vascular System that Produce Obstruction.

Syphilis. Syphilis of the pulmonary arteries is an uncommon occurrence. The extent to which it produces obstructive lesions is controversial. Brenner (1935) found that the most pronounced changes were in the pulmonary trunk and its major branches; the smaller intrapulmonary branches were minimally involved. Associated atherosclerosis was extremely common.

Syphilis of the pulmonary artery has been mentioned as a common cause of Ayerza's disease. Ayerza's disease as originally described (from White (1951) and Brenner (1935)) was a clinical syndrome without a definite pathologic basis; cyanosis was the most prominent sign. The syndrome is similar to that seen with chronic pulmonary obstruction with right heart failure. In some instances the foramen ovale may have been forced open secondary to increased pressure in the right atrium. Cyanosis would thus be increased by the right to left shunt. Syphilis has rarely been proved to be a cause of pulmonary obstruction, and Ayerza's syndrome probably has no single etiologic basis.

On the other hand, syphilis of the pulmonary trunk and its branches is often associated with some degree of dilatation and it may be the cause of a pulmonary aneurysm.

Schistosomiasis. These parasites may invade the lungs in large numbers and attack the smaller branches of the pulmonary artery. The pathologic lesion in the lungs is a widespread obliterative arteriolitis caused by repeated infection of the arterioles by the ova (Marchand et al., 1957). Rupture of these vessels and hemorrhage may occur. Many of the smaller branches may be obliterated, and cor pulmonale may develop. The most important radiographic finding is dilatation of the pulmonary artery segment in the face of anemic peripheral lung fields, indicative of pulmonary arteriolar hypertension. Increased pulsations of the pulmonary trunk and its main branches were also found in all patients studied by Cavalcanti et al. (1962).

An aneurysm of the aorta or a pulmonary or mediastinal neoplasm may partially or completely obstruct the right or left pulmonary artery (Fig. 84). The lung on the involved side will show marked decrease in the size and number of the vascular markings.

DILATATION

A. Due to increased pressure
   1. postcapillary pulmonary hypertension
   2. precapillary pulmonary hypertension
B. Due to increased flow
   1. congenital left-to-right shunts
   2. congenital arteriovenous fistula of the lung
   3. rupture of sinus of Valsalva aneurysm into the right ventricle or pulmonary artery
C. Due to turbulent flow
   1. distal to valvular pulmonary stenosis
   2. coarctation of the pulmonary artery
D. Due to degeneration of the arterial wall
   1. atherosclerosis
   2. syphilis
   3. subacute bacterial endocarditis with formation of mycotic aneurysms
   4. Marfan's syndrome
E. Miscellaneous
   1. congenital dilatation of the pulmonary artery
   2. varicosities of pulmonary veins

It has been seen that obstructions are a common cause of dilatation of the pulmonary arteries. This represents the response of an elastic arterial wall to an increased intraluminal pressure and is dynamic in nature, at least early in the course of the disease. With sustained elevation of the pulmonary arterial pressure, whether due to pre- or postcapillary causes, permanent changes in the arterial wall develop; thereafter the dilatation is unlikely to recede completely even if the cause is corrected. The same is true, though to a lesser extent, of pulmonary artery dilatation secondary to congenital shunts from left to right. That the arterial wall is relatively unchanged is supported by the observation that the caliber of the vessels returns to normal when the cause of the abnormal hemodynamics of the circulation is corrected, for example after ligation of a patent ductus arteriosus. However, dilatation of long-standing may persist despite correction of the underlying cause if permanent changes have developed in the vessel wall.

The pulmonary artery and its right and left branches are regularly and predictably dilated in patients with congenital left to right shunts if the ratio of pulmonary to systemic blood flow is in the range of 2–3 to 1. In such cases the entire pulmonary vascular system is dilated. The main pulmonary artery may be markedly dilated, simulating an aneurysm. To be authentic, however, an aneurysm must be more or less circumscribed, and organic degeneration of the vessel wall must be demonstrated. According to this definition, the dilatation found in congenital left to right shunts does not qualify as a true aneurysm even though the enlargement may be marked.

Congenital arteriovenous fistula of the lung produces dilatation of the involved pulmonary vessels and markedly increased flow. This lesion is discussed in detail in the section on congenital malformations.

An aneurysm of the sinus of Valsalva or ascending portion of the aorta may rupture into the right ventricle or pulmonary trunk. This occurrence may be fatal, or, if the patient survives for any length of time, the pulmonary arterial system dilates in its entirety due to the markedly increased flow and pressure which the pulmonary circuit must now sustain. The right ventricle enlarges and eventually fails.

Dilatation of the pulmonary artery due to turbulent flow is commonly encountered distal to valvular pulmonic stenosis. Poststenotic dilatation may produce striking enlargement of the pulmonary trunk and its left branch (Fig. 125), but the right pulmonary artery does not ordinarily participate in this dilatation. Flame-shaped dilatations of the pulmonary artery branches distal to areas of peripheral coarctation are also thought to be due to turbulent flow.

Atherosclerotic degeneration of the arterial wall is usually secondary to increased pressure and/or flow in the pulmonary circuit. It may ultimately produce enough structural change to lead to a permanent but mild degree of dilatation. Well localized areas of dilatation of the pulmonary artery and its major branches may also be produced by syphilis. Numerous small localized areas of vascular dilatation probably qualify as mycotic aneurysms in patients with subacute bacterial endocarditis (Calenoff, 1964). The surrounding lung is frequently involved in an infectious process or abscess formation. Radiographically the small mycotic aneurysms produce rounded or triangular-shaped opacities. As many

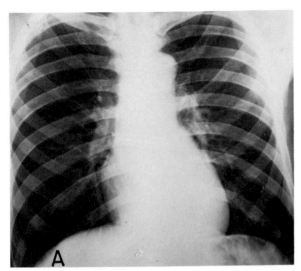 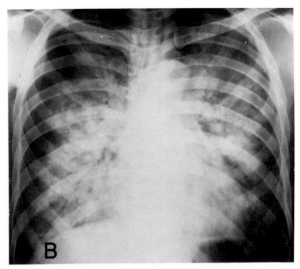

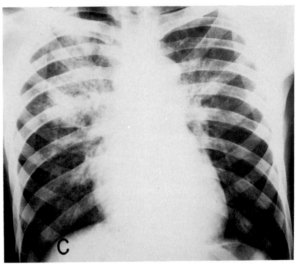

FIG. 83. PERIARTERITIS NODOSA IN 33-YEAR-OLD MAN

Patient complained of fever, myalgia, and weakness. Subcutaneous nodules were found on physical examination; blood pressure was 170/130. The diagnosis was established by skin biopsy. (A) 9/10/57. The chest x-ray was negative. (B) 9/18/57. Clinically, the patient sustained a pulmonary embolus on 9/17/57 which precipitated acute left ventricular failure. (C) 9/22/57. The patient improved greatly following digitalization. The density in the right upper lung is thought to represent changes due to a large pulmonary infarct.

as a dozen may be scattered through each lung. They may be demonstrated by pulmonary arteriography.

Larger aneurysms of the pulmonary trunk and its branches are quite rare. Deterling and Clagett (1947) found 8 such aneurysms recorded in a review of 109,571 autopsies taken from the literature. In a thorough study, these authors were able to obtain a detailed description of only 36 proved cases. The site of involvement was as follows: pulmonary trunk, 32 cases; right pulmonary artery, 3 cases; left pulmnary artery, 1 case.

Syphilis was the etiologic agent in 31% of the cases, and the aneurysm was either congenital or associated with a congenital lesion in 47%. Other causes were mycotic infection of the arterial wall and atherosclerosis.

Radiographically, an aneurysm of the pulmonary trunk or its major branches is seen as a mass that presents along the left midheart border or in either hilus. Its border is usually smooth and rounded or it may be slightly lobulated. The shadow of the aneurysm is continuous with that of the pulmonary artery in all projections. Pul-

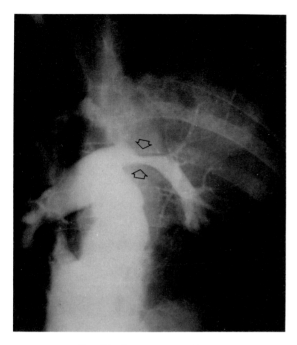

FIG. 84. CARCINOMA OF LUNG

The patient was a 59-year-old man with the complaints of hoarseness, weakness, cough, and weight loss. Posteroanterior chest films show the presence of a large area of pulmonary consolidation in the left upper lung adjacent to the hilus. Intravenous pulmonary arteriography was performed, and a selected frame from the serial films exposed is reproduced above. It shows marked narrowing of the left pulmonary artery, suggesting extensive encroachment upon the hilar and mediastinal structures by what was presumed to be a malignant tumor. This encroachment upon the main pulmonary artery at its origin suggests nonresectability. Lung biopsy revealed the presence of squamous cell carcinoma.

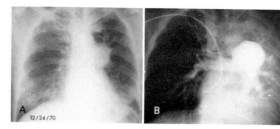

FIG. 85. ANEURYSM OF THE LEFT PULMONARY ARTERY

The patient was a 56-year-old male who complained of sudden onset of hemoptysis. Later (B) the aneurysm compressed the left main stem bronchus producing chronic atelectasis and required pneumonectomy. The cause of the aneurysm was undetermined, but the pathologist suggested a congenital anomaly.

sations of the aneurysm are common, but all aneurysms do not pulsate. Angiocardiography is the method of choice in establishing the diagnosis.

The cystic medial necrosis of the ascending aorta so characteristic of Marfan's syndrome (Marfan, 1896) may also be found in the pulmonary trunk (Marvel and Genovese, 1951). Under such circumstances massive aneurysmal dilatation of the pulmonary artery may ensue (Tung and Liebow, 1952), and the disease may be complicated by pulmonic insufficiency or even by rupture of the dilated pulmonary trunk (Wagenvoort et al., 1962).

Other localized areas of dilatation of the smaller intrapulmonary arterial branches are fairly common and are related to degeneration of the arterial wall secondary to infection. They occur where an artery runs in the wall of a tuberculous cavity (Rasmussen aneurysm) or adjacent to a chronic infectious process such as bronchiectasis or lung abscess.

Congenital dilatation of the pulmonary trunk and its branches is not well understood. The vessel wall is often thinner than normal, and the dilatation is usually strictly limited to the pulmonary trunk or its major branches. There is no hemodynamic cause for the dilatation since the pulmonary pressure and flow are normal or decreased. Nor is there any structural deficiency in the arterial wall. Several of these cases were studied by Green et al. (1949). The pressure in the pulmonary artery was decreased although the right ventricular pressure was normal. The pulmonary trunk was considerably larger than the aorta. One theory proposes that this difference in size is due to an unbalanced division of the primitive truncus arteriosus. The enlarged pulmonary trunk and its branches pulsate normally. The patients have no symptoms (Fig. 341), and the condition is important because it may be confused radiographically with a patent ductus arteriosus or other serious cardiac anomaly or disease.

Varicosities of the pulmonary veins are another form of dilatation of the pulmonary vascular system. They are commonly not associated with heart disease and represent areas of venous dilatation without overall hemodynamic significance. They may develop secondary to obstructing lesions on the left side of the heart, and Hipona and Jamshidi (1967) have reported a patient in whom the varix enlarged over the course of 7 years as the patient's heart disease progressed (mitral insufficiency), with regression of the varix after corrective operation.

ALTERATIONS IN VASCULAR PERMEABILITY

A. Due to inhalation or circulation of noxious agents
1. near-drowning
2. smoke inhalation
3. aspiration pneumonia
4. uremia

B. Due to pulmonary hypersensitivity
1. transfusion reactions
2. drugs

C. Due to necrotizing vasculitis
1. periarteritis nodosa
2. Wegener's granulomatosis
3. lupus erythematosus
4. rheumatoid lung; scleroderma
5. idiopathic pulmonary hemosiderosis
6. Goodpasture's syndrome
7. drugs

D. Due to hypoxia ("shock lung")

E. Due to central nervous system abnormalities

Pulmonary opacities are commonly seen on chest films in patients who have nearly drowned. The densities are produced by transudation of fluid into the alveoli through pulmonary capillaries whose vascular permeability has been altered by the fluid aspiration. Thus, the appearance is that of pulmonary edema as described in an earlier section in this chapter (Fig. 66D). The opacities clear rapidly if the patient survives.

The pulmonary densities seen in the lungs of patients injured by inhalation of smoke are due to vascular injury with altered permeability leading to transudation of fluid into the alveolar spaces, a form of pulmonary edema. If infection does not develop, general supportive measures are generally all that are required, and the fluid is usually rapidly absorbed. If permanent injury to the supporting structures of the lung has occurred, fibrosis may ensue.

Although most of the densities seen in the lungs in patients with aspiration pneumonia are the consequence of infection, some of the perifocal opacities which develop early are doubtless due to fluid transudation into the vicinity of the lung into which infective material was aspirated. These localized patches of pulmonary edema are likely due to increased vascular permeability, and they clear rapidly as the micro-organisms are brought under control.

Uremic pulmonary edema is incompletely understood. It may be due in part to the effect of circulating toxins on pulmonary vascular permeability, but cardiac failure is a frequent accompaniment and may contribute to the densities seen on the chest film. The appearance, previously described, is distinctive but not diagnostic (Fig. 66A).

Allergic reactions may occur in the lungs following blood transfusions and may produce patches of pulmonary edema which appear as ill-defined areas of infiltration. The development of pulmonary opacities in some patients receiving therapeutic doses of various drugs is believed to represent a hypersensitivity response mediated by antibodies, sensitized lymphocytes, or both (Rosenow, 1972). Altered vascular permeability is probably the underlying mechanism, and the densities clear rapidly upon withdrawal of the offending drug. Alveolitis with interstitial and alveolar fluid transudation is the pathological equivalent of the radiographic appearance (Brettner et al., 1970).

The collagen diseases, insofar as they affect the pulmonary vascular system, have in common the production of necrotizing pulmonary vasculitis (Levin, 1970). The pulmonary effects are produced, for the most part, by pulmonary hemorrhage, but pulmonary infarction and pulmonary edema are also found.

Periarteritis nodosa is a disease of the walls of the smaller arteries and arterioles throughout the body. The lesions are focal in nature. Necrosis of the vessel wall may be found, with rupture and hemorrhage, or one may see thrombosis with vascular occlusion. The disease may be mild and persist for months or years, but in the usual case vascular involvement of one or more vital organ systems develops. The prognosis is poor.

The pulmonary vascular system is not commonly involved (once in the 17 autopsied cases studied by Griffiths and Varol, 1951) by the vascular lesions of periarteritis, but certain x-ray changes are commonly seen in the lungs at some time during the course of the disease (Doub et al., 1954). Though the changes in the chest film are quite variable, one most often sees bilateral opacities of moderate size, perihilar in distribution and of homogeneous density; they are rather typical of pulmonary edema. They may give no symptoms and are often discovered during filming of the chest for heart size or some other unrelated reason. Occasionally only one lung or a single lobe will be involved. The opacities may be spotty and tend to follow the vascular markings. More extensive or severe lesions may cause infarction and gross hemorrhage. In some cases the lesions are fleeting in character, and, in the absence of pre-existing cardiac enlargement or nephritis, this suggests that they may have an allergic origin. Certainly a localized area of sensitivity of the pulmonary vessels with a change in capillary permeability is a possible cause of these evanescent roentgen shadows.

If the kidneys are primarily involved, nephritis and uremia may eventually develop. Changes of pulmonary edema similar to those seen in uremia may then appear in the lungs. Systemic hypertension may be present or the periarteritis may involve the coronary arteries leading to myocardial infarction. This may be followed by left ventricular failure, pulmonary edema, and some degree of chronic passive congestion of the lungs. Congestive heart failure is a common cause of death.

Wegener's granulomatosis may be limited to the lungs (7 of 12 patients reported by Israel and Patchefsky, 1971). The pulmonary changes are variable but are thought to be secondary to necrotizing vasculitis as in the other connective tissue diseases. Localized nodular lesions, localized and disseminated areas of pulmonary hemorrhage, and pulmonary edema may all be found.

Disseminated lupus erythematosus is a disease of the small arteries and arterioles. Edema and fibrinoid degeneration of the media with endothelial proliferation and thrombosis characterize the pathological lesion. Fibrosis in the myocardium and endocardium is common. Changes in the lungs are not specific. Evidence of pleuritis and pleural effusion are often found. Infarction or pulmonary edema associated with heart failure may occur (Garland and Sisson, 1954).

Vasculitis of the pulmonary vessels may also be seen in rheumatoid lung while arteriolar intimal hyperplasia is found in scleroderma. In general, however, granulomatous lesions predominate in the former and fibrosis in the latter. Evans (1959) described a case in which the specific tissue of scleroderma produced peripheral pulmonary arterial obstruction leading to pulmonary hypertension.

Idiopathic pulmonary hemosiderosis probably also qualifies as a condition resulting from necrotizing pulmonary vasculitis. The pulmonary lesions are due to spontaneous alveolar and interstitial hemorrhage, and the resultant pulmonary infiltrations are in no way distinctive except for their association with hemoptysis. When the kidney is also involved, Goodpasture's syndrome is said to be present (Goodpasture, 1919). The principal alterations are focal necrosis of alveolar walls, intra-alveolar hemorrhage and damage to the alveolar-capillary basement membrane (Robbins, 1967). When acute vasculitis is seen, the concomitant diagnosis of periarteritis nodosa may be justified.

Some drugs exert their effect on the lungs by production of an allergic angiitis. The pulmonary lesions seen on chest films are due to focal edema, hemorrhage and inflammatory cell infiltration. Sulfonomides are the drugs most commonly implicated in the production of such a vasculitis; others that are known to do so include penicillin, thiouracil, hydralazine, phenylbutazone, quinidine, promazines, and hydantoins.

The precise cause and pathogenesis of "shock lung" are as yet undetermined, but hypoxia is a likely contributory factor. Altered vascular permeability leads to pulmonary edema, and the radiographic appearance of fluffy alveolar opacities is striking but not diagnostic. Superimposed upon the presumed vascular insult one often finds atelectasis, infection, intra-alveolar hemorrhage, fibrinous exudates, and alveolar hyaline membranes. Oxygen toxicity commonly complicates the clinical and roentgenographic picture (Joffe, 1970; Hall and Margolin, 1972).

Pulmonary capillary permeability and blood pressure may be partly under central nervous system control. Certainly one can see pulmonary edema in patients with increased intracranial pressure and following seizures when there is no obvious primary pulmonary abnormality. Whether the lung changes are the consequence of neurogenic alterations, hypoxia or humoral influences is unknown.

SEQUESTRATION

A variable-sized portion of the lower lobe of either lung may derive its blood supply from an artery which originates from the descending aorta either above (85%) or below (15%) the diaphragm (Salvioni and Goldin, 1960). The branches of this anomalous artery may anastomose freely (Wyman and Eyler, 1952) with the normal pulmonary and bronchial arteries, and in the involved portion of the lung may be areas lined with bronchial epithelium. It is thought by some (Pryce et al., 1948) that the aberrant artery is the cause of this condition and produces its

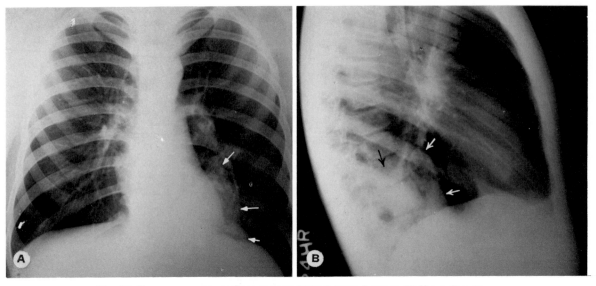

FIG. 86. SEQUESTRATION OF SEGMENT OF LEFT LOWER LOBE IN 12-YEAR-OLD GIRL
The patient had had signs and symptoms of pulmonary infection for many years. A systemic artery originating from the lower thoracic aorta entered the involved portion of lung.

effect by traction and strangulation of the growing bronchial buds. On the other hand, Smith (1956) favors the view that the primary lesion in intralobar sequestration is some failure of the pulmonary artery in fetal life to supply the segment of the lung involved. Because of this defect the systemic supply to the fetal lung persists, and as a result of the systemic pressure the lung changes arise after birth in the area of the lung to which this supply is distributed. The condition may be silent for long periods of time and be detected on a routine chest film exposed for some unrelated reason. In other instances the abnormal, usually cystic, lung may be the site of recurrent infection and thus produce symptoms.

The presence of the condition may be suspected after viewing a conventional chest film, although a high index of suspicion and familiarity with the lesion are required. Two different types of pulmonary shadows may be found. In one type there is a well-defined, somewhat elongated homogeneous mass in the lower lobe. Wyman and Eyler (1952) indicate that the mass may present a finger-like projection which points towards the dorsal aorta, and this is the site of entry of the aberrant artery into the mass. Such an appearance is highly suggestive of intralobar sequestration of the lung. The homogeneous density of the mass is due to the presence of mucoid or gelatinous material within the cystic area. In the other type, the lung shadow is not so distinct and well defined. It is due to thin-walled cysts which vary in size and density from time to time. The cystic lung segment is subject to recurrent infections, and it may be during a period of exacerbation that the lesion is first noticed. The cysts may contain fluid levels with air above, particularly during a period of infection. In some instances the cysts are quite numerous and the greater portion of the lower lobe may be involved.

The abnormal bronchopulmonary mass may lie within the confines of a lobe (intralobar sequestration) or may lie beyond lobar confines (extralobar sequestration). Differences between the two include the following: (1) Extralobar sequestration shows a very marked left preponderance. (2) The venous drainage with extralobar sequestration is usually to the hemiazygos vein, with intralobar sequestration to the normal pulmonary vein. (3) An association exists between extralobar sequestration and diaphragmatic hernia which has not been noted with the intralobar type. (4) Infection is common in intralobar sequestrations and uncommon in the extralobar lesion (Pryce, 1946).

Other lung lesions such as lung abscess, congenital cystic disease, bronchiectasis, or even bronchial carcinoma may give a similar appearance. Aortography may give a precise diagnosis and has been used for this purpose (Simopoulos *et al.,* 1959). The characteristic aortographic finding is opacification of the anomalous blood supply to the sequestered pulmonary segment (Nielsen, 1964; Ranniger and Valvassori, 1964). The anomalous systemic vessel has also been demonstrated by diagnostic pneumoperitoneum (Hill et al, 1964).

10

Rheumatic Heart Disease

Rheumatic fever is a generalized disease that affects predominantly the connective tissues and blood vessels. Changes in the heart are a common manifestation of this generalized process, and frequently the heart is the only organ that shows permanent residual damage.

The incidence of rheumatic heart disease varies in different geographical locations in the United States. White (1953) found an incidence of 23.5% of all kinds of heart disease encountered in New England, whereas Hutcheson *et al.* (1953) found an incidence of 7.5% of all types in an 18-month period (1952–53) at The University of Texas Medical Branch in Galveston, Texas. Its frequency and severity have shown a gratifying decrease during the past 20 years, and it is now much less common than hypertensive or arteriosclerotic heart disease (Shaffer and Silber, 1975).

ACUTE RHEUMATIC CARDITIS AND VALVULITIS

Many cases are mild or obscure and are not recognized clinically. In a number of others the diagnosis is made from the history, clinical signs, electrocardiogram, and course of the disease. It is generally conceded that 60–70% of children with a first attack of acute rheumatic fever will have associated carditis. Over 95% of those with a first attack of acute rheumatic fever who have no murmur during the course of that illness will have no murmur when examined five years later. Thus, the severity of the initial attack (and of the subsequent attacks, if any) is a potent factor in determining the subsequent development of chronic disease. Radiologic signs may be minimal or absent, and even when present, the radiologic findings are not too specific. They consist mainly of symmetrical enlargement of the heart in a child or young adult. The enlargement is due to (1) myocarditis with weakening of the cardiac muscle followed by dilatation, (2) valvular dysfunction (caused by acute valvulitis and/or acute left ventricular dilatation), and (3) occasionally, pericardial effusion. The usual segmental divisions of the heart are less definite or obliterated, and the heart has a smooth, rounded contour. Fluoroscopy demonstrates diminished pulsations of all contours and frequently a rapid rate.

The lungs are clear and typically without congestion even in patients with marked cardiac enlargement. Occasionally, spotty, sizeable areas of increased density will appear rather suddenly. They are homogeneous, often bilateral, and suggest the presence of pulmonary edema. These are probably the same shadows which have been described as rheumatic pneumonia.

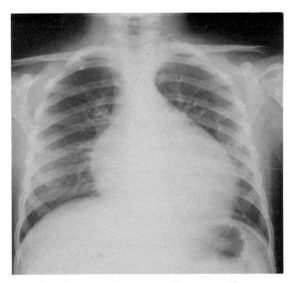

FIG. 87. ACUTE RHEUMATIC FEVER IN A CHILD
There is generalized cardiac enlargement. The lungs are clear. There may be a small pericardial effusion.

Extensive myocardial involvement may take several weeks to produce striking enlargement, in contrast to sudden enlargement due to pericarditis with effusion. Pericarditis is a serious complication, particularly in childhood (Keith *et al.*, 1958).

Serial films are valuable in following the course of the disease, and a progressive decrease in heart size is a favorable prognostic sign. A rapid decrease is usually associated with the resolution of pericardial fluid. Persistent enlargement is an indication for continued bed rest and further treatment.

In acute rheumatic fever with carditis, some of the valvular dysfunction is caused by acute valvulitis, but "functional" mitral regurgitation may also be the result of fairly acute left ventricular dilatation. In addition to dilatation of the mitral valve ring, left ventricular dilatation may interfere with the function of the chordae tendineae and papillary muscles in maintaining normal valve function.

When organic valvular disease occurs during childhood, mitral insufficiency is by far the commonest lesion (mitral stenosis is found in only 5–6% of cases with valvular disease (Keith *et al.*, 1956)). Moreover, the natural history of the disease may be quite brief, progressing from acute carditis to intractable cardiac failure due to mitral regurgitation in a period of months (Fig. 102). Although 20–30 years are sometimes required for the development of full-blown signs and symptoms of rheumatic valvular disease, the course may be very rapidly progressive in children. Death from rheumatic mitral insufficiency within months of acute carditis is not rare. The course of the disease may be accurately followed by serial cardiac volume determinations, and when the volume of the heart places the child in Group III, valve replacement should be considered (Fig. 102) p. 156.

CHRONIC RHEUMATIC HEART DISEASE

In the chronic disease the acute myocarditis has healed leaving numerous small scars. These are rarely sufficiently extensive to impair the functional capacity of the ventricular myocardium, although a recurrence of the acute process may occur at any time. The scars may, however, weaken the left atrial wall and may involve the endocardium and serve as a nidus for thrombus formation. Atrial fibrillation is common, particularly in association with mitral stenosis. It can usually be detected at fluoroscopy but rarely causes any significant change in the cardiac contour, although apparently it may contribute to dilatation of the left atrium. It is the valvular lesions, however, that are of the greatest importance, and it is the hemodynamic consequences of these changes which are most influential in producing the characteristic radiologic changes in the contour and activity of the heart. The distribution of moderately severe valvular lesions as recorded in 282 cases studies by Wallach and Angrest (1958) was: mitral, 59%; aortic, 12%; and combined valvular lesions, 29%. In addition, 5.7% had tricuspid stenosis. The mitral valve was involved in about 85–90% of all cases of rheumatic valvular disease, although it was not necessarily the predominant lesion. It is our experience that a substantial minority of patients with chronic rheumatic valvular heart disease who are under consideration as candidates for surgical correction have more than one lesion. The combination of mitral and aortic valvular disease is most frequent.

MITRAL VALVULAR DISEASE

Mitral stenosis is more common than mitral insufficiency, but some degree of insufficiency may be found even in cases selected for commissurotomy. In 150 cases, McAfee and Biondetti (1957) found 20% of their patients to have insufficiency; in 12 patients the insufficiency was predominant and in 6 there was no stenosis. Severe mitral stenosis and severe mitral insufficiency cannot exist together; intermediate degrees of each condition, however, may. Mitral commissurotomy will relieve mitral stenosis. A much more extensive surgical procedure, such as valve replacement or valvuloplasty, is necessary for relief of insufficiency. Furthermore, commissurotomy may aggravate an already existing insufficiency, and this is poorly tolerated by an already damaged heart.

Mitral Stenosis

Stenosis of the valve is due to scarring and thickening of the valve cusps which usually begin in the region of the commissure. This may be followed by fusion of the valve commissures, resulting in a slitlike opening somewhere near the central portion of the valve, and this opening may lie at the bottom of a funnel-like passageway. Calcium may be deposited in the scarred tissues and serve to bridge and rigidly fuse the commisures. This may render the procedure of commissurotomy technically much more difficult and increase the possibilities of calcific emboli. In more advanced lesions a central rigidly fixed opening may result, leaving the valve in a permanent condition of insufficiency and stenosis.

The normal mitral valve opening is large, usually 4–6 cm^2 in the adult. The effective valve area must be severely reduced in size before it seriously interferes with cardiovascular hemodynamics. Mitral stenosis may produce symptoms with moderate exertion when the valve area is in the range of 1.6–2.0 cm^2. When the valve area has been reduced to 1.0 cm^2 the patient will usually experience symptoms with only mild exertion, and in operative cases the opening may be of the order of 0.5 cm^2. The minimal size compatible with life is 0.3–0.4 cm^2 (Schlant, 1970).

Mitral stenosis is considerably more common in women than men, whereas insufficiency is found with about equal frequency in the two sexes. The radiologic signs of mitral stenosis are as follows:

1. Enlargement of the left atrium.
2. Enlargement of the pulmonary trunk.
3. Small size of the aorta.
4. Characteristic pulmonary vascular pattern.
5. Parenchymal lung changes.
6. Mitral valvular calcification.
7. Right ventricular enlargement.
8. Right atrial enlargement.
9. Left atrial calcification.
10. Absence of changes in left ventricular contour.

Enlargement of the Left Atrium. This is the most common radiologic evidence of mitral stenosis and is best demonstrated by observing the contour of the barium-filled esophagus in the extreme right oblique or lateral projection in both inspiration and expiration. An anterior impression in the region of the atrium during inspiration is good evidence of enlargement. In a heavily exposed film in the posteroanterior projection the esophagus may be deviated to the right around the atrium. The enlarged atrium forms an oval-shaped shadow of increased density superimposed on the base of the heart which is easily identified on films of proper density. The atrium, if sufficiently enlarged, may become border-forming on the right side and in conjunction with the right atrium form a double convexity. The left main bronchus may be elevated and compressed; the angle of the carina is normally about 75°, and this may be increased to 90° or more with atrial enlargement. With aneurysmal dilatation, the left atrium may form the entire right border of the heart (Fig. 91). It may extend almost to the right lateral thoracic wall and severely compress the right lung root. Aneurysmal dilatation, however, may occur with predominant insufficiency as well as predominant stenosis, although Best and Heath (1964) found it to be more common with pure stenosis.

The left atrial appendage normally accounts for a short segment of the left cardiac border between the left ventricular curve below and the pulmonary trunk above. The appendage dilates quite early in most cases of mitral stenosis and can be detected as a rounded convexity on the left border of the heart (Fig. 89A). Jacobson and Weidner (1962) have described a procedure for increasing the prominence of the left atrial appendage. By having the patient perform a strong Valsalva maneuver and then releasing the glottis, the left atrial appendage can be made to distend beyond its usual size. This distention can be detected by rapid filming of the left border of the heart. They regard this as one of the more sensitive indicators of left atrial enlargement. The present authors have had no experience with this procedure, but certainly a convexity due to the left atrial appendage can often be detected on the left border of the heart although the left atrium is only minimally enlarged.

The left atrial appendage ordinarily forms no recognizable border of the cardiovascular silhouette in normal persons. However, a slight separate bulge between the pulmonary trunk and the left ventricle may at times be seen in the PA view in normal people, and this probably represents a prominent but not pathologically enlarged left atrial appendage. Therefore, mere visualization of this bulge on the left heart border may not be considered certain evidence of enlargement of the left atrium in the absence of other radiologic or clinical signs.

Enlargement of the Pulmonary Trunk. The lateral border of the pulmonary trunk usually forms the middle segment of the left heart border on the PA view; its contour may merge imperceptibly with that of the descending branch of the left pulmonary artery. This shadow should not be confused with the enlarged left atrial appendage. The dilated pulmonary trunk is seen above and to the (patient's) left of the air shadow of the left main bronchus. The bulge of the atrial appendage is seen below this point. When both

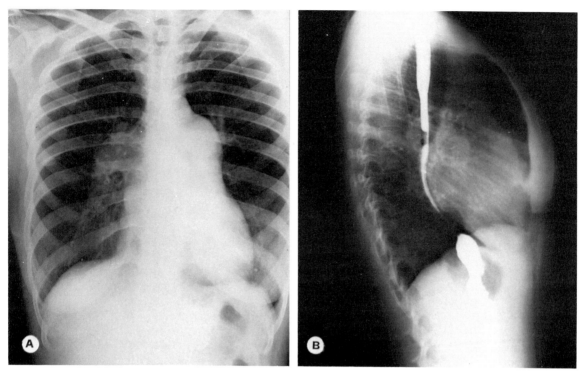

FIG. 88. "PURE" MITRAL STENOSIS AS DETERMINED AT TIME OF MITRAL VALVULOTOMY
(A) In the posteroanterior projection the left ventricular contour is rather steep. (B) In the lateral view the convexity of the left atrium above is in contrast to the rather slight curve of the small left ventricle below.

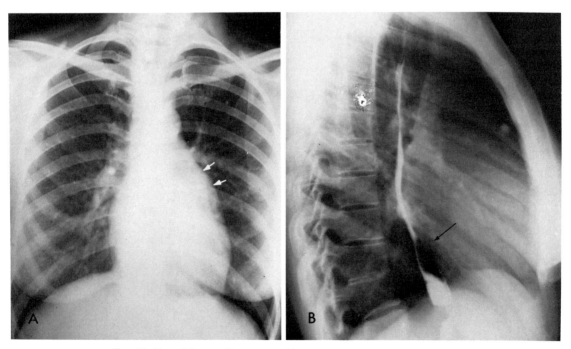

FIG. 89. PURE MITRAL STENOSIS AS DETERMINED AT COMMISSUROTOMY
(A) White arrows indicate dilated left atrial appendage. (B) Block arrow in lateral view indicates off-set between enlarged left atrium and normal sized left ventricle.

the pulmonary artery (trunk) and left atrial appendage are separately visible, four bulges will be seen comprising the left heart border; the aortic knob, the pulmonary trunk, the left atrial appendage and the left ventricle (from above to below). The pulmonary trunk is also brought into contour in the right anterior oblique position where it forms a separate convexity just below the aortic shadow and above the shadow of the right ventricle.

Measurement of the diameter of the pulmonary trunk is best made on an overexposed chest film or preferably a film exposed at a high kilovoltage (190 kv). The measurement is the distance from the superior and lateral margin of the left main stem bronchus to the most distant point on the pulmonary trunk. Measurements from conventional chest films are rather gross; however, there is some correlation with the pulmonary artery pressure. Milne (1963) concluded that there is a considerable correlation between estimated size of the pulmonary artery as seen on the chest film and the pulmonary artery mean pressure, although generally there was a tendency to overestimate the pulmonary artery pressure. The work of Moore *et al.* (1959) is noteworthy in that they described an objective measurement consisting of the distance from the midline of the thoracic spine to the farthest lateral extension of the pulmonary artery segment divided by the distance of ½ the maximum transthoracic diameter multiplied by 100, which gave a ratio that correlated quite well with the mean pulmonary artery pressure ($r = 0.89$). It appears that in uncomplicated mitral stenosis the size of the pulmonary artery segment as seen on the conventional chest film is often related to the pulmonary artery pressure. An apparently normal-sized artery, however, does not exclude some degree of pulmonary hypertension (Whitaker and Lodge, 1954). Marked enlargement, such as is seen in many cases of interatrial septal defect, is decidedly uncommon in mitral stenosis.

Angiography is a much more reliable means of measuring the size of the pulmonary artery than the conventional chest film. Soloff *et al.* (1957) found by angiographic methods that the pulmonary artery is enlarged in almost all cases severe enough to have an elevation of the mean pulmonary artery pressure (exceeding 25 mm Hg).

Small Size of the Aorta. The aortic knob is typically small and inconspicuous. It may appear relatively small because of the adjacent enlarged pulmonary artery segment. Actually the aorta is often decreased in size, particularly in association with a decreased cardiac output and particularly if the stenosis has been present since childhood.

Systemic hypertension may appear in patients with long standing mitral stenosis and particularly after the age of 40 years. Atherosclerotic changes in the aorta are occasionally seen, and either of these conditions may cause the knob to become more prominent. The ascending aorta is almost never identified in mitral stenosis on a conventional posteroanterior film.

Characteristic Pulmonary Vascular Pattern. The primary branches of the right and left pulmonary arteries and the secondary or hilar branches are frequently and typically dilated and like the pulmonary trunk show a rough relationship to the pulmonary artery pressure. Schwedel *et al.* (1957) measured the descending branch of the right pulmonary artery near the hilus in 105 patients with predominant mitral stenosis. In 90% of normal persons this segment measured in the range of 9–13 mm. In patients with mitral stenosis a measurement of 14 mm or more occurred in about 65% of all cases. Almost without exception a large artery was associated with a mean pulmonary artery pressure greater than 25 mm Hg, and the size of the artery correlated to a considerable degree with the pressure. On the other hand, about 15% of patients had pulmonary hypertension with arteries of 13 mm or less in

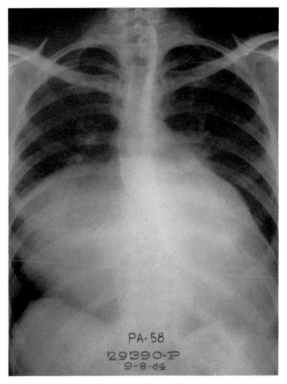

PA·58
29390-P
9-8-64

FIG. 90. GIANT LEFT ATRIUM
Postmortem study showed predominant mitral insufficiency.

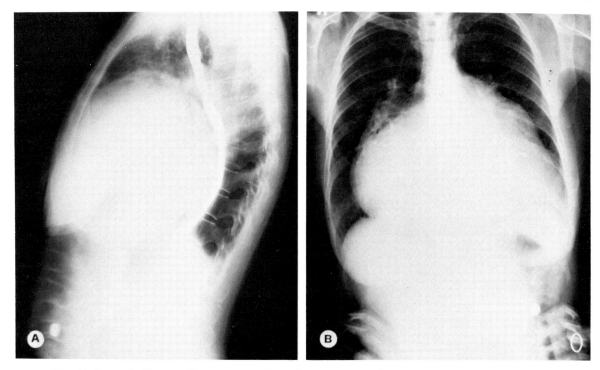

FIG. 91 A AND B. MARKED DILATATION OF LEFT ATRIUM IN LONG-STANDING MITRAL VALVULAR DISEASE
The left atrium forms the entire right border of the heart. Mitral insufficiency was probably the predominant lesion.

size. Consequently, as in the case of the main pulmonary artery, pulmonary hypertension of moderate degree cannot be excluded by inspection or by measuring the size of the major branches of the pulmonary arteries.

Davies *et al.* (1953) studied the intrapulmonary arterial system in mitral stenosis by angiography, and their description has led to the frequent recognition of a similar pattern on conventional films. When the pulmonary artery pressure was normal or only slightly elevated, the hilar and intrapulmonary arteries were normal in size or only slightly dilated, bifurcated in a normal fashion and extended well toward the periphery of the lungs. When the pressure elevation was due mainly to increased venous pressure (producing only moderate degrees of pulmonary arterial hypertension), the arterial system was slightly dilated. When the pulmonary artery pressure was elevated (due for the most part to increased peripheral pulmonary resistance) the vascular pattern was often strikingly changed. The central arteries were dilated but tapered or narrowed quite rapidly. The peripheral arteries were tortuous and a fine peripheral network could often be seen. On conventional chest films the peripheral network may not be identified, but the rapid tapering and tortuosity of the larger central arteries are easily seen and indicate a

considerable increase in pulmonary artery pressure. Fleischner and Sagall (1955) followed patients with mitral stenosis for years during which the vascular pattern changed from normal to one in which the hilar arteries were much enlarged and gave the appearance of a plump tumor with a truncated or amputated appearance of the smaller adjacent arteries. They state that this pattern is reversible, at least to some degree, although superimposed atherosclerosis may produce a permanent increase in pulmonary resistance and narrowing of the peripheral arteries. The underlying structural and functional causes for the radiologic changes have not been satisfactorily explained in every respect, but part may be due to vasoconstriction and part to intimal thickening of the smaller arteries (Parker and Weiss, 1936). Luminal obliteration of these arteries will result in decreased blood flow to the affected areas, thus accentuating the disparity between the larger central arteries and the smaller-than-normal peripheral vessels.

The upper lobe veins are almost parallel but lateral to the arteries and curve smoothly upward with convexity downward and laterally. Near the hilus their shadows fuse with those of the pulmonary arteries which they cross—but their point of entry into the left atrium is rarely identified on plain films. The lower lobe veins are

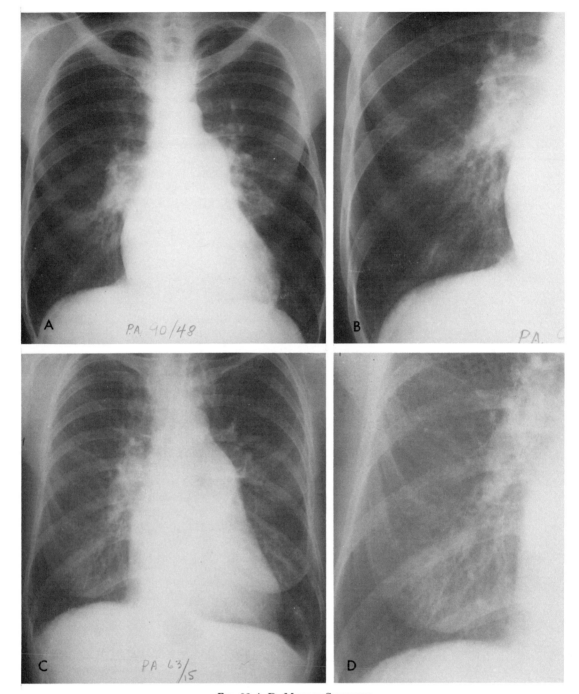

FIG. 92 A–D. MITRAL STENOSIS

Two cases of predominant mitral stenosis with increased pulmonary resistance and tapering and truncation of the pulmonary arteries. This pattern is highly suggestive of increased pulmonary resistance.

almost straight and run at an angle to the arteries which they cross as they approach the hilus at a point about 3–4 cm below the pulmonary arteries. The veins in the right lower lobe can be identified almost without exception in normal persons. The identification of pulmonary veins can be greatly improved by practice and com-

parison with pulmonary angiograms in which the veins are clearly opacified.

In mitral stenosis the venous pressure is increased (greater than 10 mm Hg) in all but the mildest cases. The veins might be thought to be passive structures with little elasticity, but their walls are approximately as thick as the arteries.

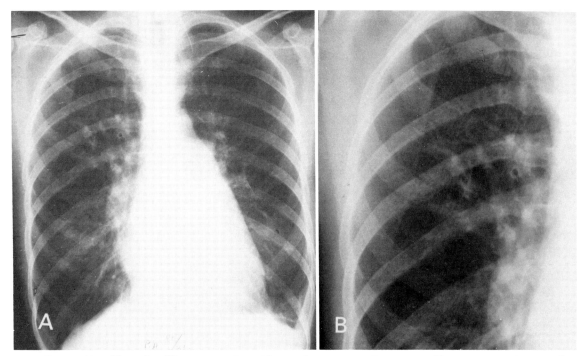

FIG. 93. THIRTY-NINE-YEAR-OLD WOMAN WITH PURE MITRAL STENOSIS AND PULMONARY HYPERTENSION (AUTOPSY CASE)
(A) There is moderate dilatation of the right upper lobe veins and also evidence of pulmonary hypertension with truncation of the pulmonary arteries to the lower lobes. (B) Enlargement of the right upper lung field.

There seems little doubt that they are under some sort of vasomotor control. Some degree of venous dilatation is visible in many cases of mitral stenosis, but the pattern is distinctive in that the upper lobe veins are selectively dilated or more prominent than the lower lobe veins in a considerable number of cases. This may be associated with increased hydrostatic pressure in the lower lobe veins in the erect position. Simon (1958) has reported that venous dilatation increases up to a pressure of about 25 mm Hg. Further increments are followed by a decrease in size probably due to reflex vasoconstriction, the mechanism of which is not well understood. Some estimate of the pulmonary venous pressure is possible from conventional chest films, although a sharp film is necessary for the veins to be seen to best advantage. Pulmonary infiltrations, edema, and large branching arteries tend to obscure the veins. Body section radiographic studies are very helpful.

Parenchymal Lung Changes. These may be divided into the following identifiable components: Kerley's B lines or costophrenic septal lines, localized nodular shadows (usually diffuse and attributed to hemosiderosis), calcific nodules, blotchy ill defined densities ascribed to pulmonary edema, and congestion.

B lines (Kerley, 1951), intrapulmonary septal lymphatic lines (Fleming and Simmons, 1958),

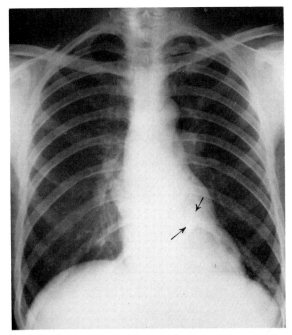

FIG. 94. PREDOMINANT MITRAL STENOSIS WITH DENSE CALCIUM (ARROWS) IN MITRAL VALVE

and costophrenic septal lines (Bruwer et al., 1955) are names for the same type of shadow. As seen on conventional chest films these are linear shadows 1–3 cm in length and about 1 mm in width. They do not branch or bifurcate and are most frequent in the lung bases and are almost never seen in the upper one-third of the lung. The number may vary from 1–2 in one base to 20–30 in each lung. Although they were undoubtedly seen for years by radiologists, Kerley was the first to give them specific recognition in 1951. A and C lines were also described but are rarely seen and are of distinctly less practical importance.

These lines are probably produced by the combination of edema of the interlobular septa of the lung and superimposed distended lymphatic channels. They can appear and disappear in a period as short as 24–48 hours after medical management and particularly after successful commissurotomy or valve replacement.

These lines are almost always associated with elevated pulmonary venous pressure in patients with heart disease. It should be remembered that these lines can vary from day to day, and a determination of pulmonary venous pressure may not be valid 2–3 days before or afterward. It is clear on the other hand that elevation of venous pressure is not always followed by the appearance of Kerley's lines. They are less common in pure or even predominant mitral insufficiency. The pulmonary artery pressure is almost always elevated when the lines are present, but conversely the pulmonary artery pressure may

be quite high without septal lines. Pulmonary edema is not common in the pressence of lines, and pleural fluid is distinctly uncommon. Prompt disappearance of the lines after commissurotomy is a favorable prognostic sign (McAfee and Biondetti, 1957). Similar appearing lines have been seen in other conditions (see page 111).

Some degree of pulmonary parenchymal infiltration is common with mitral stenosis. The present authors have frequently seen irregular small blotchy shadows scattered through the central portion of the lungs often associated with an overall increase in density. These shadows may become confluent and they may regress. We have attributed this change to pulmonary congestion and edema, although we have little support for this interpretation other than that the appearance is reversible. We differentiate this pattern from that due to hemosiderosis. In hemosiderosis collections of macrophages containing hemosiderin form nodules that are up to 3 mm in size, and these appear on chest films as focal lesions. In the more advanced cases these shadows may coalesce or be superimposed so as to give the appearance of a reticular network through the lung (Fig. 95). These small nodules do not resolve according to Esposito (1955), and our own experience confirms this impression. We recognize that this may not be the only manifestation of hemosiderosis and that many of the other opac-

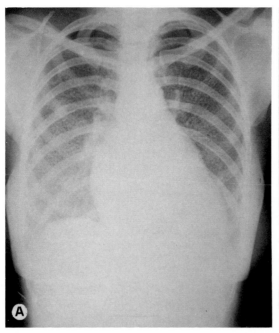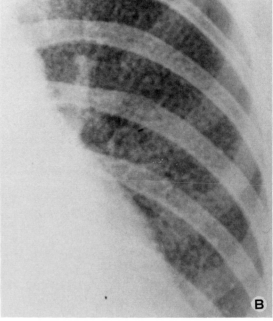

FIG. 95. PULMONARY HEMOSIDEROSIS IN LONG-STANDING CASE OF MITRAL VALVULAR DISEASE (A AND B)
The miliary opacities remained unchanged for at least 6 years. (B) Enlargement of left upper lung field.

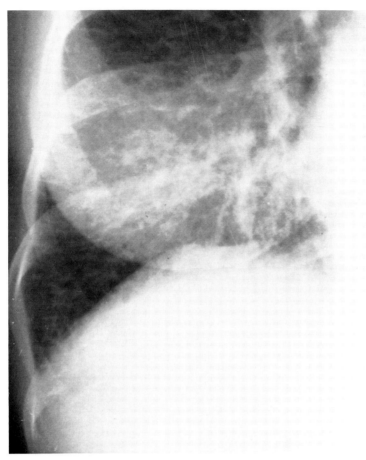

FIG. 96. COSTOPHRENIC SEPTAL LINES (KERLEY'S B LINES)
IN BASE OF RIGHT LUNG IN CASE OF MITRAL STENOSIS

ities seen in the lungs with mitral stenosis may be due to hemosiderin. The punctate type that we have described is uncommon in the present authors' experience, which coincides with that of McAfee and Biondetti (1957) in which only 1 patient out of 150 with mitral valve disease was found to have this condition. Hemosiderosis is more common in patients with hemoptysis and pulmonary hypertension. Hemosiderosis has not been described with pure mitral insufficiency.

Calcific nodules that may progress to ossification are found occasionally in mitral stenosis and appear to be more common in association with hemosiderosis. The nodules are rounded and are more often found in the lower portions of the lungs.

Pulmonary edema may be acute and rapid in onset and resemble acute edema due to a variety of other lesions. It is likely to occur when the venous pressure is high and the pulmonary arterial resistance is low, and an increase in pulmonary resistance may be a protective reaction.

The acute edema may clear rapidly and may have largely disappeared by the time a chest film is taken. Some degree of chronic edema may be manifest by an overall increase in density of the lungs.

Mitral Valvular Calcification. Calcium can be identified by the surgeon in 33–40% of cases coming to commissurotomy (McAfee and Biondetti, 1957; Bailey and Morse, 1957). About one-half of these can be positively identified preoperatively by the radiologist. The more heavily calcified valves are seen in a high percentage of cases by careful fluoroscopy. Small deposits in the commissures may be overlooked, but these deposits are not as significant as the more massive calcifications. Careful fluoroscopy using image amplification systems and cinefluorography should improve this yield (see Chapter 21, p. 549).

McAfee and Biondetti (1957) found that 43% of their cases that came to commissurotomy with some degree of mitral insufficiency had calcifi-

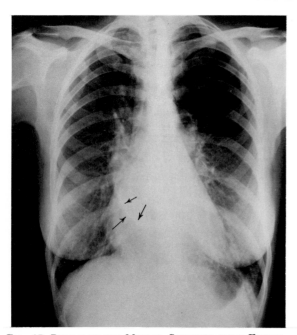

FIG. 97. PREDOMINANT MITRAL STENOSIS WITH EXTEN-
SIVE CALCIFICATION IN LEFT ATRIAL WALL (AUTOPSY
CASE)

At operation the left atrium contained a large amount of
thrombus.

cation, although the predominant lesion was stenotic. On the other hand, only 10% of their cases
with pure stenosis had calcification. Wood (1954)
found that 62% of surgical cases with some degree
of mitral insufficiency had calcium in the valves
and states that 50% of cases with significant
insufficiency will have heavy calcification. These
experiences suggest that heavy calcification is
usually found with mixed insufficiency and stenosis with stenosis as the predominant lesion.
The authors' experience would confirm this
impression. Another aspect of the problem is
that insufficiency is often made worse by commissurotomy since it is frequently impossible to
split the commissures so as to leave good diastolic apposition of the leaflets. Thus, massive
calcification is an indication for valve replacement. Furthermore, the hazard of breaking off
fragments of the calcified mass which may then
act as emboli is very considerable.

Calcification of the mitral valve is more often
associated with clinical and hemodynamic evidence of severe disease (Wynn, 1953), although
mild symptoms and disability are occasionally
seen.

Right Ventricular Enlargement. Enlargement of the right ventricle eventually occurs in
most cases of mitral stenosis. In the earlier stages
the ventricle hypertrophies only and exerts very
little effect upon the cardiac contour. In the later
stages as the ventricle begins to dilate, it may
extend into the retrosternal space and increase
that portion of the cardiac shadow which is in
close relation with the sternum anteriorly.

From angiographic studies, Grishman *et al.*
(1944) concluded that the right ventricle does
not form any part of the left heart border in the
posteroanterior projection in mitral valvular disease. The straightening or convexity of the left
midheart border is due to enlargement of the
pulmonary artery trunk.

Right Atrial Enlargement. Enlargement of
the right atrium is a late occurrence in mitral
stenosis and appears only after the right ventricle
begins to fail. Enlargement usually indicates relative tricuspid insufficiency due to the dilatation
of the valve ring. Structural tricuspid stenosis,
however, is considerably more common than suspected and probably occurs to a significant degree in about 5% of all cases. Organic tricuspid
insufficiency also is occasionally seen, and both
of these lesions are described in the section on
tricuspid valvular disease.

Left Atrial Calcification. Left atrial calcification is uncommon but not rare (see section on
Cardiac Calcification, p. 549). Vickers *et al.*
(1959) found 42 reported cases, but many have
not been reported, including at least 10 cases
observed by the present authors. Calcium may
be deposited in or underneath the endocardium
or within a mural thrombus. Laminated calcium
is characteristic of a thrombus. Left atrial calcification must be differentiated from pericardial
calcification.

Calcification in the left atrium is found in long-
standing cases, and it may be associated with
either stenosis or insufficiency. It is considerably
more frequent with atrial fibrillation. In about
50% of cases the calcium is in the body of the
atrium, and in the other 50% it is in the appendage. Atrial calcification has considerable weight
in evaluating the patient for surgery as it greatly
increases the hazards of opening the atrium. Entering the left atrium may be difficult, and
thrombus material is likely to be encountered.
Great care must be taken to prevent embolization. Extensive calcification may also prevent the
insertion of a transseptal catheter during diagnostic workup.

Calcium in the left atrium is best detected by
careful fluoroscopy in various projections. Sometimes it may be so faint that it can be seen only
on good quality overpenetrated films made with
a high speed Bucky diaphragm. The calcium may
be visible in one projection or through a narrow

range of projections. In the authors' experience it has been most often confused with linear calcification in a rib cartilage or rarely with calcium in a hilar or mediastinal lymph node. This difficulty can usually be rapidly resolved by fluoroscopy.

Left Ventricular Contour. In pure or predominant mitral stenosis the left ventricle is normal or even reduced in size in contrast to the considerable dilatation and enlargement seen in mitral insufficiency. The determination of left ventricular size is thus often of crucial importance. In the conventional posteroanterior projection the left heart border in mitral stenosis is steep and approaches the vertical. The roentgenographic cardiac apex is usually 1–4 cm above the diaphragm in contrast to the low apex of left ventricular enlargement. The right anterior oblique and lateral views with barium in the esophagus may demonstrate a considerable overhang or offset in the posterior contour of the heart where the enlarged left atrial shadow joins the curve of the left venticle (Fig. 98B). Eyler *et al.* (1959) suggested that when the left ventricular curve projected posterior to the vertical shadow of the inferior vena cava in the lateral projection by a distance of 15 mm or more enlargement was quite likely. When a notch or indentation between the left atrium and left ventricle is present, it has been in our experience a reliable and useful sign of mitral stenosis. On the other hand, its absence does not exclude stenosis. On occasion the left atrium may be so large that it intrudes on or overlaps the left ventricle. Also, the posterior border of the left ventricle may not be clearly visible due to a high diaphragm or barium in the esophagus. Nevertheless, the lateral view admittedly is most helpful in mitral valvular disease in the assessment of the size of the left ventricle.

Mitral Insufficiency

Insufficiency of the mitral valve may be due to scarring and shortening of the mitral leaflets. The most severe changes are found in the posterior leaflet which may be rolled and retracted with ensuing dilatation of the left atrium which causes tension on the valve and pulls the valve ring upward and backward so as to increase the insufficiency. Shortening of the chordae tendineae may also prevent proper closure of the valve. Scarring and calcification may occur and fix the valve in a permanent position of insufficiency. Insufficiency may also be due to a rupture

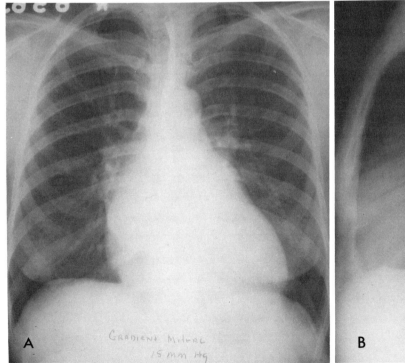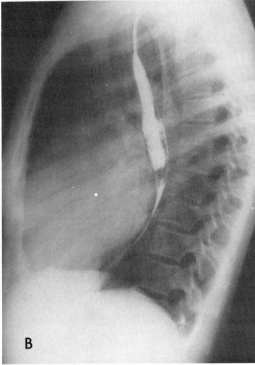

FIG. 98. PURE MITRAL STENOSIS AND MINIMAL AORTIC STENOSIS AND INSUFFICIENCY (A AND B)
The lateral view shows an indentation as the left atrial contour joins that of the left ventricle. This is highly suggestive of predominant or pure mitral stenosis.

of a chorda tendinea or rupture of a papillary muscle. Of course, congenital anomalies of the papillary muscles must be differentiated from rheumatic valvular disease.

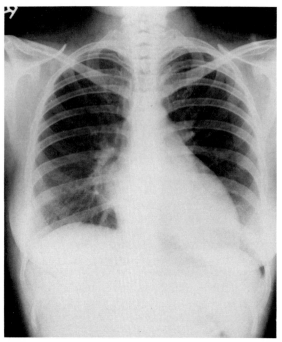

FIG. 99. PROBABLE "PURE" MITRAL INSUFFICIENCY AS DE-TERMINED AT OPERATION

The left ventricular curvature is longer and somewhat less steep than in figure 76.

Hemodynamically and anatomically the main differences between stenosis and insufficiency are found in the left ventricle, left atrium, and pulmonary veins. With predominant insufficiency, during each systole some of the blood which under normal circumstances would have departed through the aorta is expelled backward through the mitral valve. Consequently, if the heart is to maintain its normal output, the left ventricle must dilate so as to accommodate a larger volume of blood and hypertrophy in order to expel the blood. Thus, in predominant or pure mitral insufficiency the left ventricle is dilated and hypertrophied. The left atrium, in most cases, is considerably larger than in mitral stenosis (Edwards, 1961). The mean pulmonary venous pressure is not as high as in mitral stenosis, although the V waves from the atrial wedge pressure tracings may be higher than in mitral stenosis. In mitral insufficiency as seen on the conventional posteroanterior chest film, the heart is usually larger than in stenosis, and the left border is longer, more oblique, and with a low cardiac apex (Fig. 101A). The left atrium as seen through the heart shadow is large and is usually borderforming on the right. Giant left atria are seen with insufficiency and occasionally are of enormous size (DeSanctis et al., 1964). The left atrium may extend to the right chest wall and compress the right middle lobe bronchus, producing atelectasis. The pulmonary trunk and the primary and secondary branches

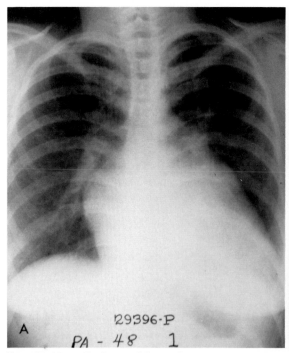

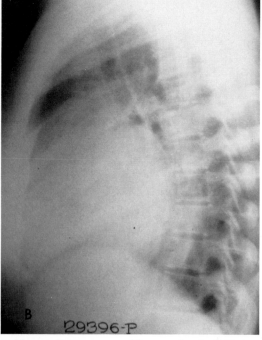

FIG. 100 A AND B. SEVERE MITRAL INSUFFICIENCY, MINIMAL MITRAL STENOSIS, AND MINIMAL AORTIC STENOSIS

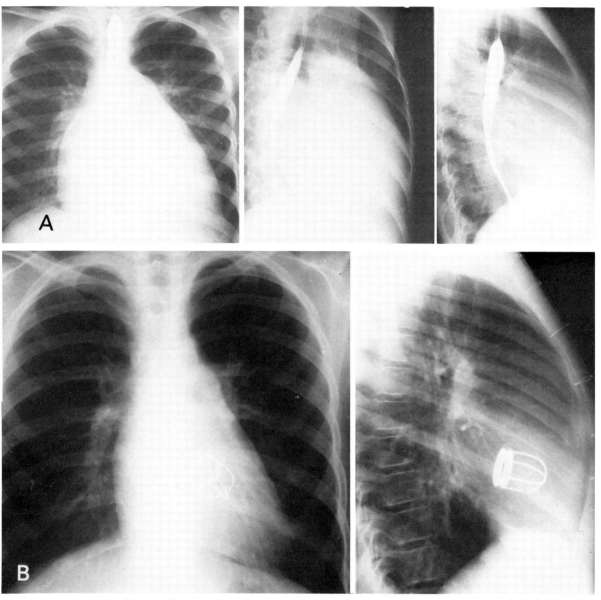

FIG. 101. TWELVE-YEAR-OLD BOY WITH RHEUMATIC MITRAL INSUFFICIENCY

(A) Posteroanterior, right anterior oblique, and lateral films made 1 month preoperatively show prominence of the pulmonary artery, gross cardiac enlargement with marked left atrial enlargement. The aorta is small. The pulmonary vascularity is normal, though the upper lobe veins may be slightly enlarged. (B) Posteroanterior and lateral films of the chest made 3 months after replacement of the mitral valve with a Starr-Edwards prosthesis. The heart has decreased markedly in size, and the shape is almost normal. The patient experienced marked amelioration of symptoms after the operation.

of the pulmonary arteries in the lungs are usually enlarged as in mitral stenosis; however, tapering and truncation of the hilar branches are uncommon. Kerley's B lines and the splotchy or granular infiltrates of mitral stenosis are rarely seen. In general, the pulmonary parenchyma is clear, although pulmonary edema secondary to left heart failure can occur.

In the lateral view, the left atrium produces a long indentation in the anterior surface of the

esophagus indicating considerable enlargement, and it merges imperceptibly with the left ventricle below. If the left atrium becomes considerably enlarged, it does not extend backward so much as to the right.

Calcium is rarely found in the valve in pure or high grade insufficiency, although moderate to marked calcification is often found with some degree of insufficiency associated with stenosis. It is in these cases that commissurotomy may greatly increase the insufficiency (Wood, 1954).

In mitral insufficiency a considerable volume of blood refluxes into the left atrium, and pressure tracings obtained from the left atrium show the V wave to be steep and much greater than the A wave. Expansion of the left atrium with ventricular systole does occur and is visible at fluoroscopy. This is best demonstrated by studying the pulsations of the barium-filled esophagus in the extreme right anterior oblique position as it courses over the posterior lateral surface of the left atrium; it also may be seen where the left atrium is enlarged sufficiently to be borderforming on the right. At fluoroscopy, the shutters should be momentarily opened sufficiently to allow observation simultaneously of both the atrial and ventricular borders in order to appraise the timing of the pulsations. These findings must be interpreted with some reservations because (1) the left atrium expands somewhat during ventricular systole without mitral insufficiency due to the inflow of blood from the pulmonary veins. In the normal left atrium the magnitude of this expansion is considerable. When the atrium is already dilated and tense, the effect of the inflow of blood from the pulmonary veins is lessened but still must be considered; (2) positional changes of the heart during ventricular systole may cause a posterior displacement of the esophagus which resembles atrial expansion. This is most likely with a well digitalized heart in which the rate is slow and the beat is forcible. In a number of cases seen by the present authors, expansion of the left atrium appeared quite definite during ventricular systole; yet at operation there was mitral stenosis and no detectable insufficiency.

Nghiem *et al.* (1967), in a careful study of 305 normal children, established normal values and ranges for cardiac volume from birth to 19 years. Their study of 27 children with mitral insufficiency disclosed that patients could be grouped according to cardiac volume and that therapy and prognosis could be based in part upon such groupings. Children with rheumatic mitral insufficiency and normal cardiac volumes (Group I) were asymptomatic and required observation only. Those whose cardiac volumes were greater than the upper limit of normal but less than twice the upper limit of normal (Group II) had moderate mitral insufficiency with signs of intolerance to moderate or marked exertion. They could be managed medically. Those in Group III, with cardiac volumes greater than twice the upper limit of normal (in the absence of overt evidence of cardiac decompensation or acute carditis) required valve replacement. None of the hearts of the children in Group III grew smaller without operation, and unless they underwent valve replacement, all of the children in Group III died. Thus, mitral insufficiency, the predominant expression of rheumatic mitral valve disease in children, can be accurately assessed and followed by the cardiac volume technique (Fig. 53 and Table 6).

Physical examination of the heart by a skilled cardiologist provides most useful evidence of either mitral stenosis or insufficiency and is helpful in differentiating between the two. The typical murmurs, however, may be modified by ar-

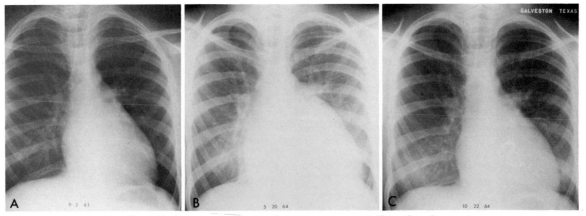

FIG. 102. RHEUMATIC MITRAL INSUFFICIENCY IN 11-YEAR-OLD GIRL

Frame A shows the appearance of the heart in September, 1963. Frame B is a reproduction of a posteroanterior chest film on May 20, 1964, 2 months prior to surgery. Frame C shows the appearance of the heart 2 months after replacement of the mitral valve with a Starr-Edwards prosthesis. The patient experienced marked improvement and amelioration of symptoms after surgery.

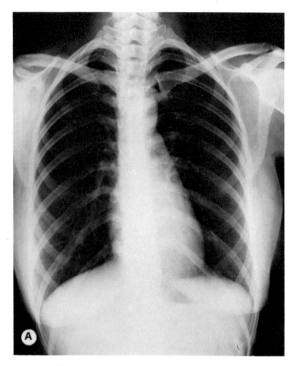
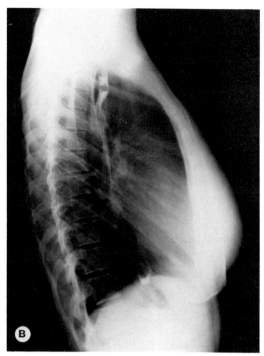

FIG. 103 A AND B. A 33-YEAR-OLD WOMAN WHO HAD HAD ATTACKS OF DYSPNEA FOR 2 YEARS

There is suggestive enlargement of the right ventricle, but otherwise the cardiac contours are entirely within normal limits. At operation there was marked mitral stenosis.

rhythmias or cardiac failure; in early cases they may be faint and difficult to elicit. It is in these cases in which murmurs are atypical or absent that roentgen findings may be helpful. Sosman (1940) has observed a number of cases of "sub-clinical mitral stenosis" in which the typical murmurs were either absent or could not be heard until searched for by an experienced cardiologist. In all of these cases there was dilatation of the left atrium, and in some there was radiologic evidence of lung stasis and/or calcification in the mitral valve. The present authors, however, believe that in general auscultation by experienced observers is a more sensitive test for the presence of mitral stenosis than the conventional radiologic examination. Figure 103 shows a patient in whom the radiologic changes were minimal and could be found only in retrospect; yet this patient had mitral stenosis of moderate severity. In one patient recently seen by the authors, dyspnea had been present for 2 years; yet there was no evidence of lung stasis. At operation a very high degree of mitral stenosis was found. Pariser *et al.* (1951) found that in 30 patients with clinical mitral stenosis in whom the diagnosis was confirmed at autopsy 6 showed no left atrial enlargement. Also, McAfee and Biondetti (1957) found 6 patients out of 150 who underwent commis-

surotomy in whom the cardiac contour was entirely normal. Consequently, it is believed that the conventional radiologic examination cannot be relied upon to rule out significant mitral stenosis.

Mitral valvular disease as seen on a conventional radiologic examination resembles a number of other conditions and must be differentiated from them. These are as follows:

1. Myxomas of the left atrium, when they obstruct the mitral valve, cause left atrial dilatation and are often diagnosed as atypical mitral disease. A high index of suspicion is necessary to diagnose these tumors. Selective angiography is most helpful in diagnosis.

2. Dilatation of the left atrium may occur in any condition which produces left ventricular failure, such as hypertension or myocardial infarction. Chronic myocarditis (Fig. 430) with some degree of left ventricular enlargement may resemble mitral stenosis to a marked degree. Left atrial catheterization or a valid pulmonary wedge pressure may be necessary for differentiation.

3. Emphysema, silicosis, marked right-sided scoliosis, and extensive fibrosis of the lung and stenosis of the pulmonary veins will produce enlargement of the pulmonary artery and right ventricle and thus result in a partial similarity to

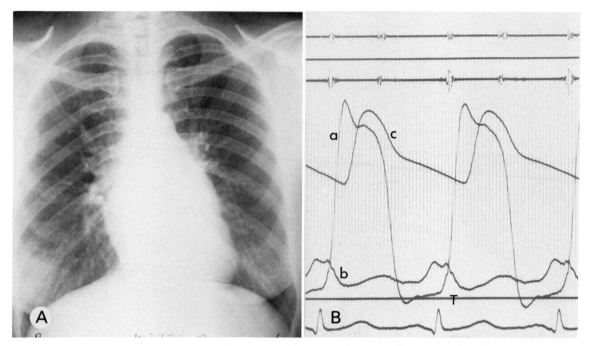

FIG. 104. PURE MITRAL STENOSIS OF MODERATE SEVERITY (OPERATIVE CASE)

Right ventricular pressure was 48 mm Hg. (A) Conventional chest film. (B) Simultaneous pressure tracings from the left ventricle (a), left atrium (b) and right brachial artery (c). During the entire period of ventricular diastole a gradient is seen between the left atrium and ventricle with accentuation at the "a" wave (atrial systole). No evidence of regurgitation.

mitral valvular disease. These conditions, how-ever, are rarely associated with left atrial enlarge-ment. Differentiation from purely radiologic findings is sometimes difficult.

4. Thyrotoxicosis may be associated with straightening of the left border of the heart, occasional enlargement of the left atrium, and atrial fibrillation. The jerky rapid pulsations of the thyroid heart, however, are different from those of mitral disease; also, evidence of pulmo-nary stasis is usually lacking. Dilatation of the left atrium is minimal.

5. Left-to-right shunts may resemble mitral heart disease because of the prominence of the pulmonary artery, increased pulmonary vascular volume and ventricular enlargement. In patent ductus arteriosus and ventricular septal defect, left atrial enlargement may add to the difficulty of differentiation. Cardiac catheterization will usually be required for complete diagnosis, though many clues can be gained from radiologic studies, auscultation and history.

6. Pulmonary hypertension of any etiology may produce prominence of the pulmonary trunk and a cardiac contour which specifically resem-bles that of mitral valvular disease.

7. Valvular pulmonary stenosis may display enlargement of the main pulmonary artery and

radiographic and electrocardiographic evidence of right ventricular hypertrophy, simulating mi-tral heart disease. The auscultatory findings are characteristic, and the left atrium is not enlarged.

Right or left heart catheterization and angiog-raphy may be necessary simply to detect the presence of mitral valvular disease. It is more usual, however, that these methods of examina-tion are used to quantitate the extent of the disease and to differentiate between stenosis and insufficiency, and, further, to detect associated aortic disease.

Although present day practice varies from in-stitution to institution, the best practice requires cardiac catheterization, often supplemented by angiography, prior to the institution of therapy, particularly surgical therapy.

Right Heart Catheterization

Right heart catheterization with catheteriza-tion of the pulmonary artery may lead to evalu-ation of pulmonary hypertension and estimation of the intrinsic pulmonary resistance. This is in turn an indication of the change in the pulmo-nary vasculature associated with mitral stenosis. Diminished cardiac output and particularly fix-ation of cardiac output after exercise or the use of drugs, such as Isuprel, provide strong supporting evidence of fixed obstruction at the mitral valve. The contour of the wedge pressures may be of some value in differentiating between predominant stenosis and insufficiency, although these tracings are very definitely inferior to those obtained from the left atrium, particularly when estimating the severity of each lesion.

Left Heart Catheterization

A catheter may be placed in the left ventricle by the transaortic route. The technique described by Ross (1959) and refined by Brockenbrough *et al.* (1960) may be used to advance the catheter from the right atrium through the interatrial septum into the left atrium and thence into the left ventricle. Ideally the mitral valve is best studied with catheters in both the left atrium and left ventricle through which simultaneous pressure tracings can be obtained. Such tracings, when free of technical artefacts, give reliable evidence of stenosis, and the magnitude of gradient across the valve leads to some quantitation of the severity of the lesion (Fig. 104b). Certainly the gradient in mitral stenosis is a good indication of the severity of the obstruction although it is a function of the cardiac output or flowrate across the valve; however, in the presence of stenosis, the degree of associated insufficiency may be more difficult to assess. After the hemodynamic studies, angiography of the mitral valve may be carried out.

Angiography of the Mitral Valve

Mitral stenosis is best studied after the injection of 0.6–0.8 ml of contrast substance per kg by a pressure injector into the left atrium. We have routinely made the injection through a Brockenbrough catheter placed into the left atrium through the transseptal route. The patient is placed in about 60° of left posterior obliquity, and filming is carried out at 4 frames/sec or with cinefluorography at 60 frames/sec. We have used cinefluorography because it was readily available to us. We do not attempt to defend its use but feel that complex changes in valve motion and contour are better shown than with direct filming, although detail may be lacking when any one film is viewed separately. Also, the simplicity of this method and the ease with which it is used have led to its routine use in our hands.

Angiographic Anatomy of Normal Mitral Valve. LEFT ATRIAL INJECTION. The normal mitral valve during early ventricular diastole has a funnel shape, and as diastole progresses this quickly changes to a large orifice with a rapid flow of contrast substance into the left ventricle. The left atrium empties rapidly and is not enlarged. In ventricular diastole the cusps of the normal mitral valve cannot be seen, and the contrast substance passes from the atrium into the ventricle through a large orifice.

In systole after the injection of contrast substance into the ventricle, the mitral valve bulges and is convex toward the atrium forming a dome (Fig. 105). The normal mitral valve is completely competent. The papillary muscles are rarely identified. Movement of the valve cusps is seen, and this is particularly noticeable in early ventricular diastole when the cusps can be seen protruding downward, although they quickly

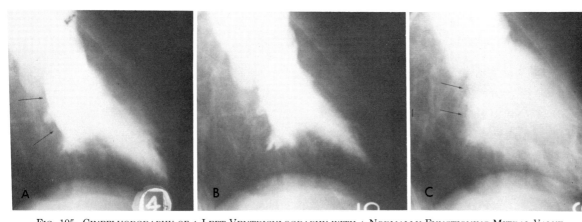

FIG. 105. CINEFLUORGRAPHY OF A LEFT VENTRICULOGRAPHY WITH A NORMALLY FUNCTIONING MITRAL VALVE
(A) Mid-systole. The cusps are in apposition and are slightly convex toward the left atrium. (B) Late systole. The small central protrusion represents a slight ballooning of a posterior scallop without hemodynamic significance. (C) Diastole. The valve leaflets are obscured by the contrast substance.

Left atrial and left ventricular catheterization showed no evidence of mitral stenosis or insufficiency, although there was evidence of aortic stenosis and insufficiency.

vanish in the large flow of contrast substance into the ventricle from the atrium.

In stenosis, the fused anterior and posterior leaflets form a funnel-shaped orifice. It remains fixed for the greater part of ventricular diastole. In the more advanced cases, the valve is almost completely fixed and unchanged in contour over the course of the cardiac cycle. Kjellberg *et al.* (1961) found the range of motion of the anterior leaflet in mitral stenosis was 4–9 mm and the posterior cusp was 0–24 mm. An interesting observation was that those cases with markedly diminished motion had combined stenosis and insufficiency. Since most of our studies were made with cinefluorography, we have not had an adequate opportunity to measure valve cusp movement. The left atrium is enlarged, and the contrast substance stagnates. The time necessary for clearing of the contrast substance averages between 5 and 10 sec. (Kjellberg *et al.*, 1961). Also, reflux into the pulmonary veins with each ventricular systole is almost invariable and usually strikingly increased over the normal. A left ventricular injection through a transaortic catheter may show mitral stenosis by outlining the ventricular phase of the valve. A stenotic valve is seen as a radiolucent dome protuding into the opacified left ventricle (Fig. 107). Some degree of fixation of the valve may be noted, and a stiffened

valve usually does not show the convexity toward the atrium such as occurs in ventricular systole in a normal valve.

Insufficiency is best demonstrated by a slow injection (3–5 sec) of 1 ml of contrast substance per kg of body weight into the left ventricle. The catheter is preferably inserted through the aortic valve using a percutaneous technique. We have used either a Teflon or a Kifa catheter with 4 side holes. Electrocardiographic monitoring is essential to time and record ventricular extrasystoles since the mitral valve shows minor degrees of incompetence with extrasystoles. On occasion a left ventricular injection has been accomplished through a transseptal catheter inserted through the left atrium and thence across the valve; however, this is undesirable since the catheter may interfere with the valve competence. A normal mitral valve is completely competent, and the cusps can be seen to bulge toward the left atrium during ventricular systole.

Insufficiency following left ventricular injection is characterized by a regurgitant jet into the atrium. This is best seen at the first systole after opacification of the ventricle, and as the atrium becomes progressively more opaque the visibility of the jet decreases. The size of the jet and the degree of opacification of the atrium provide a basis of rough quantitation of the insufficiency.

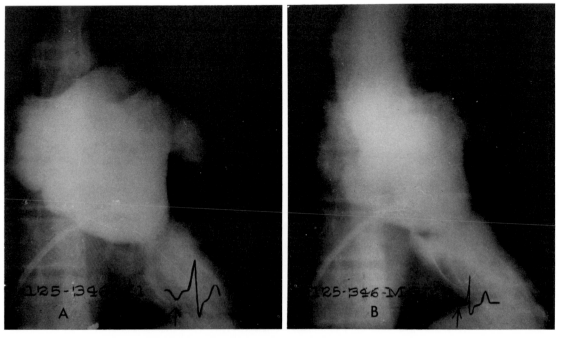

FIG. 106. MITRAL STENOSIS. LEFT ATRIAL INJECTION THROUGH TRANS-SEPTAL CATHETER

(A) Atrial systole showing reflux into left pulmonary veins and convexity downward of the valve cusps. (B) Two heart cycles later the mitral valve is unchanged in contour.

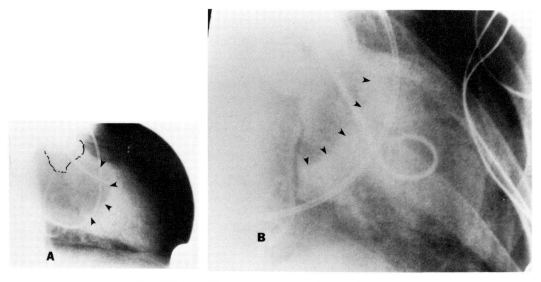

FIG. 107. LEFT VENTRICULOGRAM IN MITRAL STENOSIS

(A) RAO projection in a case of pure mitral stenosis with still pliable valve cusps (arrowheads). The outline of the aortic root has been outlined. (B) RAO projection showing pure mitral stenosis. The valve shows very little evidence of irregularity or scarring but did not descend normally into left ventricle and remained distinctly visible during diastole.

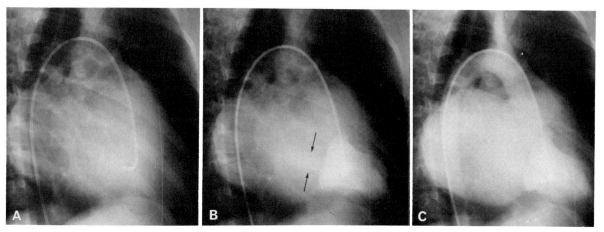

FIG. 108. MITRAL STENOSIS AND INSUFFICIENCY (A–C)

(A) Before injection of contrast substance. (B) Following left ventricular injection a central regurgitant jet is seen (arrows). The mitral leaflets are straight instead of showing the usual convexity toward the atrium. (C) Ventricular diastole. The mitral valve leaflets are unchanged in position and contour indicating marked rigidity.

The location of the jet is difficult to determine precisely, although incompetency of the mitral valve usually involves the posterior cusp (Edwards, 1961). Rupture of a chorda tendinea usually produces gross incompetence without any evidence of a valve structure. In pure mitral incompetency, likewise, the cusps are very indistinct (see Chapter 17, page 000).

The left ventricle is large with thickening of the walls and a large cavity. The left atrium is likewise dilated and contrast substance may reflux into the pulmonary veins.

Left atrial thrombi, particularly if they are 2–3 cm in diameter, may be demonstrated by left atrial angiography (Fig. 109). Failure of the left atrial appendage to fill should not be taken as conclusive evidence of a mural thrombus.

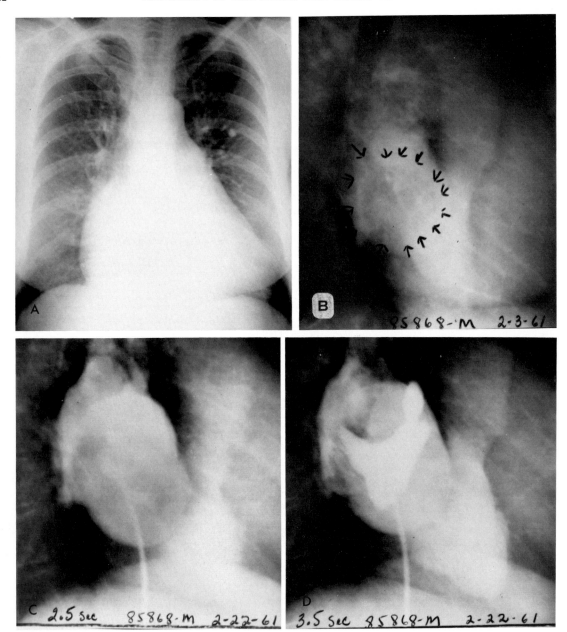

FIG. 109. MITRAL STENOSIS AND TRICUSPID INSUFFICIENCY WITH LEFT ATRIAL THROMBUS (SURGERY AND AUTOPSY)
(A) Conventional frontal projection showing cardiac enlargement and dilatation of the left atrium. (B) Venous angiocardiogram in lateral projection showing 4-cm diameter rounded thrombus in left atrium. (C) Selective left atrial injection (early systole). Radiolucency is again seen as well as mitral valve cusp. (D) Ventricular diastole 1 sec later. The valve cusps are unchanged in position and contour. The anterior leaflet appears thickened. Contrast substance has extravasated into the interatrial septum. This was absorbed in about 20 min, and no detectable untoward results were noted.

AORTIC STENOSIS AND CALCIFIC AORTIC STENOSIS

On an anatomical and etiologic basis, aortic stenosis may be divided into acquired and congenital types. These types differ not only in their etiology but to a degree in the history of onset and the obstruction as revealed by angiography, left ventricular catheterization, and surgery. The congenital group is considered in the section on congenital heart disease. Division of the acquired group according to etiologic agents is not rewarding or useful in diagnosis. A detailed discussion of the evidence as to whether "calcific aortic stenosis" is always preceded by rheumatic involvement of the valve or is due to separate disease processes is beyond the scope of this work. Aortic valvular disease due to rheumatic fever is almost always associated with a significant lesion of the mitral valve or other evidence of rheumatic fever. Rheumatic aortic valvular disease may calcify, but the majority of calcified valves seen by the radiologist do not have associated evidence of rheumatic fever (Roberts, 1970, 1971). Perry (1958) has advanced evidence that brucellosis may cause calcific aortic stenosis. Also, healed bacterial endocarditis may cause fibrosis and scarring with secondary deposition of calcium. Congenital aortic stenosis may calcify, but this is uncommon before the age of 20 years (Campbell and Kauntze, 1953). Edwards (1962) proposed that a larger proportion of cases of "calcific aortic stenosis" was superimposed on a congenital bicuspid valve. Specimens removed at operation or at autopsy, although badly scarred, tended to confirm the presence of this underlying anomaly. Atherosclerosis may be a cause of calcific aortic stenosis in the elderly (Roberts, 1970). Consequently, we believe that although the etiology of "calcific aortic stenosis"

is not always evident in the majority of cases it is superimposed on an anomalous and usually a bicuspid valve. Although these cases might be considered as congenital in origin, they are included here under the general term of "calcific aortic stenosis." Since the differences from a hemodynamic and therapeutic point of view are undetectable, all types of aortic stenosis except those of clear congenital origin will be considered here.

Just as in the case of the mitral valve, pure stenosis without insufficiency is uncommon. This has been emphasized and demonstrated by the frequent use of angiography after supravalvular and intraventricular injections of contrast substance. On the other hand, aortic insufficiency due to syphilis is almost never accompanied by stenosis, and in many instances of rheumatic insufficiency no significant stenosis is found.

In aortic stenosis, two basic processes can be recognized: (1) fusion of the cusps at their commissures; and (2) calcification of the leaflets without fusion of the cusps. Of course, both processes may combine to produce extensive deformity, fixation, and stenosis, and this is the commonest form of the disease. Calcification begins in the valve cusp, but as the calcium increases it extends to the valve ring or annulus. Also of great importance is the frequent upward extension of

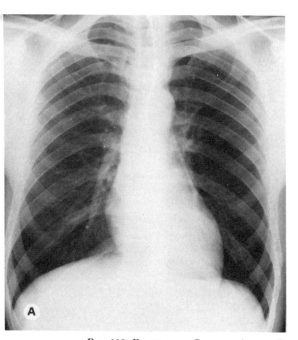 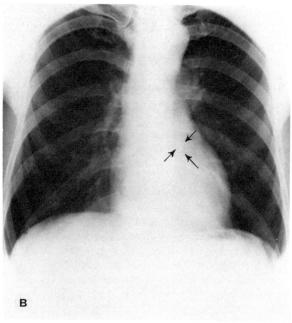

FIG. 110. RHEUMATIC CALCIFIC AORTIC STENOSIS (AUTOPSY CASE) IN 23-YEAR-OLD MAN

The heart was not enlarged, and there were only minor changes in the cardiac contour although the patient was having attacks of loss of consciousness and was severely incapacitated. (A) Conventional film. (B) Heavy exposure at ⅟₆₀ sec to show dense calcium in aortic valve which was easily visible at fluoroscopy.

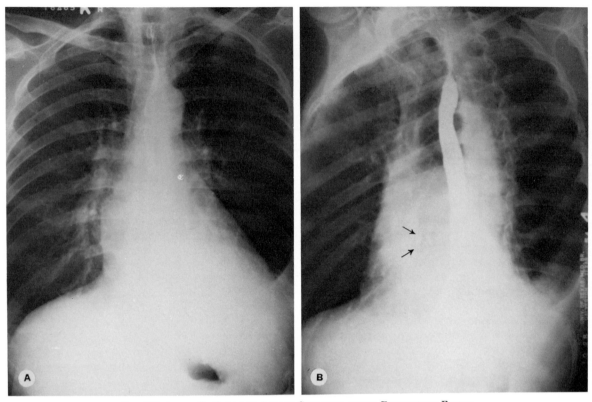

FIG. 111 A AND B. CALCIFIC AORTIC STENOSIS AFTER RHEUMATIC FEVER

The films were exposed when the patient was in a moderate degree of heart failure. Calcium (arrows) in the aortic valve was easily seen on original films.

the calcium into the sinuses of Valsalva. These extensions may be rough and irregular and form bony spurs and knobs and may obstruct the coronary orifices. The calcium may extend inferiorly into the interventricular septum or into the anterior leaflet of the mitral valve. Fusion of the cusps is most frequently due to rheumatic fever, but congenital bicuspid valves may calcify and at times differentiation may be difficult.

Calcification in the annulus of the aortic valve is ordinarily an extension from calcification of the valve leaflets and thus has the same significance as calcification of the cusps, namely aortic stenosis. This is in striking contrast to calcium deposited in the mitral annulus. Such calcification is rarely hemodynamically significant, is found mostly in aged women and is unrelated to rheumatic heart disease (see page 555).

In the early stages of the disease, the left ventricle hypertrophies. This adds very little to the overall volume of this chamber since the concentric hypertrophy is largely at the expense of the lumen. It is only after the left ventricle begins to fail that it dilates and its total volume increases. It is at this time that the changes in

the cardiac contour become evident. The root and the first part of the ascending aorta are often dilated, and this can be confirmed by angiography. The dilatation of the aorta typically extends to the origin of the innominate artery, and this differs from the dilatation of aortic insufficiency which tends to involve the entire arch.

As seen on conventional posteroanterior chest films, the changes in heart contour are often unremarkable, particularly in the earlier stages. The heart typically is not enlarged. The left ventricular contour becomes more rounded, and the upper portion of the ventricular curve more nearly approaches the horizontal. This may give an appearance of narrowing of the waist of the heart and deepening or increased concavity of the pulmonary artery segment. The lateral border of the left ventricle is usually rounded indicating hypertrophy. The lateral border of the ascending aorta may present to the right of the mediastinal shadow and have an increased sweep. The most definitive finding is the identification of calcium in the valve. The radiologic appearance of a calcific aortic valve is described in the section on cardiac calcifications. It will be summarized here again. The calcium is best detected by fluoroscopy in either the posteroanterior or left anterior oblique projection. There may be one or several separate densities. They move downward toward the apex with ventricular systole, although their course is usually elliptical or oval. In the posteroanterior projection, the calcium lies somewhat higher than the mitral valve and just to the left of the midline; part of the calcium may be superimposed on the vertebral column in the posteroanterior projection and above a line drawn from the right cardiophrenic angle to the point of opposite pulsations on the left side of the heart. The densities may also be demonstrated by high speed roentgenography and cinefluorography.

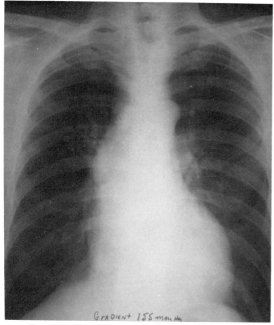

FIG. 112. SEVERE AORTIC STENOSIS AND MILD INSUFFICIENCY

The ascending aorta is dilated to about the region of the innominate artery but not beyond. The aortic valve was heavily calcified but cannot be seen on the film reproduction.

Aortic Insufficiency

Aortic insufficiency results from two basic processes: (1) retraction and deformity of the valve leaflets; and (2) widening of the commissures with dilatation of the valve ring. The first process is associated with rheumatic fever and the second with syphilis. Syphilitic aortic insufficiency is becoming increasingly uncommon and is considered in the section on syphilitic heart disease. Other causes of aortic insufficiency are the Marfan syndrome with dilatation of the aortic ring, rupture of a cusp due to bacterial endocarditis and subluxation of a cusp associated with a high ventricular septal defect. The angiographic demonstration of aortic insufficiency is not significantly different in the various etiologic types, although associated radiologic findings may permit differentiation.

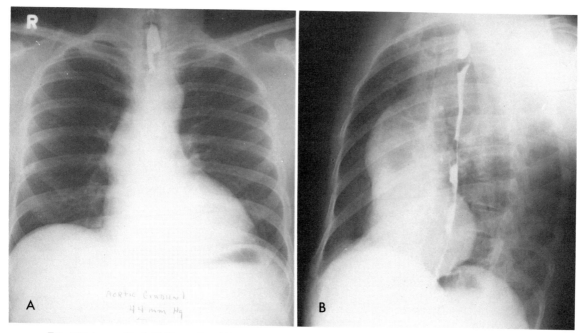

FIG. 113 A AND B. A 31-YEAR-OLD MAN WITH MODERATE AORTIC STENOSIS AND MILD INSUFFICIENCY
The left ventricle is enlarged, and the ascending aorta is dilated.

With significant aortic insufficiency there is regurgitation of a variable amount of blood from the aorta into the left ventricle during diastole. This usually takes the form of a jet, and thickening of the subvalvular endocardium is often seen at the site of impingement of this jet. In addition, blood enters the left ventricle through the normal mitral valve so that the diastolic volume of the left ventricle is increased. Therefore, both dilatation and hypertrophy appear early and are often progressive, thereby producing asymmetrical cardiac enlargement. An additional factor is the decreased coronary artery blood flow which follows a drop in the diastolic blood pressure. This may be conducive to earlier failure of the ventricular myocardium. When the left ventricle is sufficiently dilated or begins to fail, relative mitral insufficiency occurs and the train of events is started which produces an increased pulmonary artery and right ventricular pressure and finally right ventricular failure with dilatation of all of the cardiac chambers. Thus, a heart of enormous size may be found at autopsy

with predominant dilatation of the left ventricle (cor bovinum).

Even in the earlier stages of aortic insufficiency the heart is often slightly enlarged. In the posteroanterior projection there is lengthening of the left ventricular contour extending from the pulmonary artery segment above to the diaphragm below. The lower portion of this segment is increased in convexity, is rounded and the cardiac apex often descends below the level of the diaphragm. The lateral wall of the ascending aorta may appear slightly more convex and prominent than usual as the aorta is typically dilated. The aortic dilatation typically involves the entire arch, and the knob is usually enlarged. As the condition progresses, the left ventricle enlarges posteriorly so that in the left anterior oblique position there is an increased convexity posteriorly and a higher degree of obliquity is necessary for the left ventricle to clear the spine. The ascending aorta may show striking dilatation in this view.

At fluoroscopy pulsations of the left ventricle

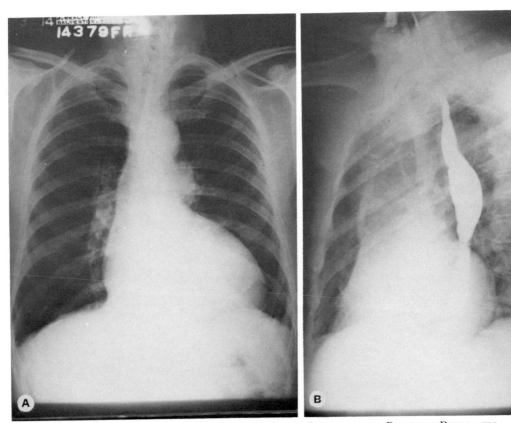

FIG. 114 A AND B. PREDOMINANT AORTIC INSUFFICIENCY, PROBABLY RHEUMATIC

There was a double aortic murmur. The abnormal contour in the region of the left hilus is due to a tortuous descending aorta. BP, 170/60–250/100.

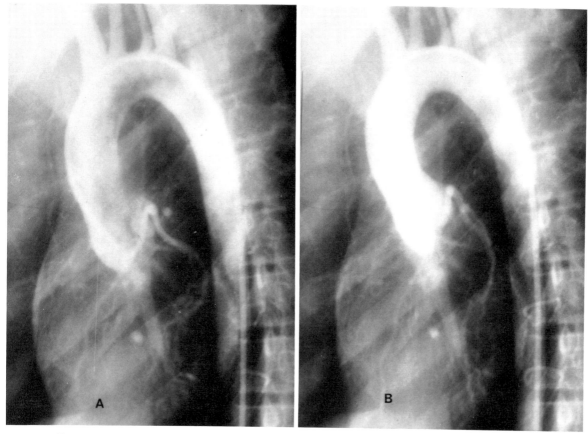

FIG. 115. SUPRAVALVULAR INJECTION SHOWING NORMAL AORTA (A) IN SYSTOLE; (B) IN DIASTOLE

In (A) some contrast substance remains in the valve sinuses, but a broad column of radiolucent blood extends almost to the descending aorta. In (B) there is no evidence of reflux, and the valve sinuses are distended. The right and left sinuses are superimposed. The left vertebral artery arises directly from the arch of the aorta. See also Figs. 49 and 50.

and the ascending aorta are noticeably increased unless the left ventricle has begun to fail. The most pronounced movement is near the apex; positional changes in both the heart and aorta are exaggerated so that there is some pendulum motion of the heart with each cardiac cycle. Pulsations in the aorta are most striking in the ascending portion and are visible along the right mediastinal border in the posteroanterior projection or anteriorly just above the right atrial appendage in the left anterior oblique projection.

Conventional radiographic and fluoroscopic examinations are most helpful in suggesting and confirming a diagnosis of aortic valvular disease. In calcific aortic stenosis, the diagnosis can usually be made from these examinations alone; however, they give at most only a crude quantitation of the severity of the lesion and almost nothing can be determined about the anatomy of the valvular obstruction or the presence of insufficiency. Furthermore, in overt or frank disease of the mitral valve or in combined valvular dis-

ease, changes due to the aortic valve lesion may be obscured or overlooked. Consequently, nowadays with the availability of reliable means of left heart catheterization and with the availability of surgical correction of many of these valvular lesions, contrast visualization of the aortic valve is widely employed.

Contrast Visualization of the Aortic Valve

Constrast material may be deposited in the ascending aorta just above the aortic valve following catheterization from a number of peripheral arteries. Percutaneous catheterization of the femoral artery is ordinarily employed, but the brachial or axillary (or even the carotid) arteries may also be used. Access to the left ventricle for contrast injection may be gained by direct puncture (rarely used), by retrograde catheterization via the transaortic route or by transseptal left atrial catheterization with passage of the catheter into the left ventricle through the mitral valve.

Transvalvular catheterization of the left ventricle is the simplest of all of the techniques. Aker *et al.* (1964) found that in aortic stenosis of the acquired type catheterization of the left ventricle could be accomplished in no more than 50% of cases. This is a serious drawback since data concerning the gradient across the aortic valve cannot be obtained and the essential left ventricular injection cannot be made. Our preference is to use the transseptal left atrial route as described by Brockenbrough and Braunwald (1960). It is true that there is a distressing tendency of the catheter to reflux from the left ventricle into the left atrium. Even a left atrial injection, however, will allow successful contrast visualization of the aortic valve. In the majority of cases that we encounter there is a question of combined valvular disease, and catheterization of the left atrium is necessary to study this possibility.

For supravalvular injections of contrast material, we employ about 60 ml of contrast agent, injecting at the rate of 20–30 ml/sec. Left ventricular injection of the same volume is introduced at the rate of 15–20 ml/sec in an attempt to avoid premature ventricular contractions. Electrocardiographic monitoring is carried out in all cases.

After the injection of contrast substance into the supravalvular area of the aorta or into the left ventricle, filming is carried out in the far right posterior oblique position. Cinefluorography at 60 frames/sec has been our routine procedure, although occasionally we have used a film changer at 4–6 frames/sec.

Normal Aortic Valve

In the far right posterior oblique projection after a supravalvular injection during ventricular diastole, the sinuses of Valsalva are distended or ballooned. The valve cusps form the inferior or caudal border of the sinuses and are convex downward. The right and left sinuses are seen more or less in contour and are symmetrical. (See Fig. 200 for nomenclature used in describing the aortic sinuses.) The noncoronary sinus is seen en face and thus appears larger than the other two, and its most caudal part extends below the level of the other two valve cusps. The normal aortic valve is completely competent to this type of injection with certain exceptions. Lehman *et al.* (1962) found that in momentary asystole a small wisp of contrast substance may reflux across the normal valve, and they also cautioned against the use of open end catheters. Certainly reflux under any other circumstance is indicative of insufficiency and valve incompetency. During

ventricular systole, the valve cusps readily fold upward against the interior of the aorta and lay parallel with the aortic lumen. Consequently, they remain visible only for a brief instant at the beginning of ventricular systole and are then lost to view, although occasionally the right cusp may be seen lying along the anterior aortic wall. The opaque column of contrast substance in the root of the aorta is rapidly diluted and swept out by a broad stream of radiolucent blood that leaves the left ventricle.

After left ventricular injection of contrast substance during ventricular diastole, the left ventricle fills out and has a somewhat elliptical shape. The outflow tract as seen in the right posterior oblique position is limited anteriorly by a nontrabeculated portion of the left ventricle and posteriorly by the anterior leaflet of the mitral valve. With the onset of systole, the outflow tract fills and tends to protrude upward and to a slight extent overlies the aortic valve area. With the use of cinefluorography, this protrusion of the outflow tract is easily identified and is very temporary and fleeting in appearance. The maximum diameter of the outflow tract occurs in early systole and the minimum diameter in early diastole with the anterior leaflet of the mitral valve producing a posterior impression (Tsioulias, 1965). The aortic valve cusps open rapidly and fold back against the interior of the aorta and present a smooth surface that cannot be usually distinguished from the interior of the aorta. Contrast substance passes through the valve in a broad front, and although there is some turbulence in the root of the aorta, there is nothing resembling a jet. During the ensuing diastole, the valves close and frequently the very thin radiolucent cusps can be distinctly seen surrounded by contrast substance in both the aorta and the left ventricle. As seen on sharp radiographs, the cusps are less than 1 mm in thickness. The root of the aorta and the left ventricle are normal in size, and the myocardium of the left ventricle is about 1 cm thick. The coronary arteries may be expected to fill following either a left ventricular or supravalvular injection. The course of the arteries may give some indication as to the thickness of the myocardium and the size of the ventricles.

Aortic Regurgitation

This is best studied by supravalvular injection. During the first ventricular diastole after the beginning of the injection, the contrast substance refluxes into the left ventricle. This reflux in all but the most severe cases takes the form of an eccentrically placed jet that progresses quite rapidly into the ventricular cavity, impinging on the ventricular wall. The site of impingement of the jet no doubt corresponds to the areas of endocardial thickening that are often found, usually fairly high up in the outflow tract of the left ventricle in this condition. The contrast substance then diffuses through the nonopaque blood. In less severe cases, two or more diastoles may occur before the ventricular cavity becomes quite opaque, and with minimal regurgitation the ventricular cavity may not become completely opaque. In the severe cases, the entire ventricular cavity becomes opaque after the first diastole. Furthermore, several heart beats are necessary to clear the contrast substance from the left ventricle as there is a continuing exchange between the ventricle and the aorta. The regurgitant jet is usually so placed as to suggest predominant involvement of one of the cusps, although we have not had an opportunity to correlate this finding with operative or autopsy observations. Our observations confirm more or less those of Odman and Philipson (1958). The aortic valve orifice appears wider than normal, and there is no thickening or disturbance of the movements of the valve. The aortic sinuses are somewhat larger and deeper than in the normal aorta. This is particularly noted during ventricular diastole. The ascending aorta is rather uniformly dilated, and this is particularly noticeable in ventricular systole. Changes in diameter of the aorta during the cardiac phase are quite striking.

Lehman *et al.* (1962) placed a quantitative grading system on the degree of aortic regurgitation of 1+ to 4+. We report our findings in terms of minimal, moderate, and severe aortic regurgitation. This evaluation is based mainly on the rapidity and volume of the reflux into and the duration of opacification of the left ventricle.

Pure aortic insufficiency occurred only in a small minority of cases we have examined. In the majority of cases, insufficiency is combined with stenosis, and the findings in stenosis will be discussed below. In insufficiency with stenosis, however, the valve cusps are often thickened and their motion is impaired.

Left ventricular injections do not demonstrate aortic insufficiency in a satisfactory fashion.

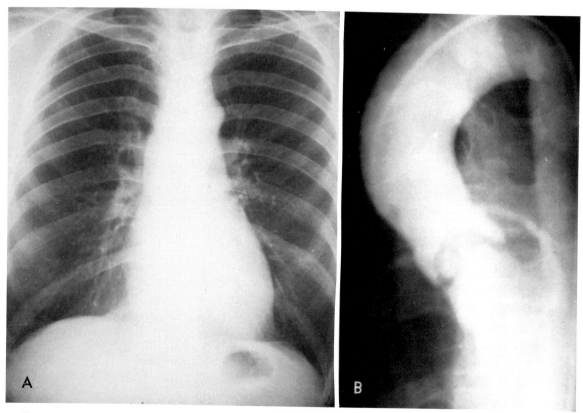

FIG. 116. AORTIC STENOSIS AND INSUFFICIENCY IN 48-YEAR-OLD WOMAN WITH ANGINA AND SYNCOPAL ATTACKS
Left heart catheterization showed a gradient across the aortic valve of 55 mm Hg. (A) Conventional chest film. (B) Supravalvular aortic injection. The valve cusps are thickened and irregular. Three plus reflux into the left ventricle.

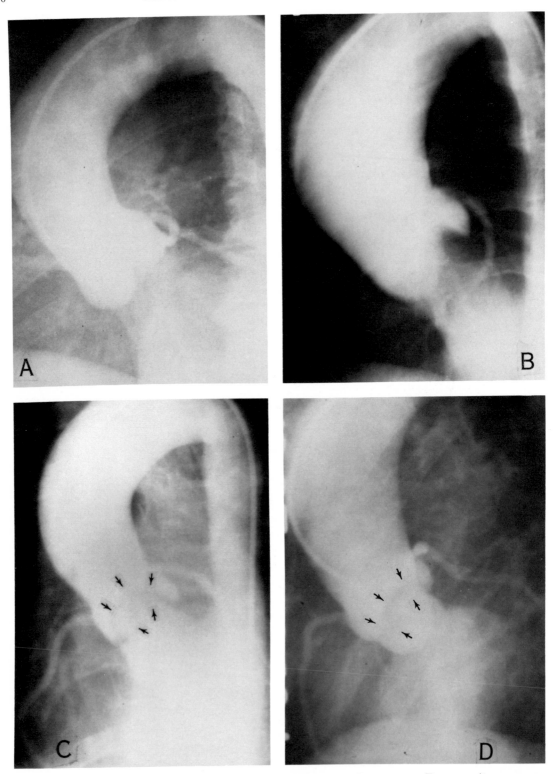

FIG. 117. AORTIC INSUFFICIENCY AND STENOSIS DEMONSTRATED BY RETROGRADE THORACIC AORTOGRAPHY
In each case the catheter tip was placed in the ascending aorta via a retrograde femoral approach. All four films were exposed in ventricular diastole and show regurgitation of contrast material into the left ventricle (films exposed in LAO position). (A) 54-year-old woman with long history of rheumatic heart disease. Catheterization showed mitral stenosis and insufficiency but no evidence of aortic stenosis. The aortic sinuses are symmetrical. (B) 27-year-old woman with aortic systolic

Aortic Stenosis

After supravalvular injection, contrast substance may reflux through the valve and thus outline the ventricular surface of the valve and indicate its thickness. Odman and Philipson (1958) were able to note thickening of the valve, and we can confirm these observations. Furthermore, the motion of the valve may be diminished in that the valve cusps do not approximate the interior of the aorta. During ventricular systole, the valve orifice may be eccentric, and this is shown by the radiolucent, nonopaque blood ex-

pelled from the ventricle. One of the most important signs is that of a radiolucent jet which may be clearly defined by the surrounding radiopaque contrast substance. This is most likely to be seen where the stenosis is dome-shaped or parachute-shaped with a central, well formed rounded orifice. This, of course, occurs in congenital stenosis. In our experience with acquired stenosis, the radiolucent jet has been very poorly defined. Instead it is replaced by marked turbulence, and occasionally an impression of a radiolucent jet directed against the anterior wall of the aorta is seen. Aker *et al.* (1964) found that

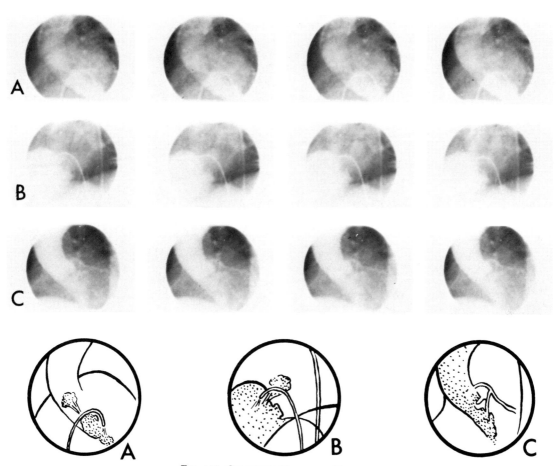

FIG. 118. COMBINED VALVULAR DISEASE

Aortic stenosis (gradient 120 mm Hg) and minimal mitral and aortic insufficiency; 16-mm cinefluorography at 60 frames/sec. (A) Left ventricular injection. Right posterior oblique projection. Radiopaque jet above aortic valve is seen. (B) Left ventricular injection. A small puff of contrast substance enters the left atrium. This is of questionable significance, particularly since the catheter crosses the valve from the left atrium. Systolic pressure in left ventricle, 200 mm Hg. (C) Supravalvular aortic injection. Moderate aortic insufficiency.

---

and diastolic murmurs. No systolic pressure gradient across the aortic valve was found at catheterization. The aortic sinuses are asymmetrical. (C) 48-year-old woman with aortic systolic and diastolic murmurs. Fluroscopy showed the aortic valve to be densely calcified, and a 50 mm gradient across the valve was found at catheterization. Arrows point to the thickened and fixed aortic valve. (D) 51-year-old man with markedly calcified aortic valve seen at fluoroscopy. At catheterization a gradient of 100 mm Hg across the valve was found. Arrows point to the irregularly thickened and deformed aortic valve. Right and left coronary arteries are well shown.

the diameter of the radiolucent jet correlated well with the diameter of the congenitally stenotic valve orifice. Whether this observation can be transferred to the acquired stenoses in which the orifice is more irregular in shape remains to be seen, but certainly it gives a gross estimate of the size of the valve orifice.

Ventricular injections have been most helpful. Contrast substance enters the ventricle over a period of 3–4 sec. During the first systole, the outflow tract of the ventricle is distended and the contour of the undersurface of the valve cusps is seen, and these may appear roughened. The motion of the valve cusps is diminished. The most important finding is that of radiopaque jet expelled through the narrowed orifice. The radiopaque jet in our experience has been more definite and easier seen than the radiolucent jet after the supravalvular injection. This jet usually impinges on the ascending aorta. The ascending aorta, particularly that part from the valve ring to the innominate artery, is dilated, and at times the impression is given that the anterior wall of the aorta is the most involved in the dilatation. Certainly, the diameter of the radiopaque jet gives some estimate of the size of the valve

orifice. In the more severe degrees of stenosis, a considerable delay in the clearing of the contrast substance from the left ventricle occurs. In many of these cases the estimate of this delay has been complicated because of the presence of mitral insufficiency. Where the mitral valve is competent and normal, a delay involving 6–7 heart beats is obviously greatly abnormal. The valve sinuses are typically small, and often they can be seen to be irregular in contour, suggesting thickening or calcification in the region of the sinuses. The myocardium of the left ventricle is thickened.

Some thickening of the valve cusps and decrease in movement have been observed by Bjork *et al.* (1961) and by Figley (1964) even though no gradient across the valve could be determined by cardiac catheterization. This is particularly likely in the presence of mitral valvular disease and left ventricular failure. We have demonstrated aortic stenosis by this method when such has not been clearly demonstrated at left heart catheterization. We thus regard left ventricular injection with contrast visualization of the aortic valve as one of the most sensitive procedures in the evaluation of aortic stenosis.

COMBINED OR MULTIPLE VALVULAR DISEASE

Tricuspid Stenosis

Although autopsy studies suggest that significant multiple valvular lesions occur in no more than 30% of cases (Wallach and Angrist, 1958), after the more extensive use of left atrial and left ventricular catheterization and angiography, multiple lesions seem more common than originally thought. Tricuspid stenosis occurs in 5–14% of all cases of rheumatic valvular disease (Garvin, 1943; Gibson and Wood, 1955; Goodwin *et al.*, 1957; Wallach and Angrist, 1958).

Bailey and Morse (1957) found 22% of 175 cases of mitral stenosis in which commissurotomy was done from the right side of the thorax had some degree of tricuspid stenosis, and in 10.5% the stenosis was severe. Tricuspid stenosis of the acquired variety does not occur as an isolated lesion and thus must be considered as a form of combined valvular disease. Tricuspid regurgitation either secondary to dilatation of the valve ring or due to structural changes in the valve was found in 20 of the 175 cases in the series of Bailey and Morse (1957).

In acquired tricuspid stenosis, the valve cusps are fused at the commissures so as to markedly reduce the size of the orifice to a critical area of

somewhere around 1.3 cm^2 or less. The gradient across the valve normally is low and in the neighborhood of 1–2 mm Hg. In stenosis, this gradient may increase to 15–20 mm Hg, and this can be best determined by right heart catheterization.

The conventional posteroanterior chest film in tricuspid stenosis shows that the right border of the heart is full and convex toward the right (Tillotson and Steinberg, 1962). This is, of course, due to right atrial enlargement and is one of the most consistent radiologic signs. Since other chambers of the heart are usually enlarged secondary to lesions of the valves on the left side of the heart, the entire heart is large and has a globular appearance. The contour may suggest pericardial effusion. The right atrium may become quite large and deviate the esophagus toward the left. Other evidence of right atrial enlargement is seen in the right oblique view. In this projection, the right atrium may appear strikingly convex and part of the contour is due to dilatation of the atrial appendage. Associated enlargement of the left atrium is common, and an attempt should be made to differentiate the outlines of each. The left atrium, however, is rarely greatly enlarged in association with tricuspid stenosis.

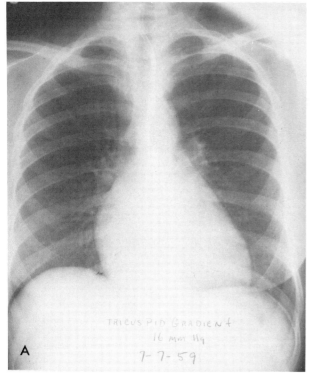
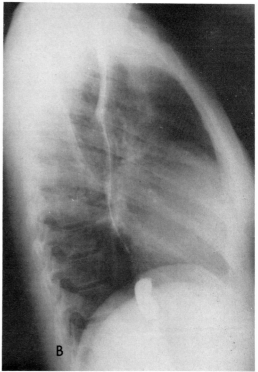

FIG. 119 A AND B. TRICUSPID AND MITRAL STENOSIS AND MIMIMAL MITRAL REGURGITATION

The right heart border is longer and more convex than normal indicating right atrial enlargement. Tricuspid valve orifice estimated to be about 1 cm^2 at surgery.

Right atrial angiography will demonstrate the dilated atrium and exclude a pericardial effusion. The atrium remains opacified for 10–12 sec, and there is corresponding slow filling of the right ventricle. The tricuspid valve is typically displaced toward the left (Fig. 121C). The cusps appear as rather thin translucent shadows, and these are convex toward the ventricle. Lung changes are dependent on the severity of the lesions: often the lungs are clear, particularly if the tricuspid valve lesion is severe.

Tricuspid insufficiency, either functional or structural, likewise causes dilatation of the right atrium and is often associated with a large heart. In the conventional posteroanterior chest film it cannot be differentiated from tricuspid stenosis, and, of course, the two may occur together. Pressure tracings obtained from the right atrium and ventricle provide a diagnosis, although considerable information can be obtained from right atrial angiography. Dotter *et al.* (1953) pointed out that the regurgitant jet associated with tricuspid insufficiency was visible and diagnostic in the early stages of angiocardiography.

The detection of significant tricuspid stenosis is of considerable value in the preoperative eval-uation of a patient for mitral commissurotomy. Tricuspid stenosis may require commissurotomy for relief of signs of right sided heart failure, and mitral commissurotomy may not improve the patient's status in the presence of tricuspid stenosis. The radiologist may direct attention to the possibility of tricuspid disease from inspection of the conventional chest film. The diagnosis, of course, is made by right heart catheterization as indicated above.

Combined Aortic and Mitral Valvular Disease

Combined aortic and mitral valvular disease was found in 29% (Wallach and Angrist, 1958) in a review of postmortem material, and White (1951) found a similar incidence in a review of clinical material. The incidence of minor abnormalities in one valve associated with gross changes in the other may be even higher. The changes in the heart and the circulatory dynamics often suggest only a single valvular lesion and tend to mask the less severe abnormality. Thus, mitral stenosis may so diminish the amount of blood entering the left ventricle that the gradient across the aortic stenosis may be regarded as

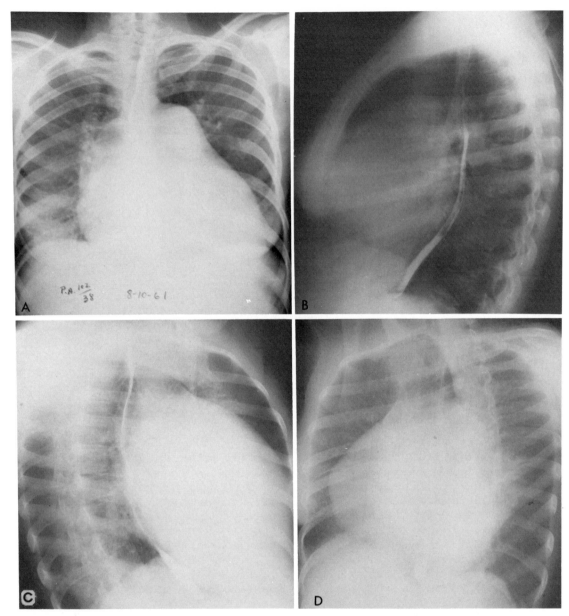

FIG. 120. A–D. TRICUSPID INSUFFICIENCY

A 26-year-old woman with tricuspid insufficiency, probably organic, and predominant mitral stenosis and pulmonary hypertension. Right atrial enlargement is striking in the PA and LAO projections. The upper lobe veins, particularly on the right, are dilated.

inconsequential, and the physical signs of stenosis may be minimal or absent. Similarly the gradient across the aortic valve in mitral insufficiency may be small due to the reflux into the left atrium, although this combination often brings on rapid heart failure. Again rather mild mitral regurgitation may be more striking and severe following the onset of aortic stenosis. Failure to diagnose or evaluate the presence of aortic

stenosis has been mentioned as a cause of poor results following mitral commissurotomy (Bailey and Morse, 1957). In fact, mitral stenosis may tend to offer some protective compensatory benefits in the presence of aortic stenosis, and a patient with both lesions may run a rapid downhill course following relief of the mitral stenosis. Consequently, the detection and evaluation of combined aortic and mitral disease is of greatest importance, and it is probably in this area that angiography of these valves has the most to contribute.

Conventional radiologic examination (fluoroscopy and films) is of variable value from case to case in the detection of combined valvular disease. The heart is usually enlarged, although the presence of a normal sized heart does not exclude a double valve lesion. The pattern of the enlargement is far from specific. A significant lesion of the mitral valve is likely to dominate because it is proximal to the aortic valve. Likewise, a tricuspid lesion may mask a mitral or aortic lesion.

Left atrial enlargement is common but is often overshadowed by the enlargement of the other chambers. The left ventricle also is frequently enlarged and may be the predominant chamber. In a large heart the usual difficulties in determining chamber size are encountered. Also, aortic disease may be found in a heart with a typical mitralized contour. Usually in these cases the aortic lesion is not severe but may be sufficient to become symptomatic following the relief of the mitral stenosis. Detection at fluoroscopy of calcium in both the aortic and mitral valves is, of course, a finding of greatest importance and is

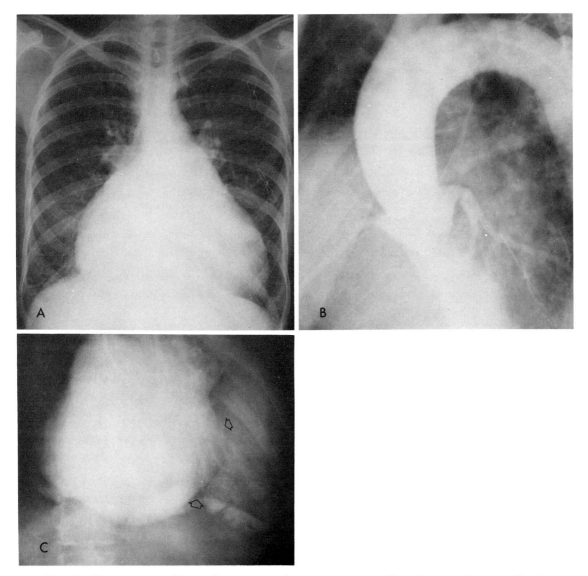

FIG. 121. TRICUSPID AND MITRAL STENOSIS AND INSUFFICIENCY WITH MILD STENOSIS (AUTOPSY CASE)
Well-marked septal lines. PA pressure, 50/24. (A) Markedly enlarged heart with enlargement of right atrium and left ventricle. (B) Grade II reflux through aortic valve. (C) Tricuspid valve (arrows) displaced toward left and slightly funnel-shaped.

diagnostic of a significant lesion in both. Although calcium in the aortic valve is diagnostic of significant stenosis, calcium in the mitral valve may be associated with either insufficiency or stenosis.

Left heart catheterization with pressure tracings obtained from the left atrium, left ventricle, and aorta are necessary to diagnose the combined valvular lesions and assess their severity;

however, angiography of both of the valves is necessary for complete evaluation because of the false pressure data that may be obtained when the hemodynamics are disturbed by one valvular lesion. The anatomy of the valves such as the aortic valve may be demonstrated by angiography, and this is essential when valve replacement is considered.

RADIOLOGIC CHANGES AFTER SURGICAL PROCEDURES ON HEART VALVES

Mitral Commissurotomy

In the immediate postoperative period, the radiologic examination is limited to portable films. Consequently, changes in heart size are difficult to estimate. Often, however, the impression is given that the heart is somewhat larger than preoperatively. Some of the enlargement may be due to pericardial fluid, although the amount is never large since the pericardial sac is only partially closed so as to permit easy drainage into the pleural space. A small amount of pleural fluid is occasionally seen. In a few cases, a rapid enlargement of the heart appeared to be associated with the onset of atrial fibrillation.

At the end of the first week, when conventional films are again available, the heart is often slightly larger than preoperatively. In estimating heart size, we often determine the frontal area, although a simpler maneuver is to superimpose the preoperative and postoperative films. The determination of the cardiothoracic index is perhaps of the least value in estimating heart size after commissurotomy. Even in the favorable cases no significant change in the size of the heart is seen before the end of the third week, and heart size is rarely stabilized until the end of the third month. No significant change in heart size has been found in over one-half of the cases followed for a period of up to several years (McAfee and Biondetti, 1957). Since 75–80% of patients are either greatly or moderately improved (McAfee and Biondetti, 1957; Ellis and Harken, 1955), it is evident that the change in heart size is not a prerequisite for a good result. A decrease in heart size of 10% (frontal plane area), however, is almost invariably associated with a good result and is thus a very favorable prognostic sign. McAfee and Biondetti (1957) found that only a very small percentage of the patients with an increase in heart size had a greatly improved or moderately improved clinical result. An increase in heart size, particularly if the increase is progressive and if it involves the

left ventricle, is almost always associated with a poor result and is suggestive of significant mitral insufficiency.

The larger preoperative hearts tend to show the most striking decrease in heart size. It should be remembered that medical management may also cause a reduction in heart size so that an immediate preoperative chest film should always be used for comparison when evaluating the postoperative film. Patients with normal sized or only slightly enlarged hearts preoperatively had almost uniformly excellent clinical results.

The change in heart size is due in most instances to a decrease in size of the right ventricle, and the size of the pulmonary artery and particularly of the left atrial appendage may contribute to the change. The hump on the left heart border due to the left atrial appendage is noticeably missing on the postoperative film as the appendage is usually amputated. The pulmonary artery decreases in size in at least one-third of the cases (Otto *et al.*, 1955).

When Kerley's B lines are present preoperatively, they may be of considerable value in prognosis. If the lines disappear promptly or within a few weeks, a good result almost invariably occurs. If the lines persist, however, some improvement can occur, but a good result is unlikely (McAfee and Biondetti, 1957). Grainger and Hearn (1955) found that the presence of Kerley's B lines preoperatively was a favorable prognostic sign, but this was not confirmed by McAfee and Biondetti (1957). Although the presence of these lines always indicates pulmonary venous hypertension, their absence does not exclude hypertension.

Changes in size of the left atrium have not been dramatic. These are probably best evaluated in the lateral view. McAfee and Biondetti (1957) found that the left atrium became smaller in only 17% of cases, larger in 7%, and, of course, in the vast majority it was unchanged.

Otto *et al.* (1955) found little correlation of changes in the transverse diameter of the heart

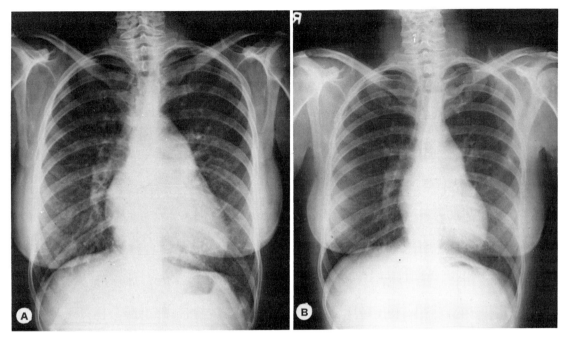

FIG. 122. MITRAL STENOSIS

(A) Mitral stenosis, preoperative. Frontal area of the heart is 121 cm.^{2} Extensive linear shadows in both lungs due to chronic stasis. (B) Eight months after mitral commissurotomy. Frontal area is 97 cm.^{2} Note regression of evidence of lung stasis.

with postoperative results as evaluated clinically. On the other hand, they found a good correlation between "postoperative x-ray change" and symptomatic improvement, although they do not state the criteria for determining x-ray changes. Presumably, they evaluated a number of findings, such as frontal heart area, Kerley's B lines, pulmonary artery size, and size of the left atrium.

Failure of commissurotomy to produce a satisfactory result is usually attributed to one or more of four different causes (Ellis and Harken, 1955):

1. Aortic disease which is unmasked by successful commissurotomy. In these cases, the left ventricle may enlarge, and this may be rapid, particularly if the aortic lesion is stenosis.

2. Poor technique with dilatation rather than fracture of the commissures resulting only in temporary improvement.

3. Conversion of stenosis to insufficiency. This may be evidenced fairly early in the postoperative period by progressive enlargement of the left ventricle.

4. Refusion of the commissures. The incidence of this occurrence is undetermined as yet, but an increasing number of second operations is now being performed. When a good result has been obtained for a period of a year or more followed by recurrence of signs or symptoms of stenosis, refusion of the commissures is a likely possibility.

Valve Replacement

Since 1962, replacement of the aortic and mitral valves with various artificial valves has become increasingly popular. Replacement of the mitral valve is carried out for predominant insufficiency and also any type of lesion with massive calcification. In the aortic valve, both stenosis and insufficiency are indications for replacement. In some cases, both valves have been replaced at a single operation, and this seems advisable in combined valvular disease.

As a practical matter, most surgeons prefer to perform an "open" operation and assess the status of the diseased valve by direct inspection and palpation. Diseased aortic valves are always treated surgically by replacement with a prosthesis. Diseased mitral valves may be treated by commissurotomy or, rarely, by valvuloplasty, but increasing numbers of patients are being managed by prosthetic valve replacement for both mitral stenosis and insufficiency.

Immediately after operation, the usual postoperative changes are noted. In a few cases of replacement of the aortic valve, we have noted a considerable reduction in heart size beginning about 1 month postoperatively.

The motion of the prosthetic valve may be studied fluoroscopically as all are opaque. The movements of the caged ball may be easily seen, but many of the discs in the low-profile valves are made of Teflon and are not opaque. Floppy and asymmetrical movements of the prosthesis suggest that the artificial valve ring has been imperfectly sutured in place or has become loosened with partial disruption at the suture line. Angiography may then show mitral or aortic insufficiency, the leak occuring at the loosened margin of the valve ring. Angiography may also show interference with movements of the anterior mitral leaflet if too large an aortic valve prosthesis has been used, particularly in a child. Care must be exercised not to allow the catheter to become tangled in the moving parts of the valve and interfere with its motion during catheterization and angiography.

Thromboembolism and valve disruption are common causes of poor late results from valve replacement (See Fig. 526, page 633).

The classification in Table 7 is provided the reader for completeness. In many of the rare causes of valvular disease, the radiologic features resemble those of the more common causes, and a separate detailed description would be repetitious. Calcific aortic stenosis is probably due to a number of causes but was described in the section on rheumatic heart disease, although rheumatic fever is not the most common cause. Likewise aortic regurgitation was described in connection with rheumatic heart disease, although a host of other causes can produce similar changes.

Some of the disease entities listed in addition to producing changes in the valves also affect the myocardium, the pericardium, and the aorta and merit a more complete description.

TABLE 7

CAUSES OF CARDIAC VALVULAR DISEASE

Rheumatic fever
Congenital
  See section on Congenital Heart Disease
Atherosclerosis
  Calcific aortic stenosis of elderly (Roberts, 1970)
  Ischemic heart disease
    Papillary muscle ischemia and infarction
      Malfunction
      Rupture
Infections
  Syphilis
  Bacterial endocarditis
Collagen diseases
  Scleroderma
  Lupus erythematosus
  Rheumatoid arthritis
  Ankylosing spondylitis
Cardiomyopathies
  Idiopathic hypertrophic subaortic stenosis
  Endocardial fibroelastosis
  Other (see section on Myocardiopathies)
Metabolic
  Genetic or inherited trait
    The Marfan syndrome
    The Hunter-Hurler syndrome (Krovetz et al., 1968)
    Ehlers-Danlos syndrome (Neill, 1968)
    Osteogenesis imperfecta (Criatielto et al., 1965)
  The carcinoid syndrome
Mucoid or myxomatous degeneration
  Prolapse or billowing of mitral valve (floppy
  valve syndrome)
  Rupture of chordae tendineae
  Rupture of aortic cusps

11

Congenital Anomalies of the Heart and Great Vessels

INTRODUCTION

The modern era in the surgical treatment of congenital cardiovascular anomalies began with the report of Gross and Hubbard (1939) of the first successful ligation of a patent ductus arteriosus. In 1945 Crafoord successfully excised a short segment of coarcted aorta and re-established continuity by an end to end anastomosis. At about the same time Blalock and Taussig (1945) described a method of producing an artificial ductus arteriosus that was effective in the treatment of many patients with congenital pulmonic stenosis. During the ensuing 20 years reports of successes in the treatment of other anomalies have appeared at a rapid rate. Among the most noteworthy accomplishments were the applications of the techniques of hypothermia and particularly those of the heart lung devices to the uses of open heart surgery. At present the list of anomalies not susceptible to surgical treatment is short and steadily diminishing.

Partly from the stimulus of this amazing surgical progress and partly as a culmination of the efforts of several workers over the preceding years, the diagnostic approach to congenital heart disease has been greatly improved. Abbott (1936) in her atlas had already collected and described the anatomical features of most of the major anomalies including many of the almost innumerable minor variations. Her work has been admirably extended by the following generation of pathologists, most notably Edwards and his group and Lev and his group. However, the recognition of congenital anomalies in the living requires not only a knowledge of the abnormal anatomy but also of the physiologic consequences and their effects on the clinical course and appearance of the patient. Taussig (1960) in her book, *Congenital Malformations of the Heart,* attempted to correlate the anatomical,

physiologic, and clinical data into a coherent whole and thus provide a logical basis for a diagnostic approach. Taussig's approach was predominantly clinical and radiologic, and, following her descriptions and methods, it is remarkable how much can be deduced by these means. Under the impetus of surgical achievement and its resultant publicity, however, an increasing number of patients appeared which could not be placed into previously well recognized categories. Some of these had anomalies not previously described; many, however, represented variants or exaggerations of previously described entities. Also, the surgeon was no longer satisfied with a simple classification of the patient's anomaly. More precise information was needed concerning the nature and size of areas of stenosis, the exact location of abnormal openings, and the size and course of the great vessels. Consequently, simple radiologic and clinical studies even in the most experienced hands could not meet these new and more exacting needs.

Angiocardiography and cardiac catheterization, while relatively new procedures, were technically standardized and easily modified to meet the needs of diagnosis in congenital heart disease where most of the patients were children. Castellanos (1938) and his associates had found that children were good subjects for angiocardiography because of their smallness which considerably improved radiographic contrast so that in some cases septal defects could be clearly visualized. This procedure was further perfected by Robb and Steinberg in 1939 and since then has been widely used in congenital heart disease where it provides information which is unobtainable by any other method of study.

Certain inadequacies of angiocardiography soon became noticeable, particularly in relation to the more minute detail of the interior of the cardiac chambers and of the aorta. Thus, selective angiocardiography and the extensive use of cardiac catheterization have largely displaced the use of venous angiocardiography.

Cournand (1945) was among the first to obtain an extensive experience with cardiac catheterization which included observations on congenital heart disease. Others, such as Bing *et al.* (1947) in Baltimore and Dexter *et al.* (1947) in Boston had the advantage of clinics in which relatively large numbers of patients with congenital heart disease were encountered and therefore were able to correlate their findings with those obtained at operation and autopsy. During the ensuing years cardiac catheterization laboratories became an integral part of every clinic which devoted itself to the diagnosis and surgical treatment of congenital heart disease.

Echocardiography in recent years has brought added information concerning the size and location of the great vessels, the adequacy of valve motion, and at times chamber size in patients with congenital heart disease (Feigenbaum, 1976). This modality is of particular value because of its noninvasive characteristics as an initial survey procedure, although in several anomalies it is capable of providing a firm diagnosis. It is also helpful in following the patient's course following diagnosis and treatment.

Dynamic studies using nuclear materials have been useful in the study of intracardiac shunts and the pulmonary circulation (Kriss *et al.*, 1972; Greenfield and Bennett, 1973; Rosenthall and Mercer, 1973; Muroff and Freedman, 1976).

It should be emphasized that no one method of examination is sufficient to provide a complete diagnosis in all cases; rather it is the correlation of the findings from all available diagnostic studies that is likely to produce a satisfactory degree of accuracy. Even the limited inspection permitted at operation is not entirely trustworthy, particularly with regard to the internal structure of the heart. Only a careful autopsy study can be regarded as providing a reliable and complete diagnosis.

CLASSIFICATION

Congenital cardiovascular defects may be considered as (1) obstructions, (2) abnormal openings or abnormal persistence of embryologically normal openings, (3) malpositions or abnormal relationships of the great vessels to the cardiac chambers, (4) positional changes of the heart and great vessels in relation to the surrounding organs, (5) enlargement or hypertrophy of a specific vessel or chamber (these may be functional and secondary to other defects), and (6) hypoplasia or atresia of a specific vessel or chamber (these may likewise be secondary). Further attempts at a precise anatomical classification are difficult because of the frequency of multiple defects. Where there are multiple defects, however, one is usually predominant in its effects, and the others may be compensatory. Also, the nature of the functional consequences of such a predominant defect can be predicted with considerable certainty, and the associated anomalies serve mainly to increase or decrease the extent of the fundamental disturbance of the circulation. In some instances it is admittedly difficult to determine which of two anomalies is more significant in its effects; also, if the patient survives for a considerable period of time, certain secondary changes may occur which may modify the original hemodynamic pattern.

Actually, the altered course and function of the circulation in congenital heart disease are produced by two fundamental factors, namely, (1) shunts and (2) obstructions. A shunt is an abnormal diversion of blood from the venous to the arterial circulation or vice versa. ("Right-to-left" will be used synonymously with venous-arterial; "left-to-right" will be used with arterial-venous shunts.) It presupposes an abnormal opening or communication and a difference in pressure between the chambers or vessels involved. Pressure differences normally exist between the right and left atria, the right and left ventricles, and the aorta and pulmonary artery, but these may be greatly modified by the presence of obstructions so long as the myocardium is capable of responding to abnormal pressure changes.

Shunts have a pronounced effect on the efficiency of the circulation and consequently on the clinical course and appearance of the patient. A left-to-right shunt overloads the pulmonary circulation and/or the left ventricle; the right ventricle may eventually fail or the lung vascular system may develop secondary changes with a resultant pulmonary arterial hypertension. Meanwhile, the systemic circulation receives an insufficient blood flow which is manifest by underdevelopment, weakness, and poor exercise tolerance of the patient. A right-to-left shunt on the other hand may cause a large amount of blood to bypass the lungs and enter the systemic circulation; consequently, clinical cyanosis appears and there is an inadequate oxygen supply to the tissues. All shunts are not harmful, however, and under certain circumstances improve the circulatory efficiency, *e.g.,* a left-to-right shunt through a patent ductus arteriosus associated with a tetralogy of Fallot increases the pulmonary blood flow with a consequent betterment of the clinical status of the patient. Furthermore, in a complete transposition of the great vessels, a constantly reversing shunt is essential if life is to continue, since venous blood must first be directed to the lungs for aeration and then reshunted to the aorta for distribution to the systemic circulation. Indeed, the duration of life in transposition is improved by the presence of one or more large communications between the systemic and pulmonary circulations. It becomes evident, therefore, that an understanding of the production of shunts and their functional consequences is fundamental in the diagnostic approach to congenital heart disease.

No entirely satisfactory classification of congenital heart disease has been devised, largely because of the great number of possible combinations of anomalies. In addition, some anomalies produce cyanosis at one time and not at another, and some evolve with time into more severe and some into less severe abnormalities. Mild and atypical cases are about as difficult to work into a comprehensive classification as unusually complicated ones. These factors considered, we may nonetheless arrange the commoner typical varieties of congenital heart disease into a classification based upon two signs, one physical and the other roentgenographic, namely, the presence or absence of cyanosis and the radiographic appearance of the pulmonary vascularity. Such a classification has the advantage of establishing a point of departure for consideration of the detailed anatomy of the lesion based on information which is generally not difficult to obtain and which is usually the first kind of information sought by the radiologist faced with a diagnostic challenge. Cyanosis is meant to indicate abnormal skin or mucous membrane coloration visible to the naked eye, and the pulmonary vascularity is assessed on conventional chest films.

In the classification which is given in Table 8, only the commoner typical examples are included. It is intended as an aid to the grouping together of similar lesions based on these two signs so that important diagnostic possibilities will not be omitted in the preliminary analysis of a patient with congenital heart disease. Although this classification is helpful as an initial point of

TABLE 8
CLASSIFICATION OF CONGENITAL HEART DISEASE
(TYPICAL EXAMPLES)

ACYANOTIC

I. Normal Pulmonary Vascularity
  A. Aortic stenosis.
  B. Anomalies of the aortic arch.
  C. Coarctation of the aorta.
  D. Dextrocardia with situs inversus (mirror-image dextrocardia).
  E. Endocardial fibroelastosis.
  F. Anomalous origin of the left coronary artery.
  G. Aneurysms of the sinus of Valsalva or coronary arteries.
  H. Congenitally corrected transposition of the great vessels.
  I. Congenital dilatation of the pulmonary artery.

II. Increased Pulmonary Vascularity
  A. Interatrial septal defect.
  B. Interventricular septal defect.
  C. Patent ductus arteriosus.
  D. Aortic-pulmonary window.
  E. Partial anomalous pulmonary venous return.
  F. Persistent atrioventricularis communis.
  G. Coronary artery fistula to right chamber.
  H. Rupture of aneurysm of sinus of Valsalva into right chamber.
  I. Congenital mitral stenosis or insufficiency.
  J. Truncus arteriosus (pulmonary arteries from main trunk).

III. Decreased Pulmonary Vascularity
  A. Ebstein's malformation with intact atrial septum.
  B. Valvular pulmonary stenosis.
  C. Infundibular pulmonary stenosis.
  D. Absence of one pulmonary artery.

CYANOTIC

I. Normal Pulmonary Vascularity
  (No uncomplicated congenital cyanotic heart lesion typically produces normal pulmonary vascularity.)

II. Increased Pulmonary Vascularity
  A. Eisenmenger's syndrome.
  B. Transposition of the great vessels.
  C. Taussig-Bing syndrome.
  D. Single ventricle (pulmonary artery from common chamber).
  E. Mitral and aortic atresia (hypoplastic left heart syndrome).
  F. Total anomalous pulmonary venous return.
  G. Obstructions of the pulmonary veins.

III. Decreased Pulmonary Vascularity
  A. Tetralogy of Fallot.
  B. Tricuspid atresia.
  C. Truncus arteriosus.
  D. Ebstein's anomaly with interatrial septal defect.
  E. Single ventricle (pulmonary artery from rudimentary chamber).
  F. Pulmonary stenosis (with opening of foramen ovale or right heart failure).
  G. Pulmonary stenosis with interatrial septal defect.
  H. Primary pulmonary hypertension.

departure for the radiologist when confronted with a chest film, it does not lend itself to an orderly description of the various entities. Conditions that vary widely in structure are lumped together, and many of the entities because of a variation in some minor aspect or due to the patient's age would have to be considered under two or more headings. The classification as given in Table 9 has no special merit except that it has been helpful in arranging material for this presentation.

Before proceeding with the roentgen examination in congenital heart disease, the roentgenologist is entitled to the answers to the following questions:

1. Is there a history of cardiac signs and symptoms which dates to infancy or childhood? In other words, does the history suggest the diagnosis of congenital heart disease?

2. Is there a history or evidence of rheumatic fever or some other disease which might complicate the congenital anomaly?

3. Is there cyanosis? If so, when was it first noticed? Is it intermittent or constant? What is its distribution?

4. Are there significant or important murmurs such as that of patent ductus arteriosus (PDA)? Murmurs are often of little importance in congenital cyanotic heart disease (Taussig, 1960).

5. What is the blood pressure and nature of the pulse in each of the four extremities?

6. Are there significant deformities of the bony thorax?

7. What is the axis deviation of the electrocardiogram? Is there an arrhythmia?

OBSTRUCTIONS

On the Right Side of the Circulation

1. Valvular Pulmonic Stenosis with Intact Ventricular Septum

a. Without an interatrial communication (no right-to-left shunt)

b. With an interatrial communication

The incidence of congenital stenosis of the outflow tract of the right ventricle with an intact ventricular septum is four out of 10,000 live births, representing 8% of all cases of congenital heart disease (Samman, 1972).

Separation of cases of pulmonic stenosis into those with and without an interatrial communication is of practical importance because of differential diagnostic possibilities. In those cases with a communication, the shunt is from right to left and cyanosis is persistent, whereas in those in which there is no interatrial communication, the patient is acyanotic unless there is heart failure. Peripheral cyanosis may be seen during exercise in cases where no atrial communication is present due to the decrease in cardiac output, but persistent central cyanosis usually indicates a septal communication. The main symptom of right ventricular obstruction with an intact ventricular septum in the presence of an interatrial communication is dyspnea on exertion.

The valve covering the foramen ovale is usually closed because pressure in the left is greater than that in the right atrium. In pulmonic stenosis with intact ventricular septum, the pressure in the right ventricle is elevated and may become quite high. This increased pressure eventually is transmitted to the right atrium and may cause the valve over the foramen ovale to open producing a right-to-left shunt. The foramen ovale itself may enlarge and increase the shunt. In some cases, a true atrial septal defect is found, and the right-to-left shunt may then be quite large. The reader should remember that in uncomplicated atrial septal defect the shunt is from left to right, and it is often a large shunt. In association with a large shunt, mild to moderate pulmonic stenosis as determined by right heart catheterization is a frequent accompanying finding. The gradient is rarely greater than 10–20 mm Hg. This may be associated with a large flow through the pulmonary conus and pulmonary valve and a relative obstruction due to the normal size of the valve ring. Some hypertrophy of the infundibulum may contribute to the stenosis. In the anomaly considered here the pulmonic obstruction is the predominant lesion and is sufficient to reduce the flow to the lungs in most instances. At any rate, when it occurs with an interatrial communication the shunt is uniformly from right to left. It is rare that the differentiation of these two conditions becomes a practical point. It is customary to repair the interatrial defect at the time that pulmonic stenosis is treated. In atrial septal defect with left-to-right shunt, it is rarely necessary to treat the relative pulmonic stenosis by surgical means. It usually regresses when the large pulmonary flow is reduced following closure of the atrial defect.

The histories of many patients suggest that some time elapses before the right-to-left shunt becomes well established as evidenced by the appearance of cyanosis. It is during these earlier years that the pressure in the right atrium is presumably increasing secondary to increased right ventricular pressure. Occasionally, a patient is cyanotic from infancy.

Anatomy. In 90–95% of all cases of pulmonic stenosis, the obstruction is at the level of the pulmonary valve. The anatomy of the lesion is

TABLE 9

CLASSIFICATION OF CONGENITAL HEART DISEASE

I. Obstructions

   A. On the right side of the circulation

      1. Valvular pulmonic stenosis with an intact ventricular septum

         (a) Without an interatrial communication

         (b) With an interatrial communication

      2. Supravalvular pulmonic stenosis

         (a) Single (usually in the pulmonary trunk)

         (b) Multiple (usually in the pulmonary artery branches: "coarctations" of the pulmonary arteries)

      3. Subvalvular pulmonic stenosis

         (a) As an isolated anomaly—infundibular stenosis

         (b) Associated with idiopathic hypertrophic subaortic stenosis (IHSS)

         (c) Obstructing muscle bands in the right ventricle (see two-chambered right ventricle)

      4. Ebstein's anomaly of the tricuspid valve

         (a) Acyanotic, without an interatrial communication.

         (b) Cyanotic, with an interatrial communication.

      5. Uhl's anomaly

   B. On the left side of the circulation

      1. Coarctation of the aorta

      2. Complete interruption of aortic arch

      3. Bicuspid aortic valve with

         (a) Aortic stenosis

         (b) Aortic regurgitation

      4. Unicommissural aortic valve

      5. Valvular aortic stenosis

      6. Subvalvular aortic stenosis

         (a) Discrete membrane

         (b) Fibromuscular

         (c) Idiopathic hypertrophic subaortic stenosis (see Myocardiopathies)

      7. Supravalvular aortic stenosis

      8. Aortico-left ventricular tunnel

      9. Hypoplastic left heart syndrome

    10. Mitral stenosis

    11. Congenital mitral regurgitation

    12. Cor triatriatum

    13. Congenital stenosis of the pulmonary veins

II. Abnormal or persistent openings between the right and left sides of the circulation

   A. Usually associated with a left-to-right shunt

      1. In the great vessels

         (a) Patent ductus arteriosus (PDA)

         (b) Aortic-pulmonary window

         (c) Rupture of an aneurysm of the sinus of Valsalva into the right side of the heart

         (d) Partial anomalouus pulmonary venous connection (PAPVC)

      2. In the atria

         (a) Atrial septal defect (ASD)

      3. In the ventricles

         (a) Ventricular septal defect (VSD)

         (b) Eisenmenger complex

      4. Involving both atria and ventricles

         (a) Endocardial cushion defect

         (b) Left ventricular-right atrial communication

   B. Usually associated with right-to-left shunt and combined with (1) an obstruction, (2) malposition of one or both great vessels, or (3) both

      1. Tetralogy of Fallot and variations

         (a) Pseudotruncus arteriosus or extreme tetralogy

         (b) Tetralogy of Fallot with absence of the pulmonary valve and pulmonic regurgitation

         (c) Two-chambered right ventricle—obstructing muscle bands in right ventricle

      2. Tricuspid atresia

         (a) Without transposition of the great vessels

         (b) With transposition of the great vessels

      3. Transposition of the great vessels

TABLE 9—*continued*

    4. Truncus arteriosus
- (a) Type I (Collett and Edwards, 1949). The ascending aorta and a single pulmonary trunk arise from the truncus
- (b) Type II. The right and left pulmonary arteries arise close together form the dorsal wall of the truncus
- (c) Type III. One or both pulmonary arteries arise independently from either side of the truncus
- (d) Type IV. Absence of the pulmonary arteries; circulation to the lungs by means of the bronchial arteries
- (e) Type V. Partial persistence of the truncus arteriosus with a localized defect in the trunco-conal septum and a communication between the aorta and pulmonary artery—see Aortic pulmonary window
- (f) Anomalous pulmonary artery arising form ascending aorta (Hemitruncus, Taussig, 1960)

    5. Total anomalous pulmonary venous connection (TAPVC)

    6. Double outlet right ventricle
- (a) Type I—defect below crista
- (b) Type II—defect above crista (Taussig-Bing anomaly)

    7. Common ventricle
- (a) With transposition and inversion of ventricles
- (b) Without transposition and inversion of ventricles
- (c) With transposition and noninversion of ventricles
- (d) Without transposition and noninversion of ventricles

    8. Pulmonary valvular atresia with normal aortic root

III. *Congenital malposition of the heart or the relationship of the cardiac chambers to each other*
- A. Dextrocardia
  - 1. Extrinsic
  - 2. Intrinsic
    - (a) Without situs inversus
      - (1) Without chamber inversion (rotational dextrocardia)
      - (2) With chamber inversion (dextrocardia plus corrected transposition of great vessels)
    - (b) With situs inversus
      - (1) Without chamber inversion
      - (2) With chamber inversion
    - (c) With indeterminate situs
      - (1) Asplenia
      - (2) Polysplenia
      - (3) Anisosplenia
      - (4) Situs inversus and levocardia
- B. Anomalies of systemic venous return
- C. Congenitally corrected transposition of the great vessels

IV. *Anomalies of the aorta without significant circulatory changes*
- A. Double aortic arch
- B. Left aortic arch
  - 1. Normal branching and minor variations
  - 2. Aberrant right subclavian artery
  - 3. Isolation of right subclavian artery from aorta
- C. Right aortic arch
  - 1. Mirror-image branching
  - 2. With aberrant left subclavian artery
  - 3. Isolation of left subclavian artery from aorta
- D. Cervical aortic arch
- E. Pseudocoarctation of aorta

V. *Pulmonary vascular anomalies*
- A. Anomalous left pulmonary artery (pulmonary sling)
- B. Congenital dilatation of the pulmonary artery
- C. Proximal interruption of a pulmonary artery
- D. Coarctations of pulmonary artery

VI. *Pulmonary arteriovenous aneurysm*

simple. The valve is a thin membrane with a small round hole in the center resembling a parachute. The hole is often eccentric. A slightly thickened linear area may suggest the site of a commissure, but there is a failure of division into cusps. The conus is usually wide, although there may be evidence of hypertrophy of the crista supraventricularis as a part of right ventricular hypertrophy. The hypertrophy of the wall of the conus constitutes a minor obstruction itself, but it is thought to regress after relief of the valvular obstruction, although it is difficult to determine preoperatively whether this will take place. The pulmonary trunk beyond the stenotic valve is typically dilated, although this is not invariable. When the pulmonary trunk is dilated, the wall is thin. The dilatation extends to the bifurcation of the pulmonary artery, and in a considerable percentage it extends to involve the left pulmonary artery and its major branches. The right pulmonary artery on the other hand is almost never dilated and is usually smaller than normal. The dilatation of the pulmonary trunk is most likely secondary to the turbulence produced by the jet effect of the blood in its passage through the nozzle-like opening of the valve into a low pressure area. It certainly may be compared with the post-stenotic dilatations that are found elsewhere in the arterial system at the site of a localized constriction (coarctation of the aorta and acquired stenosis of the renal arteries).

An atypical form of valvular pulmonic stenosis is produced by dysplasia of the pulmonary valve. In this condition the dysplastic valve is tricuspid, its commissures are unfused, the valve cusps are markedly thickened and inflexible and are literally "stuffed-up" a hypoplastic pulmonary annulus (Jeffery et al., 1972; Bharati and Lev, 1973; Schieken et al., 1973). The importance of recognizing this curious form of pulmonic stenosis lies in the fact that pulmonary valvulotomy, ordinarily entirely satisfactory for the treatment of typical valvular pulmonary stenosis, will be unsuccessful in relieving stenosis due to a dysplastic valve. Successful approaches have required valvotomy plus insertion of a right ventricular outflow tract patch or excision of the thickened dysplastic valve leaflets.

Physiologic Considerations. The degree of stenosis and the response of the heart to it is quite variable. Right ventricular pressure may vary from a mild systolic elevation of 40–50 mm Hg to 250 mm Hg. The systolic pressure in the pulmonary artery may be low (10–15 mm Hg) or normal (15–25 mm Hg). Thus, the gradient between the right ventricle and the pulmonary

artery may vary from 15 to 225 mm Hg or more. The right ventricular pressure is one of the important criteria of the need for surgical treatment. Patients with pressures of 50 mm or less usually do not need surgical relief of the stenosis, whereas those with a systolic pressure of over 100 mm Hg almost invariably need treatment. This leaves an indeterminate group in which the pressure is 50–100 mm Hg and in which surgical treatment is recommended only after complete evaluation.

In pure valvular stenosis an abrupt change in the pressure tracings from those of the pulmonary artery to those of the right ventricle is usually produced by withdrawing the catheter slowly across the valve. In the presence of combined infundibular and valvular stenosis, an intermediate pressure area can be recognized. This represents the pressure in the infundibular chamber in which the systolic pressure approximates that of the pulmonary artery and the diastolic pressure approximates that of the right ventricle. However, when the infundibular stenosis is due to a long narrow channel, the pressure tracings show a very gradual and sometimes rather poorly defined increment of pressures and changes in contour as the catheter is withdrawn over a considerable distance between the valve and the main cavity of the right ventricle. This may offer difficulties in interpretation.

A right-to-left shunt at the atrial level occurs frequently and tends to be progressive and produce cyanosis. On the other hand, it may decompress the right side of the heart and prevent overloading of the right ventricle. The problems of polycythemia, however, eventually arise.

Radiologic Findings. A considerable number of mild cases have no radiologic findings and are recognized when right heart catheterization is performed because of an incidental murmur (Dow et al., 1950; Healey et al., 1950). Perhaps in the majority of cases, and certainly in most cases with definite clinical signs and symptoms, the diagnosis can be suspected from a single well exposed chest film, particularly if the patient is over 1 year of age. The heart may or may not be enlarged, but marked cardiac enlargement is seen with some frequency. This is one of the conditions in which marked cardiac enlargement can occur in infancy and childhood; however, just as there is a wide variation in the gradient between the pulmonary artery and the right ventricle, likewise there is a wide variation in heart size. We do not know of any close correlation between the heart size and right ventricular pressure. In quite large hearts the gradient may be lower due

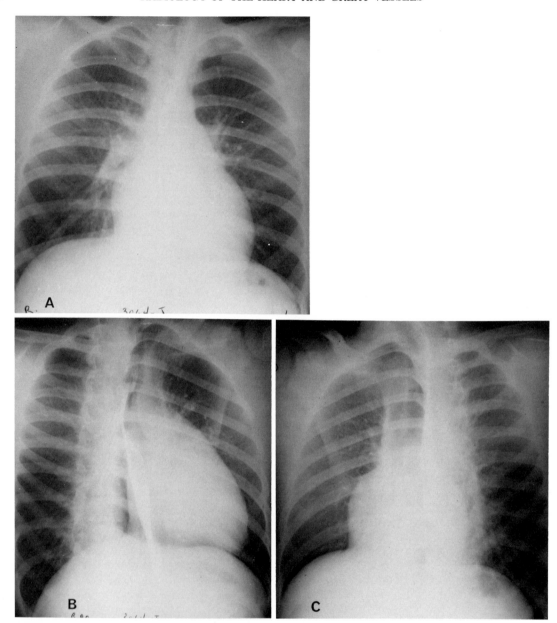

FIG. 123. A 14-YEAR-OLD BOY WITH VALVULAR PULMONIC STENOSIS (OPERATIVE CASE)
RV pressure, 145/5; PA pressure, 20/10. Patient was acyanotic but had a very poor exercise tolerance. The pulmonary arterial system was only slightly diminished in size. The right atrium was dilated and is best seen in the LAO projection (C). At operation the infundibulum showed marked hypertrophy and was dilated. It was not resected.

to heart failure. Enlargement of the heart is due predominantly to enlargement of the right ventricle. The right ventricle may be hypertrophied with very little increase in size. When it begins to dilate, cardiac enlargement will appear. Even though the enlargement of the heart radiographically is due to the right ventricle, elevation of the apex is decidedly uncommon. In the lateral view, the segment of the anterior surface of the heart that is in contact with the posterior part of the sternum is increased. Right atrial enlargement frequently follows right ventricular enlargement, and the atrial appendage also impinges upon the retrosternal space and may increase the contour of the heart in this area. Atrial enlargement, however, is better seen in the PA projection and also in the left anterior oblique projection where a considerable convexity is ev-

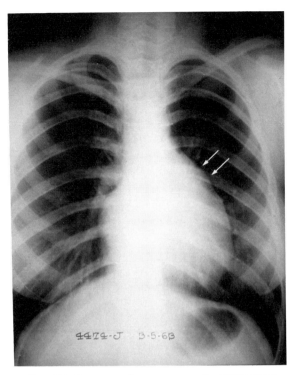

FIG. 124. PULMONIC STENOSIS WITH INFUNDIBULAR
CHAMBER

At operation using cardipulmonary bypass the infundibular obstruction appeared to be the sole cause of the pulmonary obstruction. The preoperative pressure gradient between the RV and PA was 120 mm Hg. The convexity of the
left upper heart border (arrows) was thought to be due to the
infundibular chamber.

ident. Pulsations of the right atrial border as
seen in both of these projections may be increased, although in impending or actual heart
failure the pulsations are decreased or absent.

Although not invariably present a striking
finding is poststenotic dilatation of the main
trunk of the pulmonary artery, and this is seen
as a convexity of the left mid heart border. The
dilatation may extend to the bifurcation of the
pulmonary artery and often extends on into the
left pulmonary artery to the point where it
crosses the left main stem bronchus. In a considerable percentage of cases the greater part of the
left pulmonary artery, including the primary
branches, is dilated. On the other hand, the right
pulmonary artery dwindles rapidly, and the
shadow of the descending branch in the right
hilus is abnormally small. Thus, on a posteroanterior chest film, this combination of findings is
strongly suggestive of valvular pulmonary stenosis: enlargement of the main and left pulmonary arteries with a normal or small right pulmonary artery (Fig. 125). The pulsations of the

left pulmonary artery are normal or often increased in amplitude. This disparity of pulsations
is a diagnostic feature and is highly suggestive of
valvular pulmonic stenosis (Gay and Franck,
1960).

The smaller or secondary and tertiary arteries
within the lung parenchyma are usually smaller
than normal, and the peripheral portions of the
lungs are quite clear and avascular. In many of
the milder cases the vasculature may be within
normal limits.

The aortic knob and the aorta are identified
with considerable difficulty and are usually
small.

There is no specific change in the cardiac
contour that would suggest the presence of a
right to left shunt at the interatrial level. The left
atrium does not enlarge under this circumstance.

CARDIAC CATHETERIZATION. Even in those
cases where conventional radiologic studies are
atypical, right heart catheterization is essential
for confirmation and evaluation as to the need
for surgical treatment. The most valuable infor-

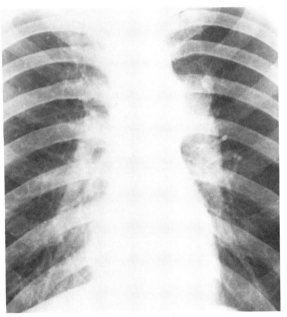

FIG. 125. ISOLATED PULMONIC STENOSIS

Conventional frontal film of the chest shows a heart of
normal size and shape in spite of the fact that the electrocardiogram recorded right ventricular hypertrophy. The main
pulmonary artery is greatly enlarged, the result of poststenotic dilatation. This dilatation extends into the left pulmonary artery and its descending branch. The right descending
pulmonary artery is normal or small in size in contrast to the
dilated left pulmonary artery and its branches. This combination of enlarged pulmonary trunk and left pulmonary
artery with a normal or small right pulmonary artery is
characteristic of valvular pulmonic stenosis.

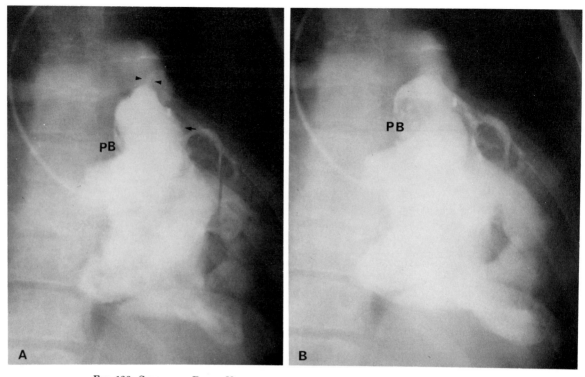

FIG. 126. SELECTIVE RIGHT VENTRICULAR ANGIOGRAM OF CASE SHOWN IN FIG. 127

(A) A faint jet is seen projecting through the slightly irregular domeshaped structure that represents the valve cusps. The large parietal band of the crista is seen (PB). (B) Exposure approximately ½ sec after A. The right ventricle is in partial diastole. A number of large muscle bundles is seen in the body of the ventricle. The parietal band has partially relaxed.

mation is obtained by the pullback of the catheter across the valve and the outflow tract of the right ventricle. This should be done under fluoroscopic vision with precise determination of the location of the catheter. An abrupt change in the contours of the pressure tracings from those of the pulmonary artery to those of the right ventricle gives an almost unequivocal diagnosis of valvular pulmonic stenosis. This combined with the determination of pressure in the right ventricle is often sufficient to allow a decision for surgical treatment with some confidence. In cases such as these selective right ventriculography may be helpful in that it provides a study of the contour of the outflow tract of the right ventricle and also may permit an estimate of the size of the opening in the valve. When contrast substance is injected with a pressure injector into the right ventricle followed by rapid serial filming correlated with the electrocardiogram, the contour of the infundibulum can be studied with some benefit. In early systole the infundibulum reaches its maximum dilatation, but in late systole it undergoes contraction. Thus, it is only with precise electrocardiographic monitoring that the observations on the contour of the in-

fundibulum are valid. The contrast substance is expressed through the pulmonary valve in a jet that often impinges on the superior wall of the pulmonary trunk. The size of the jet is roughly indicative of the size of the opening in the valve.

In cases with a well-formed infundibular chamber and valvular stenosis the pressure tracings during the pullback show a rather abrupt change from the pulmonary artery to an intermediate pressure area, namely that of the infundibular chamber. Upon further withdrawal of the catheter, and this may involve a considerable distance if the infundibular chamber is large, an intermediate pressure is encountered, and finally as the catheter tip reaches the right ventricle the right ventricular pressures are recorded. This can lead to a rather reliable diagnosis of infundibular and valvular stenosis, and under most circumstances this is a reliable guide to this diagnosis. Selective right ventricular angiography will demonstrate the infundibulum (Figs. 129 and 130).

Clear-cut pressure tracings are not always obtained due to a number of circumstances. In those cases in which the infundibular stenosis consists of a long narrow channel, a gradual transition from pulmonary artery pressures to those of the right ventricle will appear. Also, in certain cases where the infundibular chamber is quite small the change in pressure may be abrupt, and the small chamber may be completely overlooked. In a very slow pullback the catheter tip may rest in the right ventricle during diastole and in the pulmonary artery during systole; in other words, it seesaws backward and forward across the valve ring. This may give a confusing pressure tracing in which the systolic pressures are those of the pulmonary artery and the diastolic pressures are those of the right ventricle. This may suggest the presence of an infundibular chamber when one is not present. The zone of intermediate pressure may be in some cases surprisingly long. The catheter may be withdrawn a distance of 3 or 4 cm before it encounters the true right ventricular pressure. The occurrence of extrasystoles during the pullback may also make interpretation of the pressure curves more

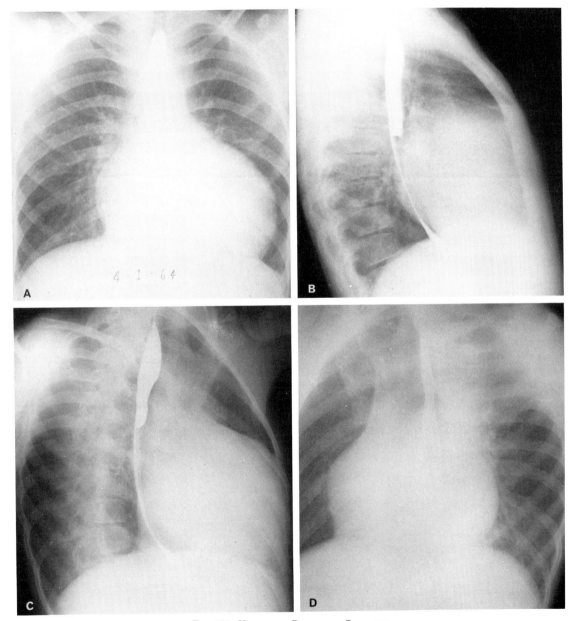

FIG. 127. VALVULAR PULMONIC STENOSIS

A 17-year-old patient had a right ventricular pressure of 120 mm Hg and a gradient across the valve of 90 mm Hg. The pulmonary trunk was not dilated (see angiogram in Fig. 126). The right ventricle and right atrium are considerably dilated as indicated by C (right oblique) and D (left oblique) views. The lungs show a diminished vascularity.

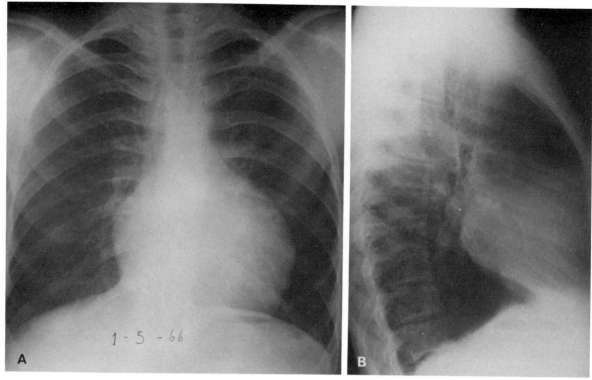

FIG. 128. SAME CASE AS IN FIG. 126, APPROXIMATELY 8 MONTHS AFTER PULMONARY VALVULOTOMY
The heart has decreased significantly in size. The pulmonary vasculature was not significantly changed. The patient was symptomatically much improved.

difficult. Difficulties in the pullback pressure tracings have been discussed by Kirklin *et al.* (1953) and Kjellberg *et al.* (1958). We regard these potential shortcomings of the pullback tracings as an additional need for the use of selective right ventricular angiocardiography in determining the anatomy of the outflow tract.

SELECTIVE RIGHT VENTRICULAR ANGIOGRAPHY. This procedure is carried out by placing a catheter into the right ventricle with the tip near the outflow tract. After the injection of contrast substance in the amount of 40–50 ml for an adult, filming is carried out at the rate of 6 per second. This rate is necessary if a detailed study of the outflow tract of the right ventricle and valve is to be obtained. It is essential to obtain films in both systole and diastole in order to determine the change in anatomy of the infundibular and valvular structures. Simultaneous biplane angiograms are usual and some angiographers prefer 16 or 35 mm cine studies. The latter have the advantage of allowing more careful study of the dynamic changes in the outflow tract during contraction and relaxation of the right ventricle.

The most striking sign of valvular stenosis is that of a jet of contrast substance projecting through the narrowed valvular orifice. This is associated with an upward protuberance of the valve cusps forming a dome or an inverted funnel-shaped appearance. The jet may be eccentric or central corresponding to the location of the valve orifice. It is usually round but may be slightly divergent or spraylike in shape. It may be seen in the AP projection but is best studied in the lateral projection. The jet may extend for a considerable distance into the dilated pulmonary artery and impinge on its anterior surface. In other cases it appears dampened and much smaller. The pulmonary artery opacifies relatively slowly and may require two or more heart beats before becoming opaque. In diastole the dome may flatten or recede toward the ventricle indicating pliability of the valve. Also, it is during diastole that the sinuses of Valsalva may bulge and thus become readily noticeable. After the pulmonary artery opacifies, both sides of the valve cusps may be visible and their thickness estimated. The cusps are usually thicker than those of a normal valve, although occasionally they are quite thin and in diastole may resemble a normal valve. Thickening and lack of mobility indicate rigidity of the valve.

The pulmonary artery distal to the valve is typically dilated, but in a small proportion of cases it may be normal or even reduced in size. The dilatation, if present, may extend into the

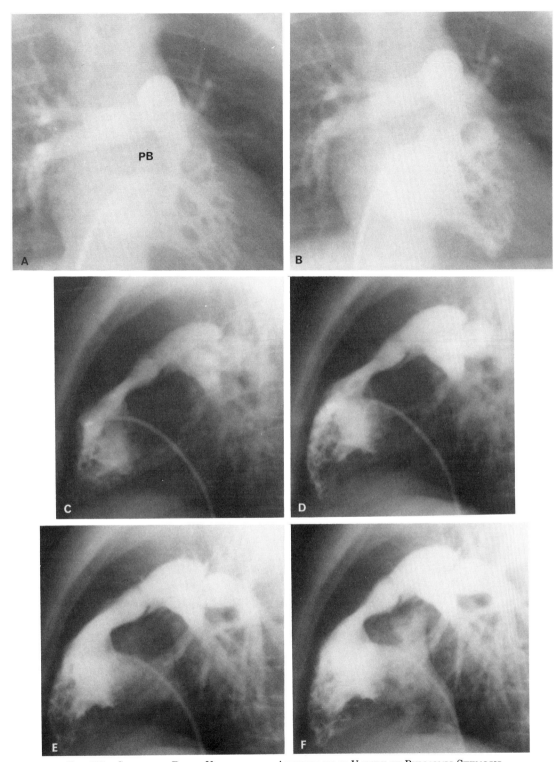

FIG. 129. SELECTIVE RIGHT VENTRICULAR ANGIOGRAM IN VALVULAR PULMONIC STENOSIS

Frontal views A and B show a prominent parietal band (PB) and large muscle bundles in the body of the ventricle. The films in the lateral view were taken ⅙ sec apart and are consecutive. A rounded jet is seen in C. The domelike protrusion of the valve in systole is shown in C and D. In D the valve sinuses are partially filled indicating the distance the valve has protruded into the pulmonary artery. The ratio of the least diameter of the infundibulum in systole/diastole can be determined from E and F. The ratio is about 0.5, and infundibular obstruction was thought to be insignificant. (Angiocardiograms presented through the courtesy of the Cardiac Clinic, Texas Childrens Hospital, Houston, Texas.)

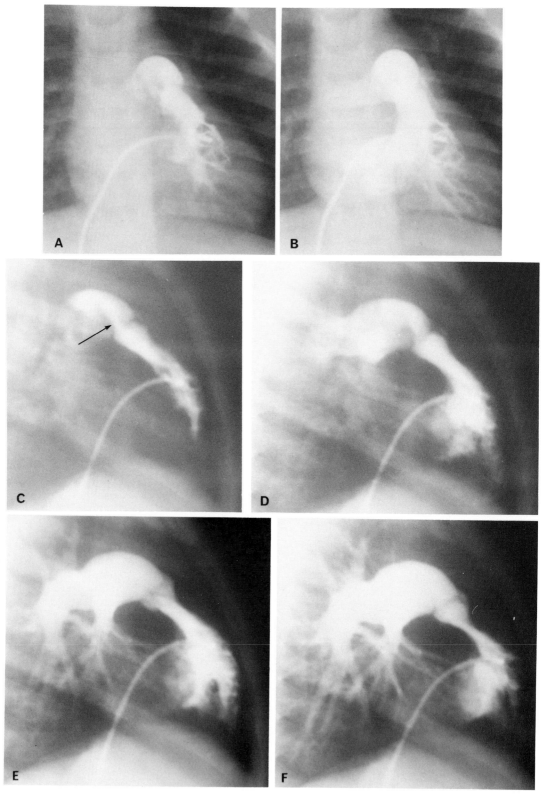

FIG. 130

left pulmonary artery or the artery may decrease abruptly in size at the point where it crosses the left main stem bronchus or at the pericardial reflection. The right pulmonary artery is almost invariably reduced in size. The contrast substance clears rather slowly from the pulmonary artery indicating a sluggish flow.

The infundibular canal may show impingement from large muscle bundles. These are the septal and parietal bands of the crista supraventricularis. During late systole these bundles may appear to greatly narrow the outflow passage and bring up the question of structural stenosis. Multiple films in systole and diastole are essential if this possibility is to be correctly evaluated (see below). No definite third ventricle can be recognized as a rule. Other hypertrophied muscle bundles may be seen lining the main ventricular cavity. Contrast substance may penetrate in between the muscle bundles and extend into the myocardium for a considerable distance (Fig. 126) suggesting the presence of myocardial sinusoids. The interventricular septum is usually bowed toward the left ventricle.

One of the more difficult diagnostic problems which as yet seems to be only partially solved is that of determining whether infundibular stenosis in a given case is due to secondary hypertrophy associated with valvular stenosis or whether it represents a primary obstruction that requires treatment. Follow-up right heart catheterizations performed following valvulotomy show that the reduction in right ventricular pressure does not occur immediately but takes place gradually over a period of months. During the same period of time the gradient of the outflow tract to the right ventricle may show a gradual reduction, and this is interpreted as showing that there is a regression in the muscular hypertrophy of the right ventricular outflow tract. On the other hand, in those cases where a considerable gradient persists the obstruction has often been due to an intrinsic infundibular change. Kirklin *et al.* (1953) advised a careful study of the thrill noted at the time of operation and also recommended that pressure tracings be made at the operating

table during a careful pullback of a small catheter across the valve and also careful measurements of the gradient at the operating table following valvotomy. In this manner they hoped to detect intrinsic infundibular obstruction. Gilbert *et al.* (1963) after a careful follow-up of some 40 cases of pulmonary valvulotomy found that in 5 of these cases in which significant obstruction persisted infundibular deformities could be demonstrated on the preoperative selective right ventricular angiocardiograms. These authors in comparing the width of the infundibulum in systole with the width of the valve ring found that those cases in which the infundibulum was less than one-half of that of the valve ring invariably had persistent unrelieved outflow obstruction. Consequently, they recommend that in cases in which this occurs infundibular resection should also be attempted. Little *et al.* (1963) in attempting the same evaluation used the ratio (diameter (narrowest) of infundibulum during systole)/(diameter of base of pulmonary artery). The normal ratio was 0.63 ± 0.08. A ratio <0.45 was considered as critical and a probable indication for infundibular resection.

Lester *et al.* (1965) proposed an additional ratio, namely, diameter of infundibulum in systole/diameter in diastole. When this ratio was >0.3 and the index of Little *et al.* <0.45, the obstruction was considered to be permanent rather than reversible (Figs. 129 and 130). It should be emphasized that the normal infundibulum contracts in late systole and that it is in early systole that it reaches its maximum diameter. It is at these phases of the heart cycle that measurements of infundibular diameter should be made. Measurements are made in the lateral projection using large films after selective injection of contrast substance into the right ventricle.

The angiographic signs of pulmonary valve dysplasia differ considerably from those of atypical congenital valvular pulmonic stenosis. Incomplete, imperfect and irregular doming of the pulmonic valve in ventricular systole is seen, and the valve leaflets are found to be irregularly and excessively thick and to lie within and partially

FIG. 130. SELECTIVE RIGHT VENTRICULAR ANGIOGRAM IN VALVULAR PULMONIC STENOSIS WITH INTACT VENTRICULAR SEPTUM

Consecutive films made ⅙ sec apart showing changes in contour of infundibular structures, valve and pulmonary trunk. (A and B) Frontal view showing large muscle bundles in body of ventricle. The anatomy of the valve is not well seen due to foreshortening. (C–F) Lateral view. An eccentric jet is seen in C (arrow). In D the infundibulum has relaxed and is presumably near maximum size and can be compared in diameter with F where it is presumed to be in systole and in its most constricted state. The ratio, minimal infundibular diameter during systole/diameter of the base of the pulmonary artery, is <0.45 indicating some infundibular obstruction (Little *et al.,* 1963). However, the ratio, diameter of infundibulum in systole/diameter in diastole, is about 0.3, suggesting that the obstruction was dynamic and probably reversible. (Angiograms presented through the courtesy of the Childrens Cardiac Clinic, Texas Childrens Hospital, Houston, Texas.)

obstruct a hypoplastic annulus. Very little change is seen between the diastolic and the systolic configuration of the dysplastic valve, though at times the appearance in ventricular diastole may be nearly normal. The sinuses of the pulmonary valve are narrowed, and post-stenotic dilatation is uncommon.

In severe pulmonic stenosis the right atrial pressure is often elevated and particularly the atrial "a" waves are elevated. Contrast substance injections into the right atrium with sampling from the brachial artery may show evidence of a right-to-left shunt, thus indicating an interatrial communication.

Differential Diagnosis. At first glance a number of conditions resemble pulmonic stenosis as seen on conventional chest films. Atrial septal defect can usually be differentiated on the basis of pulmonary vascularity and also the Eisenmenger complex for the same reason.

In infancy and early childhood the differentiation from the tetralogy of Fallot depends on the heart size. Enlargement of the heart and progressive enlargement tend to exclude tetralogy. A right aortic arch is rare with valvular pulmonic stenosis. Post-stenotic dilatation also may be a helpful feature. Selective right ventricular angiography may be necessary for differentiation.

Ebstein's anomaly offers the greatest difficulty. The right atrial border is usually larger in Ebstein's anomaly than in pulmonic stenosis. Post-stenotic dilatation is not seen in Ebstein's anomaly. Venous angiocardiography may be necessary and quite helpful.

Primary pulmonary hypertension usually has large proximal pulmonary arteries, both right and left. Right heart catheterization with insertion of the catheter into the pulmonary artery or selective angiocardiography may be necessary for differentiation.

Other Congenital Conditions Associated With Pulmonic Stenosis With Some Frequency

Single or multiple coarctations of the pulmonary artery or its branches occur occasionally associated with valvular pulmonic stenosis. In the series of cases reported by Gay *et al.* (1963) 30% had valvular pulmonic stenosis. Of course, the coarctations can be diagnosed both by catheterization or angiocardiography. Aortic valvular or subvalvular or combined aortic stenosis may be associated with pulmonary stenosis (Nadas *et al.* 1962). The patient may even arrive at the operating table with one of these lesions undiagnosed, and this can be a cause for failure of surgical treatment. Some degree of pulmonic stenosis is quite common with subaortic stenosis due to hypertrophy of the outflow tract of the left ventricle. Congenital pulmonary stenosis may also be associated with ventricular septal defect, transposition of the great vessels, tricuspid atresia with patent foramen ovale and atrial septal defect.

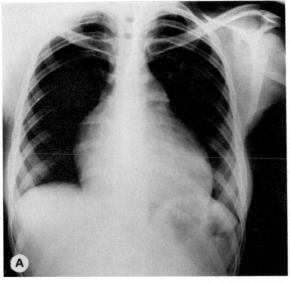 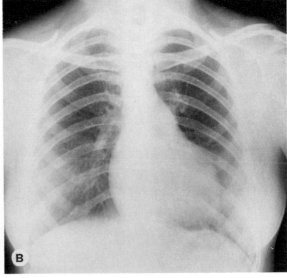

FIG. 131. PULMONIC STENOSIS WITH INTACT VENTRICULAR SEPTUM

(A) Conventional film. The heart is markedly enlarged, and there is a convexity of the pulmonary artery segment. The lungs are quite radiolucent. (B) Three years after pulmonary valvulotomy. There has been a definite decrease in heart size. The typical contour of pulmonic stenosis with intact ventricular septum has been maintained.

Radiologic Appearance After Operative Treatment. After successful valvulotomy for valvular stenosis, the enlarged heart may gradually decrease in size (Figs. 127 and 128) (Bravo et al. 1971). The change is rarely noticed until several months postoperatively. Mild to moderate cardiac enlargement may remain unchanged even though symptomatic improvement is definite and right heart catheterization shows a diminished or absent gradient. Post-stenotic dilatation of the pulmonary artery does not change, at least in the authors' experience, and this is in agreement with the findings of Mirowski et al. (1963). Also, there has been very slight change in the pulmonary vascularity. Where the heart was only minimally enlarged at the beginning, change in size may not take place. Postoperative right heart catheterization may show even in successful cases a gradient of 20–30 mm Hg between the right ventricle and the pulmonary artery. Where the gradient is in excess of 20–30 mm Hg, the possibility of an incomplete valvotomy or persistent infundibular stenosis must be considered. In such instances there may be no change in the radiologic appearance. A marked decrease in heart size on the other hand is excellent evidence of a satisfactory functional and hemodynamic result.

Johnson et al. (1972), following an analysis of 21 patients with asymptomatic uncomplicated pulmonic stenosis without surgical correction, concluded that surgical correction is indicated only in the presence of symptoms or complications of pulmonic stenosis since all of the 21 patients had a benign course during the follow-up period of 5–24 years (average 15 years) after diagnosis. Mild pulmonic stenosis (right ventricular systolic pressure less than 50 mm Hg) was present in 12, moderate stenosis (pressure 50–99 mm Hg) was present in 7, and severe stenosis (pressure greater than 100 mm Hg) was present in 2. These authors concluded that the following are indications for surgical correction: failure to grow and develop normally; definite cardiac enlargement; fatigue and exertional dyspnea of noteworthy degree; anginal pain; syncopal episodes; the onset of congestive heart failure, and cyanosis.

The experience of Nadas (1972) completely supports the conclusions of Johnson and his colleagues regarding mild pulmonic stenosis. This author does not agree with Johnson's conclusions regarding moderate and severe stenosis, believing that medical management of asymptomatic patients with moderate and severe pulmonary stenosis is fraught with danger from the long term point of view. He emphasizes that the sur-gical alternative, a very effective operation, may be offered for children with a very low risk. The last word on this subject has plainly not been spoken.

2. Supravalvular Pulmonic Stenosis

a. Single (usually in the pulmonary trunk)

b. Multiple ("coarctations" of the pulmonary artery branches)

Single or multiple stenoses of the pulmonary artery and branches are encountered with increased frequency as right heart catheterization and pulmonary angiography are increasingly utilized in cardiac diagnosis. Gay et al. (1963) have developed an anatomical classification, but we prefer to remember that the constrictions may be single or multiple. Single constrictions commonly involve the pulmonary trunk or the right or left branches near their origins while multiple constrictions are usually peripheral. In addition, there may be a combination of a central and peripheral constriction. The constriction may be quite short and consist only of a diaphragm or it may be elongated. Poststenotic dilatation is quite common in association with multiple peripheral coarctations, but it may also occur with central stenoses though it is less common in that circumstance. According to Gay's review in 1963, only about 40% of the cases of supravalvular pulmonic stenosis occurred as isolated lesions, the majority being associated with other significant cardiac abnormalities. The isolated lesions may rarely cause dyspnea and hemoptysis. The obstruction may cause an ejection type murmur with radiation toward the periphery of the chest and the interscapular region. Rarely a continuous murmur may be present and mimic that of patent ductus arteriosus. In many instances the signs and symptoms have been due to the associated cardiac malformation, and the presence of the peripheral obstructions in the pulmonary arterial system has not been suspected until after pulmonary arteriography or in some cases until after operation or autopsy.

The conventional chest film usually shows no changes that are suggestive of the diagnosis. In a few cases the stenosis has involved the peripheral arteries to such an extent that a nodular vascular pattern was evident on the ordinary chest film. This pattern should be susceptible to recognition when present.

The condition may be easily overlooked even following right heart catheterization and even though the catheter is inserted into the pulmonary artery. Hemodynamic measurements may not always show a pressure difference across the narrowing in the pulmonary artery, particularly if the withdrawal of the catheter is too rapid. A pressure gradient should be demonstrated if the tip of the catheter can be passed beyond the stenosis and slowly and carefully withdrawn.

The diagnosis is best made by pulmonary angiography preferably with the injection of contrast substance being made into the outflow tract of the right ventricle. Frontal and lateral or oblique projections are necessary to detect the sites of narrowing, particularly those involving the main and left pulmonary arteries. An indentation in the main or left pulmonary artery due to a reflection of the pericardium should not be confused with a coarctation, although such a reflection may reduce the size of the artery. Pulmonary angiography not only provides a diagnosis but also delineates the anatomy of the obstruction and is thus essential in planning surgical treatment (Fig. 132).

Although isolated or uncomplicated peripheral pulmonary coarctation may be a significant lesion in itself, it is of particular importance when it occurs in association with other important cardiac malformations. It has been most frequently associated with valvular pulmonic stenosis (Fig. 133) but has also been noted in cases of tetralogy of Fallot and atrial and ventricular septal defects. In these cases it is often over-looked and thus may prevent a good surgical result following the treatment of the primary lesion. The possibility of the presence of this lesion is a good indication for the routine preoperative use of pulmonary angiography in all cases of apparent pulmonary obstruction.

A familial predisposition to the development of supravalvular stenoses of the pulmonary arteries has been remarked upon, and the lesion has been found in association with maternal rubella (Arvidsson *et al.,* 1961). Roberts and Moes (1973) have described a syndrome of supravalvular pulmonary stenosis and an abnormal facial appearance in 15 children. These children demonstrated hypertelorism, a flat nasal bridge, a prominent upper lip and low-set ears. Angiography showed a diaphragm-like localized area of narrowing in the main pulmonary artery about 1 cm distal to the pulmonary valve. The diaphragm varied from 2–3 mm in thickness, and central jetting of contrast material could be observed through the diaphragm-like area. Mild to moderate poststenotic dilatation of the main pulmonary artery was seen in each case. Peripheral artery branch stenosis was not observed. Additional cardiac defects were present in one-third of the children, and the associated anomalies

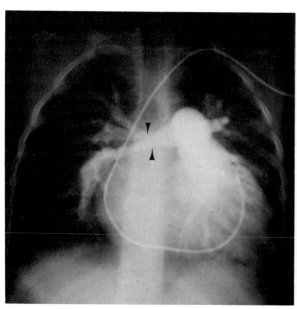 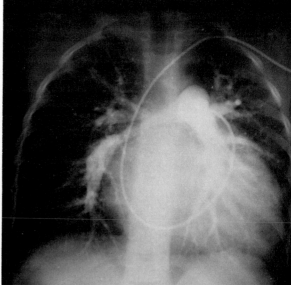

FIG. 132. STENOSIS (COARCTATION) OF RIGHT PULMONARY ARTERY IN 6-YEAR-OLD WHITE BOY WITH INTERATRIAL SEPTAL DEFECT

Selective pulmonary arteriogram shows narrowing of the right main pulmonary artery just proximal to its division into upper and lower lobe branches. Mild poststenotic dilatation is also shown. The pulmonary trunk is enlarged.

At the time of surgical repair of the IASD the right pulmonary artery was found to be constricted by adhesions and compressed by the ascending aorta against which it was tightly pressed apparently as a result of the slight forward displacement of the enlarged pulmonary trunk. Repair of the septal defect and the lysis of adhesions abolished the thrill and murmur in this area and relieved the incomplete obstruction to flow.

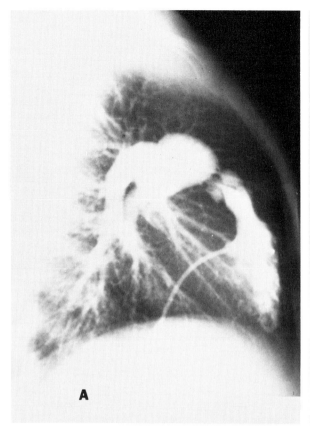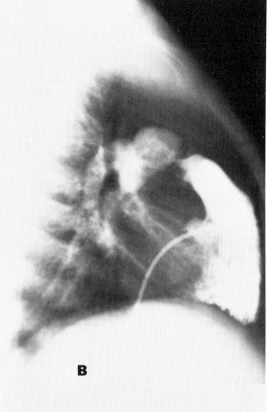

FIG. 133. SUPRAVALVULAR PULMONARY STENOSIS

Selected frames from a selective right ventriculogram in ventricular systole (A) and diastole (B) display a slightly thickened, incompletely opened and probably dysplastic pulmonary valve. About 2 cm distal to the valve is an area of pronounced supravalvular stenosis, just distal to which is an area of post-stenotic dilatation which involves only the pulmonary trunk. The right and left pulmonary arteries are not dilated. Supravalvular pulmonary stenosis may exist as an isolated lesion or be combined with other forms of congenital heart disease, in this case with mild to moderate valvular pulmonary stenosis.

included atrial septal defect, partial anomalous pulmonary venous return and ventricular septal defect.

3. Subvalvular Pulmonic Stenosis
a. As an isolated anomaly
b. Associated with other anomalies

Infundibular stenosis without valvular stenosis is rare. There are two types: (a) The infundibular chamber is well developed although it may be small. The line of division between the main cavity of the right ventricle and the infundibular chamber is sharp and well defined, forming a sort of ostium. The infundibular chamber may be large and dilated and protrude as a well-localized bulge on the anterior surface of the heart. The valve leaflets are well developed and are normal; poststenotic dilatation of the pulmonary artery is uncommon but may be present and similar to that seen in true valvular stenosis. (b) The infundibulum is shrunken with thick muscular walls forming a funnel-shaped or irregularly shaped

channel. The septal and parietal bands of the crista supraventricularis are displaced ventrally and to the left. The anatomy is often variable, and a true infundibular chamber as such may not exist. Instead there may be a long funnel-shaped passageway. Dilatation of the pulmonary artery beyond the valve may be seen but is uncommon.

Mild to moderate hypertrophy of the infundibular muscle is common secondary to the outflow obstruction produced by valvular stenosis. In some postmortem specimens, however, the infundibular deformity was of such magnitude and contour that it seems likely that it was not secondary to the valvular stenosis but rather a primary deformity. This particularly applies to the instances in which the infundibulum is a long narrow channel, and it seems unlikely that the muscular walls would regress significantly following relief of the valvular stenosis. The practical point to be determined before surgical treatment is whether or not the infundibular stenosis is of sufficient magnitude to require attention at the time of valvulotomy. While this recurrent problem has not been solved, certain angiographic clues to the possible need for infundibular resection at the time of pulmonary valvulotomy have been described and are discussed in the preceding section on valvular pulmonary stenosis.

Radiologic Findings. The cardiac contour is more variable and less characteristic than that of valvular stenosis, although in a number of reported cases and in one of our cases (Fig. 124), a definite localized convexity along the left heart border in the region of the infundibulum was noted. When the infundibular chamber is large and bulges so as to produce such a shadow, the radiologist can suggest the presence of infundibular stenosis with some confidence. In other instances, however, the chamber may be small and completely unnoticeable. Poststenotic dilatation is much less common with infundibular stenosis but certainly does occur and is of little differential value (Blount et al., 1959). Differential pulsations between the right and left pulmonary arteries such as are found in valvular stenosis are said not to occur in infundibular stenosis (Gay and Franck, 1960). The pulmonary vascularity is usually decreased, similar to the appearance seen in valvular stenosis.

The findings on cardiac catheterization and at the time of angiography are discussed in the preceding section on valvular pulmonic stenosis.

Infundibular pulmonic stenosis in the absence of valvular pulmonic stenosis is most often seen accompanying other anomalies. It is the characteristic form of right ventricular outflow obstruction seen in tetralogy of Fallot though in that condition it may also occasionally be associated with valvular pulmonic stenosis. Surgical treatment of the infundibular obstruction, along with closure of the ventricular septal defect, is critical to the total correction of this severe anomaly. Infundibular pulmonic stenosis has also been reported, in the absence of valvular stenosis, associated with congenital idiopathic hypertrophic subaortic stenosis (Neufeld et al., 1960; Nghiem et al., 1972). In such patients, gross muscular hypertrophy of the ventricular septum may produce outflow obstruction on both sides of the heart, and surgical correction requires resection of obstructing bands and hypertrophied muscle, often from both sides of the ventricular septum.

4. Ebstein's Anomaly

a. Acyanotic, without an interatrial communication

b. Cyanotic, with an interatrial communication

The normal tricuspid valve consists of large anterior and posterior leaflets and a somewhat smaller medial or septal leaflet. These are attached at their bases to the annulus fibrosus of the valve ring, the anatomical dividing line between the right atrium and ventricle. Chordae tendineae attached near the margins of these leaflets limit their retrograde motion and keep them in apposition during ventricular systole.

The basic anatomical defect in Ebstein's malformation (Ebstein, 1866) is downward displacement of an abnormal tricuspid valve (Seckel and Bensey, 1974). The anterior leaflet is usually the largest and is partially attached to the annulus fibrosus, while the posterior and medial cusps arise from the wall of the right ventricle and interventricular septum. Wide pathologic variation is shown by the valve leaflets; they may be large, rudimentary, or absent, adherent to the endocardium, thick and nodular or thin with multiple perforations. Stubby papillary muscles with short chordae tendineae closely connect the valve to the ventricular wall. These malformations result in the production of a membranous valvular structure which extends downward like a pocket into the right ventricular cavity. The right atrial cavity is thus enlarged to include this pocket which in turn encroaches upon the ventricular cavity to a significant but variable extent so that the functional portion of the right ventricle is decreased in size. Tricuspid insufficiency, tricuspid stenosis and inflow right ventricular stenosis result in inadequate right ventricular diastolic filling and poor systolic ejection. Thus, the primary disturbance of cardiovascular physiology is decreased output of the right ventricle resulting in low pulmonary blood flow.

An important feature of this anomaly is the striking thinness of the myocardium in the "auricularized" portion of the right ventricle. In contrast, the right ventricular outflow tract distal to the deformed and misplaced valve has a myocardial wall of normal thickness and is thus able to maintain a semblance of ventricular activity. Because of this thinning and resultant muscular weakness of the inflow portion of the right ventricle, the atrium and ventricle balloon out, forming, in effect, a single large dilated chamber.

In about two-thirds of the observed autopsied cases there has been functional patency of the foramen ovale; Vacca et al. (1958), in a complete review of 108 cases of Ebstein's anomaly, found defects in the interatrial septum in 46 of 57 autopsied cases (81%). In this same series, 81 of

108 patients had clinical cyanosis (75%). A study of these cases indicates that cyanosis was due almost entirely to a venous-arterial shunt through the opening in the interatrial septum.

Watson (1974) summarized data from 61 centers in 28 countries on 505 cases of Ebstein's anomaly. Catheterizations were carried out on 363 patients. Necropsy was carried out in 93 cases. Forty-eight percent of those catheterized and 81% of those coming to necropsy had associated congenital cardiac malformations. If defects in the interatrial septum are excluded, the figures are 12 and 42%, respectively. Associated anomalies included ventricular septal defect, pulmonary stenosis, coarctation of the aorta and patent ductus arteriosus.

Clinical Findings. Dyspnea, cyanosis, and excessive fatigue are the commonest findings. The average age of onset of cyanosis is about 4 years (Vacca *et al.,* 1958). When it begins in the neonatal period, cyanosis may decrease or disappear with the passage of time only to recur later in life (Schiebler *et al.,* 1959). Palpitations are a frequent complaint and are almost always related to arrhythmias of various types. They may be associated with dizziness, syncope, convulsions and chest pain. Palpitations in a cyanotic child should always raise the possibility of Ebstein's anomaly (Bialostozky *et al.,* 1972). All 20 of the patients studied by Hansen and Wennevold (1971) had normal blood pressures. A systolic precordial murmur and thrill are commonly found, and the diastolic murmurs and gallop rhythm have been frequently heard. All 65 patients reported by Bialostozky *et al.* (1972) had third or fourth heart sounds, and they declare that a cyanotic cardiopathy in the absence of heart failure associated with a third or fourth heart sound should raise the suspicion of Ebstein's anomaly. Growth features have been normal.

The electrocardiogram is rarely normal in Ebstein's anomaly. The commonest finding is complete or incomplete right bundle branch block. Other common findings include enlarged, peaked and occasionally prolonged P waves, paroxysmal atrial tachycardia, low voltage QRS complexes in the right precordial leads, right axis deviation, and premature ventricular contractions. Four of eleven patients reported by Sinha *et al.* (1960) had atrial fibrillation, and 5 of 23 patients described by Schiebler *et al.* (1959) showed the Wolff-Parkinson-White pattern. Hernandes *et al.* (1958) have described what they feel are diagnostic findings on the intracavitary electrocardiogram with simultaneously recorded pressures.

Lundstrom (1973) has examined 19 patients between the ages of 4 days and 40 years by echocardiography. He describes the echo from the anterior tricuspid leaflet as having an abnormal pattern of movement with an abnormally anterior position during diastole. The abnormal pattern of movement of the echo from the anterior tricuspid leaflet, associated with late tricuspid closure, has not been found in any other patient examined.

During cardiac catheterization it is common for the catheter to coil in the huge right atrium. Documentation of the location of the tricuspid valve far to the left of its normal position may be accomplished by pressure determinations. Tricuspid stenosis and/or insufficiency may be shown, or normal valve function may be demonstrated.

Because of the hazards of cardiac catheterization and angiocardiography, mostly related to the high incidence of arrhythmias, patients with Ebstein's anomaly have not been routinely studied by these techniques. Bialostozky (1972) reports two fatalities among 27 patients subjected to catheterization or angiocardiography or both. Watson (1974) reports 13 deaths and 6 cardiac arrests in a collected series of 363 patients who were catheterized. Hansen and Wennevold (1971) comment on the high mortality that has been reported in connection with cardiac catheterization and angiocardiography in patients with Ebstein's disease but say that in their experience the risk was not increased.

Radiologic Findings. During infancy the heart is normal in size, but enlargement occurs early and is progressive in most cases though in a few enlargement may be slight. The enlargement is due to massive distention of the right atrium and thin-walled portion of the right ventricle. This chamber may become so large as to be border-forming in all projections and may even form the posterior heart contour in the lateral projection (Hanson and Rosenbaum, 1964). The right-sided enlargement displaces the remainder of the heart to the left and posteriorly, and the left heart border characteristically bulges almost horizontally toward the left chest wall giving the heart a symmetrical, globular or box-like silhouette. Oblique and lateral views show pronounced extension into the retrosternal area. Along the right heart border cardiac pulsations are diminished or absent.

Radiologically determined heart size is not helpful in predicting the outcome for individual patients, especially as they get older. While gross cardiomegaly is an unfavorable sign, numbers of patients have survived for many years with hearts that practically fill the thorax.

It must be emphasized that mild forms of this anomaly exist, and a heart of normal size and configuration is compatible with the diagnosis.

Because the functional portion of the right ventricle is reduced in size and there is ordinarily some degree of obstruction to the flow of blood into this chamber, and because of shunting of blood from right to left through a patent foramen ovale, pulmonary blood flow is decreased. This is seen radiographically as diminished pulmonary vascularity, and the lung parenchyma appears unusually radiolucent. Decreased pulmonary vascularity is well correlated with cyanosis, but even in acyanotic patients the pulmonary vessels tend to be lower limit of normal in size. The

pulmonary artery and aorta are small and difficult to identify in any projection.

Pulmonary congestion and pleural effusion are absent, and left atrial enlargement does not occur. According to Amplatz *et al.* (1959), enlargement of the left atrium and accentuated pulmonary vasculature definitely exclude Ebstein's malformation.

Angiocardiography may be of considerable help in the diagnosis of Ebstein's anomaly and is the diagnostic procedure of choice. Contrast material enters the distended atrioventricular chamber and remains there for an abnormally long time until dilution renders it invisible. The pulmonary artery fills poorly and when outlined is seen to be small. If the foramen ovale is open, the left atrium, ventricle, and aorta fill quite

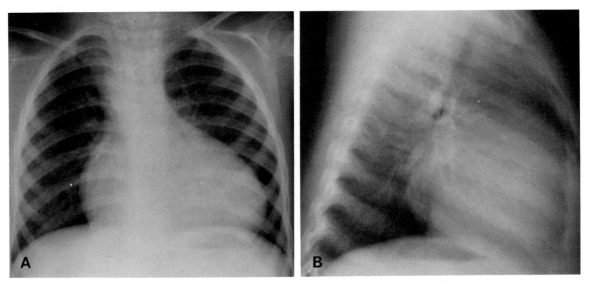

FIG. 134 A AND B. EBSTEIN'S ANOMALY WITHOUT ATRIAL COMMUNICATION IN 2-YEAR-OLD CHILD
The lungs show a diminished vascularity, and there is a right aortic arch.

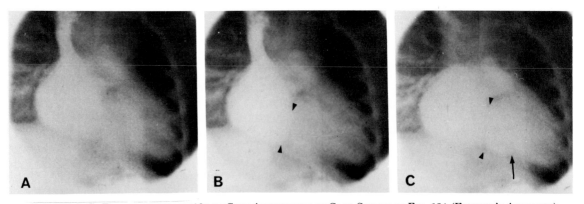

FIG. 135 A–C. REPRODUCTION OF 16-MM CINE ANGIOGRAM OF CASE SHOWN IN FIG. 134 (EBSTEIN'S ANOMALY)
The right atrium is dilated, and an indentation (arrows ▲ in B and C) indicates the tricuspid valve ring. A second indentation (→ arrow) in C presumably represents the limit of the downward extension of the abnormal fenestrated membrane that forms the atrialized portion of the right ventricle.

early with contrast substance, confirming the presence of a venous-arterial shunt and explaining the cyanosis. At times the thinness of the wall of the auricularized portion of the right ventricle may be demonstrated, excluding pericardial effusion as a cause of the cardiac enlargement.

During biplane venous angiocardiography, Soloff et al. (1951) showed a narrow nonopacified band near the apex of the heart in the RAO position which was thought to represent a tricuspid valve leaflet separating the functional right ventricle from the auricularized part. Kistin et al. (1955) reported a case in which the division of the right ventricle into a proximal atrialized portion and a distal functioning portion was seen as an inconstant deep notch on the inferior border of the heart near the apex during angiocardiography. Ellis et al. (1964) show several excellent angiocardiographic examples of the abnormally placed tricuspid valve leaflets. It would appear that this finding, in the presence of a compatible clinical and radiologic picture, is quite specific for Ebstein's malformation.

The location of the right atrioventricular sulcus on the surface of the heart bears a close relation to the location of the tricuspid valve ring. The right coronary artery normally courses through this sulcus, and opacification of the right coronary artery during aortography will thus locate the position of the ring. Displacement of the tricuspid valve leaflets from this location, shown by angiocardiography, is strong evidence in favor of the diagnosis of Ebstein's anomaly (Ellis et al., 1964).

The condition most likely to be confused with Ebstein's anomaly is pulmonic stenosis with intact ventricular septum when marked cardiac enlargement is present. Differentiation of these two conditions has been discussed under pulmonic stenosis. Pericardial effusion and congenital or acquired tricuspid stenosis must also be considered.

A rare variety of this malformation occurs in association with congenitally corrected transposition of the great vessels in which the left atrioventricular valve is anomalous in its origin, morphology, and function (Van Mierop et al., 1961; Becu et al., 1955; Dekker et al., 1965).

Operative treatment for Ebstein's anomaly may be palliative or definitive. A superior vena cava to right pulmonary artery shunt was introduced by Glenn in 1954 as a palliative procedure. The current value and indications for that operation are debated. Mannix and Berroya (1971) believe the Glenn operation may be indicated for some infants and very young children, while Wat-

son (1974) declares that palliative operations are not helpful, that they carry a high mortality and have no place in treatment and are probably contraindicated. Scattered reports may be found in the literature of patients who were operated upon and improved by partial right heart bypass (Scott et al., 1963; Balkoura-Christopoulus and Kittle, 1973). As early as 1958 a plastic procedure for the correction of this anomaly by realigning the downward displaced tricuspid leaflets to the normal annulus was proposed, and Bahnson et al. (1965) have reported some success with this operation.

Total surgical correction of Ebstein's anomaly with a prosthetic valve was first described by Barnard and Schrirre in 1963, and several centers have reported success with this form of surgical therapy (Lillehei and Gannon, 1965; Mannix and Berroya, 1971; Balkoura-Christopoulus and Kittle, 1973).

The average age at the time of death in 60 cases reported by Vacca et al. (1958) was 23 years; however, the natural history of the disease varies widely from death in infancy to maintenance of good health until late in life. One patient who survived to the age of 79 although four-fifths of the right ventricle was auricularized is on record (Adams and Hudson, 1956). While the mild forms may produce no symptoms on normal daily activity, cardiac reserve is probably reduced even in these patients, and a tendency to cardiac arrhythmias may be present (Kezdi and Wennemark, 1958).

Bialostozky et al. (1972), believing the overall prognosis to be poor, advocate consideration of the surgical approach, with few exceptions, in every patient with Ebstein's malformation of the tricuspid valve. In sharp distinction to this position is the conclusion reached by Watson (1974) after lengthy consideration of the natural history of Ebstein's anomaly in 505 cases collected from throughout the world. He points out that 71% of the children and adolescents and 60% of the adults included in this study had little or no disability and were classified as cardiac grade I or II. So many of these patients remain in grades I or II throughout childhood or adolescence and even beyond it and the number of deaths from natural causes compares so favorably with surgical mortality that there is reason to wonder if surgery is indicated in such patients whatever their age. Watson was unable to uncover evidence that successful valve replacement in any way diminished the risk of sudden death, and it may well be that operation should be delayed and advised only when increasing disability makes it difficult to pursue normal activities.

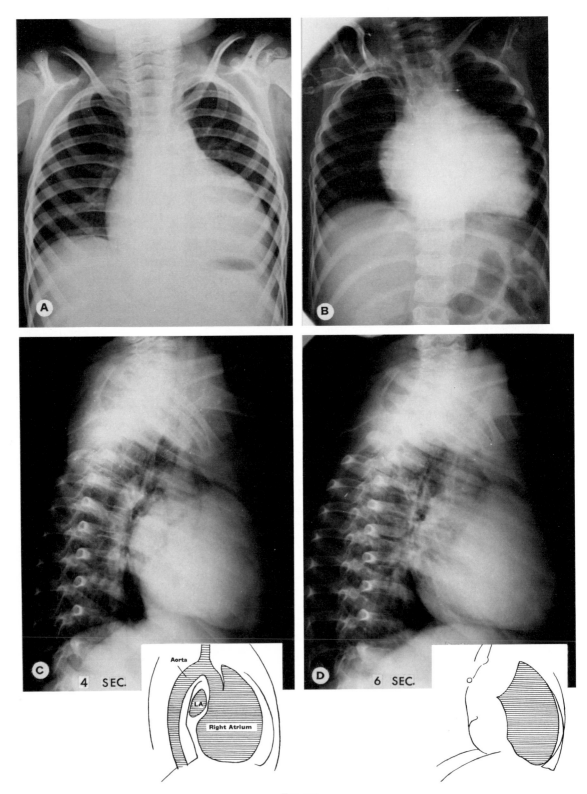

Fig. 136

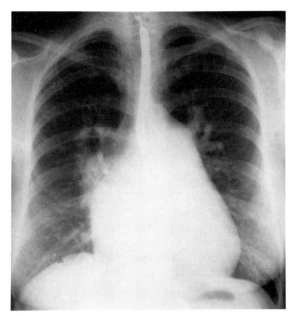

FIG. 137. RHEUMATIC MITRAL STENOSIS AND EBSTEIN'S DEFORMITY OF THE TRICUSPID VALVE IN A 40-YEAR-OLD MALE

The Ebstein's deformity was mild and an unexpected finding at autopsy.

When operation is performed replacement of the malformed tricuspid valve is ordinarily indicated. The operation should be delayed, if possible, until the patient's heart is large enough to take an adult-size prosthesis or homograft.

5. Congenital Aplasia or Marked Hypoplasia of the Myocardium of the Right Ventricle (Uhl's Anomaly)

As described by Uhl (1952) the right ventricular wall had no myocardium except for two very short segments near the tricuspid valve ring and another near the conus. The remainder of the ventricular wall was composed of thickened endocardium and fibrous tissue. Other authors (Zuberbuhler and Blank, 1970; Cote *et al.,* 1973) have found varying degrees of deformity or almost complete absence of the tricuspid valve in association with the marked hypoplasia or aplasia of the right ventricular myocardium. The condition may be considered as a severe form of Ebstein's anomaly, although it differs from the original description because of the marked dim-

inution in the right ventricular myocardium. The practical aspect of differentiation is that Uhl's anomaly could not possibly benefit from replacement of the tricuspid valve because the fundamental defect is an absence of pump power of the right ventricle.

Most of the patients succumb during infancy, although several patients have lived to adulthood (Gould *et al.,* 1967; Rowe and McDonald, 1964).

Differentiation from Ebstein's anomaly is difficult. The almost parchment thinness of the right ventricular myocardium may be suspected from the right ventricular angiogram which shows a complete absence of trabeculation and a very thin wall. The secondary indentation in the right ventricle indicating the distal margin of the misplaced tricuspid valve as occasionally seen in Ebstein's anomaly may be lacking. Differentiation from pericardial effusion and pulmonic stenosis must also be considered.

On the Left Side of the Circulation

1. Coarctation of the Aorta (Introduction). Coarctation of the aorta is a congenital malformation in which a segment of the aorta is constricted, narrowed, or obliterated. Because of the constriction, blood flow to the lower portion of the body is usually decreased, and systolic hypertension in the upper portion of the body appears after a variable period of time. The incidence of coarctation is about 1 in 16,000 in children under 14 years (Keith *et al.,* 1967). It is found about twice as often in male as in female patients (Hamilton and Abbott, 1928; Reifenstein *et al.,* 1947). Keith *et al.* (1967) state that more than one-half of the cases of coarctation will have signs or symptoms during the first year of life, and of this group about 40–50% will succumb, usually by the end of the first year. Of course, in many of those who die during infancy complications are severe, and associated cardiac defects play a role. This group presents the most difficult diagnostic problems, and it is also in this group that prompt diagnosis and treatment may be most fruitful. In the authors' experience in a general hospital, the majority of cases are encountered during the second decade, often when symptoms are minor. It has been shown, however, that even the asymptomatic cases have a

FIG. 136. EBSTEIN'S DEFORMITY OF TRICUSPID VALVE (AUTOPSY CASE)

(A) Conventional film. The heart is considerably enlarged, and pulsations of the cardiac borders were diminished. There is an increase in radiolucency of the lungs. (B) Angiocardiogram, anterposterior projection at 4 sec. Almost the entire heart is opaque and remained so for several seconds. (C) Angiocardiogram, lateral view at 4 sec. LA, left atrium. There is a large dilated chamber consisting of the right atrium and that portion of the right ventricle which is associated with the deformity of the tricuspid valve. The left atrium filled through a patent foramen ovale. (D) Contrast substance continues to stagnate in this large chamber.

shorter life expectancy than that of the population at large (Reifenstein *et al.* 1947).

Classification

The use of the terms infantile and adult in the classification of coarctation is of very little value. A more exact anatomical classification is now possible. The significant anatomical features are (1) the location and length of the coarcted area, (2) the patency of the ductus (all cases have either a ligamentum or a patent ductus), (3) the relationship of the coarctation to the ductus (pre- or postductal), and (4) the presence of significant associated cardiovascular defects, such as VSD,

ASD, transposition of the great vessels, etc. The degree of development of collateral circulation is also of practical importance, but it seems to be connected to a degree with the variations listed above and therefore does not need to be mentioned separately. The following classification takes the above-mentioned features into account.
A. Coarctation distal to or at the ligamentum arteriosum.

1. With proximal limb of ample length and width (Fig. 138A).

2. With proximal limb long but somewhat narrowed (Fig. 138B).

3. With proximal limb quite short and the

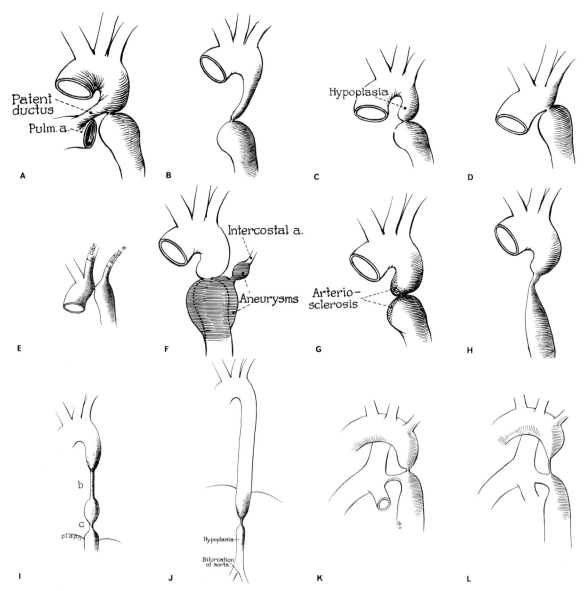

FIG. 138 A–L. COMMON AND UNCOMMON VARIATIONS IN ANATOMY OF COARCTATION OF AORTA
For further description see text.

coarctation very near or at the site of the left subclavian artery (Fig. 138D).

4. Marked narrowing of the proximal limb involving a considerable length of the aorta (Fig. 138C).

5. Constriction between the left carotid and left subclavian artery (Fig. 138E).
B. Same as above but with patent ductus proximal to coarctation (Fig. 138A).
C. Same as above with some added complicating defects, such as VSD, ASD, AI, or AS.
D. Coarctation proximal to patent ductus arteriosus (preductal) (Fig. 138, K and L).

1. Without other significant complicating associated cardiovascular disease.

2. Associated with significant cardiac abnormalities, such as transposition of the great vessels, single ventricle, endocardial fibroelastosis, etc.
E. Coarctation of unusual length or unusual site not included above.

1. Hypoplasia of the thoracic aorta (Figs. 138I and 139).

2. Coarctation of the lower thoracic and abdominal aorta (Figs. 138J and 139).

Atresia of the ascending aorta is described as a separate condition.

Each of the above categories has its own significance with regard to diagnosis, surgical treatment, and prognosis. The variations in length and width of the proximal limb as indicated in the various subheadings in category A are nowadays of minor importance. Formerly, when end to end anastomosis was the main technique of repair, these variations were more significant in that the diameter of the anastomosis was sometimes considerably less than that of the aorta on one or both sides of the coarcted segment. By

the use of grafts and also with considerable experience, surgeons nowadays have little difficulty in establishing a satisfactory passageway despite the size or length of the proximal limb. Even a considerable length of atretic aorta can be successfully bypassed, although the prognosis as to the return of the blood pressure to normotensive levels may not be quite as good as with the more ample segments.

A patent ductus as listed in category B is a frequent finding and occurred in 13 of 41 cases cited by Keith et al. (1958). The ductus is often small, and its effects on the hemodynamics of the circulation are thus minimal. Occasionally, however, it is large, and the blood flow is as usual from the aorta to the pulmonary artery. This may lead to cardiac enlargement and pulmonary plethora. About 98% of all operative cases fall into categories A and B due in part to selection of cases.

The most common cardiac defects associated with categories A and B are VSD and bicuspid aortic valve, although ASD is occasionally seen. Keith et al. (1958) found 25% of 29 cases to have a bicuspid valve, and Reifenstein et al. (1947) found an incidence of 43%. A ventricular septal defect, particularly when it is of significant size, may tend to obscure the usual hemodynamic pattern (Newcombe et al., 1961) in that it tends to equalize the pressure between the two ventricles and thus to reduce the pressure in the head and the upper part of the body. When seen in combination with a patent ductus arteriosus, the diagnosis is most difficult. A bicuspid aortic valve may be a site for bacterial endocarditis, and this may ultimately result in either AI or AS. Aortic stenosis either superimposed on a bicuspid aortic valve or due to other causes such as rheumatic fever may be found in 5–10% of coarctations (Smith and Mathews, 1955; Reifenstein et al., 1947). In the presence of aortic and subaortic stenosis the blood pressure in the upper extremities may be normal.

Categories D, 1 and 2 encompass in a general way those cases formerly considered as the infantile type. The majority of cases have signs and symptoms during the first year of life, although the cause of the symptoms is the severe cardiac malformations that accompany this type of coarctation with considerable frequency. (The postductal cases listed in categories A and B may also cause signs and symptoms of heart failure during the first year of life and seem to be the more common type diagnosed and treated by surgery.) Where the ductus is widely patent and the coarctation is of moderate to severe degree, blood flow is from the pulmonary artery to the

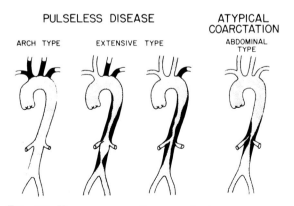

PULSELESS DISEASE

ARCH TYPE   EXTENSIVE TYPE

ATYPICAL COARCTATION

ABDOMINAL TYPE

FIG. 139. VARIATIONS OF TAKAYASU'S ARTERITIS THAT PRODUCE ATYPICAL COARCTATION OF THE AORTA AND ITS MAJOR BRANCHES
(Courtesy of Drs. A. Lande and Y. M. Berkmen and *Radiologic Clinics of North America.*)

descending aorta. Thus, the circulation to the lower portion of the body is maintained by the right ventricle and to the upper portion by the left ventricle. These patients are quite susceptible to heart failure in early infancy. The inference from the paper of Bahn *et al.* (1951) is that the heart failure is due to a lack of collateral circulation, and this becomes of considerable importance if the ductus is reduced in size or closes. It seems unlikely, however, that the presence or absence of systemic collaterals play such an important role in the development of heart failure. As cited by Keith *et al.* (1958), collaterals can be demonstrated by angiography even though the coarctation is preductal and the ductus is open. Furthermore, a fatal outcome due to heart failure is rather common in the preductal group even though the ductus remains open. Failure is probably due to overloading of the right ventricle and has nothing to do with the adequacy of collaterals. Another complicating feature in this group is that the coarctation is often somewhat longer and may extend into the arch of the aorta. Severe cardiac malformations, such as transposition of the great vessels, single ventricle, and endocardial fibroelastosis are frequent. It should be mentioned that in a preductal coarctation with transposition of the great vessels the lower portion of the body may have a normal color whereas the upper portion will be cyanotic. This is the reverse of a normal arrangement of the great vessels in which case the upper portion of the body has a normal color and the lower portion is cyanotic.

In group E we have those cases in which the coarctation is of unusual length or is at an unusual site. Hypoplasia of the descending aorta was found in about 1% of the total cases treated by surgery as reported by Schuster and Gross (1962). It was found only in women. The present authors have seen a case of a 17-year-old girl in whom a segment, some 10 cm in length, was diffusely narrowed (Bahnson *et al.*, 1949) and another case in which a 6-cm segment of the lower thoracic aorta was calcified and greatly narrowed. Some of these may be due to an inflammatory process.

Brust *et al.* (1959) reviewed 17 cases where the coarctation was below the diaphragm and involved the origin of the renal arteries. The renal arteries are not necessarily involved, although there is usually hypertension in the upper portion of the body. Several cases have been associated with Takayasu's arteritis or pulseless disease. The coarctation is typically just above the renal arteries. Coarctation of the abdominal aorta should be suspected when the hemodynamic changes suggest coarctation but pulsations of the aorta in the epigastrium can be felt and there is an absence of rib notching and no evidence of a figure of three sign.

Turner's syndrome is associated with chromosomal abnormalities and is characterized by sexual infantilism, webbed neck, and cubitus valgus. About 25% of these cases have coarctation of the aorta at the usual site.

Radiologic Findings. In discussing the radiologic evidence of coarctation it is useful to divide the signs into three groups: (1) findings in older children and adults which form the bulk of the cases for elective surgery, (2) findings during infancy, and (3) findings in those cases in which the coarctation is not at the usual site.

In older children and adults, conventional radiologic examination (chest films with barium swallow and occasionally fluoroscopy) often suffices not only to confirm a diagnosis of coarctation but to determine the location with some degree of accuracy.

RIB NOTCHING. Rib notching remains the single most important radiologic sign of coarctation. The significance of the notches along the costal grooves as demonstrated radiologically was reported by Roesler (1928) and independently by Railsback and Dock (1929) the following year. A hundred years before this, however, the tortuous intercostal arteries, their significance as collateral channels, and the fact that they eroded ribs and had been clearly noted in pathologic and anatomical dissections (Fig. 140) (Meckel, 1827). Notching is most commonly demonstrated in the fourth to the eighth ribs inclusive, the third and ninth ribs infrequently, and the remaining ribs rarely. The incidence of detectable rib notching increases with age, and in general it is only above the age of 20 years that it is found in the great majority of patients (Fig. 141). Fairly extensive right-sided notching has been noted in cases where the origin of the left subclavian artery is involved in the coarctation (Bayley and Holubeck, 1940). On the other hand, left-sided notching occurs where the right subclavian artery is aberrant and originates from the descending aorta below the coarctation (Grollman and Horns, 1964). In such circumstances, the blood may actually flow in a retrograde direction in the right subclavian artery and be part of a collateral pathway involving the vertebral arteries. Absence of notching in older patients is most frequently associated with poorly developed collateral circulation and is presumptive evidence of a mild coarctation.

A slight variation in exposure and projection may change to a surprising degree one's ability to identify a given notch on a rib, and when

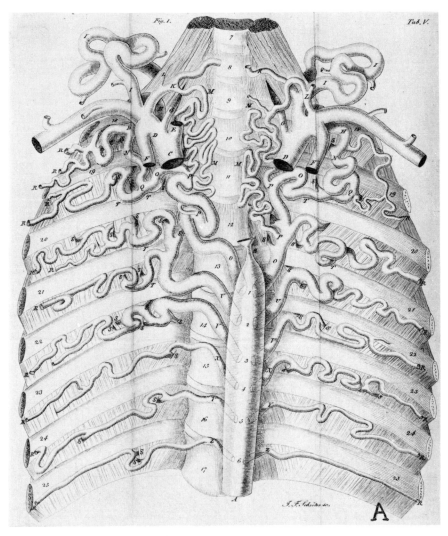

FIG. 140. RIB NOTCHING

Illustration from *Meckel's Archives of Anatomy and Physiology* published in 1827. The tortuous intercostal arteries and their significance as collateral channels are well shown. Note that the artist depicted notching of the superior borders of several ribs. (Courtesy of *Radiology*, 61: 706, 1953.)

attempting to evaluate objectively the presence of notching, it should be recalled that there is no sharp dividing line between the normal irregularities seen along the costal groove and early notching nor does the absence of notching mean that the intercostals are not entering into the collateral circulation pathways. Notching may rarely occur on the superior surface of a rib (Sloan and Cooley, 1953). Rib notching, of course, is not specific for coarctation as many other conditions are associated with enlarged dilated intercostal arteries, such as the tetralogy of Fallot, cases of pulmonary emphysema, thrombosis of the superior vena cava, thoracic wall hemangiomas, and neurofibromatosis (Boone *et al.*, 1964). From a practical clinical

viewpoint, however, these other causes can usually be differentiated from coarctation so that notching remains a reliable sign. Other evidences of dilated collateral circulation may be seen in erosion of the lateral scapular margin producing a scalloped effect and also the increased scalloped soft tissue density visible in the lateral view just beneath the sternum (Odman, 1953; Figley, 1954). This soft tissue shadow is due, of course, to the enlargement of the internal mammary arteries.

INDENTATION OF DESCENDING AORTA OR FIGURE "3" SIGN. Fray (1930) noted a defect or break in the continuity of the distal aortic arch in the left oblique position in 2 cases of coarctation. In 1937, Wolke commented on a double aortic curve

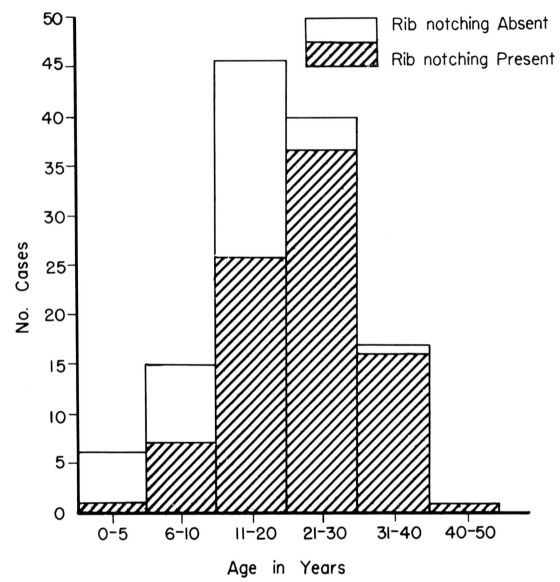

FIG. 141. RELATIONSHIP BETWEEN AGE AND DETECTABLE RIB NOTCHING IN 125 CASES OF COARCTATION

in the PA projection in the region of the coarctation and an indentation seen in the left anterior oblique projection in the same area. More recently, Bruwer and Pugh (1952) and Figley (1954) have again called attention to this sign. In the majority of cases of coarctation, some deviation in the upper part of the descending aorta can be detected, and more striking manifestations consist in the PA projection of a tuck or indentation somewhat in the form of the numeral "3" along the left border of the mediastinum just below the aortic knob. Surgical inspection and contrast vascular studies have shown that the indentation itself usually indicates the site of the coarctation. The distal portion of the curve delineates the

poststenotic segment of the aorta. The proximal or superior segment may represent either the left subclavian artery in those cases where the coarctation is just distal to the origin of this artery, or the segment of aorta proximal to the coarctation, namely the aortic knob. Occasionally, two indentations may be identified, one indicating the intersection of the contour of the left subclavian artery with the aortic arch, and the second indicating the intersection of the contour of the proximal with the distal limbs of the coarctation.

In the LAO projection, a normal distal aortic arch presents a smooth posteriorly convex contour. In coarctation, an indentation or tuck in the aorta may be noted on well exposed films and in effect produces a contour similar to the figure "3" sign in the PA projection.

An indentation or tuck is not always striking or well developed. In some cases, as pointed out by Figley (1954), a slight bulge in the aorta producing a slight lateral rounded convexity is noted just below the aortic knob.

This sign, or one of its variations, can be detected in about one-third to one-half of all cases of coarctation in adults, particularly if several films of different densities and degrees of obliquity are obtained. Its demonstration is of considerable practical significance since it not only substantiates the diagnosis but also indicates the site of the coarctation. In the authors' experience, it has always been associated with a rather short area of coarctation. Failure to demonstrate the figure "3" sign, however, does not mean that the coarctation is located elsewhere.

CONTOUR DUE TO LEFT SUBCLAVIAN ARTERY. In a normal chest film the superior mediastinum on the left above the aortic knob is concave. In contrast, in coarctation this concavity is effaced due to the position and also the dilatation of the left subclavian artery. In a considerable proportion of cases, this band of density continues on into the region of the aortic knob, and, in some cases, it forms a convex contour that may be mistaken for the knob or it may actually blend with the aortic knob, increasing its apparent size. As mentioned above, there may be an actual indentation where it joins the aortic knob, and, when this is seen, in addition to the indentation due to the coarctation, we have the two indentations referred to above.

CONTOUR OF THE AORTIC KNOB. Absence or marked decrease in size of the aortic knob in the PA projection has been frequently mentioned as one of the signs of coarctation, and this occurs in about one-half of the cases. While occasionally this absence is rather striking, particularly in adults where the ascending aorta is prominent, in younger persons the absence of the knob cannot be considered as remarkable. In about one-half of the cases one will demonstrate a rounded prominence that cannot be distinguished from a normal or slightly prominent knob.

Several factors probably play a role in obscuring the aortic knob in coarctation. In some cases hypoplasia or diminution in size of the aortic arch may be the cause, although absence of the aortic knob cannot be taken as an indication of aortic diameter. In many instances the diameter of the arch in the segment from the innominate to the coarctation is small, but this must be determined by contrast vascular studies. In the classical coarctation, there is definite anterior and medial displacement of the aorta at the site of insertion of the ligamentum arteriosum, tending to draw the distal arch deeper into the mediastinum. Finally, the left subclavian artery may be abnormally prominent along the left upper mediastinal border, tending to fuse imperceptibly with the aortic contour, and thus give the appearance of diminished size of the aortic knob.

ESOPHAGEAL DISPLACEMENT. The normal esophagus is in close relationship to the right lateral aspect of the distal aorta about 3 cm below the uppermost extension of the aorta. At this point the esophagus is normally deviated slightly to the right and anteriorly. Consequently, any change in size of the aorta may

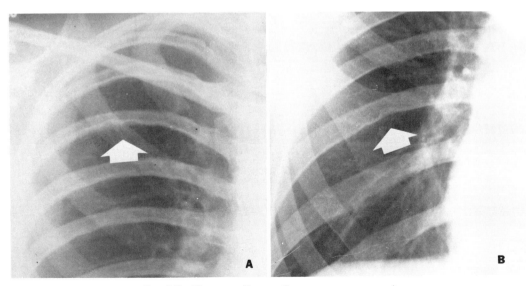

FIG. 142. NOTCHED RIBS IN COARCTATION OF THE AORTA

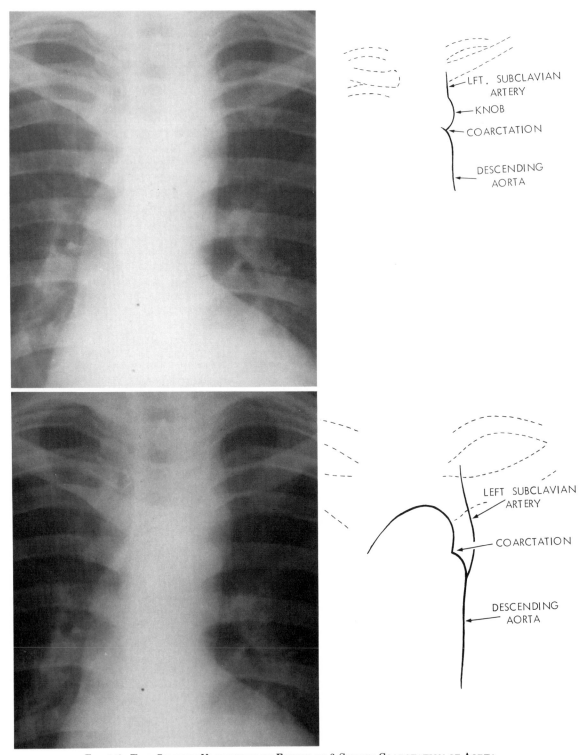

FIG. 143. TWO COMMON VARIATIONS OF FIGURE OF 3 SIGN IN COARCTATION OF AORTA

produce some changes in the course of the esophagus. Fleischner in 1949 demonstrated that the usually dilated poststenotic segment may displace the esophagus to the right and anteriorly.

This is best seen in the LAO projection with about 30° rotation and with the esophagus adequately distended with barium. Figley (1954) estimates that it can be seen in about 50% of cases

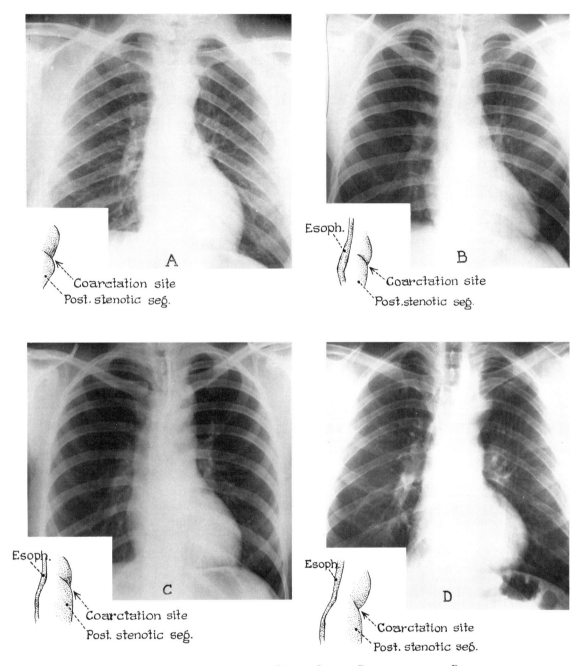

FIG. 144 A–D. EXAMPLES OF FIGURE OF 3 SIGN AS SEEN IN POSTEROANTERIOR PROJECTION
The indentation indicates the site of the coarctation. The distal portion of the curve delineates the poststenotic segment; the proximal or superior segment, either the left subclavian artery or the segment of aorta proximal to the coarctation. (Courtesy of *Radiology, 61:* 707, 1953.)

in the frontal view if the esophagus is adequately distended with barium. It is a valuable sign when present because it likewise indicates the site of the coarctation in addition to confirming the diagnosis.

CARDIAC SIZE AND CONTOUR. The heart is normal in size in about one-half of the cases, and, if

we exclude those cases occurring in infancy, the heart is rarely grossly enlarged. This is particularly so in uncomplicated coarctation. Of course, where some associated severe cardiac malformation is present, the heart may be enlarged. Since systolic hypertension proximal to the coarctation is almost invariably present, left ven-

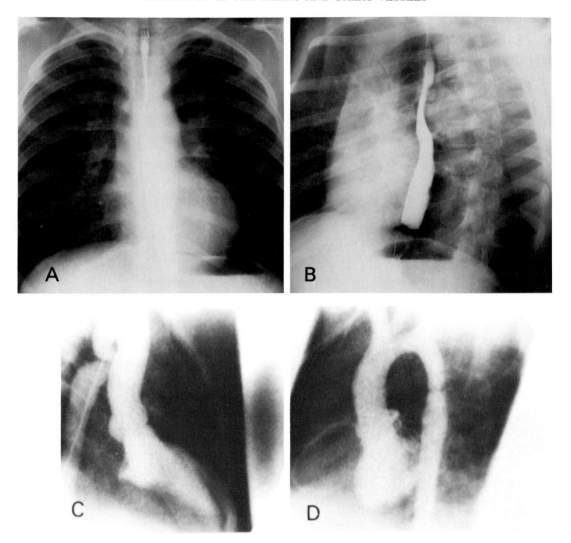

FIG. 145. COARCTATION OF AORTA WITH DEVIATION OF ESOPHAGUS TO RIGHT (A) AND ANTERIORLY (B) DUE TO
DILATATION OF DISTAL LIMB
(C) Aortogram showing anterior deviation of knuckle formed at site of coarctation and the cause for the indentation on the
esophagus. (D) Postoperative aortogram showing slight narrowing at site of repair.

tricular enlargement secondary to the hypertension is the most common abnormality detected in the cardiac contour. The left lower border of the heart is usually rounded with a rather low apex. In a significant percentage of cases the radiologic contour of the heart will not be significantly abnormal, and in general there is nothing typical about the contour which in itself would lead one to suspect the presence of coarctation.

CONTOUR OF ASCENDING AORTA. Frequently the ascending aorta is unremarkable in appearance on routine radiographic studies. In about one-third of the cases, however, obvious dilatation or tortuosity is seen, and occasionally this

may be so marked as to be aneurysmal. It has been suggested (Hamilton and Abbott, 1928) that there may be a congenital weakness of the media in such cases and that one cannot always correlate the degree of dilatation with the duration or severity of the hypertension or the width of the pulse pressure. Certainly, however, at fluoroscopy the ascending aorta often exhibits unusually vigorous pulsations.

PULMONARY VASCULARITY. This is usually normal, but when it is increased in prominence one should be suspicious of an associated patent ductus or interventricular septal defect.

RADIOLOGIC FINDINGS IN INFANCY. In contrast to those in older children and adults, the radiologic findings in infancy and particularly those in patients with symptoms of dyspnea and evidence of heart failure are nonspecific but often quite striking. The heart enlarges rapidly and may be quite large when the first film is made. Heart failure may ensue and some degree of dilatation of the lung vasculature is common, although the hilar shadows are usually obscured by the rapidly enlarging heart. The hilar shadows, of course, may be enlarged either secondary to heart failure or to an associated PDA or both. The heart is usually globular in shape and gives scant if any clue as to the specific chamber enlargement. Likewise, the outline of the aorta is usually invisible; occasionally the dilated distal limb may displace the esophagus to the right. Consequently, an esophagram with barium is always indicated. The shape of the heart is variable; it

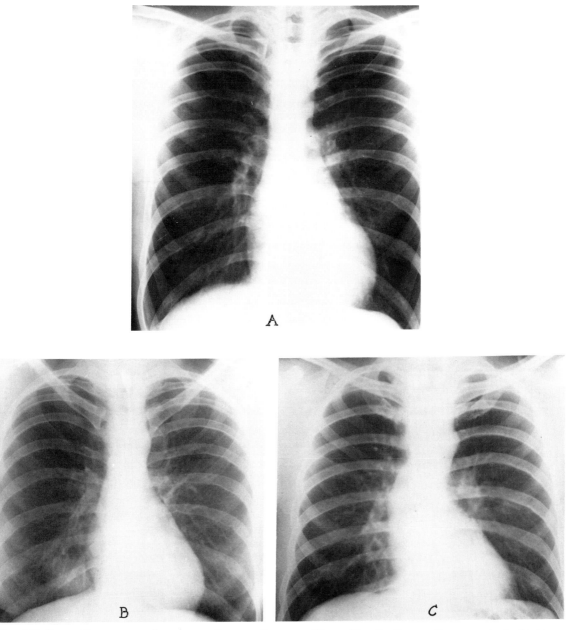

FIG. 146. OTHER EXAMPLES OF AORTIC AND CARDIAC CONTOURS WHICH MAY BE SEEN IN COARCTATION OF AORTA
Classically there is said to be an absence of the aortic knob in the posteroanterior projection. While on occasion this absence may be striking (A), one may also find in typical coarctations a rounded prominence that cannot be distinguished from a normal or slightly prominent aortic knob (B and C). (Courtesy of *Radiology, 61:* 708, 1953.)

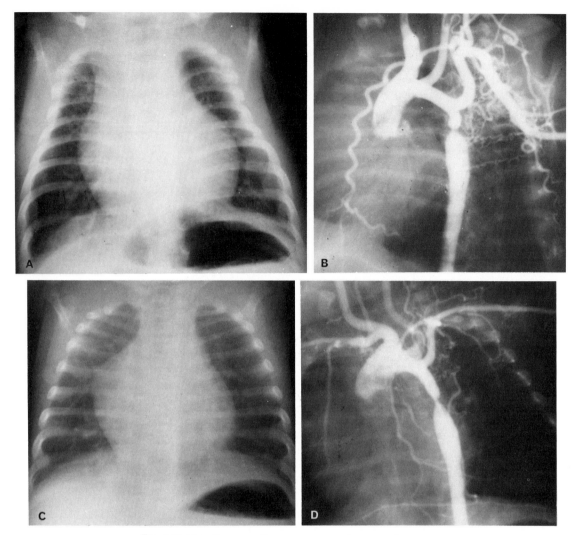

FIG. 147. TWO CASES OF COARCTATION OF AORTA IN INFANCY
(A and B) One-month-old female infant with shortness of breath. BP, right arm, 200 systolic by flush technique; right leg, 110 systolic. The heart was enlarged and globular in shape. (B) is a retrograde brachial aortogram. The distal aortic arch is reduced in size. Rich collateral circulation is demonstrated. A small ductus entered the aorta distal to the coarctation. This was not demonstrated by the aortogram. At autopsy ovarian hypoplasia was found (Turner's syndrome). (C and D) Two-month-old white male infant with symptoms of heart failure. The heart is enlarged, and right atrial contour is convex. There is no evidence of collateral circulation.

is usually symmetrically enlarged, although the apex may be somewhat full and rounded. If the radiologist is faced with a large heart with a nonspecific contour and congested lungs, he should suspect a coarctation; however, because surgical treatment may occasionally be lifesaving, contrast visualization, preferably aortography, is essential in these cases.

CONTRAST VASCULAR STUDIES. Contrast vascular studies must be used in infancy to establish the diagnosis of coarctation, and occasionally an unsuspected diagnosis is made in this way. In older children and adults the diagnosis in the

vast majority of cases is established from clinical and conventional radiologic examinations. The contrast vascular studies are used as a preliminary to surgical treatment in order to better outline the anatomical pattern of the coarctation and to make the task of the surgeon simpler and safer. Surgeons with extensive experience in the treatment of coarctation (Schuster and Gross, 1962; Bailey et al., 1959) are of the opinion that contrast vascular studies are seldom necessary and certainly should not be a routine preoperative procedure. Instead, they reserve these studies for those patients in whom careful physical and conventional radiologic examinations suggest an atypical length or location or some other complication. Some of the relative indications are absence of the typical figure "3" sign or indentation of the upper part of the descending aorta, absence of notching or atypical notching, and the presence of pulsations in the epigastrium despite the typical pressure changes in the upper and lower extremities. Schuster and Gross (1962) recommend aortography in women with absence of the figure "3" sign or notching of the ribs because of the possibility of hypoplasia of the descending aorta. Jonsson *et al.* (1951) recommend aortography routinely because it gives the surgeon a detailed picture of the coarctation, thus leading to better surgical planning. It may

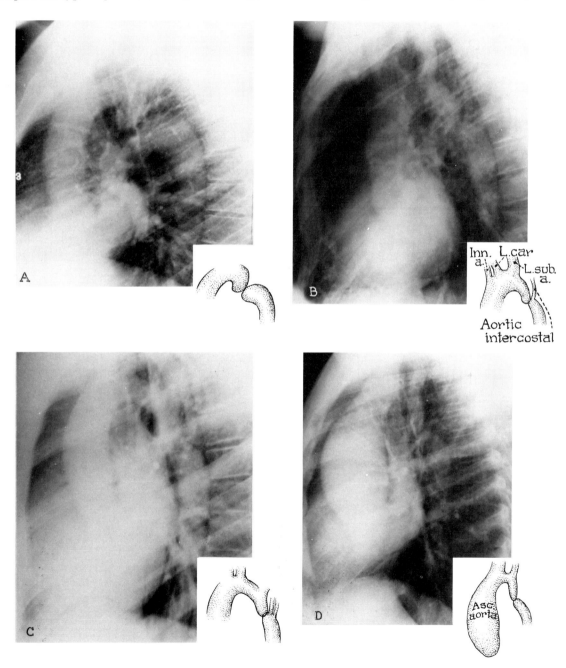

FIG. 148 A–D. COARCTATION OF AORTA

Examples of angiocardiograms in which the diagnosis is not only confirmed but, in addition, satisfactory visualization is secured of the exact site and extent of the constriction. (Courtesy of *Radiology, 61:* 712, 1953.)

show aneurysms of the intercostal arteries, patency of the ductus arteriosus, and it permits an appraisal of the adequacy of the collateral circulation. It may be of considerable value in the mild cases in demonstrating the presence of collaterals and also the size of the lumen of the aorta at the site of the coarctation. Despite these valuable contributions the present authors agree that contrast vascular studies should not be a routine procedure because they are often unnecessary, carry a slight risk, and are expensive. We recommend aortography in the absence of the figure "3" sign and particularly when notching is atypical or absent. We recommend it routinely in infancy.

ANGIOCARDIOGRAPHY. When adequately performed angiocardiography will confirm the diagnosis of coarctation in a large majority of cases. All too frequently, however, the extent and exact anatomy of the coarctation are incompletely demonstrated for diagnostic purposes (Jonsson *et al.*, 1951; Sloan and Cooley, 1953). It is not unusual to obtain an adequate concentration of the contrast medium in the ascending aorta only to find that there is insufficient medium within the distal arch or segments immediately adjacent

to the coarctation to permit adequate visualization. In such instances the radiographic appearance may suggest that the coarctation is of considerably greater length than is actually the case. It is for reasons such as these that we have largely abandoned the use of angiocardiography in older patients and adults. On the other hand, angiocardiography in small children and infants may be quite satisfactory alone or as a supplement to aortography, particularly when a complicating cardiac lesion is suspected. In fact one of the advantages of angiocardiography is that it gives a clue to the direction of flow through a patent ductus or to the presence of some other complicating defect in the heart.

AORTOGRAPHY. This is the preferable procedure. In older children and adults the arterial system of the upper extremity is well developed and is usually lacking in sclerotic changes and therefore affords easy entrance for a catheter into the ascending aorta. We prefer to insert a catheter percutaneously into the right brachial artery and place the tip in the ascending aorta. In infants, we use a left retrograde brachial injection. When followed by serial filming the entire coarctation and the arterial branches of the

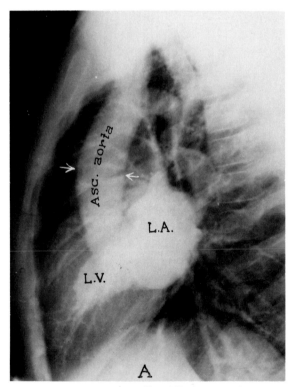
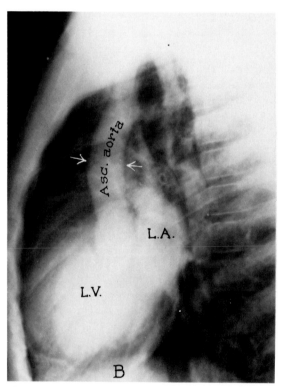

FIG. 149. ANGIOCARDIOGRAMS OF COARCTATION OF AORTA

At fluoroscopy the ascending aorta may exhibit unusually vigorous pulsations. In these angiocardiograms the variation in contour of the ascending aorta and aortic arch with systole (A) and diastole (B) is well shown. (Courtesy of *Radiology, 61:* 710, 1953.)

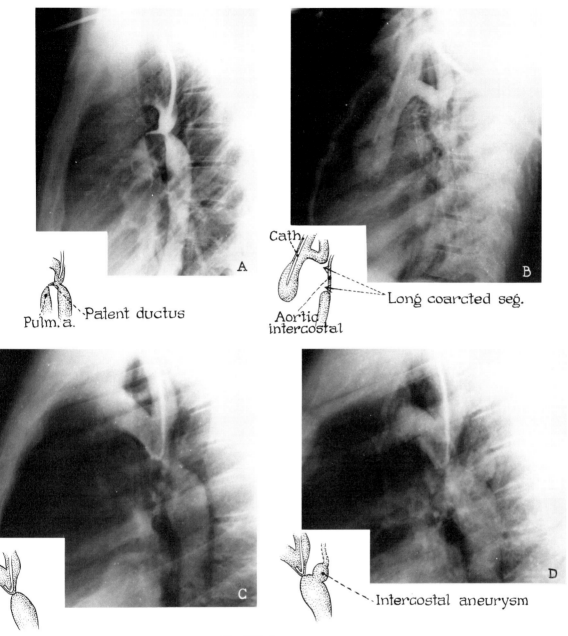

FIG. 150. AORTOGRAMS

(A) An aortogram demonstrating the presence of a small patent ductus just proximal to the coarctation. (B) An aortogram demonstrating a long coarcted segment. In this case the catheter was passed through the right arm with its tip being placed in the ascending aorta. (C and D) Aortograms demonstrating a good-sized aneurysm of an aortic intercostal adjacent to the poststenotic segment. The aneurysm did not opacify until late in the series (D), indicating that filling is taking place by way of collaterals and not from the adjacent aorta. (Courtesy of *Radiology, 61:* 715 (Fig. 11), 1953.)

aortic arch are well outlined as well as the collateral vessels and the extent of the collateral circulation. Patency of the ductus may be determined if the flow is in the usual direction from the aorta to the pulmonary artery. Intercostal aneurysms may be noted. The severity of the coarctation may be appraised in that the size of the area of constriction can be determined along with the extent of the collateral circulation. This, of course, requires rapid serial filming, but this may be of some use in determining the necessity for operation because mild cases of coarctation occur. Certainly, the demonstration of absence of collateral circulation with very mild obstruc-

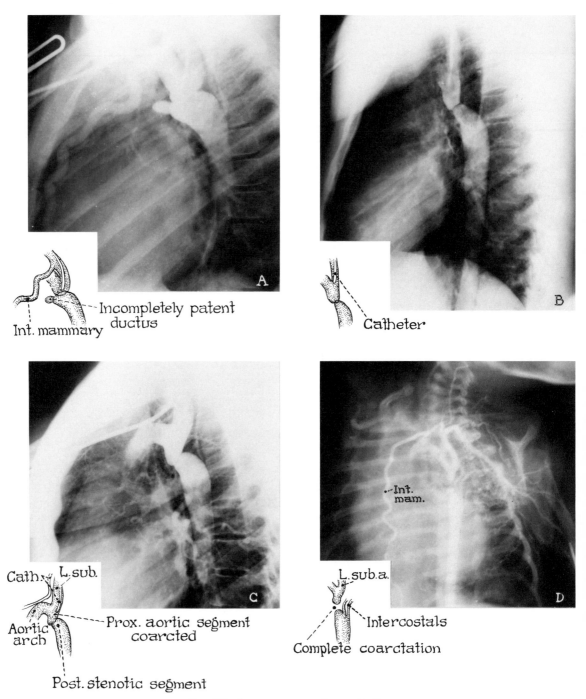

FIG. 151. COARCTATION OF AORTA (A–D)

Examples of aortograms in which there is excellent visualization of the coarctation site and the adjacent aortic segments. D is an aortogram on a 10-week-old baby in whom the opaque medium was injected in a retrograde manner through a cannula placed in the left brachial artery. Note the dilated and tortuous intercostal arteries. (Courtesy of *Radiology, 61:* 714, 1953.)

tion is a relative contraindication to operation. As indicated above, aortography will not give information concerning cardiac abnormalities.

Radiology of Postoperative Coarctation. The immediate postoperative changes are similar

to those of a thoracotomy for any reason. A mediastinal hematoma may follow leaking or weakening of the suture line, and this may occur in the immediate postoperative period. Widening of the mediastinum at a later time or some months after operation, however, suggests aneurysm formation at the suture line or leaking of the suture line.

Following successful repair the continuity of the descending aorta is re-established, and the lateral indentation or tuck just below the aortic knob is usually effaced. In other words, the descending aorta may have a normal appearance on a postoperative roentgenogram.

Rib notching may disappear following successful repair of the coarctation. This is not a frequent occurrence and failure of the notching to disappear does not mean that a satisfactory repair has not been accomplished.

The present authors have had very few opportunities to perform postoperative angiography following end to end anastomosis of the aorta. In each case the anastomotic site was visible and was obviously narrower than the adjacent proximal or distal aorta, although much wider than preoperatively. These were adult patients. It is probable that the diameter of the postoperative aorta correlates to some degree with the reduction in the hypertension. A question remains as to the size of the anastomotic site in those cases repaired during infancy and childhood in relation to the increase in diameter of the aorta due to natural growth.

2. Complete Interruption of the Aortic Arch. In this anomaly the aortic arch is completely obstructed and is discontinuous for a variable distance. The exact site of the obstruction is variable (see below) but involves part of the aortic arch. Another variation which is sometimes considered under the same heading is known as "aortic atresia" in which a fibrous remnant connects the distal arch and the descending aorta. These cases might be considered as a severe form of coarctation of the aorta. Patients with these anomalies present with two different types of signs and symptoms. The difference depends mainly on the presence or absence of associated anomalies, such as ventricular septal defect and patent ductus arteriosus. The condition is rare, but about 200 cases have been reported, and in the great majority these two additional defects have been present. Everts-Suarez and Carson (1959) suggest that cases with these additional defects should be considered as a well defined trilogy (interruption of the aortic arch, patent ductus arteriosus, and ventricular septal defect). Most of the patients with this condition have a rapid onset of symptoms in the neonatal period, and about 75% are dead by the end of the first month unless surgical treatment is used (Jaffe, 1975). The condition may be considered as one of the manifestations of the hypoplastic left heart syndrome and is one of the commonest causes of death in the neonatal period due to congenital heart disease. In a minority of reported cases, often referred to as aortic atresia (Dische et al., 1975; Gokcebay et al., 1972; Kauff et al., 1973; Morgan et al., 1970; Pillsbury, 1964), a PDA and VSD were not present or too small to be consequential, and the signs and symptoms were those of a severe coarctation of the aorta. Many of these patients survived until the second decade and were successfully treated by surgical means.

Celoria and Patton (1959) have suggested an anatomical classification of this condition according to the site of the interruption or atresia of the aortic arch. These are:

Type A—occlusion just distal to the left subclavian artery; Type B—occlusion between the left common carotid and left subclavian artery; and Type C—interruption distal to the innominate artery or the right carotid artery. In a total of 184 cases extracted from the literature, Van Praagh et al. (1971) found the distribution of the various types as follows: Type A—42%, Type B—53%, and Type C—4%. Other variations are: Aberrant right subclavian artery originating from the descending aorta distal to the obstruction with an incidence of about 20%; origin of right subclavian artery from a right ductus arteriosus with a possibility of a right subclavian steal syndrome. Moller and Edwards (1965) described a mirror image of this latter arrangement in which there was a right aortic arch with the left subclavian artery originating from a left ductus arteriosus. A very unusual and extremely rare arrangement was that described by Zetterqvist (1967) in which both subclavian arteries originated beyond the interruption, and there was an absence of the innominate artery and only one carotid artery, and all of the blood to the body was carried through the vertebral arteries into the subclavian arteries.

Other associated major anomalies are common (40 of 105 cases reviewed by Moller and Edwards (1965). These are complete transposition of the great vessels (Buckley et al., 1965), persistent truncus arteriosus, (Sundararajan and Molthan, 1972), aorticopulmonary septal defect (Moller and Edwards, 1965), and anomalous venous connection (Barratt-Boyes et al., 1972). A very high incidence of bicuspid aortic valve has been reported in these cases.

Figure 152 taken from the paper of Blake et al. (1962) shows 9 theoretical variations in the distribution of the brachiocephalic vessels that could result from an interruption at one point of each of the primitive double aortic arches. It

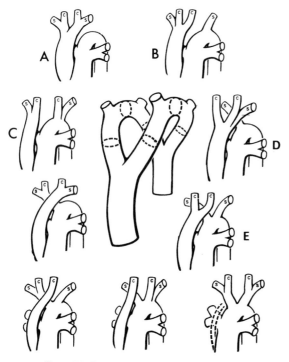

FIG. 152. INTERRUPTION OF AORTIC ARCH

Central drawing demonstrates diagrammatically the prim-itve double aortic arch with dotted circles indicating the three possible sites of interruption of each arch. Atresia of the isthmus is due to an interruption of both arches. Conse-quently, nine theoretical combinations are possible as shown. In the review by Moller and Edwards (1965) the A (43 cases) pattern was the most common with B (33 cases), E (11 cases), C (4 cases), and D (1 case) occurring in this order. These authors also reported 3 cases in which the right subclavian artery arose from the right pulmonary artery through the interposition of a ductus arteriosus. (Courtesy of Drs. Blake, Manion, and Spencer, Armed Forces Institute of Pathology; *Journal of Thoracic and Cardiovascular Surgery;* and C. V. Mosby Co.)

should be remembered that in the normal ar-rangement only one of the arches is interrupted (the distal portion of the right fourth arch). Only 4 of the possible variations have been encoun-tered (A, B, C, and D).

In the group with VSD and PDA, the blood supply to the lower portion of the body passes through the PDA into the descending aorta. Col-lateral circulation is poorly developed or absent in contrast to those cases with aortic atresia in which collaterals are present at birth and in-crease with age. In the former group (with VSD and PDA), the blood pressure in the upper and lower extremities does not differ appreciably at birth, although if the patient survives for a few months, some difference can be detected (Mur-phy *et al.,* 1971). This difference can be accen-

tuated if the patent ductus is narrowed or begins to close.

Since mixed venous blood is shunted to the lower portion of the body, the trunk and lower extremities should show some evidence of cy-anosis. A reverse situation would occur with transposition of the great vessels in which highly oxygenated blood would be shunted through the ductus to the lower part of the body and extrem-ities. Only a relatively small proportion of the cases has shown such differential cyanosis, and when present, it has not been very striking. The interventricular septal defect permits consider-able mixing of the blood with a considerable left to right shunt so that the difference in saturation between the blood in the ascending and descend-ing aorta is usually not very great.

Patients with the trilogy of complete interrup-tion, VSD, and PDA require early diagnosis if effective treatment is to be instituted. The diag-nosis depends heavily on radiologic findings, and the rapid investigation of these patients by the pediatric cardiologist and the radiologist offers a considerable challenge.

Radiologic Findings. Conventional chest films exposed on the neonate during the first few weeks of life are often nonspecific but on occasion may be quite helpful (Jaffe, 1975). The nonspe-cific changes are slight to moderate cardiac en-largement involving the right atrium and ventri-cle with dilatation of the pulmonary artery and increased vascularity of the lungs. Such changes suggest a hypoplastic left heart syndrome or more rarely a complete transposition of the great vessels. On well-exposed chest films, more spec-ific changes may occasionally be seen. In com-plete interruption of the aortic arch, the trachea is squarely in the midline if the patient is well positioned, and this is in contrast to the slight deviation to the right which is seen with a normal aortic arch. Also, the usual impression of the aortic arch on the posterolateral aspect of the barium-filled esophagus is absent. In addition, the pulmonary artery is enlarged, and the aortic knob is absent. Occasionally in a well-penetrated film, the descending aorta is seen to terminate at the level of the pulmonary artery and this, of course, is a quite specific finding. A good lateral view should always be obtained. In the lateral view, the hypoplasia of the ascending aorta is suggested by a large substernal clear space (Fig. 153B) and since the descending aorta is contin-uous with the ductus, this gives the appearance of a low aortic arch.

Although the diagnosis can occasionally be strongly suspected from an examination of con-

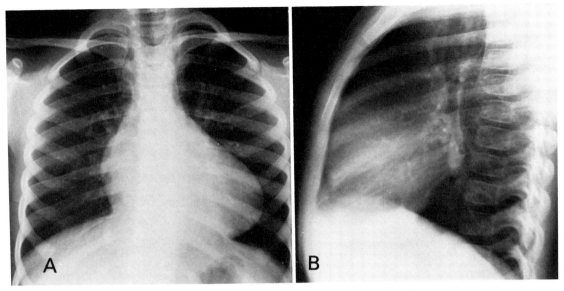

FIG. 153. INTERRUPTION OF AORTIC ARCH IN A 3-YEAR-OLD

(A) The elevation of the cardiac apex is suggestive of right ventricular enlargement, and the aorta is inconspicuous. (B) The lateral view is suggestive because of the large clear space posterior to the upper portion of the sternum suggesting a small ascending aorta. (Courtesy of Children's Cardiac Clinic, Texas Children's Hospital, Houston, Texas.)

ventional films, cardiac catheterization and selective angiography should be used immediately to establish the diagnosis. Right heart catheterization will show that the pressures in the right ventricle are approximately equal to those in the left ventricle and usually equal to those in the upper part of the body, although this may be variable depending on the origins of the subclavian arteries. Some step-up of oxygen content is found usually in the right ventricle indicating a left to right shunt, and often the shunt is of substantial proportions in early life. The catheter may pass through the pulmonary artery and the patent ductus into the descending aorta clearly delineating this portion of the abnormality. Pressure tracings on withdrawal will show whether there is a narrowing of the ductus arteriosus. Aortography is necessary to delineate the anatomy of the aortic arch. Retrograde aortography through the femoral artery should be the first procedure in order to determine the origin of the subclavian arteries, and this will demonstrate the distal portion of the complete interruption. Where the right subclavian artery is seen to originate from the descending aorta, demonstration of the ascending aorta and aortic arch may be difficult and should depend if possible on a left ventricular injection at the time of cardiac catheterization. If the right subclavian artery is not identified, then an approach to the aortic arch through the right subclavian artery should be made and the arch anomaly demonstrated.

Right and left ventriculography should be attempted in most instances because of the possibility of other associated lesions as indicated above. However, initial palliative treatment may not require a complete delineation of all of the cardiac abnormalities. In those patients without significant intracardiac lesions, the diagnostic procedures are similar to those used in coarctation of the aorta, and aortography frequently will suffice.

Surgical Treatment. Van Praagh *et al.* (1971) have indicated that the greatly increased pulmonary blood flow with associated right heart failure is the major cause of death in the neonatal period. Successful treatment during this period has been enhanced by banding procedures on the main pulmonary artery or one or both branches (Tyson *et al.*, 1970; Murphy *et al.*, 1971). Ligation of the ductus with repair of the obstructed aorta may be accomplished at the same time or reserved for a later date depending on the condition of the patient. Likewise, the repair of the interventricular septal defect or other associated intracardiac lesions may be deferred.

In the older patients, and particularly those without a PDA and VSD, establishment of aortic continuity is similar to that in coarctation of the aorta, namely the use of grafts or in some cases by using the enlarged left subclavian artery.

3. Bicuspid Aortic Valve. The incidence of this anomaly is not precisely known. It is said to occur in association with coarctation of the aorta

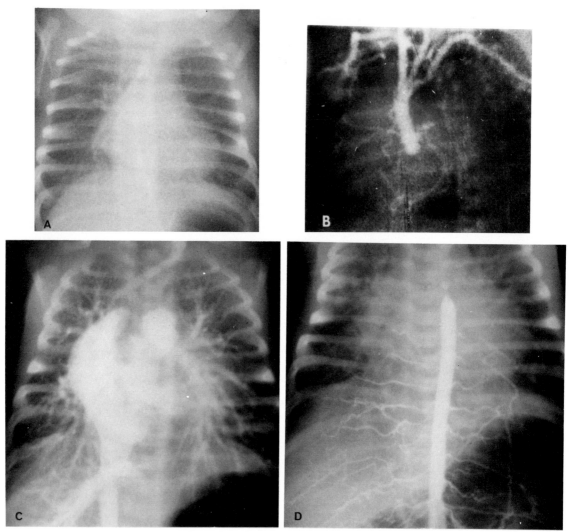

Fig. 154. Complete Interruption of Aortic Arch in 4-Week-Old-Infant (Operative Case)
(A) Conventional film. The lungs are congested. (B) 16-mm cine frame from a countercurrent aortogram made by injection into the left brachial artery. The aorta is interrupted just beyond the origin of the left subclavian artery. There is some evidence of collateral circulation. (C) Venous angiocardiogram. The pulmonary artery is dilated and communicates directly with the descending aorta. The ascending aorta was not distinctly identified on this seris of films. (D) Retrograde thoracic aortogram. The thoracic aorta tapers to a point of obstruction at the fourth thoracic vertebra.

in about 85% of the cases (Edwards, 1961; Roberts and Elliott, 1968), but this seems higher than that observed by the authors. A bicuspid valve is compatible with normal function and a long asymptomatic life. On the other hand, over a period of years it is subject to changes in structure which may lead to serious hemodynamic consequences. The reasons why some bicuspid valves remain relatively unchanged and functionally adequate and others progress to severe stenosis and insufficiency are not always clear. Minor variations in the size of the two cusps and also associated bacterial endocarditis are obviously two important considerations.

The two cusps of the valve are often of unequal size. The single commissure is oriented either from right to left or front to back dividing the valve into right and left or posterior and anterior cusps as shown in Figure 155 (Roberts, 1970). A false raphe is common, and when present, is incorporated into either the right or the posterior cusp, depending on the direction of the commissure. The larger of the two cusps may become redundant and after a period of time prolapse and become insufficient. This is perhaps the most common complication.

After a variable period of time and with advancing years, the cusps then become thickened,

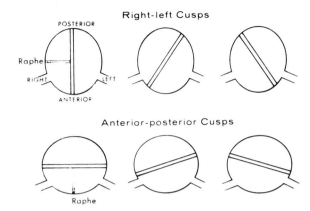

Right-left Cusps

POSTERIOR

Raphe

RIGHT   LEFT

ANTERIOR

Anterior-posterior Cusps

Raphe

FIG. 155. DIAGRAM SHOWING THE TWO BASIC TYPES OF
CONGENITAL BICUSPID AORTIC VALVES
See text for explanation. (Courtesy of Dr. W. C. Roberts
and the *American Journal of Cardiology*, 26: 79, 1970.)

irregular, and less mobile. The progress of this process is quite variable. Occasionally, the process is limited to a situation where a systolic murmur suggestive of aortic stenosis is heard. The ascending aorta is often dilated, and the heart may show a slight left ventricular contour with a low apex. The ascending aorta is often dilated. This may not be well appreciated in the frontal view but is often seen in the lateral projection. Left ventricular catheterization may fail to show a gradient, and the hemodynamic consequences are minimal.

In other instances, the thickening of the valve progresses and is followed by variable deposits of calcium producing calcific aortic stenosis. Edwards (1961) believes that the majority of cases of calcific aortic stenosis are due to anomalies of the aortic valve, and the most frequent of these is the bicuspid valve. There is an increased susceptibility to bacterial endocarditis, and this has become of increased importance in those persons who use intravenous drugs.

This anomaly is best demonstrated by a well-performed aortogram using a supravalvular injection. The posterior cusp is the lower in the right to left oriented commissure, and the right cusp is the lower in the anterior to posterior oriented commissure (Simon and Reis, 1971). The two cusps can usually be identified, particularly if the valve has not undergone significant distortion or thickening (Fig. 156). In the case shown in Figure 157, the valve had already become insufficient, and there was a mild gradient.

4. Unicommissural Aortic Valve. This anomaly is considerably less common than the bicuspid variety. The orifice is a single cleft opened posteriorly and elsewhere is surrounded by the single cusp (Fig. 158, B and C). Differen-

tiation from bicuspid valve is of some importance since the unicommissural variety is not subject to successful valvuloplasty but usually requires valve replacement. According to Simon and Reis (1971), when the unicommissural valve is stenotic, a supravalvular aortogram shows the jet is posterior and in contact with the aortic wall. The commissure is usually directed in the sagittal plane. Furthermore, there is no evidence of a sinus of Valsalva posteriorly, although two different sinuses may be seen, one on each side. Cine angiograms (35 mm) will show motion of the anterior portion of the leaflet but no motion posteriorly. Thus, differentiation from the bicuspid valve is usually possible.

Congenital obstructions in the region of the aortic valve may be classified as valvular, subvalvular, and supravalvular. This group of lesions

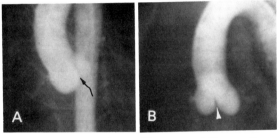

FIG. 156. BICUSPID AORTIC VALVE IN A 2-MONTH-OLD
INFANT
(A) Frontal view. Arrow indicates commissure with smaller left-sided cusp. (B) Far LAO view. White arrow represents deep raphe in large right cusp. A systolic murmur was present but no significant gradient.

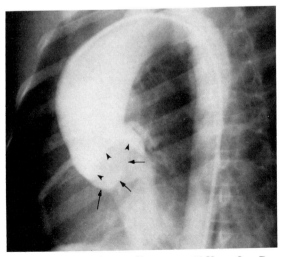

FIG. 157. BICUSPID AORTIC VALVE IN A 12-YEAR-OLD BOY
There was mild insufficiency and a 27 mm gradient across the valve. The patient came to operation several years later, and a bicuspid valve was confirmed. Arrowheads outline one cusp and arrows the other.

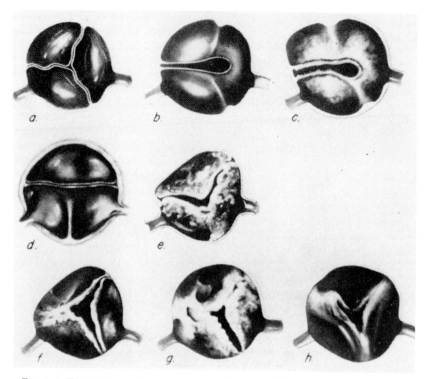

FIG. 158. EXAMPLES OF CONGENITAL AND ACQUIRED TYPES OF AORTIC STENOSIS
(a) Normal tricuspid aortic valve. (b) Unicommissural valve and (c) after calcification. (d) Bicuspid aortic valve and (e) after calcification producing a common form of calcific aortic stenosis. Acquired fusion (f) of one commissure (g) two commissures and (h) three commissures as may be found with rheumatic fever. (From Edwards, J. E., *Circulation, 31:* 590, 1970.)

accounts for about 3–5% of all congenital heart disease (Bernhard *et al.*, 1973).

5. Valvular Aortic Stenosis. Valvular stenosis is much more common than the other two types and comprises about 60–70% of all cases of congenital aortic stenosis. The stenotic valve can be classified into three anatomic types: tricuspid valve with partial fusion of the commissures, bicuspid valve, and unicommissural valve. The bicuspid valve is the most common and in most series comprises more than 50% of the cases. As indicated above, all bicuspid valves are not stenotic at birth. Most are not stenotic but in later life due to turbulence develop degenerative changes and ultimately calcification and thus become an important cause of calcific aortic stenosis. This will be discussed under that heading. On the other hand, in a group of 24 symptomatic patients less than one year of age Bernhard *et al.* (1973) found 10 that had stenotic bicuspid valves. Aortic insufficiency is common with the bicuspid valve and increases the strain on the left ventricle. The congenital tricuspid valve is stenotic because it has a partial fusion of its commissure. The orifice may be centrally located but is usually eccentric. It may be located posteriorly (25 of 33 cases) or anteriorly (4 of 33

cases) (Ellis and Kirklin, 1962). The stenotic tricuspid valve may be subject to the splitting of the partially fused commissures and valvuloplasty, although this may be approached with great caution since a flail segment may easily occur followed by significant insufficiency (Edwards, 1965). The unicommissural valve is the least common and is of importance because it almost always requires replacement by an artificial valve.

Studies of the natural history of congenital aortic stenosis suggest that the stenotic orifice in the vast majority of cases is fixed in size at birth. Only a minority of patients shows signs of the disease during the first year of life, and these form a special group. The majority of patients are asymptomatic until their teens or much later. The assumption is that the stenotic orifice does not grow in size with the patient to any significant degree. Consequently, with the increase in cardiac output due to natural growth, the stenosis becomes relatively more severe (Cohen *et al.*, 1972; El-Said *et al.*, 1972). In some instances, there is evidence that the orifice is absolutely reduced in size presumably due to the trauma and turbulence of the blood flow. Calcification may eventually occur but is unusual before the age of 30 years (Campbell and Kauntze, 1953). At operation, the valve cusps are often thickened to 2 mm or more indicating reaction to the trauma and turbulence of blood flow (Spencer et al., 1960). A further factor is a hypoplastic valve ring which is occasionally encountered and adds to the problems of successful relief of the stenosis. Simultaneous occurrence of both valvular and subvalvular stenosis occasionally occurs (3 of 46 cases of Spencer et al., 1960). Also, underdevelopment of the left side of the heart has been occasionally described.

Cases in which symptoms develop during the first year of life form a special group. Other congenital anomalies, such as coarctation of the aorta, endocardial fibroelastosis and mitral valve anomalies, are quite common and contribute to the early appearance of the symptomatology. Heart failure is a common manifestation and may be sufficient to require surgical treatment, although the results at this age do not seem to be as good as later.

Dilatation of the ascending aorta is a common finding, particularly in the older cases (Klatte et al., 1962), and is attributed to turbulence in this segment of the aorta and possibly due to impingement of a jet on the anterior wall of the aorta. This portion of the aorta frequently shows increased pulsations as seen at fluoroscopy.

The left ventricular myocardium responds by hypertrophy, but the total volume of this chamber is rarely increased until the later stages of the disease when the ventricle begins to fail. The changes in the myocardium such as fibrosis may contribute to heart failure.

Patients with congenital aortic stenosis are frequently asymptomatic and are often "discovered" during an examination for some other condition (Wood, 1958). Sudden death in otherwise asymptomatic patients is not rare (Wagner and Vlad, 1974; Morrow et al., 1958). The most common symptoms are angina, syncope, dyspnea on exertion and rarely congestive heart failure. When the symptoms appear, they usually progress rapidly. The most striking physical finding is a high systolic murmur, most intense at the base of the heart and transmitted upward toward the neck and is usually accompanied by a thrill. The electrocardiogram may or may not show left ventricular hypertrophy and/or left ventricular strain depending on the severity and duration of the lesion.

Radiological Findings. The conventional chest films including oblique views are often entirely normal. The earliest change is usually dilatation of the ascending aorta. This may be unnoticed in the frontal projection and is best detected in the lateral film or in 30–40 degrees of left anterior obliquity. Increased pulsations of this segment of the aorta may be seen at fluoroscopy. When the dilatation is well developed it can be positively identified in the frontal view, and the contour can often be followed downward inside the cardiac contour. The left ventricular myocardium is commonly hypertrophied, but this contributes very little to the size of this chamber. The left border may show slight rounding assuming a left ventricular contour with elongation and lowering of the cardiac apex. When definite cardiac enlargement appears, the left ventricle is usually beginning to fail. At this stage symptoms are usually well developed and the disease is in its later stages.

Calcification in the aortic valve can be identified at fluoroscopy and is almost pathognomonic of aortic stenosis. It is a rare finding, however, and is almost never seen in patients under 20 years of age (Campbell and Kauntze, 1953).

The diagnosis is established by supravalvular aortography and left ventriculography with associated pressure recordings. The transaortic route is preferable since it permits pullback tracings across the outflow tract of the left ventricle and is thus helpful in detecting and verifying the site of the stenosis. Entrance to the left ventricle cannot always be effected by this route, and the transseptal left atrial route should be considered. In many instances recorded in the literature, direct left ventricular puncture has been employed. The supravalvular aortic injection should outline the sinuses of Valsalva and the superior surfaces of the valve cusps. It is very useful in documenting and in evaluating the extent of the regurgitation. This is an important factor in successful treatment of this lesion. Regurgitation may occur in 25–50% of all cases and is particularly common in the subvalvular stenoses (Bernhard et al., 1973). The contour of the valve cusps and particularly the large cusps associated with bicuspid valves may be clearly delineated and lead to a diagnosis (Fig. 159, C and D). A radiolucent jet leads to a positive diagnosis of stenosis but is not uniformly present. When present, the size of the jet as measured by Friedenberg et al. (1964) correlated well with the size of the valve orifice as found at operation. Assuming that the jet is circular, its cross-sectional area can be calculated. If it is less than 10% of the aortic area, the stenosis is thought to be severe. If less than 15%, it was a positive indication for operation (Taubman et al., 1966). There are many inconsistencies between the presence and the size of the jet and the severity of the stenosis. Certainly, the size of the orifice is more reliably measured

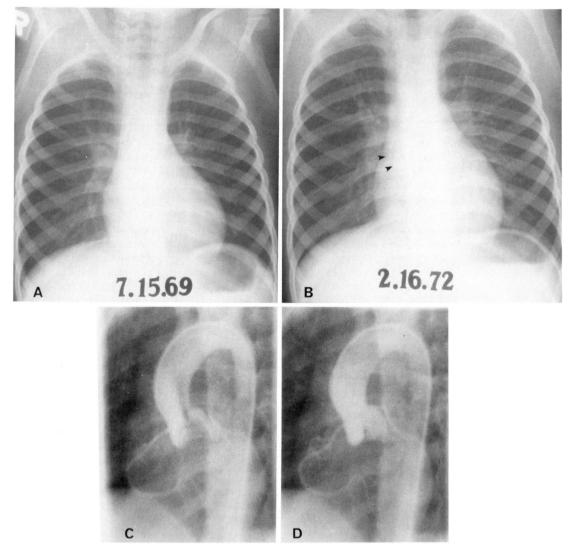

FIG. 159. VALVULAR AORTIC STENOSIS

(A) Chest film from a 3-year-old male with valvular aortic stenosis. (B) Film exposed 3 years later. The patient was still asymptomatic, but the systolic gradient was 105 mm Hg. The ascending aorta has increased prominence (arrowheads). (C and D) 35 mm cine films from a supravalvular aortic injection. The left frame (C) shows the eccentric negative systolic jet. The right frame (D) exposed in diastole shows a bicuspid valve with sagittal commissure. This was confirmed at operation.

by the use of the Gorlin formula, the determination of cardiac output and the pressure readings from the left ventricle and the aorta. A systolic gradient of greater than 50 mm Hg and a valve orifice as calculated of 0.5 cm^2/m^2 of body surface area are positive indications for surgical treatment (Bernhard *et al.*, 1973). Failure to see a radiolucent jet does not exclude the diagnosis of aortic stenosis. The jet may be absent or poorly seen in patients with mitral insufficiency, a low cardiac output and some degree of heart failure. Dilatation of the ascending aorta can also be confirmed by the supravalvular injection.

Left ventriculography may show a positive jet, and, of course, may show the contour of both the upper and inferior surfaces of the aortic valve. In some cases there is a dome effect with a definite central jet, and this is thought to represent a tricuspid type valve with some fusion of the commissures. Frequently, the thickness of the valve cusps can be appraised, and some idea of their mobility is presented. Cine recordings (35 mm) are preferable for this evaluation. The left ventriculogram will also show the volume of the left ventricular cavity and the thickness of the muscular wall. It is also useful in documenting

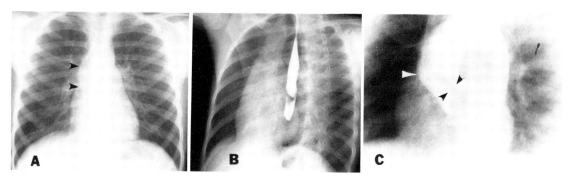

FIG. 160. VALVULAR AORTIC STENOSIS

Eight-year-old asymptomatic boy. No restriction in exercise tolerance. Gradient across aortic valve, 41 mm Hg. (A) Frontal view shows dilatation of ascending aorta (arrowhead). (B) LAO showing very minor prominence of ascending aorta. (C) Supravalvular aortogram (cinefluorogram) shows systolic jet (arrowheads) and impingement on lateral wall of ascending aorta (white arrowhead).

anomalies of the mitral valve with associated insufficiency.

6. Subvalvular Aortic Stenosis. According to Edwards (1965) congenital subaortic stenosis may be divided into intrinsic and extrinsic lesions. The extrinsic lesions consist of localized or diffuse muscular hypertrophy known as idiopathic hypertrophic subaortic stenosis, anomalies of the anterior leaflet of the mitral valve often associated with endocardial cushion defect, excess mitral valve tissue and abnormal insertions of the papillary muscle. These will be discussed elsewhere.

The intrinsic lesions are the second most common cause of congenital aortic stenosis. Operative experience suggests that about 15–30% of cases are subvalvular (7 of 23 cases, Takekawa *et al.*, 1966; 11 of 46 cases, Ellis and Kirklin, 1962; 16 of 46 cases, Spencer, 1960; and 34 of 180 cases, Bernhard *et al.*, 1973). There is also an increased frequency of associated anomalies such as coarctation of the aorta and ventricular septal defect.

The intrinsic subvalvular lesion represents a spectrum which has been classified in 2–4 different groups according to various authors (Deutsch *et al.*, 1971; Edwards *et al.*, 1965; Kelly *et al.*, 1972; Slezak *et al.*, 1965; Lundquist and Amplatz, 1965). The commonest form is the discrete fibrous diaphragm-like obstruction which is variable in location from any point just below the aortic valve to a point 1.5–2 cm below in extreme cases. In many instances, the diaphragm is only about 1 mm thick, and in others it is somewhat thicker and well below the aortic valve. This probably comprises both type I and type II as described by Deutsch *et al.* (1971). Another less common variation consists of a fibromuscular ridge often irregular in contour extending to involve the anterior leaflet of the mitral valve. It

may be associated with localized hypertrophy of the ventricular septum and frequently produces some degree of mitral insufficiency in addition to the aortic stenosis. It may be nodular in outline. Another rare variation, type IV of Deutsch *et al.* (1971) consists of an irregular fixed tunnel-like formation which is entirely fixed in contour and may be 1 to 2 cm in length. It is frequently associated with anomalies of the mitral valve. Associated changes in the aortic valve leaflets are quite common with subvalvular stenosis. Part of this change is undoubtedly due to trauma from increased turbulence. It is thus a secondary change. Aortic insufficiency is considerably more common with the subvalvular obstructions than with the valvular obstructions (Bernhard *et al.*, 1973). Dilatation of the ascending aorta occurs but is less common than with valvular aortic stenosis.

The diagnosis is established by a combination of carefully documented hemodynamic findings correlated with left ventriculography and supravalvular aortography. Withdrawal of the catheter from the left ventricle across the aortic valve into the aorta may show an intermediate chamber with the systolic pressure equal to that in the aorta, but the diastolic pressure is equal to that in the left ventricle. Ventriculography may then show a separate discrete chamber with the diaphragm below and the aortic valve above (Fig. 164). Frequently the fibrous diaphragm is thin and of the order of 1 mm in thickness and may be within 1–5 mm of the aortic valve and is thus overlooked both at the time of catheter withdrawal and at ventriculography. In some cases, the only sign of the subvalvular obstruction is a subvalvular jet as described by Lundquist and Amplatz (1965). This may be seen either with aortography or ventriculography. Excellent ra-

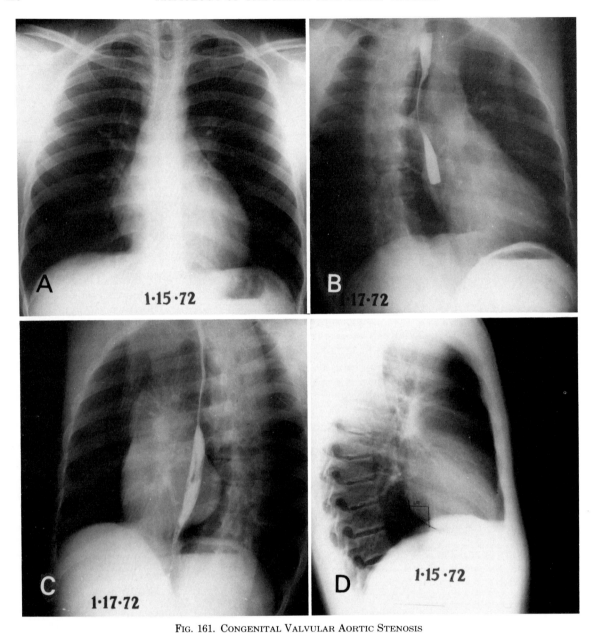

FIG. 161. CONGENITAL VALVULAR AORTIC STENOSIS

Patient was a 15-year-old symptomatic boy. Gradient across aortic valve, 64 mm Hg. (A, B, C, and D) Conventional chest films show increased prominence of ascending aorta and some left ventricular enlargement well seen in C and D.

diographic technique is required, and 35 mm cine angiography is a desirable way to look for this sign. The diaphragm may be seen in either the frontal or the left anterior oblique view but rarely in the lateral view. On the other hand, the right anterior and lateral views are helpful in looking for mitral insufficiency which occasionally accompanies this lesion. Hemodynamic evidence of aortic stenosis which is unaccompanied by doming of the aortic valve leaflets but decreased motion of these leaflets is suggestive supporting

evidence for a thin subvalvular diaphragm. The thicker fibrous and fibromuscular rings 1–2 cm below the valve offer much less difficulty in diagnosis. The more irregular-shaped fibromuscular obstruction frequently involves the anterior leaflet of the mitral valve. They may also be associated with considerable hypertrophy of the interventricular septum. The subvalvular chamber both with a discrete diaphragm and with a more irregular nodular area of obstruction may be well shown by supravalvular injection since the aortic valve is often insufficient. The smooth aspect of the right border of the subvalvular chamber due to septal hypertrophy may be well shown by supravalvular injection (Fig. 166). The subvalvular tunnel, the rarest of all the groups, may be shown by either aortography or ventriculography.

Preoperative differentiation of the various types is of practical importance to the surgeon. The simple subvalvular diaphragms can be re-sected usually through a transaortic approach and with good results (Shariatzadek *et al.*, 1972). The irregular fibromuscular obstructions, particularly those involving the anterior leaflet of the mitral valve, usually require an approach through either the left ventricle or left atrium, and there is considerable danger of permanent damage to the mitral valve. In a number of instances, the mitral valve was replaced by an artificial prosthesis. Differentiation of the more

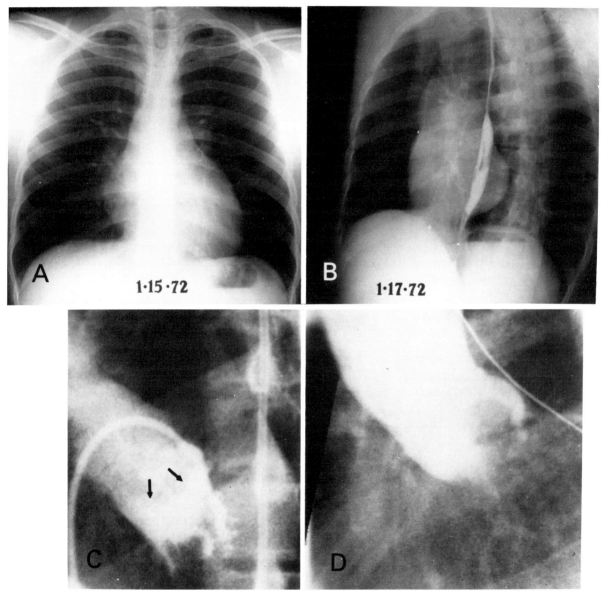

FIG. 162. CONGENITAL VALVULAR AORTIC STENOSIS

(A and B) Congenital valvular aortic stenosis in a 16-year-old male who denied symptoms and had a good exercise tolerance. The systolic gradient was 64 mm Hg. At operation a deformed bicuspid valve was found with a rudimentary commissure. (C) Supravalvular aortic injection. Contrast substance is momentarily trapped above one of the cusps (arrows). (D) In systole the commissure is open posteriorly but is not in contact with aortic wall.

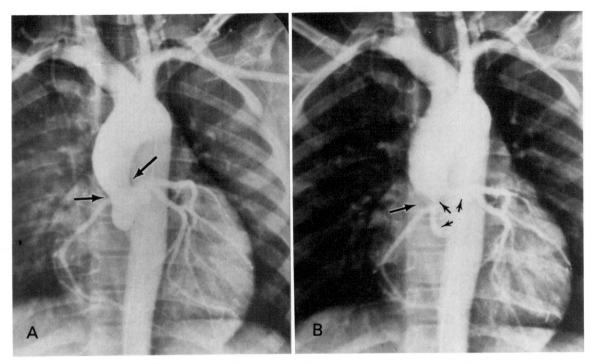

FIG. 163. CONGENITAL VALVULAR AND SUPRAVALVULAR AORTIC STENOSIS
Percutaneous transfemoral catheterization with supravalvular injection of contrast material. (A) Ventricular diastole. Mild supravalvular aortic narrowing is seen (arrows). The coronary arteries are well filled and appear normal. The ascending aorta is slightly dilated, and the innominate artery is considerably enlarged. (B) Ventricular systole. The stenotic aortic valve (small arrows) is domeshaped and appears to be ballooned upward. An eccentrically directed jet of radiolucent blood issues from the apex of the dome (large arrow) and impinges on the anterior aortic wall. A significant pressure gradient across the aortic valve was considerably reduced by operation. (By permission of *Circulation* and the American Heart Association; from Dotter *et al.* (1961.)

discrete forms of subvalvular stenosis from the diffuse type associated with idiopathic hypertrophic subaortic stenosis is important since surgery for the latter condition is much less satisfactory and controversial and may require a different approach.

7. Supravalvular Aortic Stenosis. Supravalvular aortic stenosis is the rarest of the forms of aortic stenosis (14 of 180 cases of Bernhard *et al.*, 1973; 1 of 46 cases of Spencer *et al.*, 1960). The aortic lumen is narrowed at or just above the sinuses of Valsalva. Rarely, this is due to a thin membranous band that partially or completely encircles the aorta. Much more common is the more diffuse thickening of the aortic wall with a subsequent reduction in the diameter of the aorta. The length of the involved segment may vary from less than 1 cm to several cms, and in a few cases the entire arch of the aorta has

been of diminished diameter. The reduction in diameter is due to thickening of the aortic wall. Microscopic examination shows medial hypertrophy and intimal proliferation. Usually the sinuses of Valsalva are dilated, and an abrupt and maximal constriction occurs at the upper margins. Beyond this the lumen gradually widens and resumes its normal width near the origin of the innominate artery. In a few cases, the aorta showed a poststenotic dilatation. In a minority of cases (Kurlander *et al.*, 1966), the sinuses of Valsalva are small (type II of Kurlander *et al.*, 1966), and the adjacent valve leaflets are thickened and sometimes fused producing an additional valvular stenosis. In some cases, a portion of a valve cusp may be adherent to the aorta resulting in insufficiency. Dysplastic changes in the aorta around the coronary ostia or adhesions of a valve cusp over the orifice may partially or

FIG. 164. SUBVALVULAR AORTIC STENOSIS DUE TO A DIAPHRAGM. GRADIENT VARIABLE FROM 70–100 MM HG
(A and B) The LAO projection (B) shows enlargement of left ventricle. (C) LAO and (D) RAO projections in diastole show diaphragm (arrowheads), valve ring and cusps indicated by arrows. (E and F) Systole—the diaphragm is largely obscured. F shows massive enlargement of papillary muscles indicating ventricular hypertrophy (arrowheads).

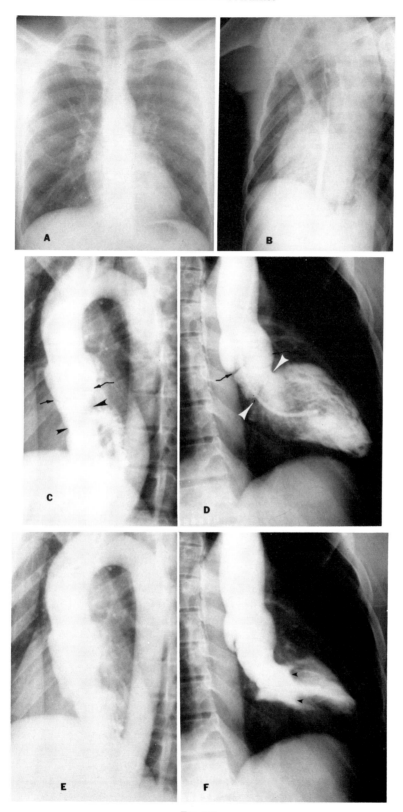

FIG. 164

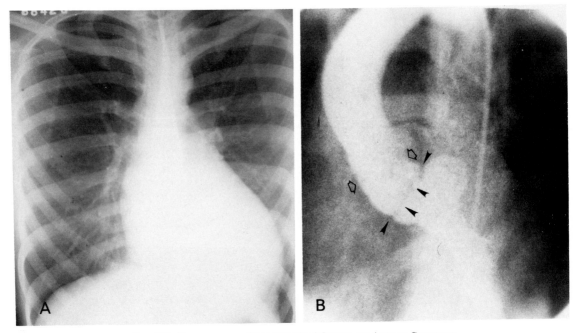

FIG. 165. SUBVALVULAR FIBROUS AND MUSCULAR AORTIC STENOSIS

This 26-year-old woman had only moderate exertional dyspnea. Systolic gradient between the low left ventricle and the subvalvular segment was 100 mm Hg, and this increased to 200 mm Hg following administration of isoproterenol. (A) Conventional chest film showing left ventricular enlargement but no evidence of enlargement of ascending aorta. (B) Cine left ventricular angiogram near end of systole. The obstruction (arrows) was about 1.5 cm below the aortic valve ring (open arrows). The hump-shaped area just below the obstruction probably represented an anomaly of anterior leaflet of mitral valve with ballooning into atrium.

completely occlude coronary blood flow (Pansegrau *et al.*, 1973; Price *et al.*, 1973). The coronary arterial bed is subject to increased pressure, and consequently the arteries are usually dilated. This may be followed by thickening of the media and fibrous intimal thickening. In some instances, the arterial walls are noted to have been thin and delicate but with enlarged lumens, and in many instances the blood flow to the myocardium is undoubtedly increased. The increased coronary flow merely compensates for the accompanying myocardial hypertrophy, and in older persons angina may be a prominent part of the symptomatology (Pansegrau *et al.*, 1973). In those cases with partial or complete obstruction of an orifice of one of the coronary arteries, myocardial ischemia may be pronounced. Kurlander *et al.* (1966) proposed a classification based primarily on the length of the segmental narrowing, the relative length of the ascending

aorta, and the state of the sinuses of Valsalva (dilated or contracted) (Fig. 167).

A substantial minority of cases of supravalvular aortic stenosis may be part of a syndrome characterized by mental retardation and peculiar facies with protruding mandible, flattened bridge of the nose, large epicanthal folds, and generous puckered lips (Williams *et al.*, 1961; Beuren *et al.*, 1962). A precursor or associated syndrome is the occurrence of infantile hypercalcemia, osteo and otosclerosis in combination with the above described facies (Black and Bonham-Carter, 1963). These patients have a high incidence of vascular stenoses, such as narrowing of the pulmonary artery and/or its peripheral branches, coarctation of the aorta, stenoses of renal and brachiocephalic arteries (22 of 122 cases reviewed by Kupic and Abrams, 1966), and also aneurysm formation of the aorta or one of its major branches (Wyler *et al.*, 1973; Morrow *et al.*, 1959;

FIG. 166. FIBROMUSCULAR SUBAORTIC STENOSIS IN A 21-YEAR-OLD MALE

(A) Marked enlargement of left ventricle with some redistribution of pulmonary circulation. (B) Ventriculogram—RAO showing well-marked mitral regurgitation. Arrowheads indicate mitral valve ring. (C) Small subvalvular chamber indicated by asterisk and arrows. (D) Pressure tracing showing intermediate pressure chamber. (E) RAO projection shows small subvalvular chamber.

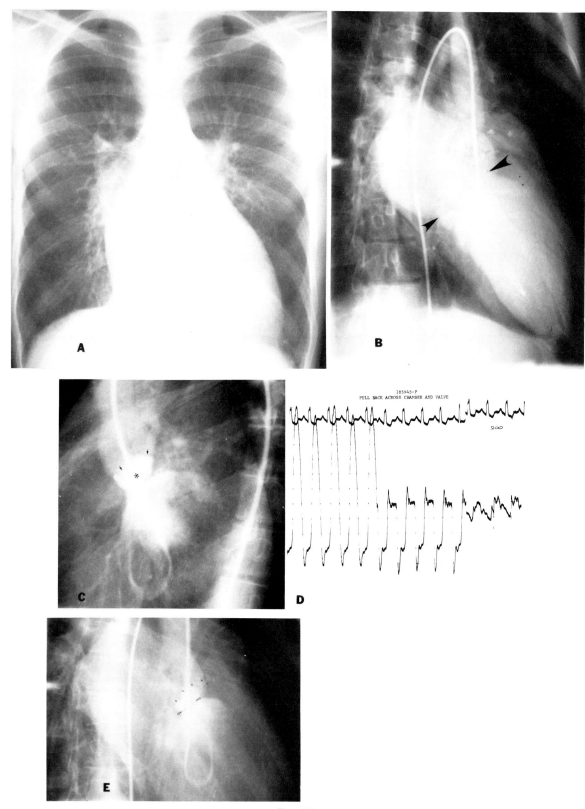

185945-P
PULL BACK ACROSS CHAMBER AND VALVE

F<small>IG</small>. 166

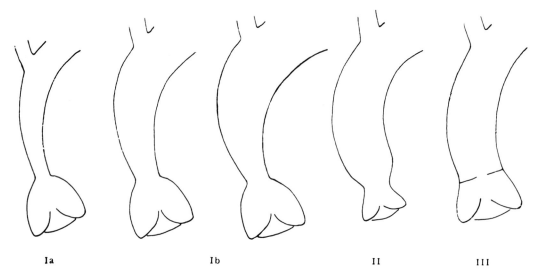

Ia   Ib   II   III

FIG. 167. SUPRAVALVULAR AORTIC STENOSIS

Diagrammatic representation of the three types of supravalvular aortic stenosis according to Kurlander *et al.* (From the *American Journal of Roentgenology, 98:* 784, 1966, with permission). Stenoses of Type Ib were the most frequent and Type III the rarest (see text).

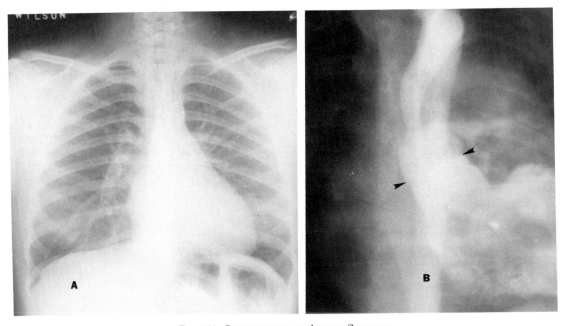

FIG. 168. SUPRAVALVULAR AORTIC STENOSIS

(A) The upper contour of the right atrial border extends to the barium-filled esophagus, and there is no evidence of the ascending aorta. (B) Aortogram showing abrupt narrowing of aorta above the valve ring (arrowheads) and extending to origin of innominate artery. (Courtesy of Dr. Leonard E. Swischuk.)

Scheinin *et al.*, 1969). The vascular changes have been attributed to the effects of the hypercalcemia.

In another substantial minority of cases, a familial incidence of supravalvular aortic stenosis has been observed (Kurlander *et al.*, 1966; Kupic and Abrams, 1966). The trait is a manifestation of an autosomal dominant gene and is not usually accompanied by mental retardation, although facial aberrations similar to those of the hypercalcemic syndrome may be noted. Another substantial group has been observed in which there is neither hypercalcemia, mental retardation, or a familial incidence.

The majority of reported cases have been in children and adolescents, but the condition may

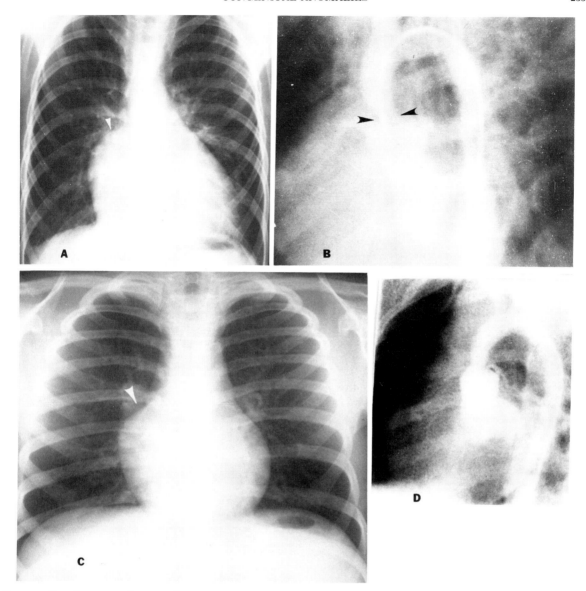

FIG. 169. TWO SEPARATE CASES OF SUPRAVALVULAR AORTIC STENOSIS WITH SHELF-LIKE CONTOUR OF UPPER PORTION OF
RIGHT ATRIAL CONTOUR DUE TO INCONSPICUOUS ASCENDING AORTA

(A) Ten-year-old child with hypercalcemia and mental retardation. Catheterization showed evidence of peripheral pulmonic stenosis. (B) Cinefluorogram showing obstruction. (C) Five-year-old child with evidence of mild pulmonic stenosis. (D) Cinefluorogram showing aortic stenosis.

be encountered in adults to age 70 (Pansegrau *et al.*, 1973). Many cases are asymptomatic. In children, symptoms are frequently those of diminished exercise tolerance, weakness, and dyspnea followed by heart failure. Associated lesions, such as obstruction of peripheral and pulmonary arteries, may contribute to the symptomatology. In adults, angina and congestive heart failure are the common presenting signs and symptoms. Typically a harsh systolic murmur is heard over the right second to fourth intercostal space with radiation into the neck accompanied by a thrill.

The pulses in the neck and arms may be unequal. The ECG frequently shows left ventricular hypertrophy and/or a strain pattern.

Radiologic Findings. The heart is often of normal size and contour. When enlargement occurs, the contour is typically left ventricular enlargement with rounding of the left border and descent of the apex. The heart size does not correlate with the observed aortic gradient similar to the relationship seen in other types of valvular stenosis (Klatte *et al.*, 1962). Left atrial enlargement indicates left ventricular failure as mitral insufficiency is not customarily seen with SVAS. The most striking finding when present is an empty space just above the right atrium due to the diminished size of the ascending aorta (Figs. 168 and 169). Fluoroscopy may show an absence of the usual pulsations of the ascending aorta. Dilatation of the right ventricle and/or atrium may accentuate the change and usually indicates increased pressure in the right ventricle secondary to pulmonary stenosis. Rarely the ascending aorta may be dilated and show increased pulsations (Kurlander et al., 1966). The pulmonary vasculature is usually normal unless there is an associated left-to-right shunt, such as an ASD. In a few cases, localized dilatation of segments of the pulmonary artery was identified secondary to localized stenoses (Kurlander et al., 1966). As indicated, enlargement of the right side of the heart with prominence of the right border can be associated with left heart failure, an associated left-to-right shunt such as atrial septal defect, or more often secondary to associated pulmonic stenosis either proximal or distal.

Although the diagnosis can often be strongly suspected from clinical findings, such as a typical systolic murmur, peculiar facies or the shape of the cardiac contour, diagnosis is established by left heart catheterization and angiocardiography. Pressure tracings with withdrawal of the catheter from the left ventricle to the aorta will establish the presence of obstruction but cannot delineate the exact site or the important anatomical details. The important details are (1) the site and length of the stenosis; (2) the degree of associated valvular stenosis and/or insufficiency; (3) the presence or absence of adhesions of the valve cusps to the region of the coronary ostia or other causes of coronary obstruction; and (4) evidence of obstruction of large brachiocephalic arteries. These details are best shown by a combination of left ventriculography and supravalvular aortography. Hemodynamic data permit the determination of the systolic gradient and the cross-sectional area of the aorta, and these are of some importance in determining the necessity for operation. However, the length of the supravalvular stenosis is of considerable importance in relation to attempts at surgical treatment. In 5 of 14 cases of supravalvular aortic stenosis reported by Bernhard et al. (1973), diffuse hypoplasia was present and was inoperable. Rastelli et al. (1966) suggest that the long or diffuse stenoses offer formidable problems in repair and might well be avoided. When the sinuses of Valsalva are small and the valve cusps are thickened or adherent, valve replacement should be seriously considered (Kurlander et al., 1966). The indications for surgical treatment are similar to those of other types

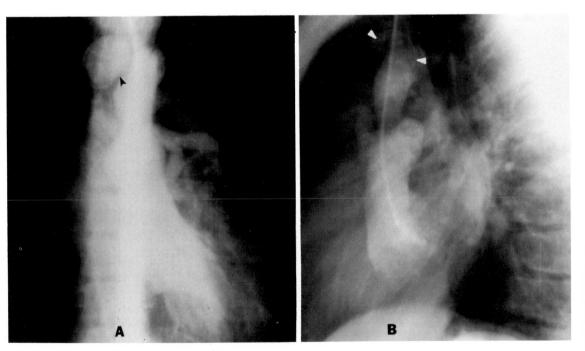

Fig. 170 A and B. Supravalvular Aortic Stenosis with Saccular Aneurysm Originating in the Proximal Aortic Arch

Note large coronary arteries. (Courtesy of Dr. Andrew Morrow and The National Institutes of Health.)

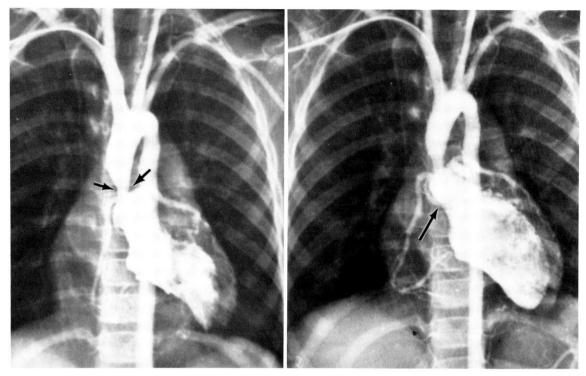

FIG. 171. CONGENITAL SUPRAVALVULAR AORTIC STENOSIS

Brachial artery catheterization with left ventricular injection of contrast material. A pronounced constriction of the ascending aorta is present at and just above the origin of the coronary arteries (small arrows). The region of the aortic sinuses is slightly dilated (single arrow points to aortic valve), and the left ventricle is enlarged. Distal to the constriction the aorta and brachiocephalic vessels appear normal. Pressures recorded at the time of surgery were as follows: left ventricle, 165/10; aorta (above constriction), 100/50. An Ivalon graft was used to restore the caliber of the aortic lumen, and the postoperative result was considered excellent. (By permission of *Circulation* and the American Heart Association; from Dotter *et al.* (1961).)

of congenital aortic stenosis, namely a gradient of greater than 50 mm Hg, marked valvular insufficiency, electrocardiographic evidence of left ventricular strain, and symptoms of dyspnea, weakness, and angina. The results of surgical treatment, although often satisfactory, seem to be less certain than in other types of aortic stenosis, particularly in symptomatic adults (Pansegrau *et al.*, 1973).

8. Aortico-Left Ventricular Tunnel. This unusual anomaly resembles and may be confused with congenital aneurysm of the sinus of Valsalva with rupture into the left ventricle. In this anomaly, a channel or tunnel extends from the ascending aorta downward into the myocardium in the region of the ventricular septum and opens into the left ventricular outflow tract below the aortic valve. This channel has a smooth interior, but it may be tortuous and show localized aneurysmal dilatation. Levy *et al.* (1963) were the first to clearly describe both the clinical and anatomical features of this condition in 3 patients, 2 of whom were successfully treated. These authors stated that 4 previous cases of this entity had been described. However, it appears from the reports that 3 of these (Tasaka *et al.*, 1960; Warthen, 1949; Hart, 1905) represent aneurysms of the right sinus of Valsalva with delayed rupture into the left ventricle. The differential anatomical feature is the higher origin of the opening of the aortico-left ventricular tunnel above the orifice of the right coronary artery. Congenital aneurysms are below the orifice of the right coronary artery. Also, the early onset of distinctive murmurs and other signs of aortic insufficiency suggest a condition different from ruptured aneurysm of the sinus of Valsalva. The tunnel often produces mild pressure on the right ventricular outflow tract, and this may be sufficient to produce some degree of stenosis. Also, aortic stenosis due to narrowing of the aortic valve ring has been a complication in 2 of the reported cases. The ascending aorta is markedly dilated.

The onset of symptoms is typically in infancy or early life. Usually there are systolic and diastolic murmurs and thrills with wide transmission. The murmurs are said to be easily differentiated from those of PDA.

The heart may be normal in size at birth but enlargement is rapid. As seen on the conventional chest film, the left ventricle is enlarged and the aorta rapidly dilates. The changes are similar to those of aortic insufficiency. In the case shown in Figure 172, the heart enlarged rapidly over a few months time and became huge.

Right heart catheterization may show evidence of pulmonic stenosis due to pressure on the right ventricular outflow tract. The definitive procedure is aortography with injection of contrast substance into the ascending aorta. This will show rapid reflux of the contrast substance into the left ventricle. Very shortly thereafter, contrast substance can be identified in a structure adjacent to the left heart border in the region of the outflow tract of the right ventricle. However, the peripheral pulmonary arteries do not fill with contrast substance, and it thus can be deduced that the contrast substance is in an abnormal cavity or tunnel. In our case shown in Figure 173, the catheter was introduced into the tunnel and contrast substance was injected directly into the tunnel. The aneurysmal dilatation is well shown. There was an associated aortic stenosis. It is of great importance to determine the condition of the aortic valve before attempting to obliterate the tunnel by surgical means. In our case, the aortic stenosis was so severe that when the tunnel was closed the left ventricle failed. In 1 of the cases reported by Levy *et al.* (1963) aortic commissurotomy was performed.

In summary, the diagnosis of aortico-left ventricular tunnel should be suspected in an infant or child with the blood pressure changes of aortic insufficiency and a large left ventricle. The diagnosis can be made by selective aortography with injection of the contrast substance into the supravalvular region followed by rapid serial filming.

9. Hypoplastic Left Heart Syndrome. The common characteristic of these anomalies is a marked reduction in the size of the ascending aorta, although this is rarely the only abnormality (Lev, 1952). Much more often an associated obstructive lesion is found in the left side of the heart, such as mitral stenosis or atresia or aortic stenosis or atresia, and these lesions are properly considered here. The left atrium and left ventricle are diminished in size in the great majority of cases (90% in the material of Keith *et al.*, 1958), although it cannot be said with certainty whether the underdeveloped chambers or the obstructive lesions are the primary cause of the anomaly. The left ventricle is variable in size but is usually small and may be so diminutive that it is found only after serial sections of the heart. In a few instances the left ventricle has been approximately normal in size, and in these cases there is usually an associated ventricular septal defect (Roberts *et al.*, 1976). Endocardial fibroelastosis is frequently found inside the left ventricle in those cases in which the mitral valve is open. A ventricular septal defect is usually in the membraneous septum and is usually small. Rarely the aorta may be transposed or override the ventric-

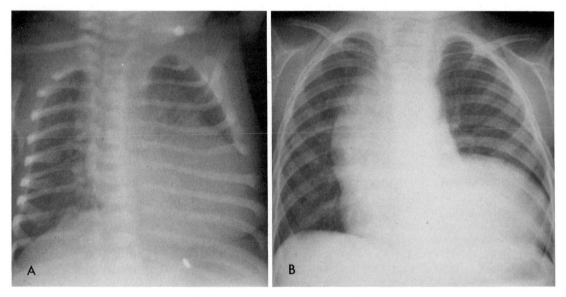

FIG. 172. AORTICO-LEFT VENTRICULAR TUNNEL
Conventional chest film at 2 days of age (A) and at 11 months of age (B). (Reproduced from *Circulation, 31:* 565, 1965.)

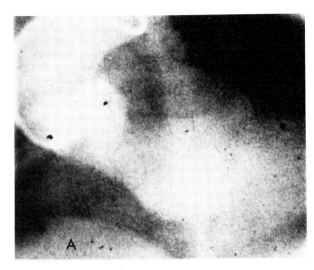
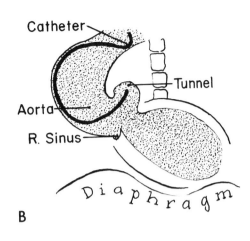

FIG. 173. AORTICO-LEFT VENTRICULAR TUNNEL

(A) A 16-mm movie frame taken in the right posterior oblique position showing the tip of the transaortic catheter in the tunnel with massive reflux of contrast substance into the left ventricle. None of the contrast substance entered the pulmonary artery indicating that the communication was not with the right side of the heart. (B) Line sketch of A. (Reproduced from *Circulation, 31:* 567, 1965.)

ular septal defect (Noonan, 1968). The ascending aorta is typically quite small, is patent just above the atretic aortic valve, and serves to carry blood in a retrograde fashion to the coronary arteries.

Because of the small size of the aorta and particularly the obstructions often present at the mitral or aortic valve, aerated blood must be shunted to the right side of the heart usually through a patent foramen ovale, an atrial septal defect, a ventricular septal defect or a combination of these. A patent foramen ovale is by far the commonest site of the shunt. The valve is usually herniated through the foramen permitting a signficant shunt from the left to the right atrium, and the pressure in the left atrium is usually substantially higher than that in the right. In addition, when the mitral valve is patent, blood can reach the right ventricle through a ventricular septal defect if such is present. When the mitral valve is atretic blood must reach the right side of the heart through the interatrial communication or rarely by retrograde flow in a left-sided superior vena cava (3 cases; Watson, 1962) or through bronchial veins (Abrams, 1958). When the interatrial communication is small increased pulmonary venous pressure follows, and this may be sufficient to cause pulmonary congestion and edema.

Aerated blood reaching the right side of the heart mixes with systemic venous blood and is expelled by the right ventricle through the pulmonary artery. Part of this blood reaches the lungs and part passes through a persistent PDA

into the descending aorta where it flows usually in both directions toward the head and feet. Thus, the blood supply to the head, arms and coronary arteries comes mainly from the retrograde flow in the aortic arch. It can be seen that a reverse flow through a patent ductus is an essential feature of this condition. Because the abnormal circulation increases the load on the right ventricle during fetal life, it enlarges, and this is one of the few anomalies in which the heart may be considerably enlarged at birth.

Associated congenital anomalies are common and occurred in about 37% of the cases reported by Noonan and Nadas (1958). These are coarctation of the aorta, interruption of the aortic arch, auriculoventricularis communis, anomalous right subclavian artery and bicuspid aortic valve.

Hypoplastic left heart syndrome is the most common cause of death due to heart disease during the first week of life (Roberts *et al.*, 1976). Watson (1962) found that 23% of the deaths during the first week of life due to cardiac malformations were cases with the hypoplastic left heart syndrome. The syndrome is characterized by dyspnea, pallor, feeble pulses, mild cyanosis and an enlarging heart and a considerable frequency of pulmonary edema.

Radiologic Findings. Chest films usually show moderate to marked cardiac enlargement. If the heart is normal in size at birth it usually enlarges rapidly. In the frontal projection it is globular in shape, although the bulk of the en-

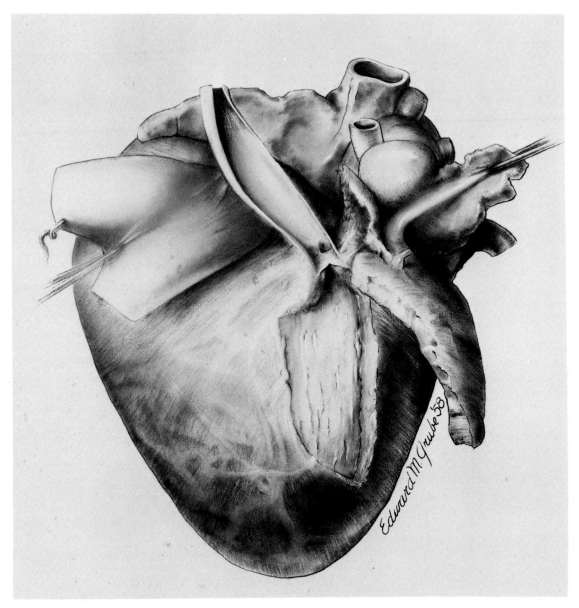

FIG. 174. SEMISCHEMATIC DRAWING OF CASE OF ATRESIA OF AORTIC VALVE WITH MARKED DIMINUTION IN SIZE OF ASCENDING AORTA

The anterior wall of the left ventricle has been reflected so as to show the diminutive chamber. Blood reached the ascending aorta through a patent ductus.

largement is due to the right atrium and right ventricle. Actually the heart extends farther to the left than to the right. The large heart tends to obscure the hilar shadows, although in most of the reported cases the pulmonary artery is enlarged. In cases with pulmonary stenosis, which are in the minority, the lung vasculature may be dimininished and the heart may be small. In the other cases after a few days there is evidence of increased pulmonary vascularity.

Pulmonary edema and congestion are seen in a sizeable proportion of cases. The edema may present as the usual appearance associated with heart failure with a diffuse alveolar pattern. Often, however, it has a reticular appearance indicating a considerable interstitial element. The presence of such an appearance (Fig. 176) suggests an obstruction to venous return usually associated with a small interatrial communication. The condition at times must be differentiated from the respiratory distress syndrome of the newborn. The enlarged or rapidly enlarging heart and associated increased pulmonary vascularity and pulmonary edema should suggest a cardiac etiology.

Cardiac catheterization and selective angiography are usually indicated, although the diagnosis can be strongly suspected from the skillful use of echocardiography (Meyers and Kaplan, 1972). The size of the ventricular chambers and the presence and activity of the mitral and aortic valves can often be appraised by this method.

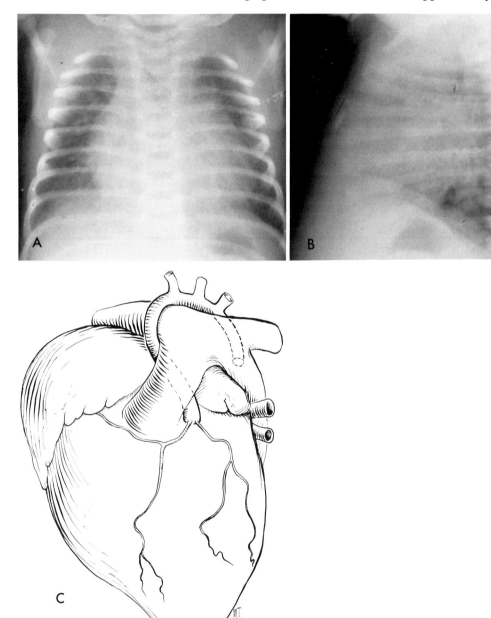

FIG. 175. AORTIC ATRESIA WITH UNDERDEVELOPMENT OF LEFT VENTRICLE WITH SEVERE MITRAL AND AORTIC STENOSIS
(A and B) Chest films exposed 24 hr after birth showing globular cardiac enlargement. The pulmonary vessels just beyond the right heart border appear enlarged suggesting increased pulmonary vascularity. The patient died 2 days later. (C) Drawing (semidiagrammatic) of exterior of heart as seen from in front. The ascending portion and arch of the aorta were tiny and gave origin to two normally placed coronary arteries and the brachiocephalic vessels. The aorta widened as it joined the large ductus which was a continuation of the pulmonary artery. Blood flowed in a retrograde direction in the aortic arch to supply the upper portion of the body and coronary arteries.

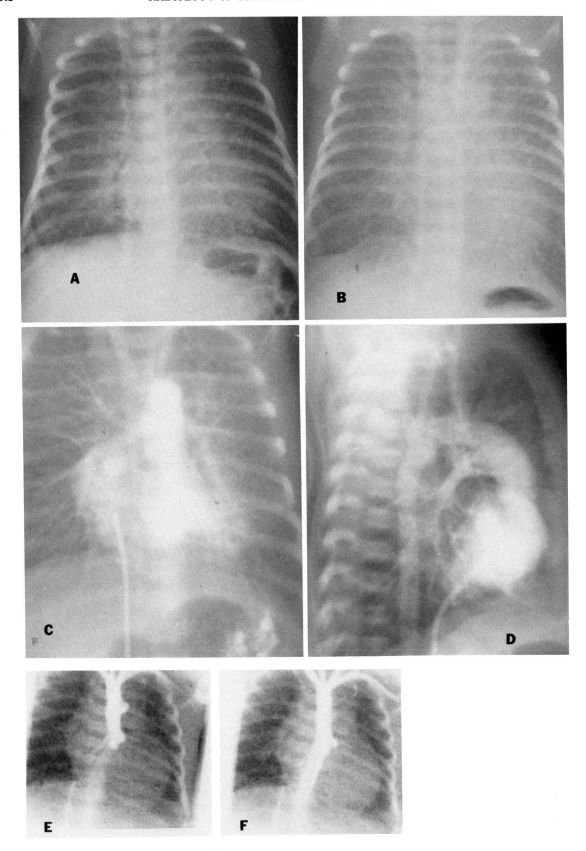

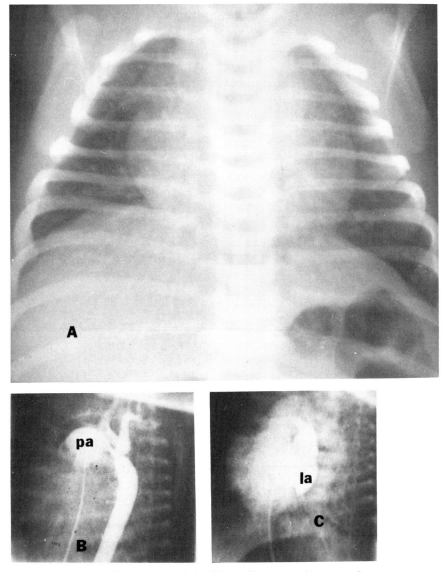

FIG. 177. HYPOPLASTIC LEFT HEART SYNDROME (AUTOPSY CASE)
Mitral atresia, small high VSD, hypoplasia of aortic valve and ascending aorta. (A) Conventional chest film at 2 days of age. (B) Injection into dilated pulmonary artery (pa) showing a narrow ductus (arrowhead), a small aortic arch, and brachiocephalic vessels. (C) Left atrial (la) injection showing rapid passage into the right side of heart and pulmonary artery.

Until recently the condition has been considered as unsusceptible to surgical treatment. Recently palliative surgery seems to be useful (Cayler *et al.*, 1970) in certain cases, particularly those with a larger left ventricle and good pulmonary flow. Cardiac catheterization and selective angiogra-

phy would still seem to be indicated as preoperative measures despite their risks and hazards in the newborn infant.

Cardiac catheterization rarely provides a definitive diagnosis. Blood drawn from the right atrium shows an increase in oxygen content over

FIG. 176. HYPOPLASTIC LEFT HEART SYNDROME. ATRESIA OF AORTIC AND MITRAL VALVES IN A NEWBORN
(A) Chest film at 2 days of age showing diffuse interstitial pulmonary edema. (B) Forty-eight hours later—edema has increased. (C and D) Frontal and lateral angiograms with injection into right atrium. A large ductus connects with the descending aorta. There is faint filling of the brachiocephalic vessels. (E and F) Aortogram showing filling of ascending aorta which is small. (Courtesy of Dr. Leonard E. Swischuk.)

that in the vena cavae. The right ventricle is large and the pressure is above the systemic pressure as a rule. The catheter can often be passed from the right ventricle through the pulmonary artery and into the descending aorta demonstrating the patent ductus. Injections of contrast substance into the right ventricle or pulmonary artery show a prompt flow through a patent ductus into the descending aorta. The ductus may be narrowed, and a pressure gradient between the pulmonary artery and the aorta is often demonstrated. Contrast substance injected through the ductus may reflux into the aortic arch and occasionally all the way to the atretic aortic valve. This is the crucial diagnostic procedure. A left atrial injection should be attempted in an effort to show the condition of the mitral valve and the left ventricle.

A retrograde aortogram with injection into the descending aorta may cause sufficient reflux to demonstrate the tiny ascending aorta. Rosengart et al. (1976) have recommended the exposure of a single portable film following the injection of contrast substance through a catheter placed in the descending aorta via the umbilical artery. This may well outline the diminutive ascending aorta and tend to confirm a clinical diagnosis. It would seem, however, that for those cases that do not seem to be operable that echocardiography should be the initial procedure and possibly followed by cardiac catheterization and angiography if operation seems feasible.

Surgical treatment in selected cases has consisted of anastomosis of the ascending aorta to the right pulmonary artery and banding of the distal pulmonary arteries. If the interatrial communication is stenotic, it should be enlarged, although the Rashkind procedure might be considered as hazardous because of the small size of the left atrium and the danger of avulsing the pulmonary veins.

Conditions which should be thought of during the first weeks of life and which should be differentiated from hypoplastic left heart syndrome are (1) severe aortic stenosis, (2) total anomalous pulmonary venous return, (3) patent ductus arteriosus, and (4) transposition of the great arteries.

10. Mitral Stenosis. Isolated congenital mitral stenosis is rare (Baker et al., 1962). In the large majority of cases it has been associated with other cardiac anomalies. These may be listed in an approximate order of frequency as patent ductus arteriosus, coarctation of the thoracic aorta, aortic stenosis, ventricular septal defect, hypoplasia of the aortic arch, and patent foramen ovale (Humblet et al., 1971; Ferencz et

al., 1954). Patent ductus arteriosus was found in 6 of 17 patients reported by Hilbish and Cooley (1956), in 3 of whom flow was reversed. In that series, 6 of 17 patients had aortic coarctation. Daoud et al. (1963) found reports in the literature of 30 patients with the isolated lesion. In this group, the diagnosis was made clinically in 8, confirmed at autopsy in 9, and 13 other patients underwent mitral valvotomy.

Detailed anatomical studies (Rosenquist, 1974; Rosenquist et al., 1975; Davachi et al., 1971) demonstrated a variety of anatomical aberrations that may cause stenosis or insufficiency or both. These are a supravalvular ring, accessory valvular tissue, Ebstein's malformation usually seen in corrected transposition, accessory orifice of the mitral valve, commissural fusion, cleft anterior leaflet of the mitral valve, short or long chordae tendineae, abnormally placed or deformed papillary muscles and the variations of a single papillary muscle associated with a "parachute mitral valve." The tetrad complex described by Shone et al. (1963) consisting of a parachute mitral valve, supravalvular ring in the left atrium, subaortic stenosis and coarctation of the aorta will be considered separately below. Endocardial fibroelastosis involving the left ventricle and extending into the left atrium is quite common.

Severe mitral stenosis is usually symptomatic in infancy and is ordinarily associated with a poor prognosis; frequently the outcome is fatal

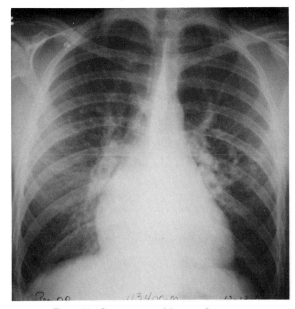

Fig. 178. Congenital Mitral Stenosis
Patient was a 15-year-old boy. Valve ring reduced in size at operation.

during the first 2 years of life. Mild cases may survive for a long time depending on the severity of the lesion. The common symptoms are dyspnea, repeated pulmonary infections, atelectasis, congestive heart failure, pulmonary edema, and poor physical growth. Pallor, sweating, syncopal episodes, and cyanosis may also be found. The diagnosis should be suspected in an infant or child with an enlarging heart, an apical diastolic rumbling murmur, signs of pulmonary hypertension, and left atrial enlargement.

The electrocardiogram commonly shows right ventricular hypertrophy with abnormal P waves.

On the conventional chest film the heart may enlarge, but the most crucial chamber is the left atrium, although enlargement of this chamber may not be very striking. Evidence of increased pulmonary venous pressure and some redistribution of the pulmonary circulation is to be expected but is not always clearly shown in the chest films of infants and children.

Right heart catheterization shows elevated pulmonary artery and wedge pressures. If the catheter can be inserted into the left atrium, a gradient may be detected across the mitral valve. Angiography offers the most definitive information concerning not only the presence of stenosis but a considerable degree of the anatomy. Injection into the pulmonary artery may demonstrate an enlarged left atrium with delayed emptying (Hilbish and Cooley, 1956). A more detailed study of the mitral valve and left ventricle is obtained by a left ventriculogram with filming in the frontal and lateral and at times the right oblique projections. Although Carey et al. (1964) were doubtful that the exact anatomy of the stenosis could be demonstrated by angiography, others have had considerable success in demonstrating supravalvular rings (Macartney et al., 1973) and the several variations of the parachute mitral valve (Deutsch et al., 1974; Schachner et al., 1975; Simon et al., 1969; Zamalloa et al., 1969). The changes associated with endocardial fibroelastosis and shortening of the chordae and fused commissures were demonstrated with less certainty, but the findings were helpful in determining if valvular resection would be necessary.

The changes in the left ventriculogram due to a parachute mitral valve are an absence of the negative shadows due to the two normal papillary muscles. The anterior and posterior papillary muscles are identified in about 50–60% of normal persons (Macartney et al., 1973; also see the description of the normal left ventriculogram). A single large negative shadow may be seen anchored to the anterior or posterior wall (Prado et al., 1965; Zamalloa et al., 1969; Ma-

cartney et al., 1973) or at the apex (Simon et al., 1969). Films exposed during the different phases of the cardiac cycle show that the motions of the valve leaflets are limited. The anterior leaflet of the mitral valve may be tethered in an anterior position and obstruct the outflow tract of the left ventricle producing subaortic stenosis similar to that seen in IHSS (Simon et al., 1969).

A supravalvular ring appears as a thin crescentic filling defect between the left atrium and ventricle seen best in the lateral projection following a left atrial injection. Some degree of mitral insufficiency is a common finding and may suffice to show the supravalvular ring.

Surgical correction of congenital mitral stenosis is difficult due to the marked and variable deformity of the mitral valve and its attachments and the frequent presence of severe endocardial fibroelastosis. Parachute mitral valve, although extremely rare, as an isolated lesion (Prado et al., 1965) requires valve replacement. Mitral insufficiency postoperatively following commissurotomy or other plastic procedures is common. Because of the marked deformity of the valve, surgery under direct vision using cardiopulmonary bypass is advocated.

The differential diagnosis includes cor triatriatum, stenosis of the common pulmonary vein, atrial myxoma and infradiaphragmatic total anomalous pulmonary venous return. In infants with congestive heart failure and evidence of pulmonary hypertension, the common left to right shunts must also be excluded. Congenital mitral stenosis may easily be overlooked when associated with coarctation of the aorta and aortic or subaortic stenosis (Jacobson et al., 1953).

The "Parachute Mitral Valve" Complex. In 1963, Shone et al. (1963) described 4 cases in which there was a tetrad of associated anomalies, namely coarctation of the thoracic aorta, supravalvular left atrial ring, parachute mitral valve, and subaortic stenosis. In 4 other cases, at least 2 of these anomalies were present, and these were considered as "form fruste" of the fully developed complex. In 2 of the cases, the obstructing mitral valve anomaly was not recognized until after the coarctation had been resected. Recognition of each of these anomalies is of great importance in the evaluation for and the carrying out of surgical treatment. Macartney et al. (1973) using left ventriculography recognized the large negative shadow of the single papillary muscle and in some cases the supravalvular ring (there is usually some degree of mitral regurgitation with filling of the left atrium). The coarctation (often preductal) is easily demonstrated by aortography. The associated subvalvular aortic stenosis may be more difficult to document fully since the anomaly of the mitral valve and papillary muscle may in itself cause an obstruction of the outflow tract of the left ventricle. Deutsch *et al.* (1974) also confirmed that the complex is susceptible to diagnosis using clinical, hemodynamic and most important angiographic findings.

11. Congenital Mitral Regurgitation. Some degree of mitral regurgitation is a common accompaniment of congenital stenosis. Isolated regurgitation is quite rare (Husson *et al.*, 1964; Carney *et al.*, 1962). Some cases have been attributed to endocardial fibroelastosis with shortening and thickening of the valve cusps and chordae tendineae (Talner *et al.*, 1961). Other cases are due to dilatation of the valve ring. In other cases, the cleft of the anterior leaflet of the mitral valve may have been a factor. Associated abnormalities have consisted of common atrioventricular canal, patent ductus arteriosus, corrected transposition of the great vessels, and transposition of the great vessels.

Symptomatology includes easy fatigability, exertional dyspnea, and other symptoms of left ventricular failure. An apical systolic thrill and a prominent apical pansystolic murmur are prominent physical findings. Electrocardiographic evidence of left ventricular hypertrophy is extremely common; other electrocardiographic abnormalities include left atrial enlargement and right ventricular hypertrophy. The pulmonary wedge pressure is usually elevated, and the right ventricular pressure may also be increased.

The commonest radiographic findings are enlargement of the left atrium and left ventricle with associated pulmonary venous congestion. Selective left ventriculography is the most definitive diagnostic procedure (Husson *et al.*, 1964). Properly exposed films show regurgitation of the contrast material from the left ventricle to the left atrium. Care should be taken to look for associated lesions, such as patent ductus arteriosus and associated endocardial cushion defects.

Congenital mitral regurgitation may be effectively treated by annuloplasty (Talner *et al.*, 1961). If a cleft valve leaflet is found, repair is indicated. Patients with associated patent ductus have usually benefitted by closure of the ductus.

12. Cor Triatriatum. Cor triatriatum is a rare congenital anomaly in which the left atrium is divided into a proximal and a distal chamber. The proximal chamber receives one or more of the pulmonary veins, and the distal chamber is in direct communication with the left ventricle through the mitral valve. In its most common

form all of the pulmonary veins empty into the proximal chamber which is usually placed dorsally and medial to the distal chamber. The proximal chamber usually empties into the distal chamber through an opening of variable size. The opening may consist of a hole in a diaphragm-like structure or there may be a funnel or tubular-shaped structure. The size of the opening between the proximal and distal chambers is crucial and is usually stenotic. The foramen ovale usually is found between the right atrium and the distal left atrial chamber but occasionally may be between the right atrium and the proximal chamber. In some instances, the foramen ovale is patent, and rarely there is an interatrial communication.

The cause of the anomaly is thought to be a faulty absorption of the common pulmonary vein into the left atrium. The common pulmonary vein arises just to the left of the septum primum as a dorsal appendage of the developing atrium in early fetal life (27–30 days) (Ellis *et al.*, 1964). Normally this common venous channel becomes incorporated into the left atrium as its dorsal wall, and in this manner the four pulmonary veins normally come to join the left atrium. In cor triatriatum, the common pulmonary vein may be only partially incorporated into the left atrium, and there may be a stenosis at the junction of the vein and the left atrium. This obstruction results in dilatation of the common pulmonary vein in such a way that it often bulges into the proper left atrial cavity producing the appearance of a separate dorsal atrium.

The classic type of cor triatriatum just described is by far the most common variety, but a number of other variations exist, most of which suggest a close similarity to PAPVR (Lucas and Schmidt, 1968; Marin-Garcia *et al.*, 1975; Thilenius *et al.*, 1976). These variations are shown diagrammatically in Figure 179. In the total variety (Fig. 179A), the proximal chamber receives all of the pulmonary veins, but the proximal chamber may empty (1) totally into the distal chamber of the left atrium, (2) into both the right atrium and the distal left atrium, or (3) through an anomalous venous return to the right atrium. Other rare variations (Fig. 179, B and C) occur where the proximal chamber does not empty directly into the distal chamber but a left-to-right shunt occurs either through an anomalous venous connection or through a communication with the right atrium. In most of these cases the coronary sinus is occluded (Thilenius, 1976). In the subtotal variety some of the pulmonary veins, usually two in number, communicate with the

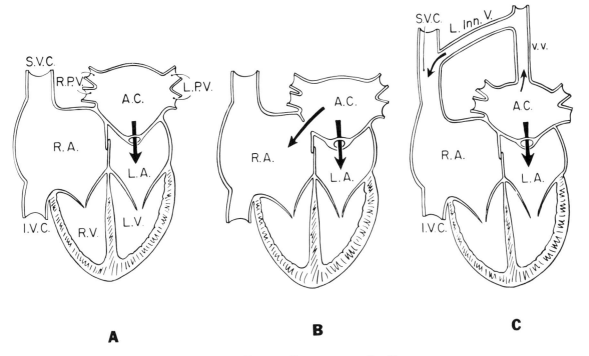

FIG. 179. DIAGRAM OF SEVERAL VARIATIONS OF COR TRIATRIATUM

A represents the most common arrangement. B represents the arrangement in the case shown in Figure 180 in which an ASD communicates with the proximal chamber. C represents the same condition as A plus an associated anomalous pulmonary venous connection. (From Lucas, R. V. and Schmidt, R. E. in *Heart Disease in Infants, Children and Adolescents.* Moss, A. J. and Adams, F. H. (eds.), The Williams & Wilkins Co.)

proximal chamber and the others with the distal chamber or the proximal chamber may communicate entirely with the right atrium. This rather bewildering number of variations is mentioned because of their similarity to some cases of partial anomalous pulmonary venous return on the one hand and stenotic lesions of the left side of the heart on the other. The classic form of Figure 179A is by far the most common. In this variety the clinical manifestations depend on the size of the opening in the left atrial membrane. If it is large, no symptoms may be produced; however, the orifice may be so small as to produce death in early infancy or may be large enough to support life for a longer or variable time. Thus, the clinical picture of the patient with cor triatriatum is not characteristic; it depends mainly upon the development of pulmonary hypertension with subsequent right ventricular failure. Dyspnea, cyanosis, hemoptysis, signs of congestive heart failure, and failure to thrive are among the prominent clinical manifestations (Grondin *et al.*, 1964). Various types of murmurs may be heard, and both systolic and diastolic murmurs have been described (Niwayama, 1960). The common-

est electrocardiographic finding has been right ventricular hypertrophy.

Radiologic Findings. In the typical case, conventional chest films show right ventricular hypertrophy, enlargement of the main and branch pulmonary arteries, and signs of longstanding pulmonary venous obstruction. The chronic lung stasis may be characterized by diffuse interstitial edema, such as Kerley's A and B lines and diffuse reticular pulmonary markings that fan outward from the pulmonary hilus particularly toward the lower lung fields. There is often considerable redistribution of the pulmonary blood flow with enlargement of the upper lobe vessels. Occasionally alveolar pulmonary edema is seen with patchy or more confluent homogeneous opacities.

Appropriate films exposed following the administration of barium by mouth may show posterior displacement of the esophagus in the region of the enlarged dorsal atrial compartment (the common pulmonary vein). Such a finding may be indistinguishable from that seen in left atrial enlargement due to the other causes of obstruction on the left side of the heart.

CARDIAC CATHETERIZATION. Right heart catheterization usually shows a considerable increase in right ventricular and pulmonary artery pressure. A crucial finding is an elevation of the pulmonary wedge pressure, and this is usually found to be in the neighborhood of 28–40 mm Hg (Marin-Garcia *et al.*, 1975). This places the site of the obstruction on the left side of the heart. If the catheter can be placed into the left atrium and a normal or reduced pressure is obtained, then the site of the obstruction can be predicted with confidence.

Angiography offers the best possibility of a specific diagnosis, although a precise preoperative diagnosis has been made infrequently in the past. Selective injection of contrast substance into the pulmonary artery with filming in the frontal and lateral projections is the recommended procedure. The contrast substance returns to the proximal atrial compartment in sufficiently high concentration to outline it, and serial filming will show that the contrast substance stagnates and the proximal compartment becomes quite dense. The shape of the proximal compartment is often different from that of the normal atrium and should arouse suspicion that an accessory chamber is present. The lower compartment fills slowly and is obviously proximal to the mitral valve. Occasionally the membrane separating the two compartments is visualized (Ellis *et al.*, 1964; Miller *et al.*, 1964; Abdulla *et al.*, 1970). By this finding the diagnosis can be made with assurance. In the absence of visualization of the membrane or recognition of the distal chamber and if a normal pressure has not been measured in the lower atrial compartment at cardiac catheterization, congenital mitral stenosis may be incorrectly diagnosed. Selective angiography may be of particular help in detecting associated conditions, such as partial anomalous pulmonary venous return (PAPVR), the subtotal variety of cor triatriatum and the other causes of obstructions in the left side of the heart.

Differential Diagnosis. In children, the differential lies within the group of congenital anomalies that produce pulmonary venous obstruction. These include stenosis of the individual pulmonary veins, supravalvular stenosing ring in the left atrium, congenital mitral stenosis, total anomalous pulmonary venous connection with obstruction (type IV), congenital mitral stenosis and congenital mitral insufficiency.

In adults, the differential includes rheumatic mitral stenosis, left atrial tumor and left atrial thrombus.

The diagnosis is of great importance since the anomaly is susceptible to surgical correction and cure. The surgical procedure consists of excision of the obstructing membrane (Lam *et al.*, 1962; Jegier *et al.*, 1963). The rare deviations from the classic cor triatriatum, particularly those in which there is a shunt into the right atrium, may

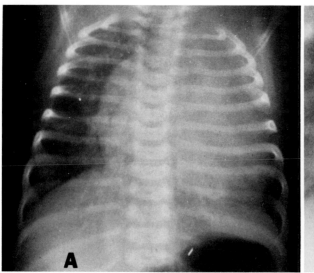 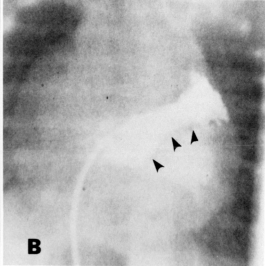

FIG. 180. COR TRIATRIATUM IN A 6-WEEK-OLD INFANT

An atrial septal defect communicated with proximal left atrial chamber. (Autopsy case.) (A) A huge heart with some pulmonary engorgement. The atrial defect decompressed the left side of the heart and overloaded the right side. (B) Injection into proximal left atrial chamber. Arrowheads show obstrucing membrane.

cause special problems for the unsuspecting surgeon.

13. Congenital Stenosis of the Pulmonary Veins. Congenital stenosis of the individual pulmonary veins of sufficient severity to be a cause of symptoms is quite rare with 20 cases reported in the world literature (Henry et al., 1975). The congenital obstructions can be divided into two types, the short segmental obstruction occurring at or near the junction of the individual veins with the left atrium and a more diffuse obstruction characterized by hypoplasia of the veins (Nakib et al., 1967). The most common variety has been a short segmental narrowing due to thickening of the walls of the individual veins. The length of the obstructing segment has rarely exceeded 5 mm. The exterior of the vein has almost invariably been of normal caliber, and the narrowing has been due to an impingement on the lumen by a greatly thickened wall in which there are found smooth muscle bundles and an increase in elastic tissue (Shone et al., 1962; Sherman et al., 1958; Henry et al., 1975). A second much rarer type of obstruction was due to a "membranous diaphragm" at the orifice of one of the veins, and this was only visible from inside the left atrium (Emslie-Smith et al., 1955; Kawashima et al., 1971). In both of the above types the exterior of the veins had a normal appearance and might be easily overlooked at the time of surgery. Dilatation of the veins distal to the point of obstruction was variable, but in only one case was the obstructed vein sufficiently dilated to be recognized on the chest film (Henry et al., 1975). In all of the reported cases where there was pulmonary hypertension, there were associated changes in the pulmonary arterial system characterized by thickening of the arterial walls. The alveolar walls were often infiltrated with some fibrous or collagenous tissue and were thickened. In one case numerous thrombi were found in the arteries and veins of the involved lung (Bernstein et al., 1959).

About 60% of the reported cases have been associated with other cardiac defects, such as PDA, ASD, VSD and mitral atresia.

This condition is often a diagnostic problem. Symptoms usually appear in infancy or childhood. The symptoms are failure to thrive, dyspnea, cyanosis, weakness, and in several cases persistent hemoptysis.

Radiologic Findings. The conventional chest films usually show some degree of cardiac enlargement with prominence of the right atrium and right ventricle. The cardiac enlargement is progressive if the patient is followed over a period of years. The pulmonary artery segment is prominent and convex. The aorta is relatively small. The left atrium is not enlarged. The most suggestive finding is the presence of a diffuse reticular pattern in the lungs. This is due to an extensive and severe interstitial edema. Kerley's B lines may be present. At times an overall increase in density indicates the presence of an additional alveolar edema. Not all cases have shown the extensive parenchymal changes in the lungs. In the case described by Contis et al. (1967) the proximal pulmonary arteries were large and prominent and tapered rapidly towards the periphery, and the pulmonary parenchyma was quite clear. The changes in that case were highly suggestive of primary pulmonary hypertension. Associated cardiac defects, such as PDA, may modify the appearance of the lungs by providing an escape valve.

CARDIAC CATHETERIZATION. Right heart catheterization shows a moderate to marked increase in pressure in the right side of the heart and in the pulmonary artery. A wedge pressure should be obtained if possible in which case it will be found to be elevated. This, of course, would localize the obstruction either in the pulmonary veins or the left side of the heart. Every effort should be made to place the catheter in the left atrium. If the left atrial tracings are within normal limits, the mitral valve can be excluded as the site of obstruction and the possibility of a venous obstruction is suggested.

ANGIOGRAPHY. A selective injection into the right ventricle or preferably the pulmonary artery may demonstrate the pulmonary veins. Shone et al. (1962) in retrospect noted an unusual tortuosity of the pulmonary arteries and the pulmonary veins in the involved lobe of the lung and a constriction at the venoatrial junction. This was associated with a stagnation of the contrast substance in the distal portion of the involved veins. Singshinsuk et al. (1966) were also able to visualize the actual site of narrowing of the pulmonary veins. In the case of Henry et al. (1975) a localized dilatation of the right upper lobe vein suggested the presence of a severe stenosis.

The condition is susceptible to surgical correction (Kawashima et al., 1971). This condition can be confused with any of the obstructive lesions on the left side of the heart or anomalies of the pulmonary venous return, such as total anomalous venous return with subdiaphragmatic connection. Since it usually runs a fatal course and is susceptible to surgical correction, every effort should be made to arrive at a diagnosis.

ABNORMAL OR PERSISTENT OPENINGS BETWEEN RIGHT AND LEFT SIDES OF CIRCULATION

Usually Associated with Left-to-Right Shunt

1. In the Great Vessels
   a. Persistent Patency of the Ductus Arteriosus
      (1) Uncomplicated with Left to Right Shunt
      (2) Complicated with Reverse Flow

Patent Ductus Arteriosus. The ductus arteriosus is a normal structure during fetal life. It is the distal segment of the sixth aortic arch that persists after the proximal portion has united with the vascular system of the lungs. Thus, it may rarely be bilateral, although most often it is unilateral and on the left side (see section on anomalies of the aortic arch). In fetal life it performs a useful function in that it shunts blood from the pulmonary artery into the descending aorta thus bypassing the lungs. Shortly after birth the pressure gradient between the pulmonary artery and the aorta changes so that the shunt is reversed, and at about this time (1–2 days postpartum) the ductus normally begins to close. The reasons for closure are uncertain but seem related to the muscular structure of the walls of the ductus, responses to neurotransmitters such as acetylcholine, changes in the O_2 content of the pulmonary blood and perhaps some mechanical torsion of the ductus. Likewise, the reason why the ductus remains open in some instances is not known. Functionally the ductus is closed in the majority of persons at the end of 48 hours. When a significant opening persists beyond the first few weeks of life, it should properly be called a persistent patency of the ductus arteriosus (PDA).

A PDA is a short blood vessel that typically connects the left pulmonary artery just beyond the bifurcation of the pulmonary trunk with the descending aorta just beyond the origin of the left subclavian artery. A number of variations have been described often in association with a right or double aortic arch, and these are mentioned in the section on anomalies of the aortic arch. The ductus varies from 0.5–3 cm in length, and rarely it may be quite short and little more than a window between the two great vessels. The diameter is likewise variable, although in patients with symptoms it is rarely less than 5 mm. Occasionally, particularly in infancy, it is as large as the aorta.

PDA occurs occasionally with other major congenital anomalies, such as the tetralogy of Fallot, transposition of the great vessels, interruption of the aortic arch, pulmonary valvular atresia, and hypoplastic left heart syndrome. In these anomalies it often provides a compensatory shunt that may improve the efficiency of the circulation. In this section, however, we will deal in detail only with isolated PDA.

HEMODYNAMICS OF THE CIRCULATION. By the third week of life both the systolic and diastolic pressures in the aorta are well above those in the pulmonary artery. Consequently, in the usual case of PDA a continuous flow of blood from the aorta into the pulmonary artery occurs, and the flow rate is dependent on the size of the ductus and the pressure gradient between the two great vessels. Turbulence associated with the continuous flow of blood through the ductus is the cause of the typical Gibson murmur of uncomplicated PDA.

Burwell *et al.* (1940) measured the flow rate through the shunt in a number of symptomatic cases using blood samples obtained at operation. They found that 40–75% of the blood entering the ascending aorta was shunted into the pulmonary artery. Thus, the blood flow through the pulmonary vascular system was 2–3 times that of the systemic flow. The pulmonary vascular bed, however, has a large reserve capacity so that the pulmonary artery pressure is usually normal or only slightly elevated. It is only when the shunt is quite large and the pulmonary blood flow is 3 times that of the systemic flow that the pressure in the pulmonary artery begins to rise. Ligation of the ductus in these cases is followed by a return of the pulmonary artery pressure to a normal range. This hemodynamic pattern may be characterized as the usual one and is found in a large majority of cases of PDA.

The large increase in pulmonary blood flow greatly augments the flow of pulmonary venous blood to the left side of the heart. The left atrium is often dilated. The major burden of the circulation is on the left ventricle, and it is usually the chamber that enlarges, dilates and finally begins to fail in symptomatic cases. Associated with the greatly increased left ventricular output the ascending aorta and aortic arch are often dilated and show increased pulsations. The work of the right ventricle is not increased until pulmonary hypertension appears due either to left ventricular failure or increased pulmonary resistance or both. Right ventricular failure associated with PDA is thus a late occurrence. In the great majority of cases of PDA symptoms are due to a large increase in pulmonary blood flow associated with decreased pulmonary compliance and eventually left ventricular failure. This is associated with dyspnea and susceptibility to pulmonary infections. Pulmonary edema and congestion following left ventricular failure represent the final embarrassment to the pulmonary circulation and may be a cause of death, particularly in premature and young infants. The diminished systemic blood flow is often a cause of poor or delayed growth, susceptibility to infection, and lack of vigor.

Pulmonary hypertension in association with PDA should be considered as a complication, particularly when it approaches systemic pressure and when it is persistent. Pulmonary hypertension has been observed during infancy, and it has been known to spontaneously regress and often returns to normal following ligation of the ductus. In other cases, however, the pulmonary vascular resistance persists and pulmonary hypertension progresses to the point where the pulmonary artery pressure exceeds the aortic pressure. At this point a reversal of the shunt

through the ductus may occur. Also, cases have been observed in which the pulmonary artery pressure was normal during early life but later increased until it approached systemic levels. In all of these cases hemodynamic studies indicated an increase in resistance of the pulmonary vascular system, and this was associated with structural changes in the pulmonary arteries and arterioles.

Chapman and Robbins (1944) and Dammann *et al.* (1953) described patients with PDA in whom there was a marked increase in peripheral pulmonary resistance due to marked intimal proliferation of the media and small pulmonary arteries, muscular hypertrophy of the vessel walls, and numerous organized thrombi in many of the small arteries. A striking feature was the extensive recanalization of the thrombi resulting in numerous thin-walled vascular channels. All of these patients were adults, and the mean pulmonary artery pressures varied from 69–107 mm

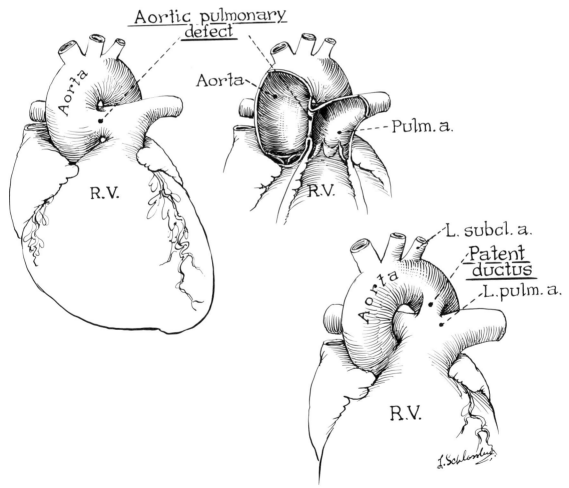

FIG. 181. PERSISTENT PATENCY OF DUCTUS ARTERIOSUS
Anatomical arrangements of patent ductus arteriosus and aortic-pulmonary defect.

Hg. Two etiologic factors seem likely, namely, a reaction of the pulmonary vascular system to the long period of increased blood flow and also damage due to the multiple pulmonary emboli or thrombi. These changes in the pulmonary vascular system are irreversible. The histories of these patients indicated that they had been asymptomatic during early life but cyanosis had supervened, usually in the second decade, and a reversed shunt through the ductus had occurred. Swan *et al.* (1954) were of the impression that large shunts to which the pulmonary artery is subjected and the dynamic factors involved in the production of the aortic pulse are likely to produce reactive changes in the pulmonary vascular system.

A somewhat comparable condition is seen in infants and young children with a PDA without a continuous murmur. Meyers *et al.* (1951) and Dammann and Sell (1952) studied a number of such cases, in all of which there was an elevation of pressure in the pulmonary artery. Some of these patients were slightly cyanotic while struggling or crying, and it is likely that there was a momentary reversal of the flow through the ductus. In this connection, Civins and Edwards (1951) studied the detailed structure of the intrapulmonary and intralobular arteries from late fetal life through the first 20 years. They found that at birth the ratio of the diameter of the lumen to that of the arterial wall in both the elastic and muscular arteries and arterioles was always < 1. Changes occurred in the arterioles beginning immediately after birth so that the lumens became progressively much wider. Changes in the other arteries occurred progressively to 20 years of age. These authors postulate that the reduction in pulmonary artery pressure normally is associated with changes in these arteries, and failure of these changes in the arterial walls may be associated with persistent hypertension.

Obstructions on the left side of the heart, such as mitral or aortic stenosis or obstruction of the pulmonary veins, may cause an increased pulmonary arterial pressure. Whatever the cause of the pulmonary hypertension, this may lead to a reversal of flow through the ductus and thus provide a distinctive, although not too easily diagnosed, entity (Taussig *et al.*, 1960). Abrams (1958) has aptly described all of these entities as "persistence of fetal ductus function after birth." Since venous blood reaches the descending aorta, some degree of cyanosis may occur in the lower portion of the body and even in the left arm.

The question as to the cause of pulmonary hypertension in association with PDA is of great practical importance. If the hypertension is due to irreversible changes in the pulmonary vascular bed with marked increased pulmonary resistance, ligation of the ductus may be disastrous since it acts as an escape valve. On the other hand, if the changes in the vascular bed are reversible or if the increase in pressure is mainly due to increased flow, then ligation may be followed by a reduction of pressure and beneficial results. In like manner, if the obstruction on the left side of the heart is the cause of the reverse flow, ligation of the ductus without correction of the primary defect would produce an unfavorable result. Selective angiography (injections into the pulmonary artery and aorta) and hemodynamic and electrocardiographic studies may aid in the resolution of these problems.

The radiologic signs of PDA vary in extent and degree in proportion to the severity of clinical manifestations and also to the age of the patient. Consequently, patients with PDA may be divided into the following clinical and radiologic groups:

1. those without symptoms. Attention is drawn to the anomaly because of the typical continuous murmur which may or may not be accompanied by a thrill. Radiologic signs are minimal or absent (Fig. 182).

2. full-term neonates and young infants in

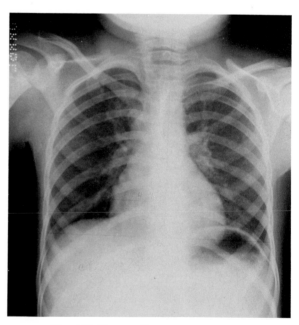

FIG. 182. PATENT DUCTUS ARTERIOSUS

This 7-year-old boy was completely asymptomatic, but there was a moderately loud continuous murmur just to the left of the sternum. The heart contour is normal, and there is only minimal enlargement of the lung vessels. (Operative case.)

whom the pulmonary blood flow is excessive and is followed by left ventricular failure and pulmonary edema. Prompt diagnosis is necessary, and surgical treatment may be indicated.

3. premature infants in whom the pulmonary blood flow remains excessive and is followed by heart failure. Of particular importance is the frequent association of PDA, respiratory distress syndrome, and prematurity. The abnormal pulmonary blood flow may be a crucial factor in the survival of the patient (Edmunds *et al.*, 1973; Thibeault *et al.*, 1975; Neal *et al.*, 1975; Lees, 1975).

4. older patients with symptoms of palpitation, dyspnea, delayed development and poor exercise tolerance. The diagnosis is made mainly on the basis of a continuous murmur. Radiological signs are often typical and helpful in confirming the diagnosis.

5. older patients without a typical murmur often with some evidence of cyanosis. This group comprises the so-called reversed ductus group and represents a distinct entity.

6. patients with evidence of subacute bacterial endocarditis presumably originating in and around the pulmonary artery end of the ductus. Radiological signs of embolism to the lungs may be present in addition to the usual signs of PDA.

7. postoperative cases in which some complication has developed, such as an aneurysm of the ligated ductus or recanalization.

Although the distribution of patients among the above-mentioned groups has changed during the past 30 years, in the authors' experience the majority of patients seen with a question of operative treatment fall into groups 2 and 3. Patients in group 4 might be designated as the typical symptomatic but uncomplicated PDA and are much less commonly encountered than previously apparently due to the impact of the wide availability of surgical treatment.

RADIOLOGIC FINDINGS. In premature, term and young infants the conventional chest films are much less specific than in older patients and adults with PDA. The most important observations are made on a series of frequently exposed chest films which show progressive cardiac enlargement, increased pulmonary vascularity and finally pulmonary edema. The heart is often globular in shape, although some left ventricular preponderance may be suspected. The intermediate convexity of the left heart border due to the enlarged pulmonary artery is often prominent. The left atrium is often moderately dilated, but this may be difficult to ascertain when associated with a large heart in an infant. The en-

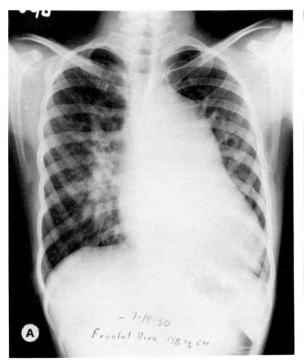 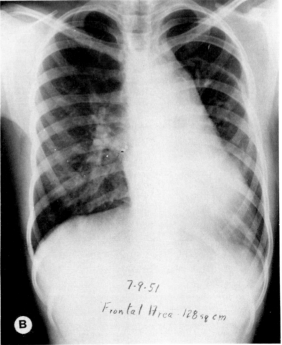

FIG. 183. PATENT DUCTUS ARTERIOSUS

(A) Preoperative appearance of a large patent ductus arteriosus. (B) Approximately 1 year postoperative. There has been a decrease in the size and a change in contour of the heart; also a marked decrease in pulmonary engorgement.

larged hilar arteries are frequently obscured by the enlarged heart and are thus difficult to evaluate.

In premature infants with the respiratory distress syndrome, the character of the pulmonary changes over a period of days may suggest a change in the circulatory dynamics. Initially the pulmonary vascular system is dilated due to the marked increase in blood flow. This inhibits respiratory motion and decreases pulmonary compliance. In a later stage left ventricular failure appears, and this is followed by pulmonary edema. A reticular pattern associated with the respiratory distress syndrome may be replaced by a more homogeneous pattern of alveolar pulmonary edema.

Echocardiography may be useful in detecting dilatation of the left atrium and ventricle and, combined with the progressively enlarging heart and the changes in the lungs, are highly suggestive of the diagnosis.

The condition of these infants is often precarious, and cardiac catheterization and aortography are a moderate risk. The most useful diagnostic procedure is retrograde aortography, and often this can be accomplished through a catheter inserted retrograde through one of the umbilical arteries and with the tip in the descending aorta near the orifice of the ductus. Thibeault *et al.* (1975) used this route and a single portable film exposed in the nursery. When the contrast substance injected into the descending aorta reached the peripheral pulmonary arteries in a sizeable quantity as shown on the single film the hemodynamic pattern of the ductus was verified. This procedure, although causing minimal risk to the patient, would seem to be subject to considerable technical variability and might easily fail to demonstrate a sizeable left to right shunt. The standard retrograde aortogram using serial filming will establish the diagnosis but is more hazardous.

Right heart catheterization also implies some hazards and is not always successful in demonstrating the volume of the shunt and the necessity for ligation of the ductus.

An increase in size of the left atrium as determined by echocardiography may confirm the impression that the shunt through the ductus has increased and is an important factor in the precarious condition of the patient (Capp, 1977).

In older children and young adults with symptoms of palpitation, dyspnea, delayed development and poor exercise tolerance (group 4) the radiologic signs are more specific. Nowadays, however, with the wide availability of diagnosis and surgical treatment the changes are rarely

striking. In frontal chest film the heart is usually enlarged but is rarely markedly enlarged. The left border is longer with a low apex. The pulmonary trunk and its major branches are dilated, and this produces a convexity of the left mid heart border. The degree of enlargement of the pulmonary trunk is usually less than that seen in ASD and may consist only of straightening of the left border. The lung vascularity is increased, and the hilar vessels may show some increased pulsations. Donovan *et al.* (1943) found that a hilar dance was found in about one-third of their clinical cases. In our experience this sign is infrequent and certainly much less common than with ASD.

An enlarged left atrium may produce an oval-shaped shadow superimposed on the base of the heart. It is almost never large enough to be borderforming on the right. The left atrial appendage is rarely noticeably dilated but occasionally contributes to a minor convexity on the left border of the heart. The best evidence of left atrial enlargement is the typical indentation or deviation of the barium-filled esophagus as seen in the far right oblique or lateral view. Enlargement of the left atrium indicates a low pulmonary resistance and a large flow.

A less frequent sign is increased prominence of the ascending aorta and the aortic knob. This is seen as a convexity to the right of the sternum and may be particularly well seen at fluoroscopy. In the authors' experience this finding occurs in no more than 20 percent of the cases depending somewhat upon the age of the patient and the volume of the pulmonary blood flow. When present it is of considerable diagnostic value in differentiating PDA from ASD and VSD and PAPVC (Table 10).

At the site of insertion of the ductus the descending aorta is often dilated with a funnel-shaped protrusion directed medially. This diverticulum-like structure can best be seen at aortography. The associated localized dilatation of the aorta is visible on plain films and has been designated as the infundibulum sign by Jönsson and Saltzman (1952). It consists of a convexity just below the aortic knob in the region where the aorta normally is straight (Figs. 184 and 185) as seen in the PA projection or in a slight degree of LAO. In the authors' experience this sign is infrequent, and Keats and Steinbach (1955) found it in approximately 25% of their cases. The infundibulum sign may be present, although the ductus is closed.

Careful postmortem examination shows that calcium is frequently found in the closed ductus (ligamentum arteriosum) (Jager and Wollenman,

TABLE 10

DIFFERENTIAL FEATURES THAT MAY BE DETECTED FROM CONVENTIONAL CHEST FILMS OF TYPICAL EXAMPLES OF COMMON CONDITIONS WITH LEFT-TO-RIGHT SHUNTS

	Atrial Septal Defect (ASD)	Ventricular Septal Defect (VSD)	Partial Anomalous Venous Return (PAVR)	Patent Ductus Arteriosus (PDA)
Right atrium	Enlarged fairly early	Not enlarged	Enlarged early	Not enlarged
Right ventricle	Enlarged early	Enlarged	Enlarged early	Not enlarged until after left ventricle is enlarged
Left atrium	Small	Often enlarged	Small	Often enlarged
Left ventricle	Small	Often enlarged	Small	Enlarged early
Ascending aorta and knob	Small	Small	Small	Normal or slightly enlarged
Pulmonary artery	Large, even aneurysmal in size	Large	Large	Large—rarely as large as in ASD
Hilar pulsations	Increased	Increased	Increased	Increased
Hilar dance	Common	Uncommon	Uncommon	Frequently—less common than ASD
Occasional specific findings			Abnormal venous shadows in lungs	Infundibulum, descending aorta

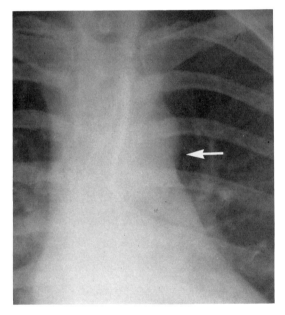

FIG. 184. INFUNDIBULUM OR SLIGHT LOCALIZED DILATATION OF AORTA ASSOCIATED WITH PERSISTENT PATENT DUCTUS ARTERIOSUS

The presence of an "infundibulum" has been inconstant in association with this condition.

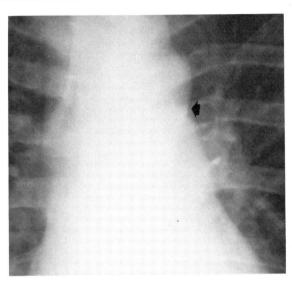

FIG. 185. INFUNDIBULUM (ARROW) OR SLIGHT BULGING OF AORTA AT SITE OF PERSISTENT PATENT DUCTUS ARTERIOSUS

Some prominence of the aortic knob is often seen, but presence of a typical infundibulum is unusual and not specific for a patent ductus.

1942). The amount is usually too small to expect detection by radiologic means. Weiss (1931) reported the presence of a curvilinear plaque of calcium in the aorta at the site of insertion of a patent ductus. A bacterial endocarditis was implanted at the pulmonary artery end of the ductus. Weiss (1931) suggested that the presence of calcium might be a useful radiologic sign of PDA. Dalith (1961) in an extensive study of the pattern of calcification in the region of the aortic arch found that the site of insertion of the ligamentum arteriosum had a different structure from the adjacent aorta and was the most frequent site of a calcified plaque.

Childe and McKenzie (1945) found a linear calcium deposit at postmortem examination approximately 1 cm long in an obliterated ductus in a 9-month-old child. They observed similar deposits on chest films in 3 other infants that seemed to be in a ligamentum as there was no evidence of a patent ductus. Currarino and Jackson (1970) surprisingly found a small deposit of calcium in the region of the ductus in the chest films of 75 children, and in 2 of these the presence of calcium was verified at operation for a PDA. The other 73 had no clinical evidence of a PDA. The calcium was often in the shape of a small dot 1–3 mm in diameter or less often a streak a few mm in length. Observation over a period of years in a few cases indicated that the calcium tended to decrease in size.

Other reports of calcium in a patent ductus are those of Keys and Shapiro (1943), 6 cases; Ruskin and Samuel (1950), 4 cases; and Margulis et al. (1954), 3 cases. All of these cases were in young adults predominantly females. The calcium was in the form of a segment of a circle, curvilinear, and usually a centimeter or more in length with the concavity facing upward and medially or occasionally laterally. The plaque was quite similar to those seen often in the aortic arch in patients over 50 years of age. Where there is a solitary plaque in a person under 30 years of age, it may have some significance as an indicator of either a PDA or a ligamentum arteriosum. The conclusions of Shapiro et al. (1963) seem justified. The presence of calcium in the region of a ductus even in a young person does not permit the assumption that the ductus is patent. The calcium may be in the aortic end of an obliterated ductus as was reported as a frequent occurrence by Dalith (1961).

Graham (1940) found calcium in an aneurysm of the ductus and reported on the unusual surgical hazards due to the presence of the calcium.

At fluoroscopy the heart is often unusually active, and the left ventricular and aortic pulsations are exaggerated. Steinberg et al. (1943) found occasional elevation of the main and left pulmonary arteries and attributed this to traction by the ductus. Keats and Steinbach (1955) found suggestive evidence of this sign in only 5 of their 100 cases, and the present authors feel that this is a sign of little consequence.

In the great majority of cases falling into group 4, the diagnosis of PDA can be made from the physical examination alone, and conventional chest films suffice to provide confirmatory information. Occasionally further studies, such as right heart catheterization and angiography, are indicated to detect or rule out associated defects, such as ASD or VSD, or to determine if pulmonary hypertension is present and sufficient to be a factor in surgical treatment. In neonates and infants where the physical signs are often indefinite, these procedures may be quite necessary for diagnosis.

Right Heart Catheterization. At right heart catheterization it is necessary to catheterize the pulmonary artery and obtain blood samples. These should show an increase in oxygen content of 1.5–2 volumes percent. Unfortunately, streamlining of blood flow from a high ventricular septal defect may produce an apparent increase in oxygen concentration in the pulmonary artery as compared with that in the right ventricle. Thus, this finding is not completely reliable. Also, some insufficiency of the pulmonary valve may cause

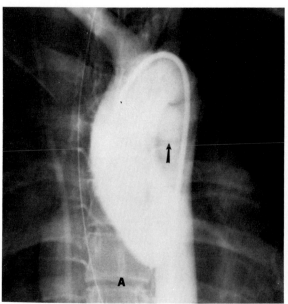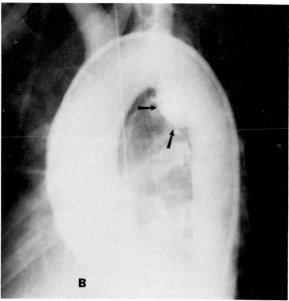

FIG. 186. DUCTUS DIVERTICULUM

An unusually large ductus diverticulum with a closed ductus in a young girl. A diverticulum of this size can be confused with an aneurysm.

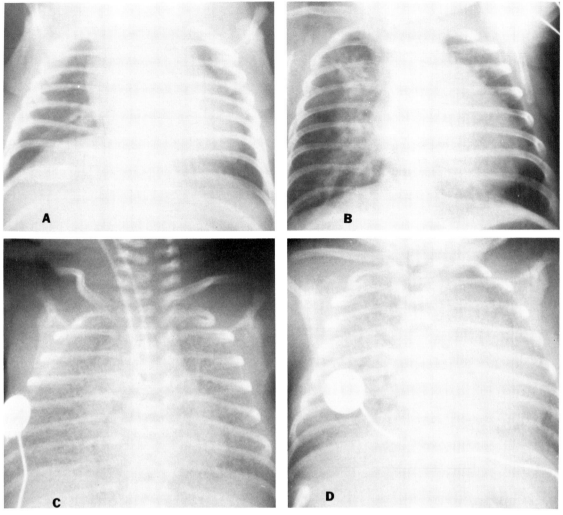

FIG. 187. RESPIRATORY DISTRESS SYNDROME
Respiratory distress syndrome in two premature infants complicated by persistent patency of the ductus arteriosus. (A) Chest film the day after birth in a premature infant with respiratory difficulty. (B) Three days later the heart has enlarged, and the increase in vascularity in right lung is striking and is suggestive evidence that a large shunt through the ductus contributes to patient's respiratory problems. (C) Chest film on day of birth of a premature infant with respiratory distress. (D) Two days later the heart has increased significantly in size, and the arterial system in right lung is dilated indicating a large flow through the ductus. (See text for discussion of confirmation of diagnosis.) (Courtesy of Dr. Leonard E. Swischuk.)

regurgitation of pulmonary artery blood into the right ventricle, and this may cause an increased oxygen content in samples aspirated from the outflow tract of the right ventricle. Dye dilution curves obtained from a peripheral artery during injection into the pulmonary artery may show a break indicating a left-to-right shunt, but the site is undetermined. The most definitive information is obtained by passing a catheter through the ductus into the descending aorta. Gas analyses of blood samples, both from the aorta and pulmonary artery, and pullback pressure tracings usually suffice to confirm the course of the catheter and establish the diagnosis unequivocally.

Angiography. Forward or venous angiocardiography is often misleading and should be rarely used. It will demonstrate a reverse flow through a ductus, but it rarely shows the left side of the heart sufficiently to evaluate possible associated anomalies. Goetz's (1951) sign, a clear radiolucent area seen in the apex of the opacified pulmonary artery, is highly suggestive of a PDA but is too inconstant to be of much use. It is due to dilution of the contrast substance in the pulmonary artery by the incoming nonopacified blood from the ductus.

A selective injection into the pulmonary artery is of some value in the complicated cases with reverse flow through the ductus. Enough contrast substance may reach the left side of the heart to permit evaluation of possible obstructive lesions which are an occasional cause of the reversed shunt.

The procedure of choice is aortography. Preferably the catheter tip should be placed in the descending aorta near the orifice of the ductus.

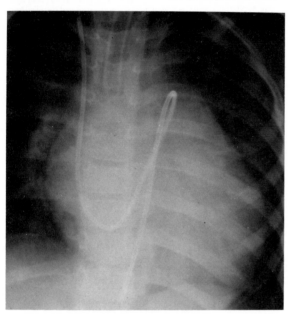

FIG. 188. TYPICAL APPEARANCE OF CATHETER THAT HAS PASSED THROUGH PERSISTENT PATENT DUCTUS FROM PULMONARY ARTERY INTO AORTA

The retrograde route through the femoral artery is preferable, although the brachial artery may be used, or in newborns, the umbilical artery. The injection of an appropriate amount of contrast substance (1 ml/kg) and serial filming in the right posterior oblique projection should be carried out. In the uncomplicated cases with a left to right shunt the ductus can often be visualized directly, and the opacification of the pulmonary vascular system confirms the shunt. Also, the density and extent of the opacification permit a gross evaluation of the volume of the shunt. A further attempt should be made to visualize the ascending aorta in order to exclude an associated aortic pulmonary window.

If there is evidence of a left-sided obstructive lesion, a left atrial, or if possible, a left ventricular injection should be done. Associated defects, such as ventricular septal defects which occur in about 10% of the cases, can be demonstrated by a left ventricular injection or occasionally strongly suspected from the hemodynamic studies and oxygen content of right ventricular blood.

Group 5 consists of patients with PDA with pulmonary hypertension and reverse flow. This condition is occasionally seen during infancy, but most of the cases have been over one year of age and frequently the patient is an adult. These patients have dyspnea, weakness, and ECG changes indicative of right heart hypertrophy and strain. Mild cyanosis may be noted, and this may be more intense in the lower portion of the body.

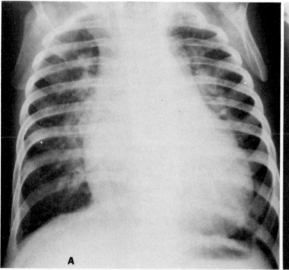

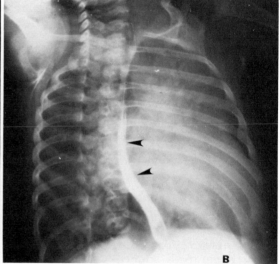

FIG. 189. PATENT DUCTUS

Patent ductus in a 2-year-old child with marked shortness of breath and heart failure. The left atrium is considerably dilated (Note deviation of esophagus).

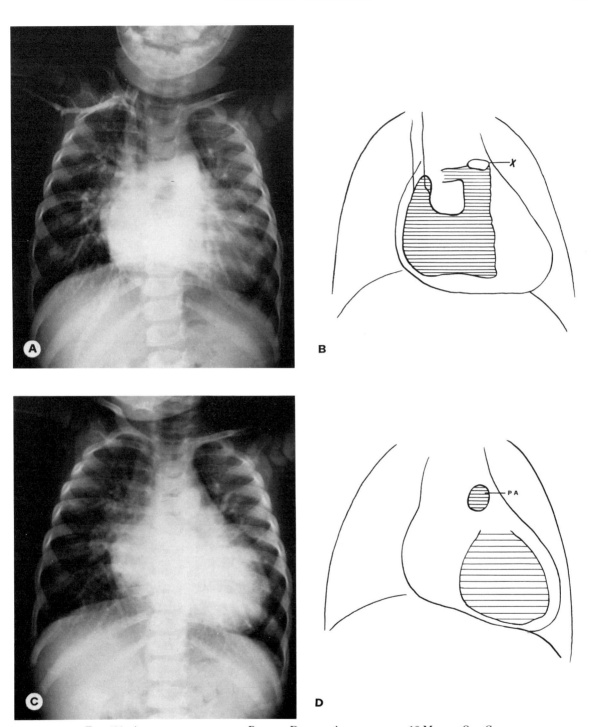

FIG. 190. ANGIOCARDIOGRAMS OF PATENT DUCTUS ARTERIOSUS IN 16-MONTH-OLD GIRL

There was a moderately loud systolic murmur in the third and fourth left interspaces but no diastolic component. (A) Film exposed at about 2 sec after injection of contrast material. There is a definite radiolucent area within the contrast substance in the pulmonary artery (Goetz's sign). (B) Sketch of A. X-radiolucent area as seen in A. (C) Film exposed at about 6 sec. There is reopacification of the pulmonary artery. (D) Sketch of C. PA, pulmonary artery. At operation the ductus was 1.4 cm in diameter.

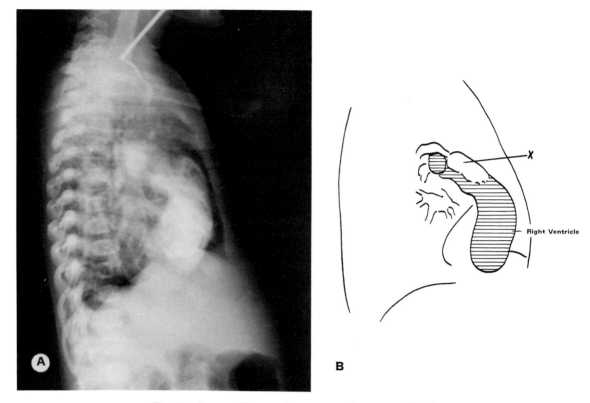

FIG. 191. PATENT DUCTUS ARTERIOSUS (OPERATIVE CASE)

(A) Lateral angiocardiogram (2 sec) showing radiolucent area in the pulmonary artery. (B) Sketch of A. X-area of radiolucency in the pulmonary artery.

Conventional chest films show that the heart is not very large, and frequently it may be normal in size. There is a considerable convexity of the left mid heart border indicating dilatation of the pulmonary artery. The right border of the heart is convex, and the lateral view may show intrusion of the cardiac shadow into the retrosternal space suggestive of right ventricular enlargement. The hilar branches are often large. The peripheral portions of the pulmonary vascular system are small, and truncation of the larger pulmonary arteries may be seen.

Right heart catheterization shows pulmonary hypertension that approaches that of the systemic circulation. Consequently, there may be very little increase in oxygen content in the pulmonary arterial blood. Again, passage of the catheter through the ductus with blood samples obtained from both the aorta and pulmonary artery are extremely helpful. A helpful diagnostic procedure is the simultaneous sampling of blood from the right radial artery and the femoral artery. It is not sufficient to draw blood from the left radial artery because blood passing through the ductus in a reverse direction may enter the left subclavian artery. If the oxygen content is significantly higher in the right arm than in the leg, then evidence of reverse flow through the ductus is strongly supported.

A selective injection into the right ventricle or pulmonary artery may show a reverse flow through the ductus. At times, however, the shunt is so well balanced that the flow in either direction through the ductus is minimal. The differential diagnosis in these cases rests between primary pulmonary hypertension, the Eisenmenger syndrome associated with ASD or VSD, and a few cases of transposition of the great vessels.

Group 6 consists of patients with subacute bacterial endocarditis. When endocarditis is engrafted upon a patent ductus it is usually localized near the opening of the ductus into the pulmonary artery. Consequently, infected emboli may be swept out into the pulmonary capillaries in large numbers where they cause small areas of inflammation and infarction. As seen on the conventional chest film, there may be many small areas, irregular, rounded or flame-shaped, and scattered through both lungs. When this occurs in the presence of pulmonary engorgement and cardiac enlargement, the radiologist is justified in suggesting endocarditis as a possibility.

Aneurysm of the pulmonary artery in association with a patent ductus is thought to occur in 1–2% of all cases (Keith *et al.*, 1958). In our experience this has been a rare complication.

Group 7 consists of patients with postoperative patent ductus arteriosus. Occasionally, an aneurysm may form in a ligated ductus. This will produce a shadow adjacent to the left upper heart border. It may not be sharply defined but continues to increase in size. A hematoma may produce a similar appearance, but it appears in the immediate postoperative period and should organize and shrink in a period of weeks. Angiography may be helpful in demonstrating the aneurysm (Fig. 197).

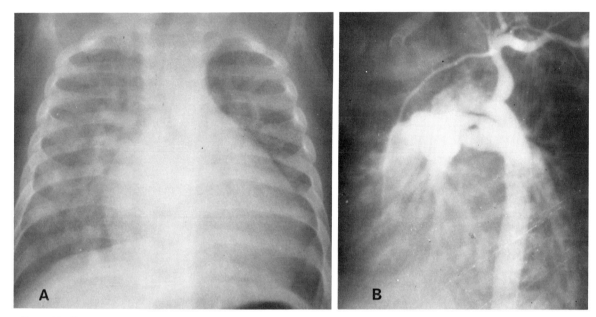

Fig. 192. Countercurrent Left Brachial Aortogram Showing Persistent Patency of Ductus Arteriosus
It is unusual to see the ductus so completely outlined.

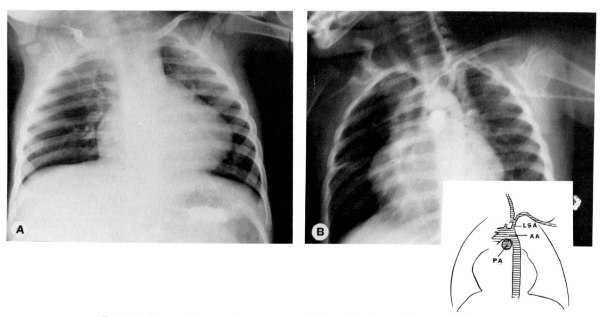

Fig. 193. Patent Ductus Arteriosus in 1-Year-Old Child (Operative Case)
The patient was having attacks of respiratory difficulty, and there was an atypical systolic murmur. (A) Conventional film. There was slight globular enlargement of the heart and only mild engorgement of the lung vascular system. (B) Countercurrent aortogram (left brachial artery). There is contrast substance in both aorta and pulmonary artery indicating a shunt between these two vessels. LSA, left subclavian artery; AA, aorta; PA, pulmonary artery.

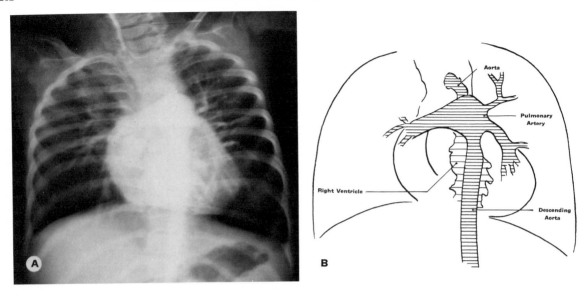

FIG. 194. PATENT DUCTUS WITH REVERSAL OF FLOW AND CONGENITAL MITRAL STENOSIS

Patient was 16-month-old child with cyanosis of the lower portion of the body and slight cyanosis of the left hand. (Autopsy case.) (A) Angiocardiogram at 2 sec. The contrast substance has passed from the right ventricle simultaneously into the pulmonary artery and descending aorta. A short segment of the aorta proximal to the ductus has also filled. (B) Sketch of A.

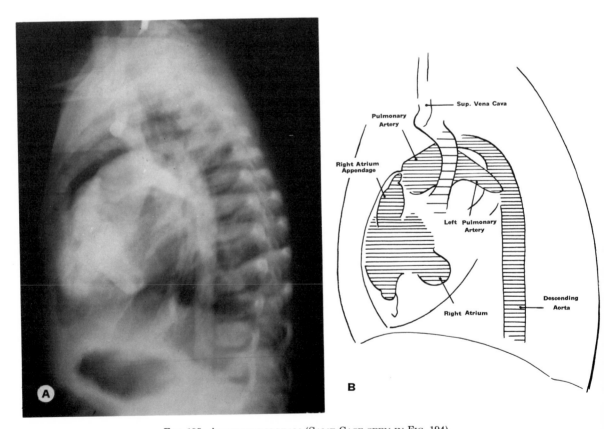

FIG. 195. ANGIOCARDIOGRAM (SAME CASE SEEN IN FIG. 194)

Lateral view showing filling of descending aorta and pulmonary arteries. Insufficient contrast material reached the left atrium to permit visualization.

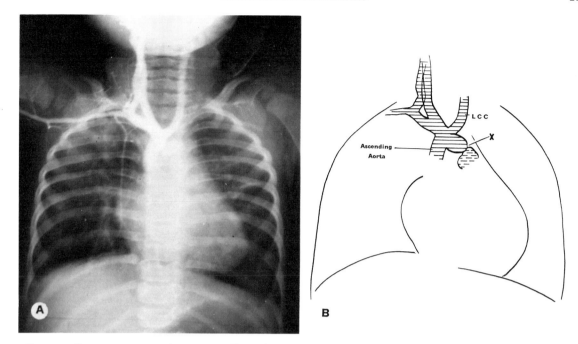

FIG. 196. COUNTERCURRENT AORTOGRAM USING RIGHT BRACHIAL ARTERY (SAME CASE AS FIGS. 194 AND 195)

The proximal portion of the left subclavian artery is not seen, but the brachial artery contains contrast material. The sudden change in density (X) in the contrast substance in the aorta led to an erroneous diagnosis of coarctation of the aorta. This appearance was due to the inflow of blood into the aorta from the patent ductus arteriosus.

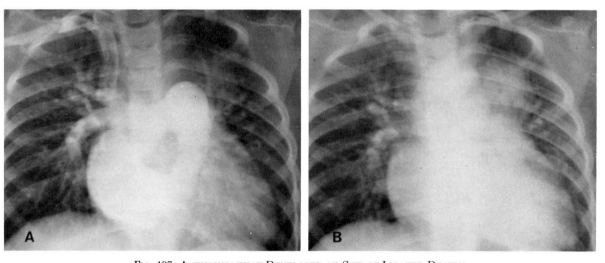

FIG. 197. ANEURYSM THAT DEVELOPED AT SITE OF LIGATED DUCTUS

(A) Right-sided angiocardiogram showing a mass adjacent to the pulmonary trunk. (B) Left-sided angiocardiogram showing faint opacification of the mass at the same time as the descending aorta.

POSTOPERATIVE CHANGES. Division of the ductus is the preferable procedure, although ligation may be appropriate in premature and young infants where the operation should not be prolonged and the condition of the patient is precarious. Following ligation or division of the ductus, a small amount of fluid commonly collects in the left pleural space but is rapidly absorbed. The left diaphragm rarely is elevated due to some paresis or paralysis of the phrenic nerve. If present, it usually improves in 6–8 weeks.

In the more clinically significant cases, there is definite radiological evidence of improvement of the cardiac status. Within a few days the pulse rate slows, and the ventricular pulsations become more nearly normal in amplitude and character. Moderately enlarged hearts usually show the greatest decrease in size. The decrease continues for several months and is accompanied by a decrease in lung vascularity. Donovan *et al.* (1943) have emphasized that the decrease in the transverse diameter of the heart postoperatively is not nearly so great as the decrease in the frontal area. This is due not only to the shape of the heart in PDA but also to the fact that the frontal area provides a more reliable estimate of heart size than the transverse diameter. The change in the clinical status and also the size of the heart and the pulmonary infiltrates in newborns and prematures are often striking. This may occur within a few days following ligation of the ductus.

Aortopulmonary Septal Defect. This entity is also known as aortopulmonary window, aortopulmonary fenestration and aortopulmonary defect. The anomaly is rare; Neufeld *et al.* (1962) found 60 cases reported in the literature and added six of their own.

ANATOMY. This anomaly is due to incomplete formation of the truncoconal septum that normally divides the primitive truncus into the pulmonary artery and aorta. The defect is a window which is usually 3–10 mm above the aortic valve ring and near the level of the orifices of the coronary arteries. In a case reported by Fletcher *et al.* (1954) the opening was higher in the first part of the aortic arch and in the case reported by Baronofsky *et al.* (1960) two defects were present. In the reported cases the openings have been oval or circular and varied in diameter from 5–30 mm or even larger. Anatomically, the condition resembles truncus arteriosus; however, it differs in that there is a normal pulmonary valve and an otherwise normal pulmonary artery. Also the interventricular septum is usually intact. In two of the cited cases (Morrow *et al.*, 1962) the right coronary artery originated from the pulmonary trunk.

Associated congenital defects as found in the 66 cases reviewed by Neufeld *et al.* (1962) were patent ductus arteriosus, 8 cases; coarctation of the thoracic aorta, 3 cases; bicuspid or fenestrated aortic valve, 2 cases; and one case each of ventricular septal defect, pulmonic stenosis, and atrial septal defect. An unusual variation was the association of aortopulmonary window with atresia of the aortic arch (Bellon *et al.*, 1974; Rosenquist *et al.*, 1974).

HEMODYNAMICS. The dynamics of the circulation are similar to those of PDA, but the deviation from normal is usually more severe. The shunt is typically from left to right, but because of the size of the window and its location in the ascending aorta the shunt is often quite large. All of the more recently reported cases have had a considerable elevation of the pulmonary artery pressure, and in two instances (Bosher, L.H., Jr. and McCue, 1962; Morrow *et al.*, 1962) a right-to-left shunt was demonstrated and a mild degree of peripheral desaturation was found. Thus, the dynamics may be compared with those of PDA with a reverse flow and those cases with the Eisenmenger syndrome. In the cases treated by surgical closure of the defect the pulmonary hypertension receded promptly indicating that a large flow was the cause of the hypertension. In two cases with a reversed flow, the evidence for permanent increase in pulmonary resistance was sufficient to suggest that surgical closure of the defect was inadvisable.

The age of the reported cases has varied from infancy to young adulthood. Survival beyond the age of 30 years is rare. The clinical profile may resemble PDA although Morrow *et al.* (1962) found a basal systolic murmur to be more common than the typical continuous murmur. Before the advent of the use of retrograde aortography confusion with patent ductus arteriosus was rather common (Gasul *et al.*, 1951).

RADIOLOGIC FINDINGS. Conventional chest films almost uniformly show some degree of cardiac enlargement. The left ventricle is the first chamber to enlarge but this is usually followed by enlargement of the right ventricle as the pulmonary artery pressure increases. The heart is therefore often globular in shape. The pulmonary trunk and pulmonary arteries are dilated indicating an increased pulmonary blood flow. The left atrium is often moderately enlarged. Bosher and McCue, (1962) make a point that only the ascending aorta is dilated in aortopulmonary septal defect in contrast to PDA where the entire aortic arch is dilated. This difference is seldom sufficient to permit a satisfactory differentiation however.

Cardiac catheterization. The hemodynamics are so similar to those of PDA that differentiation by right heart catheterization is seldom possible. Pulmonary insufficiency was found in two cases cited by Neufeld *et al.* (1962). This possibility makes precise location of the site of the left-to-right shunt even more difficult. At times the diagnosis can be strongly suspected from the course and position of the catheter seen during right heart catheterization. Dexter *et al.* (1947) were able to make the diagnosis in this manner. The catheter may pass from the right ventricle through the pulmonary valve and then through the ascending aorta and into the right carotid artery. This course is different from that taken by the catheter when it passes through a PDA in which case it may enter either the descending aorta or the left carotid or subclavian arteries but never the innominate or right carotid artery. It must be remembered that the catheter can enter the aorta from the right ventricle through the high ventricular septal defect and careful monitoring of pressures is necessary to be sure that the catheter has entered the aorta from the pulmonary artery rather than the right ventricle.

Angiography. Right ventricular injections are not usually diagnostic unless there is a reversal of the usual right-to-left shunt. The pulmonary artery may reopacify but this does not serve to differentiate the condition from PDA. The diagnostic procedure of choice is retrograde aortography with serial filming. Contrast substance injected into the root of the aorta will pass immediately into the pulmonary artery (Fig. 198). If countercurrent aortography is used in infants and young children the contrast substance must reflux backward to the region of the aortic valve for the examination to be satisfactory. The use of a catheter where it is possible is advantageous because the root of the aorta can be flooded with contrast substance with greater reliability. Also, in four cases cited by Morrow *et al.* (1962) a catheter was passed retrograde through the defect, and in three of these it was possible to enter the right ventricle. It should be remembered that contrast substance can enter the pulmonary artery very rapidly through a number of routes when contrast substance is injected into the ascending aorta. One of these is reflux through an incompetent aortic valve and then it may pass through a high septal defect into the outflow tract of the right ventricle. Also, the contrast substance may enter the pulmonary artery through a PDA. Consequently it is essential to have rapid serial filming in order to be sure that the contrast substance does not take one of these alternate routes instead of going through the supposed aortic pulmonary septal defect. Differentiation from truncus arteriosus at times is difficult. Cooley *et al.* (1967) make the point that the enlarged valve sinuses and a large orifice indicate a truncus arteriosus. In all cases where possible the catheter should be withdrawn to the descending aorta and a second injection should be made in which the contrast substance does not reach the ascending aorta. Thus an additional PDA may be diagnosed or ruled out. Lateral and left anterior oblique projections are preferred.

As indicated above the condition must be dif-

ferentiated from PDA, truncus arteriosus with an increased blood flow to the lungs, high ventricular septal defect and rupture of an aneurysm, the sinus of Valsalva into the outflow tract of the right ventricle. Before the advent of cardiopulmonary bypass procedures with hypothermia the repair of an aortopulmonary septal defect was a formidable procedure (Gross, 1953; Scott and Sabiston, 1953). Using modern surgical techniques the defect can be repaired with an acceptable mortality (Cooley *et al.*, 1957; Morrow *et al.*, 1962).

Aneurysm of a Sinus of Valsalva with Rupture into an Adjacent Cardiac Chamber. Congenital aneurysms of the sinuses of Valsalva were formerly thought to be rare. They are readily susceptible to radiologic diagnosis, however, particularly following rupture into one of the surrounding cardiac chambers. Likewise, they are susceptible to surgical treatment and cure. Under this stimulus, the number of reported cases in recent years has increased.

Some ambiguity has occurred in papers describing aneurysms of the sinuses of Valsalva due to differences in nomenclature. Figure 200, taken from Sakakibara and Konno (1962) compares the nomenclature that has been used through the years. We prefer the terms right, left, and noncoronary sinuses. The drawing in Figure 200 is also a good way to begin the study of the relative positions of the sinuses to the other cardiac chambers, although the reader is referred to the excellent papers by Edwards and Burchell (1957) and Sakakibara and Konno (1962) for a better understanding of the relationships that are necessary to understand the pathways that the aneurysms may take when they rupture. Also, a study of the isolated heart at autopsy is recommended.

The underlying defect is a failure of the medial coat of the aorta to meet or to be anchored in the aortic ring, thus leaving a weakened area in the aortic wall (Edwards and Burchell, 1957). The systemic blood pressure over a period of years causes the weakened area to bulge and eventually rupture. Abbott (1919) apparently was the first to propose that the origin of the aneurysm, particularly of the right and noncoronary sinuses, had a sound embryologic basis in that they occurred in an area of improper fusion and development of the right and left bulbar ridges associated with the division of the primitive truncus into the pulmonary trunk and the aorta. Sakakibara and Konno (1962) often observed in the normal heart an area of thinning and irregularity in the myocardium just beneath the right coronary and noncoronary cusps. The

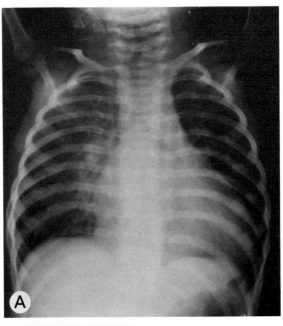

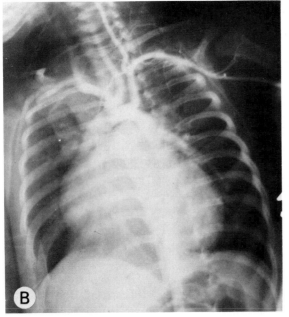

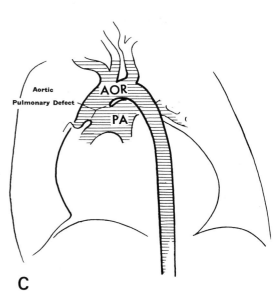

FIG. 198. AORTIC-PULMONARY DEFECT IN 18-MONTH-OLD BOY (OPERATIVE CASE)
(A) Conventional film showing slight cardiac enlargement and some engorgement of the lungs. (B) Countercurrent aortography (left brachial artery). (C) Sketch of B. AOR, aorta; PA, pulmonary artery.

slight irregularity in the tissue in this region often could be followed on into the base of the aorta and undoubtedly represented the site of fusion of the endocardial cushions and the dextro-dorsal and sinistroventral ridges. This explanation of the origin of the weakened area in the aorta also fits well with the other data collected by Sakakibara and Konno (1962) in which 20 of 52 aneurysms collected from the literature were associated with a VSD. They particularly refer to 19 of 40 aneurysms of the right coronary sinus which were associated with a high VSD. Since the left coronary sinus does not originate from the tissues that form the bulbar ridges, congenital aneurysms of this sinus should be quite rare or nonexistent. In their review, Sakakibara and Konno (1962) mentioned 4 such cases, but there is considerable doubt that these were of similar

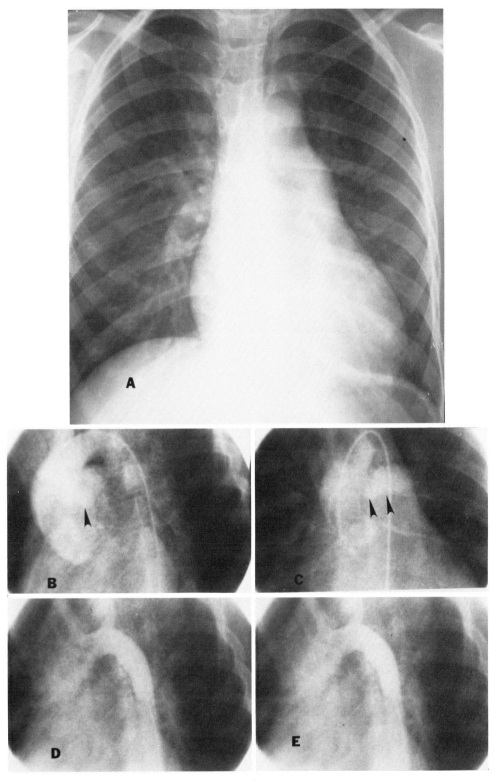

Fig. 199. Aorticopulmonary Septal Defect in a 10-Year-old Female with Moderate Limitation of Activity
(A) Left ventricle is considerably enlarged with low apex, and there is increased pulmonary vascularity. (B and C) Injection into ascending aorta shows rapid shunting into pulmonary arteries. (D and E) Injection into descending aorta does not show a shunt confirming the site of the shunt in the ascending aorta.

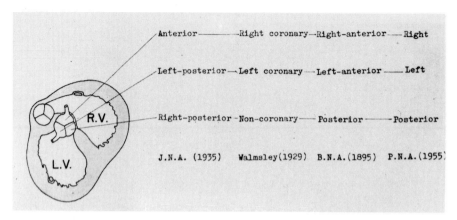

FIG. 200. NOMENCLATURE USED IN DESIGNATING CORONARY SINUSES

We prefer the nomenclature right coronary, left coronary, and noncoronary. (From Sakakibara and Konno (1962).

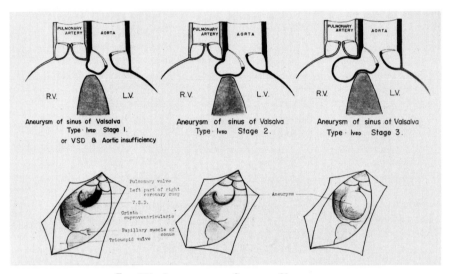

FIG. 201. ANEURYSM OF SINUS OF VALSALVA

This shows the relationship of a high ventricular septal defect with an aneurysm of the sinus of Valsalva and subluxation of the corresponding valve cusp. (From Sakakibara and Konno (1962).)

structure and origin to those reported in the right and noncoronary sinuses. A high VSD beneath the right coronary sinus or the noncoronary sinus prevents an adequate support for the corresponding aortic valve cusp. This is often followed by subluxation of the right valve cusp and aortic insufficiency.

Dilatation of the sinuses of Valsalva and the aortic root associated with Marfan's syndrome may likewise be considered as an aneurysm of the sinuses of Valsalva, but in such cases all of the aortic sinuses are usually dilated, and the aneurysm or aneurysms are not specifically limited to the sinuses and may involve the ascending aorta. The fundamental defect here is again in the aortic media but consists of cystic medial necrosis rather than an absence of the media. Aortic sinus aneurysms associated with coarcta-

tion of the aorta should also be mentioned since they may be considered as congenital in origin. We are unaware of any detailed study of the wall of the aorta in such cases, but the evidence suggests that the aneurysms are secondary to the marked increase in blood pressure. They are undoubtedly more susceptible to rupture than the normal aorta; however, they are somewhat different from the strictly congenital aneurysms that have been described in the literature.

The site of the aneurysm obviously determines to a considerable degree the location and direction of the fistula that follows rupture. It is convenient to divide each sinus into three parts. Aneurysms with the openings in each of the three parts of each sinus have a predilection for rupture into certain structures and chambers, although this can by no means be certain in any particular case. The common sites of rupture are listed as follows:

Right Coronary Sinus

Anterior one-third into the left ventricle (quite rare) or outflow tract of right ventricle above the crista supraventricularis and below the pulmonary valve.

Middle one-third into the right ventricle.

Posterior one-third in right ventricle or right atrium.

Posterior or Noncoronary Sinus

Anterior one-third into the right ventricle or right atrium.

Middle one-third into the right or left atrium.

Left one-third into the left atrium.

The left coronary sinus, anterior or right one-third, is in relation to the interventricular septum and may rupture into the right ventricle. The middle one-third is not related to any cardiac structure and would most likely rupture into the pericardium. The posterior one-third is in relationship with the mitral valve. These latter aneurysms may be atypical in their origin and may actually be false aneurysms.

Earlier reports (Abbott, 1919; Morrow, 1957; Sakakibara and Konno, 1962) suggested that aneurysms of the sinuses of Valsalva produced no symptoms until rupture occurred and that this was often delayed until the second or third decade. Also, rupture was thought to usually produce dramatic signs and symptoms of precordial distress and weakness followed by pulmonary congestion and heart failure. More recent reports (Howard *et al.*, 1973; Morgan *et al.*, 1972) indicated that a considerable proportion of the cases may be asymptomatic, and in a number of those reported the only physical sign was that of a heart murmur. Several of the patients of Morgan *et al.* (1972) are known to have had murmurs since early life, and presumably the fistula between the aneurysm and the heart chamber was present during this period. Also, associated lesions are quite common and may dominate the clinical picture and physical findings. Nine of the 26 cases reported by Howard *et al.* (1973) had a membranous ventricular septal defect, and 4 had aortic insufficiency. In addition, in 4 cases in which the aneurysm had ruptured, it was considered an incidental finding. Only 5 of the 26 cases had anything resembling a sudden onset of symptoms.

In the uncomplicated case with a typical rather abrupt onset of symptoms (Fig. 203), the diagnosis may be easy. A to-and-fro systolic-diastolic murmur is often present to the right of the sternum associated with a bounding pulse and increased pulse pressure. The differential diagnosis includes coronary artery right ventricular fistula, patent ductus arteriosus, some cases of truncus arteriosus, and some cases of high VSD with aortic regurgitation.

RADIOLOGIC FINDINGS. Since the sinuses of

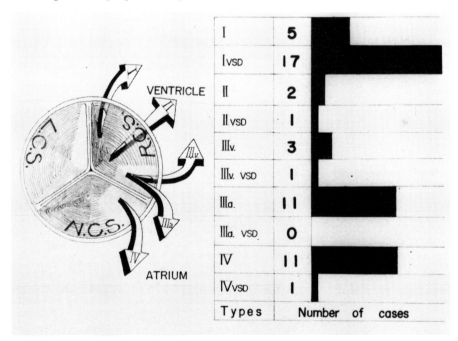

FIG. 202. ANEURYSM OF SINUS OF VALSALVA

Site of 42 cases of congenital aneurysms of the sinuses of Valsalva and the chamber into which they ruptured. The incidence of associated high ventricular septal defect is also shown. (From Sakakibara and Konno (1962).)

Valsalva lie deep within the heart, aneurysms of these structures produce no change in the cardiac contour until rupture occurs or unless there is another associated lesion. After rupture, depending on the size of the shunt, the heart enlarges, the pulmonary blood flow is increased, and the lungs become engorged. The right heart receives the shunted blood and enlarges; later the left ventricle is also overloaded and may be enlarged. The rapidity of development of cardiac enlargement depends considerably on the presence of associated defects and, of course, the size of the shunt. After a variable period of time, the heart may enlarge and fail and produce typical congestive changes in the lungs.

Right heart catheterization will show an increase in oxygen content between the vena cava and the right atrium or right ventricle, depending on the site of the rupture. This does not establish the diagnosis since the same findings can occur with an ASD or VSD or a coronary artery fistula. The most definitive procedure is supravalvular retrograde aortography with rapid direct filming or cine recording. Frontal and lateral projections are satisfactory, but we prefer at least one view in the LAO at about 45° of rotation. This projection brings the ventricular septum into profile and is thus useful in detecting small accompanying VSDs. With the supravalvular injection an aneurysm is usually distended, and a jet will often demonstrate the site of the rupture and the chamber into which the rupture has occured. Morgan *et al.* (1972) indicated that a catheter could be passed through the sinus and into the right side of the heart or in a reverse direction from the right side of the heart into the sinus, but this procedure is not necessary or recommended.

When an aneurysm of the sinus of Valsalva is associated with insufficiency of the right or posterior aortic cusp and/or a high ventricular septal defect, the diagnosis becomes much more difficult, and unfortunately a considerable proportion of cases are of this type. Thirty-five millimeter cine angiograms with filming at 60 frames/sec are desirable. Left ventriculography in the left anterior oblique projection will show the high ventricular septal defect accentuated usually in systole and visible before the sinuses of Valsalva have been filled with the contrast substance. This should clearly establish the diagnosis of ventricular septal defect. However, a shunt through a ruptured sinus of Valsalva may then be difficult to identify after contrast substance has already entered the right ventricle through the ventricular septal defect. Consequently, a subsequent supravalvular injection is needed to detect or rule out an associated rupture of the aneurysm of the sinus. This may, however, show the sinus, but if there is an accompanying insufficiency, it is often difficult to tell whether the contrast substance entered the right ventricle through a sinus between the aneurysm and the right ventricle or through a high ventricular septal defect. In the presence of all three lesions, it may be difficult to be sure that a ruptured sinus of Valsalva is present or to exclude this possibility. The surgeon should be warned that a repair of all three lesions may be required. Ventriculography and aortography exclude the other diagnostic possibilities, such as PDA and coronary artery-right ventricular fistula.

Repair of a ruptured sinus of Valsalva by surgical means is usually quite satisfactory (Morrow *et al.*, 1957; Howard *et al.*, 1973; Szweda *et al.*, 1962). The more complicated cases with associated VSD and aortic insufficiency present more formidable problems in surgical management.

Other lesions which complicate a ruptured sinus of Valsalva are pulmonic stenosis, coarctation of the aorta, tetralogy of Fallot, subaortic stenosis, and unicommissural aortic valve.

Partial Anomalous Pulmonary Venous Connection (PAPVC). During the early development of the embryo, the trachea, bronchi, and lungs are part of the primitive foregut and receive a common blood supply from the splanchnic plexus. The venous connections of this plexus are numerous and involve the anterior and posterior cardinal, umbilical, and omphalomesenteric veins. As development continues an out-pouching of the left atrium occurs and extends so as to connect with the venous radicles of the adjacent splanchnic plexus. This out-pouching of the left atrium is known as the common pulmonary vein, and normally as development continues, it is entirely incorporated into the left atrium. As blood begins to flow from the splanchnic plexus into the left atrium, the connections with the systemic veins atrophy so that in the definitive condition four or sometimes five veins carry all (except that carried by the bronchial veins) of the pulmonary blood into the left atrium. With the development and involution of so many vascular structures required for normal development, the possibilities for anomalous return of the pulmonary venous blood to the heart, systemic or portal veins are quite large.

The most severe anomaly occurs when the common pulmonary vein fails to unite with the venous plexus. All of the pulmonary blood must then return to the right side of the heart either by a circuitous route through the systemic, hepatic or portal venous system or directly to the

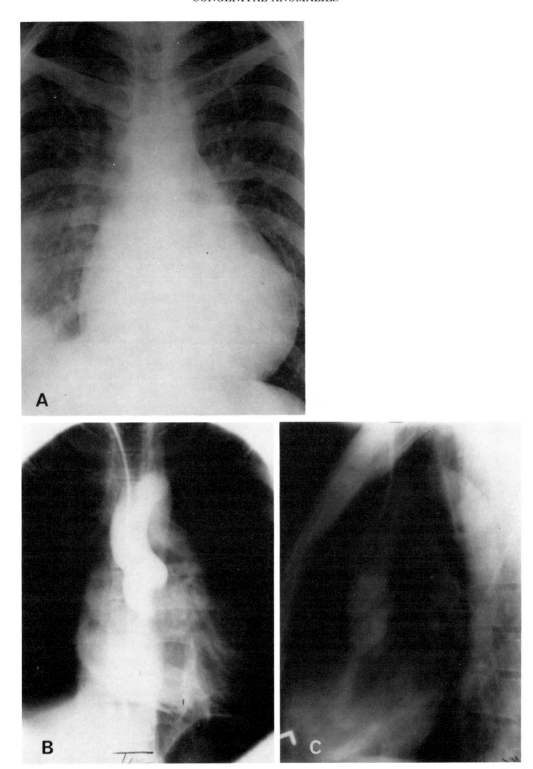

FIG. 203. ANEURYSM OF RIGHT SINUS OF VALSALVA WITH RUPTURE INTO RIGHT ATRIUM (OPERATIVE CASE)
The patient was 27 years old with signs and symptoms of heart failure. (A) Preoperative chest film showing cardiac enlargement involving both ventricles. (B and C) Aortograms after the supravalvular injection of 60 ml of contrast substance. The aneurysm of the right sinus is filled with contrast substance, and a jet is seen entering the right atrium. (From Dr. A. G. Morrow, *Circulation, 16:* 533, 1957.)

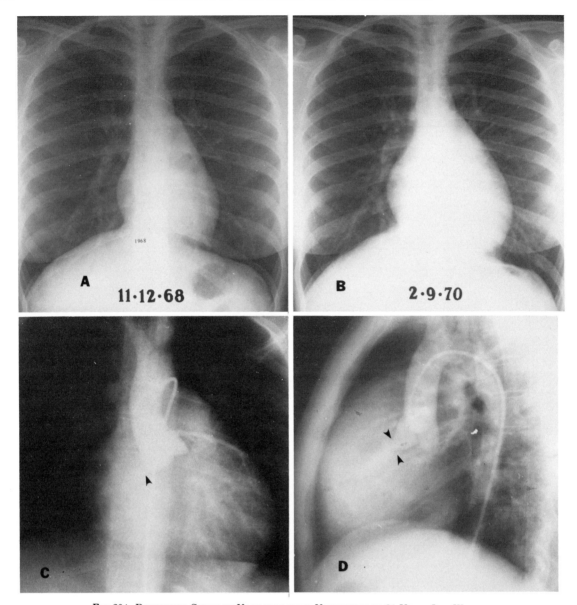

FIG 204. RUPTURED SINUS OF VALSALVA INTO VENTRICLE IN 21-YEAR-OLD WOMAN
(A) Film exposed before rupture. (B) Five days after onset of mild symptoms of dyspnea and discomfort in chest. (C and D) Frontal and lateral aortic root injections showing shunt from aortic sinus into right ventricle.

right atrium. This produces a condition known as total anomalous pulmonary venous connection (TAPVC), and this will be considered in a separate section (see page 356). Although TAPVC is anatomically similar to PAPVC, hemodynamically it is different in that it is associated with a variable but usually substantial right to left shunt in addition to a left to right shunt.

PAPVC because of the numerous anastomoses of the primitive venous plexus has a wide range of possibilities. Anomalous connections of the veins of the right lung are considerably more common than those of the left lung (Brody, 1942;

Dotter et al., 1949). A common arrangement is drainage of the right upper and middle lobe veins into the superior vena cava or more rarely the azygos vein. Another common arrangement is the separate entry of two or three veins from the right lung into the posterior wall of the right atrium and usually near the junction with the superior vena cava.

Veins from the left lung often enter a left-sided vertical vein (this may be the remnant of the primitive anterior cardinal vein) which drains into the left innominate vein. A less common variation is drainage into a left-sided superior vena cava or directly into the coronary sinus. An isolated venous connection from the left lung is rare (Kalke *et al.*, 1967). A rarer arrangement of special interest is the drainage of all or most of the veins of the right lung into a single channel which enters the inferior vena cava. This produces the "scimitar syndrome" (Neill *et al.*, 1960) and will be discussed below. A single case of drainage of the veins of the left lung into the inferior vena cava has been described (D'Cruz and Arcilla, 1964).

The incidence of PAPVC varies from 0.4–0.7% of cases of congenital heart disease (Healey, 1952; Hughes and Rumore, 1944; Kalke *et al.*, 1967). It was found in 14.5% of cases of secundum atrial septal defect in the series of Kalke *et al.* (1967). In the same series an ASD or PFO was found in 51 of 57 of the cases of PAPVC.

Anomalous connection of one or more pulmonary veins produces a left to right shunt. Oxygenated blood that normally would be returned to the left atrium and ventricle and distributed to the systemic circulation is instead recirculated through the right side of the heart and the lungs. Since the right ventricle must propel this increased minute volume of blood, it dilates and hypertrophies, and this is usually followed by dilatation of the right atrium. Changes in the heart and clinical signs and symptoms are proportional to the volume of this left to right shunt which, in turn, depends upon the size and number of the anomalous veins.

Since the large majority of patients with PAPVC have an associated ASD, the left to right shunts due to each defect are additive. Physiological studies (Dexter, 1950; Friedenberg, 1959) indicate that up to one-half of the pulmonary venous blood could be shunted to the right side of the heart without increasing the pulmonary artery pressure. Consequently, where only one or two veins or even the entire drainage from one lung is returned to the right atrium, there has been little clinical evidence of the anomaly. However, since a functional ASD is a common associated anomaly, a large majority of reported cases have had symptoms (Kalke *et al.*, 1967). The symptoms are similar to those of ASD, namely shortness of breath, easy fatigability, frequent upper respiratory infections, failure to thrive and occasionally cyanosis upon exertion. Even though the individual with the isolated anomaly may be completely asymptomatic, its presence can be a threat to health or life. Atelectasis, pneumothorax, extensive disease or surgical removal of the opposite or sound lung may bring severe disability or death.

PAPVC is occasionally seen in association with other major cardiac anomalies, such as PDA and tetralogy of Fallot (Dalith and Neufeld, 1960; Kiely *et al.*, 1967).

RADIOLOGIC FINDINGS. Conventional chest films are rarely specific except in the rarer cases with the "scimitar syndrome." In symptomatic patients the right atrium, ventricle, and pulmonary outflow tract are enlarged. The changes are identical to those seen in ASD. The proximal pulmonary arteries are dilated. The peripheral arteries are also enlarged unless pulmonary hypertension or the Eisenmenger syndrome supervenes. A localized increase in vascularity in the portion of the lung which has the anomalous connection has been reported (Dalith and Neufeld, 1960) but is an inconsistant finding. The left atrium is not enlarged and in most instances is smaller than normal. The aorta is relatively small.

A localized widening of the superior vena cava beginning at the site of entry of the anomalous veins or a localized bulging near the junction of the superior vena cava with the right atrium may suggest the diagnosis. Localized enlargement of the azygos vein may suggest the diagnosis. Where the right lower lobe veins enter the right atrium, a disorganized vascular pattern with increased obliquity of the vascular structures has been reported (Dalith and Neufeld, 1960). Tomography in frontal and oblique projections may show these structures to better advantage and increase the suspicion of the presence of PAPVC, but these findings are not diagnostic. Widening or convexity of the left upper mediastinum may indicate the presence of a left superior vena cava or a vertical vein and in the appropriate circumstances may raise a suspicion of anomalous connection of the veins of the left lung.

Where the anomalous connection is with the innominate vein or the superior vena cava, careful sampling from various sites along the route to the right atrium may show a substantial increase in oxygen content (1.5 to 2 volumes percent) and is highly suggestive of the diagnosis. Occasionally the catheter may enter one or more such veins, and the diagnosis is thus firmly established. Where the anomalous connection is with the right atrium and is associated with an ASD, confirmation of the diagnosis is difficult. Occasionally a catheter placed in the right atrium will pass into a pulmonary vein (Fig. 209). This finding must be interpreted with caution since the catheter may have entered the left atrium before entering the pulmonary vein.

Venous angiography may occasionally cause reflux of the contrast substance from the vena cava into an anomalous pulmonary vein. Selec-

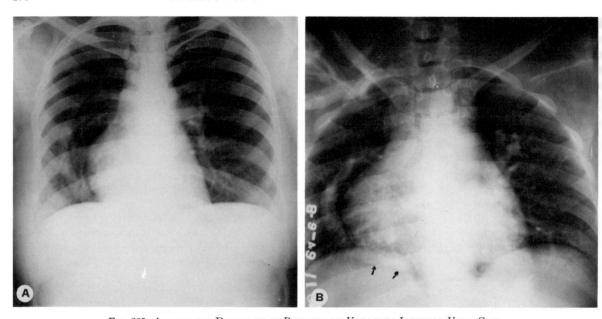

FIG. 205. ANOMALOUS DRAINAGE OF PULMONARY VEIN INTO INFERIOR VENA CAVA
The large vessel coursing in the shape of a sickle through the right lung presumably is carrying oxygenated blood into the inferior vena cava. (A) Conventional film. (B) Angiocardiogram about 5 sec after injection of contrast substance. (Courtesy of Dr. Victor A. McKusick.)

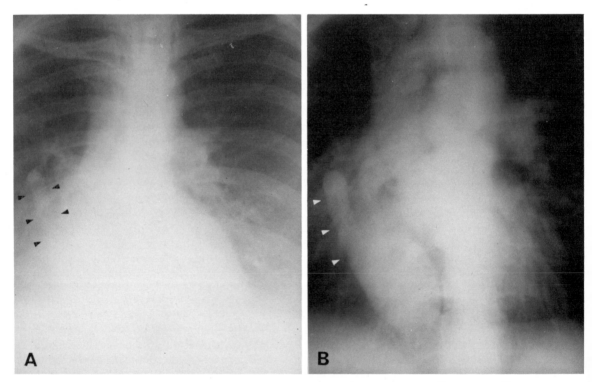

FIG. 206. PARTIAL ANOMALOUS VENOUS RETURN, QUESTIONABLY ASSOCIATED WITH CONGENITAL PULMONARY ARTERIOVENOUS FISTULA (UNPROVED)
(A) Posteroanterior roentgenogram of a 35-year-old woman with no symptoms referable to the chest. Black arrows point to an abnormal vascular structure in the right lower lung. (B) Venous angiocardiogram in the frontal projection. The left chambers and aorta are filled. White arrows point to an anomalous pulmonary vein returning blood and contrast material to and reopacifying the right atrium. This venous channel filled early, before filling of the other pulmonary veins, raising the additional possibility of pulmonary arteriovenous fistula.

tive angiography, preferably with injection into the right ventricle or pulmonary artery, may demonstrate the anomalous venous connection where they enter at a site remote from the right atrium, such as the superior vena cava or left vertical vein. Where the connection is with the right atrium, the findings are often inconclusive. In association with ASD, selective injections of dye into the right and left pulmonary arteries with peripheral sampling must be interpreted with caution because of the selective shunting of blood from the right lung through the ASD (Swan *et al.*, 1953). The same applies to selective injections of contrast substance at angiography. Fortunately, preoperative diagnosis is not quite as crucial as previously since surgical correction is usually possible at the time of repair of ASD using cardiopulmonary bypass (Bahnson *et al.*, 1958).

The Scimitar Syndrome. Anomalous venous drainage of the right lung into the inferior vena cava has special features that require separate consideration. The anomaly was first recognized and diagnosed prior to surgery or autopsy by Dotter *et al.* (1949). The term "scimitar syndrome" was used by Neill *et al.* (1960) because of the frequency of a number of associated anomalies and the resemblance of the band-like shadow adjacent to the right heart border to a scimitar.

The anomalous vein, which is a major feature of this syndrome, receives blood from one, two or often three major pulmonary veins. It descends in the major pulmonary fissure more or less parallel to the right heart border and joins the inferior vena cava usually after piercing the diaphragm or less often it may join the cava just above the diaphragm.

The special features are the frequency of dysplasia of other elements of the right lung. The entire right lung is usually decreased in size. The right pulmonary artery is frequently reduced in size and may supply only a portion of the right lung, usually the upper part. Systemic arteries arising from the thoracic or upper abdominal aorta and bronchial arteries may supply the remainder of the lung parenchyma. The bronchial pattern is often distorted. The middle lobe bronchus may be absent so that there is a resemblance to the arrangement of the left lung (Halasz *et al.*, 1956). Major bronchi may be absent or compressed or distorted. Occasionally diverticula or cystic changes of the bronchi with resultant cavities have been found.

Differential pulmonary function studies and oxygen content of blood obtained from various sources including the anomalous vein in a few cases (Kiely *et al.*, 1967; McKusick and Cooley, 1955) indicate that the blood flow through the dysplastic lung is diminished. The lung still continued to function substantially as a gaseous exchange organ although in reduced amount.

RADIOLOGIC FINDINGS. The hallmark of this syndrome is a band-like shadow adjacent to the right heart border as seen on conventional chest films. In the lateral view the shadow may be identified more commonly in the middle one-third of the thorax but occasionally in the anterior one-third (Dalith and Neufeld, 1960). The scimitar shadow is not always readily identified on the chest film. It may be quite close to the right heart border or atypical in its course or aeration of the dysplastic lung may be diminished so that contrast is insufficient to make the vein visible. Tomography may be helpful (Dalith and Neufeld, 1960; Koch and Silva, 1960). The heart and trachea are often displaced to the right probably due to the small size of the right lung. The right hilar shadow is often small or atypical in appearance indicating the small size of the pulmonary artery. The right diaphragm is often unusually high.

Angiography with injection into the right ventricle or pulmonary artery will demonstrate the vascular pattern of the right lung, and the opacification of the anomalous vein confirms the diagnosis. Later films may show systemic arteries supplying a portion of the right lung.

Right heart catheterization with selective sampling of blood drawn from the inferior vena cava

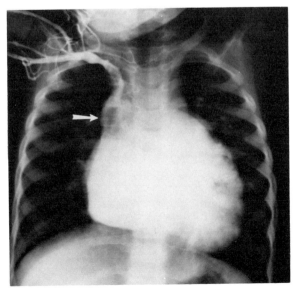

FIG. 207. PARTIAL ANOMALOUS VENOUS CONNECTION Venous angiogram showing abrupt widening of superior vena cava and radiolucent streamlining of nonopaque blood from the large anomalous vein.

may show an increased oxygen content, but this finding is often difficult to evaluate because of streamlining of blood from the kidneys. Occasionally the catheter may enter the anomalous vein and demonstrate its course. The blood in the vein has always been fully saturated (Kiley et al., 1967).

Patients with the scimitar syndrome have had an increased incidence of major associated cardiovascular defects, namely tetralogy of Fallot, patent ductus arteriosus, and coarctation of the thoracic aorta (Jue et al., 1966).

Patients with this condition are usually in their teens or adults. A majority have had symptoms, although these are often mild. The most common symptoms are dyspnea on exertion and increased fatigability. Surgical treatment has been reported but is seldom indicated (Koch and Silva, 1960; Goor and Lillehei, 1975).

Atrial Septal Defect (ASD). An atrial septal defect is commonly associated with many other congenital anomalies such as transposition of the great vessels and pulmonic stenosis; often it serves a compensatory function. In this section, however, only the changes associated with an isolated atrial septal defect will be considered.

The recorded incidence of atrial septal defect varies but is approximately one case of ASD in every 2,000 live births (Moss and Siassi, 1971). It accounts for 6–7% of all congenital heart defects and is the commonest congenital defect in adults. Ventricular septal defect is the commonest congenital heart lesion in children but is relatively rare in adults, probably because of spontaneous closure of defects in the ventricular septum in a sizeable proportion of patients. Spontaneous closure of atrial septal defects is distinctly uncommon. The average life expectancy for patients with ASD is 36–49 years, but in the absence of pulmonary hypertension it may be 50–60 years. The oldest recorded age of a patient with an atrial septal defect is 84 years. It is clear that progressive disability occurs with advancing age in a significant proportion of patients with ASD (Moss and Siassi, 1971).

Some degree of "probe patency" of the foramen ovale is found at autopsy in 20–25% of adults (Edwards, 1953). Because of the normally slightly greater pressure in the left as compared with the right atrium, the valve flap is held against the margins of the foramen ovale producing a functional closure. At times, the valve is anatomically incomplete or absent leaving a small opening. In the majority of these cases, however, there will be no definite evidence of a disturbance of the heart or circulatory dynamics.

Distention of the right atrium may stretch the foramen ovale and its valve so that it becomes patent, or it may enlarge an already small opening. This change is usually secondary to some mechanical obstruction in the right side of the heart and is considered elsewhere.

Anatomical classification of atrial septal defects is of considerable practical importance because of differences in the approach to surgical treatment. In addition, the clinical and electrocardiographic findings vary somewhat with each type. The following classification is modified from Ross (1956):

1. Ostium secundum defects.
2. Sinus venosus defects.
3. Ostium primum defects.
4. Common atrium.

The anatomy of atrial septal defects is variable, and two or more defects of different types are common. The reader is referred to the section on embryology for a review of the development of the interatrial septum and the foramen ovale.

OSTIUM SECUNDUM DEFECTS. The majority of atrial defects are of this type (DuShane et al., 1960; Lewis et al., 1955). The reader should remember that the septum secundum is to the right of the septum primum and that the foramen ovale is due to an opening in the septum secundum that is covered by an upper extension of the septum primum. The majority of defects of this type are adjacent to or involve the foramen ovale and are classified by some (Kjellberg et al., 1958) as foramen ovale defects. A common arrangement is for the foramen ovale to extend upward and posterior so that the valve is insufficient to cover the opening. Another arrangement is a resorption of the septum primum so that a fenestrated valve results leaving a sizeable effective opening, particularly when associated with some underdevelopment of the septum secundum. Rarely the defect may extend downward and posterior so that it lies near the opening of the inferior vena cava, and defects of this type offer special problems in closure.

Most symptomatic defects are 2 cm or larger in diameter, and defects smaller than this are often of minor significance. Multiple defects are common, and several smaller defects, both above and below the foramen ovale, produce the same hemodynamic changes as a large single defect.

SINUS VENOSUS DEFECTS. The recognition of these defects is important because of their frequent association with partial anomalous venous return and the care required in the surgical correction. The anatomy of these defects is very well shown by drawings of Lewis et al. (1955). The primitive sinus venosus is usually incorporated entirely into the right atrium. A portion of the sinus venosus, however, may extend farther to the left than usual and receive the pulmonary veins (a condition found in fish) (Hudson, 1955). Further development leads to a retraction of the sinus venosus toward the right so that some of the right-sided veins are drawn into the right atrium near or opposite the orifice of the superior vena cava. This arrangement requires a special technique for repair, and Ross (1956) suggests that patients with this condition develop symptoms earlier than with the usual ostium secundum defect.

OSTIUM PRIMUM DEFECTS. In its simplest form, this defect is in the lowermost portion of the septum in the region of the primitive ostium primum. The lower margin of the defect is the upper margin of the interventricular septum. Actually the defect may be due in part to faulty development of the lower part of the septum secundum. The low position of the defect is not necessarily of great hemodynamic importance, but often there is an associated defect or cleft in one of the leaflets of the atrioventricular valves. It is commonly in the anterior leaflet of the mitral valve. Finally, at the other end of a spectrum of malformations is the common atrioventricular canal with common atrioventricular valve leaflets and a continuous defect involving both the atrial and ventricular septa. These more extensive defects are best designated as an endocardial cushion defect and will be considered as a separate entity in the following section.

Simple septum primum defects deserve separate consideration because of the technique of repair. When they are associated with malformed or cleft valves, however, regurgitation from the ventricles into the atria complicates the simple left to right shunt. Left axis deviation in the ECG often accompanies septum primum defects and is thought to be due to an anomaly of the conduction system. Repair of the more extensive defects involving the atrioventricular valves is a more difficult surgical undertaking.

COMMON ATRIUM. No exact border or division between a large defect and a common atrium is drawn, but where the margins of the defect are scarcely perceptible the designation of common atrium is justified. In a review of 14 anatomically proved cases by Hung et al. (1973) all were found to be associated with persistent atrioventricular canal. Left ventriculograms in 8 cases showed typical gooseneck deformity of the left ventricular outflow tract. A single large lobular atrial structure was demonstrated in 5 cases after the injection of contrast material into the right ventricle or directly into the atrium. Repair of such a defect is a considerably more formidable undertaking than repair of a simple uncomplicated ASD.

HEMODYNAMIC CONSIDERATIONS. Following the advent of right heart catheterization, Cournand et al. (1947) demonstrated that the pressure in the normal left atrium was consistently higher than in the right and furthermore that this differential was maintained in most cases of interatrial septal defect so that an effective pressure gradient existed between the left and right atrium of about 2–4 mm Hg. Consequently, the predominant hemodynamic abnormality is a left-to-right shunt. This increases the volume of blood passing through the right side of the heart and the pulmonary vascular system, and the pulmonary blood flow in exceptional cases may reach 20 L/min, or roughly 5 times the usual systemic flow. The majority of patients with signs and symptoms show pulmonary-to-systemic blood flows of the order of 2:1–3:1.

A small right-to-left shunt was detected in 3 of 32 adult patients studied by Kjellberg et al. (1958). One of these had a septum primum defect, one had pulmonary hypertension, and another had a defect near the orifice of the inferior vena cava. Occasionally evidence of a small right-to-left shunt is demonstrated by angiocardiography, although it is possible that the small gradient between the right and left atrium is modified by the rapid injection. Lind and Wegelius (1953) believe that by using rapid filming evidence of such small shunts could be obtained frequently. The present authors have seen evidence early in the course of the examination of a right to left shunt in cases of single atrium. Banas et al. (1971) have described a technique for detecting small defects in the atrial septum which utilizes a Valsalva maneuver to cause right atrial pressure to exceed the pressure in the left atrium. This reversal of the normal interatrial pressure gradient causes a transient right to left shunt which is detected by noting an early appearance deflection in the indicator-dilution dye curve performed by injecting indocyanine green dye into the inferior vena cava during the Valsalva maneuver.

Despite the increased pulmonary blood flow, pulmonary hypertension occurs in no more than 15% of cases (Wood, 1952) and large shunts are tolerated for years. Wood (1952) mentions cases, however, in which the pulmonary artery pressure was quite high with reversal of the shunt through the defect producing cyanosis. These cases resemble the Eisenmenger syndrome. Occasionally, pulmonary hypertension is seen in childhood, but the right ventricular systolic pressure rarely exceeds 50 mm Hg (Krovetz, 1968). Dimisch *et al.* (1973) declare that they have not observed a severe degree of pulmonary hypertension in infancy attributable to ASD.

Where a large flow is present, a gradient across the pulmonary orifice may be observed at cardiac catheterization, and this may amount to 20–30 mm Hg. Such a gradient is due to high flow through a normal-sized pulmonary valve, causing relative pulmonic stenosis. Furthermore, some degree of right heart hypertrophy may lead to mild degrees of anatomic stenosis associated with infundibular hypertrophy. These changes are considered as an intrinsic part of interatrial septal defects and usually regress following adequate repair.

CLINICAL CONSIDERATIONS. Atrial septal defects may produce no symptoms. When the heart is unable to increase its output so as to be adequate to the demands of exercise, diminished effort tolerance results. Increased susceptibility to pulmonary infections in childhood is also noted. A crescendo-decrescendo pulmonary flow murmur is often heard due to the increased flow of blood through the pulmonary valve. The cardinal physical sign of atrial septal defect is fixed wide splitting of the second heart sound. In the normal heart inspiration, by augmenting venous return to the right heart more than to the left, pulmonary closure is delayed relative to aortic closure so that the separation of these two sounds, called splitting, increases on inspiration. With ASD, inspiration affects venous return to both sides to an equivalent extent, and the two sounds move in phase (Garbode and Carr, 1971).

The mode of deterioration in atrial septal defect is related to the development of pulmonary hypertension, congestive heart failure and arrhythmias. Early changes in right ventricular compliance combined with atrial septal defect can lead to early diastolic overloading of the right ventricle causing cardiomegaly and heart failure at an early age (Dimisch *et al.*, 1973).

RADIOLOGIC FINDINGS. The changes seen on conventional chest films and fluoroscopy vary with the age of the patient, the size of the defect, the size of the shunt, and an imponderable factor, namely the reaction of the heart and pulmonary vascular system to the abnormal circulatory dynamics. In a large majority of patients, radiologic changes are minimal during the first few years of life and do not become striking until the second or third decade. Exceptions are due to quite large defects, ostium primum defects with associated mitral valvular insufficiency, and associated anomalous venous return with a sinus venosus defect. Early onset of pulmonary hypertension may contribute to cardiac enlargement.

The contour of the heart is roughly triangular in the majority of cases due to straightening of the left border and some right atrial enlargement. Some degree of enlargement of the pulmonary artery and its central and peripheral branches is almost invariably found in symptomatic atrial septal defects. The enlargement is usually progressive as the patient grows older. The pulmonary trunk and the right and left pulmonary arteries may become huge and suggest the presence of an aneurysm. The more peripheral branches likewise enlarge and are mildly to moderately tortuous. Fouche *et al.* (1963) found that the upper lobe arteries were the first to distend, and usually some degree of correlation can be drawn between the flow and the size of the pulmonary arteries. Certainly the dilatation of both the central and peripheral arteries is more striking in older patients with large shunts. Furthermore, distinctively increased pulsations can be seen in the pulmonary arteries at fluoroscopy, and the amplitude of these may be such as to jusify the term "hilar dance." "Hilar dance" refers not only to an increased amplitude of pulsations in the hilar vessels but the pulsations extend outward toward the periphery in severe cases, and there is a rhythmic change in density of these vessels. Hilar dance is seen in other conditions that produce large left to right shunts such as PDA but is much less frequent than with ASD. Hilar dance is not an early sign, however, and since the use of fluoroscopy has diminished, it has been infrequently mentioned as a sign of ASD.

With the onset of pulmonary hypertension the peripheral arteries diminish in size, and a disparity is noted between their size and the large hilar vessels. These arteries may become somewhat tortuous and in some ways resemble the changes seen in pulmonary hypertension associated with mitral stenosis. This change is rather rare in ASD even with well-established hypertension. Kjellberg *et al.* (1958) did not find this change in any of 94 patients with ASD, although 77 of these were children. We have seen this change occasionally in older persons (Fig. 211).

Cardiac enlargement is common and may become striking in older patients with a significant shunt. It is due primarily to dilatation and hypertrophy of the right ventricle and atrium. The heart contour may appear normal for some years because enlargement of the right ventricle is difficult to detect, particularly in the PA projection. Also, considerable right atrial dilatation can occur before the right heart border becomes strikingly convex. Roesler (1934) writes of displacement of the tricuspid orifice toward the left

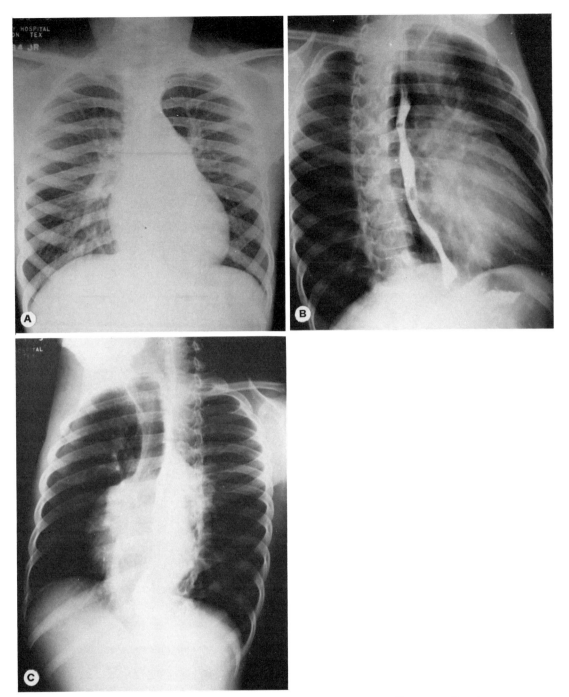

FIG. 208. INTERATRIAL SEPTAL DEFECT IN 14-YEAR-OLD BOY (OPERATIVE CASE)

The patient was having attacks of respiratory distress and was underdeveloped. (A) Posteroanterior projection. The heart was borderline in size. There was an increased convexity of the pulmonary artery segment and an increased prominence of the pulmonary vascular structures. (B) Right anterior oblique projection. There was no left atrial enlargement and a minor convexity in the region of the infundibulium of the right ventricle. (C) Left anterior oblique projection. The right atrial and ventricular borders are more convex than usual. At fluoroscopy there was an increase in amplitude of pulsations in the right hilar vessels amounting to a hilar dance.

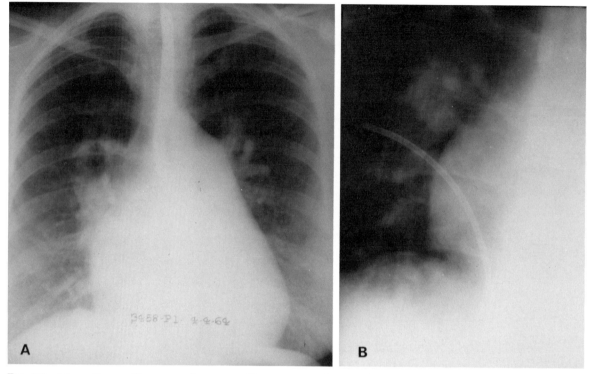

FIG. 209. ATRIAL SEPTAL DEFECT OF SECUNDUM VARIETY WITH PARTIAL ANOMALOUS VENOUS DRAINAGE FROM RIGHT LUNG (OPERATIVE CASE)

(A) Conventional film of atrial septal defect. (B) Catheter inserted through the inferior vena cava into the right atrium passed readily into a pulmonary vein as evidence of anomalous venous connection. Such a finding must be interpreted with caution since the catheter may enter the left atrium before entering the pulmonary vein.

which tends to diminish the prominence of the right border, but the present authors cannot vouch for this as a significant factor. Enlargement of the right atrium is best demonstrated in the left anterior oblique projection, and enlargement of the right ventricle is best appraised in the lateral projection where an increased segment of the heart in contact with the posterior surface of the sternum is seen. In the more advanced cases, the right ventricle may be partially borderforming on the left, but the left border is often steep and it is difficult from the PA projection to determine whether the right or left ventricle is enlarged, although a heart of triangular shape with a straight left border suggests right ventricular enlargement. The apex of the heart is usually low, although on sharp films a very shallow notch may be visible in the lower left border marking the division between the right and left ventricle. Elevation of the apex as seen in the tetralogy of Fallot does not occur. Enlargement of the right ventricle may become extreme so that the heart weight is greatly increased.

Based on the size of the aortic knob and its impression on the barium-filled esophagus in the oblique views, the aorta appears normal or decreased in size. The adjacent enlargement of the pulmonary artery tends to obscure the aortic shadow so that it regularly appears small and inconspicuous.

Differentiation of the various types atrial septal defect on the basis of the conventional radiologic examination is not possible, but certain changes may be suggestive. Evidence of left ventricular in addition to right ventricular enlargement is suggestive of an ostium primum defect with valvular insufficiency. Early or rapid enlargement is suggestive of either an ostium primum defect or a sinus venosus defect with partial anomalous venous return.

Atrial septal defect must be differentiated from partial and total anomalous venous return, VSD, and PDA. Partial anomalous venous return presents by far the most difficulties. In complete anomalous pulmonary venous return, peripheral unsaturation is common, and this does not typically occur in ASD. Also, with anomalous venous return the dilatation of the right atrium and ventricle occurs early and is usually greater than that with ASD alone. VSD is differentiated pri-

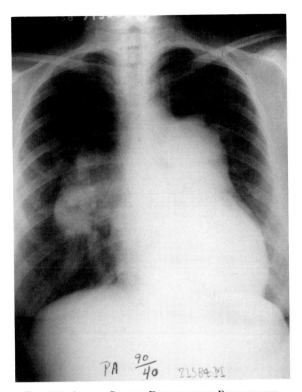

FIG. 210. ATRIAL SEPTAL DEFECT WITH PULMONARY
HYPERTENSION IN 56-YEAR-OLD WOMAN

The huge proximal pulmonary arteries contrast sharply
with the rapidly tapering distal branches and the relatively
avascular peripheral portions of the lungs.

marily on the basis of enlargement of the left
atrium and the early onset of symptoms. The left
atrium is not as a rule enlarged in ASD. Also, in
VSD the ascending aorta may be somewhat more
prominent. Differentiation from PDA likewise
depends upon demonstration of enlargement of
the left atrium and dilatation or enlargement of
the ascending aorta. The differential features are
summarized in Table 10. see page 255.

Although conventional radiologic studies are
quite helpful in narrowing the diagnostic possibilities, they are not sufficient to permit satisfactory evaluation in relation to surgical treatment.
Right heart catheterization is always necessary,
although this procedure while giving strong cir-
cumstantial evidence as to the site of a left-to-
right shunt does not provide anatomical details.
Essentially right heart catheterization will show
an increase in oxygen content in the right atrium
as compared with the inferior and superior vena
cavae. Curves following the injection of dye respectively into the pulmonary artery, right ventricle, and right atrium and monitoring from a
peripheral artery will show a washout curve consistent with a left-to-right shunt, but the site

cannot be precisely determined. Selective injection in the right and left pulmonary arteries
usually shows curves of quite different contour.
In simple atrial defect blood from the left pulmonary veins is shunted predominantly through
the defect into the right atrium, whereas blood
from the right pulmonary veins is shunted
through the mitral valve into the left ventricle
(Wakai et al., 1956). This selective shunting does
not occur in persistent common atrioventricular
canal. The use of the hydrogen electrode, however, can often localize the shunt at the atrial
level. The platinum tipped catheter is placed in
the right atrium, the patient is asked to breathe
hydrogen, and hydrogen ions can be detected
immediately in the right atrium. Furthermore,
films and fluoroscopic observation of the passage
of the catheter from the right to the left atrium
may give some indication as to the size and
location of the defect, although it is often surprisingly easy to pass a catheter through an
insignificant foramen ovale. It must be remembered that the unsupported detection of even a
significant increase in O_2 concentration between
samples of vena cava and right atrial blood does
not suffice to substantiate the diagnosis since the
same finding may be due to (1) anomalous pulmonary venous return, (2) a ventricular septal
defect with tricuspid insufficiency, (3) left ventricular right atrial defect, (4) left atrial coronary
sinus defect, and (5) an aneurysm of the sinus of
Valsalva with rupture into the right atrium. Tricuspid insufficiency can usually be ruled out at
the time of right heart catheterization by a study
of the pressure curves from the right atrium. The
catheter can be passed from the right atrium into
a pulmonary vein, and this serves to confirm the
presence of some degree of anomalous pulmonary venous return, but even this observation
may be in error since the catheter may have
passed through an atrial septal defect before
entering the pulmonary vein. Left ventricular
right atrial communications may be suspected
on clinical grounds and be proven by left ventricular angiography.

The differentiation of septum primum defects
preoperatively is important because of the increased technical difficulty in repair and frequency of associated valvular abnormalities. Cardiac catheterization may show evidence of mitral
insufficiency (pressure curves taken from the left
atrium). A low position of the catheter as it
passes through the interatrial septum may suggest an ostium primum defect, but this is not
reliable. If the ECG and vectorcardiogram show
left axis deviation with other evidence of ASD,
the probablity of an ostium primum defect is

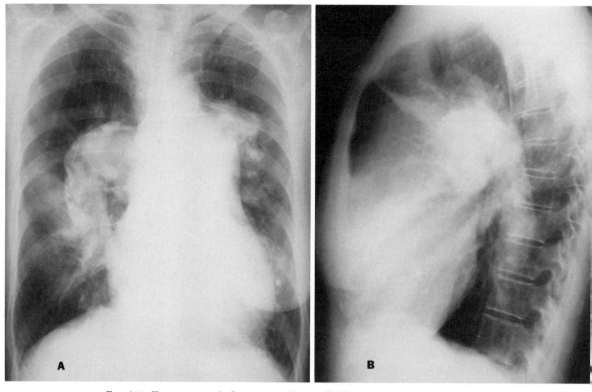

FIG. 211. EISENMENGER'S SYNDROME (A AND B, FRONTAL AND LATERAL FILMS)

Pulmonary arterial hypertension and atrial septal defect coexist in this adult patient. The heart is slightly but definitely enlarged, and the pulmonary trunk is greatly increased in size. The right and left pulmonary artery branches are huge, but the peripheral pulmonary vasculature is relatively sparse. Long-standing pulmonary hypertension has produced degenerative intimal changes in the pulmonary arteries, and they have become densely calcified.

considerable. In a series of 77 patients with ASD, Kjellberg *et al.* (1958) found left axis deviation in 8, and in 7 the presence of an ostium primum defect was confirmed. On the other hand, left axis deviation was lacking in 5 patients with proved ostium primum defects. For further consideration of ostium primum defects with cleft mitral valve, see the following section on endocardial cushion defects.

ANGIOCARDIOGRAPHY. Where the left-to-right-shunt has been of significant proportions, venous angiocardiography has not been helpful in the authors' hands. The contrast substance is rapidly diluted in the right atrium. Consequently, the density is so much reduced that the right ventricle and pulmonary artery are poorly opacified. Evidence of recirculation into the right atrium under these circumstances is quite uncertain and is rarely convincing. We have not observed temporary reversal of the shunt during the period of injection as reported by Lind and Wegelius (1953). Figley *et al.* (1956) occasionally obtained a pattern of nonopaque turbulence in the right atrium due to the incoming blood from the defect. The evidence of turbulence in the

atrium is often great, but we have not observed a significant pattern that would enable us to differentiate interatrial septal defect from anomalous venous return.

Kjellberg *et al.* (1958) advocate the passage of a catheter through the defect into the left atrium followed by the rapid injection of contrast substance and rapid filming in the right posterior oblique position. In this manner the diameter of the defect may be evaluated and perhaps something determined about its location. It requires very rapid filming immediately following the injection of contrast substance. Injection of a large volume of contrast material into the pulmonary artery may also be adequate to display grossly the morphology of an ASD after circulation through the lungs.

If an anomalous pulmonary vein is identified or suspected by main pulmonary arteriography, selective injection of the ipsilateral pulmonary artery will more clearly demonstrate it. If the pulmonary artery opposite the side of the anomalous pulmonary venous connection is injected with contrast material, the presence or absence of an associated atrial septal defect can be nicely

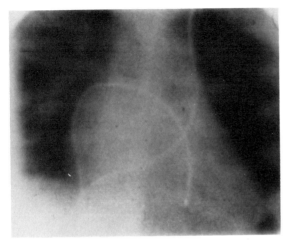

FIG. 212. ATRIAL SEPTAL DEFECT OF SINUS VENOSUS TYPE. REPRODUCTION OF 16-MM MOVIE FRAME

One catheter enters the heart through a left SVC, traverses the coronary sinus to the RA and leaves via the IVC. A second catheter inserted through the IVC passed easily through a septal defect into the LA and LV. The high position of this catheter in relation to the atria suggests that the defect was high and of the sinus venosus type.

displayed. Sos *et al.* (1974) studied 22 patients with partial anomalous pulmonary venous return. In 8 patients, the absence of an associated ASD was established by this method.

In summary, an ASD can be strongly suspected from clinical and conventional radiologic studies. Cardiac catheterization will confirm the presence of a left-to-right shunt into the right atrium and also give evidence of complicating factors such as pulmonary hypertension and pulmonic stenosis. The differentiation from anomalous venous return, either as a sole functional abnormality or as a complicating factor, is rarely made with satisfaction. Also, the anatomy, size, and location of the defect may remain in doubt, although some quantitation of the shunt can be determined from the various dye curves and the increase in oxygen content in the atrium. Injection of contrast substance into the left atrium through a catheter has given the most definitive information concerning the location and size of the defect. Ostium primum defects can be suspected in certain cases from radiologic findings of rapid enlargement of the heart and particularly where there is evidence of left axis deviation as shown on the ECG. In a considerable proportion of cases, the diagnosis as to the location of the defect and its extent is made only at the operating table, and the surgeon in general must be prepared for a number of variations and complications. For this reason, the availability of cardiac bypass techniques is essential.

POSTOPERATIVE APPEARANCE. Spontaneous functional closure of atrial septal defect occurs rarely (Cayler, 1967) and some have advocated a conservative approach to early surgical closure of ASDs because of this possibility. There is general agreement that the child with symptoms or with cardiomegaly due to atrial septal defect should be treated surgically and that operative repair, when indicated, is best carried out after the age of 2 years if successful medical management can be achieved (Hunt and Lucas, 1973). Eighty-two percent of 185 pediatric cardiologists surveyed by Moss and Siassi (1971) did not currently advise closure of very small ASDs (pulmonary-to-systemic flow ratio less than 1.5 to 1). Seventy percent recommended operation if the shunt were 1.5 to 1 or greater, and 96% favored operative intervention if the shunt were 2.0 to 1 or greater. In general, it seems prudent to consider withholding operation for the patient with a small ASD, one in which the child is asymptomatic, cardiomegaly and pulmonary hypervascularity are not seen radiographically, pulmonary hypertension is absent and the pulmonary-to-systemic flow ratio is low.

Operative mortality in uncomplicated ASDs in experienced hands is in the neighborhood of 1%. Current practice for surgical therapy is to employ cardiopulmonary bypass. Small defects may be closed by continuous suture, but a pericardial or prosthetic patch may be necessary for larger defects or for those where undue tension would be produced by direct suture (Garbode and Carr, 1971). Althaus *et al.* (1974) have recently described a circumclusion technique for closure of ASDs which requires neither hypothermia nor cardiopulmonary bypass, and King and Mills (1974) have developed an experimental technique and apparatus for transvenous closure of the defects using a pair of interlocking umbrella-like components made of stainless steel and Dacron and introduced through a catheter.

Once symptoms appear in adult patients with atrial septal defects, rapid progression to functional disability or death from congestive heart failure often occurs. Numerous recent reports attest to the appropriateness of operation for closure of an ASD in the adult since the mortality and morbidity of the procedure are low and symptomatic improvement is significant (Hairston *et al.*, 1974; Knight and Lennox, 1972; Rees *et al.*, 1973). Robb (1973) suggests that middle-aged patients with atrial septal defects should be offered surgical therapy even if they are asymptomatic since the hospital mortality rate of 5% for patients over the age of 40 undergoing closure of an atrial septal defect compares well with the annual mortality rate of around 6% in patients treated conservatively.

The usual postoperative changes are seen radiographically, mainly some haziness of the lungs and small collections of pleural fluid. Young (1973) found that 46 of 71 children who underwent operation for closure of atrial septal defects showed return of heart size to normal by x-ray study. Complete or partial reversion of radiographic abnormalities occurred within 1½–2 years postoperatively, and no change was seen thereafter. A decrease in pulmonary vascularity may be seen within a few weeks, and Pieroni *et al.* (1973) found that the pulmonary vascular markings decreased in almost all of the 34 patients they studied, whether or not residual shunts remained. In their experience, chest films were not helpful in identifying patients with residual shunts, and the main pulmonary artery size and cardiothoracic ratio decreased whether or not surgery was completely successful. In older patients with marked pulmonary dilatation, a large pulmonary trunk may persist indefinitely.

Persistent postoperative cardiac enlargement may be due to incomplete repair or persistent hemodynamically significant arrhythmias occurring as a complication of surgery. Primarily it is the result of failure of myocardial disease to regress and can be considered a cardiomyopathy of volume loading (Young, 1973). Thus, although early closure of an atrial septal defect is curative for most, residual myocardial disease in some

may ultimately result in a less than normal life expectancy. Cardiac catheterization usually shows a considerable decrease in pulmonary artery flow, and if there has been mild pulmonary hypertension, the pulmonary artery pressure usually falls to normal. The gradient between the right ventricle and pulmonary artery disappears.

LUTEMBACHER'S SYNDROME. The anatomic basis of Lutembacher's syndrome is mitral stenosis and an interatrial communication. The mitral stenosis may be congenital or acquired. Some of the proved cases have had a double mitral lesion, such as stenosis and insufficiency, and even those cases with a rare anomaly of the papillary muscle with mitral insufficiency might be included in this category. In the vast majority of the proved cases, the mitral stenosis was secondary to rheumatic fever. In the majority of cases the interatrial communication apparently consisted of a patent foramen ovale although in the case described by Lutembacher (1916) the commmunication was a true atrial septal defect. Whatever the nature of the interatrial communication, it must be of the order of 1 cm in diameter and permit a considerable shunt in order to produce the syndrome.

Lutembacher's syndrome undoubtedly has been diagnosed frequently without sufficient reason as its incidence at autopsy does not support the frequency with which it has been diagnosed (Edwards, 1953). Roesler (1934) found evidence of rheumatic involvement of the mitral valve in

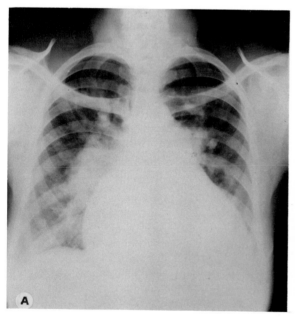 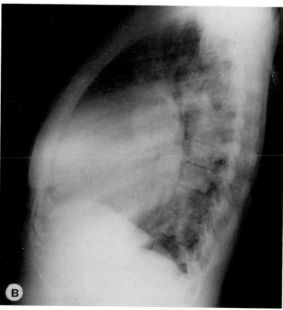

FIG. 213. LUTEMBACHER'S SYNDROME

A 37-year-old woman who was well until 1½ years before death. There was a prominent bilateral hilar dance. At autopsy the interatrial septal defect measured about 2 cm in diameter, and there was an obstruction at the mitral valve.

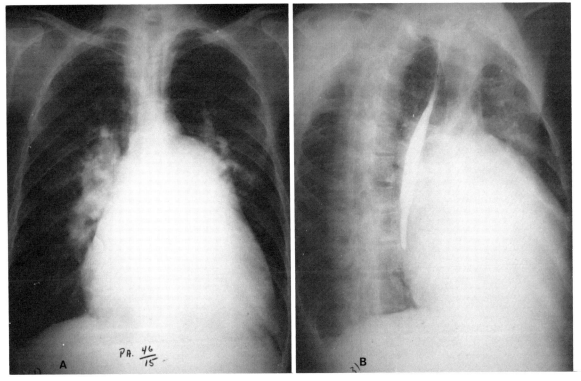

FIG. 214. ATRIAL SEPTAL DEFECT

A 48-year-old man with evidence of atrial septal defect and mitral insufficiency, probably rheumatic in origin. The changes are similar to the Lutembacher's syndrome.

66% of 62 cases of ASD, and in 30 of these (48%) the change in the valve was sufficient to produce obstruction. On the other hand, Espino-Vela (1959) could find only 12 proved cases after many years' experience in a large clinic where 40% of the patients suffered with rheumatic heart disease. The same author accepted cases in which there was a double mitral lesion, namely stenosis and insufficiency. Nadas and Alimurung (1952) found that only 2 of 19 cases of ASD examined at autopsy had significant mitral stenosis. Slight thickening of the endocardium of the valve cusps that occurs with aging and which hemodynamically is of little significance should not be attributed to rheumatic fever (Edwards, 1953).

The predominant hemodynamic effect of the mitral stenosis is to obstruct the blood flow to the left ventricle and increase the left to right shunt through the ASD. Thus, it is believed that patients with Lutembacher's syndrome tend to have more severe symptoms at a relatively earlier time than those with a simple ASD.

Radiologic Findings. In older patients with a well-developed syndrome, the heart is moderately to greatly enlarged. In early life, as in atrial septal defect, the heart may be almost normal in contour. Patients are most commonly seen in the third and fourth decades. Enlargement is usually symmetrical, although the left ventricle as a rule is not enlarged unless there is an associated mitral insufficiency or a lesion of the aortic valve.

One of the most striking changes is the dilatation of the pulmonary artery. This may be so great as to suggest the presence of an aneurysm and was a prominent feature of the case presented by Lutembacher (1916). In a minority of cases, however, the pulmonary artery segment may not be particularly prominent. Espino-Vela (1959) attributed this lack of pulmonary convexity to rotation of the heart secondary to marked right-sided enlargement. Marked cardiac enlargement may also tend to obscure the contour of the greatly enlarged pulmonary artery. The smaller secondary and tertiary arteries in the lungs are also dilated and show markedly increased pulsations with changes in density (hilar dance). The left atrium is often not enlarged, and it seems that the atrial septal defect would prevent a significant increase in left atrial pressure. However, a minor degree of enlargement is not unusual (Espino-Vela, 1959) and may be detected on films made in the RAO and lateral views with barium in the esophagus. The reason for the left atrial enlargement is not always clear and cannot be finally determined until more data concerning left atrial pressure have been accumulated. There does not seem to be a good correlation between the left atrial size and the size of the atrial septal defect.

The right atrium is moderately to greatly enlarged and forms most of the right heart border. It extends farther to the right than normal, and this tends to give the heart a symmetrical appearance in the frontal projection. The right ventricle is also enlarged and often dilated and actually extends farther toward the left than to the right. The greater part of the total cardiac enlargement is due to the right ventricle, although the appearance of the heart in the frontal projection may suggest left ventricular enlargement. In older patients calcific plaques may be seen in the pulmonary arteries indicating atherosclerosis.

Lutembacher's syndrome is considerably more common in women than in men. It may be suspected in any case of atrial septal defect in which there is considerable dilatation of the pulmonary artery and an unusually large heart for an uncomplicated secundum ASD (Tandon et al., 1971). The typical crescendo murmur of mitral stenosis is rarely present in this condition because the atrial septal defect usually prevents an increase in pressure in the left atrium during ventricular diastole. Likewise, catheterization of the left atrium and even the left ventricle with pressure measurements does not always give definitive information because the usual gradient of mitral stenosis is diminished.

Since the effect of the mitral stenosis is to increase the shunt through the atrial septal defect, relief of the valvular stenosis by surgical means is indicated and has usually been helpful (Muller et al., 1966).

Ventricular Septal Defect (VSD). Isolated ventricular septal defect is one of the commonest of cardiac anomalies and is estimated to occur in 20–30% of children with clinical congenital heart disease (Engle, 1972). Ventricular septal defect is a frequent finding in association with other often complicated anomalies, such as the tetralogy of Fallot and complete transposition of the great vessels. In this section we will deal only with ventricular septal defect as the predominant abnormality in the heart. Essentially it consists of an opening in either the muscular or membranous portion of the ventricular septum that permits a usually intermittent (systolic) flow of blood from the left to the right ventricle.

From an anatomical and angiographic viewpoint, ventricular septal defects may be classified as follows (after Baron et al., 1963):

BULBAR (SUPRACRISTAL OR SUBPULMONIC) SEPTAL DEFECTS. These are located high in the right ventricular outflow tract just below the posterior cusp of the pulmonary valve and in very close relation to the coronary cusp of the aortic valve. These defects comprise about 5% of all isolated VSDs (Steinfeld et al., 1972).

MEMBRANOUS DEFECTS. The membranous portion of the ventricular septum on the right ventricular aspect lies just below the crista supraventricularis and underneath the septal leaflet of the tricuspid valve. Defects here often extend into the adjacent muscular portion of the ventricular septum. This is by far the commonest defect encountered at surgery.

MUSCULAR DEFECTS. These may be divided into anterior and posterior varieties. The posterior variety is closely related to the septal and posterior leaflets of the tricuspid valve and the medial commissure of the mitral valve. The anterior variety is not closely related to any of the valves and may occur anywhere else in the muscular septum other than the posterior part. These defects may be multiple (10% of defects in the muscular septum according to Breckenridge et al., 1972).

MEMBRANOUS ATRIOVENTRICULAR DEFECTS. The development of the endocardial cushions and atrial septum is such that a portion of the membranous septum separates the left ventricle from the right atrium. A defect in this septum produces a left ventricular right atrial communication, and this will be considered in a separate section.

The practical implications of such a classification are of considerable importance. Bulbar defects may be missed at right heart catheterization unless care is taken to obtain samples high in the outflow tract of the right ventricle. Also, membranous atrioventricular septal defects are a special situation as mentioned above. Muscular defects may be hidden by the leaflets of the tricuspid valve and overlooked. However, the size of the defect, the presence of and extent of pulmonary vascular resistance with their resultant effects on the size of the intracardiac shunts are the more important considerations and have led to the hemodynamic classification given below. Where the defect is small and consequently the shunt is small, the increased pulmonary flow is well tolerated and the anomaly runs a benign course and is often known as the maladie de Roger. On the other hand, larger defects associated with larger shunts may be followed by a series of complicating circumstances that threaten life and raise the question of surgical treatment. Two of the more common complicating circumstances are (1) pulmonary hypertension, either primary or secondary to increased pulmonary blood flow, and (2) pulmonic stenosis, either due to a relatively narrow pulmonary orifice which, however, is of normal diameter or to a developing secondary muscle hypertrophy of the outflow tract of the right ventricle. Other associated anatomical abnormalities occasionally occur and are listed below:

1. Adherence of a cusp of the tricuspid valve to the margins of the defect producing tricuspid incompetence (Marquis, 1950).

2. Incompetence of the aortic valve due to deformity or prolapse of one or more of the valve cusps (Ellis et al., 1963; Nadas et al., 1964; Steinfeld et al., 1972).

3. Associated subaortic stenosis (Lauer et al., 1960).

4. Hypoplastic aorta.

Another most interesting facet of the problem of ventricular septal defect is the recent accumulated evidence that shows that a significant minority of even sizeable defects close spontaneously during early childhood years (Evans et al., 1960; Nadas et al., 1961; Hoffman and Rudolph, 1963). There is general agreement that the incidence of spontaneous closure of VSDs varies between 21 and 45% of all children born with such defects (Engle, 1972; Bonchek et al., 1973; Hoffman, 1968). According to Alpert et. al. (1973), 58% of VSDs diagnosed at birth, 40% of the ones diagnosed after one year, and 35% of those diagnosed after two years would be expected to close by age 5. Since few deaths occur in persons with VSD after the age of 2 years, spontaneous closure of VSDs affects the incidence of the anomaly. In the congenital heart disease population, the incidence of VSD is about 30% at birth, 20% in childhood and less than 10% in adulthood.

Spontaneous closure of VSDs is accompanied by a decrease in heart size and a return of pulmonary blood flow to normal levels.

Current usage considers the term "ventricular septal defect" as applying not only to the septal defect but the associated and ensuing complications mentioned above, particularly where the defect is the predominant abnormality. Thus, a considerable spectrum of clinical and radiologic changes may be considered under this heading varying from evidence of a marked left-to-right shunt with lung plethora and a large heart at one extreme to a normal sized heart with relatively clear lungs and a right to left shunt at the other.

Conditions bordering on the tetralogy of Fallot, namely pulmonic stenosis with ventricular septal defect, are considered under this heading. The criterion of separation is the predominant direction of the ventricular shunt; those cases with a predominant right-to-left shunt and pulmonic stenosis are considered as the tetralogy of Fallot, whereas cases with a left-to-right shunt and a gradient between the right ventricle and pulmonary artery of 30 mm or less are considered primarily as ventricular septal defects. Gasul et al. (1957), Taussig (1960, Page 696) and Kjellberg et al. (1958) have followed cases of ventricular septal defect with hypertension and left-to-right shunts in which after a period of years pulmonic stenosis supervened so that a left-to-right shunt was reversed producing a clinical and hemodynamic picture of the tetralogy of Fallot. One can speculate upon the origin of the pulmonic stenosis, but in most of these cases the obstruction was in the infundibulum, and it seems logical to suspect that it represents a reaction of the infundibular musculature to increased work.

Eisenmenger Complex. The Eisenmenger complex (Eisenmenger, 1897) which was originally described as a high ventricular septal defect and dextroposed aorta with no obstruction to the pulmonary flow is considered also as a variation of ventricular septal defect. The question of anatomical overriding of the aorta in a child's heart with a high ventricular septal defect may at times be difficult to determine, but there is no question that a ventricular defect may effectively shunt blood from the right ventricle into the aorta whether there is overriding or not. Taussig (1960) recommends the term "Eisenmenger syndrome" for those cases of ventricular septal defect with pulmonary hypertension and a predominant right-to-left shunt.

A detailed discussion of the origin and evolution of pulmonary hypertension in association with ventricular septal defect is not within the scope of this section. It is well known that pulmonary flows of 2–3 times systemic flow may be accommodated by the pulmonary vascular system without hypertension. The flow, however, may serve as a stimulus, leading to intimal proliferation or, more often, thickening of the muscular walls of the small arteries in the lung with an ultimate increase in pulmonary resistance. Another factor in the early development of hypertension, particularly in infancy, is the persistence of the fetal character of the pulmonary vasculature. For further information on this subject, the reader is referred to the work of Dammann et al., 1960, Lucas et al., 1961, and Wagenvoort *et al.*, 1961. The extent and rapidity of development of the hypertension are variable and often unpredictable. Certainly in many cases the hypertension is mild and stationary for long periods, whereas in other cases it is found a few weeks after birth and is severe in its consequences. If pulmonary hypertension progresses, and particularly if the pulmonary resistance increases, the pulmonary flow will decrease, and this may in turn bring an improvement in both the clinical and radiologic appearance of the patient. Certainly the presence of pulmonary hypertension and its cause, whether due to increased flow or increased resistance or a combination of the two, is of great importance in considering surgical closure of the defect or a palliative banding procedure.

The following classification is a hemodynamic and functional one. Consequently, patients may change from one group to another over a period of years due to changes in circulatory dynamics.

Classification of Ventricular Septal Defects (Modified from Kjellberg *et al.* (1958), Singleton *et al.* (1959) and Capp *et al.* (1968).) Group I. Small left-to-right shunt with normal pulmonary artery pressure. Right ventricular pressure is below 35 mm Hg, and the left-to-right shunt is less than 40% of the total blood flow to the lungs. The defect is small, usually less than 1 cm in diameter and often in the muscular septum. The patient is usually asymptomatic and may be considered as an example of maladie de Roger. Prognosis is excellent.

Group II. Pulmonary artery pressure 50–85% of systemic pressure with a moderate to large left-to-right shunt and with a pulmonary blood flow of 2–4 times systemic flow. Cases in this group may progress to Group IIIA or regress to Group I. Many infants with heart failure fall into this group.

Group IIIA. Pulmonary artery pressure 85–100% of systemic pressure with a left-to-right shunt usually smaller than in Group II with an occasional reversal.

Group IIIB. Right ventricular systolic pressure 85–100% of systemic pressure with pulmonic stenosis and a right ventricular pulmonary artery gradient not exceeding 30 mm Hg. Some of these cases progress to the point where the shunt is predominantly right to left and are then considered as examples of the tetralogy of Fallot.

Group IV. Pulmonary artery pressure equal to or greater than systemic with a right to left shunt and peripheral unsaturation (the Eisenmenger syndrome).

Group V. A miscellaneous group in which one of the above groups is combined with some other anatomical defect, such as PDA, aortic insufficiency, or subaortic stenosis.

RADIOLOGIC CHANGES. Conventional films and occasionally fluoroscopy are helpful in the evaluation and follow-up of patients with known ventricular septal defect since they correlate to a considerable degree with the above stated groups. The diagnosis in all cases, however, depends on a careful right heart catheterization complemented at times by selective left ventriculography and retrograde aortography.

Group I. In these cases the heart is not enlarged generally, and the contour is usually within normal limits except for left atrial enlargement in some patients (Fig. 215). Occasionally, the middle convexity of the left heart border is more prominent or more convex than usual, and the left pulmonary artery and its branches may be a little larger than expected. This is noticed often in retrospect after reviewing other evidence indicating the diagnosis. The patients are usually asymptomatic.

Right heart catheterization shows a normal right ventricular pressure and little if any increase in oxygen content between the right atrium and right ventricle. Left ventriculography is probably the most sensitive means of demonstrating these small defects, although it is not recommended as a routine procedure. Following the injection of contrast substance into the left ventricle, a jet may be seen extending across the ventricular septum into the right ventricle (Fig. 218), and this may occur when differences in oxygen saturation in the right ventricle are not evident (Nadas *et al.*, 1961). Venous angiocardiograms or selective right ventricular angiograms are usually of little value, although theoretically they might show a little blanching or dilution of the contrast substance in the right ventricle or some evidence of recirculation. Usually the shunt is so small that neither of these signs is recognized.

Group II. Many patients in this group are under the age of 14 months and may appear in incipient or actual heart failure. The heart is uniformly enlarged with both ventricles participating in the enlargement, although the left ventricle may predominate. From radiographs made in the conventional projection, the left ventricle may appear larger, although it is often difficult or impossible to ascertain which ventricle predominates. The left atrium is usually (75–80% of cases) enlarged and can be identified in the right oblique and lateral films with barium in the esophagus. Rarely, the left atrial appendage will produce a small convexity on the left upper heart

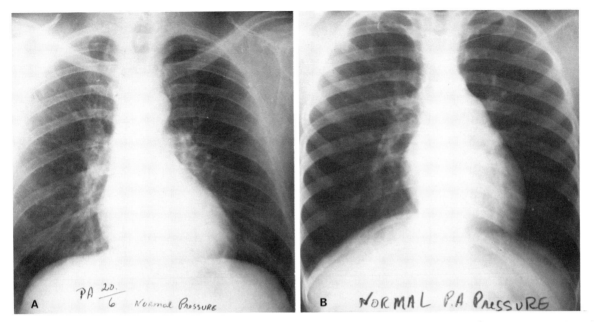

FIG. 215. CONVENTIONAL CHEST FILMS OF 2 ASYMPTOMATIC PATIENTS WITH EVIDENCE OF VENTRICULAR SEPTAL DEFECT (RIGHT HEART CATHETERIZATION) AND NORMAL PULMONARY ARTERY PRESSURES

(A) Age 39. (B) Age 7.

border indicating enlargement. Caution must be exercised not to confuse a posterior deviation of the esophagus due to a large heart or be misled by a film exposed in expiration. The left atrial size is roughly proportional to the pulmonary blood flow and as such is a valuable indicator.

The pulmonary vascularity is increased as indicated by dilatation or enlargement of the peripheral pulmonary arteries. The larger pulmonary arteries are often obscured by the enlarged heart, and it is difficult to judge their size. The dilatation of the peripheral arteries is usually definite but not striking. In infants and young children in incipient or actual heart failure, radiographs of the lungs may show an overall increase in density suggesting fluid or edema, and this seems to coexist with evidence of increased vascularity and regresses with improvement in the circulatory state.

The diagnosis is established by right heart catheterization where there is a step-up of one and usually two volumes percent in the oxygen content of the right ventricular as compared with the right atrial blood. The determination of pulmonary pressure, and if possible of pulmonary blood flow, is helpful in forming a baseline for future comparison and also in the grouping of patients. In some of these patients, the pulmonary hypertension increases, and the pulmonary blood flow decreases. This seems at times to be accompanied by improvement or stabilization of the patient's condition. On the other hand, some infants in this group lapse into intractable heart failure, and the question of surgical intervention at an early age is raised. In general, it is desirable to postpone surgery until the patient is at least several years of age.

Venous or selective angiography will show a blanching of the contrast material as it is diluted in the right ventricle. Also, after a good technical injection of the contrast substance, reopacification may clearly be demonstrated in the right ventricle. These signs are often fleeting, and while they are quite suggestive of the diagnosis, they usually do not provide any information that cannot be determined from cardiac catheterization. Left ventricular angiography shows the defect to good advantage but is rarely indicated if right heart catheterization is completely satisfactory. It should be mentioned, however, that an apparent increase in O_2 saturation in the right ventricle as compared to the right atrium must not be taken as unequivocal evidence of ventricular septal defect since pulmonic insufficiency with a large pulmonary flow secondary to PDA may permit highly oxygenated blood to regurgitate into the right ventricle. Left ventriculography and retrograde aortography may be indicated if there is any doubt as to the site of the shunt.

Group IIIA. This group merges imperceptibly with Group II, and the conventional roentgen

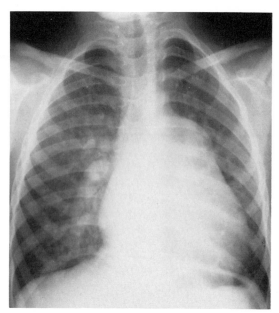

FIG. 216. VENTRICULAR SEPTAL DEFECT IN A CHILD

The heart is enlarged and somewhat triangular in shape. The pulmonary trunk is very large and overshadows the normal sized aorta which, by comparison, seems small. The pulmonary artery branches in the hilus and in the periphery of the lung are enlarged, and the pulmonary vascular volume is increased. Biventricular and left atrial enlargement were verified by electrocardiography and barium swallow.

changes are similar. Since the pulmonary flow is less, the arteries in the mid lung fields may be smaller and the vascularity less marked. Also, the left atrium may be smaller or normal. A survey by Singleton *et al.* (1959) of patients in this group indicated that the heart in general is somewhat smaller than it is in Group II. The radiologist when confronted with a slightly enlarged heart and only slightly increased or normal lung vascularity in a patient with known or suspected ventricular septal defect may postulate the presence of considerable pulmonary hypertension. This position may be strengthened, particularly if there are films exposed over a period of time showing a regression of the pulmonary vascularity. It should be remembered, however, that regression of pulmonary vascularity does not always mean pulmonary hypertension. In some cases there is actually regression or decrease in pulmonary blood flow associated with rather normal pulmonary artery pressures, and this is presumptive evidence of spontaneous decrease in size or closure of the defect. It is in this group, however, that the most difficult decisions regarding the advisability of surgical closure of the defect arise. This decision revolves around the question as to whether the pulmonary hy-

pertension is due to increased and possibly fixed pulmonary resistance or to increased flow. The logical approach is to measure the flow and determine the pulmonary resistance, if possible, by right heart catheterization, although this is technically difficult in young children. There seems little doubt (Nadas *et al.*, 1961; Kjellberg *et al.*, 1959) that the heart actually gets smaller as the pulmonary hypertension increases.

Group IIIB. Pulmonic stenosis and ventricular septal defect with left to right shunt is not an unusual combination. Usually the heart is smaller than that found in Group II and IIIA, and the pulmonary vascularity is normal or decreased. The development or presence of pulmonic stenosis does not necessarily produce decreased pulmonary vascular markings. Even a sizeable pulmonary gradient may be accompanied by normal vascularity. The left atrium is usually not enlarged. There is a preponderant enlargement of the right ventricle and a number of these cases have an upturned apex indicating definite enlargement of the right ventricle, and this may serve to differentiate them from the preceding groups. Differentiation from the Eisenmenger syndrome at this stage would depend on differences in vascularity of the lungs, although the diagnosis depends mainly on the findings obtained from right heart catheterization. Differentiation from tetralogy of Fallot, as stated above, depends on the predominant direction of the shunt. Some of these cases have been classified as "pink" tetralogies. However, if the shunt is predominantly from right to left and if the pulmonary gradient is in excess of 30 mm Hg, the condition is properly classified as a tetralogy of Fallot. Selective right ventricular angiography may demonstrate the anatomy of the outflow tract of the right ventricle and clearly demonstrate an infundibular chamber or a valvular stenosis and provide the correct diagnosis. Of course, one of the more difficult questions to answer is whether the pulmonary stenosis will remain as a significant factor after closure of the ventricular septal defect.

Group IV (The Eisenmenger Syndrome). In the more classical form of the Eisenmenger complex, the heart is slightly enlarged, although in some instances marked enlargement may occur. The right ventricle is usually the predominant chamber so that the left border of the heart may be slightly elevated, although there is a great variability in the contour of the left border of the heart. In some cases the border is rather straight with a low apex. The right oblique and lateral views, however, show that the right ventricle is uniformly enlarged. The pulmonary trunk and

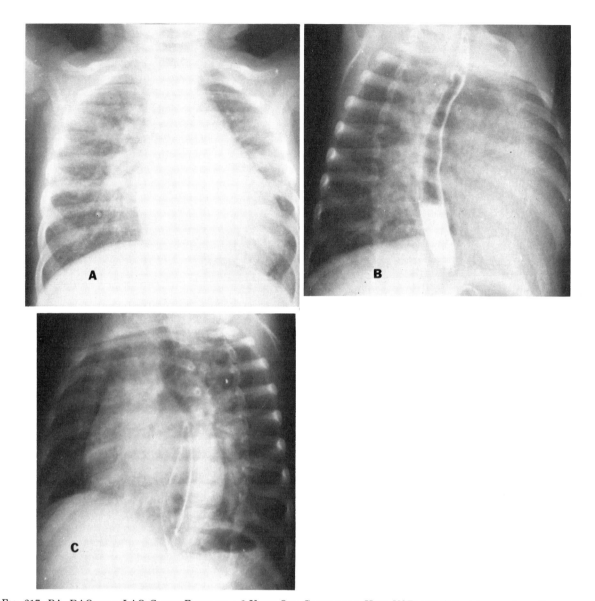

FIG. 217. PA, RAO, AND LAO CHEST FILMS OF A 2-YEAR-OLD CHILD WITH HIGH VSD AND SYMPTOMS OF LEFT VENTRIC-
ULAR FAILURE. THE LEFT ATRIUM AND LEFT VENTRICLE ARE ENLARGED

the main pulmonary arteries are greatly enlarged, and the lung vascularity is variable. In
the majority of cases (Kohout *et al.*, 1955) the
larger pulmonary arteries are increased in size,
but the extreme peripheral arteries are smaller
than normal. Thus, the main pulmonary artery
and right and left branches are enlarged out of
proportion to the peripheral artery size (Capp *et
al.*, 1968). In patients with right to left shunts
with ventricular septal defect the heart is typically not as large as in those with marked left-to-
right shunts, and the pulmonary vascularity may
be normal.

Venous angiography may show overriding of
the aorta in the Eisenmenger complex or some
degree of right-to-left shunt in the Eisenmenger
syndrome. The diagnosis depends for the most
part, however, on the hemodynamic findings
after right heart catheterization. In general, differentiation of this group from Group IIIA and
the other groups of ventricular septal defect can
be suggested from conventional radiologic findings.

Excessive pulmonary blood flow is the consequence of a large shunt from left to right through
a defect in the ventricular septum, and left-sided

heart failure occurs frequently due to volume overload on the left ventricle. Capp *et al.* (1968) have clearly shown that the increased cardiac size in children with larger shunts is due to increased left ventricular volume. As right ventricular and pulmonary artery hypertension develop because of marked pulmonary vascular obstruction, bidirectional shunting exists. When the pulmonary resistance is at obstructive levels equal to or higher than the systemic resistance, the pulmonary blood flow diminishes, and the volume overload on the left side of the heart subsides. The work of the left ventricle is now normal, and the left atrium and ventricle decrease in size, becoming normal. A pressure overload on the right ventricle now develops, and it enlarges from hypertrophy and dilates if right-sided failure is present. Thus, the spectrum of hemodynamic events from a small ventricular septal defect with small left-to-right shunt through the development of the Eisenmenger syndrome determines the size and shape of the heart, the pulmonary vascular volume and the shift from left to right ventricular volume overload, dilatation, and failure.

Ventricular septal defects falling into Groups I, II, and III from the radiologic point of view must be differentiated from all those other forms of acyanotic heart disease that have an increased pulmonary vascularity as shown on the conventional chest film. This includes, of course, atrial septal defect, partial anomalous pulmonary venous return, and patent ductus arteriosus. Table 10, page 255, outlines the major differential features. In the authors' experience, a precise differentiation from conventional radiologic findings was possible in no more than one-third of the cases. Even then the certainty of differentiation is not sufficient to permit a consideration of surgical treatment. As a result the great majority of these patients come to cardiac catheterization and selective angiography.

The Eisenmenger complex and syndrome must be differentiated from other forms of ventricular septal defect and also from patent ductus with pulmonary hypertension and reverse flow and the Taussig-Bing anomaly. Differentiation on the basis of any one set of films is usually most difficult. In the Taussig-Bing anomaly the pulmonary artery is usually not so large and yet the pulmonary vascularity is more pronounced than is usual with the Eisenmenger syndrome.

Group V (Miscellaneous Group). Patients with clinical and hemodynamic evidence of ventricular septal defect may have a complicating patent ductus arteriosus. Twenty such cases were found by Walker *et al.* (1965) in a series of 415 cases of ventricular septal defect, and Sasahara *et al.* (1960) described the findings in 22 such cases. These cases should be considered separately from those cases that have the typical findings of patent ductus arteriosus and which also have a small ventricular septal defect. This latter group seemingly have a better prognosis (Sasahara *et al.*, 1960). An unsuspected persistent patent ductus discovered at the time of surgical repair of a ventricular septal defect may constitute a considerable hazard due to flooding of the operative field by flow through the ductus. The diagnosis is difficult and requires a high index of suspicion. The heart is invariably enlarged and may be greatly enlarged, but there is no definite deviation or distinctive feature noted in the cardiac contour as seen in the conventional chest film. Right heart catheterization with deliberate attempts to pass the catheter through the ductus is helpful and is diagnostic when successful. The usual criterion of step-up in O_2 concentration in going from the right ventricle to the pulmonary artery is not too reliable since there may be streamlining or turbulence from a high ventricular septal defect that will produce a false positive increase in O_2 in the pulmonary artery.

Retrograde thoracic aortography also may be diagnostic and is indicated in doubtful cases. Although the mean pulmonary artery pressure in most of these cases is elevated, the shunt is from the aorta into the pulmonary artery and this can be clearly demonstrated by thoracic aortography.

Aortic regurgitation is a serious complication of ventricular septal defect and difficult to correct by surgical means. Also, it may offer a difficult diagnostic problem and must be differentiated from aneurysm of the sinus of Valsalva with rupture into the right ventricle or coronary right ventricular fistula and rheumatic aortic insufficiency. In a number of instances patients with this condition have been operated upon with a diagnosis of persistent patency of the ductus arteriosus (Keck *et al.*, 1963).

The ventricular septal defect is typically high in the membranous or bulbar portion of the septum above and anterior to the crista supraventricularis. The right coronary cusps have been involved in almost all of the reported cases, although the posterior or noncoronary cusp may be involved to some extent. Insufficiency of the cusp or cusps seems to develop over a period of time since no cases have been observed in patients under 1 year of age. The right coronary cusp is typically deformed, and its leading edge may become fibrous and thickened. Some observers have described the cusp as shortened,

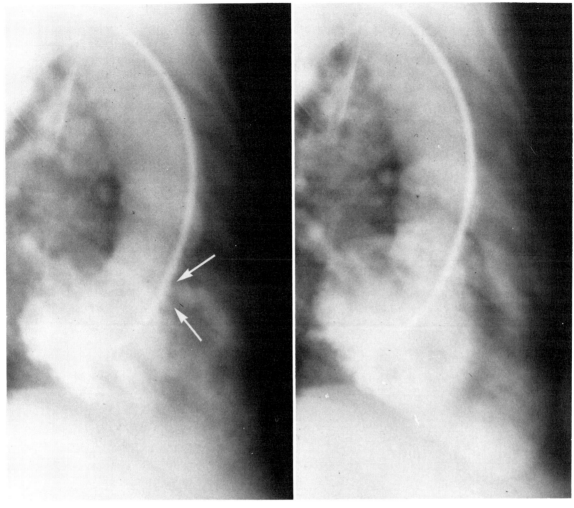

FIG. 218. VENTRICULAR SEPTAL DEFECT

The patient is an 8-year-old girl. A catheter was introduced into the right femoral artery, and its tip was advanced past the aortic valve into the left ventricle. Contrast material was injected into the left ventricle, and serial filming was performed in anteroposterior and lateral projections. The films reproduced here are selected lateral frames. That on the left shows contrast material pouring through a small high interventricular septal defect from the left ventricle anteriorly into the right ventricle. Arrows point to the location of the defect, and contrast material can be seen passing into the right ventricle between the arrows. The film reproduced on the right was made a moment later and shows contrast opacification of the right ventricle and the pulmonary outflow tract.

whereas others have found the leading edge of the cusp to be elongated. In many instances the ventricular septal defect has been immediately below the cusp, and this may be a factor in allowing the valve to recede or prolapse downward. In other cases this does not seem to be a factor, and the reason for the development of the insufficiency is obscure. A sizeable proportion (50% in the series of Keck *et al.*, 1963) of cases has had a significant pulmonic stenosis of the infundibular type with a gradient in excess of 15 mm Hg. Otherwise, pulmonary hypertension is the rule.

The significant clinical findings are those of aortic insufficiency with increased pulse pressure and ECG evidence of overloading of the left ventricle.

The radiologic changes as seen on conventional chest films are not distinctive. The heart is invariably enlarged and may be huge (Fig. 222). The left contour of the heart is long and the apex is low indicating left ventricular enlargement. The right border is also prominent and convex indicating enlargement and dilatation of the right atrium and right ventricle. Thus, the contour does differ to a degree from that of

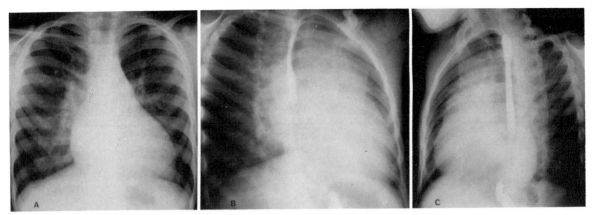

FIG. 219. VENTRICULAR SEPTAL DEFECT
VSD (1 cm) with moderate left to right shunt and PA pressure of 53/21. There is biventricular enlargement with the left ventricle being predominant. The left atrium is questionably enlarged. (Operative case.)

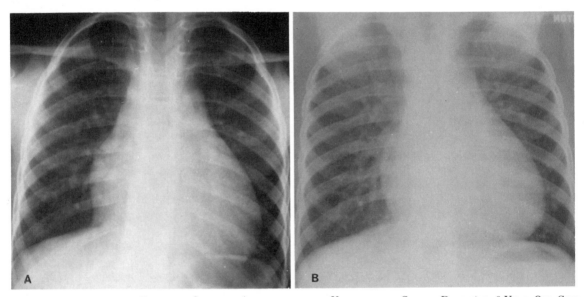

FIG. 220. DEVELOPMENT OF PULMONIC STENOSIS ASSOCIATED WITH VENTRICULAR SEPTAL DEFECT IN 6-YEAR-OLD GIRL
Right heart catheterization in 1958 showed a pulmonary artery pressure of 60/22 and a pulmonary-over-systemic flow ratio of 1.95/1. (A) Film exposed 3½ years later. The right ventricular pulmonary artery gradient is now about 20 mm Hg. (B) Film 2 years later. The gradient is now about 40 mm Hg. The heart is smaller, the apex is elevated, and the contour is more suggestive of a tetralogy of Fallot. This is now classified as an atypical tetralogy of Fallot. A right aortic arch is present.

uncomplicated aortic insufficiency. In about one-half of the cases reported by Keck *et al.* (1963) the left atrium was enlarged, although this was not present in 3 cases seen by the present authors. The peripheral arteries in the lungs are dilated even in the cases with pulmonic stenosis indicating increased pulmonary blood flow.

Left and right heart catheterization may show evidence of a ventricular septal defect with left-to-right shunt and reflux of contrast substance from the aorta into the left and usually the right ventricle. However, the mechanism and route of the shunt cannot be determined by this proce-dure. Retrograde thoracic aortography with injection of contrast substance just above the aortic valve is the crucial examination. The contrast substance refluxes into the left ventricle demonstrating a much enlarged and dilated chamber. The valve cusps are rarely seen sufficiently well to recognize a prolapse. In the 3 cases seen by the present authors the contrast substance as it refluxed was directed toward the left side of the ventricular cavity suggesting insufficiency of the right coronary cusp. Also, the contrast substance may be seen to enter the right ventricle through a septal defect confirming the presence of this anomaly (Fig. 222C). Contrast substance may be later identified in the pulmonary arteries. Even after a technically good aortogram showing contrast substance in both the left and right ventricles some doubt may remain as to the course of the contrast substance and the nature of the defect. Cineangiography, according to the authors' experience, is the method of choice in these cases because of the fleeting characteristics of the shunts.

Selective left ventriculography is the examination of choice for the demonstration of the defect in the ventricular septum located just beneath the pulmonic valve with which aortic insufficiency is commonly associated. On the frontal view of a selective left ventriculogram,

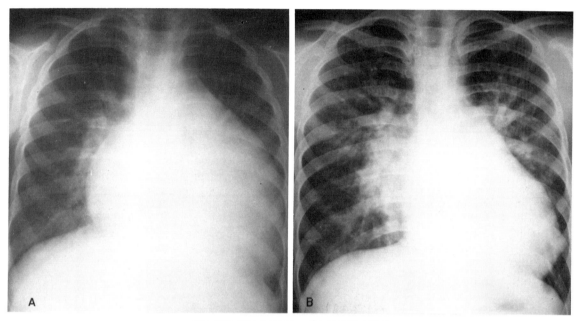

FIG. 221. VENTRICULAR SEPTAL DEFECT

(A) Conventional chest film of a 6-year-old girl with a membranous septal defect and aortic insufficiency. (B) Conventional chest film of a 14-year-old boy with a 3-cm membranous ventricular septal defect and subluxation of the right coronary aortic cusp. (Operative case.)

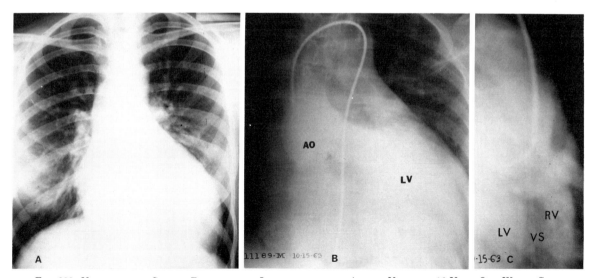

FIG. 222. VENTRICULAR SEPTAL DEFECT WITH INSUFFICIENCY OF AORTIC VALVE IN 16-YEAR-OLD WHITE GIRL

(A) Conventional chest film showing marked cardiac enlargement with predominance of the left ventricle. (B) Retrograde aortogram showing reflux into the left ventricle. (C) Lateral view showing contrast substance in both right and left ventricles. AO, aorta; RV, right ventricle; LV, left ventricle; VS, ventricular septum.

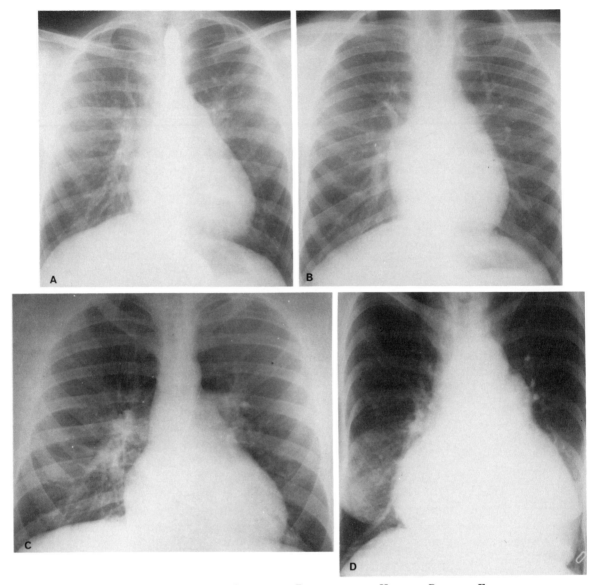

FIG. 223. FOUR CASES OF EISENMENGER COMPLEX AS DETERMINED BY HISTORY, PHYSICAL EXAMINATION, AND CARDIAC CATHETERIZATION

(A) Eleven-year-old boy with a heart murmur since early life, minimal cyanosis, and a pulmonary artery pressure equal to systemic pressure. Symptoms of limited exercise tolerance appeared during past year. (B) Thirteen-year-old boy with a heart murmur but little impairment of activity and no cyanosis, peripheral saturation of 90%, pulmonary artery pressure 109/60, systemic 112/70. (C) Nineteen-year-old male patient with frank cyanosis. PA pressure 119/57, brachial artery pressure 120/70. Marked right to left and minimal left to right shunt at ventricular level. The pulmonary trunk appears only minimally dilated. (D) Forty-year-old woman, cyanotic since 3 years of age. Marked limitation of activity. PA pressure 118/79, systemic 122/70.

such a defect is seen as a jet of contrast material arising from beneath the left aspect of the aortic valve and extending into the subpulmonic region of the right ventricle. It should be remembered that opacification of the right ventricular outflow tract alone, and not the body of the right ventricle, is not reliable evidence of such a defect because the jet of contrast material passing through a membranous septal defect may be directed upward and fill primarily the infundibular region. Recognition of a subpulmonic ventricular septal defect in the lateral view depends upon identification of the crista supraventricularis and location of the opacified shunt above it or across it (Steinfeld et al., 1972).

Surgical repair of the high ventricular septal defect will not suffice in these cases. The prolapsed and deformed valve cusps must be treated in some manner that restores the integrity of the valve, and this taxes the ingenuity of the surgeon (Spencer *et al.*, 1962; Ellis *et al.*, 1963; Trusler *et al.*, 1973). San Fellipo *et al.* (1974) recommend early closure for VSDs associated with mild aortic insufficiency. With severe aortic insufficiency, VSD closure and valve plication are preferred, although valve replacement may be necessary either at the primary operation or at some future date. In adults, replacement with a prosthesis is indicated for the patient with severe aortic insufficiency.

Lauer *et al.* (1960) reported on 10 cases of ventricular septal defect in which there was a muscular subaortic stenosis or bandlike subaortic stenosis or an abnormality of the anterior leaflet of the mitral valve. In all of these cases there was an obstruction to the exit from the left ventricle. The presence of such an obstruction would prevent a good result following repair of an interventricular septal defect, and the possibility of such an obstruction should be considered. These obstructions are demonstrated by left ventricular angiography.

SURGICAL CONSIDERATIONS. Almost all infants and babies with ventricular septal defects improve on modern medical management, and spontaneous closure of some defects may make subsequent consideration of surgical treatment unnecessary. Recurrent cardiac decompensation despite optimal medical therapy or the inability of the baby to gain weight and grow normally indicate failure of medical management and suggest the need for early cardiac repair.

Surgical alternatives include palliative banding of the pulmonary artery and definitive closure of the septal defect at open heart surgery. Pulmonary artery banding in order to diminish pulmonary blood flow and tide the young patient over a difficult period has been quite popular and has doubtless been extremely beneficial in many patients. The risks of banding include an immediate mortality of 20–25% on the average (Engle, 1972), the production of a right-to-left shunt by too tight banding and the difficulty of removing the band and repairing the defect at a second operation. In addition, the results of banding are poor when the ratio of pulmonary flow to systemic flow (Qp/Qs) is less than 2.0 (Utley, 1973). In addition, the mortality from the two-stage surgical management (banding followed by definitive repair at a later date) is considerably in excess of the mortality reported for primary closure (Patel *et al.*, 1973; Cordell *et al.*, 1972; Henry *et al.*, 1973; Coleman *et al.*, 1972). Some advocates of pulmonary artery banding have found an increased incidence of spontaneous closure of VSDs in this group of patients when compared with the rate of closure of large VSDs without pulmonary artery banding (Mesko *et al.*, 1973), but others believe that the banding procedure probably does not influence spontaneous closure

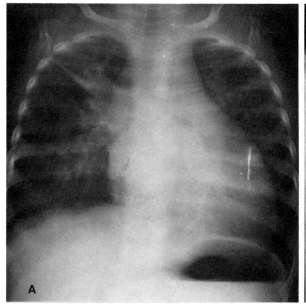 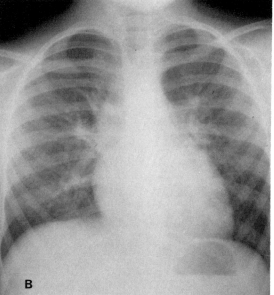

FIG. 224. VENTRICULAR SEPTAL DEFECT WITH PULMONARY HYPERTENSION (61/17) AFTER BANDING PROCEDURE
(A) Preoperative film. (B) Three years postoperative. The heart had decreased in size, and the pulmonary vasculature was less prominent. There had been a corresponding improvement in the patient's condition.

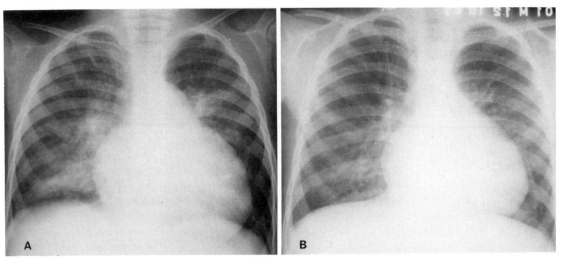

FIG. 225. VENTRICULAR SEPTAL DEFECT WITH PULMONARY HYPERTENSION AFTER BANDING PROCEDURE
(A) Preoperative film. (B) Two years postoperative. The heart is slightly smaller, and the pulmonary vascularity is within normal limits.

(Bonchek *et al.* 1973). While some continue to advocate the two-stage surgical management of large VSDs as a satisfactory alternative to early primary closure (Girod *et al.*, 1974), most authors now advocate primary closure of ventricular septal defects in symptomatic infants and consider this to be the procedure of choice in dealing with infants who fail to respond to medical management (O'Donovan *et al.*, 1972; Nicoloff *et al.*, 1971; Henry *et al.*, 1973; Hoffman, 1974; Griep *et al.*, 1974). Most authors now declare that pulmonary artery banding may still be the procedure of choice in some children with complex lesions or in those for whom no definitive operation is currently available or in patients with unusual problems such as multiple muscular defects and associated complicating lesions or because of the extremely small size of the infant. Its routine use in children whose primary lesion is a ventricular septal defect is probably no longer justifiable.

The overall results of surgery in ventricular septal defect associated with a high level of pulmonary vascular resistance are unfavorable. Efforts should be made to interrupt the natural history of the disease before significant pulmonary vascular obstructive changes have occurred, and that can be achieved by surgical closure at an early age (Friedli *et al.*, 1974). A transventricular approach is ordinarily employed, but trans-atrial and transaortic approaches have also been described and used (Galioto *et al.*, 1973).

The single most important criterion employed by pediatric cardiologists in determining the suitability of a patient with an uncomplicated ventricular septal defect for operation is a large pulmonary blood flow. According to Moss (1970), 95% of pediatric cardiologists polled by him would not advise operation for the person with uncomplicated small VSD, but 90% would recommend operation if the Qp/Qs were 2.1 to 1, and all would refer for operative closure patients with Qp/Qs of 2.5 to 1 or greater.

Radiologic Changes after Surgical Repair of Ventricular Septal Defect. The postoperative appearance varies according to the preoperative appearance of the chest, such as heart size, extent of pulmonary vascularity and length of the postoperative period. At the end of 1–2 weeks, when conventional chest films are possible, the heart is commonly larger than it was preoperatively, and the smaller hearts often show the largest increase in size. The enlargement appears to be due to some degree of heart failure after cardiotomy. Over the ensuing year a gradual decrease in heart size is usual with the larger heart showing the greatest decrease in size. Rarely, however, does the heart become normal in size, particularly if it was considerably enlarged preoperatively. Ho *et al.* (1973), reporting on pre- and postoperative chest films on 42 patients, found approximately the same degree of cardiac enlargement as that before surgery. In their experience, most patients with severe pulmonary hypertension (5 of 6) and previous pulmonary artery banding (5 of 8) had persistently abnormal cardiothoracic ratios following surgery.

The size of the main pulmonary artery segment changes little if at all though over the ensuing year following operation the segment

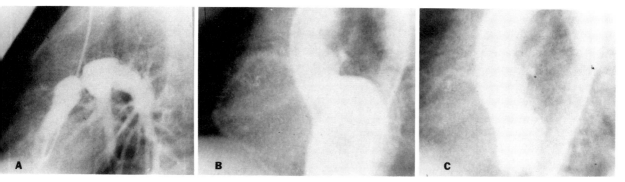

FIG. 226. SPONTANEOUS CLOSURE OF VENTRICULAR SEPTAL DEFECT FOLLOWING PULMONARY ARTERY BANDING
(A) Lateral film from a selective right ventriculogram shows the narrowed area in the pulmonary trunk which marks the site of the band applied to the pulmonary artery to reduce the increased pulmonary blood flow in this child shown by cardiac catheterization to have a ventricular septal defect. (B) Selective left ventriculogram. The catheter was introduced into the left ventricle across the aortic valve. The left anterior oblique position was employed, and this frame was exposed in ventricular diastole. No abnormality is seen. The interventricular septum is seen end on in this view. (C) At the height of ventricular contraction, no contrast material traverses the interventricular septum to opacify the right ventricle and pulmonary artery. It was concluded that the defect previously demonstrated by cardiac catheterization had closed spontaneously.

may gradually become somewhat reduced in size in the successful cases. The majority of patients show increased pulmonary vascularity in the immediate postoperative period, and part of this may be due to the venous congestion that attends open heart surgery. It tends to disappear after a few weeks. In the series reported by Ho et al. (1973), the central and mid portions of the lungs showed the most striking changes following operation. Fifteen of the 21 patients who had increased vascularity in the midlung fields before surgery showed a reduction in these markings. Return toward normal in the size of the left atrium is unpredictable following operation.

Tricuspid regurgitation may develop after repair of ventricular septal defect and may be due to operative injury to the tricuspid valve or may be the consequence of right ventricular dilatation (Fisher et al., 1973). When incapacitating right heart failure is caused by primary tricuspid regurgitation it can usually be effectively relieved by tricuspid valve replacement. Complete right bundle branch block, probably the result of the ventriculotomy, has also been reported (Ziady et al., 1972), and recurrence of the defect (usually due to failure of the sutures to hold securely in the perimeter of the defect) occurred in 22 of 370 patients reported by Dobell et al. (1972). Since the accuracy of roentgenograms in predicting the severity of a ventricular septal defect has been shown to be poor (Ho et al., 1973), it is not surprising that the completeness of surgical closure of the VSD could not be predicted by this means.

Endocardial Cushion Defects. GENERAL CONSIDERATIONS. Endocardial cushion defects consist of a spectrum of anomalies with simple primum defects of the atrial septum at one end and a complete persistent common atrioventricular canal at the other. The common denominator in all of these conditions is that the defects occur in those structures that develop from the endocardial cushions.

For a detailed discussion of the anatomy and embryology of these defects, the reader is referred to the excellent articles by Rogers and Edwards (1948) and Van Mierop et al. (1962). In reference to the section on embryology (page 44), it can be seen that at approximately the 7-mm C-R length stage the primitive cardiac tube is divided into three chambers, namely the atrium, the ventricle, and the bulbus cordis. Corresponding to the infoldings on the exterior the endocardial cushions appear on the interior of the heart in the region of the common atrioventricular canal. If the superior surface of the diaphragm is considered to be in a horizontal plane, then the cushions are arranged in a vertical plane. At about the 9-mm C-R length stage the cushions have developed so that the atrioventricular canal is a slitlike opening with vertical extensions on each end and the entire opening resembles somewhat the contour of an I-beam. At this stage four cushions are recognized, namely superior, inferior, and right and left lateral cushions. The superior and inferior cushions fuse centrally dividing the primitive canal into two parts. Also, at about the same time these two cushions arch superiorly and posteriorly and proliferate to join the margin of the septum primum and thus close the ostium primum. Meanwhile, the ventricular septum grows superiorly and anteriorly and deviates somewhat toward the right to join the endocardial cushions and complete the interventricular septum. The lateral portions of the endocardial cushions develop into the mitral and tricuspid valves. Thus, the endocardial cushions are the precursors of the mitral and tricuspid valves, the membranous ventricular septum, and the inferior portion of the atrial septum. The left lateral cushion is the precursor of the posterior leaflet of the normal mitral valve. The left portion of the superior cushion forms the anterior one-half of the anterior leaflet of the mitral valve, and the corresponding portion of the inferior cushion forms the posterior one-half. When these two precursors fail to fuse normally, the anterior leaflet shows a partial or complete cleft. Similarly, the anterior one-third of the medial or septal leaflet of the tricuspid valve is formed by the right part of the superior cushion and the middle one-third by the right part of the inferior cushion, and failure of fusion produces a cleft in the tricuspid valve. A partial or complete cleft of the anterior leaflet of the mitral valve is a frequent finding in association with a septum primum defect and may cause some degree of mitral insufficiency. A cleft in the medial leaflet of the tricuspid valve is less common and is usually associated with a defect in the membranous ventricular septum.

In the normal heart the mitral valve ring or line of attachment is at a higher level than that of the tricuspid valve. Because of the lower position of the tricuspid valve a part of the outflow tract of the left ventricle is separated from the right atrium by a thin membrane, and this provides the anatomical basis for a left ventricular

right atrial septal defect (page 305). In the more severe forms of endocardial cushion defect the mitral valve is displaced downward and lies at the same level as the tricuspid valve. Particularly in persistent common atrioventricular canal the mitral and tricuspid valve cusps are continuous through an interventricular septal defect. Of particular importance, however, is the line of attachment of the anterior leaflet. This leaflet is displaced downward and forward, its line of attachment is along the outflow tract of the left ventricle, and its margins are attached by short chordae tendineae in the upper scooped out edge of a ventricular septal defect (Baron, 1968). This anterior leaflet is thickened and cleft. Because of this combination of deformities there is impingement on and narrowing of the outflow tract of the left ventricle producing subaortic stenosis (Rogers and Edwards, 1948; Van Mierop et al., 1962; Baron et al., 1964). As will be seen, this narrowing and deformity of the outflow tract of the left ventricle may be the key to the angiographic diagnosis of the more severe forms of endocardial cushion defect.

Five lesions are possible as a result of congenital defect in the endocardial cushions: (1) a defect in the lower portion of the atrial septum, (2) a high ventricular septal defect, (3) a cleft in the anterior leaflet of the mitral valve, (4) a cleft in the septal leaflet of the tricuspid valve and (5) subaortic stenosis as a result of the anomalous insertion of chordae tendineae from the mitral valve to the ventricular septum. The two most common combinations are (1) ostium primum atrial septal defect accompanied by a cleft in the anterior leaflet of the mitral valve and (2) complete atrioventricular canal in which central fusion of the endocardial cushion derivatives has not occurred and the mitral and tricuspid valves are not clearly differentiated.

SEPTUM PRIMUM DEFECT WITH CLEFT OF ANTERIOR LEAFLET OF MITRAL VALVE. As indicated in the previous section, some degree of deformity with cleft formation of the anterior leaflet of the mitral valve is a frequent finding in association with primum defects of the atrial septum. Conventional films do not offer any specific changes that would permit differentiating this condition from septum secundum defects. Left atrial enlargement has been noted in a few cases (Kjellberg et al., 1958) and occasionally is a significant differential feature (Fig. 228D). The left ventricle is larger and more hypertrophied than with the septum secundum defects, but this is seldom detectable on conventional films. Electrocardiographic and vectorcardiographic findings and left ventriculography are

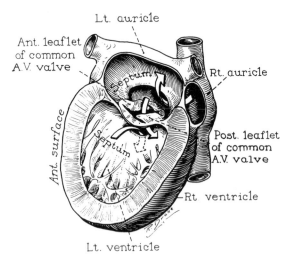

Lt. auricle

Ant. leaflet of common A.V. valve

Septum

Rt. auricle

Ant. surface

Septum

Post. leaflet of common A.V. valve

Rt ventricle

Lt. ventricle

FIG. 227. SEMIDIAGRAMMATIC DRAWING OF PERSISTENT COMMON ATRIOVENTRICULAR CANAL
(From Rogers and Edwards (1948).)

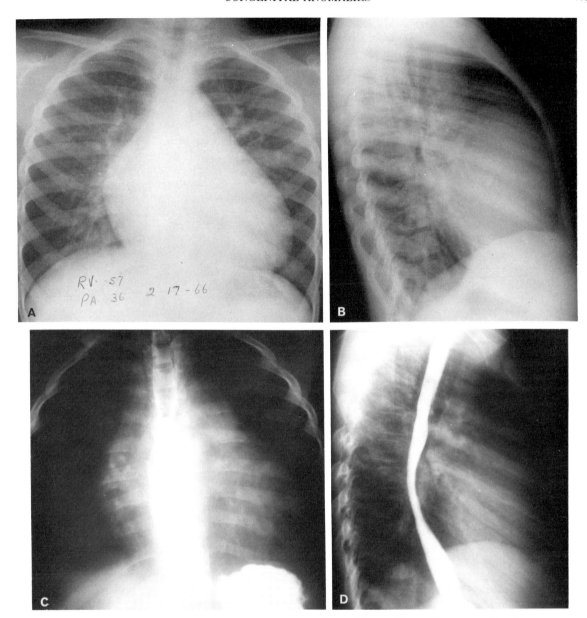

FIG. 228. LARGE SEPTUM PRIMUM DEFECT WITH CLEFT MITRAL VALVE (OPERATIVE CASE)
(A) and (B) show an enlarged right ventricle and increased pulmonary vascularity. Cinefluorography showed reflux from the left ventricle into the atria. The left atrium appears enlarged (C and D) due to the mitral insufficiency and this is of diagnostic importance. The right atrial contour is full and convex indicating marked enlargement.

the keys to the diagnosis, particularly the latter procedure. A selective injection of contrast substance into the left ventricle may show the outline of the displaced anterior leaflet of the mitral valve and the cleft best seen during ventricular systole (Baron *et al.*, 1964). In ventricular diastole the outflow tract is deformed producing a "goose neck" contour (see below). Reflux through the valve into the atrium may be noted indicating insufficiency (Grant *et al.*, 1957).

PERSISTENT COMMON ATRIOVENTRICULAR CANAL (AURICULOVENTRICULARIS COMMUNIS). This anomaly is the most severe and complete manifestation of the group of endocardial cushion defects. As indicated above, less extensive varieties may occur. The cushions may fuse to divide the A-V canal into two parts, but the atrial and ventricular septal defects persist along with a cleft in the mitral valve. This condition may be considered as a transitional type. More rarely the atrial or ventricular septum may be intact. Differentiation of these varieties of cushion defects by radiologic means is rarely possible, and we consider all of the variations under a single heading. The recognition and differentiation of these conditions from the simpler forms of atrial septal defect and other forms of congenital heart disease are of great importance since repair is most difficult.

In persistent common atrioventricular canal the atrial septum is deficient in its lower portion, usually in the form of an arched opening, the floor of which is formed by a common atrioventricular valve (Fig. 227). This common valve may have as many as five leaflets, although the major anterior and posterior leaflets are by far the largest. The smaller leaflets, which on the right side are the remnants of the tricuspid valve and on the left side are the posterior leaflets of the mitral valve, are succinctly described in the article by Rogers and Edwards (1948) and by Van Mierop *et al.* (1962). The valve leaflets are deformed, their edges are rolled, and the chordae tendineae may be shortened so that some degree of insufficiency of a portion or all of the valve is present. The underlying ventricular septum is also deficient. This usually involves the membranous portion but may extend to or involve also the adjacent muscular portion. The most important feature is the impingement of the valve on the outflow tract of the left ventricle which has been described above.

The pulmonary artery is dilated and considerably larger than the aorta unless there is an associated pulmonic stenosis. This additional anomaly of pulmonic stenosis has been noted in a number of cases (Rogers and Edwards, 1948; Abrams and Kaplan, 1956). The right ventricle is dilated and hypertrophied even more than is usual in simple atrial defect. The right atrium is also considerably dilated, and the left atrium is often enlarged secondary to insufficiency of the atrioventricular valve.

Blood is shunted left to right through both atrial and ventricular septal defects, and the blood flow to the lungs is greatly increased. Furthermore, some degree of pulmonary hypertension is usual, and rarely this may be sufficient to reverse the left-to-right shunt and produce a mild and often terminal cyanosis. The most influential factor in the production of cyanosis is the presence or absence of pulmonic stenosis, but this is an additional complicating anomaly.

This anomaly is uncommon. It constituted about 2% of all cases of congenital heart disease reported by Keith *et al.* (1958). Rogers and Edwards (1948) were able to collect a total of 55 cases from the literature. About one-third of the reported cases have been in children with mongolism. Symptoms appear early, usually during the first months of life, and are characterized by shortness of breath and heart failure. Cyanosis is rare. Keith *et al.* (1958) state that the first clues to the diagnosis are the presence of a harsh murmur to the left of the sternum and particularly an ECG pattern in which the standard leads show left axis deviation and the precordial leads show right ventricular hypertrophy. In the cases collected by Rogers and Edwards (1948), half of the patients were dead by the end of the first year.

Radiologic Findings. As seen on conventional chest films, the heart is enlarged (Fig. 229). The contour may resemble that of uncomplicated atrial septal defect except that the heart is usually larger and enlarges at a much earlier age than is usual with uncomplicated atrial septal defect. The heart is often roughly triangular in shape with convex right and straight left borders. The right atrial contour is often long and convex indicating considerable dilatation. Although the left atrium is often enlarged, it is difficult to identify it by the usual criteria. The pulmonary vasculature is increased in prominence, and the pulmonary trunk is dilated unless there is pulmonic stenosis. The right ventricle may be quite large and dilated, and Keith *et al.* (1958) state that it often produces a bulge along the left upper border of the heart.

Cardiac catheterization may be quite helpful but is rarely diagnostic. The right atrial blood shows a considerable increase in O_2 concentration as compared with that in the superior or inferior vena cava. Also, dye curves and hydrogen tests will show a left-to-right shunt. Of crucial importance is a further increase in oxygen content of blood removed from the right ventricle as compared with that in the right atrium. Wakai *et al.* (1956) reported that such an increase in oxygen content was found in 6 of their 9 cases; however, Kjellberg *et al.* (1958) regard this finding as unreliable since it is also found in uncomplicated atrial septal defect with a large left-to-right shunt due to streamlining of the blood so that it passes into the right ventricle without appreciable mixing in the right atrium.

The pressure in the right ventricle is almost uniformly elevated in contrast to that found in uncomplicated atrial defects in which the pressure is seldom elevated in early life. The catheter may be manipulated through the atrial defect usually without difficulty and may appear to enter the left ventricle through the high ventricular septal defect. Thus, the catheter may appear

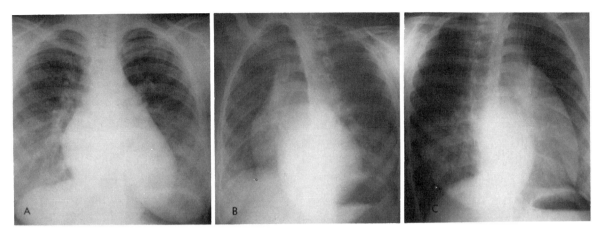

FIG. 229 A–C. ENDOCARDIAL CUSHION DEFECT (OPERATIVE AND AUTOPSY CASE)
There were atrial and ventricular septal defects and a cleft in the anterior leaflet of the mitral valve.

lower or more caudal in relation to the cardiac silhouette than is usual with secundum defects. A further differential feature was mentioned by Wakai *et al.* (1956). In simple atrial defect, as a rule, blood entering the left atrium from the left lung is shunted through the atrial defect into the right atrium, whereas blood from the right lung passes into the left ventricle. Such differential shunting is not found in persistent atrioventricular canal. Consequently, injections of dye into each pulmonary artery should give dye contours or curves of similar form in contrast to curves of different contour found in atrial septal defect.

Selective left ventriculography is the angiographic procedure of choice. The displaced and deformed anterior mitral leaflet impinges on the right lateral margin of the outflow tract of the left ventricle as seen in the frontal projection (Fig. 230). In ventricular systole, the cleft in the anterior leaflet of the mitral valve forms a radiolucent notch on the right side of the left ventricular outflow tract. In diastole the anterior leaflet balloons downward into the outflow tract causing it to be more horizontal than normal and narrowed. This deformity has a gooseneck contour (Baron *et al.*, 1964; Girod *et al.*, 1965; Cornell, 1965; Baron, 1972), and the outflow tract may be sufficiently narrowed to produce a degree of subaortic stenosis. When the typical appearance is seen in both systole and diastole, a definite diagnosis of a cushion defect can be made. According to Baron (1972) the systolic picture is more reliable because it is not encountered with any other cardiac lesion. Anatomic studies by Blieden *et al.* (1974) indicate that the inflow aspect of the left ventricle and the ventricular septum are short relative to the outflow length of the ventricular septum in this anomaly. In addition,

there is a deficiency in the subaortic aspect of the ventricular septum.

Left ventriculography may also show reflux of contrast substance into the left atrium as a manifestation of mitral insufficiency. McMullan *et al.* (1973) found that the severity of mitral regurgitation demonstrated angiographically correlated poorly with the degree of insufficiency found by auscultation, intra-atrial palpation at the time of operation and analysis of indicator dilution curves in a series of 232 patients.

Cardiopulmonary bypass is necessary for the complete repair of these anomalies; hypothermia and circulatory arrest may also be employed. The cleft mitral valve is sutured, and if the tricuspid valve septal leaflet is cleft it is also repaired. The atrial septal defect is closed using a pericardial or prosthetic patch if necessary, and the ventricular defect, if present, is closed with interrupted sutures or a separate patch. If the defect in the anterior leaflet of the mitral valve is so great as to prevent repair, the valve may be replaced with a prosthesis (Garbode and Carr, 1971). The mortality rate for repair of partial atrioventricular canal varies between 5 and 19%, but the surgical mortality for the repair of complete atrioventricular canal has varied between 30 and 73% according to Garbode and Carr (1971). McGoon *et al.* (1973) declare that corrective repair of complete atrioventricular canal in older patients can be accomplished with a mortality rate of only 7%.

McMullan *et al.* (1973) determined the cardiothoracic ratio before and after operation on 60 patients who underwent surgical treatment of partial atrioventricular canal. Forty-eight patients showed a decrease in heart size, 10 showed no change, and 2 showed enlargement. In gen-

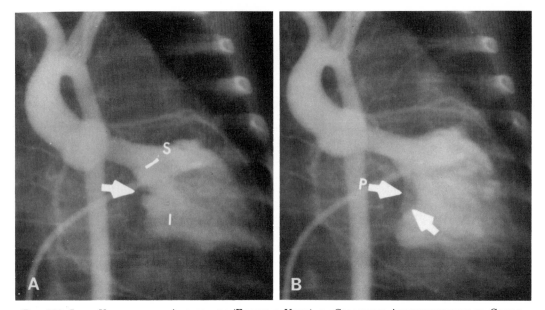

FIG. 230. LEFT VENTRICULAR ANGIOGRAM (FRONTAL VIEW) IN COMPLETE ATRIOVENTRICULAR CANAL.

(A) Early systole. The cleft (arrow) between the superior (S) and inferior (I) segments of the anterior mitral leaflet is seen along the right contour of the ventricle. There is no evidence of mitral insufficiency or an interventricular shunt. (B) Diastole. The ventricular outflow tract is narrowed and lies in a more horizontal position than is normal. The right border of the ventricle can be followed directly into the scooped out margin (arrow) of the interventricular septum. The attachment of the posterior mitral leaflet (P) is also visible because of a thin layer of contrast material trapped between the leaflet and the posterior ventricular wall. (From Baron *et al.*, 1964.)

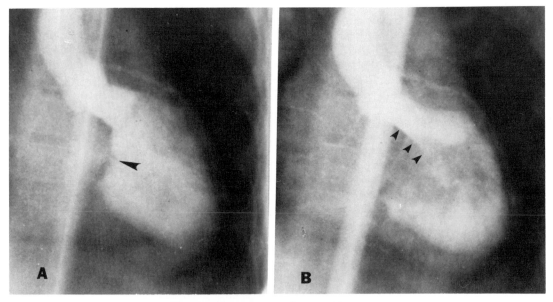

FIG. 231. ENDOCARDIAL CUSHION DEFECT

Contrast material was injected into the left ventricle through a catheter which was introduced across the aortic valve from the aorta. Filming was performed in the frontal projection. In ventricular systole (A) the right border of the left ventricle is seen to be irregular, and a notch in its border (arrow) indicates the location of the cleft in the deformed anterior leaflet of the mitral valve. A tiny puff of contrast material can be seen just to the right of this notch, representing minimal but definitie mitral regurgitation. In ventricular diastole (B) the deformed and dislocated anterior mitral leaflet encroaches upon the outflow tract of the left ventricle producing the elongated "gooseneck" deformity characteristic of this condition (arrows).

eral, successful cases will show decrease in heart size, pulmonary artery size and pulmonary vascular volume. If repair of the mitral valve is incomplete and some degree of mitral insufficiency persists, the left atrium may remain somewhat enlarged.

Surgical repair of the atrial septal defect and the cleft mitral valve in adult patients causes very little change in the characteristic angiographic picture of the left ventricle, the left ventricular outflow tract or the mitral valve. The radiolucent notch representing the cleft in the anterior leaflet was seen in 6 of 8 cases postoperatively despite suture repair in a series reported by Randall et al. (1974). The gooseneck deformity also persists after surgical treatment even if the mitral valve is replaced by a prosthesis, and Blieden et al. (1974) suggest that the gooseneck deformity which remains even following correction of the deficiency in the ventricular septum appears to be related to the short nature of the inflow part of the left ventricular wall at its diaphragmatic aspect.

Left Ventricular-Right Atrial Communication. A comunication between the left ventricle and right atrium should be considered in the differential diagnosis of both ASD and VSD. The variable anatomy of this rare anomaly has been well described by Perry et al. (1949). It exists in three general forms:

1. The upper and posterior portion of the membranous ventricular septum is in contact with the right atrial wall. Consequently, a defect may result in a communication between the left ventricle and right atrium.

2. Most defects of the membranous ventricular septum occur near the septal leaflet of the tricuspid valve. If, in addition, a defect or cleft in this leaflet of the tricuspid valve is present, blood from the left ventricle may enter first the right ventricle, then reflux into the right atrium, and, thus, in effect, produce a left ventricular-right atrial shunt.

3. The septal leaflet of the tricuspid valve may have a defect that is adherent to the margins of the defect in the ventricular septum. The flow of blood is thus from the left ventricle through the ventricular septal defect and through the substance of the tricuspid valve into the right atrium. The net effect is a left-to-right shunt of variable size, depending upon the size of the defect. Associated defects are said to be rare, but a proved case of complete transposition of the great vessels associated with a left ventricular-right atrial communication has been described by Edwards et al. (1965, page 370).

Symptoms may be mild or absent, but a considerable proportion of the reported cases have had dyspnea, palpitation, poor nutrition, and a susceptibility to respiratory infection (Gerbode et al., 1958; Braunwald and Morrow, 1960; Stahlman et al., 1955). A common and often striking finding was the presence of a loud systolic murmur and thrill just to the left of the lower portion of the sternum. On the basis of clinical examination, a ventricular septal defect was often suspected.

Right heart catheterization shows an increase in oxygen content in the right atrium and mild hypertension in the right ventricle. Also, as particularly noted in the cases of Braunwald and Morrow (1960) following right atrial catheterization through the inferior vena cava, the catheter could not be made to enter the left atrium. The above-mentioned combination of findings should lead to a suspicion of the presence of left ventricular-right atrial communication.

RADIOLOGIC FINDINGS. On the PA chest film, the heart is always enlarged, and in a few instances the enlargement has been marked. The contour is somewhat symmetrical due to increased prominence of the right atrial contour. The left midborder of the heart is convex due to enlargement of the pulmonary trunk. The right and left pulmonary arteries and the more peripheral branches are enlarged indicating increased pulmonary blood flow. In the left anterior oblique view, enlargement of the right atrium may be striking, and this involves the right atrial appendage at the base of the aorta. The left ventricle is usually enlarged as indicated by the posterior convexity in this view. In the right anterior oblique view, enlargement of the right atrium is again evident by a posterior extension, often posterior to the barium-filled esophagus. The frequency of enlargement of the left atrium seems uncertain. Kramer and Abrams (1962) found the left atrium enlarged in only 1 of 5 patients, whereas Edwards et al. (1965) found enlargement of both atria to be common and of considerable value in differentiation from both ASD and VSD as single lesions. In the single case observed by the present authors, the left atrium was definitely enlarged.

The right ventricle is enlarged, and this is best shown in the lateral projection where it bulges into the retrosternal space. Some anterior bowing of the sternum is common (Kramer and Abrams, 1962).

Although the left ventricle is uniformly enlarged in this condition, differentiation from uncomplicated ASD on the basis of left ventricular

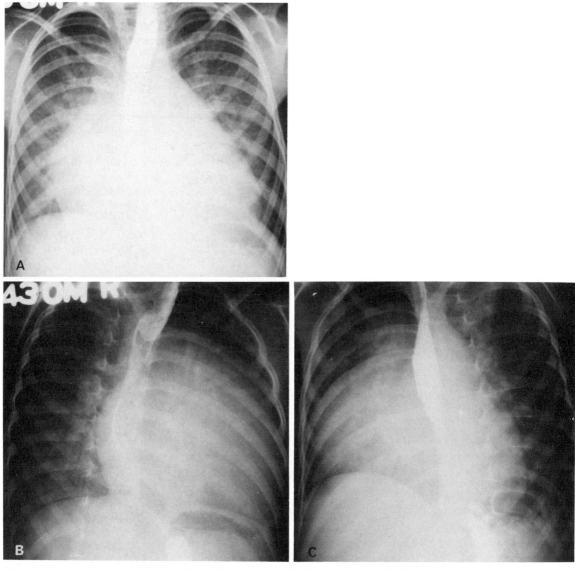

FIG. 232. LEFT VENTRICULAR-RIGHT ATRIAL COMMUNICATION

The preoperative diagnosis was ventricular septal defect, and the correct diagnosis was made after the heart was opened at the operating table. There was also a mild subaortic stenosis. Left ventriculography is the method of choice in establishing the diagnosis.

enlargement is uncertain. The most important finding on the conventional films is the increased prominence of the right atrial contour in a patient thought otherwise to have a ventricular septal defect and the presence of biatrial enlargement with other evidence of a left-to-right shunt at the atrial level.

The most definitive diagnostic procedure is left ventricular angiography (Braunwald and Morrow, 1960; Nordenström and Ovenfors, 1960). The contrast substance is shunted rapidly from the left ventricle into the right atrium, and this can be demonstrated by rapid serial filming in frontal and lateral projections. The route by which the contrast substance reaches the atrium might be subject to question, however, since a ruptured sinus of Valsalva might show early opacification of the right atrium. This difficulty was encountered by Carey et al. (1964) and was resolved by percutaneous left transaortic ventriculography and aortography. Braunwald and Morrow (1960) felt that the absence of a continuous murmur was good evidence against an aortic right atrial shunt.

Response to closure of the communication was usually objective and gratifying, and there was often a striking reduction in heart size and pulmonary vascularity (Braunwald and Morrow, 1960; Gerbode et al., 1958).

Usually Associated with Right-to-Left Shunt with (1) and Obstruction; (2) Malposition of One or Both Great Vessels; or (3) Both.

Tetralogy of Fallot. This malformation is the most common cause of congenital cyanotic heart disease. Furthermore, since it is susceptible to surgical palliative treatment either by the establishment of a systemic to pulmonary shunt (Blalock-Taussig (1945), Potts (1946), or Waterston (1962) procedure) or by total correction (Lillehei et al., 1955; Kirklin et al., 1955) it represents more than 70% of those cases of cyanotic heart disease that come to surgical treatment.

The malformation consists of the following abnormalities: (1) pulmonic stenosis, (2) high ventricular septal defect, (3) dextroposed (in relation to the interventricular septum) and overriding aorta, and (4) hypertrophy of the right ventricle.

Pulmonic stenosis is the most important of these defects and may be the primary initiating abnormality during the maturation of the embryonic heart (Van Praagh et al., 1970). In the tetralogy of Fallot, the crista supraventricularis is displaced anteriorly and to the left and thus encroaches on the outflow tract of the right ventricle. This causes a narrowing and often a distortion of the infundibulum with a variable degree of pulmonic stenosis. Much evidence suggests that the infundibular stenosis becomes relatively more severe as the heart increases in size with natural growth (Kirklin and Karp, 1970). Although displacement and hypertrophy of the crista supraventricularis is an essential feature of the tetralogy of Fallot, from a functional viewpoint it is not always easy to differentiate this abnormality from a simple hypertrophy of the infundibular musculature secondary to an increased work load. This latter condition obtains in some cases of ventricular septal defect with pulmonary hypertension and valvular pulmonic stenosis. Gasul et al. (1957) followed several cases of ventricular septal defect with pulmonary hypertension for several years. During this time pulmonic stenosis appeared and increased in severity to the point that a left-to-right shunt was reversed, although in most instances the peripheral unsaturation was insufficient to produce cyanosis. There is little doubt that borderline cases exist in which it is difficult to determine whether a tetralogy of Fallot with a congenital abnormality of the crista supraventricularis is present or whether one is dealing with a ventricular septal defect with pulmonic stenosis due to hypertrophy of the infundibulum. Where the systolic pressure in the right ventricle is equal to that in the aorta associated with a pulmonic stenosis and there is peripheral unsaturation, classification of a functional tetralogy seems justified.

The pulmonary stenosis is infundibular or a combination of infundibular and valvular or quite rarely is due to an isolated valvular obstruction. Although the crista supraventricularis is constantly enlarged and displaced, the pattern of enlargement and the anatomy of the infundibulum are variable. Both branches of the crista, namely the septal and parietal bands, may sharply divide the right ventricle into two chambers, the main chamber and a smaller outflow or infundibular chamber (the so-called third ventricle). The ostium or passageway into the infundibular chamber may be of varying length, and the chamber may be of variable size. When the passageway is long, it is usually irregular and shows a number of pits or depressions in the muscular wall. On the other hand, the chamber may be fusiform or bell-shaped or the entire outflow tract may be a long, narrow slightly irregular passageway without a distinct dilatation or chamber.

Valvular stenosis in the tetralogy of Fallot is most often due to a bicuspid or unicommissural type of valve (Jeffery et al., 1972). The valve may be thickened with rolled edges, and in some of these cases, there is associated valvular insufficiency. In some cases, the valve leaflets are small warty-like excrescences, and the valve is insufficient. In addition, in a minority of cases the valve ring is narrowed, and in a few instances, this may be the predominant cause of the stenosis. Complete obliteration of the valve ring or pulmonary atresia produces a pseudotruncus arteriosus or an extreme tetralogy. In this condition, despite the interruption in the region of the pulmonary valve, the distal pulmonary artery and its branches persist and by means of bronchial and other systemic anastomoses carry blood to both lungs (Taussig, 1960). Also, the interior of the heart shows a displacement and hypertrophy of the crista supraventricularis characteristic of the tetralogy. Pseudotruncus should be differentiated from type IV truncus arteriosus (Collett and Edwards, 1949) on the anatomical basis that in type IV truncus the pulmonary artery and its branches are absent and the blood supply to the lungs is carried by a number of systemic arteries of variable size. Also, in type IV truncus the interior of the right ventricle does not show the changes of the crista that are typical of the tetralogy of Fallot. The differentiation between the two conditions is of considerable practical importance since effective surgical treatment for pseudotruncus is often possible whereas no satisfactory treatment is yet available for type IV truncus (see below).

In a study of 95 autopsy specimens of the tetralogy of Fallot, Johns *et al.* (1953) found the following variations.

1. Pulmonary atresia (pseudotruncus)—22 cases. In 19 of these, the infundibulum terminated in cul de sac just below the level of the valve, and in the other 3, the obstruction was lower in the infundibulum and involved the crista. Despite the atresia, the pulmonary artery distal to the valve area was normal in size in 2 and small in 19, and only once was it absent. Blood reached the distal pulmonary arteries through anastomoses with systemic collateral vessels.

2. Infundibular stenosis—49 cases. The obstruction was found at varying distances below the valve. The length of the obstruction and its location below the valve determined the size of the infundibular chamber. In 18 cases, the chambers varied between 2 and 3 cms in length, and in 13, the chamber was 15–18 mm in diameter. In 18 others, it was quite small or nonexistent. The pulmonary artery beyond the valve was occasionally normal but much more frequently was reduced in size.

3. Valvular stenosis—10 cases. The most frequent abnormality was a thin diaphragm, presumably secondary to fusion of the commissures. The pulmonary artery, in contrast to those cases of infundibular stenosis, was either normal in size or dilated distal to the stenotic valve.

4. Combined infundibular and valvular stenosis—14 cases. The pulmonary artery in these cases was often of normal size.

The material studied by Johns *et al.* (1953) is probably not representative of the usual spectrum of tetralogy since it consisted of cases who had died postoperatively and was therefore heavily weighted toward the more severe cases. Muster *et al.* (1973) found an incidence of 9% of pseudotruncus arteriosus in 592 patients with a tetralogy of Fallot. Based on angiographic evidence, Kjellberg *et al.* (1958, page 295) found 24 of 67 cases had both valvular and infundibular stenosis. Also, dilatation of the pulmonary artery occurred in 13 cases, and this was not invariably associated with valvular stenosis.

The ventricular defect is in the membranous septum, and just beneath the posterior and right aortic cusps, the ventricular septal defect opens into the right ventricle typically below the crista,

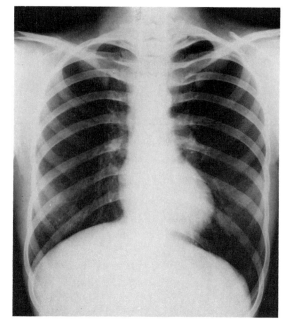

Fig. 233. A 23-Year-Old Woman with Tetralogy of Fallot (Operative Case)

There is slight elevation of the cardiac apex, but the heart is remarkably normal in contour. There is an increased radiolucency of the lungs.

although occasionally it may be intracristal, and in a few cases, it is higher in a subpulmonary location (Rao and Edwards, 1974). The defect is usually relatively large and permits free access from the right ventricle into the aorta and also into the left ventricle. The aorta is displaced to the right and overrides the ventricular septum to a variable degree. There is no doubt about the anatomical and spatial displacement of the aorta, and support for this view is the changed relationship of the aortic cusps to the mitral valve. In the tetralogy of Fallot, the anterior leaflet of the mitral valve is coextensive with the posterior cusp of the aortic valve, and this is one of the differential features between the tetralogy of Fallot and double outlet right ventricle. However, in the tetralogy of Fallot, the aortic valve cusps are rotated in a clockwise direction as seen from below so that the posterior cusp is more to the right and the right cusp more anterior than usual. The ventricular septal defect is of sufficient size to permit free exit of the blood, both into the aorta and into the left ventricle. Consequently, in the usual case systolic pressures in the right and left ventricles and aorta are approximately equal.

Although the aorta is displaced toward the right, it is posterior to the pulmonary artery. The aorta is usually larger than normal, and as a rule,

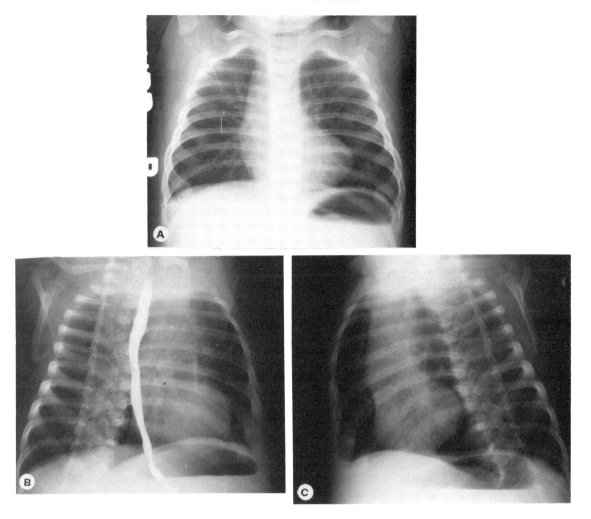

FIG. 234. TETRALOGY OF FALLOT IN 5-MONTH-OLD CHILD

The cardiac apex is elevated from the diaphragm. (A) Posteroanterior projection. (B) Right anterior projection. (C) Left anterior oblique projection.

the larger the aorta, the smaller the pulmonary artery, or vice versa. In about 25% of cases, the aorta arches toward the right over the right main stem bronchus and descends for a variable distance to the right of the midline. With a right arch the brachiocephalic vessels usually originate in a mirror image arrangement (see page 402). There are rare variations in the origin of the brachiocephalic vessels which consist of (1) right patent ductus arteriosus or ligamentum arteriosus; (2) left subclavian artery arising from the descending aorta and thus resembling the type of right aortic arch that is seen in otherwise asymptomatic patients; and (3) isolation of the left subclavian artery in which the subclavian artery originates either from the pulmonary artery or may be entirely isolated and receive its blood supply from a reverse flow through the

ipsilateral vertebral artery. This rare variation is of clinical importance because it may produce the "subclavian steal syndrome" (Fig. 338, page 408). Additional pulmonic stenosis may be due to narrowing at the origin of the left pulmonary artery or narrowing in the branches of the pulmonary artery. This is said to occur in about 2% of cases (Nagao et al., 1967).

Collateral circulation to the lungs occurs in variable degree in nearly all cases of tetralogy of Fallot but is most abundant in those with high grade pulmonary stenosis or atresia (pseudotruncus). Several pathways can be identified. The bronchial arteries, of which there are customarily two to the left lung and one to the right, become enlarged and tortuous. These arise from the undersurface of the arch of the aorta and the upper part of the descending aorta. The intercostal

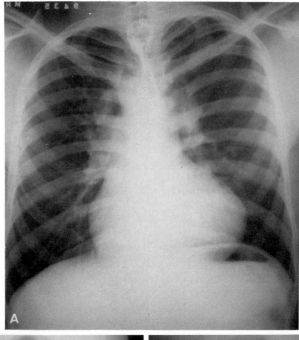

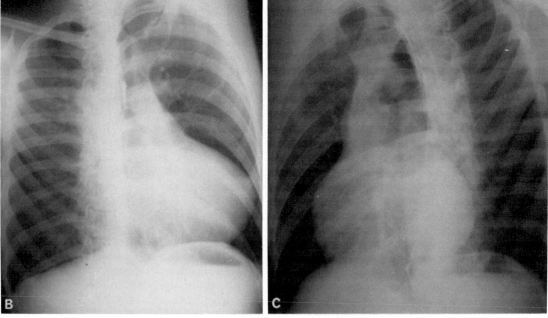

FIG. 235. TETRALOGY OF FALLOT WITH RIGHT ARCH

arteries may send numerous small twigs or branches through the pleural space via pleural adhesions. As a consequence, the intercostal arteries enlarge, and this accounts for notching of the ribs in some older patients (Fig. 239). Other large mediastinal vessels arising from the aorta may become quite large and even cause pressure defects on the barium-filled esophagus (Cooley *et al.*, 1949).

Other congenital defects that occur with tetralogy of Fallot with some frequency are as follows. Atrial septal defect (ASD) occurred in 5.4% of the cases reported by Muster *et al.* (1973), and its incidence seemed to be somewhat higher in the surgically treated cases (Kirklin and Karp, 1970). The condition is sometimes called pentalogy of Fallot. Other anomalies mentioned by Muster *et al.* (1973) with some frequency were

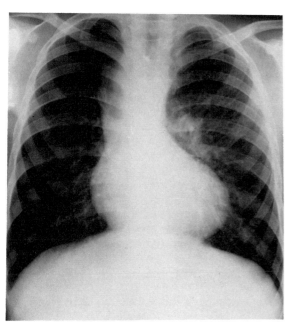

FIG. 236. PSEUDOTRUNCUS ARTERIOSUS WITH A RIGHT
AORTIC ARCH
A mass of collateral vessels in the left hilus connected with
small distal pulmonary arteries. (Operative case.)

PDA, 6%; left superior vena cava emptying into the coronary sinus, 4%; and also mentioned with less frequency were partial anomalous venous drainage, persistent AV canal, left pulmonary artery originating from aorta, and total anomalous pulmonary venous return. All of these infrequently associated anomalies can cause complications associated with surgical treatment, and preoperative diagnosis is most helpful.

The left superior vena cava must be dealt with separately in applying cardiopulmonary bypass operations.

Unilateral pulmonary atresia may affect the pulmonary artery to either lung. Typically, however, in otherwise normal hearts it affects the right pulmonary artery, whereas in the tetralogy of Fallot, the left pulmonary artery is absent (Nadas et al., 1953; Goldsmith et al., 1975). In the 4 cases reported by Nadas et al. (1953), the left artery was missing in 3, and in another case there was a dextrocardia, and the right artery was missing.

RADIOLOGIC INVESTIGATIONS. The hemodynamic features of the tetralogy of Fallot can be readily investigated by right heart catheterization. Right atrial pressures are usually unremarkable, although occasionally the "a" wave is increased in height. Right ventricular pressures are invariably elevated and typically have a systolic level approximating that in the aorta and

left ventricle. Where the ventricular septal defect is small or where an anomalous tricuspid valve partially occludes the defect, the right ventricular pressure may considerably exceed that in the left ventricle and aorta. In only about one-half of the cases is it possible to pass the catheter into the pulmonary artery where the pressure may be normal or slightly reduced. The catheter may be passed into the aorta, although this does not confirm an overriding aorta since the same appearance can result with an uncomplicated ventricular septal defect. The diagnosis of tetralogy of Fallot can be made from right heart catheterization only if both the aorta and pulmonary artery are entered and pressure tracings and blood gas determinations are made. An accompanying ASD may be detected by passing the catheter into the left atrium. The shunt through the atrial defect is usually from right to left. The predominant functional aberration or change in the blood flow in the tetralogy of Fallot is the shunting of increased amounts of venous blood into the aorta and systemic circulation associated with a decreased blood flow through the lungs.

The radiologist is responsible for recognition and confirmation of the presence of the tetralogy of Fallot and for the demonstration of anatomical details that may be helpful in surgical treatment. Most important perhaps is to determine the size of the pulmonary artery and its branches and its distribution to the lung. The morphology of the outflow tract of the right ventricle is also of some help in evaluating the difficulties that may be encountered in carrying out a complete repair. The location of the aortic arch and its branches, of course, is important when a shunting procedure is contemplated.

Conventional radiography using PA, lateral, and oblique views typically shows a normal-sized heart, although some enlargement occasionally occurs in older patients, but marked enlargement is rarely seen. In early infancy, it is difficult to detect any deviation from the normal contour of the heart. After one year of age, however, a usually typical pattern emerges. The left midheart border, representing the pulmonary artery, is concave so that the waist of the heart is narrow. The lower left cardiac border may be rounded and entirely normal in a significant proportion of cases (Fig. 234), although typically the apex is raised producing some degree of coeur en sabot contour. Occasionally, the raised or elevated apex is pointed. Careful study of the left border may occasionally reveal a notch indicating the point of division between the ventricles.

The aortic knob is difficult to identify in infancy, but by the second or third year of life it is

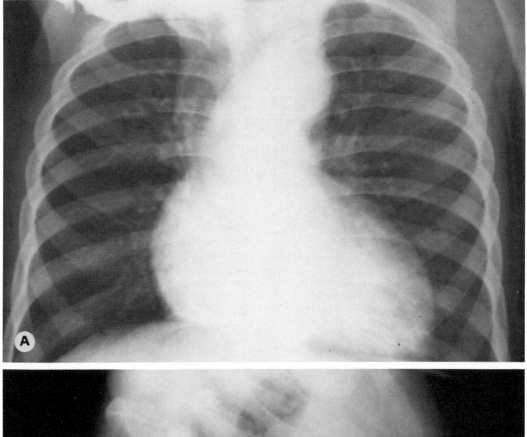

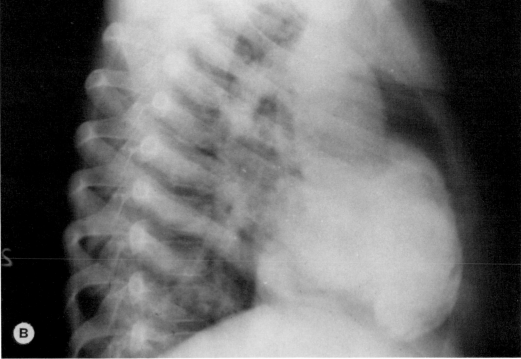

FIG. 237. PSEUDOTRUNCUS ARTERIOSUS

Angiocardiograms show no evidence of proximal pulmonary arteries. The ascending aorta is quite large. There was no systolic murmur or thrill. At operation evidence of proximal pulmonary atresia was found; however, a distal pulmonary artery on the left, 5 mm in diameter, was sufficiently large to permit a pulmonary-subclavian anastomosis. There is a mass of small collateral vessels in each hilus.

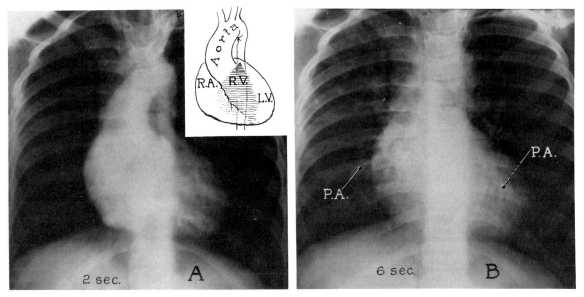

FIG. 238. PSEUDOTRUNCUS ARTERIOSUS
(A) Angiocardiogram 2 sec after injection of contrast material. The pulmonary artery is not seen. The right ventricle terminates in a pointed projection in the region of the infundibulum. (B) Six seconds after injection. Contrast substance lingers in collaterals in the lung parenchyma. (Courtesy of *Radiology, 52:* 344 (Fig. 10), 1949.)

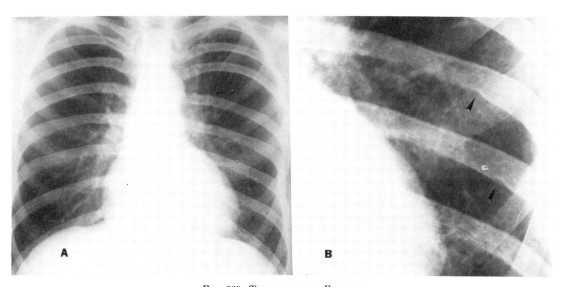

FIG. 239. TETRALOGY OF FALLOT
(A) Eighteen-year-old male patient with tetralogy of Fallot and notching of ribs. (B) Close-up of left ribs. The most striking notching is in the left 7th and 8th ribs. A Potts type procedure had been carried out 3 years previously.

visible and typically in the tetralogy of Fallot it is distinct and may be slightly enlarged and produces some indentation on the left margin of the trachea. If the impingement of the aortic arch on the left margin of the trachea cannot be identified on conventional films, the direction of the aortic arch can usually be determined by fluoroscopy and films following a barium swal-

low. In most cases, this additional procedure is not required, and fluoroscopy is not recommended as a routine procedure.

The hilar shadows should be studied carefully. The primary branches of the pulmonary artery are often seen, particularly the descending branch of the right pulmonary artery. These branches are usually reduced in size but may be normal. If they are enlarged, a diagnosis of tetralogy may be questioned, although poststenotic dilatation occurs both with and without valvular stenosis although the dilatation rarely extends to the secondary branches. Also, estimates as to the size of the pulmonary arterial branches from a conventional film are not always reliable. In high grade stenosis or atresia, the pulmonary artery to one or both lungs may not be identified. Instead, the hilar shadows may be deviated in contour due to masses of collateral vessels, and these become more noticeable after infancy. These masses of collateral vessels are usually somewhat rounded or lobulated or comma-shaped, and they may be relatively slightly higher in the mediastinum than the normal hilus. Furthermore, careful study will show branching reticular shadows extending through the lungs. At times the hilar shadows combine with the reticular branching pattern in the lung and bring up the question of increased blood flow, and care should be taken to recognize that the shadows are due to collateral circulation associated with a reduced flow through the pulmonary arteries. Typically, the lung parenchyma is avascular, although a considerable proportion of cases will have a normal vascular pattern. Estimates of minor changes in pulmonary vascularity are difficult and depend to a degree on proper exposure techniques. In a sizeable proportion of cases,

however, the increased radiolucency of the lungs leaves little doubt about the decreased vascularity.

In the right anterior oblique view, the right ventricle presents some increased convexity that is in contrast to the decreased size of the infundibulum and outflow tract, and this tends to accentuate a concavity in the left midheart border (Fig. 235 B). In some cases, however, the infundibular chamber is dilated and may present as a slight convexity, and this may be seen also in the PA projection and may lead the radiologist to strongly suspect the presence of a large infundibular chamber.

In the left anterior oblique view (Fig. 235C), the right ventricular and atrial contours present a full curve, and particularly the extent of the contour in contact with the diaphragm is increased. The left ventricular contour posteriorly may, because of its short arc, appear as a hump attached to the right ventricle. The pulmonary window is clear.

In the lateral view, the anterior extension of the right ventricle is best shown and best evaluated. Also, the anterior displacement of the aorta may be noticed in films of good contrast.

The typical case without cardiac enlargement and with the above-described contours and with cyanosis from early life can be recognized with confidence using only conventional films, al-

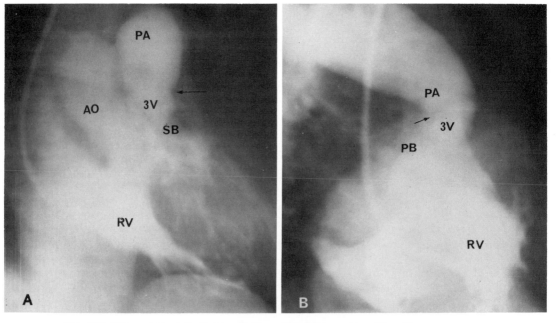

FIG. 240. TETRALOGY OF FALLOT IN 46-YEAR-OLD WOMAN WITH MILD HYPERTENSION

A selective right ventricular injection shows a small infundibular chamber (3V) and no evidence of valvular stenosis. AO, aorta; PA, pulmonary artery; PB, parietal band; SB, septal band. Arrows indicate the pulmonary valve.

though it may be confused with some cases of complete transposition with pulmonic stenosis, tricuspid atresia, and rarely with a double outlet right ventricle with pulmonic stenosis. The frequent anatomic variations, particularly in the pulmonary blood flow and in the infundibulum, mentioned above may or may not be recognizable on conventional films. Selective angiography is necessary and recommended in all suspected cases, particularly if surgical treatment is anticipated. Specifically, it gives information, often crucial, as to the anatomy and severity of the pulmonic stenosis and the distribution of blood flow to the lungs and also the presence of minor anatomic variations, such as absence of one of the pulmonary arteries or of the origin of one pulmonary artery from the aorta. Selective right ventricular angiography with the tip of the catheter in the mid portion of the right ventricle is preferable. Filming is carried out with the biplane film changer at the rate of 4–6 frames/sec in the AP and lateral projections. Film speeds of this order are necessary to properly study the anatomy of the outflow tract of the right ventricle. The outflow tract is best shown perhaps in about 25° of right anterior obliquity, but usually the frontal and lateral projections are sufficient. We have also used cinefluorography, predominantly in the AP projection, and the rapid filming is helpful in studying the morphology of the pulmonic stenosis. This technique has the disadvantage that if a lateral projection is necessary in order to study the position of the aorta or the size of the ventricular defect a second injection is necessary.

Rapid filming, particularly with ECG monitoring, permits a sequential detailed study of the outflow tract, and both projections are useful. The contour of the outflow tract of the right ventricle, and particularly the contour of the infundibular chamber, changes with the cardiac phase. The chamber is usually distended in early systole, but it shows contractile activity in late systole. Consequently, in order to determine the size and contour of the infundibular chamber, it is desirable to have films exposed in several phases of the cardiac cycle. This is one of the advantages of cinefluorography in which the contour of the outflow tract can be viewed in all phases of the cardiac cycle. A considerable proportion of cases of tetralogy have small to medium-sized infundibular chambers, often shaped like an inverted flask with the base at the valve. The neck of the chamber corresponding to the neck of the flask is formed by the parietal and septal bands of the crista supraventricularis. Usually the parietal (medial as seen on the AP

film) band is much more prominent and appears to displace the entire outflow tract lateralward. At times only a narrowed passageway may be seen with only a slight dilatation or resemblance of an infundibular chamber. The passageway may be distorted with small pits or recesses. The septal or lateral band is usually much less conspicuous, particularly in the AP projection. At times it may cast a shadow as large as the parietal band. A considerable variability in the shape of the infundibular chamber occurs in that some are triangular and others are rounded. When the valve is stenotic, a jet of contrast substance projecting through the narrow opening into the nonopaque blood in the pulmonary artery is seen. With marked pulmonary stenosis or atresia, the appearance of the infundibular region is often quite distinctive. The infundibulum may be shaped like a funnel with the apex near the valve (Fig. 238). Also, none of the contrast substance enters the proximal pulmonary artery.

With a right ventricular injection, the contrast substance almost invariably passes through the high ventricular septal defect during late diastole and early systole, thus outlining the defect. The aorta fills immediately thereafter, and although it may be partially obscured by the pulmonary outflow tract in the lateral view, its outline is usually sufficient to permit a judgment as to the degree of overriding (Fig. 241C). Usually the interventricular septum is clearly outlined in the lateral projection, and its relationship to the aortic orifice can be closely estimated. It is important to ascertain the extent of overriding and if the outflow tract from the left ventricle is sufficient to allow for the increase in flow that follows with the establishment of an artificial ductus or a total correction. Marked overriding, however, is not a positive contraindication to operation.

The size and contour of the pulmonary trunk and its branches are usually determined with exactness except in those cases with extreme stenosis or atresia. Localized or diffuse narrowing of the pulmonary artery or one of its major branches is thought to occur in about 2% of cases (Nagao et al., 1967), and these are best demonstrated by angiography. Even in cases with severe stenosis or atresia, the right and left arteries may fill through systemic collaterals and can thus be identified and their size estimated. Identification of the peripheral pulmonary arteries is essential in the preoperative diagnosis of pseudo truncus arteriosus and the differentiation from the inoperable type IV truncus.

As indicated above, absence of the left pulmonary artery is a rare additional anomaly that

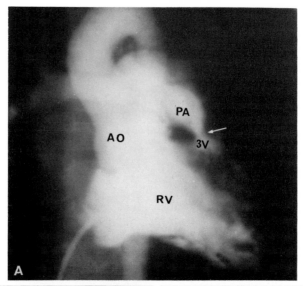

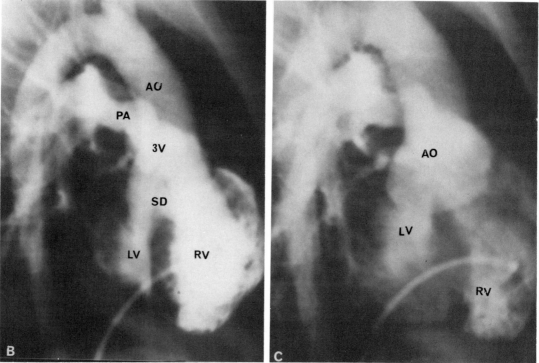

FIG. 241. SELECTIVE RIGHT VENTRICULAR ANGIOGRAM IN 3-YEAR-OLD PATIENT WITH TETRALOGY OF FALLOT WITH INFUN-
DIBULAR AND MILD VALVULAR STENOSIS

(A) Frontal projection. (B and C) Lateral projections. The aorta is much larger than the pulmonary artery and straddles the
ventricular septum. AO, aorta; PA, pulmonary artery; SD, ventricular septal defect; VS, ventricular septum; RV, right ventricle;
3V, infundibular chamber. Arrow indicates pulmonic valve.

is seen with the tetralogy of Fallot. Usually with
this condition the aorta arches toward the right
side. Although the possibility of this anomaly
can be suspected from inspection of the chest
films, angiography is necessary for definitive diagnosis. In some cases, there has been notching

of the ribs on the left side (Kirklin and Karp,
1970).

The term "pink tetralogy" has been applied to
a group of borderline cases, some of which are
true anatomical tetralogies of Fallot, and others
are closely similar conditions, such as congenital

pulmonic and subpulmonic stenosis with a ventricular septal defect. Acyanotic tetralogy of Fallot may occur in as many as 10% of all cases (Keats and Martt, 1959). In these patients, the peripheral unsaturation is insufficient to be clinically evident. The peripheral blood does show some degree of unsaturation, however. The patient may be acyanotic during early life and become cyanotic later or remain relatively acyanotic all of his life. Some of the causes for this are

1. persistent patency of the ductus arteriosus.

2. mild pulmonic stenosis associated with a small ventricular septal defect.

3. large well-developed peripheral collateral circulation to the lungs.

Closely related conditions may be cases like those reported by Gasul *et al.* (1957) in which pulmonic stenosis developed over a period of time. Cardiac catheterization, and particularly selective angiography, are necessary to properly elucidate these cases. A number of other less common congenital abnormalities may simulate the tetralogy of Fallot and should be considered in the differential diagnosis (Rao and Edwards, 1974). These are

1. double outlet right ventricle with pulmonic stenosis. In this condition, there may be an infundibular chamber that resembles that seen in the tetralogy of Fallot. The crucial procedure is to demonstrate the mitral valve by means of angiography and show that there is a lack of continuity of the valve with the base of the aorta.

2. tetralogy of Fallot with an additional endocardial cushion defect. Both the electrocardiogram and the left ventricular angiogram are helpful in diagnosis.

3. single ventricle with normally related great vessels and subpulmonary stenosis.

4. complete transposition of the great vessels with pulmonary stenosis.

5. two-chambered right ventricle.

SURGICAL TREATMENT OF THE TETRALOGY OF FALLOT. Palliative procedures are used in infants and young children to improve the blood flow to the lungs and the circulatory status pending the optimum time for complete surgical repair. This usually occurs at about 5 years of age. The

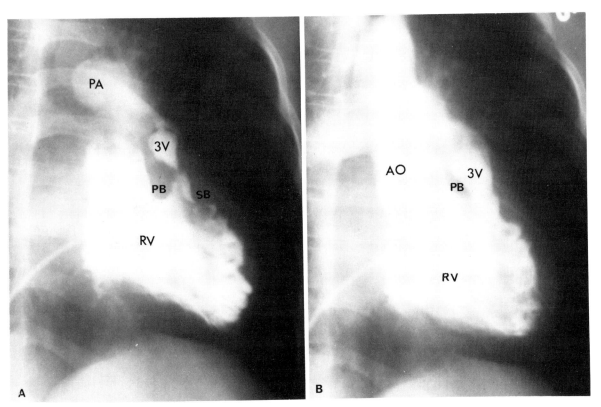

FIG. 242. SELECTIVE RIGHT VENTRICULAR ANGIOGRAM IN TETRALOGY OF FALLOT WITH VALVULAR AND INFUNDIBULAR STENOSIS

(A) Midsystole. (B) Diastole. AO, aorta; PB, parietal band; SB, septal band; RV, right ventricle; 3V, third ventricle. (Courtesy of Dr. T. E. Keats, Department of Radiology, University of Virginia.)

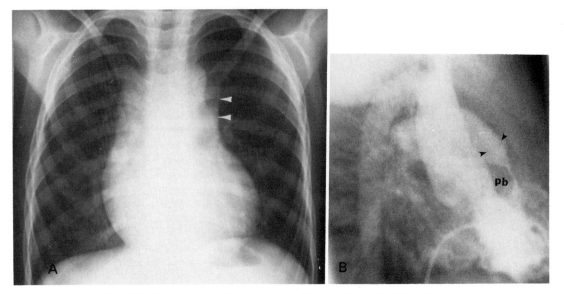

FIG. 243. TETRALOGY OF FALLOT WITH A DOUBLE SUPERIOR VENA CAVA
The left vena cava is indicated by arrows in A. (B) Cinefluorogram (RAO) showing typical infundibular stenosis and overriding aorta. pb, parietal band; arrows indicate valve cusps.

Waterston procedure (1962) consists of creating an ostium of suitable size between the posterior surface of the aorta and the anterior surface of the right pulmonary artery. The approach is through a right thoracotomy. It is the preferable procedure in the neonate and babies under one year of age and any patient in whom the subclavian artery is of insufficient size to permit an adequate anastomosis (Kirklin and Karp, 1970). The Blalock-Taussig procedure (1945) consists of an end to side (in some cases an end to end) anastomosis between the innominate or one of the subclavian arteries and the ipsilateral pulmonary artery. Preferably the innominate on the opposite side from the direction of the aortic arch is used. The Potts procedure (1946) consists of the creation of an ostium between the left pulmonary artery and the descending aorta. All of these procedures depend on the presence of a pulmonary artery of adequate size, usually at least 5 mm in diameter. In all of these procedures, except an end to end anastomosis of the subclavian to the pulmonary artery, unsaturated systemic blood is shunted to both lungs.

The Waterston procedure seems preferable in small infants because of the technical difficulties associated with the small size of the subclavian artery. Care must be taken to create an ostium of the proper size and not produce narrowing or excessive torsion of the right pulmonary artery. Also, if the shunt is taken down at the time of total repair, care must be taken to avoid a stenosis of the right pulmonary artery (Gay et al., 1973).

The Blalock-Taussig procedure is desirable for older children because the innominate or subclavian arteries are usually of appropriate size to carry a suitable amount of blood and tend to increase in size with the growth of the patient. Long-term complications of the Blalock-Taussig procedure are: (1) stenosis or closure of the anastomosis; (2) congestive heart failure; and (3) pulmonary hypertension. Pulmonary hypertension developed in 20 of 685 patients who underwent a Blalock-Taussig procedure in the series reported by Marr et al. (1974). The transverse diameter of the heart was larger in these cases than in those that did not have this complication. The most reliable radiologic sign was an increase in diameter of the descending branch of the right pulmonary artery which can usually be measured on a well-exposed chest film. The peripheral arteries remain normal in size, and when compared with the dilated central arteries, an appearance of truncation was given. The lung vasculature may resemble that seen in the "Eisenmenger syndrome." The development of pulmonary hypertension is a serious complication and may preclude total repair. It is thought to be less common with the Blalock-Taussig procedure than with the Potts procedure. Early recognition of the signs of pulmonary hypertension may be a positive indication for total repair before changes in the vascular bed become irreversible.

The creation of an ostium between the left pulmonary artery and the descending aorta (Potts procedure) has been used in infants, but the results are less predictable due to the difficulty in obtaining the proper size of the ostium. Complications are due to increased blood flow to the lungs with left heart failure, or if the increased flow persists for some time, pulmonary hypertension with fixed pulmonary resistance may ensue. In a few cases, stenosis or occlusion of the left pulmonary artery occurred after interruption of the shunt at the time of total repair.

All of these anastomotic or shunting procedures are carried out through a right or left thoracotomy. Immediately postoperatively a small amount of pleural fluid may collect on the operative side, and this is usually eliminated by means of a drainage tube. The ipsilateral lung may be partially opaque due to local edema and hemorrhage. The increased pulmonary blood flow secondary to a successful procedure is usually not apparent until the end of the first week. At the end of the second week when well-exposed films are available, the heart is usually increased

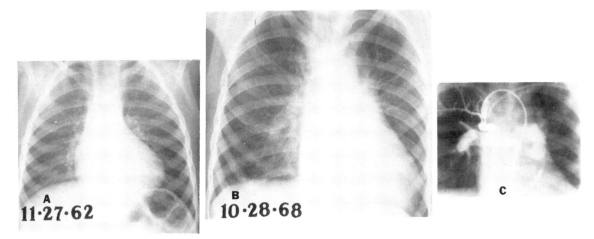

FIG. 244. PRE- AND POSTOPERATIVE TETRALOGY OF FALLOT (BLALOCK-TAUSSIG PROCEDURE ON THE RIGHT)
(A) Preoperative. (B) Six years postoperative. The patient enjoyed almost normal activity. The heart is relatively slightly larger, and the lung vascularity is more prominent. (C) Selective injection of subclavian-pulmonary shunt shows continued good function. Blood flows both ways in the pulmonary artery.

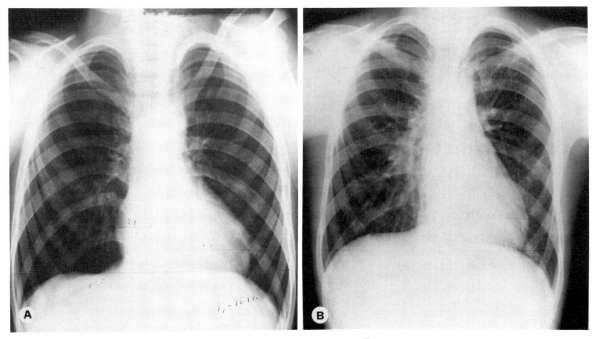

FIG. 245. TETRALOGY OF FALLOT
(A) Preoperative. (B) Eight years after establishment of a pulmonary-subclavian anastomosis on the right side.

over its preoperative size. However, it is rarely greatly enlarged. The pericardium is left partially open so that fluid does not collect in significant amounts within the pericardium. The enlargement may continue, but after few weeks the heart accommodates to the changed circulatory dynamics, and its size becomes stable even though the patient becomes active. In a minority of cases, however, the period of stabilization is prolonged. Right heart failure may be observed clinically, and the heart may continue to enlarge. Usually there is a good response to bed rest, digitalis, and the usual medical treatment. If response to such treatment is poor and if cardiac enlargement progresses, one should suspect either an error in diagnosis or the possibility of too large a shunt should be considered. Other possibilities, of course, are the presence of irreversible changes in the pulmonary vascular system.

Rarely, left-sided heart failure may develop producing signs of pulmonary edema. Films may show haziness through both lungs, more marked in the central zones and around the hilus. In general, the clinical signs of edema are more striking than the roentgen findings. Such an occurrence is thought to be due to a small left ventricle with perhaps marked overriding of the aorta. In most cases after a period of time the left ventricular function improves, and the patient's condition becomes stable.

Patients have been followed for periods of up to 20 years following the Blalock-Taussig procedure, during which time many have enjoyed relatively normal activities (Taussig *et al.*, 1973). The heart tends to maintain its preoperative contour. The lung vascular structures on the side of the artificial ductus often appear more prominent than on the opposite side (see Figs. 244 and 245). The incidence of closure of the shunt is variable. Where the shunt closes immediately, the changes in the lung vasculature are often not prominent. Where the shunt closes gradually over a period of time, the changes in the lung vasculature may be imperceptible. Patency of the shunt is best determined by means of aortography, although auscultatory and clinical findings are quite helpful.

INTRACARDIAC SURGICAL CORRECTION USING EXTRACORPOREAL CIRCULATION (LILLEHEI ET AL., 1955; KIRKLIN ET AL., 1955). The use of the pump oxygenator and hypothermia have served to make this operation a routine procedure for a properly organized surgical team. A midline sternal splitting approach is used. The right ventricle is opened usually through a transverse incision in the region of the conus. Care must be taken not to transect a major coronary artery. This particularly applies to those cases in which an anomalous anterior descending coronary artery originates either from the right sinus of Valsalva or the right coronary artery and crosses the infundibulum of the right ventricle on the way to its distribution to the anterior wall of the left ventricle.

The ventricular septal defect is closed by means of a Dacron or Teflon patch. The septal and parietal bands of the crista are dissected

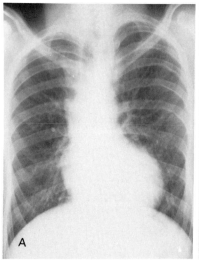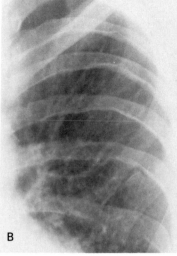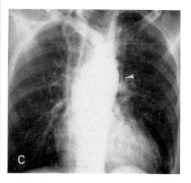

FIG. 246.

(A) Postoperative Blalock-Taussig (subclavian-pulmonary anastomosis) on the left side. Only modest improvement in exercise tolerance. (B) Notching of ribs on left. (C) Frontal aortogram showing small but functioning anastomosis (arrow).

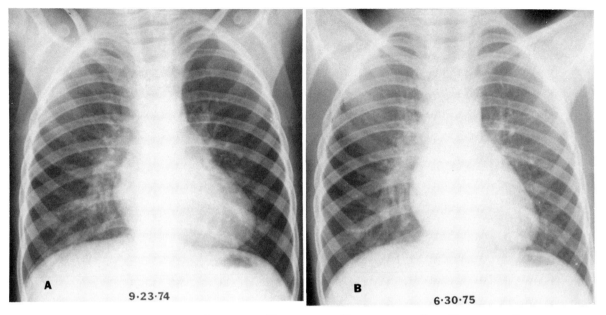

FIG. 247. TOTAL REPAIR OF A TETRALOGY OF FALLOT WITH A GOOD FUNCTIONAL RESULT
(A) Preoperative. (B) Postoperative.

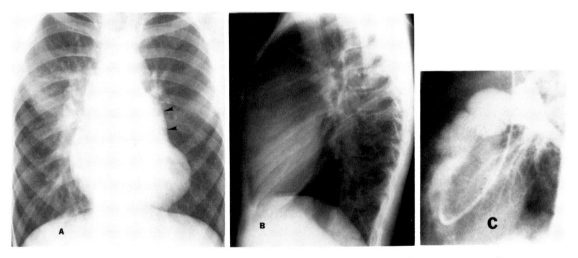

FIG. 248. COMPLETE REPAIR OF TETRALOGY OF FALLOT WITH RESULTING PULMONARY INSUFFICIENCY AS DETERMINED BY
RIGHT HEART CATHETERIZATION

(A) Arrows indicate dilated outflow tract of right ventricle. The pulmonary arteries are enlarged. (B) The dilated outflow tract fills in the substernal space. (C) Lateral view of postoperative right ventricular angiogram showing dilatation of infundibulum.

away in order to relieve the infundibular stenosis. When the valve is stenotic, the opening is stretched and if possible the fused commissures are incised. In a minority of cases, the valve ring or the first portion of the pulmonary artery is so small that the pulmonic stenosis is not relieved by the infundibular resection or the incision of the valve. The usual procedure in these cases is to widen the outflow tract by the insertion of a patch extending from the infundibulum across the valve ring and into the first portion of the pulmonary artery. In earlier cases, a Dacron or Teflon patch was used, but more recently autologous pericardium has been found to be more satisfactory. Considerable judgment is necessary in tailoring the patch to the appropriate size. If the patch is too small, the pulmonic stenosis will not be relieved. If the patch is too large, the outflow tract may become aneurysmal and be associated with a high degree of pulmonary insufficiency (Fig. 249B). Moderate degrees of pulmonary insufficiency are well tolerated, but the results of the operation on average are less satisfactory than in those cases in which a patch is not needed (Jones *et al.*, 1973; Kirklin and Karp, 1970). In some instances, combined pulmonary stenosis and insufficiency persist and greatly increase the work of the right ventricle and may be a cause of heart failure. Other causes of an unsatisfactory postoperative result are failure to close the interventricular septal defect or dehiscence of the closure, inadequate resection of the infundibular stenosis, injury to the conduction system with partial or total heart block, and injury to a large coronary artery, such as the anomalous anterior descending artery that may originate from the right coronary artery. Reoperation may be considered for an incomplete closing of the VSD or the failure to properly relieve the pulmonic stenosis (Castaneda *et al.*, 1974).

Persistent pulmonary hypertension can be an uncommon but severe complication following repair of the tetralogy of Fallot (Kinsley *et al.*, 1974). This can be due to a number of causes, such as residual ventricular septal defect, congenital absence of one pulmonary artery or an acquired occlusion of a pulmonary artery secondary to a previous anastomotic procedure, or multiple peripheral pulmonary thrombi. The conventional chest film may give evidence of such a complication, such as truncation of the pulmonary arteries with enlargement of the proximal pulmonary artery as has been described above in connection with shunting procedures. In general, those patients who have had a previous shunting procedure are particularly susceptible to the development of pulmonary hypertension (Ruzyllo *et al.*, 1974; Reid *et al.*, 1973).

A number of variants of the tetralogy of Fallot require modifications of the basic operative procedure. The most common of these is the surgical treatment of pseudotruncus arteriosus. A pseudotruncus is the most severe form of the tetralogy of Fallot in which there is a pulmonary atresia involving predominantly the pulmonary valve and proximal pulmonary artery and with a usually well-formed infundibulum. Typically, the distal right and left pulmonary arteries are intact. Systemic blood is carried to the lungs through these arteries by means of precapillary anastomoses with systemic arteries. The extent of this collateral circulation is quite variable, but in some cases, it is equal or greater than the systemic circulation, and the patient is able to enjoy

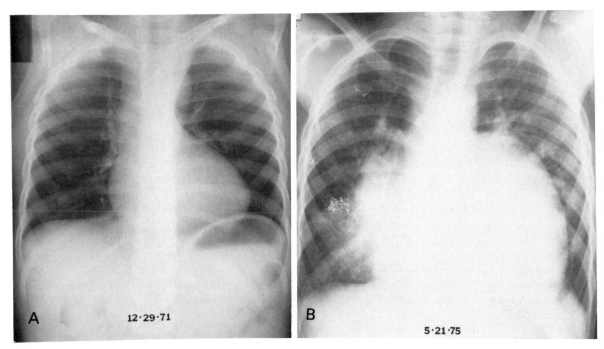

FIG. 249. TETRALOGY OF FALLOT

(A) Preoperative tetralogy of Fallot with a small muscular infundibulum. (B) Three years and five months postoperative. A graft was applied to the outflow tract in order to alleviate the stenosis. This has resulted in an aneurysmal dilatation with marked pulmonary insufficiency.

a considerable degree of activity. Surgical treatment consists of the establishment of a conduit from the outflow tract of the right ventricle to the reconstituted main or separately to the right and left pulmonary arteries (Pacifico *et al.*, 1974; Kirklin and Karp, 1970). The ventricular septal defect is repaired in the usual way. One of the crucial requirements is the presence of a pulmonary artery or arteries of sufficient size to permit the anastomosis and which will connect with an adequate pulmonary vascular bed. Levin *et al.* (1974) have emphasized the importance of outlining the systemic arterial supply to the lungs as a preliminary to the surgical treatment of pseudotruncus. Where the blood supply is through numerous smaller systemic arteries, operative treatment is not possible.

Other modifications of the surgical repair are required where one pulmonary artery arises from the aorta (Robin *et al.*, 1975; Imai *et al.*, 1975) or where there is atresia of one pulmonary artery either secondary to a previous shunting procedure or a congenital atresia as described above (Goldsmith *et al.*, 1975; Donahoo *et al.*, 1973).

CLINICAL SYNDROME OF TETRALOGY OF FALLOT WITH PULMONARY REGURGITATION OR ABSENCE OF PULMONARY VALVE. Ruttenberg *et al.* (1964) in a review found 38 cases of congenital pulmonary valvular insufficiency. In 27 of these, there was an associated ventricular septal defect, and, in 20, the anatomic features otherwise resembled the tetralogy of Fallot. The infundibulum was usually deformed and narrowed. In 2 cases studied in detail by Ruttenberg *et al.* (1964) and in 5 others reported by Miller *et al.* (1962) there was a loud coarse diastolic murmur and usually a to and fro murmur associated with systolic and diastolic thrills. The pulmonary trunk was uniformly dilated, and, in one case, it constricted the left main bronchus producing respiratory obstruction. In one of the cases of Ruttenberg *et al.* (1964), the infundibulum was dilated and contributed to bulging of the left midcardiac contour. The heart is typically enlarged, and its contour does not suggest the tetralogy of Fallot. Pressure tracings from the right ventricle show a high end diastolic pressure, and the pulmonary artery tracings do not have a dicrotic notch. A similar picture may be produced following the placing of a patch over the outflow tract and pulmonary artery during the surgical correction of the tetralogy of Fallot.

In patients with isolated valvular insufficiency, the chest films may be normal or show prominence of the main and left pulmonary arteries (Ruttenberg, 1968). Fluoroscopy shows increased pulmonary arterial pulsations and a hilar dance.

Bose *et al.* (1974) reported on 2 cases of absence of the pulmonary valve in association with absence of the thymus and parathyroids, hypocalcemia and facial anomalies (the DiGeorge syndrome).

ANOMALOUS MUSCLE BUNDLES IN THE RIGHT VENTRICLE; TWO-CHAMBERED RIGHT VENTRICLE. In the tetralogy of Fallot the site of outflow obstruction of the right ventricle is in the region of the infundibulum. In the present condition, by contrast, the obstruction is in the sinus or inflow portion of the right ventricle. One or more muscle bundles cross the sinus portion of the right ventricle and divide the chamber into two hemodynamically separate compartments and in fact produce a two-chambered right ventricle. About 73% of the reported cases have had a ventricular septal defect (Fellows *et al.*, 1977) that usually communicates with the right ventricle proximal to the obstructing muscle bundle. The shunt through the defect is usually from left to right, but occasionally it is from right to left, and the anomaly may resemble the tetralogy of Fallot (Fisher *et al.*, 1971). The anomaly may rarely coexist with the tetralogy of Fallot (Edwards *et al.*, 1965; Fellows *et al.*, 1977), and it may be difficult to determine whether the anomalous muscle bundle or the infundibular obstruction due to the tetralogy of Fallot is the more significant. Hartmann *et al.* (1962; 1964) and Fellows *et al.* (1977) emphasize that anomalous bundles in the right ventricle producing a two chambered right ventricle is not a variant of the tetralogy of Fallot. It is of some interest that 15% of the cases reported by Fellows *et al.* (1977) had a right aortic arch.

The anomalous muscle bundles may be single or rarely multiple. Frequently a single bundle divides into two limbs usually near its posterior insertion. This provides two or sometimes three narrow passageways between the proximal and distal right ventricle. These passageways typically narrow during ventricular systole, and rarely a jet is visible at angiocardiography indicating their presence (Fellows *et al.*, 1977). The muscle bundles are variable in location, some being low in the body of the ventricle, where they are often massive, and others high near the infundibulum where they are often narrow and resemble a diaphragm (Fellows *et al.*, 1977; Fisher *et al.*, 1971). An additional pulmonic stenosis, either valvular, infundibular or peripheral, was present but variable in different series, 12 of 28 patients (Fellows *et al.*, 1977), 5 of 11 patients (Warden *et al.*, 1966), and only 2 (presumably tetralogies) in the series of Fisher *et al.* (1971).

Symptomatology was relatively nonspecific

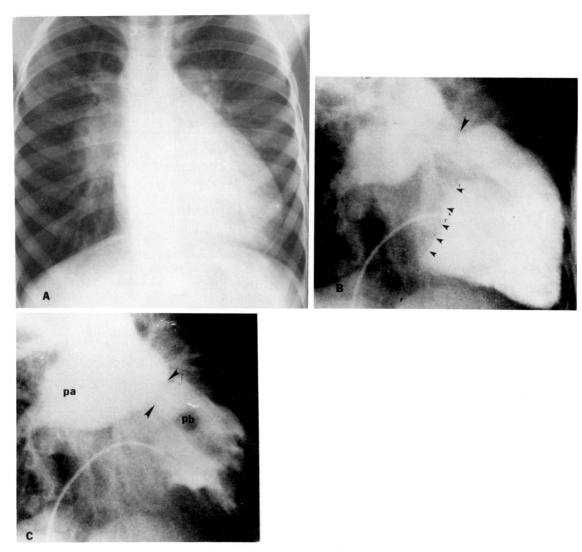

FIG. 250. TETRALOGY OF FALLOT

(A) Tetralogy of Fallot with absence of pulmonary valve. The right ventricle is dilated, and the proximal pulmonary arteries are quite dilated. (B) Right ventricle in diastole. Arrowheads indicate closed tricuspid valve, and larger arrowhead indicates site of pulmonic valve. (C) Right ventricle in systole. Arrowheads indicate valve ring. There is also some hypertrophy of the parietal band.

and consisted of dyspnea on exertion, failure to thrive, easy fatigability, and rarely, cyanosis. The most striking physical finding was a holosystolic ejection type murmur just to the left of the sternum usually accompanied by a thrill. A considerable proportion of patients were asymptomatic and were investigated because of a heart murmur. Thirty-five percent of the patients presented by Fellows *et al.* (1977) had an original diagnosis of infundibular stenosis or tetralogy of Fallot.

Conventional chest films show variable findings depending on the severity of the pulmonic stenosis, the presence of valvular stenosis, and the volume and direction of the shunt through the VSD if such was present. A majority of the cases had enlargement of the right ventricle and the pulmonary artery. In those cases where there was a significant left to right shunt, there was some increased pulmonary vascularity, and in those cases with valvular pulmonic stenosis, there was enlargement of the left pulmonary artery. A few cases had a small pulmonary artery segment and avascular lungs resembling the tetralogy of Fallot (Fisher *et al.*, 1971).

Right heart catheterization shows a significant

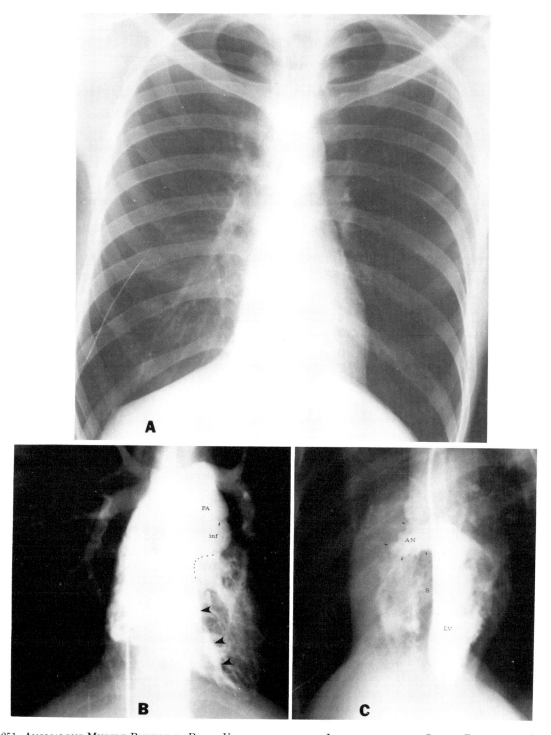

Fig. 251. Anomalous Muscle Bundle in Right Ventricle with an Interventricular Septal Defect and Aneurysm Formation (Operative Case)

(A) Chest film is within normal limits. (B) Selective right atrial injection. Right ventricle is in diastole, and anomalous
bundle is indicated by arrowheads. inf, infundibulum distal to obstructing bundle; PA, pulmonary artery. (C) Selective left
ventricular injection. S, septum, AN, aneurysm of the interventricular septum with opening at apex permitting a left to right
shunt. The opening was proximal to the obstructing muscle bundle.

increase in right ventricular pressure proximal to the muscle bundle and a gradient between the right ventricle and pulmonary artery. At times two gradients may be found where there is an additional infundibular or valvular stenosis. The exact site of this obstruction is often difficult to determine solely on the basis of the position of the catheter tip, although a suspicion may be aroused that the obstruction is not in the usual position in the outflow tract. Also, there may be evidence of a left-to-right shunt.

Right ventriculography is the most definitive procedure and is essential for diagnosis. The contrast substance should be injected into the inflow tract of the right ventricle proximal to the muscle bundle. Rapid filming in the frontal and lateral projections is recommended by Fellows et al. (1977) and in the frontal and RAO projections by Fisher et al. (1971). The present authors have found the frontal and lateral projections as usually the most helpful. Fellows et al. (1977) reported on the demonstration of anomalous muscle bundles in 28 patients and classified these into groups, those with a low obstruction and those with a high obstruction. In 14 patients the obstruction was low in the right ventricle and produced a filling defect seen in the frontal projection extending from the septum toward the tricuspid valve at an angle varying from 20–55° with the vertical. On the lateral view the filling defect was usually less conspicuous extending diagonally across the ventricle from a low position anteriorly to a high position posteriorly. The filling defects are most prominent and distinct during systole and were occasionally obscured by the surrounding contrast substance in diastole. A left ventriculogram was often helpful in those cases with a ventricular septal defect. The contrast substance in passing through the defect helped to outline the muscle bundle which was just above the defect. High obstructions were usually less massive and often resembled a diaphragm extending across the upper portion of the right ventricle just below the infundibulum and were a frequent finding in the other series (Hartmann et al., 1962; 1964; Ashcraft et al., 1973; Fisher et al., 1971; and Lucas et al., 1962) except those of Warden et al. (1966). Other associated congenital anomalies reported by Fellows et al. (1977) were pulmonic stenosis (12 patients—8 valvular; 4 peripheral), subaortic stenosis (3 patients), aortic stenosis (1 patient), and atrial septal defect (1 patient).

Lucas et al. (1962) and Warden et al. (1966) comment on the problems associated with the surgical treatment of this condition. If the surgeon is not forewarned he may mistake the passages around the muscle bundle as a septal defect and further narrow the passageway by attempting to close the defect. The true ventricular septal defect may be obscured by the muscle bundle and thus escape detection. The treatment of associated conditions, such as valvular pulmonic stenosis, is not sufficient, and proper resection of the muscle bundle is necessary. A preoperative diagnosis is most helpful in avoiding these surgical pitfalls.

Tricuspid Atresia. Tricuspid atresia is uncommon and occurs in about 3% of congenital anomalies as seen clinically or at postmortem examination (Keith et al., 1967).

A common feature of all cases is a failure of development or differentiation of the tricuspid valve. The floor of the right atrium is typically smooth and structureless with no visible remnants of valve leaflets, although a small nodule or a centrally placed scar is common (Fig. 258). This prevents any communication between the right atrium and right ventricle.

Another common feature is a functional interatrial communication which is essential if life is to continue. Keith et al. (1967) found a patent foramen ovale in 66% of their cases and a defective septum in 33%. The size of the patent foramen ovale was greater in older patients, and the opening was always larger with a defective septum.

The right ventricle is variable in size and functional activity. The chamber may be so small that it is found only by careful search at postmortem study or it may be almost normal in size. The outflow portion of the chamber may have an infundibular obstruction with a separate small chamber similar to that seen in infundibular stenosis. In other cases the valve ring is quite small and constricted, producing a stenosis. Rarely, the valve cusps are fused forming a domed diaphragm-like obstruction similar to that seen in pure pulmonic stenosis, and occasionally there may be a tricuspid pulmonary valve. Complete occlusion rarely occurs. Also, atresia of the pulmonary trunk is occasionally seen in which case blood can reach the peripheral pulmonary arteries only through a patent ductus arteriosus or bronchial arteries. Very rarely the morphological right ventricle is a left-sided chamber associated with l-transposition of the great vessels, and this will be mentioned below.

A ventricular septal defect is present in a very high proportion of cases. It may be quite small and communicate only with the upper or infundibular portion of the diminutive right ventricle. On the other hand, it may be large, over 1 cm in diameter, and so arranged that a free passage of blood from the left ventricle into the pulmonary artery can occur. This arrangement is usually associated with a sizeable pulmonary artery and may permit an adequate or an increased blood flow to the lungs. In all cases, unless there is a patent ductus arteriosus or a transposition of the great vessels, the greater portion of the blood that reaches the lungs must pass through the ventricular septal defect.

Keith *et al.* (1967, page 648) have classified tricuspid atresia mainly on an anatomical basis. I denotes tricuspid atresia without transposition of the great vessels, II with d-transposition, and III with l-transposition of the great vessels. Under each category, there are three subdivisions, namely (a) those with pulmonary atresia, (b) those with pulmonary stenosis, and (c) those with no stenosis and with relatively normal or increased blood flow to the lungs. For the radiologist the following classification is useful:

1. Tricuspid atresia without transposition
    (a) with decreased pulmonary vasculature
    (b) with normal or increased pulmonary vasculature
2. Tricuspid atresia with transposition, and
    (a) decreased pulmonary vasculature
    (b) normal or increased pulmonary vasculature

Another small group consists of cases in which the pulmonary vasculature changes over a period of time, usually decreasing in prominence. Transpositions can be divided often on a radiological basis into the d- and l-type. In the d-type, the aorta arises to the right and anterior to the pulmonary artery, and in the l-type, it arises to the left and somewhat anterior to the pulmonary artery. The l-type transposition is quite rare and comprises about 3% of all cases of tricuspid atresia.

TRICUSPID ATRESIA WITHOUT TRANSPOSITION. This type comprises about 70% of all cases. Of these, about 85% will have a decreased pulmonary vasculature. In these cases, the pulmonary artery and ventricular septal defect are usually small. The right atrium is always approximately normal in size and often is enlarged, depending somewhat perhaps on the size of the interatrial communication. The left atrium is almost always enlarged, but the enlargement is not very striking.

Radiological Findings. The heart is usually normal in size or only slightly enlarged. The cardiac contours as seen in the PA, oblique, and lateral views are rarely specific or are occasionally suggestive of the diagnosis. A highly suggestive but infrequent contour in the frontal projection is characterized by flattening or even a concavity of the right border of the heart. In most of these, the right heart border does not extend beyond the right border of the shadow of the vertebral column. If it is seen, it is flattened or concave (Fig. 252D). The left border is long and rounded with a low apex suggesting left ventricular enlargement. In the LAO view, the anterior border may be flattened, and the left ventricle projects posteriorly again suggesting left ventricular enlargement. The pulmonary vascularity is typically decreased. The aortic knob is usually normal in size, although in infancy it is inconspicuous. The incidence of right aortic arch was found by Wittenborg *et al.* (1951) to be about the same as that in the tetralogy of Fallot, but in the authors' experience with more than 50 cases, this seems too high.

In the majority of cases, the main deviation of the cardiac contour from the normal is a concavity in the region of the pulmonary artery segment. Also, the left border of the heart may be either normal in contour or have a steep left border with a more box-like appearance. In many cases the contour is suggestive of the tetralogy of Fallot with decreased pulmonary vascularity and a concave pulmonary artery segment. The right atrium is normal in size or enlarged, and the right border of the heart may be normally convex. A small secondary convexity in the mid portion of the left cardiac contour occasionally represents the enlarged left atrial appendage (Astley *et al.*, 1953). This has been a rare finding in the authors' experience. The apex of the left ventricle is rarely elevated as is seen in many cases of the tetralogy of Fallot.

Wittenborg *et al.* (1951) found 4 cases of tricuspid atresia with dextrocardia and situs solitus out of 11 cases. The electrocardiogram was said to be helpful in suggesting the diagnosis. The presence of an l-type transposition should be suspected in these cases. Cokkinos *et al.* (1974) also suggest an increased incidence of tricuspid atresia associated with dextrocardia and situs solitus.

In about 15% of cases with tricuspid atresia without transposition, the pulmonary vasculature is normal or increased. The contour of the heart is rarely suggestive of tricuspid atresia and often has a remarkably normal appearance. The pulmonary artery is normal in size or enlarged, and consequently there is not a recognizable concavity in the region of the pulmonary artery segment. Increased blood flow to the lungs is usually associated with a large interventricular septal defect that permits the left ventricle to communicate easily with the pulmonary artery.

TRICUSPID ATRESIA WITH TRANSPOSITION OF THE GREAT VESSELS. d-Transposition of the

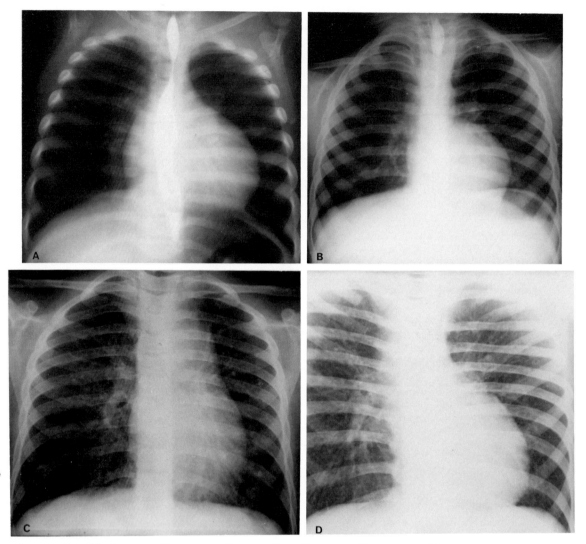

FIG. 252. VARIABLE CONTOUR OF HEART IN FOUR DIFFERENT EXAMPLES OF TRICUSPID ATRESIA

(A) represents the contour most commonly encountered. The left border is somewhat elongated and rounded. The lungs are avascular. In a lesser number of cases the left mid border is definitely concave (B). (C) represents a case with corrected transposition of the great vessels in addition to tricuspid atresia. The contour in (D) represents only a small minority of cases. The right contour of the heart is flattened.

great vessels denotes a right-sided origin of the aorta from the diminutive right ventricle. Rarely, the aorta may override the ventricular septum (Edwards *et al.*, 1965; Cooley *et al.*, 1950). The pulmonary artery originates from the large left ventricle. The pulmonary artery is usually large, and in about two-thirds of the cases, the blood flow to the lungs is increased. Pulmonic or sub-pulmonic obstruction is found in about one-third of the cases with an accompanying variable reduction in pulmonary blood flow. This obstruction may be valvular or due to an interposing bundle of muscle in the outflow tract of the left ventricle. Patients with the rare combination of

transposition with moderate pulmonic stenosis offer the best prognosis.

A peculiarity of d-transposition and tricuspid atresia is its association with juxtaposition of the atrial appendages (JAA). JAA is a rare anomaly and is most often seen with transposition of the great vessels, but over 50% of the reported cases have occurred with d-transposition of the great vessels and tricuspid atresia (Elliott *et al.*, 1968). The juxtaposition may be right or left-sided but is more often left-sided. The right atrial appendage lies in back of the great vessels and above the left atrial appendage. In this position it forms a striking convex contour along the left upper

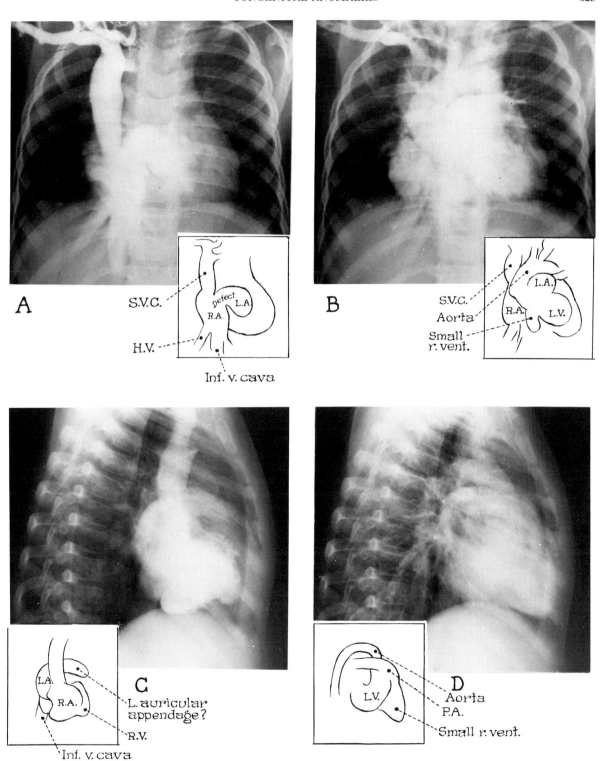

FIG. 253. TRICUSPID STENOSIS WITH SMALL BUT PROBABLY FUNCTIONING RIGHT VENTRICLE

(A) Angiocardiogram at 1 sec showing contrast substance passing from the right atrium into the left atrium through the interauricular septal defect. (B) One second later all of the heart chambers contain contrast substance. A diminutive right ventricle is seen lying over the spine and just above the diaphragm. The pulmonary arteries are small and difficult to identify. (C) Lateral view at 1 sec. Both the right and left atria are filled. (D) One second after (C). The aorta and pulmonary artery are seen as well as diminutive right ventricle. (Courtesy of *Radiology, 54:* 854 (Fig. 4), 1950.)

heart border as seen in Figure 259. The identification of this shadow is strong evidence for a transposition with tricuspid atresia.

l-Transposition with tricuspid atresia is quite rare and comprises about 3% of all cases (Keith *et al.*, 1967). This nomenclature refers primarily to the position of the aorta which arises to the left and anterior to the pulmonary artery. As pointed out by Tandon *et al.* (1974), this is usually not associated with a levocardiac loop. Only the conus in most cases is inverted, and the left ventricle is morphologically a left ventricle with a mitral valve. The importance of this rare variation is that the ascending aorta forms a considerable portion of the left heart border and presents a more bizarre contour that is not at all suggestive of tricuspid atresia (Fig. 252C).

Radiologic Findings. In transposition with tricuspid atresia, the heart is usually larger than when the vessels are normally placed, and the heart is usually enlarged (Fig. 255). The contour more often resembles that of transposition of the great vessels. The pulmonary vasculature is usually increased, the base of the heart is narrow, and the left border is convex and rounded suggestive of an "egg-shaped" appearance. The position of the aorta is often difficult to identify, and if the heart is enlarged, its contour is often bizarre, and it does not suggest any particular diagnosis. The presence of transposition is suspected much more often than that of the associated tricuspid atresia. In those cases in which there is a moderate or severe pulmonic stenosis and the pulmonary vasculature is decreased, the contour may resemble a tetralogy of Fallot.

Left axis deviation of the ECG associated with cyanotic congenital heart disease is presumptive evidence of tricuspid atresia. This finding is extremely valuable in differentiating this condition from the tetralogy of Fallot. Left axis deviation was found in 88% of 43 cases reported by Keith *et al.* (1958). A balanced axis is occasionally seen, and rarely a right axis occurs. However, a careful study with numerous chest leads almost always shows some evidence of left ventricular hypertrophy. Left axis deviation occurs also in other types of congenital heart disease other than tricuspid atresia. It is particularly likely to occur in infants with pulmonary atresia and diminutive right ventricle, and it has been found in a few cases of persistent truncus arteriosus and single ventricle. In those cases with tricuspid atresia with a balanced axis, precardial chest leads are usually helpful, and also after a period of time the elec-

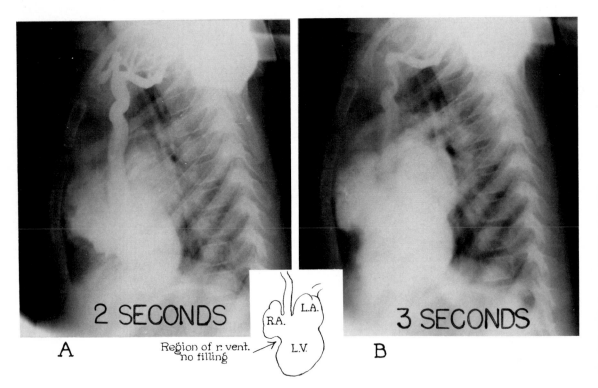

FIG. 254. TRICUSPID ATRESIA

Lateral views of angiocardiogram showing that the right ventricle fails to fill. (Courtesy of *Journal of the Faculty of Radiologists, 2:* 258 (Fig. 328), 1951.)

trocardiographic pattern may become more typical.

An increased frequency of coarctation of the aorta has been reported associated with tricuspid atresia and transposition of the great vessels (Keith *et al.*, 1967; Dick *et al.*, 1975).

Diagnosis. Cardiac catheterization is helpful in confirming the diagnosis and may occasionally document the presence and extent of pulmonic stenosis in patients with transposition. The catheter enters the right atrium but will not enter the right ventricle; instead it tends to go through the interatrial communication into the left atrium and left ventricle, and occasionally it can be introduced into the rudimentary right ventricle or in the case of transposition into the pulmonary artery.

Angiography is recommended in all cases of tricuspid atresia. Selective injections can be carried out during or in connection with cardiac catheterization. Filming is carried out in the AP and lateral projections at film speeds of 4–6/sec or using cinefluorography.

A selective injection into the right atrium will usually show most of the features of the abnormality. The right atrium is outlined and is usually larger than normal or dilated. It may extend downward and somewhat to the left in the frontal projection and occupies some of the area normally reserved for the right ventricle. Contrast substance courses immediately into the left atrium in most instances. We formerly felt that the rapidity of passage permitted an opinion as to the adequacy or the size of the septal defect and the need for further enlargement at the time of surgery. Rapid passage is the rule, however, even though collateral evidence, such as enlarged liver and a dilated vena cava, indicates that further enlargement of the defect would be beneficial. Kjellberg *et al.* (1958) point out that even though filming is carried out in two planes it is difficult to determine the size of the defect unless the septum is viewed tangentially, and this usually does not obtain in the standard AP and lateral views.

The left atrium is usually slightly to moderately enlarged and lies over the central mass of the heart in the frontal projection. The atrial appendage is border-forming on the left side of the heart and may be slightly enlarged, but in many cases this structure does not fill adequately to be recognized.

The left ventricle typically fills from 1–2 sec after filling of the right atrium and is always enlarged. As filming is carried out in diastole, the myocardium may be seen to be thickened and hypertrophied.

One of the cardinal angiographic signs of tricuspid atresia is a clear radiolucent area in the cardiac contour. In the frontal projection, this is seen just below and medial to the right atrium, and in the lateral view, it is seen anteriorly behind the sternum and above the diaphragm. This is best seen early in the course of the angiographic series when the right atrium, the left atrium, and the left ventricle have just filled. This radiolucent area represents that portion of the cardiac contour normally reserved for the right ventricle. When the right ventricle is seen in tricuspid atresia, it protrudes into this radiolucent area as a chamber of variable size. Rapid filming may increase the chances of demonstrating this chamber, but in the majority of cases following a selective right atrial injection, it is not seen. Nonvisualization may be due to the small size or to incomplete or momentary filling. A selective left ventricular injection is much more likely to show the diminutive right ventricle and often gives considerable information regarding the anatomy of the outflow tract and is helpful in differentiating tricuspid atresia from pulmonic atresia with a small right ventricle.

The pulmonary artery typically fills after the aorta and the left ventricle. Of course, delayed and poor filling of the pulmonary artery may be taken as presumptive evidence of pulmonary stenosis. However, a selective injection into the left ventricle is helpful in confirming this impression and showing the anatomy of the outflow tract of the right ventricle. Occasionally the catheter can be inserted into the right ventricle and a more detailed study obtained if this is necessary. Although most cases of tricuspid atresia have a diminished blood flow and a pulmonary stenosis, not all are so arranged. In some the interventricular defect is large, and the flow from the left ventricle into the outflow tract of the right ventricle and pulmonary artery is ample. This may be a crucial point in deciding as to the advisability of a systemic artery shunt, or in some cases a banding of the pulmonary artery might be indicated.

With complete transposition of the great vessels, the sequence of filling is the same as without transposition, but the aorta may fill after the pulmonary artery unless there is a pulmonic stenosis. The most striking finding is a markedly anterior position of the aorta, and it often overhangs the radiolucent area usually occupied by the right ventricle. The aorta may be slightly to the right of the pulmonary artery, and the valve rings are at about the same height. The pulmonary artery is more often of normal size than in tricuspid atresia without transposition, although

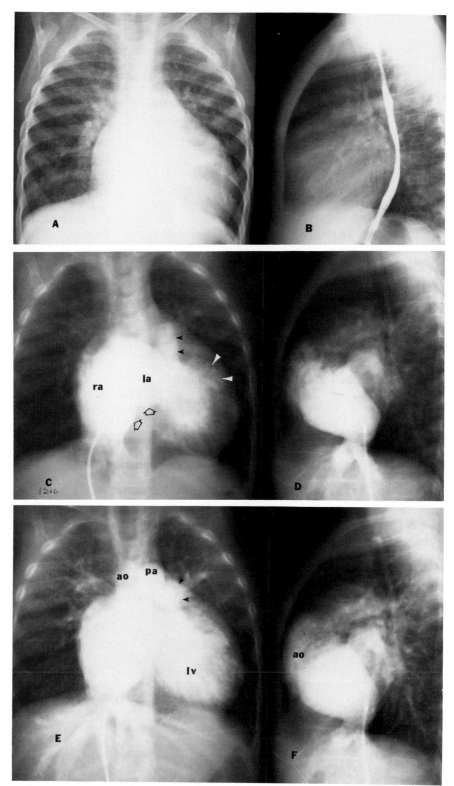

Fig. 255. Transposition with Tricuspid Atresia and Juxtaposition of Atrial Appendages

(A and B) Heart is enlarged and enlargement of left atrium is suggested. Pulmonary vascularity is slightly increased. (C and D) Right atrial injection. Black arrowheads show beginning filling of right atrial appendage. White arrow shows faint filling of left atrial appendage. Open arrow indicates space usually occupied by right ventricle (right ventricular window). (E and F) About 2 sec after C and D. Left ventricle has filled and has a quite thin myocardium (failure?). The aorta arises anteriorly, and a clear space is seen in the usual position occupied by the right ventricle.

332

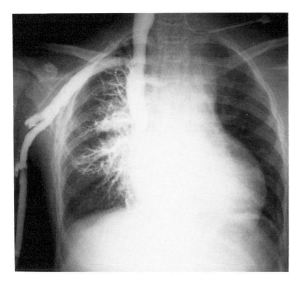

FIG. 256. ANOTHER CASE OF TRICUSPID ATRESIA

The Glenn (anastomosis of superior vena cava to right upper pulmonary artery) procedure in a patient with tricuspid atresia.

there may be a pulmonic or subpulmonic stenosis in which case the artery may be quite small. Even though the pulmonary artery is large, it is usually posterior to the aorta, and consequently in the AP projection the convexity on the left border of the heart may not be seen. A selective left ventricular injection is necessary to show in detail the pulmonary artery and the outflow tract of the left ventricle. Partial transposition of the aorta with overriding of the ventricular septum is unusual but was found in 2 of 21 cases previously reviewed by one of us and is reported by Edwards et al. (1965). In these cases, the ventricular septal defect may be of good size, and the filling of the aorta may be quite adequate.

Following venous angiocardiography or selective right atrial injection, reflux into the hepatic veins is quite common in association with tricuspid atresia. This is by no means a specific finding, however, and is often seen in other forms of congenital heart disease, such as the tetralogy of Fallot and transposition of the great vessels.

Either venous or selective angiography is capable of providing a satisfactory diagnosis unaided by other means of study, although this does not always obtain. In most cases, however, the diagnosis of tricuspid atresia is strongly suspected because of the clinical, conventional radiographic, and particularly the electrocardiographic findings. In these cases, angiography is confirmatory. Angiography is perhaps more useful in newborns and infants when the electrocardiographic patterns are not so well fixed but the patient is showing rapid deterioration. In older patients, particularly those with associated transposition of the great vessels, it may further elucidate the picture and particularly give information regarding the likelihood of improvement following the establishment of an artificial ductus.

Tricuspid atresia without transposition frequently resembles the tetralogy of Fallot from the radiologic point of view. The differentiation between the two conditions is usually easily made on the basis of electrocardiographic findings and supported by angiography. Tetralogy of Fallot with an atrial septal defect (pentalogy of Fallot) may have an electrocardiogram similar to that of tricuspid atresia, and certainly angiography is helpful in differentiation.

Underdevelopment or defective development of the right ventricle may be associated with severe pulmonary stenosis or atresia and an atrial septal defect (Taussig, 1960; Keith et al., 1967). Differentiation by radiologic means including angiography in these cases is most difficult. In newborns the electrocardiogram may not be helpful, but later the electrocardiographic pattern becomes more definite. It is quite useful to try to insert the catheter through the often stenotic tricuspid valve and into the small right ventricle and do a selective injection.

Occasionally single ventricle and truncus arteriosus will show a left axis deviation and thus be difficult to differentiate from tricuspid atresia. Angiography is quite helpful in these cases.

SURGICAL TREATMENT OF TRICUSPID ATRESIA. In patients with diminished pulmonary flow, a systemic to pulmonary shunt is usually beneficial and may greatly prolong life (Dick et al., 1975; Taussig et al., 1973). The Waterston procedure is often elected for patients under one year of age and the Blalock-Taussig procedure in older patients. The Glenn procedure (anastomosis of the superior vena cava to the distal right pulmonary artery) has also been beneficial (Dick et al., 1975) (Fig. 256).

In older patients in whom one of the shunt procedures has lost its effectiveness and in whom the heart has reached its approximate definitive size, a more extensive procedure has been used with apparent success (Fontan and Baudet, 1971; Ross and Somerville, 1973; Kreutzer et al., 1973; Sanford et al., 1973; Henry et al., 1974). This procedure basically consists of placing a xenograft with attached valve at the opening of the inferior vena cava into the right atrium. Another prosthesis or homograft containing a valve is used to connect the right atrial appendage with the right or the main pulmonary artery. The

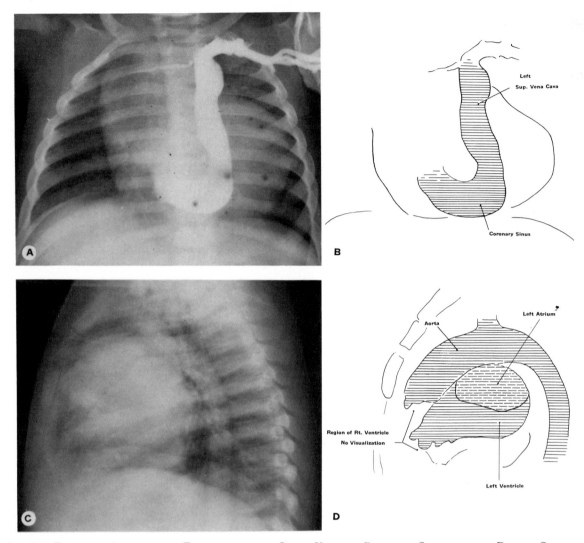

Fig. 257. Tricuspid Atresia with Transposition of Great Vessels, Pulmonic Stenosis, and Double Superior Vena Cava (Autopsy Case)

(A) Angiocardiogram at 1 sec showing a left-sided superior vena cava entering the right atrium through the coronary sinus. The heart was quite large and bizarre in shape, and the lungs were avascular. (B) Sketch of A. (C) Lateral angiocardiogram at 4 sec. The left atrium, ventricle, and aorta are filled with contrast substance. The aorta originates quite far anterior indicating a transposition; however, the chamber from which it originates either failed to fill or is too small to be seen, suggesting tricuspid atresia. (D) Sketch of C.

patent foramen ovale or atrial septal defect is closed. Thus, the right atrium is converted into a pumping chamber for the pulmonary circulation. This operation is recommended for patients who are 10 years of age or older and in whom the pulmonary resistance is still within the normal range. The early reports that have been listed above are encouraging.

In cases of tricuspid atresia with transposition and with a large pulmonary artery and increased pulmonary flow, pulmonary hypertension and increased pulmonary resistance may eventually be a threat to life. Neches *et al.* (1973) describe

such a case in which banding of the pulmonary artery was carried out with improvement. Later in the same patient when the ventricular defect threatened to close an aorticopulmonary window was created with beneficial results.

Complete Transposition of Great Vessels. Complete transposition of the great vessels is not a rare anomaly. The incidence is reported as 4.9% of autopsy cases of congenital heart disease by Abbott (1936). In this malformation the aorta originates entirely from the right ventricle and receives systemic venous blood; the pulmonary artery originates from the left ventricle and receives highly oxygenated blood. In the usual case where there is no significant rotation of the heart, the aorta is anterior and the pulmonary artery posterior in position. The unsaturated blood in the aorta is distributed to the systemic circulation and returns to the right side of the heart. The oxygenated blood in the pulmonary artery is distributed to the lungs and returns to the left side of the heart. These two circulations are thus separate except for certain compensatory communications which must be present if life is to continue.

The defects which may provide a communication between the systemic and pulmonary circulations are shown in Figure 260 and are (1) a

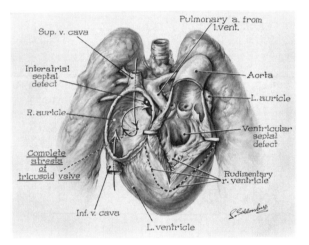

FIG. 258. DRAWING OF HEART AT AUTOPSY FROM CASE SHOWN IN FIG. 257

Right anterior view. (Courtesy of *Radiology, 54:* 849 (Fig. 1), 1950.)

patent foramen ovale (patent foramen ovale indicates any interatrial communication), (2) an interventricular septal defect, and (3) a patent ductus arteriosus. In a review of 123 proved cases of this condition, Blalock and Hanlon (1950) found that the most common single defect was a patent foramen ovale (or interatrial defect), and the most common combination of defects was a patent foramen ovale and a patent ductus arteriosus. Among the single defects, an opening in the interventricular system was associated with the longest life span and a combination of interventricular and interauricular defects gave an even greater duration of life. The explanation for this increased life expectancy is not entirely clear, but presumably the interventricular defect offers, as a rule, the best exchange of blood between the two sides of the heart. In a series of 179 personally observed cases of transposition of the great vessels without ventricular inversion reported by Van Mierop (1973), the best prognosis occurred in patients who had both a ventricular septal defect and pulmonary stenosis.

The pulmonary arteries and particularly the smaller branches in the lungs are usually dilated and their walls are secondarily thickened. These changes are more pronounced in older patients and are presumably associated with increased pulmonary artery pressure. In patients with associated pulmonic stenosis, the pulmonary artery pressure is reduced, and the smaller branches in the lungs are diminished in size.

Differences in pressure between the two sides of the heart, or between the aorta and pulmonary artery in complete transposition are minimal. Consequently, the minute volume of shunts between the two circulations is small. In 94 patients

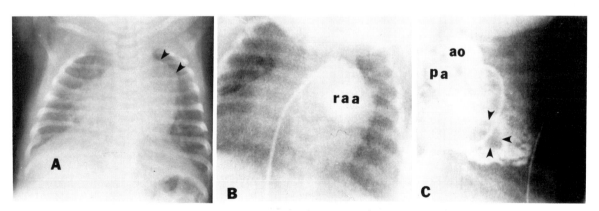

FIG. 259. TRANSPOSITION WITH TRICUSPID ATRESIA AND JUXTAPOSITION OF THE ATRIAL APENDAGES

(A) The large right atrial appendage produces a distinct and unusual convexity of the left upper cardiac contour (arrowheads). (B) Catheter inserted through large right atrium into dilated right atrial appendage (cinefluorogram). (C) Left ventricular injection (cinefluorogram). Arrowheads show eccentric AV valve. Aorta and pulmonary artery fill immediately. Juxtaposition of atrial appendages is highly suggestive of transposition with tricuspid atresia.

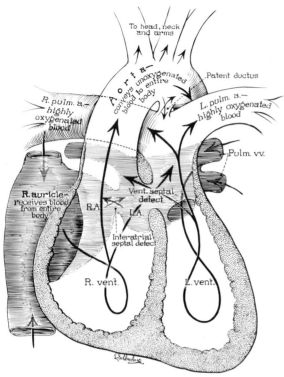

FIG. 260. DIAGRAM OF HEART AND GREAT VESSELS IN
COMPLETE TRANSPOSITION

All three commonly associated defects which may permit
an exchange of blood between the two sides of the heart are
shown. (Courtesy of *Radiology*, 58: 482 (Fig. 1), 1952.)

studied by Mair *et al.* (1971), the mean systemic
flow was 5.5 L/min/m², the mean pulmonary
flow was 9.0 L/min/m², but the effective pulmonary flow (that blood flow responsible for effective gas transport) was only 1.7 L/min/m². It is
obvious that a unidirectional shunt cannot be
maintained for more than a short time without
overloading one side of the heart. Consequently,
if only one defect is present, there must be a
periodic reversal of the shunt, dependent upon
differences in pressure between the two circulations. With an increase in the volume of blood in
one side of the heart, the pressure on that side
increases, and the shunt is thus reversed. The
presence of two openings such as an interventricular and interatrial septal defect presumably
would allow predominantly unidirectional but
opposite shunts through the two defects, and
thus there would be less tendency for the two
circulations to become unbalanced. It is because
of this small volume and frequent change in
direction that venous angiocardiography has not
proven to be a reliable means of demonstrating
shunts between the two circulations in transposition of the great vessels.

Where a sizeable patent ductus arteriosus is
associated with a complete transposition, significant amounts of highly saturated blood may
enter the descending aorta from the pulmonary
artery. Of course, the amount of this shunt would
be greatly enhanced by a coarctation proximal to
the entrance of the ductus. Thus, more highly
oxygenated blood would be distributed to the
lower trunk and extremities than to the head and
upper extremities. A consequent difference in the
degree of cyanosis between the hands and feet
may be visible and is a diagnostic sign of importance.

The coronary arteries receive highly unsaturated blood from the aorta, and the myocardium
is consequently inadequately supplied with oxygen. This, combined with the distention secondary to the constantly reversing shunts, usually
results in progressive cardiac enlargement. The
right ventricle is proportionately larger than the
left.

CLINICAL FINDINGS. Cyanosis beginning in the
neonatal period is the commonest clinical sign.
It was present in all of 16 cases reported by
Astley and Parsons (1952) and all of 44 cases
reviewed by Keith *et al.* (1953). The latter authors emphasize that cyanosis is marked and is
ordinarily much more severe than in most cases
of tetralogy of Fallot at the same age. However,
acyanotic transposition of the great vessels has
been encountered by Mehrizi and Taussig (1959).
Dyspnea, especially on exertion, and venous
congestion are common, and rapid enlargement
of the heart after birth is usual. About one-half
of the cases may be expected to have a systolic
precordial murmur, but auscultation is of little
definite diagnostic value. The electrocardiogram
may show right axis deviation, right ventricular
hypertrophy, and P pulmonale but shows no
specific characteristics. A history of congestive
heart failure was elicited in 37 of 50 patients
reported by Noonan *et al.* (1960), and failure can
be expected to develop by the age of 6 months
(Lenkei *et al.*, 1959). Poor growth and development are the rule; squatting is uncommon. The
average age at death in the series of Keith *et al.*
(1953) was 3 months. Roberts *et al.* (1962) have
reported a proved case of complete transposition
in a male who survived to the age of 21 years. A
Blalock-Taussig anastomosis, in combination
with associated valvular pulmonic stenosis, atrial
and ventricular septal defects, and increased collateral bronchial arterial circulation were
thought to be responsible for his long survival.
There are numerous other reports of survival to
school age, and varying degrees of severity of
clinical manifestations are to be expected.

RADIOLOGIC FINDINGS. Taussig's (1960) description of the typical contour is helpful and usually reliable although there are a number of variations. The heart is slightly to moderately enlarged, and enlargement is often progressive but is variable in its development. Consequently, in young children and infants, enlargement may not be a prominent feature. The heart contour is somewhat symmetrical but extends farther to the left than the right. The apex points down and out. The base is narrow, but there is no pronounced concavity of the left mid contour in the region of the pulmonary artery, such as is often seen in the tetralogy of Fallot; instead, the contour is straight and smooth. It may be formed, in part, by the transposed aorta. Although the base of the heart is narrow in the posteroanterior projection due to some superimposition of the pulmonary artery and aorta, as the patient is rotated into the left anterior oblique position under the fluoroscope the base or vascular pedicle increases in width. In the lateral view at fluoroscopy, the aorta is seen to originate quite far anterior in relation to the heart contour although this is best demonstrated by angiocardiography.

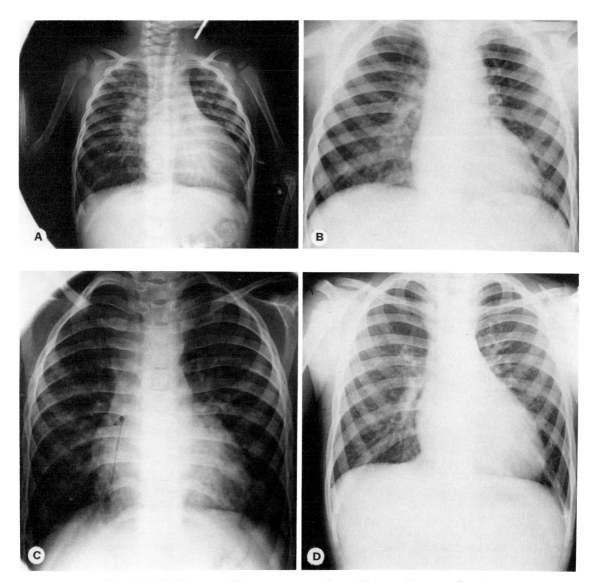

FIG. 261 A–D. COMPLETE TRANSPOSITION OF GREAT VESSELS (AUTOPSY CASES)

Conventional films of 4 different cases. The oldest (C) was 7 years, and youngest (A) was 10 months. Note that the heart is not greatly enlarged, and there is a marked increase in prominence of the pulmonary vascular structures in all cases. The base of the heart is of normal width or slightly narrowed.

Guerin *et al.* (1970) found either an anteroposterior or oblique relationship between the aorta and the pulmonary artery in 38 patients with complete transposition of the great vessels. In every case, the aorta was anterior to the pulmonary artery. In 14 cases the aorta was directly anterior to the pulmonary artery, in 19 it was slightly to the right and in 5 slightly to the left. When the main pulmonary artery was directly visualized on the left mediastinal border, the ascending aorta was always located slightly to the right of the pulmonary artery. If the pulmonary artery branches were at the same level and of the same length, the main pulmonary artery was medially placed, indicating a slightly left-sided aorta. When the right pulmonary artery was higher than the left, the ascending aorta was likewise located in the left upper mediastinum. If the left pulmonary branch was higher than the right, the main pulmonary artery was usually left-sided and the aorta ascended to the right of the main pulmonary artery. The importance of locating the ascending aorta lies in the fact that the position of the ventricles can thereby be identified according Van Praagh's loop rule (Paul *et al.*, 1968; Van Praagh *et al.*, 1964). An aortic valve located to the right of the pulmonary valve indicates a right-sided morphologic right ventricle as is seen in the usual case of complete transposition of the great vessels. An aortic valve to the left indicates a left-sided morphologic right ventricle as is ordinarily seen in congenitally corrected transposition of the great vessels.

Because of the ample blood supply, the vascular structures within the lungs are prominent. Rarely, however, is a large proximal pulmonary artery in the hilus identified. Instead, the branches in the lung parenchyma are larger and can be followed farther towards the periphery than usual. Frequently, there is a cluster of vascular shadows around the hilus, but these are continuous with sizeable arteries which can be followed into the lung parenchyma. At fluoroscopy, these shadows show an increase in pulsation which is distinctive but rarely amounts to a "hilar dance" such as is seen in an interatrial defect. It should be emphasized that it is very difficult to determine fluoroscopically whether a small baby has pulmonary plethora or not. Good film studies are essential.

Taussig (1960) has written of a rhythmic change in the fullness of the right atrial contour as seen at fluoroscopy, which is independent of respiratory phase. This she attributes to a change in the direction of the shunt through a patent foramen ovale and is therefore evidence of a transposition with such a defect.

There are a number of variations or additional defects which may alter the cardiac contour and must be evaluated. The most common of these are (1) anomalies of the great veins such as double superior vena cavae which tend to widen

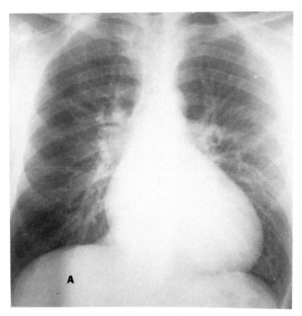 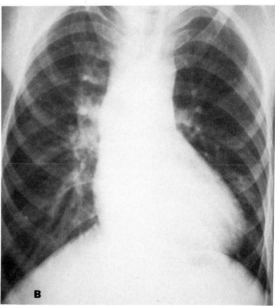

Fig. 262. Frontal Chest Films of Two Different Patients with Complete Transposition of the Great Vessels

In both patients one sees nondistinctive cardiac enlargement (more marked in A) with increased pulmonary vascular volume. That combination in an obviously cyanotic patient should suggest the correct diagnosis.

the shadow of the cardiac base; also, some or all of the pulmonary veins may enter the right atrium and one or both of the vena cavae may enter the left atrium giving a partial or completely corrected transposition; (2) pulmonic stenosis in which the pulmonary vascularity is decreased rather than increased; and (3) rotational or torsional dextrocardia with a resultant variation in the heart contour. Congenital tricuspid atresia may also occur in association with transposition of the great vessels. Generalized cardiac enlargement with pulmonary plethora was present in 2 of 3 such cases reported by Macafee and Patterson (1961). One of the 3 survived to age 5 years and 10 months. Van Mierop (1973) declares that he has never seen a patient with transposition of the great arteries who had aortic valvular stenosis.

Both cardiac catheterization and angiocardiography may supply helpful additional information. Either procedure may demonstrate a double superior vena cava or some other venous anomaly. Right heart catheterization will not provide an absolute diagnosis of transposition, even though the catheter enters the aorta, although it is of some value in indicating the location and volume of shunts. At angiocardiography, the transposed aorta fills immediately from the right ventricle with a high concentration of contrast substance. The ascending portion as seen in the lateral view is quite far anterior in relation to the cardiac contour; often, it is just underneath the sternum.

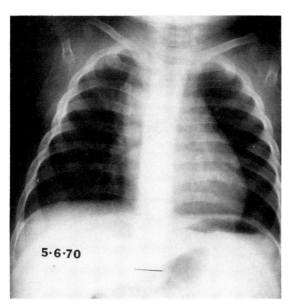

FIG. 263. TRANSPOSITION OF GREAT VESSELS, PULMONIC STENOSIS, AND A RIGHT AORTIC ARCH
Differentiation from a tetralogy of Fallot is difficult (see text).

In the anteroposterior projection, it originates from the right ventricle near the midline and arches almost directly posterior. It is an average size vessel in contrast to that seen in truncus arteriosus or tetralogy of Fallot. In a rotational dextrocardia, the right or venous ventricle is often posterior, and this may alter the relative position of the ascending aorta.

Selective injection of contrast material into the ventricle from which the transposed aorta arises will show characteristics of a morphologic right ventricle. The trabeculae show a typical pattern, being larger, coarser and fewer when compared with the numerous fine trabeculae of the left ventricle. The body of the right ventricle is separated from the outflow tract or infundibulum by a ring of muscular tissue consisting of the body of the crista supraventricularis along with its parietal and septal bands and the moderator band. The parietal band is directed forward to the right anterior wall of the ventricle, and the septal band is attached to the interventricular septum. The moderator band is contiguous with the septal band of the crista and extends from the ventricular septum to the free wall of the right ventricle in the region of the origin of the anterior papillary muscle (Barcia et al., 1967).

In the presence of a sizeable ventricular septal defect, selective right ventriculography may fill both ventricles, depending upon pressure and flow relationships at the time of injection. One may then see on the lateral series of films the precise location and the size of the VSD as well as the relationships between the ventricles and between the great vessels.

Catheterization of the left ventricle for purposes of angiography may be difficult but is regularly accomplished by experienced operators. The catheter may be passed into the left side of the heart through either an interatrial or interventricular septal defect. Injection into the ventricle from which the pulmonary artery arises will show the morphologic characteristics of a left ventricle. The ventricular body is characterized by the presence of numerous small fine trabeculae, giving the inner surface a smoother appearance than that of the right ventricle. No crista supraventricularis is present, and the anterior leaflet of the mitral valve is contiguous with the posterior cusp of the pulmonary valve.

Injections into each ventricle will enable the examiner to define the relative sizes of the two ventricles, to detect hypoplasia of either chamber, to determine the morphology and therefore the situs of the ventricles and to examine the interventricular septum for normal or abnormal

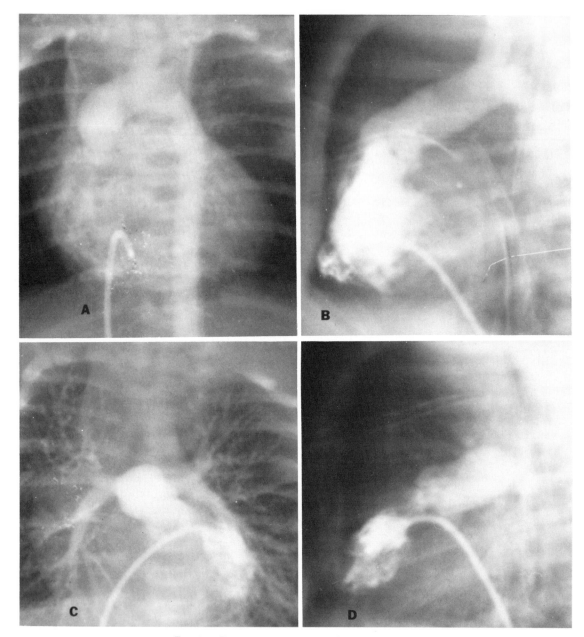

FIG. 264. TRANSPOSITION OF THE GREAT VESSELS

Frontal (A and C) and lateral (B and D) views of selective right (A and B) and left (C and D) ventriculograms in a patient with transposition of the great vessels. The pulmonary valve is located to the left of and posterior to the aortic valve, but the bodies of the two ventricles are nearly side by side.

placement and the presence of an interventricular septal defect. A ventricular septal defect was present in 52 of 60 cases of dextroposition studied by Barcia *et al.* (1967). The defect was usually located inferior to the crista supraventricularis from the right ventricular aspect, and from the left ventricular aspect the defect was adjacent to the pulmonary valve.

Selective left ventriculography is important in the evaluation of patients with transposition of the great arteries in order to search for and detect left ventricular outflow tract obstruction. Twenty-eight of 200 patients reviewed by Shaher *et al.* (1967) demonstrated narrowing of the left ventricular outflow tract. Both valvular and subvalvular types of obstruction were identified.

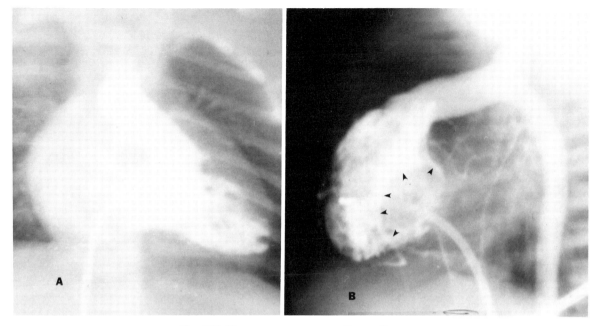

FIG. 265. TRANSPOSITION OF THE GREAT VESSELS

Frontal (A) and lateral (B) frames from a selective right ventriculogram in a patient with transposition of the great vessels. The right ventricle is large and shows prominent trabeculations. The aorta arises anteriorly, entirely from the right ventricle. No filling of the pulmonary arteries is seen. On the lateral view one can see the tricuspid valve leaflets bulging into the ventricle (arrows).

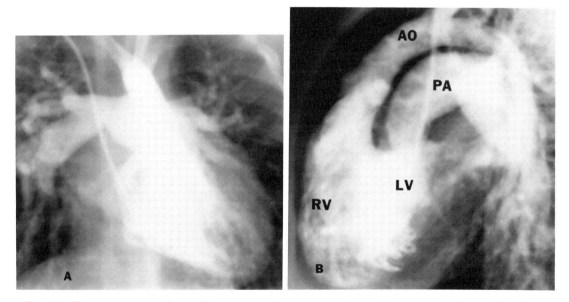

FIG. 266. TRANSPOSITION OF GREAT VESSELS WITH VENTRICULAR SEPTAL DEFECT IN A 2-MONTH OLD BOY

A and B are frames from a selective right ventriculogram. The right ventricle is situated anteriorly and to the right and communicates through a large ventricular septal defect with the left ventricle which is located posteriorly and to the left. The transposed aorta originates from the right ventricular infundibulum directly anterior to the pulmonary artery. The aortic valve is located higher and slightly to the right relative to the pulmonary valve. (With permission, from Transposition of the Great Arteries by A. Barcia, O. W. Kincaid, G. D. Davis, J. W. Kirklin and P. A. Ongley, *American Journal of Roentgenology, Radium Therapy and Nuclear Medicine, 100:* 249–283, 1967.)

Valvular pulmonic stenosis was seen in patients with and without ventricular septal defect; a fibromuscular tunnel was found only in patients with a ventricular septal defect; a fibrous ring or diaphragm was seen in patients with and without a VSD; and subvalvular muscular narrowing of the outflow tract caused by bulging of the ventricular septum into the cavity of the left ventricle was found in patients with and without a VSD. While the pulmonary vascularity may be decreased in the presence of left ventricular outflow tract obstruction in transposition of the great arteries, most of the patients reported by Shaher *et al.* (1967) showed increased pulmonary vascular volume. These authors found that when pulmonary stenosis is present in the case of complete transposition of the great vessels with a ventricular septal defect, the pulmonary valve was almost invariably involved. They also believe that a pulmonary artery smaller than the aorta is diagnostic of left ventricular outflow tract obstruction.

In patients with pulmonary valvular stenosis and normally related great vessels, post-stenotic

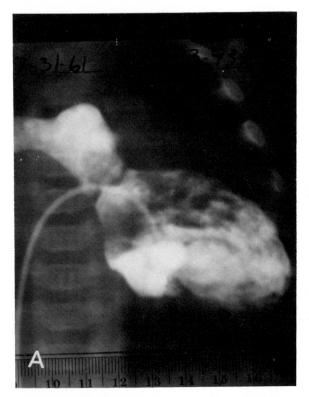 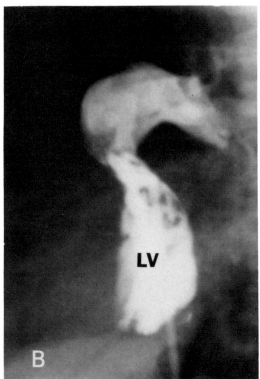

FIG. 267. TRANSPOSITION OF THE GREAT VESSELS, ATRIAL SEPTAL DEFECT AND INTACT VENTRICULAR SEPTUM IN A 5-MONTH OLD BOY

The catheter was passed via the saphenous vein through an atrial septal defect into a ventricular cavity with the morphologic characteristics of a left ventricle, situated to the left and posteriorly. A and B are frontal and lateral planes from a selective left ventriculogram showing the pulmonary artery to originate entirely from the left ventricle. The aorta was located to the right of and anterior to the pulmonary artery. The interventricular septum runs parallel to the anterior chest wall. (With permission, from Transposition of the Great Arteries by A. Barcia, O. W. Kincaid, G. D. Davis, J. W. Kirklin, and P. A. Ongley, *American Journal of Roentgenology, Radium Therapy and Nuclear Medicine 100:* 249–283, 1967.)

FIG. 268. TRANSPORTATION OF THE GREAT VESSELS, VENTRICULAR SEPTAL DEFECT, AND ATRIAL SEPTAL DEFECT IN AN 18-YEAR-OLD GIRL

A and B are frontal and lateral films from a selective left ventriculogram showing that the transposed great arteries are located side by side, the aorta to the right of the dilated pulmonary artery, the latter of which arises entirely from the left ventricle. C and D are frames from a selective right ventriculogram showing that the aorta arises entirely from the right ventricle. The tricuspid valve ring and leaflets are outlined on C and D. (With permission, from Transposition of the Great Arteries by A. Barcia, O. W. Kincaid, G. D. Davis, J. W. Kirklin, and P. A. Ongley, *American Journal of Roentgenology, Radium Therapy and Nuclear Medicine, 100:* 249–283, 1967.)

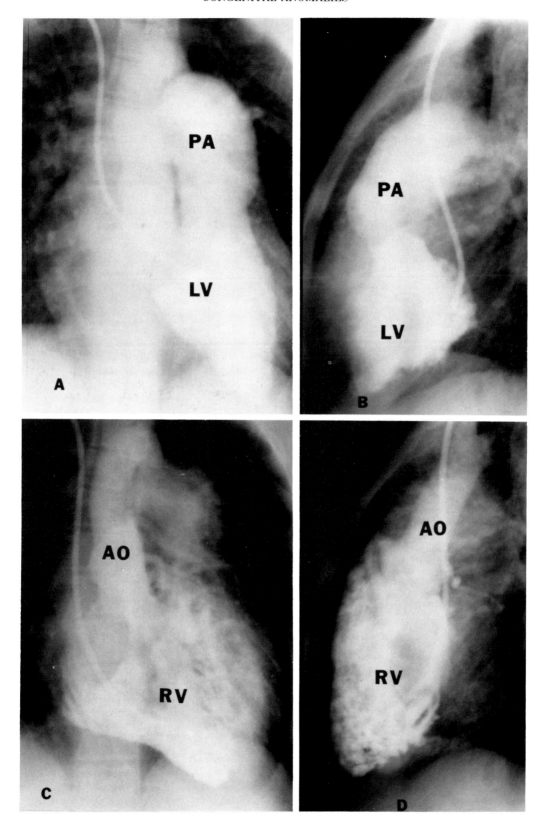

dilatation usually involves the main pulmonary artery and the left branch. In patients with transposition of the great arteries and valvular pulmonary stenosis, the right branch tends to be involved to a greater degree than the left, probably because of alignment of the right branch with the main pulmonary artery; the direction of the jet of blood is mainly to the right.

In summary, one should be able to determine from ordinary chest films of patients with complete transposition of the great arteries (d-transposition) the size of the heart, the relationships between the great vessels, the pulmonary vascular volume and the situs of the viscera and therefore of the atria. Selective right and left ventriculograms will show the relationships between the ventricles, their size and identity, the precise positions of the great vessels relative to one another and their size, the presence of an interventricular septal defect and the presence of left ventricular outflow tract obstruction.

Gramiak *et al.* (1973) and King *et al.* (1973) have described contributions of cardiac ultrasonography to the diagnosis of transposition of the great vessels.

In planning angiocardiography some thought must be given to determining the minimal volume and concentration of contrast material which will suffice to demonstrate the anatomic alterations present. Contrast material enters the cerebral circulation in high concentration, and an excessive dose may be hazardous.

Response to medical treatment with digitalis and other decongestive measures, though important, is, on the whole, disappointing (Noonan *et al.*, 1960). Several surgical procedures have been devised which have achieved a variable degree of success. Rashkind and Miller (1966) reported on a technique for creation of an atrial septal defect without thoracotomy. This technique, now known as the Rashkind procedure, is also called balloon atrial septostomy and consists of creation of or enlarging of an interatrial septal defect by pulling a balloon-tipped catheter sharply from the left atrium into the right atrium, thereby tearing the margins of a small atrial septal defect or foramen ovale and thus enlarging the communication between the atria. This permits greater mixing of blood and usually effects prompt improvement in an intensely cyanotic and seriously ill infant (Rashkind, 1974). Blalock and Hanlon (1950) surgically created or enlarged

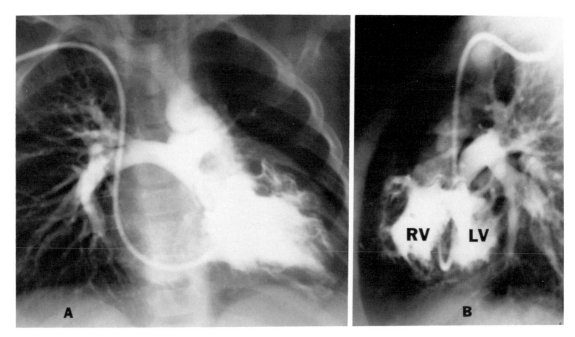

FIG. 269. TRANSPOSITION OF THE GREAT VESSELS WITH VENTRICULAR SEPTAL DEFECT
AND VALVULAR PULMONARY STENOSIS

Selective right ventriculogram in frontal (A) and lateral (B) projections shows the right ventricle to be located anteriorly and to communicate through a ventricular septal defect with the left ventricle, situated posteriorly. The aorta originates from the right ventricle and is situated anteriorly and slightly to the left of the pulmonary artery. The pulmonary artery originates from the left ventricle and shows valvular pulmonic stenosis. The septum lies in a transverse plane and is seen on end in the lateral projection. (With permission, from Transposition of the Great Arteries by A. Barcia, O. W. Kincaid, G. D. Davis, J. W. Kirklin, and P. A. Ongley, *American Journal of Roentgenology, Radium Therapy and Nuclear Medicine, 100:* 249–283, 1967.)

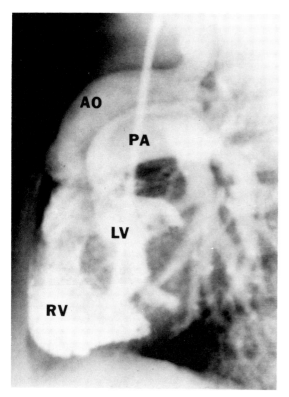

FIG. 270. TRANSPOSITION OF THE GREAT VESSELS, VEN-
TRICULAR SEPTAL DEFECT, AND SUBVALVULAR AND VAL-
VULAR PULMONARY STENOSIS IN A 4-MONTH-OLD BOY
Selective right ventricular angiocardiogram shows that
the aorta originates entirely from the right ventricle and the
pulmonary artery entirely from the left ventricle. The aorta
is located anterior to the pulmonary artery, and both atrio-
ventricular valves are seen. (With permission, from Trans-
position of the Great Arteries by A. Barcia, O. W. Kincaid,
G. D. Davis, J. W. Kirklin, and P. A. Ongley, *American
Journal of Roentgenology, Radium Therapy and Nuclear
Medicine, 100:* 249–283, 1967.)

an atrial septal defect to improve the exchange
of blood between the two sides of the heart.

Mustard in 1964 reported a method of inserting
a pericardial patch or baffle into the atria following excision of the interatrial septum in such a
manner as to redirect systemic venous blood
through the mitral valve to the left ventricle and
thence to the lungs through the transposed pulmonary artery. Pulmonary venous blood was re-
directed via the tricuspid valve to the right ventricle and thence to the transposed aorta. The
Mustard procedure has now become the standard operative treatment for correction of complete transposition of the great arteries.

Although some centers advocate elective intracardiac repair in the first year of life, it is more
usual to perform balloon atrial septostomy or a
palliative operation if any is needed in the first

year of life, with the Mustard intra-atrial baffle
repair being performed after one year of age
(Gutgesell and McNamara, 1974). Palliative operations may consist of one or more of the following: (1) Blalock-Hanlon atrial septostomy, (2)
systemic-to-pulmonary artery shunting for associated pulmonic stenosis, (3) pulmonary artery
banding for large VSDs, and (4) closure of a large
patent ductus arteriosus. With this approach one
can expect a 55–70% two-year survival (Tynan,
1971; Kidd *et al.*, 1971; Clarkson *et al.*, 1972;
Gutgesell and McNamara, 1975). This is in contrast to a mortality of 95% by age two years
among patients with transposition of the great
arteries seen before 1963.

In patients with transposition of the great vessels and ventricular septal defect, the VSD may
be closed at the time of performance of the
Mustard procedure, and Idriss *et al.* (1974) de-
clared that most of the defects can be closed
through the tricuspid orifice rather than through
a ventriculotomy. For patients with severe pulmonary vascular disease, the Mustard procedure
without closure of the VSD gives satisfactory
results and palliation.

Angiography following the Mustard procedure
shows the effects of rerouting of the systemic and
pulmonary blood flow. The intra-atrial baffle
creates a V-shaped tunnel with the apex of the V
pointing to the patient's left. The superior vena
cava empties into the upper limb of the tunnel;
the inferior vena cava and coronary sinus empty
into the lower limb. Blood is transported to the
newly created venous atrium which consists of
portions of the original right and left atrium and
is therefore a spacious chamber, bearing both
atrial appendages. This chamber empties
through the mitral valve into the left ventricle
which then transmits systemic venous blood into
the pulmonary artery for oxygenation.

The atrium receiving pulmonary venous blood
consists of the posterior wall of the original left
atrium and the major portion of the original right
atrium. It empties through the tricuspid valve
into the right ventricle, transmitting oxygenated
blood which is then pumped into the aorta and
into the systemic circulation. Rizk *et al.* (1973)
found the tunnel from the superior vena cava to
the mitral valve to be invariably narrowed, but
in spite of the angiographic appearance of stenosis, a significant pressure gradient was recorded in only one patient. As much as an 80%
narrowing of a segment of the vena cava was
usually not associated with a clinically detectable
obstruction or a significant gradient. Stark *et al.*
(1974) reported the development of systemic venous obstruction in 8 of 172 survivors of the

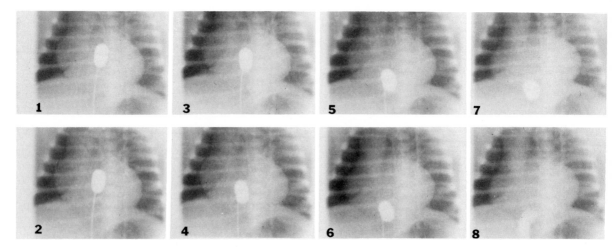

FIG. 271. CINERADIOGRAPHIC MONITORING OF THE RASHKIND PROCEDURE

A catheter is introduced into the left atrium through a small ASD or patent foramen ovale, and the balloon on the tip is then filled with contrast material (1, 2). The balloon is pulled down until it is snugly approximated to the interatrial septum (3-7). At this point the catheter is sharply withdrawn (8), producing a rent in the septum which allows for better mixing of the two otherwise separated circulations. Immediate improvement in the patient's color and general condition often occurs.

Mustard operation in whom pericardium had been used for the baffle. This complication occurred in 26 of 84 survivors with a Dacron baffle. Ruel *et al.* (1974), because of a similar experience, advocate the use of pericardium rather than Dacron for the intra-atrial baffle. In all cases in which superior or inferior vena caval obstruction was present, the azygos vein served as the largest collateral, taking the blood to the unobstructed or less obstructed vena cava. Obstruction occurred most commonly in the intracardiac portion of the venous return pathways, and venous angiography was the most helpful single investigation to demonstrate the presence and site of obstruction.

Price *et al.* (1971) report two patients with systemic venous obstruction following the Mustard procedure. They speculate that angiography might also be useful in cases of periatrial clot, a circumstance which might decrease the size of the newly created left atrium and thereby compromise pulmonary venous drainage, resulting perhaps in pulmonary edema.

The poor general health of infants with transposition of the great vessels results in thymic atrophy, and this may contribute to the narrow appearance of the waist of the heart on the posteroanterior roentgenograms. Rizk *et al.* (1972) reported rebound enlargement of the thymus after successful corrective surgery for transposition of the great vessels in 17 of 40 patients who had been treated by the Mustard operation.

Truncus Arteriosus. A persistent truncus arteriosus (PTA) is a single large vessel which carries all of the blood which leaves the heart. It is due to failure of partitioning of the truncus arteriosus into an ascending aorta and pulmonary trunk. A ventricular septal defect (VSD) is always present, and the truncus overrides the VSD and arises from both ventricles or from the right ventricle. A mixture of arterial and venous blood occurs within the ventricles or within the truncus or both, and this blood is distributed to the systemic and pulmonary circulations.

The incidence of persistent truncus arteriosus has been variously estimated at from 0.4% to between 2 and 3% of congenital cardiac anomalies (Victorica and Elliott, 1968; Rudolph, 1974; Keith *et al.*, 1967).

According to Collett and Edwards (1949), only two absolute criteria are necessary for the pathologic diagnosis of persistent truncus arteriosus: (1) the presence of only one main arterial trunk arising from the base of the heart, with no remnant of an atretic pulmonary artery or aorta, and (2) this trunk must supply branches to the coronary, pulmonary, and systemic circulations. On the basis of an analysis of 93 cases, Collett and Edwards (1949) classified persistent truncus arteriosus as follows.

Type I. The truncus gives rise to the aorta and to a single pulmonary trunk which then divides into right and left pulmonary arteries (48% of their material).

Type II. The right and left pulmonary arteries arise independently but close together from the dorsal wall of the truncus at varying levels above the truncal valve (29%).

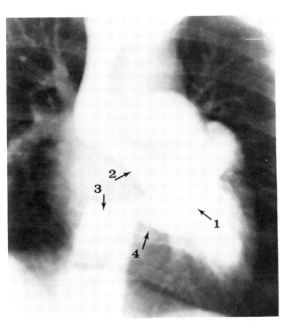

FIG. 272. INTRAVENOUS ANGIOCARDIOGRAM IN A PATIENT FOLLOWING CORRECTION OF TRANSPOSITION OF THE GREAT VESSELS BY THE MUSTARD PROCEDURE

Blood from the superior vena cava enters the body of the venous atrium (1), which is bounded inferiorly by the mitral valve, by passing through the superior limb of the artificially created tunnel (2). The inferior limb of the tunnel is also displayed (3), as is partial filling of the coronary sinus (4). (From the Angiographic Appearance of the Heart Following the Mustard Procedure by Ghassan Rizk, James H. Moller, and Kurt Amplatz, *Radiology 106*: 269–273, with permission.)

Type III. One or both pulmonary arteries arise independently from either side of the truncus (10%).

Type IV. The pulmonary arteries and the ductus arteriosus are absent; circulation to the lungs is by means of bronchial arteries (13%).

In actual practice, it may be very difficult to separate on clinical or even angiographic grounds Types I, II, and III. Unless pulmonary stenosis is present, the lungs are likely to be engorged with blood, and the pulmonary circuit is subjected to the systemic pressure of the aorta. Systemic arterial oxygen unsaturation will of course be present, but cyanosis may be absent or minimal in these patients (Victorica *et al.*, 1969). The prognosis is poorest in those patients with the largest pulmonary blood flow, and early and severe congestive heart failure is the frequent result of overloading of the left side of the circulation because of the torrential pulmonary blood flow. Pulmonary hypertension may eventually develop in those patients who survive, following which cyanosis may become more obvious.

In patients with Type IV PTA, the blood sup-

ply to the lungs is reduced, and cyanosis is a constant feature. Bronchial and mediastinal collateral arteries supply the lungs. This condition is to be differentiated from pseudotruncus or tetralogy of Fallot with pulmonary atresia. The following are the differential points:

1. No pulmonary infundibulum is present in PTA Type IV but is present in pseudotruncus.

2. No ductus arteriosus is present in PTA Type IV while pseudotruncus is associated with a ductus arteriosus, though it may be difficult to identify.

3. Pulmonary arteries are never identified in PTA Type IV, but retrograde filling of the main pulmonary arteries may be present in patients with atresia of the main pulmonary trunk (Dalinka *et al.*, 1970).

Hemitruncus is the name given to the rare variation which occurs when the blood supply to one lung originates from the aorta and that to the other lung originates from a pulmonary artery that originates from the heart. PTA Type V of Collett and Edwards, described as partial persistence of the truncus arteriosus, with a localized defect in the truncoconal septum and communication between the aorta and the pulmonary artery, is probably better classified as an aorticopulmonary septal defect rather than as a form of persistent truncus arteriosus.

COURSE OF THE CIRCULATION. Venous blood enters the right atrium from the vena cavae and passes without obstruction into the right ventricle. Mixing of venous blood from the right ventricle and oxygenated blood from the left ventricle occurs within the heart to a greater or lesser degree depending upon the size of the interventricular septal defect. Mixing also occurs in the truncus. A portion of the blood that enters the truncus arteriosus is distributed to the lungs and returns, after being oxygenated, to the left atrium and ventricle. In patients with Types I through III PTA, the volume of blood returned to the left side of the heart may be very great and may overwhelm the left ventricle, producing congestive heart failure. The remainder of the blood is distributed to the systemic circulation. The interesting finding that the pulmonary artery oxygen saturation is less than systemic oxygen saturation in some patients is doubtless due to preferential streaming of blood leaving the two ventricles. Thus, the left ventricle may preferentially eject its blood through the truncus into the aorta and the right ventricle into the pulmonary arteries (Victorica *et al.*, 1969).

CLINICAL FEATURES. Common clinical findings include dyspnea, cyanosis, growth retardation and congestive heart failure. Cyanosis varies con-

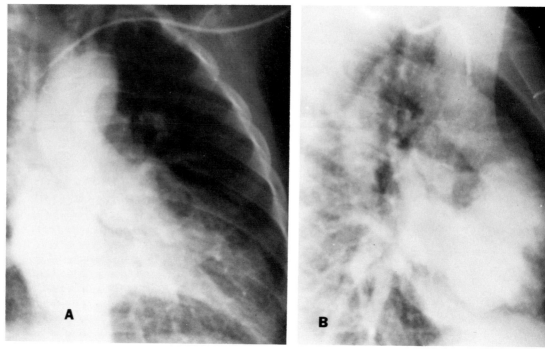

FIG. 273. LEVO PHASE OF AN ANGIOCARDIOGRAM IN A PATIENT FOLLOWING THE MUSTARD OPERATION FOR CORRECTION OF
TRANSPOSITION OF THE GREAT VESSELS

Oxygenated blood returns from the lungs to the new "left" atrium which empties into the right ventricle which then transmits oxygenated blood to the aorta. (From the Angiographic Appearance of the Heart Following the Mustard Procedure by Ghassan Rizk, James H. Moller, and Kurt Amplatz, *Radiology 106:* 269–273, 1973, with permission.)

siderably from patient to patient and depends largely upon the status of the pulmonary arteries. A patient with normal sized pulmonary arteries to each lung and normal pulmonary resistance may be practically acyanotic. On the other hand, a child with diminutive pulmonary arteries or inadequate pulmonary blood flow from whatever reason, including pulmonary vascular obstruction, may exhibit severe cyanosis. On auscultation the second sound over the pulmonic area may be increased in intensity and "pure" in quality. A loud pansystolic murmur is present at the lower left sternal border in most patients (Nadas and Fyler, 1972). Electrocardiographic findings offer little diagnostic assistance. In most patients the electrocardiogram shows left ventricular hypertrophy, alone or in combination with right ventricular hypertrophy. Isolated right ventricular hypertrophy is rare.

The prognosis is poor. The majority of 14 patients reported by Anderson *et al.* (1957) died in early infancy, but three lived to at least seven years of age. About 10% of the patients analyzed by Collett and Edwards lived to the age of 20 years or more. Nine of 20 patients followed by McCue *et al.* (1964) were living at the time of the report, the oldest being 18 years old. The critical period seems to be the first three months of life, and only 15–30% of patients can be expected to survive beyond the first year of life. A few patients have been reported to live past the age of 20, and Silverman and Scheinesson (1966) reported a case of survival to the age of 43 years of a man with persistent truncus arteriosus. The usual cause of death in infants is congestive heart failure from high pulmonary blood flow sometimes complicated by truncal valvular insufficiency and often complicated by pneumonia.

RADIOLOGIC FINDINGS. The heart may be normal in size or enlarged, but a moderate degree of cardiomegaly is the rule. Both ventricles and the left atrium are likely to be enlarged when blood flow to the lungs is increased, and the right ventricle is the most prominent chamber. Since there is no pulmonary trunk, a definite concavity is often seen in the left mid heart border. A shelf-like defect is often seen in the left anterior oblique projection, representing the right ventricle extending anteriorly from the aorta toward the chest wall. The apex of the heart may be elevated, but as the child grows older, the heart elongates, the apex descends and the shelf-like left border tends to disappear. Consequently, the heart becomes longer and more normal in ap-

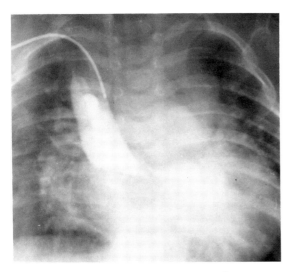

FIG. 274. SEVERE STENOSIS OF THE UPPER LIMB OF THE
TUNNEL

This developed in a patient with surgical correction of
transposition of the great vessels by the Mustard procedure.
The patient displayed a mild superior vena caval syndrome.
(From the Angiographic Appearance of the Heart Following
the Mustard Procedure by Ghassan Rizk, James H. Moller,
and Kurt Amplatz, *Radiology 106:* 269–273, 1973, with permission).

pearance, although enlargement and some concavity of the left heart border persist. Hallermann *et al.* (1969) found the mean cardiothoracic
ratio to be 0.65 (range 0.53–0.72). Victorica and
Elliott (1968) emphasized a tendency for the
upper left heart border to exhibit an obvious
straight line contour that is not ordinarily seen
in common cyanotic conditions with increased
vascularity.

The truncus resembles a large aorta; the ascending portion and arch cast a conspicuous
shadow both to the right of the vertebral column
and in the region of the knob. The aortic indentation on the barium-filled esophagus on the left
and anteriorly is accentuated. The knob of the
aorta may be quite high and very prominent. In
about 25% of cases, the aortic arch may be located on the right.

The appearance of the pulmonary vascular
structure varies with the development of the
pulmonary vascular system. In patients with
Type I, II, or III PTA, the peripheral pulmonary
vasculature is likely to be increased. These pulmonary vessels may pulsate vigorously at fluoroscopy. Diminished pulmonary vascular volume
may be a consequence of either inadequate pulmonary circulation because of the type of malformation present (Type IV PTA) or because of
the development of increased pulmonary vascular resistance (pulmonary hypertension) as a re-

sponse to the chronically increased pulmonary
blood flow. In patients with decreased pulmonary
vascularity, with the blood supply to both lungs
provided by enlarged bronchial, esophageal or
other mediastinal arteries originating from the
aorta, one may see an unusual hilar network of
collateral channels, and indeed close inspection
of the chest film may show very fine irregular
densities distributed throughout the lung parenchyma. A disparity between the vascular patterns in the two lungs may be present when one
lung is supplied by a pulmonary artery while
bronchial arteries supply the other lung.

The combination of right-sided aortic arch and
increased blood flow to the lungs in a cyanotic
infant suggests the diagnosis of persistent truncus arteriosus very strongly.

The pulmonary artery shadow on the left may
appear higher than usual and may simulate the
presence of an unusually prominent pulmonary
trunk. The density is produced by the left pulmonary artery as it courses in a more superior
position than normal following its variable origin
from the truncus.

Dalinka *et al.* (1970) have described a large
retrosternal clear space in patients with persist-

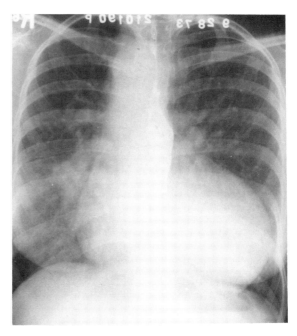

FIG. 275. FRONTAL CHEST FILM AND ESOPHAGRAM IN PER-
SISTENT TRUNCUS ARTERIOSUS

The heart is enlarged and globular, and the blood flow to
the lungs is increased. The arch of the aorta is on the right.
The combination of a right-sided aortic arch and increased
blood flow to the lungs in a patient with congenital heart
disease strongly suggests the diagnosis of persistent truncus
arteriosus (type I, II, or III).

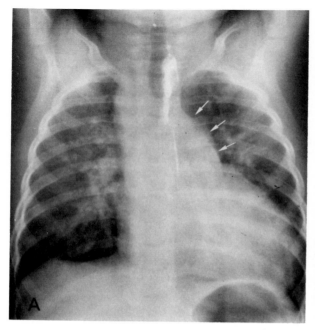
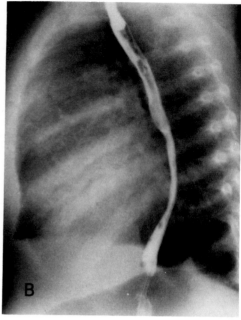

FIG. 276. PLAIN FILM FINDINGS IN PERSISTENT TRUNCUS ARTERIOSUS, TYPE I

(A) Posteroanterior view of the chest shows increased pulmonary vascularity, a right aortic arch, and a convexity along the upper left heart border (arrows) which simulates a large pulmonary trunk. This represents the left pulmonary artery coursing in a higher than normal position. (B) In the lateral view one sees posterior deviation of the barium-filled esophagus indicating the left atrial enlargement. (From the Roentgenologic Findings and Approach to Persistent Truncus Arteriosus in Infancy by Benjamin E. Victorica and Larry P. Elliott, *American Journal of Roentgenology, Radium Therapy and Nuclear Medicine 104:* 440–451, 1968, with permission.)

ent truncus arteriosus which may be seen in the lateral projection and may be due to the absence of the pulmonary outflow tract. In the presence of cyanosis and increased blood flow to the lungs, the diagnosis of truncus arteriosus may be suggested by this sign.

Complete angiographic study of persistent truncus arteriosus requires selective injection of contrast material into the right ventricle as well as a supravalvular injection of contrast agent ("aortography"). Right ventricular injection shows immediate filling of the truncus, with no contrast material in the lung vessels until the truncus is filled. The left ventricle may become opacified through an interventricular septal defect. Depending upon the pulmonary circulatory pathways present, one may see opacification of large pulmonary arteries directly from the truncus or more numerous, small and tortuous bronchial or mediastinal arteries. The persistent truncus itself may be twice the size of an ordinary ascending aorta; it becomes much smaller beyond the origin of the brachiocephalic vessels. In the lateral view the truncus will commonly be seen to override the septal defect and to be located more anteriorly than a normal aorta. The pulmonary trunk or pulmonary artery branches are visualized posterior to the truncus.

Of fundamental importance is the total absence of visualization of a right ventricular infundibulum following injection of contrast material into the right ventricle (Meszaros, 1969; Victorica and Elliott, 1968; Chessler *et al.*, 1970).

Injection of contrast material above the truncal valve permits assessment of several additional features. One can determine that a single common semilunar valve is present, and frequently one can determine the number of valve cusps (2–6, with 3 being the most common). The valve is more anterior and at a higher level than the normal aortic valve. In addition, the competence of the truncal valve can be assessed, and truncal insufficiency is a common finding. When insufficiency is sufficiently pronounced to be obvious angiographically, one will commonly see preferential regurgitation of blood into the right ventricle (Hallermann *et al.*, 1969). The semilunar valve cusps may be thickened, but this is difficult to detect angiographically.

Injection into the supravalvular area will display to best advantage the origin of the pulmonary arteries, either from a single trunk posteriorly and to the left of the truncus (Type I), posteriorly and independently from the truncus but close together (Type II), or independently from the lateral aspect of the truncus (Type III).

In actual practice it may be quite difficult to distinguish between these three types angiographically. In Type IV PTA one will discern no filling of the pulmonary arteries, the lungs being supplied by large systemic collaterals arising from the descending aorta. (Taussig *et al.*, 1973).

The coronary artery pattern can also be determined from supravalvular injection of contrast

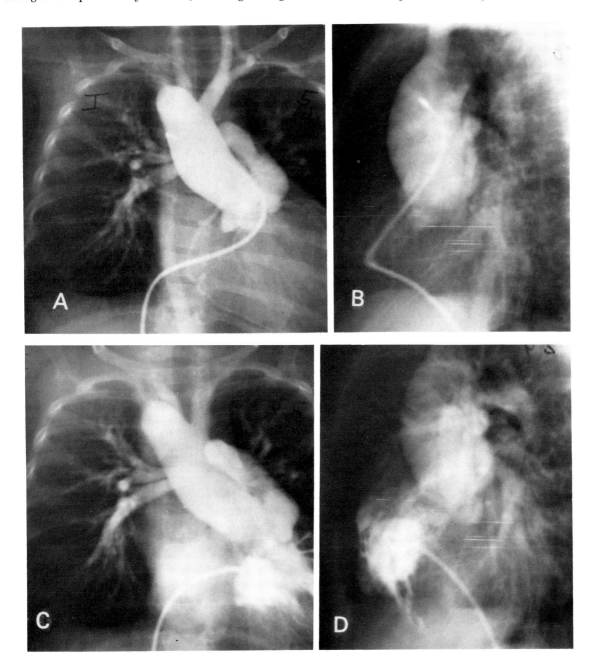

FIG. 277. PERSISTENT TRUNCUS ARTERIOSUS, TYPE I (SAME CASE AS SHOWN IN FIG. 276)

(A) Anteroposterior and (B) lateral views following injection into the truncus arteriosus. The right and left pulmonary arteries arise from the left inferior aspect of the common trunk. The left pulmonary artery forms the so-called pseudopulmonary trunk characteristic of Type I. (C) Anteroposterior and (D) lateral films from a selective right ventriculogram. The inflow portion of the trabeculated right ventricle is well opacified. There is immediate opacification of the truncus arteriosus and the pulmonary artery. Characteristic of persistent truncus arteriosus is absence of opacification of an infundibulum or outflow tract of the right ventricle. (From the Roentgenologic Findings and Approach to Persistent Truncus Arteriosus in Infancy by Benjamin E. Victorica and Larry P. Elliott, *American Journal of Roentgenology, Radium Therapy and Nuclear Medicine 104:* 440–451, 1968, with permission.)

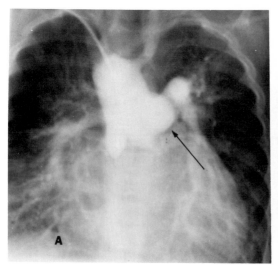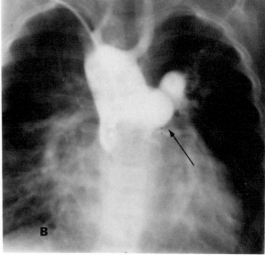

FIG. 278. PERSISTENT TRUNCUS ARTERIOSUS

A and B are serial anteroposterior views following retrograde injection of contrast material into the truncus (Type I). A right aortic arch is present. In A one sees the semilunar cusps bulging into the subvalvular portion of the ventricles. The arrow points to a bulge which represents the undersurface of the pulmonary artery. In B, exposed in ventricular systole, the true ring of the truncal valve can be identified. The bulge to which the arrow points is now recognized as a part of the single main pulmonary artery. (From Persistent Truncus Arteriosus: A Radiographic and Angiographic Study by F. J. Hallermann, O. W. Kincaid, A. G. Tsakiris, D. G. Ritter, and J. L. Tisus, *American Journal of Roentgenology, Radium Therapy and Nuclear Medicine, 197*: 827–834, 1969, with permission.)

material. This may be useful in distinguishing PTA from some form of transposition of the ascending aorta, particularly when the truncus is markedly displaced anteriorly. In PTA, the right coronary artery arises from the right or anterior cusp. In all other conditions characterized by transposition of both the aorta and the pulmonary trunk, the right coronary arises from the posterior cusp. Hence discovery of the arrangement of the coronary arteries tends to verify the angiographic diagnosis.

Other interesting and curious findings may be discovered by selective right ventriculography and by supravalvular injection of contrast material in PTA. Becker *et al.* (1970) have reported three specimens in which the ostium of the left pulmonary artery lay to the right of and above that of the right pulmonary artery. The two pulmonary arteries crossed each other as they proceeded to their respective lungs. Knowledge of this curious finding may aid in the interpretation of angiocardiograms in appropriate cases. It is interesting that in each of their cases of PTA with this pulmonary arterial anomaly, interruption or atresia of the aortic arch occurred. Interruption of the aortic arch is not a common anomaly in patients with persistent truncus arteriosus but has been reported sufficiently often that one should be alert to the possibility (Sundararajan and Molthan, 1972). The arch may be atretic or

interrupted either proximal or distal to the left subclavian artery. In either event, blood flow through the descending aorta and its branches is provided through a patent ductus arteriosus. Atrial septal defects are also common in patients with persistent truncus arteriosus.

Chung *et al.* (1973) have reported the use of echocardiography as a direct and noninvasive method of excluding the diagnosis of truncus arteriosus by demonstrating the pulmonic valve.

Cardiac Catheterization. Pressures in the right ventricle approximate those in the left, and the oxygen content of the right ventricle is increased over that of the right atrium because of the presence of a VSD. Arterial oxygen unsaturation is always present, but saturation is usually more than 80%. The saturation in the systemic artery is usually identical to that in the pulmonary artery. Left atrial or pulmonary capillary pressure may be increased, and systemic arterial pulse pressure is wide. Pulmonary resistance is variable, and pulmonic-systemic flow ratios vary enormously. If the catheter can be manipulated into the truncus, into the pulmonary arteries, and through the septal defect, oxygen saturation, pressures, and indicator dye dilution curves can be expected to be of great value in diagnosis. If not, as is frequently the case, confusion with aortic-pulmonary window, patent ductus arteriosus or ventricular septal defect with pulmonary hypertension may result. Angiography is usually required for a specific diagnosis.

TREATMENT. Supportive medical therapy for the patient in congestive failure is indicated and may be unpredictably effective. Banding of the pulmonary artery or arteries was the only palliative procedure previously available for children with the truncus deformity and increased blood flow to the lungs. The indication for this operation today is palliation of the very ill or moribund infant who would not be a candidate for open heart surgery and in preparation for later corrective surgery. In patients with truncus arteriosus Type IV, a Blalock-Taussig operation to increase

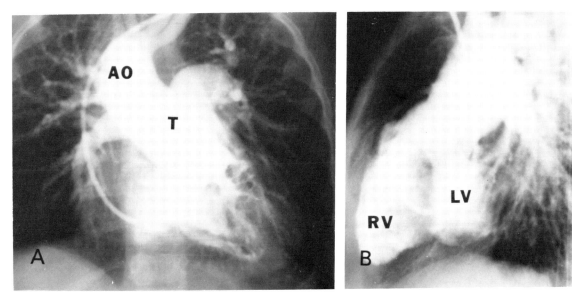

FIG. 279. PERSISTENT TRUNCUS ARTERIOSUS, TYPE I

A and B are frontal and lateral frames from a selective right ventriculogram. Both ventricles are enlarged, a ventricular septal defect is present immediately below the origin of the truncus (T), and no right ventricular infundibulum is seen. The single pulmonary trunk arises from the left lateral aspect of the truncus, and the left pulmonary artery is higher than the right. A right-sided aortic arch is present, and the brachiocephalic arteries are mirror-image to normal. The pulmonary vasculature is increased. (From Persistent Truncus Arteriosus: A Radiographic and Angiocardiographic Study by F. J. Hallermann, O. W. Kincaid, A. G. Tsakiris, D. G. Ritter, and J. L. Tisus, *American Journal of Roentgenology, Radium Therapy and Nuclear Medicine, 107:* 827–834, 1969, with permission.)

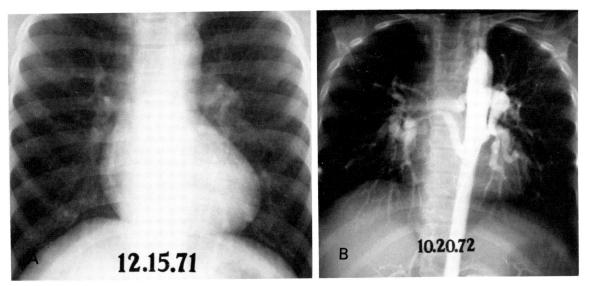

FIG. 280. TRUNCUS, TYPE IV

The greater portion of the blood supply to both lungs originated from two large arteries arising from the descending aorta.

blood flow to the lungs may provide similarly effective palliation (Taussig *et al.*, 1973).

In July of 1968, McGoon, Rastelli, and Ongley reported an operation for the correction of truncus arteriosus (McGoon *et al.*, 1968). They disconnected the pulmonary arteries from the truncus and closed the ventricular septal defect in such a way that the truncus became the true aorta. A new outflow tract from the right ventricle to the pulmonary arteries was established by the use of a homograft of ascending aorta including the aortic valve. This has become the standard operative procedure for correction of PTA, and its performance requires the use of extensive clinical, catheterization and angiocardiographic data to clarify the site of origin of the truncus, the amount of pulmonary flow, the architecture of the truncal valve and vascular tree, the coronary circulation, the size of the ventricular septal defect, and the presence or absence of associated cardiac and extracardiac abnormalities (Bharati *et al.*, 1974). A prosthetic Dacron conduit containing a porcine aortic valve is being used by some investigators because of the nearly invariable calcification of the homograft, the need to replace the homograft in some patients, progressive cardiac failure related to stenosis of the graft, and the tendency of the homograft to bend

at the level of the valve, thus distorting it (Mair *et al.*, 1974). Patients with severe truncal valve incompetence may require valve replacement, but that is associated with a significantly increased surgical mortality. Patients with markedly elevated pulmonary resistances are probably inoperable, and McGoon *et al.* (1968) estimate that about half of the patients surviving infancy are inoperable on the basis of severe pulmonary obstructive disease. Elective operation usually is deferred until a patient is about four years old.

Postoperative angiography will show filling of the pulmonary arteries from the right ventricle through the homograft or prosthetic conduit, with subsequent return of contrast material to the left atrium and ventricle, followed by its expulsion through an enlarged ascending aorta, formerly the truncus (Wallace *et al.*, 1969).

ANOMALOUS ORIGIN OF ONE PULMONARY ARTERY FROM THE ASCENDING AORTA. In this anomaly one pulmonary artery arises normally from the pulmonary trunk whereas the other arises from the ascending aorta. The most common arrangement is one where a systemic artery arises from the ascending aorta and supplies the right lung and a single pulmonary artery originates from the right ventricle and supplies the

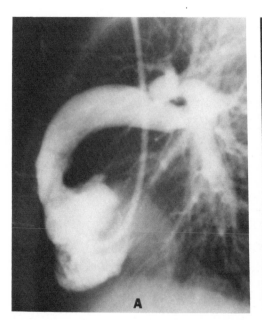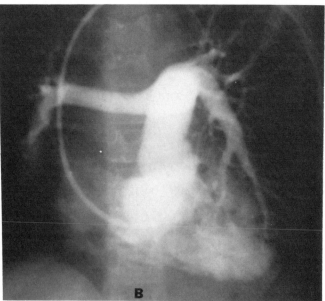

FIG. 281. POSTOPERATIVE RIGHT VENTRICULOGRAM FOLLOWING COMPLETE REPAIR IN A PATIENT WITH TRUNCUS ARTERIOSUS, TYPE IV

A homograft of aortic arch, ascending aorta, aortic valve, a portion of the ventricular septum, and the entire anterior leaflet of the mitral valve has been sutured in place. The distal end of the graft has been anastomosed to the ends of the arteries supplying the lungs, and the proximal end of the graft was anastomosed to the edges of a large window made in the right ventricle. Frontal and lateral views now show continuity between the right ventricle and the pulmonary arteries through the graft. (From Complete Repair of Truncus Arteriosus Defects by Robert B. Wallace, G. C. Rastelli, P. A. Ongley, J. L. Titus, and D. C. McGoon, *Journal of Thoracic and Cardiovascular Surgery* 57: 95–107, 1969, with permission.)

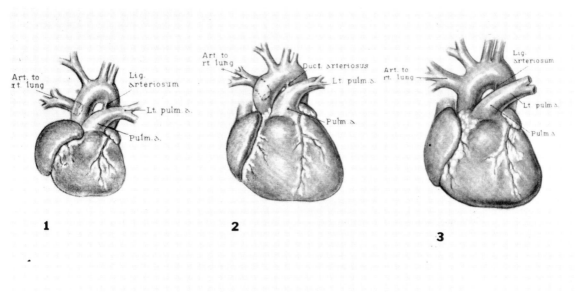

Fig 282.
Variations in the site of origin of the right pulmonary artery from aorta in the 3 cases of hemitruncus reported by Griffiths *et al., Circulation, 25*: 80, used by permission of American Heart Association. In cases 1 and 2 the origin is posterior, and in case 3 it is from the right side of the aorta.

eft lung. When no other anomalies are present, the condition has been called a "hemitruncus" (Taussig, 1960, pages 316–324). Taussig reported on 2 patients, both of whom had enjoyed good health and for whom no treatment was indicated.

Keane *et al.* (1974) in an extensive review found 44 cases (not including those of Taussig) and added 6 of their own. In a number of instances other severe cardiac anomalies were present such as tetralogy of Fallot, 6 cases; PDA, 8 cases; and VSD, 4 cases. All of the reported patients were symptomatic; about one-third of the cases succumbed in infancy or early childhood, and the remainder showed varying degrees of incapacity. The most common manifestation was congestive heart failure appearing in infancy or early childhood.

The initial significant hemodynamic change is due to the marked increase in blood flow to the lung supplied by the systemic artery. The pulmonary resistance is low so that the blood flow is excessive and overloads the left side of the heart, and this is often followed by left ventricular failure. If the patient survives for a period of time, the pulmonary vascular resistance in the "systemic" lung increases, and the flow decreases. Meanwhile, as a rule, the pressure in the right ventricle and the normal pulmonary artery increases. Keane *et al.* (1974) found substantial elevation of pressure in the right ventricle and in the normally arising pulmonary artery. The heart enlarges, and heart failure often ensues. If a ductus is present, there may be some reversal of a left-to-right shunt, and in a few cases there has been mild cyanosis.

Radiologic Findings. The conventional chest film may show a difference in vascular pattern between the two lungs. The vascular pattern in the "systemic" lung does not have the branching pattern of the normal pulmonary artery. Instead, the arterial system is often tortuous and toward the periphery may have a fine reticular pattern. The normal lung may show increased or decreased flow depending on the stage of the disease and the pulmonary resistance. The majority of the reported cases have shown an increased vascularity on the side of the normal pulmonary artery (Keane *et al.*, 1974). Cardiac catheterization shows an increased pressure in the right ventricle. The catheter will enter only one pulmonary artery, and usually the pulmonary arterial pressure is increased.

A lung scan using intravenous macroaggregates of albumin labeled with I^{131} can be quite helpful (Keane *et al.*, 1974). Only the lung with the normally arising pulmonary artery will show uptake of the nuclide, and this could be the first clue to the nature of the anomaly.

Angiography of both the right and left sides of the heart is the definitive procedure. A right ventricular injection will show the normally arising pulmonary artery and the absence of a pulmonary artery to the systemic lung. A left ventricular injection will show the systemic artery originating from the ascending aorta.

The condition is susceptible to surgical treatment (Armer *et al.*, 1961; Weintraub *et al.*, 1966; Keane *et al.*, 1974). The recommended procedure is a transplantation of the "systemic" artery from the aorta to the pulmonary trunk, and this was successful in 12 of the 18 cases reviewed by Keane *et al.* (1974). The associated conditions such as the tetralogy of Fallot, VSD, and PDA, if present should be treated in the appropriate way.

Other reports of this condition are those of DuShane *et al.* (1960), Findlay and Maier (1951), Griffiths *et al.* (1962), and Mudd *et al.* (1964).

Total Anomalous Pulmonary Venous Connection (TAPVC). Total anomalous pulmonary venous connection is an uncommon congenital cardiac defect accounting for about 1.5% of all types of congenital heart disease (Keith *et al.*, 1967). However, according to Cooley *et al.* (1966), total anomalous pulmonary venous drainage ranks fourth in frequency (after complete transposition of the great vessels, tetralogy of Fallot, and tricuspid atresia) among cyanotic congenital cardiac defects requiring operation during the first year of life. This anomaly results in the connection of all of the pulmonary veins to the right atrium or to its tributary veins. Thus, the pulmonary venous return and the entire systemic venous return enter the right side of the heart. In order for the patient to survive, an obligatory right-to-left shunt must also be present, and this ordinarily takes the form of an interatrial septal defect or patent foramen ovale.

TAPVC has been classified by Darling *et al.* (1957) according to the site of emptying of the pulmonary venous blood into the systemic circulation. Four general types are recognized.

I. *Supracardiac Type.* Pulmonary venous blood returns via a common trunk to the superior vena caval system. Usually the common pulmonary vein drains into an anomalous vertical vein (persistent left anterior cardinal vein, also called left superior vena cava) and then into the left innominate vein. Less often, the common pulmonary vein may drain directly into the right superior vena cava.

II. *Cardiac Type.* Pulmonary venous blood drains directly into the body of the right atrium or into the coronary sinus.

III. *Infracardiac Type.* Pulmonary venous

blood passes through a common pulmonary vein into a descending vein which passes through the diaphragm, usually at the esophageal hiatus, to enter the inferior vena cava, the portal vein or the ductus venosus. While associated pulmonary venous obstruction may be present in 15–40% of the patients with supradiaphragmatic TAPVC, it is invariably present in all patients with infradiaphragmatic drainage (Higashino *et al.*, 1974).

IV. *Mixed Type.* Pulmonary venous blood enters the right side of the heart by a combination of the connections previously described.

Jensen and Blount (1971) in a review of the literature analyzed a combined group of 343 patients with TAPVC. In 38% of the total number, venous drainage was via a persistent left anterior cardinal vein. Pulmonary venous blood drained into the coronary sinus in 16%, directly into the right atrium in 14%, into the right superior vena cava or its tributaries in 14%, and to an infradiaphragmatic site in 12%. The location of drainage sites was multiple or unspecified in 7% of cases.

Prognosis for survival in patients with TAPVC is extremely poor. Seventy to eighty percent of patients die within the first year of life (Burroughs and Edwards, 1960), and the chances of survival to childhood are poor if symptoms of congestive failure appear during the first six months or year of life (Cooley *et al.*, 1966). Jensen and Blount (1971) described a man 46 years of age who is reputed to be the oldest reported surviving patient with this lesion, and the present authors have seen one such patient over 40 years of age.

Cardiac enlargement, increased pulmonary vascular volume, cyanosis and fixed splitting of the second heart sound is virtually pathognomonic of TAPVC, but it is much more often present in older patients and is absent in the majority of the neonates and infants with this lesion. In the latter group one is more likely to find dyspnea, frequent respiratory infections, palpitations, irritability, failure to thrive, and feeding difficulties. Feeding difficulties may be more common in patients with infradiaphragmatic anomalous drainage and may be related to compression of the esophagus by the distended vein during feeding (Sukumar *et al.*, 1973). Physical findings include cardiomegaly (except in Type III), signs of congestive failure, a left parasternal heave, and a loud pulmonary component of the second sound. The pulmonary second sound is also often found to be widely split and without respiratory variation. Cyanosis is present in most patients, but because of the mixing of pulmonary and systemic venous blood in the right atrium, pulmonary arterial oxygen saturation may be sufficiently high that visible cyanosis may not be present. The electrocardiogram commonly shows right ventricular enlargement, right axis deviation and, in some, right atrial enlargement.

Cardiac catheterization may provide valuable information in this anomaly. One finds equal or nearly equal oxygen saturations in all four cardiac chambers, and the oxygen saturation in the pulmonary artery equals or exceeds that in the aorta. Right ventricular pressures are often equal to those on the left side but do not usually exceed them. Indicator dye dilution curves show a longer appearance time following pulmonary arterial or right ventricular injection than following right atrial or vena caval injection because of the right-to-left shunt at the atrial level. During catheterization a significant interatrial pressure gradient may be found. That is decidedly uncommon, but when present it indicates a communication that is too small, suggesting that the patient might benefit from balloon or surgical atrial septostomy.

RADIOLOGIC FINDINGS. Film findings depend upon the type of anomaly present, but cardiomegaly and pulmonary vascular engorgement are common to Types I and II. Both the right atrium and pulmonary artery are commonly enlarged. Drainage of all of the pulmonary veins into an anomalous vertical vein which connects with the left innominate vein produces a distinctive shadow in the left upper mediastinum on the conventional chest film, giving the heart a shape likened to the figure "8." The appearance has also been described as the "snowman" sign, and when it is seen in combination with enlargement of the right side of the heart and engorgement of the lungs, TAPVC to a persistent left anterior cardinal vein is quite likely. In patients in whom the anomalous common pulmonary vein drains directly into the superior vena cava or one of its tributaries, distention of the superior vena cava is likely to result in widening of the mediastinum only to the right of the mid line.

In Type II TAPVC, with drainage directly into the right atrium, the radiologic findings will be those of cardiomegaly, increased pulmonary vascular volume, and enlargement of the main pulmonary artery and the right atrium. In addition to these findings, patients with drainage via the coronary sinus may show a characteristic indentation on the barium-filled esophagus where the large coronary sinus passes anterior to it. The curvature of this indentation is smaller than that caused by left atrial enlargement and is best seen in the lateral view (Jensen and Blount, 1971). In addition, an angular out-pouching of the upper border of the right atrial silhouette as seen on the posterioranterior film may be found in patients with TAPVC to the coronary sinus. According to Darling et al. (1957), this out-pouching probably represents direct pressure on the adjacent lateral right atrial wall from the streaming of the pulmonary blood into the right atrium along a somewhat more horizontal plane than usual.

In Type III TAPVC, with pulmonary venous connection below the diaphragm, chest roentgenograms will ordinarily show a normal or only slightly enlarged heart with lung fields exhibiting a diffuse ground-glass haziness and reticulated appearance. The discrepancy between a normal-sized heart and clinical and roentgenographic features of congestive heart failure in a cyanotic newborn infant should suggest the diagnosis. The differential considerations ordinarily entertained in these patients include the respiratory distress syndrome and pneumonia. Also to be considered are cor triatriatum, stenosis of the pulmonary veins, and mitral atresia. The small size of the heart and the finely granular congested appearance of the lungs is due to partial obstruction or resistance to flow in the path of pulmonary venous return, either from an internal stenosis or external compression or from the interposition of an organ such as the liver which the pulmonary venous blood must traverse before reaching the heart (Cooley et al., 1966).

In all types of TAPVC the left atrium, the left ventricle, and the aorta are inconspicuous since they handle only a fraction of the blood which passes through the right side of the circulation.

Angiocardiography is the method of choice for studying patients with total anomalous pulmonary venous drainage. The intravenous study is likely to be thoroughly unsatisfactory because of the obligatory right to left shunt at the atrial level and the therefore simultaneous opacification of all of the cardiac chambers following right atrial filling. Selective right ventriculography or pulmonary arteriography is the method of choice. In Type I, following circulation through the lungs, the contrast material collects in a vertical vein in the left upper mediastinum at the level of the middle third of the heart. Blood and contrast material progress superiorly to a point where the vertical vein enters the left innominate vein. The opacified blood then passes into the superior vena cava and the right atrium. Thereafter the right ventricle and left atrium are simultaneously opacified, as are all of the chambers of the heart. The upper portion of the figure "8" or snowman is thus seen to be formed by a venous arc in the shape of an upside-down letter

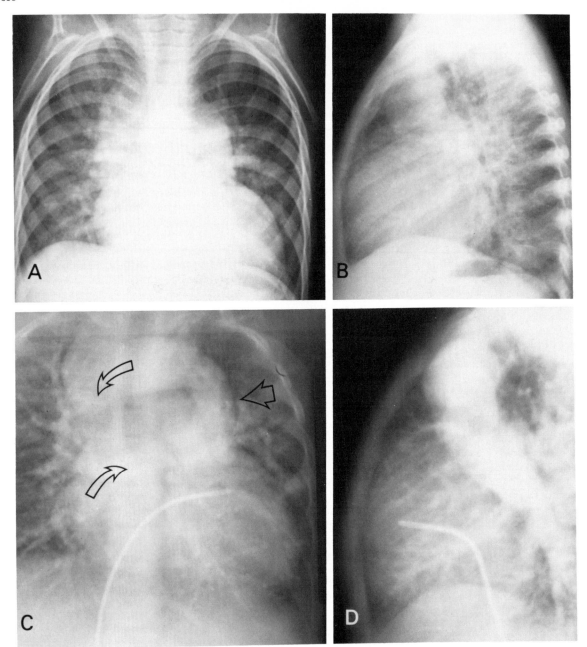

FIG. 283. TOTAL ANOMALOUS PULMONARY VENOUS CONNECTION TYPE I

A and B are frontal and lateral chest films showing cardiac enlargement, pulmonary engorgement and widening of the superior mediastinum to both right and left sides, giving the heart a "snowman" or "figure of 8" configuration. The fullness of the anterior mediastinum is due to dilatation of the left innominate vein.

C and D are frontal and lateral films from a biplane selective right ventriculogram. In C the pulmonary veins are seen draining into a persistent left anterior cardinal vein (lower arrow) which forms the left margin of the widened mediastinal shadow. Blood and contrast material then drain into a dilated left innominate vein and then into a dilated superior vena cava, which forms the abnormal right mediastinal border. (From Leonard E. Swischuk, *Plain Film Interpretation in Congenital Heart Disease,* Philadelphia, Lea & Febiger, 1970, with permission.)

"U" and composed of the persistent left anterior cardinal vein, the left innominate vein and the superior vena cava. In those instances where the common pulmonary vein joins the superior vena cava or its tributaries directly, that connection is easily visualized angiocardiographically provided that both frontal and lateral serial sequences are made.

The appearance of the heart in TAPVC in which the pulmonary veins drain into the coronary sinus is particularly well displayed by selective angiocardiography. The pulmonary veins can be seen to enter the coronary sinus which lies at the level of and just behind the left atrium in the frontal view (Lester *et al.*, 1966). The coronary sinus is often grossly dilated, and it may be mistaken for the left atrium itself. However, the long axis of the coronary sinus is directed in a supero-inferior direction, and the long axis of the left atrium is directed in a horizontal plane, allowing differentiation between the two, though this is admittedly a subtle sign.

In patients with Type III TAPVC, the pulmonary veins converge upon a common venous channel behind the heart and then drain inferiorly through a long connecting vein which traverses the diaphragm usually through the esophageal hiatus. This anomalous vein then enters the portal vein, the ductus venosus, a hepatic vein or rarely other veins. Because of the precarious clinical condition of infants with this type of TAPVC and because of their very young age,

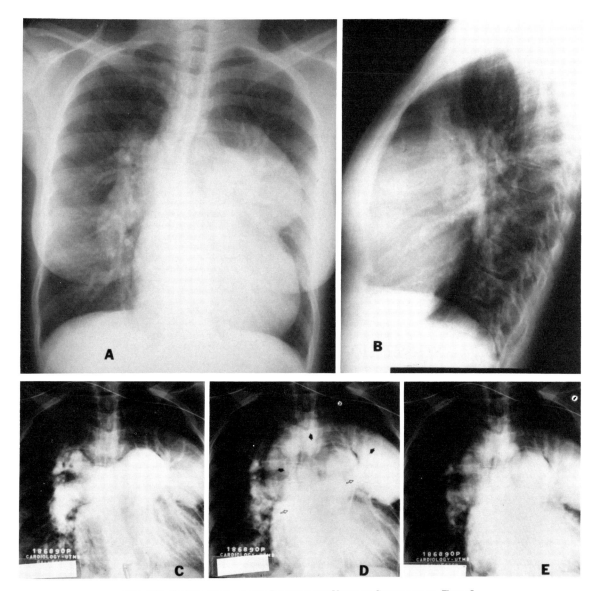

FIG. 284. TOTAL ANOMALOUS PULMONARY VENOUS CONNECTION, TYPE I

The large "mass" in the left upper mediastinum is shown by angiocardiography to represent an enormously dilated vertical vein (persistent left anterior cardinal vein or left superior vena cava) into which drain all of the pulmonary veins. The vertical vein empties into the left innominate vein which returns oxygenated blood to the right atrium via the superior vena cava (C, D, & E).

Lester *et al.* (1966) suggest that the venous approach to angiocardiography may be more appropriate in certain patients.

In all of the types of TAPVC, the left-sided cardiac chambers will be shown to be small. Coussement *et al.* (1973) have demonstrated diminished volume and abnormal shape of the left atrium in all nine of the patients with total

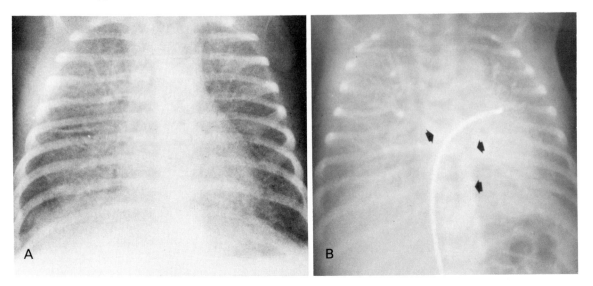

FIG. 285. TOTAL ANOMALOUS PULMONARY VENOUS CONNECTION TYPE III

In contrast to the other types of TAPVC, the heart is not enlarged. The lungs show a finely granular pattern due to pulmonary congestion related to partial obstruction of pulmonary venous return. The venous phase of a selective pulmonary arteriogram shows right and left pulmonary veins (upper arrows) converging to empty into a single retrocardiac vertical vein (lower arrow) which drains into a venous structure below the diaphragm. Partial obstruction of this descending vertical vein is a characteristic feature of this type of TAPVC. (From Leonard E. Swischuk, *Plain Film Interpretation in Congenital Heart Disease,* Philadelphia, Lea & Febiger, 1970, with permission.)

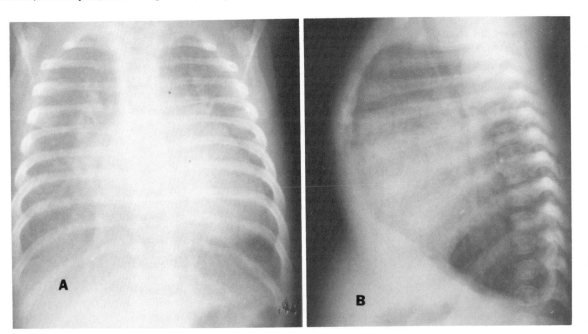

FIG. 286. TOTAL ANOMALOUS PULMONARY VENOUS CONNECTION, TYPE II

Frontal (A) and lateral (B) films show mild cardiomegaly with a nonspecific contour and increased pulmonary vascular volume. The bulging sternum and flattened diaphragm seen on the lateral view are sometimes encountered in patients with poor pulmonary compliance because of greatly increased pulmonary blood flow. In this patient the pulmonary veins drained directly into the right atrium.

anomalous pulmonary venous return which they studied by biplane cine angiocardiography and selective left atrial injection of contrast material.

Obstruction to flow through the anomalous venous pathway should be suspected when one finds delay in emptying of the right side of the heart, persistence of opacified blood in the pulmonary vascular system or failure to reopacify the right atrium. Such obstruction is the rule in infradiaphragmatic total anomalous venous drainage, but it may also be found in the supra-cardiac type.

TREATMENT. While El-Said *et al.* (1971) recommend intensive medical management and balloon atrial septostomy as effective palliative treatment in the first six months of life, to be followed by definitive surgical therapy at a somewhat later time, other authors are strong in their conviction that early surgical intervention is essential (Gersony *et al.*, 1971; Higashino *et al.*, 1974). The principles of surgical repair include the use of the pump oxygenator, the creation of the largest possible anastomosis between the common venous trunk and the left atrium, closure of the atrial septal defect, and ligation of the persistent left anterior cardinal vein, the connection to the right superior vena cava or the connection with the infradiaphragmatic venous system, whichever is present (Cooley *et al.*, 1966). Should a large ventricular septal defect complicate TAPVC in a critically ill patient with pulmonary hypertension and congestive heart fail-ure, a palliative operation, banding of the pulmonary artery, might be considered (Steeg *et al.*, 1973). Gomes *et al.* (1970) believe it appropriate to consider balloon septostomy in symptomatic infants at the time of initial cardiac catheterization if there is any evidence that the interatrial communication is small. Should the patient show a good response, with resolution of congestive heart failure, a totally corrective procedure can be delayed until the age of one year or older when it can be accomplished with lower risks.

Origin of Both Great Vessels from the Right Ventricle (Double Outlet Right Ventricle). In this uncommon cardiac anomaly, both the aorta and the pulmonary artery arise entirely from the right ventricle. A ventricular septal defect is the only means of exit of blood from the left ventricle, and according to the location of this ventricular septal defect, two types are distinguished (Neufeld *et al.*, 1962). Type I consists of those cases in which the ventricular septal defect is located posterior and inferior to the crista supraventricularis, and Type II consists of those cases in which the defect is located anterior and superior to the crista and directly beneath the pulmonary valve (Fig. 288). Type II cases are synonymous with the Taussig-Bing anomaly and are described subsequently. Type I cases will be considered here and may be further subdivided into those with and those without pulmonary stenosis.

TYPE I: WITHOUT PULMONARY STENOSIS. In

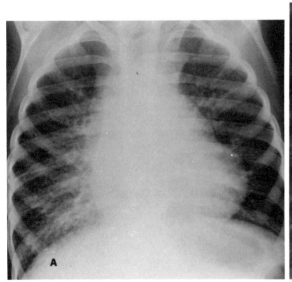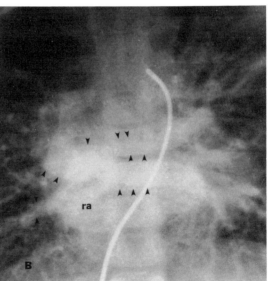

FIG. 287. TOTAL ANOMALOUS PULMONARY VENOUS CONNECTION, TYPE II WITH OBSTRUCTION AND INTERSTITIAL PULMONARY EDEMA IN A 3-YEAR-OLD

(A) Interstitial pulmonary edema is most noticeable in base of right lung. (B) Late film from injection into a common ventricle (same case as Fig. 300). The pulmonary veins (arrowheads) converge to empty into right atrium possibly through separate orifices, although there is a suggestion that at least two of the veins converge to form a single trunk. ra, right atrium. (Courtesy of Children's Cardiac Clinic, Texas Children's Hospital, Houston, Texas.)

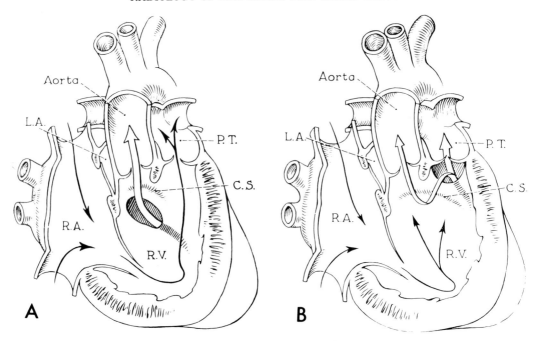

FIG. 288. DOUBLE OUTLET RIGHT VENTRICLE

(A) Origin of both great vessels from the right ventricle without pulmonary stenosis. Blood from the right ventricle exits through both great vessels which are separated by a muscular limb of the crista supraventricularis having a characteristic angiographic appearance. Blood from the left ventricle exits only through a septal defect beneath the crista. Complete mixing of left and right ventricular blood may occur in the right ventricle or left ventricular blood may stream selectively into the aorta, as shown here. (B) Transposition of the aorta with overriding of the pulmonary artery (Taussig-Bing malformation). This defect differs from origin of both great vessels from the right ventricle in that the septal defect lies above the crista supraventricularis and at the base of the pulmonary artery. The pulmonary artery consequently receives a large proportion of its flow from the left ventricle. (From Neufeld *et al.* (1962).)

this malformation the internal relationships of the great vessels are abnormal. The aorta does not originate from the left ventricle caudal, posterior and to the left of the pulmonary artery but instead arises entirely from the right ventricle and extends vertically upward. The aortic root lies to the right of the pulmonary trunk, and the aortic and pulmonary valves are at the same level in both the coronal and transverse planes. A ventricular septal defect is present below the crista supraventricularis, and a portion of the crista commonly forms the superior and anterior margin of the defect. The anterior mitral leaflet and the septal tricuspid leaflet may form the posterior boundary of the defect. The location of the crista supraventricularis is such as to separate the outflow tract of the right ventricle into two channels, one to the aorta and one to the pulmonary trunk. Blood is expelled from the right ventricle simultaneously through both the aorta and the pulmonary artery, and exit from the left ventricle is entirely through the septal defect. Streaming of blood appears to favor ejection of the bulk of the left ventricular output across the septal defect and into the aorta.

The clinical findings in patients with double outlet right ventricle without pulmonary stenosis are similar to those in patients with ventricular septal defect and pulmonary hypertension. Cyanosis is inconstant and ordinarily mild when present. Dyspnea on exertion and congestive heart failure are common findings, and cardiac decompensation was the cause of death in four of six patients reported by Neufeld and associates (1962). A systolic murmur (Grade II–IV) is usually present, with maximal intensity at the third or fourth left intercostal space and is indistinguishable in nature and location from the systolic murmur ordinarily heard in patients with ventricular septal defect. The second pulmonic sound is accentuated. The systemic blood pressure is normal in the absence of associated anomalies such as coarctation of the aorta.

Electrocardiographic findings include prolongation of the PR interval, right ventricular hypertrophy and a counterclockwise loop of the QRS vector in the frontal plane.

Cardiac catheterization shows closely similar systolic pressures in the right and left ventricles. The peripheral arterial oxygen saturation may vary from slightly below normal to normal. If mixing of systemic venous and left ventricular blood in the right ventricle is good, the oxygen saturation in the pulmonary artery may be almost equal to that in the aorta. When oxygen saturation of blood in the pulmonary trunk is lower than that in a systemic artery, one may assume that mixing in the right ventricle is incomplete or that most of the blood in the aorta is derived from the left ventricle by a streaming effect through the ventricular septal defect. A clue to the correct diagnosis of double outlet right ventricle may be obtained at cardiac catheterization by recognizing the unusual positions of the aorta and pulmonary arteries in relationship to each other by inspection of the catheter locations in frontal and lateral views. The great vessels will be noted to lie side by side, the aorta to the right of the pulmonary artery.

Plain films are similar to those seen in patients with VSD and pulmonary hypertension. Right ventricular enlargement is present and is associated with striking prominence of the pulmonary trunk and central pulmonary vasculature suggesting pulmonary arterial hypertension (Neufeld et al., 1961). Right atrial enlargement was present in 80% of the patients studied by Sukumar et al. (1972).

Selective right ventriculography shows distinctive and perhaps diagnostic findings (Carey and Edwards, 1965). Frontal and lateral serial views are essential and disclose the following findings: both great vessels fill from the right ventricle, and opacification of the pulmonary artery and aorta may be equal in intensity, though the pulmonary trunk may occasionally appear to be more opaque than the aorta. The pulmonary and aortic valves will be located at the same level in the frontal plane, the aorta being located just to the right of the pulmonary artery. A characteristic finding in the frontal view is a tongue-like filling defect at the base of the right ventricle which represents the parietal limb of the crista supraventricularis separating the outflow tract of the right ventricle into two channels, one to the aorta and one to the pulmonary artery. Lateral films disclose transposition of the aorta, and the pulmonary and aortic valves will be seen to be located at about the same level in the coronal and transverse planes. The flow across the septal defect is almost entirely from left to right in double outlet right ventricle, but the forceful injection of contrast material into the right ventricle often produces some opacification of the left ventricle, and the mitral valve can often be outlined. It is in its normal position, on the posterior aspect of the left ventricle, and it is

separated from the aortic valve by a segment of the ventricular wall. This abnormal mitral-aortic relationship is characteristic of double outlet right ventricle, and both valves should be seen on the angiocardiogram if the diagnosis is to be established with certainty (Baron, 1971; Sukumar et al., 1972). Separation of the aortic and mitral valves does not occur in other cardiac anomalies unless there is transposition of the great vessels. Selective left ventriculography in the left anterior oblique or lateral position may show an opacified stream of contrast material traversing the ventricular septal defect to the aortic root arising from the right ventricle (Steinberg and Engle, 1965). Retrograde aortography will show the anterior location of the ascending aorta, the higher than normal position of the aortic valve and its nearly horizontal plane.

WITH PULMONARY STENOSIS. In this anomaly, infundibular pulmonary stenosis is created by a vertical limb of the crista supraventricularis (Neufeld et al., 1961).

The hemodynamic, clinical, and electrocardiographic data resemble those in the tetralogy of Fallot. Patients are cyanotic from early life, and clubbing of the fingers may be present. Congestive heart failure is not a common feature. The electrocardiogram shows right ventricular hypertrophy of the type seen in the tetralogy of Fallot.

Peripheral arterial oxygen desaturation and right ventricular hypertension are expected findings at cardiac catheterization. A pressure gradient across the pulmonary valve may be shown. Indicator dilution dye curves show a large right-to-left shunt with little flow from the right ventricle directly into the pulmonary artery. Thus, the hemodynamic state is similar to that present in severe tetralogy of Fallot with cyanosis.

Plain films show only slight to moderate cardiac enlargement, and the heart may be normal in size and shape. Diminished pulmonary vascular volume is usual, commonly accompanied by a concave area along the heart border in the position ordinarily occupied by the pulmonary artery.

The appearance of the heart following selective right ventriculography in frontal and lateral planes may mimic that of tetralogy of Fallot. In a severe tetralogy, the aorta may appear to arise almost entirely from the right ventricle. Thus, the position of the aortic valve in relation to the ventricular septum as seen in the lateral view cannot be used to distinguish a double outlet right ventricle from a tetralogy of Fallot (Baron, 1971). However, no matter how far anteriorly the aortic valve is situated, in the tetralogy of Fallot it remains in fibrous continuity with the mitral

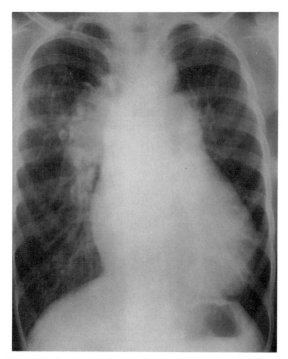

FIG. 289. ORIGIN OF BOTH GREAT VESSELS FROM RIGHT
VENTRICLE WITH HIGH VENTRICULAR SEPTAL DEFECT AND
PULMONIC STENOSIS
A Potts operation was performed 8 years before.

valve. In double outlet right ventricle, the mitral valve is separated from both the aortic and pulmonary valves regardless of the relative positions of the two great vessels. The infundibular or valvular or combined stenosis in double outlet right ventricle does not differ in angiographic appearance from that seen in other conditions.

Patients with double outlet right ventricle and pulmonary stenosis requiring surgical intervention before the age of four years may receive a systemic-to-pulmonary artery shunt with complete intracardiac repair being delayed until the patient is somewhat older. The pulmonic stenosis is relieved by the same technique as in the repair of tetralogy of Fallot. A patch of prosthetic material or pericardium is used to construct a left ventricular conduit or tunnel in such a way as to connect the left ventricle via the ventricular septal defect with the aortic orifice (Gomes *et al.,* 1971).

TYPE II: THE TAUSSIG-BING ANOMALY. The clinical features and hemodynamic pattern of the circulation in this condition were described in 1949 by Taussig and Bing following a detailed study of an autopsy case. Since then, additional cases have been seen, and the condition stands as a well-defined entity. It is considered by Neufeld and associates (1962) to be a variety of origin

of both great vessels from the right ventricle in which the ventricular septal defect lies above the crista supraventricularis. Van Praagh (1968) reexamined the case reported by Taussig and Bing and also concluded that this malformation should be viewed as one form of true double outlet right ventricle.

The characteristic features of this malformation are the following: origin of the aorta and pulmonary artery entirely from the right ventricle, semilunar valves side by side and approximately at the same height, and a large subpulmonary ventricular septal defect located anterior and superior to the crista supraventricularis. The pulmonary artery is usually dilated, and the smaller branches in the lung may show intimal changes with narrowing.

Blood enters the right atrium in the usual way from the superior and inferior vena cavae and passes without obstruction into the right ventricle. The right ventricular pressure is elevated, and right ventricular blood may leave the heart through either the aorta or the pulmonary artery. In the patient studied by Taussig and Bing the aortic flow was 3920 ml/m^2/min, of which 3210 ml came from the right ventricle. The remainder of the aortic flow (710 ml/m^2/min) represented oxygenated blood which entered the aorta from the left ventricle. These figures indicate that although the ventricular septal defect is just beneath the orifice of the pulmonary artery, it permits a considerable shunt of blood from the

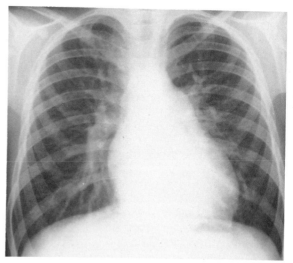

FIG. 290. DOUBLET OUTLET RIGHT VENTRICLE, TYPE II
(THE TAUSSIG-BING ANOMALY)
Mild cardiac enlargement, dilatation of the pulmonary trunk and pulmonary engorgement are the typical features. The bulk of left ventricular output is distributed to the lungs through a ventricular septal defect located above the crista supraventricularis and just below the pulmonary valve.

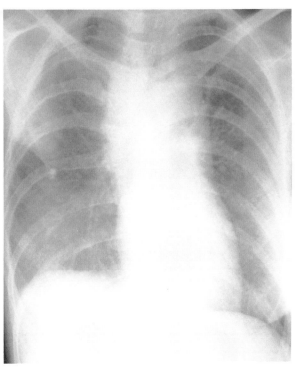

Fig. 291. Origin of Both Great Vessels from the Right Ventricle, with Pulmonary Stenosis

The heart is normal in size and shape, but the mediastinum is widened to the left. That is partly the consequence of the patient's scoliosis, but at angiography a transposed ascending aorta arising anteriorly from the right ventricle was found in this location along with a persistent left superior vena cava. The pulmonary artery also arose from the right ventricle and showed infundibular stenosis, accounting for the appearance of decreased pulmonary vascularity. The curious network of vessels in the lungs is the appearance cast by greatly enlarged bronchial arteries. A Blalock-Taussig systemic-to-pulmonary artery anastomosis had been performed on the right years earlier, accounting for the unilateral right-sided rib notching. The shunt was found to be thrombosed.

left ventricle into the aorta. Unless a patent ductus arteriosus or interatrial septal defect is present, this shunt is the sole route by which oxygenated blood reaches the aorta. The remainder of right ventricular blood which leaves through the pulmonary artery is equal in volume to that which enters the aorta from the left ventricle, namely 710 ml/m²/min in Taussig and Bing's case. This represents effective pulmonary flow and is quite small (normal is about 3,000 ml/m²/min); the remainder of the pulmonary artery flow (total 2300 ml/m²/min) comes from the left ventricle and represents re-circulation of oxygenated blood through the lungs (1590 ml/m²/min in Taussig and Bing's case). The pressure in the pulmonary artery is elevated, and the changes which have been described in the smaller pulmonary arteries are compatible with increased peripheral pulmonary resistance. Although there is doubtless considerable variation from case to case in the size of the ventricular septal defect and its relationship to both pulmonary artery and the aorta, this would cause only a variation in the volume of the shunts rather than a basic change in their direction.

Because of these alterations in their circulation, the patients are permanently and usually progressively cyanotic from birth or very early life and thus are different from those with the Eisenmenger complex in which cyanosis is commonly delayed for many years. Clubbing of the fingers and polycythemia are common and stunting of growth and failure to gain weight may be present. Right ventricular hypertrophy is usually found by electrocardiography.

The heart is normal in size or slightly enlarged. In the posteroanterior projection one sees a distinct convexity of the pulmonary artery segment due to the usually large pulmonary artery. This bulge helps to differentiate this condition from complete transposition of the great vessels in which the pulmonary artery is behind the aorta and the base of the heart is narrow in the posteroanterior projection. The pulmonary vascular markings are normal or moderately increased in prominence, and both the pulmonary trunk and its hilar branches show increased pulsations. One may see evidence of right ventricular enlargement on the oblique views of the chest, but that is usually not striking.

Selective right ventriculography offers the best opportunity to display the arrangement of the origins of the great vessels, and the right ventricle and aorta will be seen to fill immediately with a high concentration of contrast substance. The aorta originates relatively far anteriorly in relation to the heart contour and entirely from the right ventricle. The pulmonary artery is usually definitely but poorly opacified, and although the angiocardiographic pattern is similar to that of complete transposition of the great vessels, demonstration of the presence of both a subaortic and subpulmonary conus in the right ventricle will allow the distinction to be made. Because of the presence of a bilateral conus, discontinuity is present between the mitral valve and both the aortic and pulmonary valves. This is ordinarily best displayed following selective injection of contrast material into the left ventricle. Visualization of the pulmonary artery along the left upper heart border alongside the aorta also helps allow differentiation of this condition from complete transposition of the great vessels. Beuren (1960) has pointed out that physiologically the

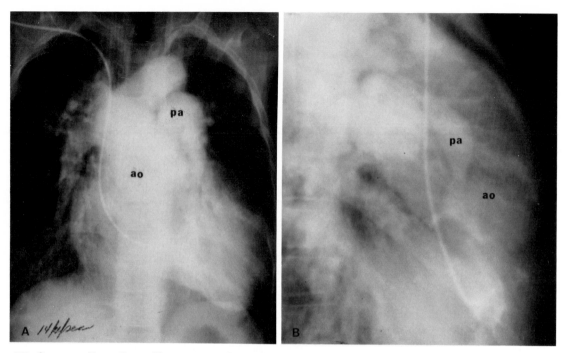

FIG. 292. ORIGIN OF BOTH GREAT VESSELS FROM RIGHT VENTRICLE AND PULMONIC STENOSIS AND VENTRICULAR SEPTAL
DEFECT ABOVE CRISTA (TYPE II DEFECT OF NEUFELD *et al.* (1962))

A Potts-type procedure had been carried out 6 years before. (A) Selective injection into the right ventricle. The proximal
portion of the pulmonary artery was small (see B—lateral view).

Taussig-Bing malformation is not so fundamentally different from the other types of transpositions as it is anatomically.

Cardiac catheterization is usually quite helpful. There is an increase in oxygen content of the blood in going from the right atrium to the right ventricle and a further increase in going from the right ventricle to the pulmonary artery. The oxygen content of pulmonary artery blood is typically higher than that of the femoral artery. Pressures in the right ventricle are elevated. It may be entirely possible to catheterize both the aorta and pulmonary artery from the right ventricle.

Associated anomalies of the aorta are common. Chiechi (1957) reviewing 10 cases verified by autopsy, found aortic coarctation in three and hypoplasia of the aorta distal to the left subclavian artery in two. Interatrial septal defect has also been reported.

Differential diagnostic considerations include complete transposition of the great vessels with ventricular septal defect, single ventricle with or without transposition, truncus arteriosus, and the Eisenmenger complex.

Operative correction consists of repair of the ventricular septal defect so that left ventricular blood is ejected into the pulmonary artery via a prosthetic tunnel. Thereafter venous return is transposed within the atria by means of a pericardial baffle (Mustard technique) (Hightower *et al.*, 1969). Alternatively, a transventricular tunnel may be constructed to transmit blood from the left ventricle through the ventricular septal defect directly to the aorta, without obstructing the right ventricular outflow tract (Agarwala *et al.*, 1973).

Common Ventricle. The terms "single ventricle" and "common ventricle" may be used interchangeably, but this can lead to further confusion in a discussion of an already complicated group of entities. A number of authors (Elliott *et al.*, 1964, 1966; Kozuka *et al.*, 1973; Hallermann *et al.*, 1966) have used the term common ventricle in reference to a condition in which a single ventricle receives blood directly from each atrium through mitral and tricuspid valves or in some cases a common atrioventricular valve. Specifically, this excludes tricuspid and mitral atresia in which a functioning single ventricle communicates with only one of the atria. These latter two conditions are considered in separate sections (page 326). Common ventricle is rare anomaly and accounts for about 3% of congenital heart disease.

Van Praagh *et al.* (1964) have classified cases of common ventricle into four types depending on anatomical details obtained from autopsy specimens. Radiological studies including detailed large film angiograms provide a positive or potential identification of the much more common Type A of Van Praagh. The other three types combined comprise about 20% of all cases, are a more heterogenous group, and offer some difficulty in classification by radiological means. They are considered as Group III, which comprises the other three groups of Van Praagh. In this section we will deal in some detail only with the more frequent forms which are generally the Type A of Van Praagh (1964) and Hallermann *et al.*, (1966) and the similar examples described by Elliott *et al.* (1963, 1964, 1968) as common ventricle with and without transposition of the great vessels. The rarer variations will be only briefly mentioned. These are really the same condition as described by Taussig (1960, page 325), as single ventricle with rudimentary outflow chamber.

Van Praagh *et al.* (1964) believe that in the majority of cases of common ventricle the body or sinus of the right ventricle fails to develop leaving only the infundibulum or that portion distal to the crista supraventricularis. The primitive parietal and septal bands of the crista form a definite septum, and Hallermann *et al.* (1966) consider this as the remnant of the interventricular septum which has been displaced upwards to the left or to the right as the case may be.

These cases may be further divided into those with an l-loop (inverted) or d-loop (noninverted) arrangement. With an l-loop the infundibulum is to the left of the midline and anterior, and with the d-loop the infundibulum is to the right of the midline and also somewhat anterior. Thus, we have two groups of common ventricle, those with a d-loop and those with an l-loop. In a reported series of cases, the l-loop or inverted infundibulum has been somewhat more common (Marin-Garcia *et al.*, 1974; Van Praagh *et al.*, 1964, 1965; Hallermann *et al.*, 1966).

A third aberration frequently associated with common ventricle is transposition of the great vessels. When the vessels are transposed the aorta is usually anterior and originates from the infundibular chamber, and the pulmonary artery is posterior and originates from the common ventricle. This does not necessarily imply that the aorta is directly in front of the pulmonary artery in all cases. In fact, this is unusual and the aorta in most instances is rotated anywhere from 30–60° either to the right or the left in the horizontal plane. Cases with transposition have outnumbered those with normally related great arteries by a wide margin (only 19 reported cases of normally related vessels by Marin-Garcia *et al.*, 1974).

Another important variation is the presence and degree of stenosis of the outflow tract of the

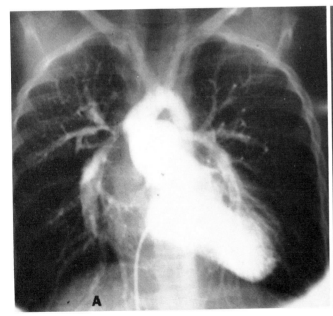
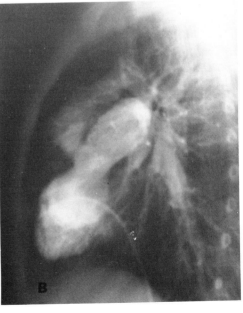

FIG. 293. DOUBLE OUTLET RIGHT VENTRICLE WITH COARCTATION OF THE PULMONARY ARTERY BRANCHES
Selective right ventriculogram in the frontal projection shows simultaneous filling of the aorta and pulmonary artery (A). The right and left pulmonary artery branches are markedly narrowed, and some secondary branches show post-stenotic dilatation. On the lateral view the aorta and pulmonary artery arise independently and entirely from the right ventricle, each from a separate conus (B). The aorta is anterior to the pulmonary artery.

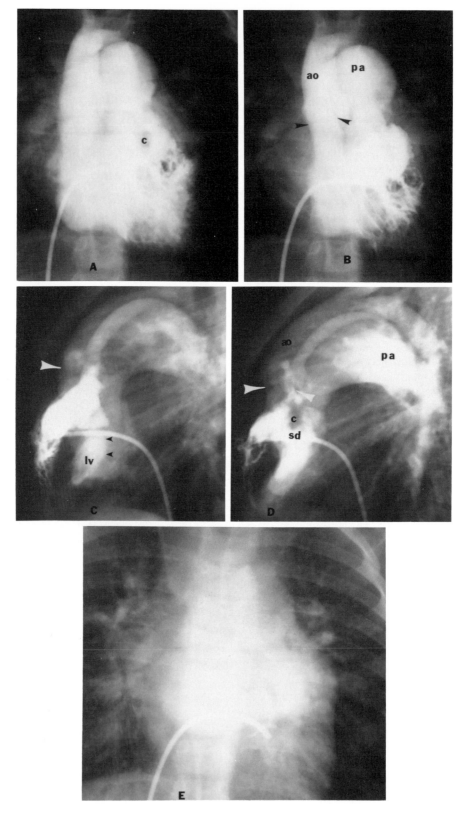

FIG. 294

aorta and pulmonary artery. Pulmonary stenosis is considerably more common than aortic stenosis even though the aorta originates from the infundibular chamber in a majority of cases. The stenosis may be subvalvular, valvular, or a combination. Pulmonary atresia is a rare variation. The presence and degree of pulmonary stenosis affect considerably the radiologic appearance and the clinical course of the patient.

Other rare variations are (1) origin of both great vessels from the infundibular chamber, (2) absence of a septum and infundibular chamber with both vessels originating from the single ventricle, and (3) cor biloculare in which there is both a common atrium and a common ventricle usually associated with asplenia. Additional malformations occur with some frequency (Hallermann et al., 1966; Elliott and Morgan, 1968) such as partial and total anomalous pulmonary venous return, patent ductus arteriosus, and interruption of the aortic arch.

The clinical course and life expectancy are quite variable depending for the most part on the adequacy of the pulmonary blood flow. With pulmonary obstruction cyanosis may appear in early life depending on the severity of the stenosis. In those without obstruction cyanosis is usually minimal until the peripheral pulmonary resistance increases to a crucial level. On the other hand, in those cases without pulmonary stenosis congestive heart failure may appear during infancy, and cardiac enlargement may appear early in life. Common ventricle can mimic many other types of congenital heart disease, and the list of differential possibilities is more extensive than that for any other congenital abnormality (Elliott and Morgan, 1968).

The electrocardiogram may be helpful in suggesting the diagnosis, and the radiologist should remember that this is one of the types of congenital cyanotic heart disease in addition to tricuspid atresia that can occasionally give a left axis deviation.

RADIOLOGIC FINDINGS. *Conventional Chest Films.* Similar to the clinical findings, the chest films are variable depending on the anatomic type of common ventricle as described above. Transposition of the great vessels with an l-loop or inversion of the infundibulum is the most common type. In the frontal view, the ascending aorta usually forms the left upper border of the cardiovascular contour similar to that seen in corrected transposition. This border is smooth and usually slightly convex but occasionally is concave. The normal aortic knob is replaced by a smooth straight shadow, and the descending aorta cannot be identified. The superior mediastinum at times is narrow. The right upper cardiovascular contour is usually flat because of the absence of the ascending aorta on the right side of the mediastinum. The normal pulmonary artery convexity is not present, and the pulmonary artery usually cannot be identified. A convexity in the left midcardiovascular contour is often present and of variable size due to the infundibular chamber. This convexity is usually slightly below that of the normally placed pulmonary artery. Hallermann et al. (1966) describe a shallow notch due to a protrusion of the lateral wall of the infundibular chamber. As shown by angiography, the infundibular chamber is variable in size and contour, and the corresponding left cardiovascular contour is variable in length and convexity. The identification of this bulge or notch in the left mid cardiac contour is quite helpful in suspecting the diagnosis.

The pulmonary vasculature in the majority of cases is increased. The proximal or hilar branches of the pulmonary artery are dilated. Elliott et al. (1964) call attention to the high transverse contour of the right pulmonary artery and its draped appearance resembling a "waterfall." The pulmonary trunk is near the midline of the cardiovascular contour. It is often large and can be dilated even though there is some degree of pulmonic stenosis (poststenotic dilatation with valvular stenosis). The pulmonary trunk is difficult to identify but may cause an indentation on the lateral aspect of the barium-filled esophagus near the carina. In cases with severe pulmonary stenosis or atresia, the pulmonary vasculature is diminished, and a reticular pattern due to collateral bronchial vessels may be present. Rarely in older patients the pulmonary arteries are truncated towards the periphery suggesting an increased peripheral pulmonary resistance.

In the lateral view, the superior mediastinum

FIG. 294. DOUBLE OUTLET RIGHT VENTRICLE WITH VSD BELOW CRISTA

A and C, beginning systole; B and D, end systole. Right ventricular injection. The aorta and pulmonary artery are almost side by side (the aorta is slightly anterior). The aortic valve is faintly seen (black arrowheads in frontal view and white arrow heads in lateral view). Small arrowheads in C indicate mitral valve, and there is discontinuity between the valve and the aorta which is characteristic of double outlet right ventricle. c, crista supraventricularis; lv, left ventricle; sd, septal defect. (E) A late film shows stagnation of contrast substance in left atrium suggesting mild mitral stenosis. The pulmonary wedge pressure was elevated. (Courtesy of Dr. Jack Henry, Spawn Hospital, Corpus Christi, Texas.)

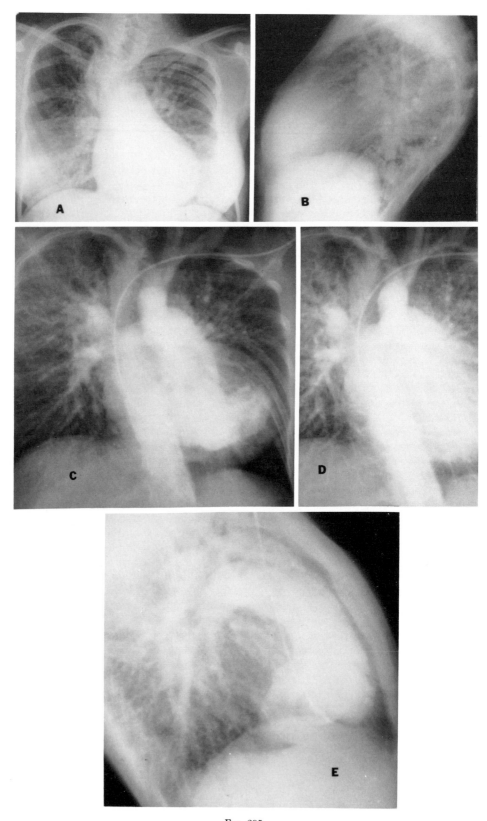

Fig. 295

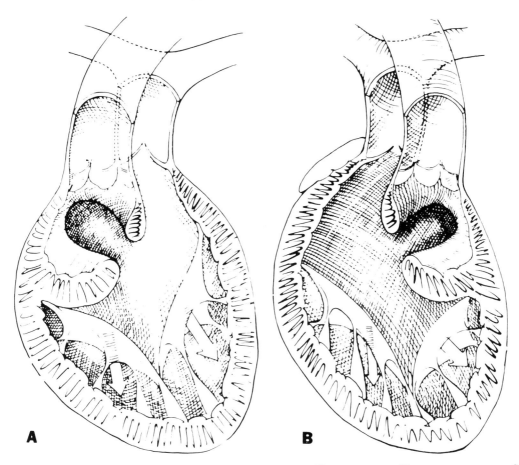

FIG. 296. DIAGRAMS OF THE MORE COMMON VARIATIONS OF COMMON VENTRICLE WITH TRANSPOSITION OF THE GREAT VESSELS

(A) Aorta arising anteriorly from noninverted (d-loop) infundibulum of right ventricle. (B) Aorta arising anteriorly from inverted (l-loop) infundibulum. This is the most common variation (see text). (Reproduced by courtesy of Drs. Elliott, Ruttenberg, Eliot, and Anderson, and *British Heart Journal 26:* 304, 1964.)

and retrosternal space are more opaque than normal due to the anterior position of the transposed ascending aorta. The left atrium is occasionally enlarged associated with an increased pulmonary flow.

The plain film findings, particularly those in which a suspicion of an infundibular chamber exists along with prominence of the ascending aorta along the left side of the mediastinum, are highly suggestive of transposition with a left-sided infundibular chamber.

In the less common variation with the d-loop (noninverted infundibulum), the cardiovascular contour is much less specific. The ascending aorta is in its usual position. The heart is frequently globular in contour, and the aortic arch and knob are in their usual position. The convexity due to the pulmonary artery is often absent since the pulmonary artery usually has a medial position. Occasionally it may be sufficiently dilated to be borderforming.

In the quite rare variation in which the great vessels are not transposed, the cardiovascular contour is nonspecific, although Elliott *et al.* (1963) found elevation of the apex, diminished pulmonary vascularity and prominence of the right ventricle as seen in the lateral view. Several cases with pulmonic stenosis have had contours

FIG. 295. DOUBLE OUTLET RIGHT VENTRICLE, TYPE I

The mediastinum is deformed because of the patient's scoliosis. The convexity in the left upper mediastinum is produced by the superimposed shadows of the aortic arch and the pulmonary trunk. Selective right ventriculogram in the frontal plane (C and D) shows simultaneous opacification of the aorta and the pulmonary artery. The lateral view (E) shows both great vessels arising entirely from the right ventricle and partly superimposed.

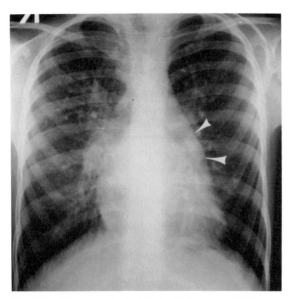

FIG. 297. COMMON VENTRICLE WITH TRANSPOSITION OF GREAT VESSELS AND INVERTED INFUNDIBULUM. THE SLIGHT CONVEXITY OF THE LEFT HEART BORDER IS DUE TO THE INFUNDIBULUM (ARROWS).

suggestive of the tetralogy of Fallot (Elliott *et al.,* 1964; Edie *et al.,* 1973). A right aortic arch was encountered in 10% of the total (including those with and without transposition) cases reported by Hallermann *et al.* (1966).

Cardiac Catheterization. The findings may vary according to the anatomic types mentioned above. A constant finding, however, is a step-up in oxygen concentration in samples obtained from the right atrium and what may be thought to be a right ventricle but which is in reality the common ventricle. Samples obtained from different sites in the common ventricle may show different oxygen concentrations due to streamlining effects. The aorta is usually anterior and may be easier to enter than the more posteriorly placed pulmonary artery. Again, oxygen concentrations in either of the great vessels may differ from that obtained in the common ventricle due to streamlining effects. A subaortic stenosis may be encountered less commonly at the entrance to the infundibular chamber or more commonly at the exit from the rudimentary chamber. If the usually posteriorly placed pulmonary artery is entered, a stenosis may be encountered either below or at the valve or both. Small injections of contrast substance under fluoroscopic observation may help to identify the two great vessels and thus lead one to suspect strongly the presence of a common ventricle and transposition. Selective angiography is necessary to establish a satisfactory diagnosis.

Angiocardiographic Findings. Venous or forward angiocardiography is usually unsatisfactory, although it can be helpful in excluding the presence of tricuspid atresia, and it can outline the main features of a typical case (Fig. 298). However, detailed information concerning the presence and location of the A-V valves, the position and precise site of origin of the great vessels, and the internal structure of the common ventricle require a selective left ventricular injection. Although cine recordings may suffice, biplane large film angiograms in the frontal and lateral projections provide more detailed information.

In the frontal view, the common ventricle most often has a triangular shape with a rounded apex. The internal trabecular structure in diastole is usually finely serrated and scarcely perceptible. In the lateral view, the ventricle occupies the greater part of the cardiac contour.

The infundibular chamber is usually well seen in the frontal view. It is quite variable in size and contour. It is often flattened and somewhat triangular in shape. In one case cited by Hallerman *et al.* (1966) it reached almost to the apex of the heart. Its interior may be irregular indicating a coarse trabecular musculature. The ventricular defect leading to the chamber is infrequently smaller than the vessel that arises therefrom, and usually this is the aorta. It is rarely the site of an obstruction. Obstruction to the pulmonary artery or the aorta may be valvular, subvalvular or a combination. The location of the great vessels and the relationship of their origin to the A-V valves are best determined from the lateral view. The valve associated with the infundibular chamber is usually higher than that of the vessel that originates from the common ventricle. Occasionally the valves are at the same level, and the great vessels may be more nearly in a side to side relationship. This may be seen in the rare type in which both vessels originate from a remnant of the right ventricle. The larger of the great vessels usually carries a greater flow, but the pulmonary artery may be dilated distal to a valvular stenosis.

Clues to the presence of other anomalies, such as patent ductus arteriosus, interruption of the aortic arch and anomalous pulmonary venous return, should be sought for.

Recent reports (Ionescu *et al.,* 1973; Edie *et al.,* 1973) indicate that surgical repair of certain types of common ventricle can be successful. Separate A-V valves should be present. The relationship of the great vessels and the presence and degree of stenosis should also be determined preoperatively. A second injection into the left

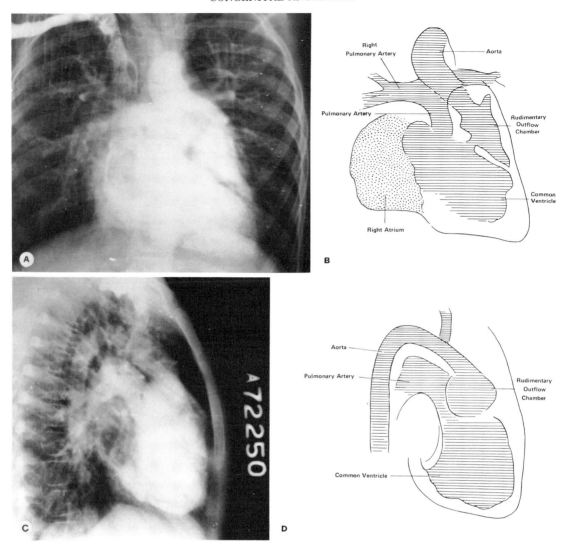

FIG. 298. ANGIOCARDIOGRAMS OF CASE SHOWN IN FIG. 297

(A) Anteroposterior projection at 3 sec. (B) Sketch of A. (C) Lateral view exposed simultaneously with A at 3 sec. (D) Sketch of C. The pulmonary trunk originated from the right ventricle, and the aorta originated from the inverted anterior infundibulum. No evidence of aortic or pulmonary obstruction, but selective angiography and hemodynamic studies are necessary to rule this out.

atrium may be of some value in determining the presence of an interatrial defect and also something concerning the anatomy of the A-V valves.

The list of conditions to be considered in the differential diagnosis of common ventricle is lengthy and depends on the type and severity of the associated abnormalities. Only a few of the entities associated with each type will be listed. Common ventricle with transposition and l-loop must be differentiated from corrected transposition with large septal defect. A d-loop and transposition should be differentiated from complete transposition of the great vessels. With d-loop transposition and pulmonic stenosis, the tetral-

ogy of Fallot is often considered. In the older cases with increased peripheral pulmonary resistance, differentiation from the Eisenmenger complex is necessary.

Pulmonary Valvular Atresia with Intact Ventricular Septum. This is an uncommon anomaly, and its incidence is estimated to be between 3 and 8% (Toledo *et al.,* 1971) of those cardiac anomalies that cause severe distress in the newborn. It is one of the most common causes of an enlarging or a large heart with avascular lungs and cyanosis occurring in the first few days of life. It has a poor prognosis, although prompt diagnosis and surgical treatment have shown promising results (Ellis *et al.,* 1972; Dhanavaravibul *et al.,* 1970).

Greenwold *et al.* (1956) classified this anomaly into two types: (1) those with a small right ven-

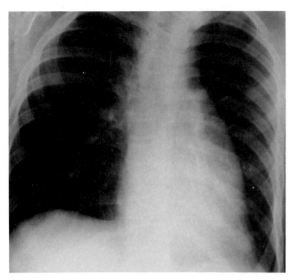

FIG. 299. COMMON VENTRICLE IN AN 18-YEAR-OLD WITH INVERTED INFUNDIBULUM AND TRANSPOSITION WITH SUBPULMONIC STENOSIS

Note convexity of left upper heart border due to infundibular chamber and avascular lung fields. The cardiac contour is not specific, and selective angiography is required for diagnosis. (Courtesy of Children's Cardiac Clinic, Texas Children's Hospital, Houston, Texas.)

tricle, and (2) those with a normal-sized or large right ventricle. Actually a spectrum of ventricular sizes occurs, and the incidence of each varies in different series (right ventricle small in 15 of 20 cases, Davignon *et al.,* 1961; 12 of 20 in the series of Kieffer and Carey, 1963; 28 of 36 cases in the series of Dhanavarabivul *et al.,* 1970).

In those cases with a small right ventricle the myocardium is usually thickened or at least of normal thickness. The tricuspid ring is reduced in size corresponding to the size of the right ventricle. The leaflets are usually well formed, but they may be shortened, rolled or deformed and thus the valve is insufficient (Elliott *et al.,* 1963). In the type 2 cases with a normal or enlarged right ventricle the tricuspid valve is frequently abnormal. The medial or septal leaflet is often displaced downward and has an appearance similar to that of an Ebstein's malformation. Furthermore, hemodynamic studies (Davignon *et al.,* 1961) show that the valve is often insufficient.

The pulmonary valve is replaced by a fibrous membrane or diaphragm that completely blocks the pulmonary artery. The pulmonary trunk is usually reduced in size, and this is an important feature in determining operability. The distal pulmonary arteries fill through a patent ductus arteriosus, and this is the only way that blood can reach the lungs. When the ductus closes, which it usually does, the patient dies.

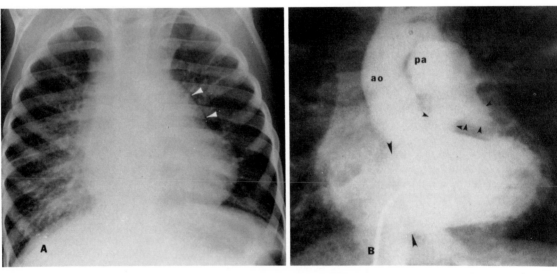

FIG. 300. COMMON VENTRICLE WITH INVERTED INFUNDIBULUM BUT NORMAL (NONTRANSPOSED) ORIGIN OF GREAT VESSELS AND TAPVC (SAME CASE AS FIG. 287)

(A) Arrows indicate convexity due to inverted infundibular chamber. Pulmonary congestion because of TAPVC with obstruction. (B) Selective injection into common ventricle. The aorta fills from common ventricle and the pulmonary artery fills from infundibular chamber. Large arrowheads mark plane of tricuspid valve, and the right atrium is faintly opaque due to return through anomalous veins. Arrowheads indicate infundibular chamber and passageway from common ventricle into chamber. It appears adequate in size but does not exclude a minor degree of pulmonic stenosis. (Courtesy of Children's Cardiac Clinic, Texas Children's Hospital, Houston, Texas.)

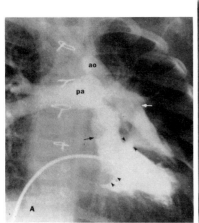
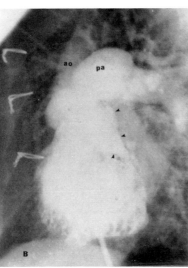
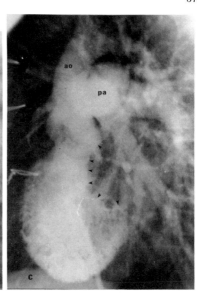

FIG. 301. COMMON VENTRICLE WITH TRANSPOSITION AND INVERSION OF INFUNDIBULUM
(A) Selective injection into common ventricle with immediate filling of infundibular chamber and the great vessels. Arrowheads indicate opening between common ventricle and infundibulum, and this varies with systole and diastole. The aortic valve (white arrow) is slightly higher than the pulmonary valve (black arrow). The difference in density between the pulmonary artery and aorta enables a rough estimate of the amount of oxygen in the blood in each vessel, although this is often better appraised in the lateral view. The tricuspid valve is seen (arrowheads). (B) Common ventricle in diastole. The aorta (ao) is slightly anterior to pulmonary artery (pa) and is less dense suggesting a lesser degree of saturation. Infundibular chamber outlined by arrowheads. (C) Later film with common ventricle in diastole showing mitral valve (arrowheads) and verifying presence of two valves. (Courtesy of Children's Cardiac Clinic, Children's Hospital, Houston, Texas.)

An interatrial communication is present in all cases, and this may be either a patent foramen ovale or an interatrial defect of the secundum type.

An added anomaly of considerable interest is found occasionally in the type 1 cases and less frequently in the type 2 cases. Sinusoids in the right ventricle which are a feature of the fetal myocardium remain open. These sinusoids may converge into one or several vessels which connect with the coronary arterial system (See Fig. 384). Cineangiographic and hemodynamic studies (Davignon et al., 1961; Anselmi et al., 1961; Sissman and Abrams, 1965) have shown that the systolic pressure in the right ventricle exceeds that in the aorta and that during a considerable portion of systole the flow is toward the coronary circulation and during diastole it is reversed and flows toward the right ventricle. This quite striking phenomenon is highly suggestive of a completely obstructed ventricular chamber.

RADIOLOGIC FINDINGS. *Conventional Chest Films.* In the type 1 cases the heart may be normal in size at birth but is often slightly enlarged (Fig. 303A). The right atrial contour, even when the heart is not enlarged, is often convex and prominent. The heart usually increases in size during the first few days or weeks of life. The left ventricular border is rounded, and the apex is low due to the usual generous size of the left ventricle.

In the type 2 cases the heart is usually large even at birth and may become quite large within a few days.

In both types the left mid-cardiac border is concave since the pulmonary trunk, although present, is usually decreased in size and rarely is as large as either of its branches (Elliott et al., 1963). The pulmonary vasculature is typically decreased, and the lungs are clear, although in a minority of cases the pulmonary vasculature may be normal or increased. The pulmonary blood flow and the pulmonary vascularity depend on the size and flow through the patent ductus.

The aorta is usually enlarged. The upper mediastinum may be widened, and this is most likely due to deviation of the superior vena cava by the large ascending aorta.

In the type 2 cases with a normal or enlarged right ventricle the left border of the heart may show a slightly elevated apex reflecting the increased size of the right ventricle.

The oblique and lateral views usually add little of diagnostic value, although the posterior convexity of the heart may suggest left ventricular enlargement.

Cardiac Catheterization. In the type 1 cases every attempt should be made to insert the cath-

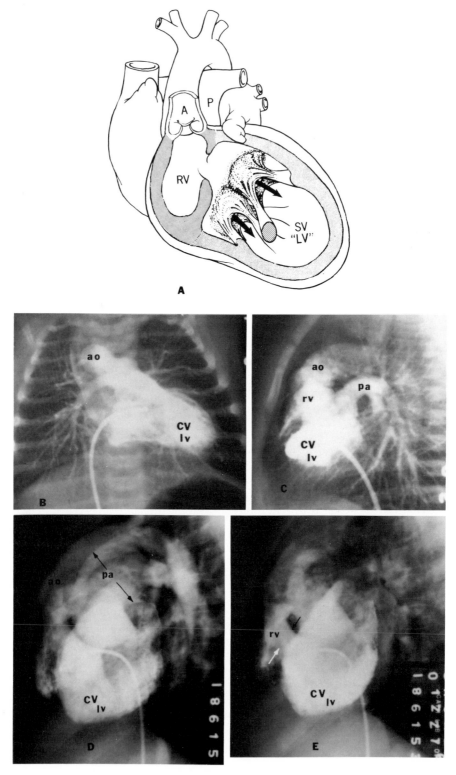

Fig. 302

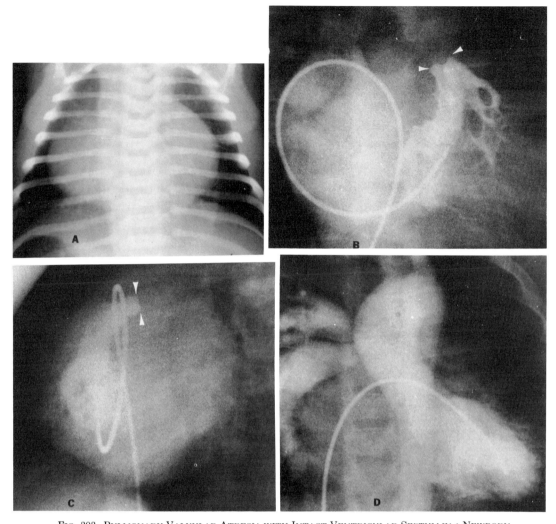

FIG. 303. PULMONARY VALVULAR ATRESIA WITH INTACT VENTRICULAR SEPTUM IN A NEWBORN

(A) Heart enlarged at birth. Enlargement due mainly to right atrium. (B) Selective right ventricular injection. Catheter has made a loop in right atrium showing enlargement. Coarse pattern of ventricle indicates hypertrophy and cavity is diminished in size and infundibulum terminates abruptly (arrows). (C) Lateral view of right ventricle and infundibulum. (D) Selective left ventriculogram. Catheter passed easily through atrial septal defect. Pulmonary arteries are large and fill through a patent ductus. (Courtesy of Children's Cardiac Clinic, Texas Children's Hospital, Houston, Texas.)

eter into the small right ventricle. This is the easiest way to exclude the presence of tricuspid atresia. It is also necessary to determine the size of the right ventricle. Pressures in the right ventricle, whether large or small, are high, and the systolic pressure usually exceeds that in the aorta. The catheter is usually easily inserted into the left atrium and the left ventricle. The blood

FIG. 302. ANGIOGRAMS OF TWO CASES OF COMMON VENTRICLE WITH NONINVERTED RUDIMENTARY OUTFLOW CHAMBER AND TRANSPOSITION

(A) Diagram of B. (B) Atrial injection with filling of common ventricle which resembles a left ventricle. Elliott now prefers the term "single ventricle" for cases of this type. A right aortic arch is present. The rudimentary chamber is obscured in this view. (C) Rudimentary noninverted ventricle (rv) is well seen in this view and has a more anterior location than in the inverted type (see Figs. 301). (D and E) Lateral angiograms of another case showing rudimentary outflow chamber (rv) in anterior position. Arrows indicate interventricular communication and suggest that there is no outflow obstruction. The rudimentary or right ventricle is a sizeable chamber. ao, aorta; pa, pulmonary artery; CV, common or left ventricle. (Courtesy of L. P. Elliott, from *Heart Disease in Infants, Children and Adolescents,* 2nd Edition. A. J. Moss, F. H. Adams, and G. Emmanouilides (eds.), The Williams & Wilkins Co.)

in both chambers is typically unsaturated due to the right to left shunt through the interatrial communication.

Angiocardiography. Venous or forward angiocardiography is usually of little help. It may show a pattern similar to that of tricuspid atresia, and the right ventricle seldom fills sufficiently to be properly identified. Selective right ventriculography is the crucial diagnostic procedure. Where the right ventricle is small or minute, it may be difficult either to enter the ventricle or maintain the catheter in the ventricle. It is desirable to outline the outflow tract which usually consists of a narrow tongue-like projection extending into the region of the pulmonary valve. If the right atrium is outlined either due to the position of the catheter or to reflux through the tricuspid valve, it will be well seen as large and may be huge. The contrast substance leaves the right atrium through the interatrial communication and rapidly passes into the left atrium and left ventricle. The left atrium is often slightly enlarged, and this is to be expected since it receives blood from both the systemic and pulmonary circulation. In some instances the left atrium is quite large.

The diagnosis can be strongly suspected from the size and contour of the right ventricle and the evidence that there is obstruction at the pulmonary valve. This impression would be further reinforced if as occurs in a minority of cases sinusoids are demonstrated connecting with the coronary circulation. Even with this information a left ventricular or left atrial injection is desirable. It is still necessary to determine the condition of the pulmonary arterial system, and this is best determined by left ventricular injection which permits the shunting of blood through the ductus into the pulmonary vascular system. Frequently the pulmonary trunk can be identified and also the pulmonary arteries. The demonstration of a proximal pulmonary arterial system is an essential part of the diagnosis and is necessary for successful surgical treatment.

Surgical treatment consists of the use of two procedures, namely (1) an aortic to pulmonary anastomosis of the Potts, Blalock-Taussig, or Waterston type, and (2) pulmonary valvotomy, or (3) a combination of these two. In a few cases the Glenn procedure (1954) has been used (an anastomosis between the superior vena cava and the distal right pulmonary artery). Valvotomy has given less than optimal results mainly due to the residual poor functional status of the right ventricle. Where the right ventricle is tiny, it is obvious that such a procedure would not be helpful. Where the right ventricle is of intermediate size, there is yet no way to determine whether the ventricle will grow and assume a satisfactory function during adolescence and adult life. Angiographic determination of right ventricular size is, of course, of some value in appraising the chances of surgical success.

The aortic pulmonary shunts have often been helpful even in patients with small right ventricles. This seems to be the procedure of choice, although Ellis *et al.* (1972) suggest that both valvotomy and an aortic pulmonary shunt are helpful and may produce the best results. In those cases that do not have valvotomy, the pressure in the right ventricle may eventually reach a very high level, and this can cause myo-

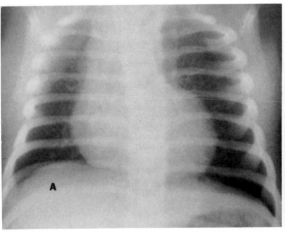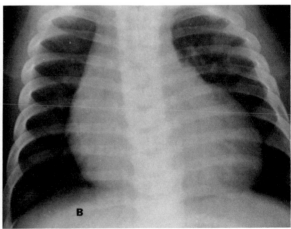

FIG. 304. PULMONARY VALVULAR ATRESIA WITH INTACT VENTRICULAR SEPTUM

(A) Chest film at 2 weeks of age. Heart is moderately enlarged. (B) Chest film 5 months later. Heart has increased in size. Enlargement is due mainly to increase in size of right atrium. Slight decrease in pulmonary vascularity. (Courtesy of Children's Cardiac Clinic, Texas Children's Hospital, Houston, Texas.)

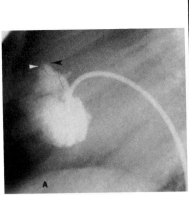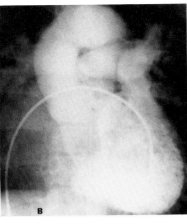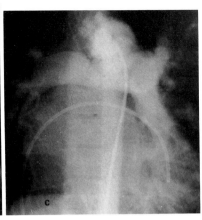

FIG. 305. SAME CASE AS FIG. 304 CINEFLUOROGRAMS

(A) Selective right ventricular injection showing small right ventricle and obstruction in the region of the pulmonary valve (arrows). (B) Selective left ventricular injection. Catheter easily passed through ASD. The pulmonary artery and branches are normal in size and fill from aorta through a patent ductus arteriosus. (C) Aortogram showing filling of pulmonary arteries through a patent ductus. (Courtesy of Children's Cardiac Clinic, Texas Children's Hospital, Houston, Texas.)

cardial necrosis. Immediate diagnosis and surgical treatment are necessary if the patient is to survive.

The differential diagnosis consists of those congenital anomalies that cause diminished blood flow to the lungs in the newborn. These are tricuspid atresia; some cases of Ebstein's anomaly; severe pulmonic stenosis with intact septum; severe tetralogy of Fallot, particularly those with pulmonary atresia (pseudotruncus); and transposition of the great vessels with pulmonic stenosis.

CONGENITAL MALPOSITIONS OF THE HEART OR OF CARDIAC CHAMBERS TO EACH OTHER

Classification

I. Dextrocardia
   A. Extrinsic—The heart is displaced to the right by a variety of conditions, such as hypoplasia of the right lung, absence of the right pulmonary artery, or congenital left diaphragmatic hernia.
   B. Intrinsic
      1. Dextrocardia with situs solitus
         a. Without inversion of ventricles
            (1) Without significant associated anomalies
            (2) With significant associated anomalies
         b. With inversion of ventricles (corrected transposition)
            (1) With significant associated anomalies
            (2) Without significant associated anomalies
      2. Dextrocardia with situs inversus
         a. With ventricular inversion (mirror image dextrocardia)
            (1) Without significant associated anomalies
            (2) With significant associated anomalies
         b. Without ventricular inversion (the atria are inverted in keeping with the situs inversus but the ventricles are not producing the equivalent of corrected transposition in a complete situs inversus)
            (1) Without associated congenital anomalies
            (2) With associated congenital anomalies
      3. Dextrocardia with heterotaxia and/or uncertain situs of the abdominal organs
         a. Asplenia
         b. Polysplenia
         c. Anisosplenia
II. Mesocardia
III. Levocardia with situs inversus
   A. Without associated congenital anomalies
   B. With associated congenital anomalies

Definitions. The literature describing congenital malpositions of the heart suffers from a multiplicity of terms which have led to confusion of an already complicated subject. Van Praagh *et al.* (1964) introduced a new classification and a series of new terms that are helpful in determining the anatomical arrangement of the cardiac chambers and the great vessels associated with the various malpositions. The use of these terms requires angiographic localization of the chambers and vessels. The general radiologist when faced with a cardiac malposition as seen on conventional films does not have the findings elicited by special procedures. Nevertheless, he should be able to place the case tentatively in one of the above classifications. Consequently, the older classifications are used in relation to the findings elicited from conventional chest films. The terms employed by Van Praagh *et al.* (1964) become useful only after the use of angiography and cardiac catheterization.

DEXTROCARDIA. The heart is located on the right instead of the left side of the body. From a radiologic viewpoint, dextrocardia is present when more of the cardiac shadow is seen to the right than to the left of the midline. In many cases of the congenital variety, however, the apex of the heart lies to the right, and the long axis of the cardiac contour is directed caudad from left to right.

MESOCARDIA. This is an atypical location of the heart in the midline of the thorax.

LEVOCARDIA. The heart is located on the left side when the other viscera are transposed. The term frequently used is levocardia with situs inversus.

INVERSION. The equivalent chambers, such as the atria or ventricles or both have exchanged places.

DEXTROVERSION. In relation to dextrocardia, dextroversion means that the ventricles have rotated around the vertical axis of the body in clockwise direction as seen from above. This term has been used by many authors as interchangeable with dextrocardia with situs solitus. Some authors have used the terms "dextrorotation" and "dextrotorsion" as synonymous with dextroversion.

SITUS SOLITUS. The viscera are in their normal position.

SITUS INVERSUS. The viscera are in an inverted position.

HETEROTAXIA. Anomalous placement or transposition of viscera or parts. Heterotaxia is usually accompanied by asplenia or other anomalies of the spleen and is distinguished from situs inversus in that the organs are not completely inverted but are not in their usual solitus position. The stomach may be in the midline or just to the right of the midline, and the pancreas may retain

its primitive mesentery. The intestines may only be partially inverted.

RIGHT ATRIUM. The morphological right atrium is the atrial chamber that contains the limbus of the fossa ovalis, receives the blood from the coronary sinus, and usually receives the inferior vena cava. It may be on the right or the left side of the body, depending upon the location of the other viscera. It is almost always concordant with the other viscera, and the only exceptions are those cases of anomalies of the spleen in which it is difficult to determine the morphology of the atria.

LEFT ATRIUM. The morphological left atrium is the atrial chamber that contains the valve flap of the foramen ovale. It is almost always the arterial atrium as it agrees with the visceral situs uniformly except in those cases of anomalies of the spleen when it is difficult to determine the morphology of the atrium.

MORPHOLOGICAL RIGHT VENTRICLE. This is the ventricle which has a coarse interior trabecular structure, a moderator band, and a well formed infundibulum with an indenting muscle mass known as the crista supraventricularis. The ventricle has a conus above the crista and empties through a semilunar valve that is higher (more cephalad) than that of the morphologic left ventricle. It communicates with the atrium through a tricuspid valve and usually has three papillary muscles. The morphological right ventricle may be either on the right or the left side of the body and may receive either venous or arterial blood.

MORPHOLOGICAL LEFT VENTRICLE. This ventricle is more elliptical in shape than the right ventricle, has a fine internal trabecular pattern, and a smooth non-trabeculated outflow tract. It ordinarily does not have a separate conal structure, and a tricuspid valve that marks its communication with the great vessels is at a lower level than that of the right ventricle. The morphological left ventricle may receive either venous or arterial blood and may be located either on the right or the left side of the body. The morphological right and left ventricles can usually be identified from a series of anteroposterior and lateral angiograms in which the ventricular cavities and great vessels are well outlined.

DEXTROVENTRICULAR LOOP (d-LOOP) (SEE FIG. 306). The primitive straight cardiac tube normally bends towards the right. The morphological right ventricle is on the right side of the body and is accompanied by the conus arteriosus and a high position of the semilunar valve which marks the exit from this chamber.

LEVOVENTRICULAR LOOP (l-LOOP). The primi-

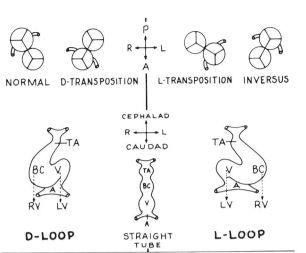

NORMAL D-TRANSPOSITION L-TRANSPOSITION INVERSUS

D-LOOP STRAIGHT TUBE L-LOOP

FIG. 306. THE LOOP RULE FOR VENTRICULAR
LOCALIZATION
(1) Normally related great arteries and (2) d-transposition
almost always indicate a d-loop. (3) Inverted normally related
great arteries and (4) l-transposition almost always indicate
an l-loop. Semilunar valves viewed from above. TA, truncus
arteriosus; BC, bulbus cordis; V, ventricle; A, atrium; RV,
right ventricle; LV, left ventricle. (From Van Praagh et al.,
American Journal of Cardiology 15: 234, 1965, by permission
of the Reuben H. Donnelly Corporation.)

tive cardiac tube bends towards the left side. The
morphological right ventricle and conus are on
the left side of the body. The morphological right
ventricle, although it is on the left side of the
body, has a higher semilunar valve than that of
the left ventricle.

NORMAL RELATION OF THE GREAT VESSELS. In
normal relation of the great vessels, the pulmonary artery is anterior and to the left of the
ascending aorta.

INVERTED RELATIONSHIP OF THE GREAT VES-
SELS. In inverted relationship of the great vessels,
the pulmonary artery is to the right and anterior
to the ascending aorta.

DEXTROTRANSPOSITION (d-TRANSPOSITION).
In dextrotransposition, the aorta is anterior and
to the right of the pulmonary artery.

LEVOTRANSPOSITION (l-TRANSPOSITION). In
levotransposition, the aorta is to the left and
anterior to the pulmonary artery.

BALANCED RELATIONSHIP OF THE GREAT VES-
SELS. This arrangement is infrequent. The great
vessels are side by side, and usually there is a
double conus arrangement, and the semilunar
valves are at approximately the same level.

LOOP RULE FOR LOCALIZING THE VENTRICLES
(VAN PRAAGH ET AL., 1965) (SEE FIG. 306). (1)
Normally related great arteries and (2) d-transposition almost always indicate the presence of
a d-loop (right ventricle right-sided). (1) Inverted

related great arteries and (2) l-transposed great
arteries almost always indicate the presence of
an l-loop (right ventricle left-sided).

CONCORDANT LOOP. The cardiac loop is towards the same side as the anatomic right atrium
and hepatic veins and opposite that of the stomach. Thus, a d-loop is concordant with a situs
solitus and an l-loop with a situs inversus.

DISCORDANT LOOP. The cardiac loop is in the
opposite direction to that of the body situs, as an
l-loop with situs solitus.

The presence or absence of significant associated anomalies is determined by the referring
physician and is based largely on the history and
physical examination of the patient. Usually it is
quite easy to determine if the patient has had
significant associated congenital anomalies because they are usually symptomatic or have been
symptomatic for some time. If the patient is
asymptomatic and without physical signs of
heart disease the chances of a significant congenital anomaly are remote.

Dextrocardia is a radiologic sign that is usually
first detected from inspection of a frontal chest
film. It does not represent a specific anatomic
entity or disease. Its evaluation and significance
depend on a multitude of accompanying signs
and clinical findings. Population surveys (Cock-
ayne, 1938; Torgersen, 1949) suggest that a majority of persons in the general population with
dextrocardia are asymptomatic and do not have
significant heart disease. On the other hand, the
majority of patients with dextrocardia who are
referred to the radiologist have evidence of associated significant heart disease. Dextrocardia
makes the diagnosis and treatment of the associated cardiac disease more complicated. The
radiologist should have an approach based on
the findings from conventional films of the chest
and abdomen combined with the history of significant heart disease. The contributions by Elliott et al. (1966) and Elliott (1967) are very
helpful in this regard. The classification presented here is based on these findings. If there
are associated congenital malformations, these
require special angiographic and catheterization
studies for precise diagnosis, and the dextrocardia is simply a complicating factor.

RADIOLOGIC APPROACH. The frontal chest film
usually permits a determination of visceral situs
by locating the stomach and main mass of the
liver. If this cannot be done from the chest film,
then a barium swallow plus an abdominal film
will be helpful. The atria for practical purposes
are always concordant with the abdominal viscera except in those cases of asplenia or polysplenia in which it is difficult to determine ana-

tomically which is the morphological right and which is the morphological left atrium. If the aorta arches towards the same side as the stomach bubble, this is a helpful confirmatory sign. If it arches in the opposite direction, a congenital abnormality in addition to the dextrocardia is usually present. Situs indeterminate or heterotaxia can usually be suspected from the frontal chest film. The stomach is not in its usual position and is often near or just to the right of the midline. The liver shadow commonly has a symmetrical appearance that can be ascertained from the chest film.

The bronchial tree is normally asymmetrical with a short epiarterial bronchus on the right side and a longer left main bronchus which bifurcates. In anomalies of the spleen, the lung and bronchial tree are frequently symmetrical. In asplenia, there are commonly three lobes (bilateral right-sidedness) and bilateral epiarterial bronchi without a typical long curved bronchus on either side. In polysplenia, there are usually two lobes with bilateral left-sided type bronchi in which there are only hyparterial bronchi (bilateral left-sidedness). In anisosplenia (one large and several small spleens), there is said to be a difference between male and female bronchial patterns (Landing, 1974). In male anisosplenia there are bilateral right lungs, often a normal visceral situs with a considerable frequency of atrioventricularis communis and pulmonic stenosis. In female anisosplenia there are bilateral left lungs, abnormal visceral situs, and congenital heart disease.

The lateral chest film may be helpful in determining the presence of the inferior vena cava which often can be seen just above the diaphragm. The absence of the shadow suggests the absence of the inferior vena cava with an azygos return. The recent article by O'Reilly and Grollman (1976) suggests that the hepatic veins may mimic the inferior vena cava, and thus this sign may not be significant. In summary, the radiologist can determine from the conventional chest films (1) visceral situs, (2) atrial situs, (3) position of the aortic arch, (4) bronchial anatomy, (5) pulmonary vascularity, increased or decreased, and (6) occasionally may determine the size of the pulmonary artery. From these findings the radiologist should be able to place the particular case into one of the major categories listed above. In many instances he can suggest the nature of the underlying congenital defect if such is present, *e.g.*, right-to-left shunts, left-to-right-shunts, pulmonic stenosis, etc.

Information to be determined from angiogra-

phy and cardiac catheterization:

1. Relative position of the aorta and pulmonary artery.
2. Location of the respective semilunar valves in each great vessel.
3. Determination of internal structure of each ventricle and therefore the location of the anatomical right and left ventricle.
4. Location of a conus structure.

From these findings, the radiologist can confirm the fundamental types of dextrocardia and be in a better position to determine the associated cardiac abnormalities, such as shunts, stenoses, etc.

Dextrocardia

1. Extrinsic—These have been often confused with dextrocardia with situs solitus without ventricular inversion. Most of these are due to hypoplasia of the right lung, absence of the right pulmonary artery, or left diaphragmatic hernia.
2. Intrinsic
   A. Dextrocardia with situs solitus
      a. Without inversion of the ventricles
         (1) Without significant associated anomalies

These cases are uncommon. The cardiac contour may be bizarre. The pulmonary vascularity is normal. The aorta usually arches towards the left and, of course, the visceral situs can be easily determined.

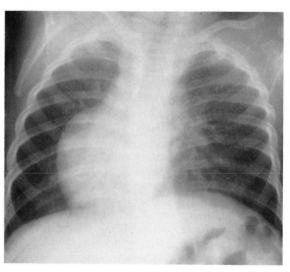

FIG. 307. DEXTROCARDIA WITH SITUS SOLITUS WITHOUT EVIDENCE OF HEART DISEASE

Presumably A a (1) without ventricular inversion. Since the patient had no symptoms referable to the heart, no further investigations were carried out. This is an uncommon type of dextrocardia.

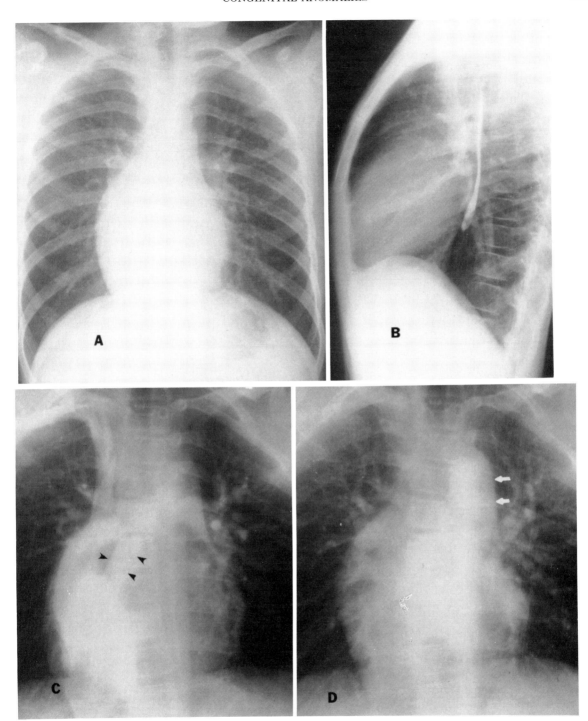

FIG. 308. DEXTROCARDIA WITH SITUS SOLITUS AND INVERSION OF THE VENTRICLES WITH A VENTRICULAR SEPTAL DEFECT

(A) The smooth long left upper segment of the cardiac contour is suggestive of the ascending aorta. (B) Lateral view suggests enlargement of left atrium. (C) The right-sided left ventricle is superimposed on the right atrial shadow but clearly does not have the contour of a right ventricle. The pulmonary artery (arrowheads) runs an oblique course and bifurcates near the midline. (D) The ascending aorta (arrows) is quite straight (arrows) and forms the left upper border of the cardiovascular contour.

(2) With significant associated anomalies

Most of these have been confused with extrinsic cases such as those with hypoplasia of the right lung or absence of the right pulmonary artery. In those which have intrinsic congenital heart disease, the pulmonary vascularity may be of value in suggesting the presence of shunts or stenoses. Because the heart is rotated toward the right, the aorta often is in a more anterior position than in the normal. Consequently, the condition may be confused with those cases in which there is a ventricular inversion with an l-loop. The aorta usually arches toward the left. However, the morphological characteristics of the ventricles should prevent this error. These cases are statistically less common than b (below).

b. With inversion of the ventricles (corrected transposition) (This is the most common type of dextrocardia with situs solitus).

(1) With significant associated anomalies (Fig. 308)

A high proportion of these cases do have associated anomalies. The commonest are ventricular septal defects and pulmonic stenosis. Tetralogy of Fallot does not occur and cannot occur with an l-transposition. The contour of the heart is bizarre. Angiography shows an l-transposition. In the conventional film, the aorta may course up the left side of the mediastinum and immediately give a clue to the presence of the l-transposition.

(2) Without significant associated anomalies. (These are quite rare, and the present authors are not sure of any verified cases.)

B. Dextrocardia with situs inversus

a. With ventricular inversion (mirror image dextrocardia)

(1) Without significant associated anomalies

This is the most common type encountered in the general population. Since most of these patients are asymptomatic, the dextrocardia is an incidental finding, and the radiologist may be the first to discover the anomaly providing he is alert enough to notice the right and left markers on the film. Otherwise, since the cardiac contour is often quite normal, the situs inversus may be completely overlooked. The ECG is useful in confirming the diagnosis in that the P, QRS, and T waves are inverted in lead I and interchangeable with lead III as seen in the normal heart. The detection of the situs inversus, of course, is important because of the surgical implications in the abdomen.

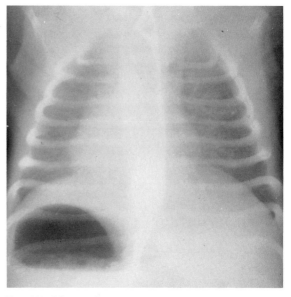

FIG. 309. MIRROR IMAGE DEXTROCARDIA B a (1) WITHOUT SIGNIFICANT ASSOCIATED ANOMALIES. THE PATIENT HAD NO EVIDENCE OF HEART DISEASE

Although these cases do not have associated cardiac anomalies, they do have a markedly increased incidence (15–25%) of bronchiectasis and sinusitis, and this triad of dextrocardia, bronchiectasis, and sinusitis is known as Kartagener's triad (1935). The bronchiectasis is thought to be due to a congenital defect in the bronchial mucosa. These patients are susceptible to acquired heart disease to the same degree as other people.

(2) With significant associated anomalies

This is also known as mirror image dextrocardia. The incidence of this type is uncertain. Keith et al. (1958) found it in 3% of cases of mirror image dextrocardia. In material collected from large cardiac clinics, the incidence is much greater, and Campbell and Reynolds (1952) and Taussig (1960) comment on the frequency of severe cardiac anomalies associated with this type of dextrocardia. Van Praagh et al. (1965) found 4 of their 6 cases had rudimentary spleens and state that the incidence of abnormality is high. Much depends on the source of the material. As stated above, it is the authors' opinion that mirror image dextrocardia without associated anomalies is more common than those with associated anomalies. Those that do not have associated anomalies are asymptomatic and are not the source of case reports and rarely come to the attention of physicians because of their heart condition. On the other hand, the cases that are reported in the literature usually come from cardiac clinics where the selection of patients with

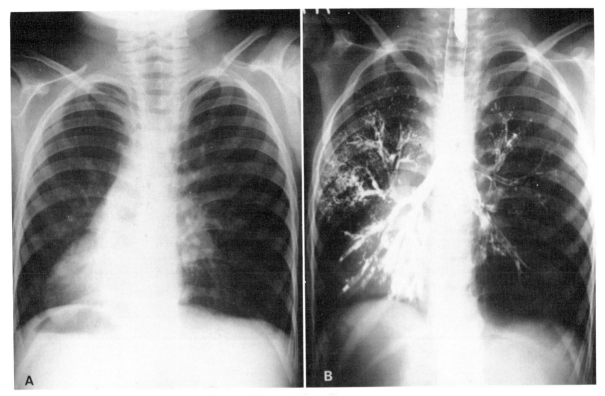

FIG. 310. MIRROR IMAGE DEXTROCARDIA

Dextrocardia with situs inversus viscerum, bronchiectasis, and sinusitis known as Kartagener's triad. The aortic arch and knob are on the right.

heart disease is obviously much higher. Also, some of these cases are confused with cases of anomalies of the spleen.

Also considered in this group are those cases of d- and l-transposition of Van Praagh. Where the aorta is clearly anterior, a transposition of the great vessels is present and the incidence of abnormality is quite high. The cardiac contour in these cases is grossly abnormal and depends considerably on the underlying cardiac defect.

    b. Without ventricular inversion
       (1) Without associated congenital anomalies

This is the counterpart of corrected transposition in a normally placed heart. It would of necessity be associated with a d-transposition, and consequently it is unlikely that this would occur without some other abnormality in the heart. The present authors have never seen such a case and it is mentioned only as a theoretical possibility.

       (2) With associated congenital anomalies

The cardiac contour is almost always abnormal and reflects the underlying defect. VSD is the single most common abnormality and, of course, the tetralogy of Fallot does not occur, although pulmonic stenosis is frequent.

C. Dextrocardia with
    a. asplenia (Ivemark's syndrome 1955)
    b. polysplenia
    c. anisosplenia
       (1) M—anisosplenia
       (2) F—anisosplenia

Formerly, all of the above-mentioned abnormalities were considered together as anomalies of the spleen. As further cases are reported, it appears that there is a pattern of anomalies that is associated with each, although there is considerable overlap. Further studies are needed to establish a clear-cut profile that would enable one to completely differentiate the three groups (Landing, 1974).

ASPLENIA. In this group, there is a tendency to symmetry of the liver and a midline or paramedian stomach. The lungs have three lobes producing what is termed bilateral right-sidedness. Howell-Jolly bodies are found in the blood. The pancreas is often freely movable, and incomplete rotation of the intestine is common. The most frequently associated anomalies of the heart are conal or truncal anomalies, such as truncus arteriosus, transposition of the great vessels, and pulmonic stenosis.

POLYSPLENIA. The lungs are symmetrical and

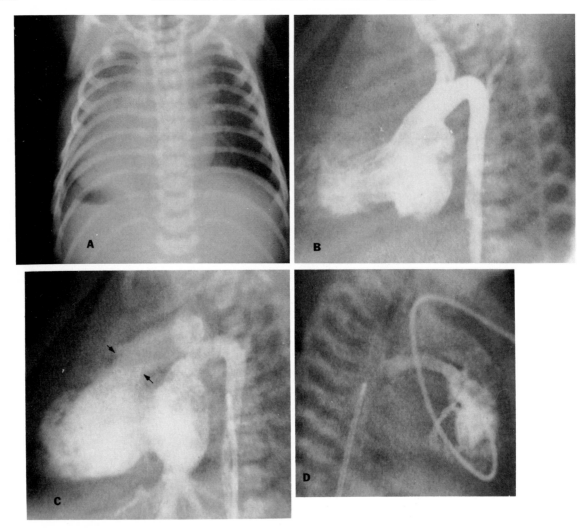

FIG. 311. DEXTROCARDIA WITH SITUS INVERSUS, TRANSPOSITION OF GREAT VESSELS, INVERSION OF VENTRICLES WITH MITRAL ATRESIA, AND INTERRUPTION OF INFERIOR VENA CAVA WITH AZYGOS CONTINUATION (AUTOPSY CASE) B a (2)

(A) Situs inversus with dextrocardia and cardiac enlargement. The aorta was thought to arch to the right. (B) Injection into azygos extension of inferior vena cava. Contrast substance refluxes into left-sided vena cava and probably an intercostal vein. The venous atrium is on left side and communicates with an anatomical right ventricle. (C) Aorta fills from right ventricle, and valve (arrows) is above a conus. Aorta is anterior. (D) Left ventricle entered through a septal defect. Pulmonary artery is posterior and originates from left ventricle.

have two lobes. Venous anomalies are common, such as double vena cavae or double inferior vena cavae or interruption of the inferior vena cava with azygos return. Also, anomalies of the pulmonary veins with return into the right atrium form a developmental complex (Ongley *et al.*, 1965). Not all patients with multiple spleens present this complex, although the vast majority do have symmetrical two-lobed lungs.

ANISOSPLENIA (LARGE SPLEEN WITH MULTIPLE ACCESSORY SPLEENS). This is a separate syndrome with a different manifestation in each sex. In the male, it is associated with bilateral right-sidedness, and in the female, with bilateral left-sidedness (Singleton *et al.*, 1972). Patients may or may not have abnormal visceral situs (see description from Landing given above).

Splenic scans and angiography may be helpful in locating and delineating the spleen. Howell-Jolly and Heinz bodies in the peripheral blood are strong evidence for asplenia.

Levocardia with Situs Inversus (Isolated Levocardia). This is a rare condition, much less common than dextrocardia. Campbell and Forgacs (1953) found an incidence of about 1.2% of all cases of congenital heart disease. It is associated with a high incidence of asplenia or polysplenia. Keith *et al.* (1958) found 74% of their

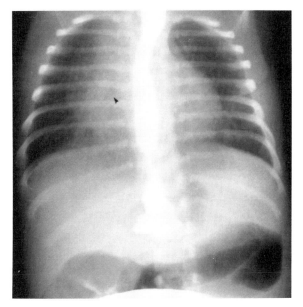

FIG. 312. DEXTROCARDIA WITH ASPLENIA AND HETEROTAXIA OF THE ABDOMINAL ORGANS (THE IVEMARK SYNDROME)

The midline stomach and symmetrical liver shadow are highly suggestive of this syndrome. The right main stem bronchus is faintly seen and appears to be of the right-sided variety (see text). Autopsy confirmed the presence of asplenia and cor biloculare.

cases had asplenia (Ivemark syndrome) and 10% polysplenia. The rule that atrial situs is concordant with and can be established by determination of visceral situs cannot be applied with certainty in these cases since the identification of the right and left atrium and also the visceral situs may be in doubt. Campbell and Forgacs (1953) suggested a classification according to (1) where the venous atrium was on the right side and was connected with a right-sided superior vena cava, or (2) the venous atrium was on the left side and connected with a left superior vena cava. Frequency of certain anomalies seemed to be associated with each type. Van Praagh (1968) does not believe this classification is useful because of the difficulty in ascertaining true atrial situs. Each case should be worked out by the combined use of the ECG, angiography and cardiac catheterization.

Less than 10% of the cases will have normal functioning hearts (for exception, see Fig. 315). A certain number of normally functioning hearts will have associated venous anomalies, such as partial anomalous venous return or azygos continuation of the inferior vena cava (Rosenbaum, 1962).

In the great majority of cases the heart shows the most severe anomalies. Single or common

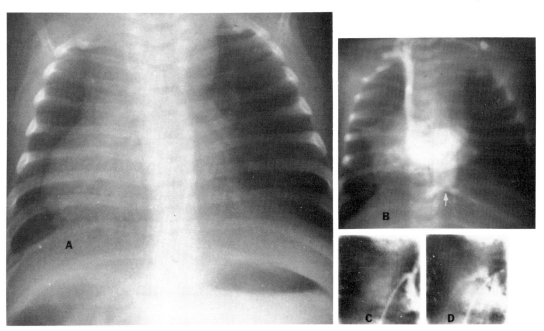

FIG. 313. DEXTROCARDIA WITH SINGLE ATRIUM AND VENTRICLE, DOUBLE SUPERIOR VENA CAVAE, INTERRUPTION OF INFERIOR VENA CAVA AND PROBABLE ASPLENIA

(A) Note symmetry of liver shadow. The stomach is to the left of the midline. Bronchial pattern cannot be determined with certainty. (B) Angiocardiogram with injection into right jugular vein and a right-sided vena cava that empties into an atrium of undetermined situs since the hepatic veins are on the left side (arrow). (C) 16-mm cinefluorogram shows catheter in hemiazygos extension and left vena cava. (D) Filling of pulmonary artery from a single ventricle. Case incompletely diagnosed but considered to be inoperable.

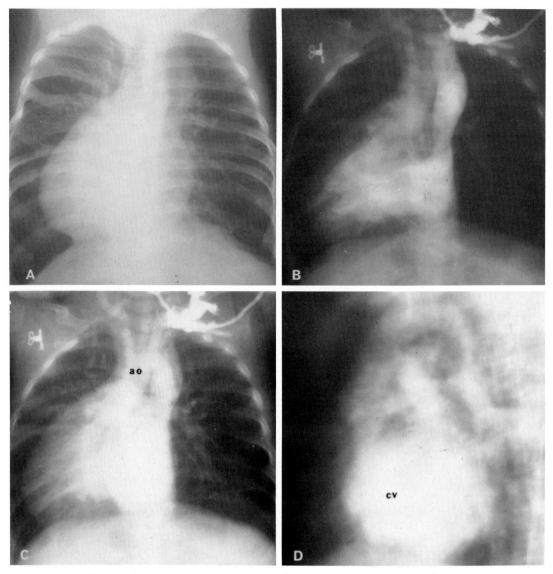

FIG. 314. DEXTROCARDIA, ASPLENIA, AND HETEROTAXIA OF ABDOMINAL ORGANS
Postmortem examination showed a cor biloculare with a persistent common atrioventricular canal and complete anomalous venous connection to the left superior vena cava. It was impossible to determine whether there was chamber inversion because there was a common atrium and ventricle. The aorta arched toward the left. ao, aorta; CV, common ventricle.

ventricle is common, often associated with transposition and pulmonic stenosis. Most cases are not susceptible to presently available methods of surgical treatment. This particularly applies to those with asplenia.

In a few cases, the contour of the heart is normal. In most instances, the contour is dependent on the underlying anomalies. Since pulmonic stenosis is common a sizeable proportion, particularly those who survive for a few months to years, will have decreased vascular markings. Evidence of anomalous venous return should be looked for, such as abnormal vascular shadows within the lungs. Interruption of the inferior vena cava with azygos return is common, and its presence may be suggested by enlargement of the azygos vein. Perhaps of some value is failure to detect the usual shadow of the inferior vena cava on the lateral view, although this shadow can be mimicked by the hepatic veins (O'Reilly and Grollman, 1976). An overexposed chest film should be used to study the bronchial pattern as this occasionally may be helpful in suggesting asplenia or polysplenia. Visceral angiography may be useful in detecting polysplenia or asplenia.

Anomalies of the Systemic Venous Return (ASVR). LEFT SUPERIOR VENA CAVA. A left superior vena cava (LSVC) is the most frequently encountered anomaly of the systemic veins. Steinberg *et al.* (1953) placed the incidence at 0.5% in the general population and Sanders (1946) found one case in every 350 routine autopsies. It is much more common in patients with congenital heart disease with an incidence quoted as follows: Abbott (1936)—3.6% of 1,000 cases of all types; Campbell and Deuchar—3% of cases of congenital heart disease and 40% incidence in patients with transposition of the heart or viscera; Wood (1956)—20% of the tetralogy of Fallot and 8% of the Eisenmenger syndrome; Fraser *et al.* (1961)—29 of 30 cases were associated with congenital heart disease. Sinus venosus defects were found in 18% of the cases reported by Fleming and Gibson (1964). Usually there are two vena cavae and a single left-sided vena cava is unusual except in patients with mirror image dextrocardia.

A LSVC is a persistent left anterior cardinal vein. In the most frequent situation it communicates distally with the left subclavian or innominate vein and also receives the first or superior intercostal vein. A communication across the midline with the right superior vena cava (usually the left innominate vein) was present in 61% of the cases reported by Winter (1954), although this communication is often smaller than normal and at times rudimentary. When there is no communication with the RSVC, the LSVC carries about 20% of the systemic venous return and is about equal in size to the RSVC. The LSVC communicates with the right atrium through the coronary sinus in about 92% of cases (Meadows and Sharp, 1965) and with the left atrium in 8%. The LSVC may receive one or all of the pulmonary veins and these anomalies have been discussed in the section on PAPVC and TAPVC. The LSVC may receive the hemiazygous continuation of the inferior vena cava and thus carry the entire systemic venous return from the lower portion of the body except that of the portal system and liver. This occurs when there is an interruption of the prehepatic portion of the inferior vena cava and will be discussed further below.

When a LSVC is an isolated anomaly and communicates with the right atrium its presence is of little consequence. It may be encountered

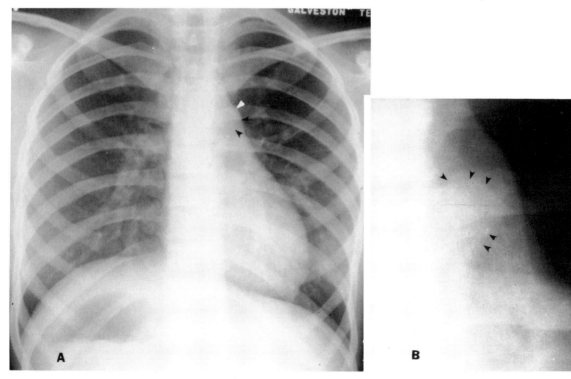

FIG. 315. SITUS INVERSUS

(A) Situs inversus with levocardia and polysplenia, interruption of inferior vena cava with azygos extension on left and double superior vena cavae. No abnormality in the heart. (Autopsy case) The opacity in the region of aortic knob (arrowheads) was the greatly dilated left-sided hemiazygos vein. (B) Close-up showing dilated hemiazygos vein emptying into a left superior vena cava.

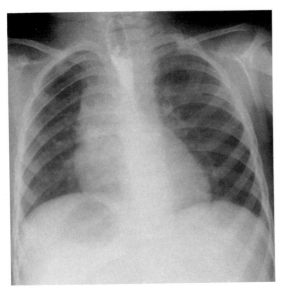

FIG. 316. SITUS INVERSUS

Situs inversus with levocardia and asplenia, transposition of great vessels, double superior vena cavae and probable absence of left pulmonary artery.

by chance when an attempt is made to catheterize the right heart or perform venous angiocardiography from the left arm. When it is associated with other anomalies such as the tetralogy of Fallot or a sinus venosus atrial septal defect it can present a number of obstacles. If catheterization is attempted from the left arm, the catheter may enter the right atrium through the coronary sinus. This directs the tip towards the lateral wall of the right atrium and it is very difficult to enter the right ventricle or pulmonary artery. Also, partial occlusion of the coronary sinus by the catheter may stimulate a supraventricular tachycardia (Fraser *et al.*, 1961). Also at the time of cannulation of the vena cavas in preparation for open heart surgery, failure to control the flow from the LSVC may be very troublesome.

When the LSVC communicates totally or partially with the left atrium the coronary sinus is usually either anomalous or obliterated. When a LSVC is an isolated anomaly it may or may not produce peripheral cyanosis (Davis *et al.*, 1959; Meadows and Sharp, 1965). In those that are

cyanotic (9 of 11 reported cases) the cyanosis may be cured by ligation of the vessel provided there is a normal RSVC and an adequate communication between the two vessels. If this is not present transplantation into the right atrium should be attempted.

Communication of the LSVC with the left atrium is more common in association with primitive cardiovascular defects such as often found in association with partial situs inversus, visceral heterotaxy and the splenic syndrome (Ivemark, 1955). In many of these cases it is difficult to determine which chamber is the anatomical left atrium.

A LSVC is usual with mirror image dextrocardia and there is an increased instance of double superior vena cava with this condition (Campbell and Deuchar, 1967).

Radiologic Findings. As seen on a conventional PA chest film the LSVC presents as a crescentic vascular shadow passing from the left upper border of the aortic arch toward the middle one-third of the clavicle. It may resemble superficially the shadow of the left subclavian artery but it extends to a lower level in the mediastinum. This evidence of a left LSVC is found in about 50% of cases (Fraser *et al.*, 1961).

The LSVC may be easily recognized when a catheter is inserted into a vein in the left arm and instead of following a course across the midline to the RSVC, it courses down the left side of the mediastinum and curves through the coronary sinus into the right atrium. Venous angiocardiography from the left arm may show the same finding and some of the contrast substance may also cross to the RSVC thus outlining the communicating vein and the adequacy of the RSVC. Occasionally, angiography from the right arm will reflux into the left innominate vein and then into the LSVC. Rarely, contrast substance will reflux into the coronary sinus from the right atrium in sufficient quantity to outline the proximal portion of the LSVC (Campbell and Deuchar, 1967).

INTERRUPTION OF THE INFERIOR VENA CAVA. IIVC occurs when the prehepatic portion fails to develop and connect with the post renal portion. In the early stages of the embryological development there are bilateral symmetrical venous

FIG. 317. VENOUS ANGIOGRAMS OF SAME CASE AS FIG. 316

(A, B, C, and D), from right arm. A large right superior vena cava empties into a larger atrial cavity that communicates with multiple hepatic veins. The great vessels are transposed, and only a single ventricular structure is seen. (E, F, G, and H) Injection from left arm shows smaller left superior vena cava, a smaller atrial structure (partially filled?) communicating with large hepatic veins and emptying into a large anterior ventricular structure. Aorta is anterior. The pulmonary artery in F appears to give off only a right branch, and the left lung is avascular.

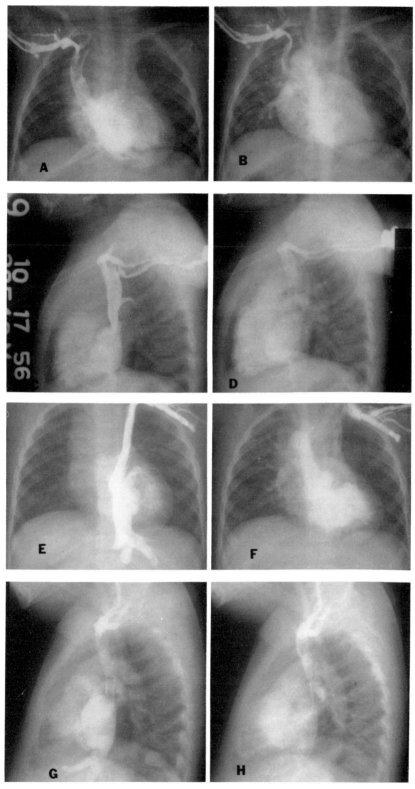

Fig. 317

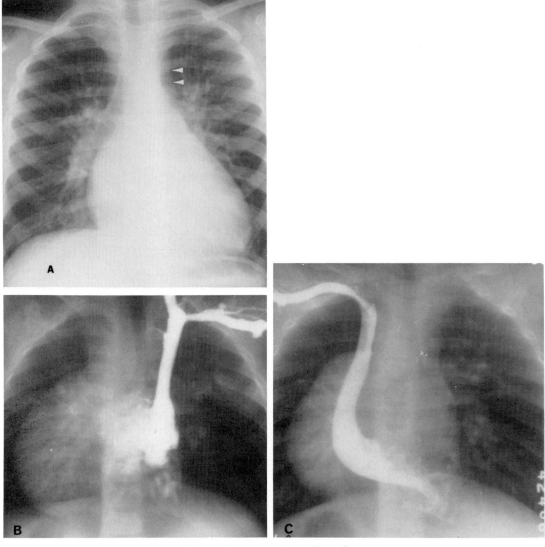

FIG. 318. LEFT AND RIGHT VENA CAVA

(A) Left superior vena cava (arrowheads) in a patient with an ASD. This was an unsuspected finding at operation. (B and C) Another patient with dextrocardia with heterotaxia of abdominal organs and bilateral vena cavas. The right vena cava enters the coronary sinus in a mirror image arrangement of a left superior vena cava with the heart in its normal left-sided position.

systems composed of the posterior cardinal and the infra and supracardinal veins. Numerous collaterals exist between each of these veins on the same side and also across the midline in the region of the kidney. Consequently, when the prehepatic portion of the vena cava fails to develop or unite with the venous system on the right side the blood seeks an alternate route to the heart. This is usually provided by the right supracardinal system which is the precursor of the azygous vein. In a minority of cases, however, the flow is shifted towards the left side and into the left supracardinal system which is the precursor of the hemi-azygous vein. In these cases the hemi-azygous vein empties into a left superior vena cava. The hepatic vein and a very short segment of the vena cava is all that remains of the prerenal part of the vena cava. For further details concerning the development of the inferior vena cava, azygous and hemi-azygous systems the reader is referred to the review by McClure and Butler (1925).

IIVC with azygous (right) or hemi-azygous (left) continuation is rare in patients with a nor-

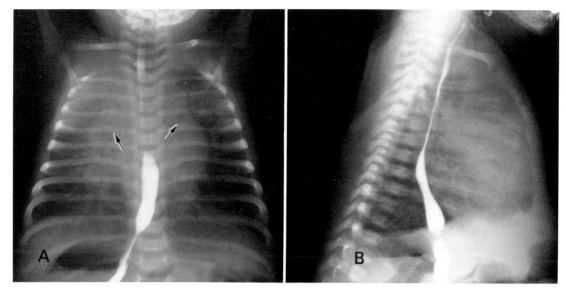

FIG. 319. INFERIOR VENA CAVA
(A) Interruption of inferior vena cava with azygos return, heterotaxia of abdominal organs and polysplenia. A symmetrical proximal bronchial tree is faintly visible (arrows). (B) In lateral view there is no evidence of the shadow of the inferior vena cava.

mal heart. Such a case however is reported by Pacofsky and Wolfel (1971) and the present authors have also seen such a case (Fig. 315).

In a study of 64 cases Campbell and Deuchar (1967) found IIVC in 1% of patients with congenital heart disease; in 20% of patients with situs inversus with congenital heart disease and 46% of patients with the asplenic syndrome and partial or complete situs inversus. A considerable incidence of IIVC is also seen with polysplenia (Landing, 1974). About one-half of these cases will have a double superior vena cava (Campbell and Deuchar, 1967).

IIVC does not disturb the hemodynamics of the return of venous blood to the heart and is an important finding only because of its frequent association with severe cardiac anomalies such as cor biloculare, endocardial cushion defects, origin of both great vessels from the right ventricle and anomalous pulmonary venous return.

Radiologic Findings. The conventional chest film may show a dilated azygous vein and this combined with the right-sided stomach bubble is highly suggestive of the diagnosis (Pacofsky and Wolfel, 1971). As has been previously indicated, the normal azygous vein is seen just above the right main stem bronchus and ordinarily does not exceed 5 mm in diameter (Shuford and Weens, 1958). In association with IIVC the azygous shadow is often much larger. The vascular nature of the shadow can be elicited by exami-

nation in the erect and recumbent positions and also by the use of inspiratory, expiratory and Valsalva maneuvers. Singleton *et al.,* (1972) mentions that failure to identify the normal inferior vena caval shadow in the lateral chest film might be suggestive of an IIVC but O'Reilly and Goldman (1976) indicate that the normal hepatic veins may mimic the vena cava and regard this finding as unreliable.

The diagnosis of IIVC by cardiac catheterization is unlikely unless the heart is approached through the saphenous or femoral vein. If this approach is used, the catheter as it enters the thorax passes into a slightly lateral and posterior location that is clearly outside of the inferior vena cava and right atrium. In the case of a hemi-azygous continuation the catheter crosses the midline and enters the thorax to the left of the vertebral column.

The definitive procedure is angiocardiography through the femoral vein. The dilated azygous vein is easily identified by its (candystick) arch seen in the lateral view. The entire vein is considerably dilated. If there is a hemi-azygous continuation the deviation to the left of the midline and entrance into a left-sided superior vena cava is diagnostic. As indicated above, the major problems are usually associated with unraveling the complex cardiac anomalies. In cases of asplenia or polysplenia there may be a high incidence of anomalies of the lung.

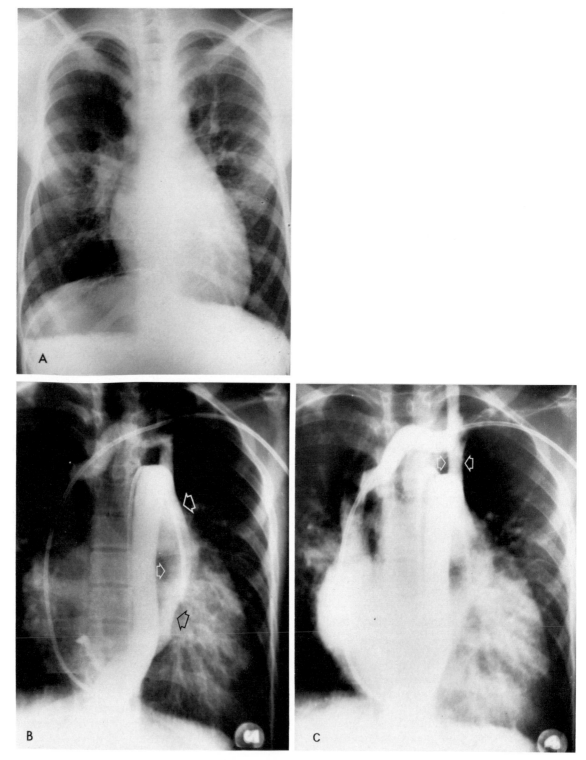

FIG. 320. INTERRUPTION OF THE INFERIOR VENA CAVA WITH HEMIAZYGOS CONTINUATION INTO LEFT SUPERIOR VENA CAVA (ARROWS)

Patient had situs inversus with levocardia. (A) Conventional chest film showing right-sided stomach. (B and C) Injection into IVC.

Congenitally Corrected Transposition of the Great Vessels. The cardinal features of this anomaly are (1) transposition of the great vessels and (2) inversion of the ventricles. Embryologically, ventricular inversion is due to leftward instead of rightward bending of the bulvoventricular loop; in addition there is an interchange in the positions of the pulmonary artery and ascending aorta which follow parallel courses without crossing over in the normal manner (de la Cruz et al., 1962; Grant, 1964). The result is that the aorta arises anteriorly from the left-sided ventricle and receives oxygenated blood, while the pulmonary artery arises somewhat posteriorly from the right-sided ventricle and receives unoxygenated blood. The atria and venous connections are normally placed. In the absence of other cardiac anomalies there is no alteration in normal hemodynamics, and a normal life span can be expected (Lester et al., 1960).

The venous or right-sided ventricle has the anatomic characteristics of the left ventricle: (1) the right-sided atrioventricular valve is bicuspid, (2) there is no infundibulum or crista supraventricularis, and (3) the internal ventricular surface is only slightly trabeculated. The arterial or left-sided ventricle is an anatomic right ventricle: (1) the left-sided A-V valve is tricuspid, (2) a well-developed infundibulum is present, as is the crista supraventricularis, and (3) the internal surface is marked by sizeable trabeculations.

The coronary arteries are more or less inverted. The usual arrangement is for the right coronary artery to originate from the right posterior sinus and give rise to anterior descending and circumflex branches while the left originates from the left posterior sinus and gives rise to a posterior descending branch.

Congenital cardiac malpositions are commonly associated with corrected transposition. Eighty percent of the cases of dextrocardia with situs solitus (dextroversion) in the series of Elliott et al. (1966) were found to have corrected transposition. In the 30 cases reported by Ellis et al. (1962) 10 had some form of cardiac malposition. Corrected transposition is also a common cause of mesocardia or midline heart.

Although corrected transposition is compatible with a normal circulation, the large majority of reported cases have had significant associated defects. The true incidence of congenital anomalies is uncertain since persons with a normal circulation may escape recognition. The most commonly reported defects were VSDs, and these were often associated with pulmonic stenosis (Ruttenberg, 1968). Other less frequent defects were PDA, ASD, MI, and AI. Although a pulmonic stenosis in association with a VSD may produce a functional tetralogy of Fallot, a true anatomical tetralogy of Fallot is not possible with a corrected transposition. Of particular interest are anomalies of the tricuspid valve associated with the inverted right ventricle. These consist of the Ebstein type of malformation and shortening and deformity of the chordae tendineae and occasionally a supravalvular ring. Some degree of mitral insufficiency is a common finding.

Abnormalities of conduction, particularly A-V block, are commonly found in association with corrected transposition of the great vessels, and the diagnosis may be suspected on this basis. A further clue may be forthcoming at cardiac catheterization when difficulty may be encountered in passing the catheter into the medially and posteriorly placed pulmonary artery (Anderson et al., 1957). Contrast visualization of the heart chambers should establish the diagnosis.

RADIOLOGIC FINDINGS. The left border of the heart may show only two convexities instead of the usual three, the upper convexity commonly displaying a more gradual slope than usually associated with the pulmonary artery of a normal heart. This convexity is produced by the ascending aorta as it arches upward from its lateral position of origin to cross over the left pulmonary artery (instead of to the right as is usually the case) before descending. The medially placed pulmonary artery is not borderforming. By virtue of its posterior location it may cause an inden-

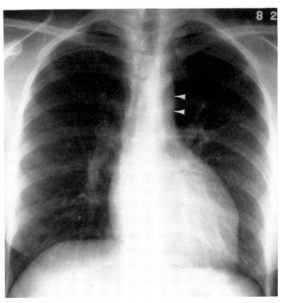

FIG. 321. CORRECTED TRANSPOSITION IN A PATIENT SUSPECTED OF HAVING ENDOCARDIAL FIBROELASTOSIS. NO EVIDENCE OF A SHUNT WAS FOUND. ARROWS INDICATE ASCENDING AORTA

tation on the barium-filled esophagus below the area of the normal indentation of the aortic arch. If some degree of mesoversion or dextroversion is present, the main mass of the heart may lie to the right of the spine. Other plain film findings will depend on the presence of complicating defects.

Selective angiocardiography is the most valuable diagnostic procedure for the identification of corrected transposition of the great vessels. The anteroposterior and lateral views are recommended. As seen in the frontal projection, the contour of the right-sided (venous) ventricle is roughly triangular in shape with the apex pointed downward and the base at the bicuspid valve ring. The apex of the triangle actually forms a tail-like projection that extends far towards the left border of the heart. The pulmonary artery originates from the superior side of the triangle and near the midline of the heart. The pulmonary valve is low, and the outflow tract is smooth without evidence of the usual conal structures. The interior of the ventricle is relatively smooth with a fine trabecular structure. The pulmonary artery courses almost straight upwards and parallel to the spine. The pulmonary valve is lower than the aortic valve. The arterial ventricle is rounded and located above the tail of the right-sided venous ventricle. The aortic semilunar valve is high and often can be identified above a definite conal structure with an indentation due to the crista supraventricularis. The aorta extends upwards and is inclined slightly towards the midline and forms the left border of the cardiovascular contour.

In the lateral view, the venous ventricle is anterior and somewhat triangular in shape with the base of the triangle above and the apex near the diaphragm. The pulmonary artery originates posteriorly and arches posteriorly. The arterial ventricle is posterior and is rounded and shows a coarse trabecular structure. A definite indentation in the outflow tract in the lateral view posteriorly is due to the crista supraventricularis, and this usually identifies a definite conus structure. Although the arterial ventricle is somewhat posterior, the ascending aorta is anterior and is anterior to the pulmonary artery. It is often just underneath the sternum.

With mesocardia and lesser degrees of dextrocardia, the contours of the ventricles are more distorted and are thus more difficult to identify. The venous ventricle is more posterior, and the arterial ventricle is more anterior. Their typical shape may be distorted, and thus identification is more difficult. With well marked dextrocardia, the arterial ventricle may form part of the right-sided apex of the heart. The ascending aorta is

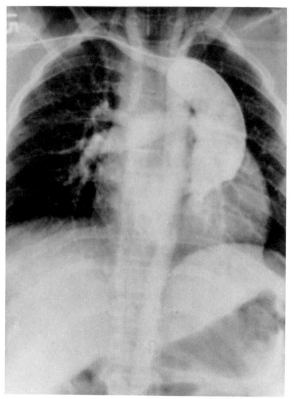

FIG. 322. CORRECTED TRANSPOSITION OF GREAT VESSELS AND VENTRICULAR SEPTAL DEFECT

(From Dotter, C. T. and *American Journal of Roentgenology, 83:* 978, by permission.) (See also Fig. 308 for example of connected transposition with dextrocardia.)

anterior, and the pulmonary artery is posterior, and both are to the right of the midline. Identification of the two ventricles is more difficult and depends on the angiographic morphology described above. Differentiation from a single ventricle (common AV valve) may be difficult, particularly when the rudimentary ventricle associated with the latter condition is a large structure.

A left ventriculogram should always be obtained because of the high incidence of anomalies of the mitral valve with resultant mitral insufficiency.

Associated congenital defects are demonstrated in the usual way using angiography and physiological data obtained from cardiac catheterization.

Surgical treatment is required only for the correction of associated cardiovascular defects (Beck *et al.,* 1961). Anomalous distribution of the coronary arteries and conduction system may offer a formidable obstacle to repair of pulmonary stenosis and interventricular septal defects via ventriculotomy of the right-sided ventricle, and in such cases a transatrial approach may be desirable (Ellis *et al.,* 1962).

ANOMALIES OF THE GREAT VESSELS WITHOUT SIGNIFICANT CIRCULATORY CHANGES

Aortic Arch

The definitive aorta and its major branches and the pulmonary trunk and its right and left branches develop from six pairs of branchial arches that connect the primitive ventral aorta and the aortic sac with the right and left dorsal aortas. The transformation from the embryonal stage takes place by a continuing series of migrations and consecutive obliterations of various segments of this primitive vascular network (Fig. 324).

The first and second arches regress early, but the anterior (cephalic) portions of the dorsal aortas persist as part of the internal carotid arteries bilaterally. The third arches bilaterally remain as part of the definitive common and internal carotid arteries. The left fourth arch, the proximal portion of the left ventral aorta, and the left half of the aortic sac persist as the definitive aorta. As the left side of the aortic sac elongates, the left common carotid artery comes to originate from the aortic arch. The right half of the aortic sac elongates to form the innominate artery, and the right fourth arch continues as a permanent right subclavian artery. The more distal portion of the right fourth arch between the origin of the subclavian and the distal fused dorsal aorta is obliterated. The fifth arches disappear completely. The proximal portions of the sixth arches remain as the right and left pulmonary arteries; the distal portion of the left arch persists as the ductus or ligamentum arteriosum,

and the distal portion of the right sixth arch usually disappears. Failure to follow this developmental pattern can theoretically produce a large number of anomalous arrangements of the great vessels and their branches.

A classification of these anomalies has been placed on a logical and embryologically sound basis by Stewart et al. (1964). Their point of departure is the primitive almost completely symmetrical aortic arch system (Fig. 325). Failure of regression or regression of one or two specific segments and one or both ductus arteriosi can produce a normal arch and most of the commonly recognized variations. When this system is applied, some 24 different arrangements can be expected. The classification listed below is modified from that of Stewart et al. (1964) in that the hypothetic and rarer forms have been

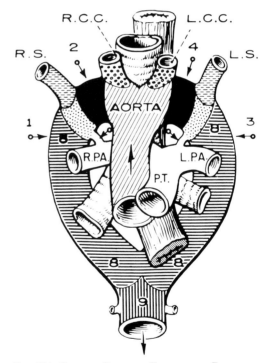

Fig. 324. Schema Showing Embryonal Basis for Origin of Vascular Rings and Related Malformations

Ventral view of Edwards' hypothetic double aortic arch and bilateral ductus arteriosi. Arrows point to the four key locations where regression occurs that leads to a normal left arch or one of the anomalous arrangements. Arrow 1 indicates the eighth segment of the right dorsal aortic root; arrow 2, the right fourth arch, arrows 3 and 4, the corresponding two positions on the left. (With permission, from J. R. Stewart, O. W. Kincaid, and J. E. Edwards, *An Atlas of Vascular Rings and Related Malformations of the Aortic Arch System,* Springfield, Ill., Charles C Thomas, Publisher, 1964.)

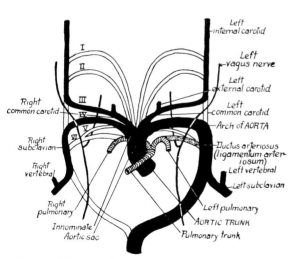

Fig. 323. Diagram Illustrates Transformation of Aortic Arches

For further description see text. (From H. E. Jordan and J. E. Kindred, *Textbook of Embryology,* New York, Appleton-Century-Crofts, Inc., 1926.)

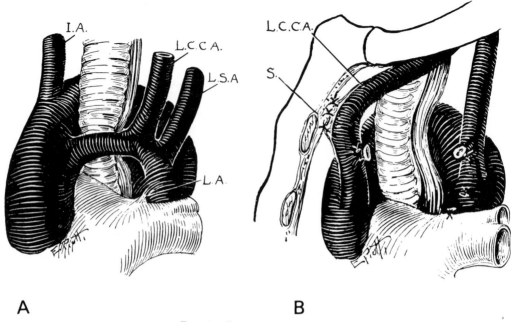

A   **B**

FIG. 325. DOUBLE AORTIC ARCH

(A) The ascending aorta divides into two limbs which subsequently join to form the descending aorta. (B) Appearance after surgical treatment. The anterior limb has been severed between the left common carotid and left subclavian arteries. IA, innominate artery; LA, ligamentum arteriosum; LCCA, left common carotid artery; LSA, left subclavian artery; S, sternum. (Courtesy of Drs. R. E. Gross and P. F. Ware, *Surgery, Gynecology and Obstetrics, 83:* 437, 1946.)

omitted so that attention is focused on the commoner and more significant variations.

Classification Modified from Stewart *et al.* (1964)

A. Aortic arch
  1. Double aortic arch
    a. Both arches patent
    b. One arch atretic
  2. Left aortic arch
    a. Normal branching and minor variations
    b. Aberrant right subclavian artery
      (1) Left ductus arteriosus
      (2) Right ductus arteriosus
    c. Isolation of right subclavian artery from aorta
  3. Right aortic arch
    a. Mirror image branching
      (1) Left ductus arteriosus
      (2) Right ductus arteriosus
      (3) Bilateral ductus arteriosi
    b. Aberrant left subclavian artery
      (1) Left ductus arteriosus
    c. Isolation of left subclavian artery from aorta
      (1) Left ductus arteriosus
  4. Cervical aortic arch
  5. Pseudocoarctation of aorta
B. Pulmonary arteries
  1. Anomalous left pulmonary artery (pulmonary sling)
  2. Idiopathic dilatation of the pulmonary artery
  3. Proximal interruption of one pulmonary artery
  4. Coarctations of the pulmonary arteries

"Ductus arteriosus" signifies either a patent ductus arteriosus or a ligamentum arteriosum.

Double Aortic Arch. a. When both arches are patent, the ascending aorta divides anterior to the trachea into two branches (Fig. 326), the right and left arches which pass around the trachea and esophagus to unite posteriorly to form the descending aorta. Each arch gives rise to a common carotid and a subclavian artery in a rather symmetrical fashion. The aorta may descend on the right or left side, although a left-sided aorta seems to be more common in the operated cases (13 of 21 cases operated upon by Gross, 1953). Typically or more frequently (Stewart *et al.*, 1964; Gross, 1953, pages 413–435) the arches are of different sizes with the left often being the smaller. A left ductus is usually present extending between the left pulmonary artery and the left arch. Although the literature constantly refers to one or the other arch as being located anteriorly, in the autopsy cases observed by the authors, it would have been difficult to say which arch was anterior (Fig. 326).

This anomaly may be symptomless and encountered in adults, but in the majority of cases it produces symptoms during the first 6 months or year of life. The symptoms may be difficulty in nursing or swallowing, regurgitation of feedings, inspiratory stridor, fits of coughing, and cyanosis. Respiratory infections are common.

The radiologic signs of double aortic arch were described by Neuhauser (1946) and Griswold and Young (1949). Neuhauser found no abnormality in the PA chest film, although in a case seen by the authors the vascular shadows at the base of the heart appeared wider than normal. Occasionally the trachea which normally is slightly deviated toward the right shows a slight deviation to the left. An enlarged thymus may obscure this area and make appraisal of supposedly abnormal shadows hazardous. A well-exposed lateral film may be quite helpful in that the trachea can often be seen to be narrowed and displaced forward at the level of the aortic arch. Fluoroscopy following barium swallow and particularly the use of cinefluorography are very helpful. When the esophagus is distended with barium mixture, a bilateral indentation at the level of the aortic arch is seen producing some degree of constriction. The indentation on one side of the esophagus may be slightly larger than on the opposite side (Fig. 328). In the far oblique and lateral projections a large posterior impression is usually seen, and typically there is a slightly smaller and higher impression anteriorly. At fluoroscopy these impressions can be seen to be due to pulsating masses which represent the bilateral arches. If the trachea can be seen to be angled or buckled in a slightly anterior direction at the same level as the anterior indentation on the esophagus, this is excellent evidence of a symptomatic vascular ring.

Neuhauser (1946) found what appeared to be erosion of one or more of the upper thoracic vertebrae at the level of the posterior arch and attributed this to pulsations from the aorta.

Although the conventional radiologic studies may strongly suggest the presence of a vascular ring, Neuhauser recommends the instillation of iodized oil into the trachea for confirmation. A tracheogram will show an indentation on the posterior surface of the trachea at the same level as the indentation in the esophagus.

Gross (1953) has had considerable experience with vascular rings and indicates that an exact preoperative delineation of the anatomy of the ring is not necessary since the surgical approach is the same for all, namely, a left-sided approach. Our experience, however, could not entirely confirm this opinion. We agree that a precise delineation of the anatomy of the constricting ring is not always possible. However, in one of our recent cases the most advantageous place for in-

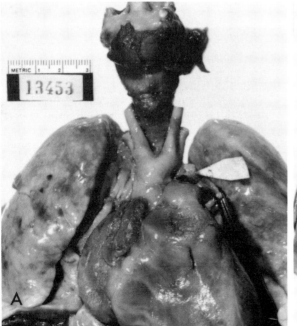 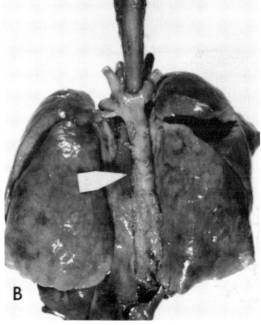

FIG. 326. DOUBLE AORTIC ARCH WITH BOTH ARCHES PATENT (AUTOPSY SPECIMEN FROM CASE SHOWN IN FIG. 327)
(A) Anterior view. The large arrow points to a severed ductus. The carotid and subclavian arteries originated in a symmetrical arrangement form each arch. (B) Posterior view. The arrow points to the esophagus which is to the left of the descending aorta.

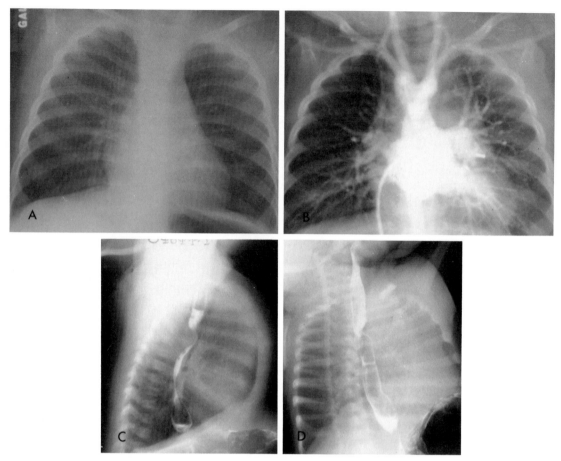

FIG. 327. A 6-MONTH-OLD GIRL WITH HISTORY OF INTERMITTENT RESPIRATORY DIFFICULTY SINCE 5 WEEKS OF AGE
(A) Conventional chest within normal limits. (B) Selective right ventricular angiocardiogram showing a double aortic arch.
Each limb is about the same size. (C and D) Esophagrams showing approximately equal-sized indentations posteriorly and on
the left side forming a ring. The trachea was indented at this same level. (Postmortem specimen is shown in Fig. 326.)

terruption of the ring was on the right side, and
this would have been most easily approached
from the right side of the thorax. We have been
much impressed by the contributions of selective
angiography in this condition. In addition to
confirming the diagnosis, angiography may give
an indication of the relative size of each arch
(Fig. 327B), and this may be helpful in preoperative planning. Surgical treatment consists of
division of the smaller arch. In the experience of
Gross (1953) this was usually the left, but in 3
recent cases seen by the authors the arches were
about the same in size and rather large.

b. When one arch is atretic it is usually the
left. In all of the reported cases (Gross, 1953; also
3 cases quoted in the Atlas of Stewart *et al.*,
1964; Shuford *et al.*, 1972) the left arch was
obliterated, and there are apparently no reported
cases of obliteration of a right arch. In the case
with obliteration of the left arch, the appearance
is similar to that associated with a right arch and

aberrant left subclavian artery or right aortic
arch with mirror image branching, and preoperative differentiation even by angiography is most
difficult.

Left Aortic Arch. (a) With normal branching
and minor variations, the predominant pattern
of the large vessels originating from the aortic
arch (the brachiocephalic vessels) is that of three
branches, namely the innominate, left common
carotid, and subclavian arteries. This pattern is
found in about 60–80% (Bosniak, 1964) of persons
in the United States, depending somewhat on
the racial extraction of the sample. As few as one
branch and as many as six vessels have been
described as originating from the aortic arch
(Gray, 1942). The common patterns are shown
in Figure 329, although this might vary from
sample to sample. As can be seen, the commonest
variation consists of a closer relationship of the
origin of the left carotid artery to the innominate,
and in about 8% the left common carotid artery

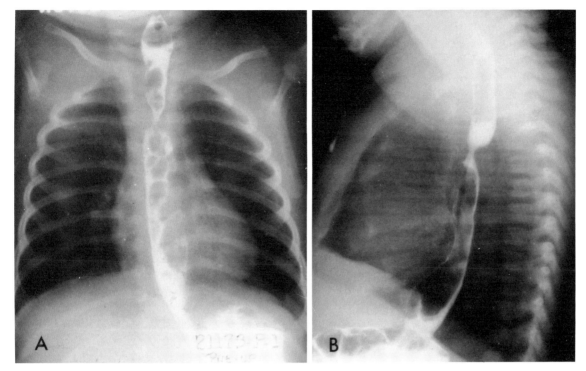

FIG. 328. ESOPHAGRAM WITH DOUBLE AORTIC ARCH
The indentations on the esophagus are of approximately equal size.

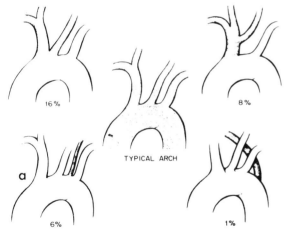

FIG. 329. ORIGIN OF BRACHIOCEPHALIC VESSELS
Incidence of common variations in the origin of the bra-
chiocephalic vessels as determined from 100 arch aortograms.
The shaded vessel in (a) is the vertebral artery. (Courtesy of
Dr. M. A. Bosniak, *American Journal of Roentgenology,
Radium Therapy and Nuclear Medicine*, 91: 1223, 1964.)

arises from the innominate. Most of these variations are of little if any clinical importance. Attempts to perform vertebral angiography from
the left side may be frustrated, however, due to
the anomalous position of the artery if it arises
from the arch. Also, statements as to occlusion
of any of the arteries at their origin or their
absence may be in error unless there is an accompanying satisfactory arch aortogram. Differences
in size of the two vertebral arteries may occur
normally in 45% of presumably normal persons
(Bosniak, 1964).

Gross (1953) operated on cases in which the
innominate artery originated from the aortic
arch somewhat farther to the left than usual so
that the artery crossed the trachea from left to
right. Apparently the crucial feature is the length
of this vessel, and if it is short and taut, it may
produce tracheal compression. This may be seen
on a good lateral or oblique film of the chest. A
similar condition occurs when the left carotid
artery originates farther to the right than usual
and winds around the anterior surface of the
trachea. Gross (1953) described this anomaly in
3 patients where there was tracheal compression
which was relieved by freeing up the left carotid
and attaching it to the sternum.

A left aortic arch with a right ductus arteriosus
is exceedingly rare. Apparently one of the patients described by Paul (1948) had such a condition, and this was associated with a right descending aorta. The ductus might conceivably
exert pressure on the posterior esophageal wall
and in effect form a ring.

(b) Aberrant right subclavian artery

(1) Left ductus arteriosus. This is the commonest anomaly in this area and is said to occur in 0.4–0.8% of bodies found in anatomical laboratories (Sprague *et al.*, 1933).

If the proximal portion of the right aortic arch (Segment 2—Fig. 324) is obliterated instead of Segment 1, then the right subclavian artery will remain attached to the distal portion of the left arch and will then become the last branch originating from the arch. This artery crosses behind the esophagus to reach its distribution in the right shoulder and arm. According to Stewart *et al.* (1964) no unquestioned or proved cases have been found in which this vessel crossed anterior to the esophagus or anterior to the trachea, although quoted reports of these two variations have been carried in the literature for years (Neuhauser, 1946; Stauffer and Pote, 1946). The point of origin is from the distal arch or the upper descending aorta, and it varies from the level of the third to the fourth thoracic vertebral segment and may be from the superior, medial, or lateral wall of the aorta. The vessel courses obliquely upward (cephalad) toward the right.

The frequency with which this anomaly produces detectable radiologic changes is undetermined since many cases must remain undetected. The site of origin of the aberrant vessel may be visible on a PA chest film, particularly if it is on the superior or lateral surface of the aorta. The most striking radiologic change is due to a cir-

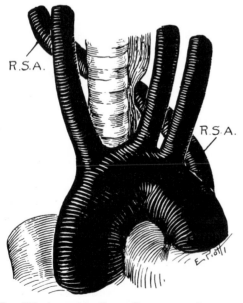

FIG. 330. ABERRANT RIGHT SUBCLAVIAN ARTERY
RSA, right subclavian artery. (Courtesy of Drs. R. E. Gross and P. F. Ware, *Surgery, Gynecology and Obstetrics,* 83: 441, 1946.)

cular indentation in the posterior surface of the barium-filled esophagus best seen in the lateral projection. Frequently in the PA projection following a barium swallow, an oblique stripe of decreased density is noted coursing obliquely upward, toward the right (Fig. 331A). The esophagus is not dilated proximal to the indentation, and there is usually no obstruction to the act of swallowing. In fact, the condition is often discovered during a routine gastrointestinal examination and fluoroscopy of the esophagus. This condition was originally described as producing "dysphagia lusoria" (Bayford, quoted from Stauffer and Pote, 1946) and Gross (1953) has reported good results following ligation of this vessel in 12 patients varying between 6 weeks and 6 years of age, all of whom apparently had some difficulty in swallowing. Stewart *et al.* (1964), however, feel that the anomaly seldom if ever can be proved to be the cause of a "lump in the throat" or dysphagia. Figure 332 shows the case of a 50-year-old woman who had complained of dysphagia. Esophagoscopy showed a pulsating indentation on the posterior esophageal wall, and the retroesophageal artery appeared dilated, probably due to atherosclerosis. This condition may be found as an incidental finding associated with other congenital anomalies, such as coarctation of the aorta and tetralogy of Fallot.

(2) Right ductus arteriosus is apparently quite rare, and only 2 cases are presented in the Atlas of Stewart *et al.* (1964). The ductus which extends from the right pulmonary artery to the descending aorta passes behind the esophagus. Also, the entire aorta may be shifted to the right or there may be a diverticulum at the site of origin of the aberrant subclavian artery so that a large impression should be seen on the posterior surface of the esophagus. Although there have been no cases reported in which this condition has been diagnosed by radiologic means, it is the mirror image of a right aortic arch with an aberrant left subclavian artery and should produce similar radiologic changes except that the position of the soft tissue shadow of the aorta should be reversed. This condition should be considered whenever there is evidence of a vascular ring with an obvious left-sided arch. For isolation of right subclavian artery from aorta see page 406.

3 Right Aortic Arch. a Mirror image branching. This anomaly is a mirror image of the normal left aortic arch and is due to a persistence of the right fourth branchial arch as the definitive aorta, whereas the left arch becomes the left subclavian artery. This arrangement is relatively common. It is the rule with mirror image dextro-

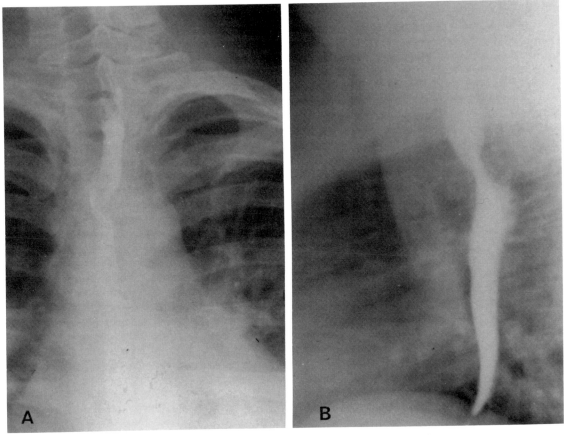

FIG. 331. ABERRANT RIGHT SUBCLAVIAN ARTERY IN ASYMPTOMATIC PATIENT

cardia and situs inversus viscerum. Also, it is seen in about 20–25% of cases of tetralogy of Fallot (Taussig, 1960), is common in truncus arteriosus, and is occasionally seen in tricuspid atresia (5%—Keith *et al.*, 1967). Agenesis of the left pulmonary artery is also occasionally encountered in association with tetralogy of Fallot.

Typically the aorta courses upward and backward over the right main bronchus and descends to the right of the vertebral column. The first major vessel to take origin from the aorta, other than the coronary arteries, is the left innominate artery which divides into the left common carotid and left subclavian arteries. The next branch is the right common carotid followed by the right subclavian artery.

The following variations in the arrangement of the ductus arteriosus may be encountered:

(1) Left ductus arteriosus. With a left ductus arteriosus and a right aortic arch, the ductus may extend from the left pulmonary artery to the innominate or left subclavian artery or to a diverticulum which represents a persistent left dorsal root of the right-sided descending aorta. This latter arrangement may form a ring (Stewart *et* *al.*, 1964) but apparently is much rarer than the arrangement where the ductus communicates with the innominate or left subclavian artery.

(2) Right ductus arteriosus. This, of course, is a mirror image of the normal in that the ductus extends from the right pulmonary artery to the aorta. This arrangement is occasionally encountered and should produce no significant symptoms.

(3) Bilateral ductus arteriosi. This arrangement is quite rare. A ring could be produced if the left ductus communicated with the descending aorta.

Usually a right-sided aorta with mirror image branching produces no symptoms per se but is often associated with some significant cardiac malformation. In establishing an artificial ductus by the Blalock technique, it is preferable to use the subclavian artery that arises from the innominate artery. Also, the Potts operation consisting of establishing an opening between the left pulmonary artery and aorta cannot be carried out unless the upper descending aorta is on the left. Consequently, it is of considerable practical importance to determine preoperatively on which

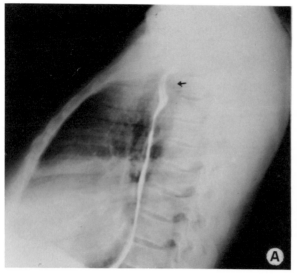
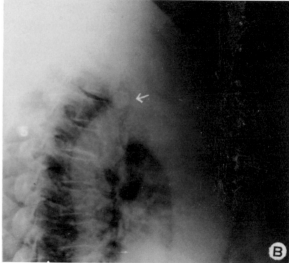

FIG. 332. ABERRANT RIGHT SUBCLAVIAN ARTERY

Fifty-two-year-old patient with symptoms of dysphagia for 2–3 months. On esophagoscopy a pulsating mass indenting the esophagus posteriorly was found and thought to be an aneurysm. (A) The indentation is slightly larger than is usually seen with a retroesophageal subclavian artery. (B) The artery fills readily in the lateral angiocardiogram.

side the aortic arch lies. In children, this is best done by fluoroscopy following a barium swallow. The aortic knob in children is often quite small and may be invisible on the conventional chest film, although careful inspection may show a shallow indentation on the trachea. This is particularly so with a right aortic arch. At fluoroscopy the pulsations of the aorta may permit its identification as a right-sided impression on the esophagus. In older patients a conventional chest film often suffices to determine the site of the aortic arch (Fig. 335A).

b Aberrant left subclavian artery

(1) Left ductus arteriosus. The incidence of this anomaly is difficult to determine, but it is probably the most common type of right aortic arch (Shuford, Sybers, and Edwards, 1970). Since it is usually asymptomatic, it is often encountered by chance in routine examinations of the chest; however, it may form a vascular ring sufficiently tight to produce symptoms. Gross (1955) noted that symptoms of esophageal or tracheal obstruction were usually later in onset than with double aortic arch. In adults symptoms may appear following elongation and dilatation of the aorta due to atherosclerosis. By referring to Figure 324, it can be seen that the anomaly is due to obliteration of Segment 4; the left dorsal arch persists as the left subclavian artery and sometimes there is an additional diverticulum. In this malforma-

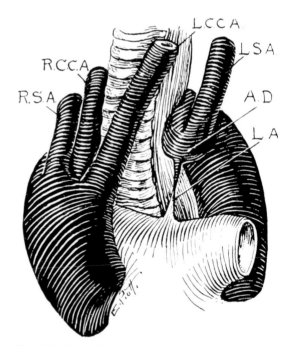

FIG. 333. RIGHT AORTIC ARCH WITH PERSISTENT LEFT AORTIC DIVERTICULUM GIVING RISE TO LEFT SUBCLAVIAN ARTERY AND LIGAMENTUM ARTERIOSUM

AD, aortic diverticulum; LA, ligamentum arteriosum; LCCA, left common carotid artery; LSA, left subclavian artery; RCCA, right common carotid artery; RSA, right subclavian artery. (Courtesy of Drs. R. E. Gross and P. F. Ware, *Surgery, Gynecology and Obstetrics, 83:* 437, 1946.)

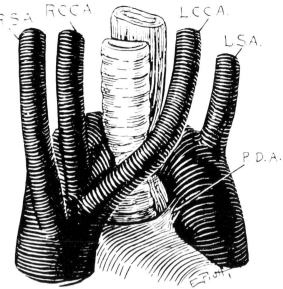

FIG. 334. RIGHT AORTIC ARCH WITH LEFT DESCENDING AORTA AND ANTERIOR ANOMALOUS LEFT COMMON CAROTID ARTERY AND SHORT LIGAMENTUM ARTERIOSUM WHICH IS ATTACHED TO LEFT PULMONARY ARTERY

LCCA, left common carotid artery; LSA, left subclavian artery; PDA, patient ductus arteriosus; RCCA, right common carotid artery; RSA, right subclavian artery. (Courtesy of Drs. R. E. Gross and P. F. Ware, *Surgery, Gynecology and Obstetrics, 83:* 437, 1946.)

tion, the first major branch of the aorta is the left common carotid artery followed by the right common carotid and then the right subclavian arteries, and the left subclavian artery is the last branch. The left subclavian artery may originate from the descending aorta which may deviate somewhat toward the right or it may originate from a diverticulum. A ligamentum arteriosum may connect the left pulmonary artery with the descending aorta or with a diverticulum thus completing a vascular ring (Figs. 333 and 334).

As seen on the conventional PA chest film, the aortic knob is on the right rather than the left side (Fig. 335A) and is usually higher (more cephalad) than expected for the age of the patient. Occasionally a rounded shadow will present to the left of the upper mediastinum and just a little below the level of the right-sided aortic knob. This represents a diverticulum or a remnant of the left dorsal fourth arch that gives origin to the left subclavian artery, or in some cases it may represent increased tortuosity of the upper part of the descending aorta. This shadow may be of such size and configuration as to suggest the presence of a left-sided aortic knob. The most striking findings occur following filming and fluoroscopy after a barium swallow. This shows a large rounded posterior indentation on

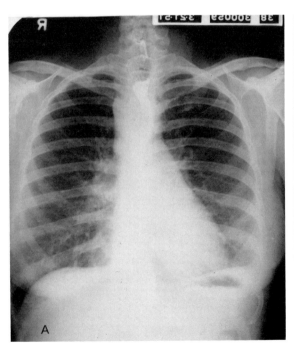

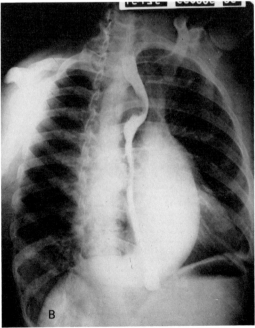

FIG. 335. POSTEROANTERIOR AND RIGHT ANTERIOR OBLIQUE PROJECTIONS OF RIGHT AORTIC ARCH WITH LEFT DESCENDING AORTA

This was an incidental finding in a 38-year-old nurse.

the esophagus just below the level of the right-sided aortic knob. The curvature of the indentation suggests the presence of a vessel 3 cm or more in diameter. Also, the esophagus may be deviated slightly toward the left. Oblique and lateral views usually show no distinct evidence of an anterior or left-sided impression, such as is seen in double aortic arch. Occasionally, as reported by Neuhauser (1946) and Felson and Palayew (1963), a double posterior indentation is seen. An upper smaller notch is due to the aberrant left subclavian artery, and a larger inferior indentation is due to the aorta or a diverticulum. The trachea is usually indented slightly on the right side and posteriorly. The aorta may descend near the midline on the right or left side. Felson and Palayew (1963) reported a predominance of right-sided descent.

The differentiation of the anomaly from a double aortic arch has not posed a problem in the authors' experience since most of the cases encountered have been in adults without symptoms. In symptomatic cases, particularly in children, a few differential signs should be looked for. In double aortic arch, the right-sided and posterior impression on the esophagus should be smaller than in the case with a right-sided aorta since the right arch in the case of double arch is smaller than the aorta itself and carries only a part of the total blood flow. Also, a double posterior impression suggesting an aberrant subclavian artery above and the aorta below is quite suggestive of a right aortic arch with an aberrant left subclavian artery. Angiography will clearly show a double arch unless one arch is quite small or atretic, in which case differentiation by any means short of surgical exploration may be impossible.

Stewart *et al.* (1964) indicate that a right arch with mirror image branching and a left-sided ductus joining the left pulmonary artery with a right descending aorta might form a ring that would be impossible to differentiate from the above conditions. This, of course, is quite rare.

c Isolation of left subclavian artery from aorta.

Either subclavian artery may be isolated from the aorta. With a left arch, the right subclavian artery may originate from the right pulmonary artery, and with a right arch, the left subclavian artery may originate from the left pulmonary artery. In each case the communication is effected through a ductus arteriosus, but this structure may be strand-like and transmit little or no blood. In the two patients reported by Shuford *et al.* (1970) and in the single case we have encountered, a right aortic arch was present with isolation of the left subclavian artery. The clinical findings resulted from relative ischemia of the left upper extremity. Aortography showed no

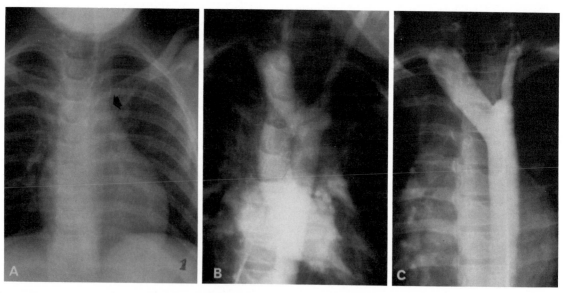

FIG. 336. RIGHT AORTIC ARCH WITH AORTIC DIVERTICULUM AND ABERRANT LEFT SUBCLAVIAN ARTERY
Nine-year-old white girl. No symptoms referable to a vascular ring. On the conventional chest film (A) the diverticulum gives the appearance of a small aortic knob (arrow). (B) Angiogram following left atrial injection. The right-sided aortic arch extends upward into the neck and is above the clavicle. (C) Retrograde aortogram showing aortic diverticulum and left subclavian artery.

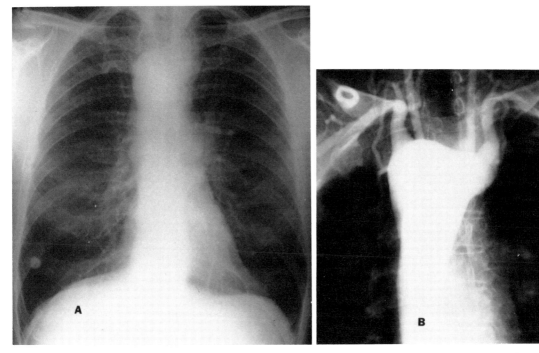

FIG. 337. RIGHT AORTIC ARCH WITH ABERRANT LEFT SUBCLAVIAN ARTERY IN AN ELDERLY MALE WITHOUT SYMPTOMS (A) Chest film showing "mass" to right of trachea. (B) Frontal aortogram. The aorta is dilated probably due to atherosclerosis. The aorta descends to the right of the midline.

evidence of a left subclavian artery arising from the aortic arch, and selective injection of the right vertebral artery showed retrograde flow down the left vertebral artery which then filled the isolated left subclavian (Fig. 338).

Most reports of isolation of the left subclavian artery have been in patients with a right aortic arch and tetralogy of Fallot, but this anomaly has also been seen in patients with no evidence of congenital heart disease.

4 Cervical Aortic Arch. In this anomaly the ascending aorta arises normally from the left ventricle and extends upward in such a manner that the aortic arch is situated high in the neck on either side. Twelve cases have been reported in the literature, two on the left and ten with the aortic arch on the right side of the neck (Shuford et al., 1972). In all cases a pulsatile mass was felt above the clavicle. In none of the reported cases has the cervical aortic arch malformation been associated with intracardiac congenital heart disease.

Widening of the mediastinum may be the only abnormality displayed on an ordinary chest film. The trachea may be displaced forward by the retroesophageal position of the distal arch, and the shadow of the aortic knob is absent. Barium swallow shows a posterior compression defect from the retroesophageal position of the distal arch. The esophagus may be displaced laterally in the neck by the cervical aorta. Aortography displays an aorta which ascends into the neck either to the right or left side, making a hairpin loop at the apex of the arch and crossing the midline behind the esophagus as the arch returns to the thorax to descend alongside the spine opposite the side of the arch.

5 Kinking or Buckling of Aorta (Pseudocoarctation). Kinking or buckling of the aorta is a condition in which the arch and the first portion of the descending aorta are elongated, usually somewhat dilated, and sharply deviated or indented. The condition appears to be congenital in origin and has been encountered in the second decade of life (Steinberg and Hagstrom, 1962) before atherosclerosis could have been a factor. Atherosclerosis in later life may increase the aortic deformity and exaggerate the radiologic features of this condition. Since the report of Souders et al. (1951), about 40 cases have been reported (Stevens, 1958; Pattinson and Grainger, 1959; Saric et al., 1960; Steinberg and Hagstom, 1962; Griffin, 1964). The importance of the condition is that it produces an

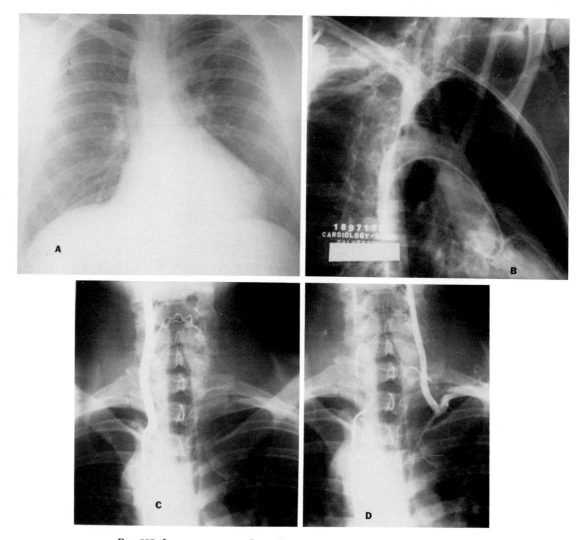

FIG. 338. ISOLATION OF THE LEFT SUBCLAVIAN ARTERY FROM THE AORTA

A right aortic arch is displayed in A. The aortogram in B shows filling of the left and right common carotid arteries and the right subclavian artery. In C the large right vertebral artery has been selectively injected, and D shows retrograde flow down the left vertebral artery, filling the isolated left subclavian artery.

easily discernible widening of the left upper mediastinum as seen on the conventional chest film, and this has been confused with a mediastinal neoplasm or enlarged mediastinal lymph nodes. The condition is benign and usually asymptomatic. The anomaly does resemble coarctation of the aorta in that the first part of the descending aorta is deviated sharply toward the midline at the site of the ligamentum arteriosum, producing a lateral indentation in the aortic contour. Slight narrowing of the aorta may occur, and undoubtedly the redundancy causes increased turbulence in this region. The narrowing is insufficient to produce a significant gradient, although a murmur may be noted over the base of

the heart, and a delay in the femoral pulse has been observed (Griffin, 1964).

In the conventional PA chest film a rounded or oval opacity presents high in the left mediastinum. It may be behind the sternoclavicular joint and extend well above this level. The opacity may be slightly less dense than the normal aortic knob, although this is certainly not a striking feature. The lower rounded margin of the opacity fuses with a denser slightly convex shadow that is continuous with the descending aorta. At the point of this intersection an indentation of the left lateral margin is seen, and this represents the site of the redundancy or infolding. The denser inferior shadow is due to the descending aorta but may be mistaken for the normal aortic knob. In some instances, the knob may appear large and not quite so high with an indentation below, and the resemblance to coarctation is thus striking. Notching of the ribs has not been found in this condition, however. The segment of aorta between the left carotid and left subclavian arteries is typically increased, and the left subclavian artery may originate below the kink. In our case (Fig. 339), the right subcla-

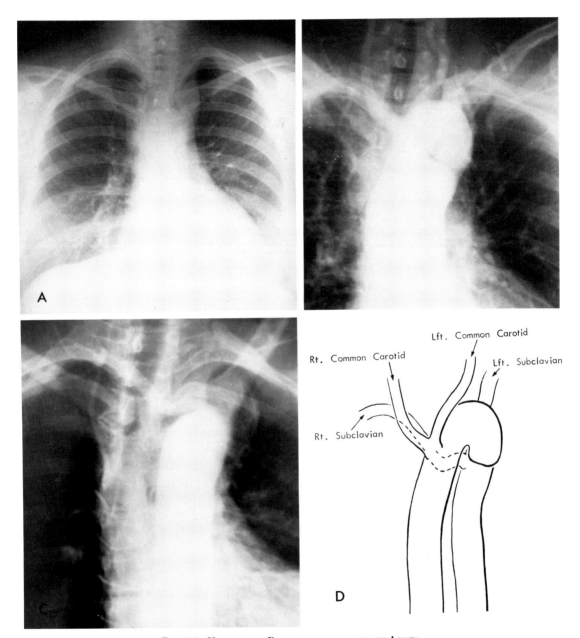

FIG. 339. KINKING OR PSEUDOCOARCTATION OF AORTA

Asymptomatic 33-year-old white woman who came to the hospital because of a mass in the left upper mediastinum discovered on a routine chest film. Blood pressure was normal in arms but was about 10–12 mm lower in legs. (A) PA chest film showing shadow in upper mediastinum with identation on lateral aspect at point where mass joined what was thought to be the aortic knob. (B) Intravenous aortogram showing indentation in aorta. (C) Retrograde thoracic aortogram with injection below area of kinking. (D) The aberrant right subclavian is demonstrated. It passed to the right behind the esophagus. At operation the aorta was drawn medially and severely kinked at the site of insertion of the ligamentum arteriosum. No gradient across the area of kinking was found.

vian was the last branch and originated below the kink. The indentation is perhaps best demonstrated by rotation of about 30° into the left anterior oblique position. Laminography may be helpful in outlining the anatomy of the region. The diagnosis can be strongly suspected from the conventional radiologic examination, but angiography is the definitive diagnostic procedure and when combined with normal hemodynamics is sufficient to establish the diagnosis.

Endocardial fibroelastosis and bicuspid aortic valve have been observed associated with this condition (Steinberg and Hagstrom, 1962).

Pulmonary Vascular Anomalies

Anomalous Left Pulmonary Artery (Pulmonary Sling). In this anomaly, the pulmonary trunk gives origin to a left-sided ductus arteriosus and then continues to the right for a considerable distance before giving origin to a sizeable vessel that serves as the left pulmonary artery. Stewart et al. (1964) feel that the left pulmonary artery in this condition is absent and that the branch from the right pulmonary artery is a collateral vessel. Other authors (Potts et al., 1954; Wittenborg et al., 1956) speak of anomalous left pulmonary artery. At any rate, a sizeable artery arises from the right pulmonary artery, crosses the right main stem bronchus and then courses between the trachea and esophagus to enter the hilus of the left lung. It often constricts the right main stem bronchus producing either atelectasis or emphysema, and pulmonary infection is common. Associated defects within the heart have also been common (Stewart et al., 1964).

The reported cases have been in infants and young children, and there has been a history of respiratory infection and stridor. The stridor is said to be expiratory instead of inspiratory as in most vascular rings.

The radiologic findings are quite helpful in diagnosis, and the angiographic findings should be specific. With barium in the esophagus, an anterior indentation is noted just above the carina and well below the aortic arch. The trachea may show a corresponding posterior impression. Differences in radiolucency between the right and left lung may be evident. In our case (Fig. 340) the difference was thought to be due to a decreased blood flow to the left lung rather than to emphysema. Angiocardiograms have demonstrated quite clearly the aberrant or anomalous left pulmonary artery (Stewart et al., 1964; Hiller and McClean, 1957). This artery could be seen forming an arch or a knob above the right pulmonary artery and coursing toward the left lung. In our case the aberrant artery was posterior,

and the blood flow to the right lung was much greater than to the left lung. In our particular case the artery also crossed under the left main stem bronchus.

This condition should be strongly suspected from the PA and lateral chest films and the patient's history. It can be confirmed by angiography. Reconstruction of the left pulmonary artery has been attempted in a number of cases with some success but with a very high operative mortality.

Isolated Dilatation of the Pulmonary Artery (Trunk). Dilatation of the pulmonary trunk and short segments of its major branches may exist as an isolated anomaly; it is occasionally associated with a diminution in size of the aorta and may be due to unequal division of the primitive truncus arteriosus communis. In other cases the course is uncertain. The Marfan syndrome with disease of the arterial wall has been postulated in some cases (Castellanos et al., 1957).

Individuals with this anomaly are healthy and usually symptom-free and often come to a physician's attention because of a murmur discovered incidentally during the course of an examination. Chest pain, sometimes associated with dyspnea, is occasionally found (Braun, 1961).

The most prominent and consistent physical finding is a systolic murmur heard best in the second or third intercostal space to the left of the sternum. The murmur is inconstant and is occasionally accompanied by a thrill. In 3 of 6 patients reported by Kaplan et al. (1953) an inconstant diastolic murmur was also heard in the pulmonic area. The second pulmonic sound is increased in intensity and is often louder than the aortic second sound. Splitting of the first heart sound at the apex was heard in 5 of 13 patients discussed by Deshmukh et al. (1960). A pulmonary diastolic murmur may be heard in about 25% of cases (Challis and May, 1969). Laboratory tests and electrocardiogram are normal.

Cardiac catheterization findings reveal no evidence of intra- or extracardiac shunts. The right ventricular and pulmonary artery pressures are normal, though there may be a small systolic pressure gradient across the pulmonary valve during the systolic ejection phase in some cases. This is thought to be due to the deceleration of blood flow in the dilated pulmonary artery (decreased resistance to flow) rather than true anatomic obstruction of the pulmonary valve. Cardiac output and arterial oxygen saturation are normal.

Plain chest films show a heart of normal size and shape with definite dilatation and promi-

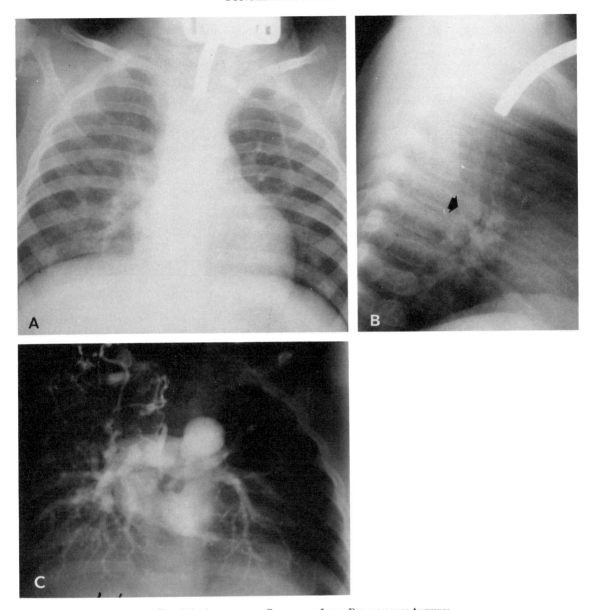

FIG. 340. ANOMALOUS COURSE OF LEFT PULMONARY ARTERY

A 10-month-old white male infant with intermittent respiratory difficulties for several months. (A) PA chest film showing avascularity of the left lung. (B) Lateral film showing opacity posterior to the carina (arrow) due to the anomalous pulmonary artery. (C) Venous angiocardiogram. A striking difference in vascularity between the right and left lung is again demonstrated. The left pulmonary artery was absent. A medium-sized artery originated from the large pulmonary artery to the right of the midline and coursed behind the trachea and over the left main stem bronchus to enter the left lung. (Operative and autopsy case.)

nence of the main pulmonary artery segment, seen best in the posteroanterior and right anterior oblique positions. Occasionally the dilatation extends to the main pulmonary artery branches, but the peripheral vessels are normal (Van Buchem *et al.*, 1955). Fluoroscopically, pulsations may be normal or slightly decreased in amplitude. Angiocardiography may demonstrate the isolated abnormality and show normal mor-

phology and circulatory dynamics otherwise, but as a rule cardiac catheterization is the procedure of choice to rule out other causes of pulmonary artery enlargement.

The diagnosis is made by exclusion and may be considered established if the following criteria are fulfilled:

1. Dilatation of the pulmonary artery without involvement of the rest of the arterial tree.

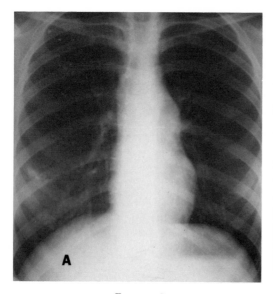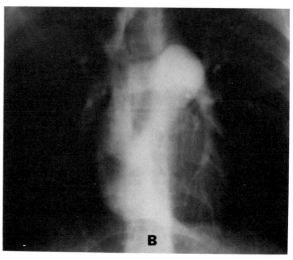

FIG. 341. ISOLATED DILATATION OF THE PULMONARY ARTERY (TRUNK)

The patient has a systolic murmur over the region of the pulmonary artery but no symptoms. (A) Convexity of left mid heart border due to dilated artery. (B) Confirmation by angiography. Right heart catheterization showed normal pressures and a very slight gradient between the right ventricle and pulmonary artery.

2. Absence of intra- or extracardiac shunts.

3. Absence of chronic cardiac or pulmonary disease.

4. Absence of arterial disease (such as lues) and no more than minimal atheromatosis or arteriosclerosis of the pulmonary vascular tree.

5. Normal right ventricular and pulmonary artery pressures.

Differential diagnosis includes chiefly valvular pulmonic stenosis and the causes of left to right shunts. Congenital dilatation of the pulmonary artery is a benign anomaly with a good prognosis. It is important that the diagnosis be established to avoid unnecessary treatment and to avoid restrictions upon the patient's physical activity that may be imposed because of the murmurs.

Proximal Interruption of One Pulmonary Artery. Proximal interruption of a pulmonary artery is the same condition that has been referred to in the literature as "unilateral absence of a pulmonary artery" and "agenesis of a main branch of the pulmonary artery" and other similar terms. Proximal interruption of a pulmonary artery as first used by Kieffer *et al.* (1965) seemed to us to be more appropriate since the distal pulmonary vasculature is often present and at least to a degree functionally adequate. As emphasized by others, this condition should be considered separately from cases of absence of the pulmonary artery associated with agenesis of the lung and also from cases of severe narrowing or coarctation of a pulmonary artery. An excellent discussion of the embryology and its possible

relationship to the development of this condition is given in the review by Pool *et al.* (1962). When the proximal portion of a pulmonary artery is interrupted, blood may reach the peripheral lung vasculature through a patent ductus arteriosus and/or bronchial arteries originating from the arch or descending aorta. Another variation occurs where the proximal right artery is interrupted and the blood supply to the right lung is supplied by a large single artery arising from the ascending aorta. This condition is then identical to one form of a hemitruncus described in the preceding section. In the review of Pool *et al.* (1962), of a total of 78 cases, 7 were found in which this latter arrangement obtained. In the review of Sherrick *et al.* (1962), 9 of 52 cases were of this type, and there were 2 additional cases in which the left lung was supplied from a single large artery originating from the ascending aorta. In 8 other cases a single artery from the innominate artery supplied the right lung. In the majority of cases, however, the blood supply to the involved lung was transmitted through bronchial arteries originating from the arch and descending aorta. It is this bronchial circulation that accounts for the lacy branching vascular pattern of the lung vasculature of the involved lung as seen on the chest film.

Proximal interruption of the pulmonary artery may be an isolated defect (32 of 78 cases—Pool *et al.*, 1962) or may occur in combination with other major anomalies of the heart and great vessels. The majority of patients with isolated lesions have few if any symptoms, and the condition may be first suspected following inspection of a routine chest film, particularly if there is a high index of suspicion. The condition is far from innocuous and is always a threat to the patient's life. Involvement of the normal lung by a pathologic process such as pneumonia or emphysema may bring on severe signs of pulmonary insufficiency. Also, in those cases that have been sufficiently studied pulmonary hypertension has been found in 19% (Pool *et al.*, 1962). Death may occur during early life secondary to pulmonary hypertension and heart failure. Threat of persistent pulmonary hypertension seems to be sufficient indication to attempt to correct the anomaly by a plastic procedure on the obstructed artery. The detection of the condition in early life before the development of vascular changes in the opposite lung would appear to be essential if surgical correction is to be effective (Pool *et al.*, 1962; Kieffer *et al.*, 1965).

In more than half of the reported cases proximal interruption of the pulmonary artery has been found in combination with other major anomalies, such as patent ductus arteriosus, ventricular septal defect, tetralogy of Fallot, patent foramen ovale, aorticopulmonary window and anomalous pulmonary venous return. The interruption of the pulmonary artery has always exerted an additional unfavorable effect. In association with ventricular septal defect and patent ductus arteriosus it has been almost invariably associated with significant pulmonary hypertension. In cases of tetralogy of Fallot the interruption has almost invariably involved the left pulmonary artery with the exception of a single case (Nadas *et al.*, 1953) in which there was a complete situs inversus and the involved artery was on the right side. Interruption of the left pulmonary artery may greatly embarrass the surgeon who is attempting to establish an artificial ductus on the left side using either the Blalock or Potts procedure. It is of some interest that combined defects are considerably more common in association with absence of the left than with absence of the right artery. The interrupted artery is more apt to be on the side opposite to the arch of the aorta, and right aortic arch has been unusually common in those cases with interruption of the left pulmonary artery.

RADIOLOGIC FINDINGS. The diagnosis can often be strongly suspected from inspection of the conventional chest film. This is particularly likely in the isolated cases. Wyman (1954) was the first to collect and describe most of the recognizable changes. The lung on the involved side is slightly hypoplastic as a rule, and this is

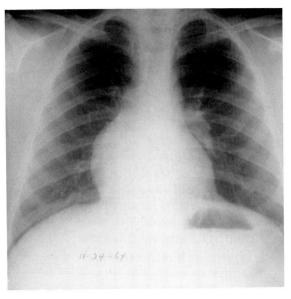

FIG. 342. PROXIMAL INTERRUPTION OF RIGHT PULMONARY ARTERY

reflected in a diminished size of the hemithorax. The rib interspaces on the involved side are narrowed. The diaphragm is often elevated, and the heart is deviated towards the involved side. If observed at fluoroscopy, the mediastinum and the heart do not shift with respiratory motion, such as might be seen with bronchial obstruction. On close inspection the pulmonary vasculature of the involved lung is nearly always different from that of the opposite normal lung. When the blood supply is predominantly through the bronchial arteries, the vascular pattern is fine and reticular or branching in character. The normal hilar vascular shadow on the involved side is absent. Where the heart is shifted the hilar area may be partially obscured, and the detection or evaluation of a hilar shadow therefore may be difficult. Where a single large vessel originating from the aorta supplies the involved lung, an abnormally shaped vascular structure may be identified near or in the hilus. In some instances the findings are identical with those of a "hemitruncus" (see page 354). In some instances the enlarged bronchial arteries originating from the aorta may produce nodular or wormlike hilar shadows. The hilus of the opposite normal lung is often larger or more prominent than normal. Rib notching on the involved side is occasionally seen, and this is secondary to enlargement of the intercostal arteries which participate in the increased collateral flow. This is one of the rare causes of unilateral rib notching. The heart is usually not significantly enlarged. However, since it may be shifted in position, its contour may appear slightly bizarre. Of course, in those cases in which there is an associated major cardiac anomaly, the shape of the heart may reflect the underlying condition.

Kieffer *et al.* (1965) encountered 2 cases in which intermittent pulmonary edema occurred on the side of the normal pulmonary artery.

Angiography. Selective right ventricular angiography is preferable to venous angiography because in addition to giving a better demonstration of the pulmonary artery it is more likely to permit visualization of the left side of the heart and aorta and thus demonstrate the systemic vessels that supply the involved lung. Retrograde aortography may be useful in demonstrating the collateral flow to the involved lung. For practical purposes of diagnosis, it seems to be rarely indicated. In a considerable number of cases there

has been a reverse flow through a patent ductus from the uninvolved pulmonary artery into the descending aorta. This, of course, has been associated with considerable pulmonary hypertension.

Proximal interruption of a pulmonary artery must be differentiated from unilateral pulmonary emphysema, bronchiectasis, coarctation of one of the pulmonary arteries, thrombosis or embolism, and agenesis of one lung.

Selective right ventricular angiography will show a pulmonary vascular system suggestive or typical of the first 3 of these conditions. Pulmonary embolism or thrombosis, particularly if massive, might not be readily differentiated by pulmonary angiography, but the history and symptoms should permit differentiation. In agenesis of the lung the absence of aerated lung is

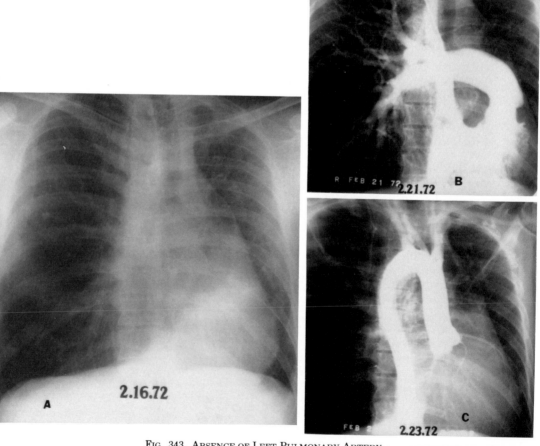

FIG. 343. ABSENCE OF LEFT PULMONARY ARTERY
The left pulmonary artery was absent in a patient with a right aortic arch and minimal respiratory symptoms. (B) Pulmonary angiogram showing large pulmonary arteries to right lung. (C) Aortogram showing right aortic arch and scant collateral blood supply to left lung.

quite different from the picture seen in proximal interruption of the pulmonary artery where the involved lung is usually quite well aerated.

Coarctation(s) of the Pulmonary Artery(ies). Single or multiple narrowings of the pulmonary artery(ies) is a better description of this condition as "coarctation" implies a congenital origin. The majority of reported cases have been associated with other congenital cardiac anomalies (Gay *et al.*, 1963) such as valvular pulmonic stenosis, ASD, VSD, tetralogy of Fallot, and supravalvular aortic stenosis. In 40% of the cases it was an isolated condition. A number of reports indicate that acquired disease may produce similar localized or diffuse narrowing of the pulmonary arteries. These are rubella (Williams and Carey 1966; Rowe, R. D., 1963) and arteritis, probably of the Takayasus type (Gotsman *et al.*, 1967).

Gay *et al.* (1963) have classified the various types according to whether they were central (Types I and II), or peripheral (Type III), or combined central and peripheral (Type IV). Type II (diffuse narrowing at the bifurcation of the main pulmonary artery) tends to occur with the tetralogy of Fallot and may complicate its surgical treatment.

The hemodynamic effects depend on the number, length, and location of the narrowed segments and the nature of the associated cardiac defect, if any. A considerable number have been incidental findings discovered during right heart catheterization or pulmonary angiography. In a majority of reported cases where right heart catheterization was carried out the pulmonary artery pressures were found to be mildly to moderately elevated (Rowe 1963; Gay *et al.*, 1963; Folkeubach *et al.*, 1959). The stenosis may be a cause of a systolic or continuous murmur that is widely transmitted (Rowe, R. D., 1963). Hemoptysis rarely occurs secondary to leaking of the thin walled post stenotic dilatations.

RADIOLOGIC FINDINGS. Since associated cardiac defects are frequent, the conventional chest film may show a cardiac contour suggestive of the cardiac lesion, such as a pulmonic stenosis or VSD. In the isolated cases borderline right-sided enlargement may occasionally be seen in association with pulmonary hypertension—also, some dilatation of the pulmonary artery. In a few instances one of the hilar shadows may be noticeably small or poorly defined in comparison with that of the other side. Difference in vascularity of the two lungs occurs where the stenosis or stenoses are predominantly on one side. This disparity in vascularity may be accentuated when there is an associated left-to-right shunt.

Rarely does the pulmonary parenchymal pattern suggest the diagnosis. The vascular pattern may show nodulation or sausage-shaped shadows

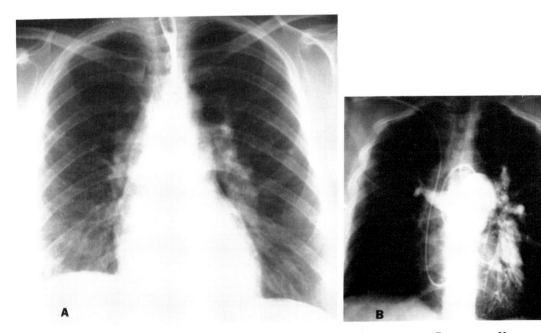

FIG. 344. MULTIPLE COARCTATIONS OF THE PERIPHERAL PULMONARY ARTERIES WITH PULMONARY HYPERTENSION
(A) The left hilus has a nodular appearance, and the descending branch of the left pulmonary artery is broad and nodular. (B) Pulmonary angiogram shows "nodular" obstruction with post-stenotic dilatation. (See also Figs. 132, 133, and 293 for other examples of coarctation of pulmonary arteries.)

due to the multiple stenoses with post stenotic dilatations. In another example the branches of the pulmonary artery were seen to narrow and disappear (Meszaros, 1969).

The diagnosis may be occasionally, and at times, unexpectedly made by right heart catheterization. Careful monitoring of the pressure as the catheter is inserted into the pulmonary artery and its branches will show a drop in pressure where a change is not expected. This should be confirmed by a "pull back" tracing.

Pulmonary angiography is the definitive diagnostic procedure and the injection is preferably made in the right ventricle. Injections into the pulmonary trunk may suffice, but an immediate supravalvular aortic stenosis may be missed. The frontal views will show the peripheral stenosis to advantage—also, the bifurcation of the pulmonary artery. A lateral view will show the pulmonary trunk to good advantage. Oblique views are occasionally indicated to show the left pulmonary artery and to identify or better locate peripheral stenosis.

Surgical treatment is occasionally indicated where the stenosis involves the central arteries and contributes to pulmonary hypertension or complicates the surgical treatment of the tetralogy of Fallot.

Pulmonary Arteriovenous Aneurysm. IN-TRODUCTION. Among those malformations capable of producing cyanosis is one involving the pulmonary vascular bed, an anomaly basically hemangiomatous in nature. This has been described under a variety of names in the literature, including pulmonary arteriovenous aneurysm, pulmonary arteriovenous fistula, hemangioma or cavernous angioma of the lung, congenital telangiectasis of the lung, and hemorrhagic telangiectasis with pulmonary artery aneurysm. While some of these terms have definite merit, congenital pulmonary arteriovenous aneurysm has been selected because of its wide usage and general acceptance. Wilkens (1917) is generally given credit for having been the first to describe the anomaly as seen at autopsy, in a case reported in 1917. It was not until 1937, however, that the diagnosis was first made during life (Smith and Horton, 1939), and the first successful surgical attack took place in 1940 (Hepburn and Dauphinee, 1942).

Frequently these pulmonary lesions have been but one manifestation of a generalized angiomatous tendency. In a significant number of the reported cases hemangiomas have been noted elsewhere in the body, the majority of these being of the telangiectatic type. Attention has also been called to the increased incidence of

pulmonary arteriovenous aneurysms in patients with hereditary hemorragic telenagiectasia (Rendu-Osler-Weber disease). On occasions, members of the same family have been found to have pulmonary arteriovenous aneurysms (Goldman, 1948; Moyer and Ackerman, 1948; Sloan and Cooley, 1953).

Of particular interest are cases of pulmonary telangiectasia occurring mainly in infants and children (Cooley and McNamara, 1954; Higgins and Wexler, 1976; Currarino et al., 1976). These patients have multiple small arteriovenous bridges between arterioles and venules often scattered widely through the lungs but with some preference for the bases. Although at times invisible on chest films, they were sufficient to produce clubbing, cyanosis, and other clinical findings typical of arteriovenous aneurysm. A majority of the patients had telangiectasia of the skin and other parts of the body, and there was an increased familial incidence of similar lesions. It is becoming increasingly clear that there is a spectrum of arteriovenous communications ranging from one or a few large or dominant lesions to a diffuse type with numerous widely dispersed but minute telangiectatic lesions. Also of some interest is the occasional association of pulmonary arteriovenous shunts with "hepatic cyanosis" (Kravath et al., 1971).

PATHOLOGIC ANATOMY. Pathologically, arteriovenous aneurysms of the lung are similar to hemangiomatous malformations found elsewhere in the body. They are composed of two basic elements: (1) vascular channels lined with endothelium and (2) a supporting connective tissue stroma. The vascular channels range from capillary-sized structures to huge tubular or saccular multilobulated dilatations with walls of varying thickness, and there may be considerable variation in the amount of associated connective tissue elements. Most of the clinically significant arteriovenous aneurysms of the lungs are fundamentally hemangiomas of the cavernous type, being composed of large tortuous and irregular channels with relatively thin walls and scant connective tissue stroma. Usually one border of these lesions presents on the pleural surface of the lung, and it apparently has been an impressive sight at surgery to see these bulging and pulsating vascular sacs with walls frequently so thin that the blood can actually be visualized swirling and streaming within their lumens. Small calcified plaques have been encountered within pulmonary arteriovenous aneurysms, but apparently phlebolith-like calcifications have not been noted (Baker and Trounce, 1949; Crane et al., 1949; Jones and Thompson, 1944). A rounded densely calcified arteriovenous aneurysm in the left lower lobe of the lung of an asymptomatic 43-year-old man was reported by Steinberg in 1961.

The vascular supply and pattern of these arteriovenous aneurysms are of considerable importance. The most satisfactory method for demonstrating this has been to inject suitable materials into the vessels supplying the area and to obtain an actual cast of the lumen of the channels within and around the anomaly (Lindskog *et al.*, 1950). Surgical and pathologic studies have revealed that the major arterial supply is usually from a branch or branches of the pulmonary artery, and the venous drainage empties into the pulmonary vein system. Frequently, the arterial and venous branches supplying the aneurysm may be considerably dilated, and this dilatation may extend for a variable distance toward the heart. Not only may these supplying trunks be dilated, but their walls may also be considerably thinner than normal. This phenomenon has been encountered in large arteriovenous aneurysms elsewhere in the body, as well as in traumatic arteriovenous fistulas involving the systemic circulation. In most of the clinically significant pulmonary arteriovenous aneurysms which have been carefully studied there have been large channels providing more or less direct communication between the afferent arterial supply and the efferent venous drainage. This shunt is parallel, as it were, permitting varying amounts of pulmonary arterial blood to be short-circuited into the pulmonary veins. Since this blood bypasses the pulmonary capillary bed, varying amounts of unoxygenated blood are returned to the left side of the heart. Some authors have suggested that the bronchial arterial system may enter into the composition of the vascular supply to pulmonary arteriovenous aneurysms (Baker and Trounce, 1949; Lawrence and Rumel, 1950), and rarely there may be anomalous arterial or venous trunks supplying these lesions (Baer *et al.*, 1950; Jones and Thompson, 1944; Lindskog *et al.*, 1950). Occasionally at surgery the arteriovenous aneurysm or adjacent lung has been found to be attached to the parietal pleura and chest wall by unusually dense vascular adhesions, suggesting the establishment of a secondary vascular supply. Several authors have reported cases of unilateral rib notching due to large and tortuous intercostal arteries which were contributing a systemic blood supply to the malformation (Stork, 1955; Wilson, 1960; Boone *et al.*, 1964), and Drexler *et al.* (1964) suggested the additional possibility that the dilated intercostal arteries may contribute collateral circulation to that portion of the pulmonary vascular bed bypassed by the large flow through the fistula.

Anatomically, pulmonary arteriovenous aneurysms may be found anywhere in the lung and frequently there are multiple lesions in the same individual with involvement of two or more lobes. In one reported case, the presence of aneurysms in all five lobes was surgically confirmed (Adams, 1951; Adams *et al.*, 1944). Also of importance is the fact that a careful search at surgery or autopsy has frequently revealed additional lesions whose presence had not been detected by clinical means. These have varied from small pinpoint angiomas to lesions of moderate size.

While it is usual to find a saccular dilatation interposed between the afferent and efferent vessels comprising the malformation, the present authors have recently encountered a case of multiple pulmonary arteriovenous aneurysms in which several of the arteriovenous connections appeared thin and tubular and no larger than the vessels supplying and draining the area (Fig. 345B). Indeed, it was impossible to determine where the artery ended and the vein began. It is presumed that this represents an early stage in the natural history of the lesion and that the pulmonary arterial pressure will, in most cases, ultimately result in dilated aneurysmal connecting channels.

Pulmonary arteriovenous aneurysms do not seem to cause any significant disturbance in the adjacent lung parenchyma. There is occasionally some minimal compression of the surrounding lung, but there have been no reports of associated atelectasis or bronchiectasis.

PHYSIOLOGIC ASPECTS. Physiologic disturbances associated with pulmonary arteriovenous aneurysms may be totally absent or quite marked, depending upon the amount of unoxygenated blood which is shunted from the pulmonary artery through the aneurysm into the systemic circulation. Relatively few of the reported cases have been carefully studied from a physiologic aspect (Baker and Trounce, 1949; Maier *et al.*, 1948; Sloan and Cooley, 1953). In those cases which have been so studied, the proportion of the right ventricular output which has passed through the shunt and bypassed the pulmonary capillary bed has been estimated as ranging from 18 (Segers *et al.*, 1950) to 89% (Lequine et al., 1950). When significant amounts of unoxygenated blood are returned to the left side of the heart, varying degrees of oxygen unsaturation occur in the systemic circulation, with resultant cyanosis and polycythemic response.

It is of some interest to speculate upon the

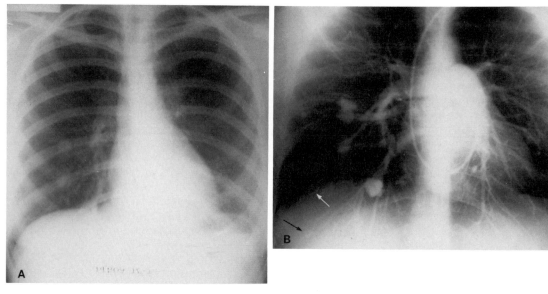

FIG. 345. MULTIPLE CONGENITAL ARTERIOVENOUS FISTULAS
The arrows point to vascular loops in which a sizeable artery merges imperceptibly with a sizeable vein.

combination of size and number of arteriovenous aneurysms necessary to produce a clinically significant shunt. In a large majority of the reported cases, one or more large aneurysms have been present. The confirmation of the cases with telangiectasia demonstrates that a large number of very small lesions can produce the same results (Brink, 1951; Moyer *et al.*, 1962; Sloan and Cooley, 1953; Currarino *et al.*, 1976; Higgins and Wexler, 1976). Also, the relapse of patients following resection of one or more large lesions suggests that there are often a number of small and latent lesions that may enlarge under the stimulus of increased local flow or after a period of time.

It is usually stated that there is no significant disturbance in the overall circulatory dynamics in cases of pulmonary arteriovenous aneurysms. The blood pressure, pulse rate and circulation time are typically unaltered. In those instances where cardiac catheterization has been performed, the right atrial, ventricular, and pulmonary artery pressures have usually been essentially normal, and the cardiac output within normal limits. These findings are in distinct contrast to congenital or acquired lesions in the systemic circulation which permit the shunting of significant amounts of arterial blood into the venous circulation. The usual explanation for the absence of such changes in lesions involving the pulmonary circulation is that the pulmonary artery pressure is normally so low that the presence of a shunt in parallel does not significantly reduce the overall vascular resistance of the lung (Fried-

lich *et al.*, 1950). While it is apparently true that the average pulmonary arteriovenous aneurysm does not cause any significant disturbance in circulatory dynamics, there is some evidence that this is not always the case (Sloan and Cooley, 1953).

It should be emphasized that all pulmonary arteriovenous aneurysms do not produce a significant degree of arteriovenous shunt or cause obvious physiologic disturbances. Most of the reported cases have had significant shunts, but this may be explained by the fact that such lesions tend to make themselves clinically apparent.

CLINICAL ASPECTS. The clinical aspects of pulmonary arteriovenous aneurysms will be discussed under the headings of (1) symptomatology, (2) physical findings, (3) laboratory data, (4) roentgenologic findings, and (5) treatment.

Symptomatology. Dyspnea, resulting from anoxemia, is by far the most common symptom. There is considerable variation in its intensity, but more often than not it is exertional in type and relatively mild. Neurologic disturbances are also relatively frequent. These are usually transitory in type, ranging in intensity from slight sensory or motor disturbances to grand mal convulsive episodes. Occasionally, permanent damage, such as hemiplegia, has been noted. It is presumed that these episodes represent cerebral insults of varying intensity due to anoxemia or thrombosis and that polycythemia plays an important role (Berthrong and Sabiston, 1951). Hemoptyses occasionally occur, varying from repeated minor episodes over a period of years to a single massive fatal hemorrhage. Vague chest pain or discomfort is occasionally noted. Epistaxes are frequent, but these are not regarded as a symptom of pulmonary arteriovenous aneurysm per se but rather as a manifestation of telangiectases in the mucosa of the nasal airways.

All patients with pulmonary arteriovenous aneurysms do not have significant symptoms, and in many symptomatic cases the degree of subjective incapacity may be minimal. Frequently, these patients are able to carry on normal activity quite well, noticing limitations only upon physical exertion. In reported cases the clinical history has often dated back many years, without significant increase in the degree of symptomatology, tending to substantiate the concept that pulmonary arteriovenous aneurysms may have a prolonged and relatively benign clinical course.

Physical Findings. Abnormal murmurs are frequently detected over the region of the aneurysm. These vary considerably in intensity and quality in individual cases but are usually either continuous in nature with a systolic accentuation or are heard only during systole. Frequently, the murmurs are noted to increase in intensity during or at the end of deep inspiration. Associated telangiectasis or hemangiomas in the skin or mucous membrane should always be searched for. In the cases with clinically significant shunts, cyanosis and clubbing of the fingers are usually present.

There are no other consistent physical findings. The patients are more often than not reasonably well developed and nourished, and save for the murmur over the arteriovenous aneurysm, the heart and lungs are usually unremarkable. The absence of cardiac murmurs tends to exclude congenital cardiac malformations as a cause of cyanosis. As noted previously, the blood pressure, pulse, and respiratory rates are usually within normal limits. The spleen is only rarely enlarged, helping to differentiate this condition from polycythemia vera.

Laboratory Data. Of the various routine hematologic studies, the red blood cell count, hematocrit, and hemoglobin are the only ones to show significant alteration with any frequency. With a significant shunt through the arteriovenous aneurysms, these figures are usually found to be elevated, but it should be recalled that hemorrhage can mask the expected polycythemic response. With control of such hemorrhage and supportive therapy, an elevation of the red cell count from anemic to polycythemic levels has been noted in several instances. The white cell

and differential counts as well as that of the platelets show no significant alterations. In cases with a significant shunt, one may expect varying degrees of systemic arterial oxygen unsaturation.

The ECG usually is within normal limits, although several instances of right axis deviation have been recorded. No consistent changes in the circulation time are noted, although occasionally this may be somewhat shortened in instances where the shunt is large.

Radiologic Findings. In almost all of the reported pulmonary arteriovenous aneurysms in which x-rays of the chest were taken, some abnormality was detected within the lung fields. The typical lesion, on routine radiography, is a rounded or lobulated homogeneous density within the lung parenchyma having relatively well defined borders and being connected to the hilar region by cordlike bands (Figs. 347 and 348). It has been suggested that this pattern is quite typical and specific, but it seems fair to say that a high index of suspicion is of considerable help in making the radiologic diagnosis. All of the lesions have not been so typical in appearance, and it is not surprising that a diagnosis of bronchiectasis, tuberculosis, and primary or metastatic neoplasm have been entertained on oc-

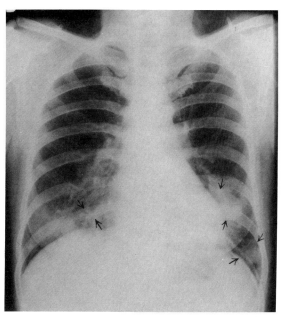

Fig. 346. Proved Multiple Arteriovenous Aneurysms Involving Both Lower and Right Middle Lobes

The rounded nature of the lesions is well shown, but the vascular channels supplying the aneurysms are not particularly prominent. (Courtesy of the *American Journal of Roentgenology, Radium Therapy and Nuclear Medicine, 70:* 199 (Fig. 6), 1953.)

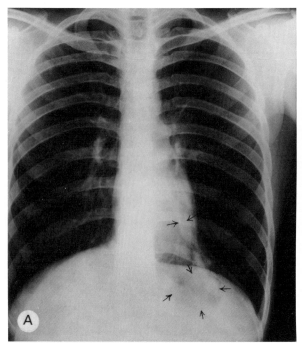
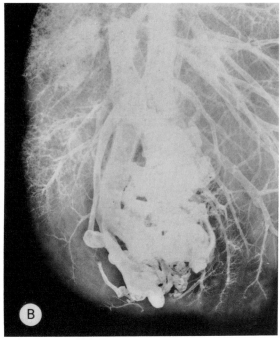

FIG. 347. LEFT LOWER LOBE BEFORE AND AFTER RESECTION

(A) A proved arteriovenous aneurysm involving the left lower lobe. There are several rounded densities at the left base, which in the posteroanterior projection are partially visualized through the gas bubble in the stomach. Prominent vessels extend downward from the left hilus into the parenchymal densities. (B) Roentgenogram of the resected left lower lobe following the injection of a barium suspension into the prominent arterial trunk supplying the arteriovenous aneurysm. The tortuous channels within the aneurysm are clearly shown, as is the large venous trunk draining the area. (Courtesy of the *American Journal of Roentgenology, Radium Therapy and Nuclear Medicine, 70:* 194 (fig. 3), 1953.)

casions. Calcification within the aneurysm is uncommon and when seen has been plaquelike in appearance. Fluoroscopic study should be performed routinely. Intrinsic pulsations are occasionally detected within the aneurysms. It has also been noted that the diameter of the aneurysm may increase with a reduction of intrathoracic pressure (Müller maneuver) and decrease with a rise in intrathoracic pressure (Valsalva maneuver). Kymography may confirm some of the fluoroscopic impressions. Not infrequently, unusually active pulsations are observed within hilar vessels, and pulsations within the communicating vessels in the lung parenchyma may be seen. Laminography frequently helps to establish the nature of the lesion; the tortuous vessels in and around the anomaly often stand out with surprising distinctness (Figs. 348B and 349, C and D).

Chest films in patients with telangiectasia have presented a variety of changes in the lung parenchyma. These have been described (Currarino *et al.*, 1976; Cooley and McNamara, 1954; Higgins and Wexler, 1976; Kravath *et al.*, 1971) as a spidery appearance of the vascular markings, tortuosity of the pulmonary vessels, hypervascularity, diffuse strand-like infiltrates and multiple tiny nodular densities. In 3 of the reported 18 patients, the chest films were normal.

By far the most definitive radiologic procedure is angiocardiography. This may be performed by the intravenous technique or preferably by selective injection via a catheter in the pulmonary artery. The large arterial and venous trunks supplying the anomaly are usually well opacified, as are the tortuous channels and sacculations within the arteriovenous aneurysm (Figs. 350 and 351). These vessels usually reach their maximum density within 2 or 3 sec after filling of the pulmonary artery. With large arteriovenous shunts, it has occasionally been noted that the vascular tree elsewhere in the lung does not opacify normally and that the opaque material may appear in the left atrium with abnormal rapidity (Fig. 352).

The minimal size of the arteriovenous aneurysm or its associated vascular channels that is susceptible to angiographic demonstration has not been established and obviously depends somewhat on the quality of the angiogram and

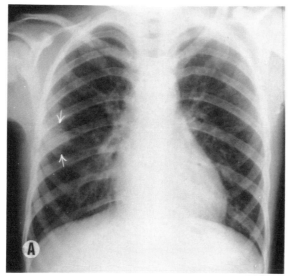

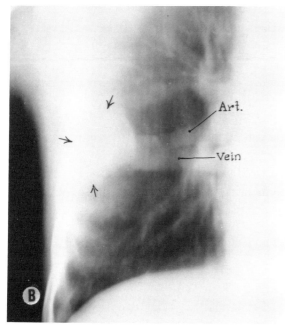

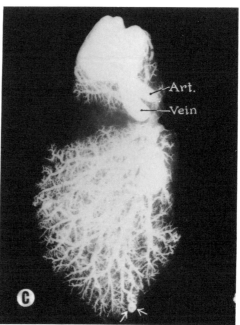

FIG. 348. ARTERIOVENOUS ANEURYSM INVOLVING RIGHT MIDDLE LOBE

(A) A proved arteriovenous aneurysm involving the right middle lobe, with additional multiple small angiomas not suspected prior to surgery. A routine film reveals the rounded density of the largest aneurysm in the lateral aspect of the right midlung field. (B) A laminogram clearly reveals the rounded arteriovenous aneurysm and the two large vessels intruding into it from the hilus. (C) The arterial tree of the resected right middle lobe was injected with a barium suspension. The specimen film reveals the large arteriovenous aneurysm, as well as the enlarged afferent and efferent vascular trunks supplying it. One of the smaller arteriovenous shunts is demonstrated at the base. It is questionable whether lesions of this small size can be demonstrated by roentgenographic means. The triangular area in which the vascular tree is not filled represents an injection artefact. (Courtesy of the *American Journal of Roentgenology, Radium Therapy and Nuclear Medicine, 70:* 202 (Fig. 8), 1953.)

the astuteness and experience of the observer. Currarino *et al.* (1976) in their review of 15 cases from the literature and 2 of his own of pulmonary telangiectasia found that in 4 instances the angiogram was interpreted as normal. In one other case only a rapid pulmonary circulation was demonstrated. The other cases showed a variety of findings. These consisted of visualization of tiny irregular vessels bridging arterioles and venules; an abnormal vascular pattern with dilatation of

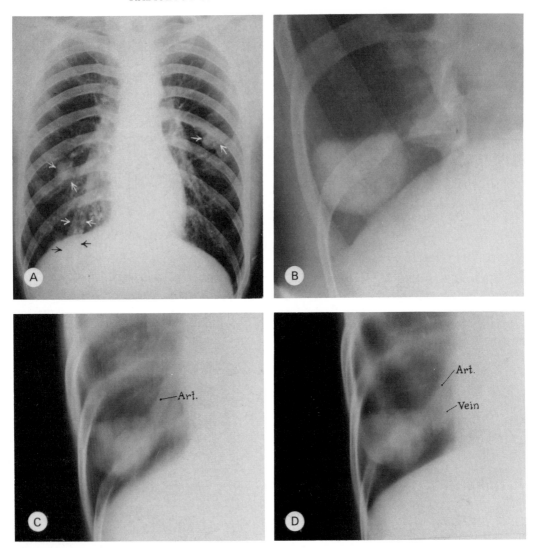

FIG. 349. PROVED MULTIPLE ARTERIOVENOUS ANEURYSMS INVOLVING RIGHT LOWER AND LEFT UPPER LOBES

(A) A routine chest film reveals the rounded parenchymal densities within both lung fields. One of the lesions is obscured behind the dome of the right diaphragm, but prominent vessels can be identified leading down to it. (B) A close-up oblique view showing the rounded density at the right base posteriorly. (C and D) Laminograms at slightly different levels reveal the lobulated nature of the arteriovenous aneurysm at the right base and demonstrate clearly the prominent afferent and efferent vascular channels supplying the lesion. (Courtesy of the *American Journal of Roentgenology, Radium Therapy and Nuclear Medicine, 70:* 198 (Fig. 5), 1953.)

small vessels and late emptying of small scattered areas suggesting dilated sinuses and a myriad of small arteriovenous fistulas scattered through both lungs and rapid right-to left atrial transit time. Although technically adequate pulmonary angiograms may be negative in an occasional case of telangiectasia, the procedure should be considered in every case in which the clinical and laboratory findings suggest the diagnosis. Even though one or more dominant lesions may be clearly visible by chest films and laminography, angiography can demonstrate small lesions not

visible by these means (Fig. 345B). Angiography is essential in any case in which surgery is contemplated.

Treatment. Three forms of specific therapy have been tried in the treatment of pulmonary arteriovenous aneurysms, two of these being of only historical interest. Pneumothorax has been attempted in the hope that the vascular channels within the aneurysm would collapse along with the lung, but in the few cases tried (Hepburn and Dauphinee, 1942; Jones and Thompson, 1944), this did not prove successful. Roentgen therapy

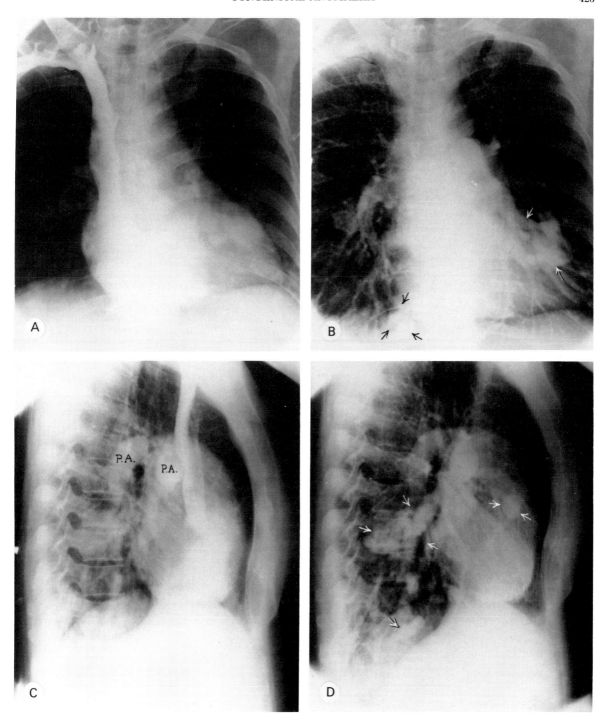

FIG. 350. SAME CASE AS SEEN IN FIG. 346

(A) An anteroposterior angiocardiogram taken at the end of one second, showing an opacified superior vena cava and right atrium. Note the soft tissue density of one of the arteriovenous aneurysms adjacent to the left heart border. (B) A film at the end of 3 sec showing the definite opacification of the aneurysm adjacent to the left heart border. The smaller arteriovenous aneurysm in the right cardiophrenic angle is partially obscured. (C) A lateral film at the end of one second demonstrating filling of the superior vena cava, right side of the heart, and the pulmonary artery and its branches with the opaque medium! (D) A film at the end of 3 sec demonstrating the opacification of the vascular channels within and adjacent to the arteriovenous aneurysms. (Courtesy of the *American Journal of Roentgenology, Radium Therapy and Nuclear Medicine, 70:* 200 (Fig. 7), 1953.)

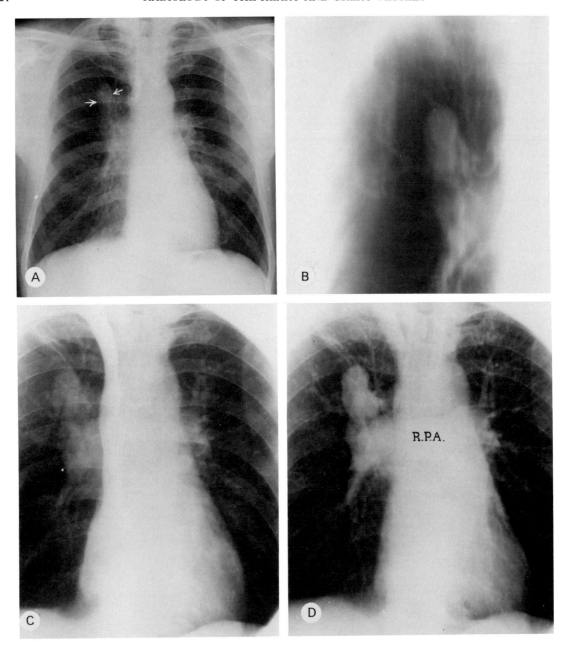

Fig. 351. Unproved but Probable Arteriovenous Aneurysm Adjacent to Upper Border of Right Hilus

(A) A routine film reveals the oval soft tissue density as well as a somewhat prominent right hilus. (B) A laminogram reveals the oval soft tissue density to be composed of a single coiled tubelike structure. (C) An anteroposterior angiocardiogram at the end of one second reveals an opacified superior vena cava and right atrium. The contrast medium has not reached the pulmonary artery. (D) A film at the end of 3 sec reveals the opacification of the soft tissue density adjacent to the right hilus and suggests that it is a single large, coiled vessel. Of interest is the fact that the right pulmonary artery (RPA) is moderately dilated. (Courtesy of the *American Journal of Roentgenology, Radium Therapy and Nuclear Medicine, 70:* 206 (Fig. 10), 1953.)

has also been utilized occasionally but without obvious benefit (Jones and Thompson, 1944; Robb and Gottlieb, 1951). Surgery appears to offer the only logical method of definitive therapy. Removal of the lesion is usually undertaken, either by lobectomy or less frequently by segmental resection or total pneumonectomy. In rare instances, the feeder vessels supplying the arteriovenous aneurysms have been ligated, the aneurysm being left in place (d'Allaines *et al.*,

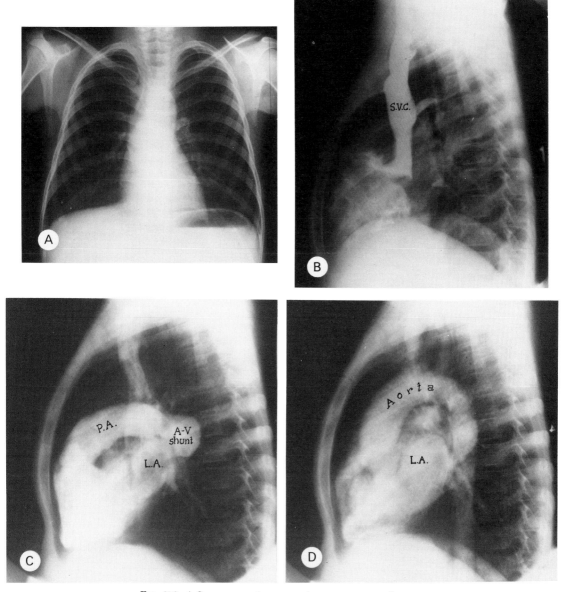

FIG. 352. A SOMEWHAT ATYPICAL ARTERIOVENOUS SHUNT

(A) A proved somewhat atypical arteriovenous shunt consisting of a large vascular channel connecting the right pulmonary artery with the left atrium. Routine chest films and roentgenoscopy were thought to be normal, although in retrospect an oval prominence can be identified in the mediastinum adjacent to the right hilus. (B) A lateral angiocardiogram taken at the end of 1 sec with the opaque medium outlining the superior vena cava (SVC) and starting to enter the right cardiac chambers. (C) At the end of 3 sec the right ventricular cavity and the pulmonary artery (PA) are well opacified as is the arteriovenous shunt. There is beginning opacification of the left atrium (LA), the peripheral portions of the lung fields are abnormally avascular. (D) At the end of 4 sec the left-sided cardiac chambers and the aorta are well visualized. The rapid appearance of the opaque medium in the systemic circulation and the avascularity of the lung fields indicate that there is a marked shunt through the anomaly. (Courtesy of the *American Journal of Roentgenology, Radium Therapy and Nuclear Medicine, 70:* 196 (Fig. 4), 1953.)

1950; Packard and Waring, 1948; Watson, 1947). In patients with bilateral lesions, two or more stage thoracotomies may be necessary (Adams, 1951; Adams *et al.*, 1944; Sloan and Cooley, 1953). The shunting of blood from larger to smaller lesions after ligation of the afferent vessels of the larger lesion may render visible at surgery small and previously unsuspected arteriovenous connections.

The indications for surgical interference have

not been completely established. All agree that surgery is justified in the patient with an isolated lesion causing hemoptysis or significant symptoms secondary to anoxemia and polycythemia or even in symptomatic cases with a limited number of lesions involving one or both lungs. The most difficult decisions occur in those patients with isolated lesions in whom symptoms are minimal or absent and in whom there is no clinical evidence of a marked shunt and in those patients with extensive and multiple lesions where successful therapy would necessitate the removal of large segments of pulmonary tissue in several stages. Surgical treatment is contraindicated in pulmonary telangiectasia.

12

Hypertensive Heart Disease

Hypertensive heart disease is due to systemic hypertension. Hypertension or high blood pressure exists when both systolic and diastolic pressures are persistently elevated above the normal range. Systemic hypertension is quite common in adults in the United States, and Lew (1973) estimated that 15% of persons between the ages of 15 and 79 years have an elevated blood pressure, and in those above 55 years of age this increases to 25%. White (1951) found that it was a factor in at least 30% of all cases of heart disease in New England.

Hypertension may be due to a variety of causes such as (1) essential hypertension, the origin of which is still not fully explained; (2) renal disease such as glomerulonephritis, polycystic kidneys, obstruction of the renal arteries, large renal infarcts, etc.; (3) endocrine factors such as pituitary adenomas, adrenal tumors and pregnancy; (4) vascular factors such as coarctation of the aorta and arteriosclerosis; (5) diseases of the nervous system such as increased intracranial pressure, emotions, etc. Of these, essential hypertension is by far the most common and is the cause of about 95% (White, 1951; Hanenson, 1976) of cases of hypertensive heart disease.

Hypertension is not invariably followed by hypertensive heart disease. The hypertension may be transient such as that which occurs during pregnancy or the menopause. Also, the hypertension may disappear when the cause is removed such as seen following the resection of a coarctation of the aorta. In conditions such as these there may be no permanent or irreversible changes in the cardiovascular system, and the heart may return to its normal status.

The reaction of the heart to hypertension is quite variable. Moderate to marked degrees of hypertension may exist for years without cardiac enlargement or evidence of cardiac insufficiency. These persons may succumb to some other disease, and it is difficult without a careful anatomical study to be sure of any significant changes in the heart.

Essential hypertension, although it may be benign in its effects for many years, tends to be progressive, and a considerable proportion of patients will eventually suffer from cardiac insufficiency in some form. Fishberg (1966) divided the natural history of essential hypertension into three stages: (1) the stage of cardiac compensation, (2) the stage of isolated left ventricular failure, and (3) the stage of combined left- and right-sided failure.

Such a classification is helpful to the roentgenologist because certain roentgen changes accompany each of three stages.

Complications of essential hypertension are frequent and may be fatal and thus prevent the disease from running its natural course. The usual complicating conditions are cerebral hemorrhage, coronary thrombosis, and renal insufficiency. Coronary arteriosclerosis is so frequent during the latter stages of hypertensive heart disease that it is often considered as an integral part of the condition.

In recent years a number of antihypertensive drugs have added to the treatment of essential hypertension. These have had demonstrable effect in lowering the blood pressure and in reducing the complications due to hypertension (Freis, 1970). The effect on the developing of atherosclerotic complications has not been so clear-cut.

CARDIAC COMPENSATION

In the stage of cardiac compensation, the cardiac output is approximately normal, and the work of the left ventricle is increased by the extent of the rise in the mean arterial pressure. In order to overcome the higher aortic pressure, the left ventricle must contract with increased force. It responds with slight dilatation followed by hypertrophy. The hypertrophy is concentric in type, which means that it is hypertrophy without dilatation. There is little change in heart volume, and consequently the cardiac silhouette shows slight if any enlargement. Left ventricular hypertrophy may cause the left lower cardiac segment to become rounded with some increase in convexity; there may be an associated apparent increase in concavity of the left midsegment. The cardiac apex remains the usual distance above the diaphragm.

ISOLATED LEFT VENTRICULAR FAILURE

In the stage of isolated left ventricular failure, dilatation of the heart is much more noticeable. Previously, the heart was hypertrophied; in this stage, it is both dilated and hypertrophied. The heart is, therefore, moderately but asymmetrically enlarged. The entire left ventricle is elongated; there is an increase in convexity with rounding of the left border so that the transverse diameter is considerably increased. As the left ventricle increases in size, it extends posteriorly into the retrocardiac space. This is best demonstrated in 45–50° left anterior obliquity where the convex curve of the ventricle extends posteriorly, often (depending on its size and the shape of the thorax) sufficiently to be superimposed on the vertebral column. The excursions of the left ventricle are variable but usually decreased in amplitude. The aorta is somewhat dilated and elongated, and the knob is prominent.

The left atrium usually has begun to show minor dilatation; this is best demonstrated in the far right oblique position with a barium swallow. The enlarged atrium produces a posterior deviation of the esophagus in its lower portion. Signs of pulmonary stasis and congestion are common. The pulmonary trunk dilates, tending to fill in the concave heart bay on the left and thus straighten the left middle cardiac contour. The hilar branches of the pulmonary arteries are dilated, and the smaller branches in the lung parenchyma are larger than normal and have a slightly irregular, fuzzy appearance. The lung parenchyma is often slightly hazy suggesting the presence of an increased amount of fluid. Septal

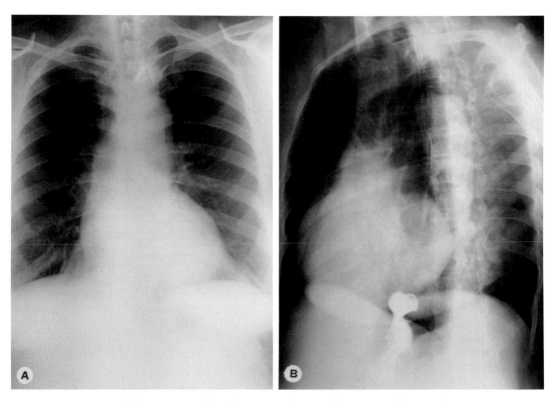

FIG. 353. MODERATE HYPERTENSION OVER PERIOD OF SEVERAL YEARS WITH MINIMAL SYMPTOMATOLOGY
The patient was moderately obese. There is evidence of left ventricular enlargement (predominantly hypertrophy), and there are well marked fat pads in both cardiophrenic angles. BP 150/90–180/90.

lines (Kerley's A, B, and C lines), both oblique and horizontal and similar to those seen in mitral valvular disease, are often seen. The interlobar fissures are thickened and thus appear widened due to subpleural fluid; they may contain small amounts of fluid and also there may be fluid in the costophrenic angles. Gross pulmonary edema is common in this stage of the disease. Consequently, there may be sizeable blotchy or homogeneous areas of increased density, often somewhat symmetrical in their distribution, scattered through the lungs or more often radiating from the hilar areas (Figs. 62A and 64).

Symptoms in this stage are quite definite although they are variable in intensity. Major symptoms are dyspnea, orthopnea, palpitation, and limitation of exercise tolerance; attacks of paroxysmal dyspnea are common. Response to medical treatment is often surprisingly good, and roentgen evidence of this is commonly seen. Following bed rest, digitalis, diet, etc., the heart decreases in size; the lung haziness disappears; the fluid in the pleural spaces is absorbed and the diaphragm appears lower (Fig. 62B). These changes may take place within a period of 2 or 3 weeks and are accompanied by a corresponding clinical improvement in the patient.

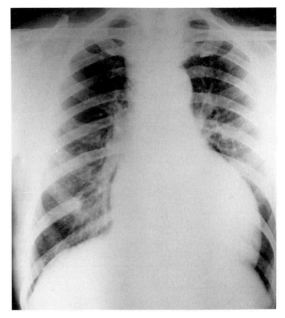

FIG. 354. MARKED HYPERTENSION FOR MANY MONTHS
(BP, 220/120)

Asymmetrical cardiac enlargement with marked dilation and hypertrophy of the left ventricle. There is probably some dilation of the other cardiac chambers.

COMBINED LEFT AND RIGHT HEART FAILURE

In the stage of combined left and right heart failure, all of the cardiac chambers are hypertrophied and dilated. In the preceding stage of left ventricular failure, the right ventricle was able to continue to pump blood against the increased pulmonary pressure. Consequently, there was congestion of the lungs with exudation and edema. When the right ventricle begins to fail, the pulmonary congestion decreases and systemic venous congestion appears; this is followed by peripheral edema.

The heart is moderately to markedly enlarged; the enlargement is usually symmetrical and the transverse diameter and frontal area are increased. The right atrium is dilated so that the heart extends almost as far to the right as to the left. The superior vena caval shadow is widened. Evidence of pulmonary congestion is usually not striking, and it may be minimal or absent. Pulsations of the heart are decreased over all contours. There may be small or moderate amounts of fluid in the pleural spaces, and there may be pericardial fluid which increases the size of the cardiac silhouette.

In this stage of hypertensive heart disease, coronary arteriosclerosis is quite common. Coronary arteriosclerosis decreases the blood supply to a laboring and hypertrophied ventricular myocardium. This impairment of nutrition and gaseous exchange is a potent factor in reducing the activity of the heart and in causing it to fail. Unless there is outright coronary thrombosis, however, there may be no specific roentgen evidence of coronary arteriosclerosis other than that of an enlarged, dilated heart. Coronary arteriosclerosis will be discussed in more detail in a following section.

It should be re-emphasized that the course of hypertensive heart disease is variable. A sizeable percentage of patients will die with combined right and left heart failure. In another very sizeable group, the disease does not complete its natural course; it may be terminated by any number of complications.

EFFECT OF DRUGS

Most patients with systemic hypertension are treated with drugs, and if therapy is effective in lowering the blood pressure in a patient with a resilient myocardium, a decrease in cardiac size

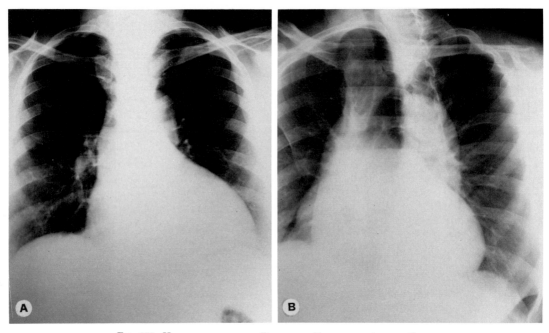

FIG. 355. HYPERTENSION AND PROBABLE RUPTURED AORTIC CUSP
(See "Syphilitic Heart Disease," p. 527). Patient was known to have hypertension for years. At the time of the above examination there was a loud "cooing" diastolic murmur. There was quite marked left ventricular enlargement.

and return to a more normal shape may occur. In a hypertensive patient with left heart failure and cardiac dilatation, dramatic decrease in the size of the heart may follow bed rest and drug therapy, especially with digitalis and diuretics.

This decrease in size must be understood as the result of the return of compensation to a dilated heart and not as change due to improvement in the magnitude of hypertension.

HYPERTENSION ASSOCIATED WITH NEPHRITIS

In acute glomerulonephritis, the blood pressure is frequently elevated almost from the time of onset. Even when the systolic pressure is not significantly changed, there is an increase in the diastolic pressure. Although the pressure rarely reaches high levels such as is sometimes seen in chronic nephritis, the heart, particularly the left ventricle, tends to fail quite early, and this is frequently a serious complication. It is probable that in addition to the hypertension, there is some other toxic factor which adversely affects the myocardium (Fishberg, 1966).

The chest film frequently shows surprisingly few changes in the heart. It is rarely enlarged unless the nephritis has been present for several weeks. There may be lengthening of the left ventricular border with rounding of the apex indicating some left ventricular enlargement. Fluoroscopy might show poor or diminished pul-

sation of the left ventricular borders, but ordinarily these patients are too sick to be disturbed. Changes in the lungs on the other hand are frequently present and often striking. They are due predominantly to pulmonary edema and have been described in the section on the pulmonary vascular system. Although extensive pulmonary edema may be asymptomatic, it is much more often associated with symptoms of left ventricular failure such as dyspnea and orthopnea.

In chronic glomerulonephritis, the blood pressure may reach quite high levels and remain persistently elevated. In a considerable percentage of patients, major symptoms will be referable to the heart. Left ventricular hypertrophy is common. Also, in the presence of uremia, pericarditis, often with a collection of fluid and occasionally with cardiac tamponade, may be seen.

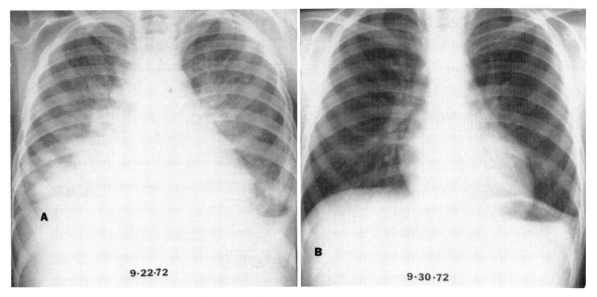

FIG. 356. ACUTE GLOMERULONEPHRITIS

Four-year-old female with shortness of breath, fever and cough. A shows diffuse cardiac enlargement with interstitial and alveolar pulmonary edema and a small amount of pleural fluid on left. B shows rapid clearing of the edema and decrease in size of the heart. (Courtesy of Dr. L. E. Swischuk.)

BERNHEIM'S SYNDROME

In this syndrome, the left ventricle is greatly enlarged; the lung parenchyma is quite clear with a relatively normal vascular pattern and without signs of congestion; yet there is peripheral venous stasis and edema. Thus, on the chest film, there is moderate to marked cardiac enlargement, usually asymmetrical with predominant enlargement of the left ventricle and elongation of the aorta associated with a rather normal pulmonary vascular system.

In the original cases observed by Bernheim (1910), the left ventricle at autopsy was markedly dilated and hypertrophied due usually to hypertension and coronary arteriosclerosis. The right ventricle on the other hand was small, not dilated, and showed no evidence of failure. The interventricular septum was markedly convex toward the right ventricle due to the marked dilatation of the left ventricle. This bulging of the septum impinged greatly upon the right ventricular cavity so that it was greatly reduced in size and near the apex was little more than a slit between the septum and the right lateral wall. It was postulated that this septal bulging interfered with right ventricular filling and thus explained the presence of peripheral venous stasis without pulmonary congestion.

This mechanism of interference with right ventricular filling has been questioned, since it may be more apparent than real. Nevertheless, in practice well marked asymmetrical cardiac enlargement is encountered with clear lungs and evidence of peripheral venous stasis. Unless there is some other better explanation these cases may be considered as "Bernheim's syndrome."

13

Atherosclerotic Changes in the Heart Coronary Arteriosclerosis Myocardial Infarction

VALVES

In older persons, atherosclerotic changes are frequent in the aortic valve and somewhat less common in the mitral valve. The valve cusps or leaflets are slightly thickened, stiffened, and often contain fatty or calcific plaques. Calcification of the annulus fibrosus or valve ring is also a degenerative change closely akin to arteriosclerosis. Furthermore, the aortic ring may be slightly dilated secondary to arteriosclerosis of the aorta, thus causing a minor degree of aortic regurgitation. These changes may produce murmurs; however, they rarely cause a significant malfunction of the involved valve and hemodynamically they are of little consequence. An exception may be the occurrence of calcification in the aortic annulus and valve cusps in the elderly. Roberts *et al.* (1971) propose that calcific aortic stenosis in patients over 65 years of age and often with preexisting hypertension may have a different clinical course from the usual case of calcific aortic stenosis in younger persons and may be a

manifestation of atherosclerosis. Many of these patients have calcifications in the mitral annulus. Calcification in the mitral annulus alone is often seen in persons over 65 years of age and is more common in women. The calcification is usually benign in its effects, although it commonly produces flow alterations resulting in the production of murmurs. Rarely it may be a cause of insufficiency and stenosis (Korn *et al.,* 1962).

Roentgen findings in arteriosclerosis of the heart valves are therefore minimal. Calcific plaques in the valves are ordinarily too thin to be seen by roentgen means. Also, since there is little, if any, change in the work performed by the cardiac chambers, there is no significant deviation of the cardiac contour. Calcification of the annulus fibrosus is easily demonstrated (see "Cardiac Calcifications," p. 554), but with the exception noted above such calcification has no special significance other than that it should not be confused with a calcified valve.

CORONARY ARTERIOSCLEROSIS

This is a widespread disease of great importance and is a major cause of death. It is particularly prone to occur during the later stages of hypertensive heart disease and in association with diabetes. It produces its untoward effects by decreasing the blood flow to the heart and particularly to the left ventricular myocardium.

The conventional roentgen examination has almost nothing to offer in the early diagnosis of this disease, and it is only after major and severe

damage to the myocardium has occurred that definite findings appear on plain roentgenograms. Areas of calcification in the coronary arteries may be detected by screen intensification systems (see "Cardiac Calcifications," p. 555). Earlier changes can be detected by coronary arteriography, (see p. 443).

Since arteriosclerotic narrowing of the coronary arteries decreases the blood supply to the heart musculature, there is a corresponding decrease in the amount of work that the heart can perform. Ordinarily, the heart has a large reserve which is more than adequate to take care of the usual needs of maintaining the circulation. Consequently, even when the blood supply to the myocardium is reduced, the heart, because of its large reserve potentialities, may carry on for long periods without evidence of dilatation. Thus, cardiac enlargement is uncommon in uncomplicated coronary arteriosclerosis. Roentgen examination may show an entirely normal heart contour; yet the patient may suffer a coronary occlusion immediately thereafter. Also, arteriosclerotic changes in the aorta are not a reliable guide to the presence of coronary arteriosclerosis as the two may exist quite independently of each other.

Calcification in the coronary arterial system can occasionally be detected by conventional chest films and much more often by image amplified fluoroscopy or cinefluorography. In certain locations and in certain age groups, its presence has considerable significance, and this is discussed in the section on "Calcifications within the Heart."

Coronary arteriosclerosis and hypertension will cause left ventricular dilatation and hypertrophy which is eventually followed by generalized cardiac enlargement and failure. Even a mild degree of coronary arteriosclerosis becomes an important factor when the heart is already hypertrophied and working under an increased load such as occurs in hypertension or aortic valvular

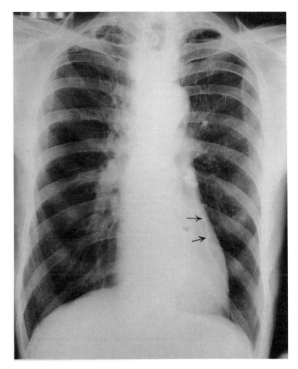

FIG. 357. EXTENSIVE DEPOSITS OF CALCIUM IN ANTERIOR DESCENDING CORONARY ARTERY (ARROWS)

disease. The left ventricle shows more pronounced changes than the other chambers because its myocardium is more active and bears the greater burden of the circulation.

MYOCARDIAL INFARCTION

Myocardial infarction in the overwhelming majority of cases is the result of ischemic heart disease secondary to coronary atherosclerosis; less common other causes are trauma and thromboembolism to the coronary arteries. Myocardial infarcts, and certainly those that are of clinical importance, are limited almost entirely to the left ventricle, the interventricular septum, and that portion of the right ventricle adjacent to the interventricular septum. The infarcts may be old or recent or acute.

Patients with acute myocardial infarcts may be divided into (1) those that are relatively asymptomatic and unrecognized, (2) those that are symptomatic and are usually admitted to a hospital or a coronary care unit, and (3) those who die rapidly without effective medical support. This latter group comprises about 35% of all cases. The radiologist is concerned primarily with the second group.

Formerly, the radiologist had little to offer in the diagnosis of acute myocardial infarction. The diagnosis was usually established by history, physical examination, electrocardiographic findings, and enzyme studies. Recently, taking advantage of the selective localization of tracer materials in normal and ischemic myocardium, imaging procedures have begun to play an active role in the diagnosis and also the determination of size and location of acute myocardial infarcts. Both cold-spot (potassium $\sim {}^{43}K$) and hot-spot techniques using stannous pertechnetate are used. A portable gamma camera is helpful. The reader is referred to current papers on these procedures (Holman, 1976; Hurley *et al.*, 1971; Bonte *et al.*, 1974, Bruno *et al.*, 1976; Parkey *et al.*, 1974).

In acute myocardial infarction, radiologic observations are limited almost entirely to portable chest films. Needless to say, films of good quality are helpful. The essential observations are related to cardiac size and contour and to the circulatory status in the lungs. In the majority of cases of acute infarction, the heart is either normal in size or only slightly enlarged. In a patient who is suffering from recurring infarction, the most recent infarct may be associated with enlargement of the heart. The most important observations are those of comparison of heart size on a day to day basis and evidence of increase or decrease in size. Particular attention should be given to evidences of aneurysm formation, such as an abnormal bulge or calcification (from previous infarcts) along the left border of the heart (Figs 358, 365, and 366).

A large minority (33% in the series of Harrison *et al.*, 1971) of patients will show changes in the chest film indicating left ventricular failure. These consist of (1) loss of definition of pulmonary blood vessels; (2) clouding of the pulmonary parenchyma either perihilar or peripheral; (3) alveolar edema; (4) septal lines (A, B or C lines of Kerley); (5) pleural effusion; (6) increased heart size; (7) venous distention; (8) increased diameter of the right descending pulmonary artery (greater than 17 mm). These changes are secondary to ventricular failure or a combination of left ventricular failure and mitral insufficiency.

The appearance of the lungs, heart, and pulmonary vasculature is a more sensitive indicator of left ventricular function than clinical observation, and the day-to-day progress of the lung changes is of considerable value in prognosis (Harrison *et al.*, 1971).

About 30% of patients with acute infarction will appear with a clinical syndrome known as "cardiac shock" or "pump failure." This is characterized by a systolic blood pressure of less than 90 mm Hg, mental confusion, decreased urinary output, and peripheral vasoconstriction. The chest film almost invariably shows signs of left ventricular failure. Cascade *et al.* (1976) suggest that from 55–76% of patients will show one or more of the above-mentioned changes in the chest film, and at least 20% will have frank alveolar pulmonary edema which is the most severe and represents the most advanced type of left ventricular failure. Where alveolar pulmonary edema persists or where it is increasing, the prognosis is more ominous. If signs of pulmonary edema appear suddenly, the possibility of some severe complication, such as rupture of a papillary muscle, can be suggested. Also, persistent alveolar pulmonary edema in the face of supportive treatment is suggestive of severe mitral insufficiency as a complication of left ventricular

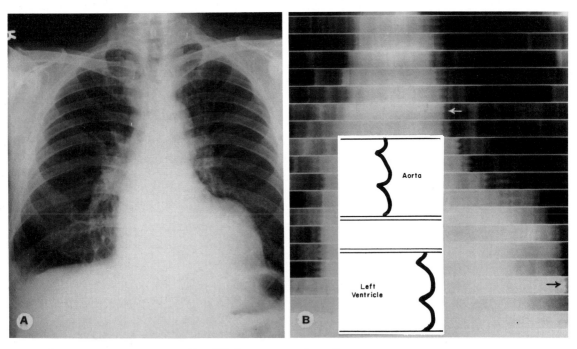

FIG. 358. ANEURYSM OF LEFT VENTRICLE

A 55-year-old diabetic who had had symptoms of coronary thrombosis 6 weeks before. There were paradoxical pulsations over the greater part of the left ventricular border. (A) Conventional film. (B) Roentgenkymography showing that pulsations of left ventricular border are approximately in phase with those of aorta.

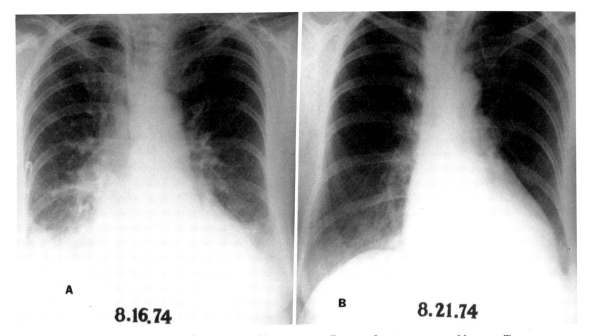

8.16.74

B 8.21.74

FIG. 359. MYOCARDIAL INFARCTION WITH LEFT VENTRICULAR FAILURE IMPROVING WITH MEDICAL TREATMENT
(A) Film exposed 3 days after a second myocardial infarct. Pulmonary interstitial edema and a small amount of fluid in each pleural space. (B) Five days later. Marked improvement although the heart is considerably enlarged.

failure. Also, a careful comparison of films made from day to day is useful in detecting the presence of other complications, such as pulmonary thromboembolism and pneumonia.

Some degree of mitral insufficiency is a common finding in patients immediately following myocardial infarction. It is manifest by a systolic murmur and evidence of pulmonary edema. It was formerly held to be due to dilatation of the mitral valve ring accompanying dilatation of the left ventricle. Burch *et al.* (1968) have pointed out that the more likely mechanism is some degree of derangement of the function of papillary muscles. With dilatation and elongation of the left ventricular wall, the site of attachment of the papillary muscles is displaced away from the mitral valve, and this tends to prevent complete closure. Also, as the cardiac wall dilates the alignment of the papillary muscles is changed with a resultant loss in mechanical efficiency. Ischemia associated with the underlying coronary atherosclerosis may reduce the contractility of the papillary muscles which is necessary for proper valve closure. Infarction may occur followed by fibrosis with consequent immobilization of the papillary muscles. The most serious complication is that of rupture of one of the papillary muscles or chordae tendineae, and this has a very serious prognosis and is discussed further in the next section.

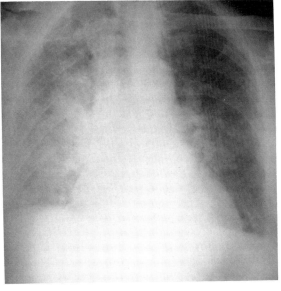

FIG. 360. CARDIOGENIC SHOCK
Film exposed 12 hours after massive posterior infarction. Patient died 24 hours later. The infarct involved the posteromedial papillary muscle.

Fluoroscopy using image amplification in the authors' opinion has little to offer during the early stages of myocardial infarction. After convalescence is established, fluoroscopy may be used, and a considerable older literature is avail-

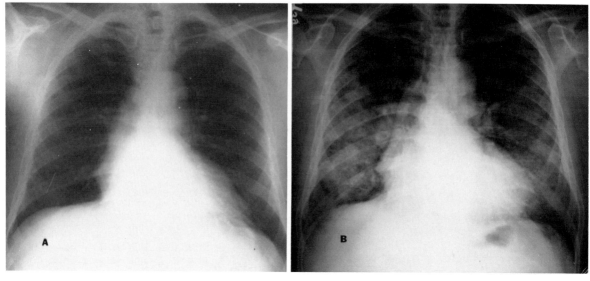

FIG. 361. CARDIOGENIC SHOCK

(A) Chest film exposed two months before B when patient was suffering from angina. (B) Chest film exposed three hours after massive myocardial infarct. There is little change in heart size but lungs show extensive edema. The patient died 24 hours later.

able concerning the detection of the sites of infarction and the activity of the left ventricular wall. Both roentgenkymography and electrokymography will show abnormalities of motion in a high percentage of cases and, of course, this offers confirmatory evidence of infarction (Sussman *et al.*, 1940; Dack *et al.*, 1950). The present authors believe that there are few indications for fluoroscopy or kymography following acute myocardial infarction. Occasionally, the presence of an aneurysm may be suspected, and fluoroscopy may be of help in further substantiating this impression. Routine fluoroscopy of patients with myocardial infarcts is not recommended.

As the infarct heals, fibrosis and scarring occur. Impairment of cardiac function depends on the relative size of the infarct in relation to the total mass of the left ventricle, location (involving conduction system or papillary muscle), and the presence of systemic hypertension. Multiple or repeated infarcts may eventually replace so much of the ventricular musculature that the heart actually loses viable muscle volume and can no longer function satisfactorily as a pump, and chronic congestive heart failure occurs.

Persistent cardiac enlargement due solely to a myocardial infarct is unusual. In a group of 489 patients who survived an acute myocardial infarction for at least 2 months, only 25 showed cardiac enlargement (Weiss and Weiss, 1957). In 15 of these, there were other commonly accepted

causes of enlargement, such as hypertension, and in 2 others, enlargement of the heart was not observed until quite late after the initial infarction. Thus, only 8 cases demonstrated enlargement due solely to the infarction. All 8 of these had associated congestive heart failure. The heart, and particularly the left ventricle, may dilate or there may be aneurysm formation, all of which will contribute to enlargement of the heart. There is rarely an increase in actual muscle mass.

The radiologist has an important role to play in the investigation of those patients with acute myocardial infarction in which surgical procedures are considered or those with threatened infarction, such as unstable angina. These patients should be investigated with coronary arteriography and left ventriculography.

The prime role of the radiologist is to detect those changes which may affect prognosis or which indicate a complication, such as the formation of a ventricular aneurysm, rupture of the interventricular septum or a papillary muscle. These complications are considered below. Every effort should be made to improve the quality of portable chest films made in the coronary care unit. Nevertheless, the radiologist should not be discouraged by the quality of the films since careful and persistent observation of less than optimal films often provides valuable information to those with a high index of suspicion.

CARDIAC ANEURYSM

Edwards (1961) defines a ventricular aneurysm as "a protrusion of a localized portion of the external aspect of the left ventricle beyond the remainder of the cardiac surface, with simultaneous protrusion of the cavity as well." This definition is difficult to apply to radiologic observations of the intact beating heart, particularly as seen during ventriculography. The outer wall may not be clearly visible and it makes no allowance for the cases in which the ventricular wall is thin but does not protrude significantly. For radiologic purposes, a ventricular aneurysm is considered to be present when there is a localized, permanent abnormal blood-filled dilatation of the left ventricle resulting from disease of the wall (Kittredge and Cameron, 1972). The presence of paradoxical pulsations, although often present, is not essential for diagnosis. The widespread use of left ventriculography in association with coronary arteriography has uncovered a much larger incidence of ventricular aneurysms than had been previously suspected.

A true cardiac aneurysm has remnants of myocardium within its walls. A false cardiac aneurysm, although communicating with one of the heart chambers, is surrounded by tissue other than myocardium, such as pericardium, adjacent pleura and reactive fibrous tissue. Most false aneurysm are secondary to rupture of the heart with containment of the hematoma by surrounding pericardium and pleura (VanTassel and Edwards, 1972).

Abrams *et al.* (1963) found aneurysms following 8–12% of myocardiac infarcts, but this incidence may be too low, depending somewhat on the judgement of the observer and also varying according to whether the observations were made following left ventricular cineangiography or at postmortem. Cheng (1971) found left ventricular aneurysms in 35 of 100 patients referred for coronary artery disease. All of the patients were distinctly symptomatic. His conclusions were based on predominantly left ventricular cineangiography performed in 20–30° in the RAO projection and 60–70° in the LAO projection. Local segments of non-contracting or paradoxical expansile myocardium were taken as evidence of aneurysm formation. Only 7 of the 35 cases showed an abnormal left ventricular bulge that could be identified on a conventional chest film. Gorlin *et al.* (1967) in a study of 24 patients with a left ventricular aneurysm found that the chest film was diagnostic in only 5 but was suspicious

in an additional 10 patients. The size of the aneurysm was usually underestimated even after ventriculography as compared with the findings confirmed at surgery or necropsy.

The overwhelming majority of ventricular aneurysms are secondary to ischemic heart disease and myocardial infarction. Other important causes are trauma either following myocardial contusion with infarction or direct injury by an object such as a knife blade or a bullet; postoperative, usually secondary to a ventriculotomy; congenital (Bertran and Cooley, 1955); rheumatic involvement of the coronary arteries and adjacent myocardium; syphilis with gumma formation and localized suppuration secondary to mycotic aneurysms.

The large majority of aneurysms are secondary to infarction involving the left ventricle or ventricular septum. In a study of 40 postmortem specimens, Edwards (1961) found 31 with involvement of the anterior wall and only 9 with involvement of the posterior or inferior wall of the left ventricle. Occasionally, the interventricular septum and portion of the right ventricle will be involved (Bjork, 1964; Singh *et al.*, 1975). The anterior inferior portion of the septum is the most susceptible part and is the most frequent site of rupture of the septum (Mundth *et al.*, 1972).

The aneurysm probably begins to develop within a week after the establishment of an infarct and becomes firm and fibrotic after several weeks. After fibrosis occurs, the aneurysm becomes relatively stable in size and may persist unchanged for many years. Rupture of a true stabilized aneurysm is unusual, and the risk is negligible. The aneurysm frequently contains clot and/or organized thrombus. Portions of this thrombus material may break away and form a systemic embolus.

A cardiac aneurysm is compatible with a long period of survival. On the other hand, they are a common cause of left ventricular failure, cardiac arrhythmias, and occasionally the site of origin of a significant embolus to the brain or other crucial organs. The presence of an aneurysm can be suspected from clinical and electrocardiographic changes with persistent arrhythmias and persistent elevation of the ST segment in chest leads and leads II and III.

Postsurgical aneurysms are usually secondary to ventriculotomies and frequently involve the right ventricle (Mirowski *et al.*, 1964; Summarrai *et al.,* 1976) and even the left atrium (Atlas *et al.,* 1976). The majority of traumatic and post-surgical aneurysms are of the false variety.

Ventricular aneurysms are now susceptible to surgical resection with acceptable mortality and good results in many cases (Cooley *et al.,* 1959; Favaloro, 1965; Lam, 1964). This places a considerable responsibility on the radiologist for the detection and delineation of this condition.

Radiologic Procedures and Findings

Formerly, conventional chest films and fluoroscopy were the dominant procedures in detecting cardiac aneurysms. The diagnosis was often confirmed by angiography, particularly in preoperative cases. Following the widespread use of coronary arteriography and associated left ventriculography, many cases of cardiac aneurysms were discovered in which the conventional study, even in retrospect, showed no abnormalities. Conventional chest films and fluoroscopy cannot exclude the presence of a cardiac aneurysm, and probably less than half are susceptible to recognition by these means.

The most common radiographic sign of a cardiac aneurysm is a deviation or convexity of the left border of the heart, particularly that portion attributed to the left ventricle. The convexity may consist of a "bump" with a short radius of curvature or a more pronounced convexity that may be difficult to differentiate from a dilatation of the left ventricle. In most cases, the abnormal convexity or protrusion is in the lower two-thirds

of the left ventricular curve. Confusion with a dilated left atrial appendage is easily avoided, usually because of the presence of associated evidence of left atrial enlargement. Other causes of deviation of the left ventricular contour are cardiac tumors, such as myomas or myosarcomas and fibromas (occasionally associated with tuberous sclerosis), pericardial cysts which are uncommon on the left side of the heart, and extrinsic tumors, such as pedunculated thymomas and dermoids.

Occasionally, lateral (Kittredge *et al.,* 1976) and oblique films show a bulge or a silhouette often rounded in contour against the background of the cardiac mass. Aneurysms of the posterior portion and diaphragmatic surface of the left ventricle are exceedingly hard to recognize on chest films. Baron (1971) recommends distention of the gastric bubble in order to better visualize the diaphragmatic surface of the heart and increase the chances of detecting an aneurysmal protrusion.

Another important finding is the presence of calcium deposited either in the wall of the aneurysm or in organized thrombus material. Most often the calcium is curvilinear and may follow the curve of the left ventricle. Localization of the calcium by fluoroscopy may be necessary for differentiation from pericardial calcification which has a different significance. Calcium associated with an aneurysm is always several mms. below the exterior surface of the heart. The deposition of calcium in the wall of the heart

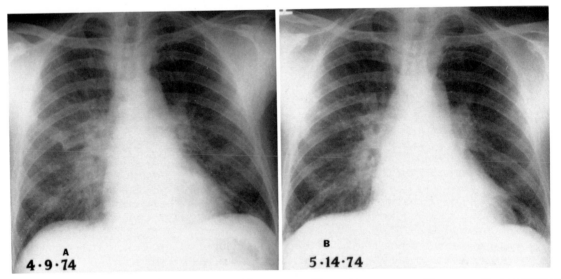

FIG. 362. RUPTURE OF POSTEROMEDIAL PAPILLARY MUSCLE WITH MITRAL INSUFFICIENCY REQUIRING REPLACEMENT OF MITRAL VALVE

Patient had angina for 8 months prior to a myocardial infarct 10 days before A. (B) Cardiac failure persisted with progressive cardiac enlargement and persistent pulmonary edema despite vigorous medical treatment.

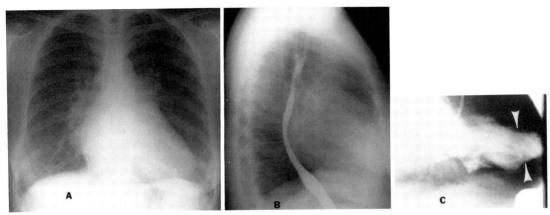

FIG. 363. ANEURYSM AT APEX OF LEFT VENTRICLE

(A and B) The heart is enlarged, particularly the left ventricle, but there is no deviation in contour that suggests aneurysm formation. (C) Left ventriculogram in RAO projection in systole. Aneurysm at apex showed slight but definite paradoxical motion. Aneurysms of this type are a fairly common finding in patients with extensive ischemic heart disease.

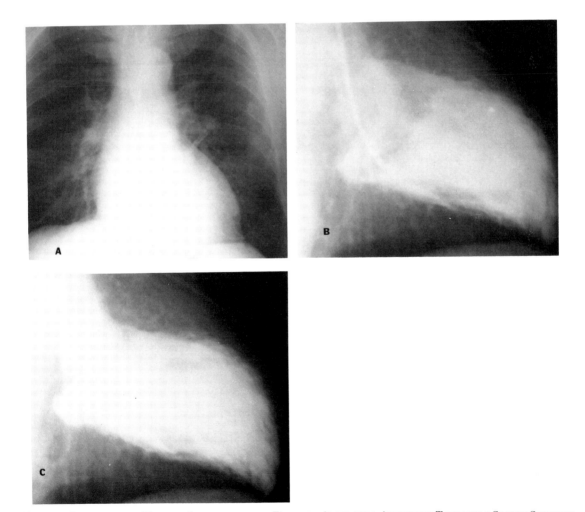

FIG. 364. PATIENT WITH MARKED AKINESIA BUT NO DEFINITE ANEURYSM, ALTHOUGH THERE WAS SLIGHT SYSTOLIC EXPANSION OF ANTERIOR SURFACE OF LEFT VENTRICLE

(A) Borderline cardiac enlargement. (B) Left ventriculogram in diastole (RAO). (C) In systole.

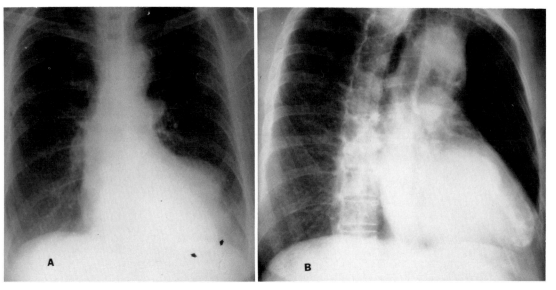

FIG. 365. MULTILOCULATED CARDIAC ANEURYSM WITH SOME CALCIUM IN WALL (ARROWS IN A)

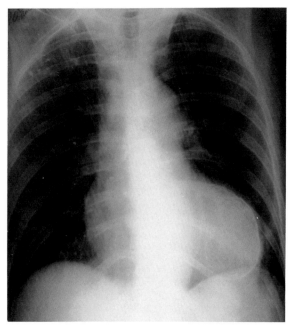

FIG. 366. LARGE CARDIAC ANEURYSM WITH CALCIUM IN WALL. PART OF THE ANEURYSM SHOWED PARADOXICAL PULSATIONS

is not pathognomonic of an aneurysm since infarcts without aneurysm formation may calcify (Baron, 1971).

The heart is often normal in size or only moderately enlarged. A markedly enlarged, and particularly a dilated heart, may obscure even a large aneurysm. The aneurysm may merge imperceptibly with the exterior surface of the dilated ventricle.

Fluoroscopy using image amplification not only is helpful in identifying calcium but because of the use of multiple projections segments of abnormal pulsation may be discovered. Paradoxical pulsations may not be present and are not necessary for the diagnosis of cardiac aneurysm. Occasionally, the aneurysm may be surrounded by active muscle and appear to contract with systole. Fresh and healing infarcts may for a time show paradoxical pulsations which usually disappear as the infarct heals. Keats and Martt (1962) emphasized that the superior portion of the posterior wall of the normal left ventricle as seen in the lateral view will show a posterior bulge during early systole. This is due to the slight difference in timing of contraction of the different portions of the ventricle and is entirely normal. In summary, paradoxical pulsations, particularly when associated with a localized protrusion of the ventricular contour, are good evidence of ventricular aneurysm. The absence of such pulsations is of no diagnostic significance. Furthermore, conventional films and fluoroscopy, even in skilled hands, cannot eliminate the possibility of even a large aneurysm.

Angiography is the definitive method in the diagnosis of cardiac aneurysm, although radioisotope gated cardiac blood pool imaging offers considerable promise (Botvinick et al., 1976). Injections of contrast substance into the right side of the heart or pulmonary artery will delineate the left ventricular cavity sufficiently to establish the diagnosis, although the detail is such that small aneurysms may be missed. Left ventriculography is much superior and when carefully performed should carry minimal additional risks. The dislodgement by the catheter of emboli from the thrombus material within the aneurysm can be avoided by monitoring of the catheter position by repeated small hand injections of contrast substance under fluoroscopic control. The danger of rupture of the aneurysm due to the force of the injection is negligible, particularly if the injection is made slowly as is the rule in left ventriculography. The RAO projection is most useful, although two projections, namely the other LAO projection, should be used. Recording by cinefluorography is desirable since it shows all phases of the cardiac cycle and is helpful in identifying extrasystoles. Care must be taken not to confuse localized and often inconstant protrusions of the ventricle which are not due to abnormalities. The anterior and superior wall of the left ventricle is a common site for momentary outward excursion either during late diastole (due to atrial systole) or most often in early ventricular systole. This protrusion is likely to be most pronounced during extrasys-

toles. Careful study of these segments of outward protrusion will show that the inner margins are serrated during systole which is due to the normal pattern of the columnae carneae. With a true aneurysm, the margins of the protrusion are usually irregular due either to scar or retained clot.

Baron (1971) mentions that some cases of hypertrophic subaortic stenosis may show apparent protrusions near the apex, but the thick wall and irregular interior and other hemodynamic findings should lead to the correct diagnosis.

The differentiation of true from false ventricular aneurysms is of considerable importance since false aneurysms often rupture whereas true aneurysms rarely do so (VanTassel and Edwards, 1972). False aneurysms typically have a narrow neck whereas true aneurysms have wide-open base with no appreciable neck or narrowing. False aneurysms often contain abundant clot, and the contrast substance may show only the neck of the aneurysm.

RUPTURE OF THE HEART, THE INTERVENTRICULAR SEPTUM OR A PAPILLARY MUSCLE

Rupture of the interventricular septum or papillary muscle follows about 2–4% of clinically diagnosed myocardial infarcts (Mundth *et al.,* 1972). Rupture of the external wall of the left ventricle occurs in about 3–4% of myocardial infarcts (Sievers, 1966). The mortality following these complications is quite high. Consequently these combined lesions are responsible for about 6–8% of deaths following transmural myocardial infarction. A large majority of patients will die within a few minutes to a few hours, but a small proportion will live for days or months or rarely for years, depending on the severity of the defect and other factors. Since all of these complications are now susceptible to surgical treatment, early diagnosis is essential. Rupture of the interventricular septum or a papillary muscle is characterized by a sudden change in the patient's condition, although occasionally a high index of suspicion is necessary to make a tentative diagnosis. Rupture of a papillary muscle is characterized by marked shortness of breath and intractable pulmonary congestion and the appearance of a harsh systolic murmur usually accompanied by a thrill. These complications occur usually within 3–10 days of the onset of a myocardial infarct. The diagnosis in each case can be confirmed by cardiac catheterization and angiography.

Rupture of the external surface of one of the ventricles, usually the left ventricle, occurs almost always within 3–10 days of the onset of a myocardial infarct (Van Tassel and Edwards, 1972). Dating of the onset of the infarct is difficult because the rupture may be a complication of several successive infarctions. As pointed out by Edwards (1961) and VanTassel and Edwards (1972), a rupture of the free ventricular wall is rarely sudden. Instead, it is characterized by a slow progress (over a few days at least) of a dissecting hematoma in the myocardium with slow but increasing leakage of blood into the pericardium. Finally, leakage into the pericardium becomes massive, and pericardial tamponade is usually the final event. However, in a number of cases the rupture is followed by the formation of a false aneurysm, and the patient may survive for months or even years, although the aneurysm tends to progress to rupture.

Infarction of a papillary muscle is not invariably followed by rupture. Infarction may impair the ability of the muscle to contract and lead to mitral insufficiency which is much more common than rupture. The mitral insufficiency may contribute significantly to pump failure. The posterior papillary muscle is much more susceptible to rupture than the anterior papillary muscle. Rupture of a papillary muscle leads to massive mitral insufficiency, and this is usually poorly tolerated.

Radiologic Findings of Rupture of a Papillary Muscle, Interventricular Septum or External Wall of Left Ventricle

Conventional chest films are nonspecific. The most striking finding is pulmonary congestion and edema. The pulmonary edema is severe and intractable and is no way different from that seen with left ventricular pump failure except it is likely to be more intractable. The left atrium is rarely significantly enlarged. This failure to dilate is undoubtedly due to the rapidity of the onset of the massive insufficiency. Unfortunately, the radiologist must depend on portable chest films for the determination of left atrial size and also minor changes in the lungs. The passage of a Swan-Ganz catheter into a wedge position followed by the observation of large V waves (in excess of 20 mm Hg) may suggest the diagnosis and is helpful in differentiating rupture of a papillary muscle from rupture of the interventricular septum. The diagnosis can be confirmed by left ventriculography. This procedure, of course, can only be applied if the patient survives any appreciable length of time in which case surgical treatment should be contemplated (Austen et al., 1965, 1968; Mundth et al., 1972).

Rupture of the interventricular septum is often abrupt in onset. If the patient survives for any significant period of time, dilatation of the pulmonary artery and pulmonary vasculature will occur secondary to the left to right shunt. The shunt must be of the order of 3:1 to produce significant early dilatation. This may be difficult to detect on a portable chest film, particularly if it is associated with any degree of pulmonary edema secondary to the original infarction. The diagnosis can be established by right heart catheterization and often left ventriculography is employed. These procedures will show increased saturation of the blood in the right ventricle and also a left to right shunt. There are several reports of successful repair of a ruptured septum, although the prognosis in such cases is still unfavorable (Buckley et al., 1971; Cooley et al., 1957).

Rupture of the external wall of one of the ventricles (usually the left) is usually characterized by a slow leakage of blood into the pericardium. The radiologist has little to offer since the detection of small amounts of blood in the pericardial cavity as seen on portable chest films is not usually possible. A significant number of ruptures are contained by false aneurysms and the radiologist may detect these in their earlier stages. They, of course, are manifest by changes in the cardiac border, usually the left border but occasionally noted inferiorly or anteriorly. False aneurysms should be treated promptly by surgical means, and the diagnosis can usually be established by angiography. Radioisotope gated blood pool imaging should be considered as an alternative method if available (Botvinick et al. 1976).

14

Coronary Arteriography

LUIS B. MORETTIN, M.D.

Dedication—To the memory of Father, the love of Mother, and my three C's.

KEY TO ABBREVIATIONS USED IN THIS CHAPTER*

A—atrial branches
LA—left atrial
RA—right atrial
AD—anterior descending
AM—acute marginal or right marginal
AVN—atrioventricular node branch
ILV—inferior left ventricular branch
D—diagonal
C, CX—circumflex
CXP—circumflex proximal segment

CXD—circumflex distal segment
CO—conal
LCo—left conal
LC or LCA—left coronary
RC or RCA—right coronary
RCo—right conal
PD—posterior descending
SN—sinus node artery
S or SEP—septal branches
OM—obtuse marginal or left marginal(L M)

* (Abbreviations are used in both capital and lower case letters.)

INTRODUCTION

The management of coronary artery disease, the leading cause of death in the United States, has undergone a drastic change, almost a revolution, that began in 1959 with the advent of selective coronary arteriography. The widespread use of direct coronary surgery is predicated upon the reliable information that coronary arteriography can provide. It can safely be said that the hard facts established by angiographic evaluation of the coronary vessels and ventricular function in ischemic heart disease have changed not only the practice of cardiology but the direction and the perspective of research in cardiology.

THE HISTORY OF CORONARY ANGIOGRAPHY

Rousthoi (1933) is widely credited as describing the earliest attempt at purposeful demonstration of the coronary tree in his experiments with rabbits. Radner in 1945 reported on his attempts at visualizing the coronary vessels in man by means of the transthoracic puncture of the ascending aorta. In 1952, DiGuglielmo and Gottadauro, working in Sweden, published a study of coronary anatomy derived from examinations performed with a large bolus of contrast injected into the root of the aorta. Numerous modifications of this technique were developed over the years in an attempt to obtain better and more consistent opacification of peripheral coronary vessels. In order to increase coronary filling, timed injections were made to coincide with ventricular diastole. Arnulf and Buffard (1959) took advantage of the transient diastolic pause that could be induced by the use of intravenous acetylcholine. Others similarly attempted to diminish cardiac output by means of increased intra-bronchial pressure under general anesthesia or by means of aortic balloon occlusion (Dotter and Frische, 1958). Paulin (1964), in an attempt to deliver a larger bolus of contrast with a better distribution, used specially designed loop catheters that deposited contrast substance in the coronary cusps in immediate proximity to the coronary ostia. All of these methods with the exception of the last, are of mostly historical interest at the present time.

Sones *et al.* (1959), motivated by the necessity of reliable and consistent evaluation of the coronary vessels demanded for the selection of patients for myocardial revascularization, introduced selective coronary angiography. His method and the modifications using percutaneous approaches are the techniques currently used.

TECHNIQUES OF SELECTIVE CORONARY ARTERIOGRAPHY

Undoubtedly the coronary arteries are best visualized by selective injections. Selective coronary arteriography, unlike aortic root injections, permits use of a smaller volume of contrast, avoids interference from the opacified aortic root and ventricular cavity (in cases with aortic regurgitation), and makes it possible to perform numerous injections in different projections without superimposition of vessels in different planes. Basically, two approaches are currently in use: the retrograde brachial and the percutaneous.

Retrograde Brachial Technique of Sones (Sones and Shirey, 1962)

This method requires a brachial artery cutdown immediately above the elbow, preferably the right. The right brachial artery is exposed, a small longitudinal incision is performed and a specially designed catheter is introduced which permits catheterization of both right and left coronary arteries and the left ventricle. The catheter (Fig. 367) is French 7 or 8 caliber and tapers to a 5.5 French diameter in the distal 5 cm. The tip is flexible and contains one end and four side holes. In order to enter the left coronary artery a loop has to be formed with the tip of the catheter in either the aortic cusps or the innominate artery. Ventriculography and pressure studies are accomplished with the same catheter. At the completion of the study the catheter is removed and the artery closed after ascertaining that the brachial artery is patent and free of clots distal to the point of entry.

Several techniques of selective catheterization of the coronary vessels using percutaneous entry have been described (Bourassa *et al.* 1969; Judkins, 1968; Ricketts *et al.* 1962; Schoonmaker, *et al.* 1974; Wilson *et al.* 1967). The most widely used is the technique of Judkins that uses preformed, separate catheters (Fig. 368) for both right and left coronary arteries and ventricular

catheterization. The femoral arteries are entered by means of the standard Seldinger technique. Catheterization of the left coronary artery can be achieved with considerable ease and stability. Intubation of the right coronary artery is a little more difficult. Several different sizes of preformed catheters are available to accommodate for different sized aortas. A "pigtail" catheter is used for studies of the left ventricle.

Several other catheter configurations have been described for percutaneous use. The catheters of Wilson *et al.* (1967) can be used via both

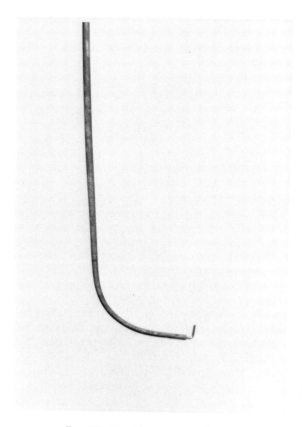

FIG. 367. THE CATHETER OF SONES

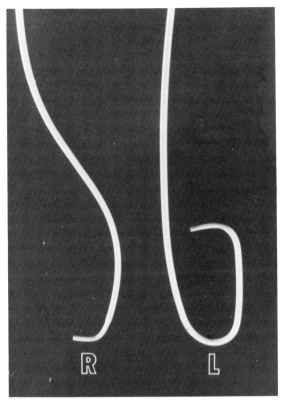

FIG. 368. THE CATHETERS OF JUDKINS
R, for the right coronary artery; L, for the left coronary artery.

the femoral or brachial arteries. Because the preceding technique requires different catheters for right and left coronaries and ventriculograms, this method has not gained wide acceptance.

More recently Schoonmaker and King (1974) reported their experience using a single catheter for coronary arteriography and ventriculography as well as for saphenous bypass injections that can be introduced percutaneously. The catheter is a French 8 size. Its tip has a gentle tapering curve of about 45° like that of the catheter of Sones. The mechanics of catheterization are similar to those of the brachial approach.

The nonselective methods of coronary arteriography (Paulin, 1964), although seldom used, are still of value in unusual cases, such as when the suspicion exists that a coronary artery or one of its branches arises independently from the aorta or when, because of technical difficulties, a complete, successful study cannot be achieved by the selective techniques, and in the evaluation of a possibly occluded aortocoronary graft.

Each one of the selective methods has its advantages and limitations and their proponents have engaged in heated arguments in defense of the value and safety of their preferred techniques. The method of Sones is preferred by cardiologists whereas radiologists prefer the percutaneous technique of Judkins. The technique of Sones has the following advantages: (1) A single catheter is used for both coronary artery injections and ventricular catheterization, as well as for catheterization of coronary bypass grafts, eliminating catheter replacements. (2) It permits catheterization of the coronary vessels in patients with obstructive disease of the aorta and iliac vessels. (3) Because of the end and side holes, contrast delivery is faster and catheter recoil is minimized. (4) The need for a brachial artery cutdown is considered by some to be a disadvantage when compared with the percutaneous method, but in fact, in experienced hands, is not more time-consuming than multiple catheter changes frequently required for the percutaneous approach.

The main disadvantage relates to the fact that the technique is a little more difficult to learn than the other methods and tortuosity of the subclavian vessels may make catheterization difficult if not impossible. In addition a clot can form in the side holes of the Sones catheter without damping arterial pressure. This clot may be dislodged during manipulation and enter the systemic or coronary circulation. Stable catheterization of the right coronary artery is easier with the Sones method.

Conversely, stable catheterization of the left coronary artery is more easily achieved with the Judkins catheters, whereas difficulties are frequently encountered in catheterizing the right coronary artery and maintaining cannulation throughout the injection. Recoil is more prominent with these catheters, and it is often difficult to regulate the degree of penetration, particularly in the right coronary artery, which is determined more by the physical properties and design of the catheter than by manipulation.

When the ascending aorta is considerably dilated and when there is clinical evidence of aortic stenosis or insufficiency and deformity of the aortic leaflets or in the presence of marked cardiomegaly we employ electively the technique of Judkins. When there is clinical evidence of aortoiliac occlusive disease or when femoral pulses are diminished, we electively use the technique of Sones. We consider that one method complements the other and recommend that proficiency be acquired, developed, and maintained by the continuous performance of both techniques.

Further discussion on the relative safety of

each method can be found in the section "Complications."

The single catheter percutaneous technique of Schoonmaker and King (1974) utilizes elements of both the Sones and the Judkins methods. As in the Sones method, it has the advantage of the use of the single catheter for both coronary injections and ventriculography but it requires much more operator training than the other percutaneous techniques using pre-formed catheters. The maneuvers necessary to catheterize the coronary arteries are similar to those with the Sones technique but without the need of forming a loop for intubation of the left coronary artery.

Radiographic Equipment and Instrumentation

For a comprehensive review and guidelines for the planning and operation of diagnostic installations for the examination of the cardiovascular system, the reader is referred to the Report of the Intersociety Commission for Heart Disease Resources (Judkins et al., 1976).

Several manufacturers produce radiographic installations specifically designed for the performance of coronary angiography. Particularly valuable are those that permit both rotation and angulation of the tube and image intensifier for the easy performance of multiple angled views: they are very useful to avoid vascular superimposition and to better define lesions of the left

main coronary artery and its proximal branches. This type of coronary dedicated unit eliminates the use of rotating cradles and simplifies the handling of the patient.

Generators and x-ray tubes should be of sufficient capacity to allow very short exposures to diminish motion blur and the lowest possible KVP for ideal contrast.

The image should be recorded by means of a 35-mm camera with rates of 60 frames/sec for ventriculography and 30 frames/sec for the coronary artery injections.

In recent years great improvements in the resolution and reliability of the new generation image intensifiers have made serial spot film cameras extremely reliable and they can replace the 35-mm cine for filming the coronary arteries (Grollman et al. 1973). Injections in the coronary arteries can be done by hand or, as we prefer, by means of a variable rate injector connected to a manifold system to permit instantaneous choice of injection, pressure monitoring, or saline perfusion. We have found this system of coronary injections very safe and it eliminates problems that arise from leaking connectors and stopcocks and syringes used for hand injections.

Equipment necessary for physiological monitoring of the patient should include a system that allows for continuous display of pressure tracings and electrocardiogram, preferably with alarm systems to indicate emergency situations.

INDICATIONS FOR CORONARY ARTERIOGRAPHY

In general it can be safely said that an indication for coronary arteriography is "the need to know" (Conti, 1977). As with most diagnostic or therapeutic methods the indications vary from place to place and change with the passage of time as the method becomes established and more widely used (Baltaxe, 1971; Gulotta, 1976; Pichard, 1976; Sones, 1972). In this context the need or benefits of the information to be gained should be weighed in relation to the relative risk in each particular setting. It can then be stated that "coronary arteriography is indicated when a problem is encountered which may be resolved by the objective demonstration of the coronary tree provided competent personnel and medical facilities are available and the potential risks are acceptable to the patient and the physician" (Sones, 1962).

The clinical circumstances in which coronary arteriography is indicated can be grouped basically into five categories:

Patients with Typical Anginal Chest Pain Who are Considered Candidates for Surgery

Since the indications for bypass coronary surgery continue to change with the passage of time and vary from institution to institution, the indications for coronary angiography are expected to vary accordingly. In this group would be included patients with progressive or unstable angina and with angina that has become incapacitating. Opinions are divided as to whether or not coronary angiography should be offered only to those who have severe functional limitation or should also be employed in patients with moderate symptoms. In the latter group it would depend upon whether or not coronary surgery would eventually prove effective in prolonging survival and diminishing the complications of coronary disease (Gulotta, 1976). It remains true that coronary arteriography should not be performed if surgery is not contemplated and if conservative medical management is satisfactory. In patients with angina complicated by acute myocardial infarction the increased risks of coronary arteriography and surgery performed in an attempt to prevent extension of an infarct should be individually evaluated on the basis of the results obtained in each individual setting.

Favaloro *et al.*, (1971), based on their experience with emergency arteriography and surgery in patients with impending and acute myocardial infarction, conclude, "Emergency coronary arteriography can be performed with a minimal risk, and when operations are performed within 6 hours of an acute myocardial infarction, most of the heart muscle can be preserved." Others (Achuff *et al.*, 1975) hold opposite views.

Patients with Chest Pain of Unknown Nature in whom Coronary Heart Disease Cannot Be Categorically Excluded By Other Means

In this group of patients the demonstration of an unquestionably normal coronary system practically excludes significant coronary disease as the probable cause of symptoms and has a very reliable prognostic value (Brusche *et al.*, 1973).

The social, economic, and psychologic consequences of the erroneous diagnosis of coronary artery disease in a normal individual are such that the value of coronary angiography is clearly justified.

Patients with Known Cardiac Disease without Angina

Coronary angiography has been used in patients with cardiogenic shock in association with acute myocardial infarction (Favaloro *et al.*, 1971), and in cases of uncontrollable cardiac failure as a preoperative means of evaluation with the intent of improving ventricular function by means of bypass or corrective ventricular or valvular surgery. Patients with repeated or increasing cardiac arrhythmia may similarly benefit from surgery. In the presence of acquired aortic or mitral valvular disease coronary angiography should only be employed in the presence of angina, to exclude associated lesions of the coronary vessels that may both complicate surgery or require a coronary bypass, (Sos and Baltaxe, 1974; Bonchek *et al.*, 1972) or when valvular dysfunction is a possible complication of myocardial ischemia.

In patients with congenital heart disease—particularly the tetralogy of Fallot, trans-

position complexes and truncal abnormalities—the information provided as to the anatomical variations in the origin and distribution of the coronary vessels may be of significant value in preventing injury to an anomalous vessel at the time of ventriculotomy. In patients with evidence of cardiac injury following serious chest trauma, coronary angiography will define the possible nature and extent of injury to the epicardial vessels.

Patients with Electrocardiographic or Laboratory Evidence of Ischemic Heart Disease, without Angina

In general, asymptomatic patients should not be considered for coronary arteriography; however, there is a group of individuals who develop ischemic electrocardiographic response to stress. With the widespread use of the treadmill exercise test, the number of patients in this group is increasing and in these individuals the presence or absence of coronary disease can only be determined by coronary arteriography. This is particularly important to those individuals who because of their occupations have the need to know with certainty (Sones, 1972).

The indications for postoperative coronary angiography are not at the present time clearly established. In most centers, routine coronary and graft angiography is not performed in all patients but is reserved only for those with persistent symptoms or complications. The objectives of immediate postoperative angiography, performed 2–3 weeks following surgery, are to establish the patency of the arterial or venous grafts, to determine flow and to demonstrate whether or not the increased regional perfusion has resulted in improvement of ventricular function (Guthaner and Wexler, 1976). Coronary angiography is also important in the evaluation of coronary injury or embolism resulting from prosthetic valvular replacement. Lesage *et al.* (1970) recommends that coronary angiography be routinely employed in patients of this type that develop postoperative angina or myocardial infarction.

A relative contraindication is the presence of circumstances which predispose to cardiac complications such as failure and serious electrolyte deficiencies, namely potassium depletion. They should be corrected. The decision whether or not to perform coronary angiography in a patient with severe disturbance of cardiac rhythm should be critically evaluated and done only when possible therapeutic conclusions are to be derived from the examination. In these circumstances the arteriogram can be performed with the aid of continuous cardiac pacing. Sones (1972) believes that coronary arteriography and ventriculography should not be performed in patients with well-established myocardial infarction if symp-toms have been present for more than 6 hours; the diminished possibilities of revitalizing the damaged myocardium by emergency bypass surgery by that time make the increased risk more important.

ANATOMY OF THE CORONARY VESSELS (Figs. 369, 370)

Many excellent works have been published on the anatomy of the coronary vessels. Fundamental studies have been contributed by Bianchi (1904), DiGuglielmo (1952), James (1961), Mc-Alpine (1975), Paulin (1964), and Smith (1962) among others. A thorough knowledge of the anatomical distribution and variations of the coronary vessels is absolutely essential in the reliable performance and interpretation of the coronary angiogram.

Both the right and left coronary arteries arise from the respectively named right and left coronary sinuses. The ostia are located in the center of the sinus of Valsalva or slightly posterior, immediately below the supravalvular ridge. Their placement varies considerably and according to Vlodaver et al., (1975) they may be situated above the ridge in as many as 30% of the cases for the left, 8% for the right ostium, and 6% bilaterally.

The Left Coronary Artery From its origin in the left sinus of Valsalva, the main coronary artery courses between the root of the pulmonary artery and the left atrium to appear on the surface of the heart. Its average caliber is 4.9 mm and it varies considerably in length (Vieweg et al., 1976). It may be very short or absent, resulting in apparent separate origin of its branches from the sinus (Fig. 378) or may be as long as 5 cm. Its average length is 2 cm (Fig. 372). Patients with dominant left coronary arteries tend to have shorter main left coronary arteries than those with mixed and right dominant systems (Vieweg et al., 1976). At the upper portion of the interventricular groove under the left atrial appendage, it divides into its two main branches, the anterior descending and the circumflex. The main coronary artery runs in a course that mostly parallels the frontal plane of the body. It is best seen in the frontal or slight left anterior oblique projection. The anterior descending artery, which is the most constant in origin and distribution of all the coronary vessels, is the direct continuation of the main left coronary artery. It courses to the left of the pulmonary valve and runs along the anterior interventricular sulcus to its end where it may encircle the apex of the heart and extend in the posterior interventricular groove (Fig. 373) to a length determined by the length of the posterior descending branch of the right coronary artery. In its course the anterior descending gives origin to several branches. A few small branches are given off to the anterior surface of the right ventricle which are variable in size and number. The first is the left conal branch that courses over the surface of the outflow tract of the right ventricle where it anastomoses with the right conal branch of the right

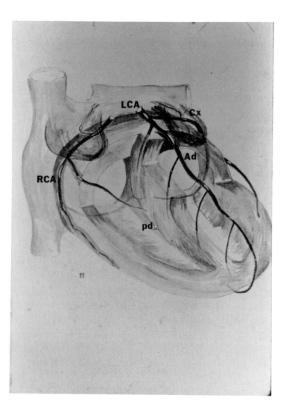

FIG. 369. SEMI-SCHEMATIC CUT-AWAY REPRESENTATION OF THE HEART

This illustrates the distribution of both coronary arteries and their branches and their relationships to the atrioventricular and interventricular grooves, the interventricular septum, and the atrial appendages. The anterior walls of both ventricles, the aorta and the pulmonary artery are removed (see description in text).

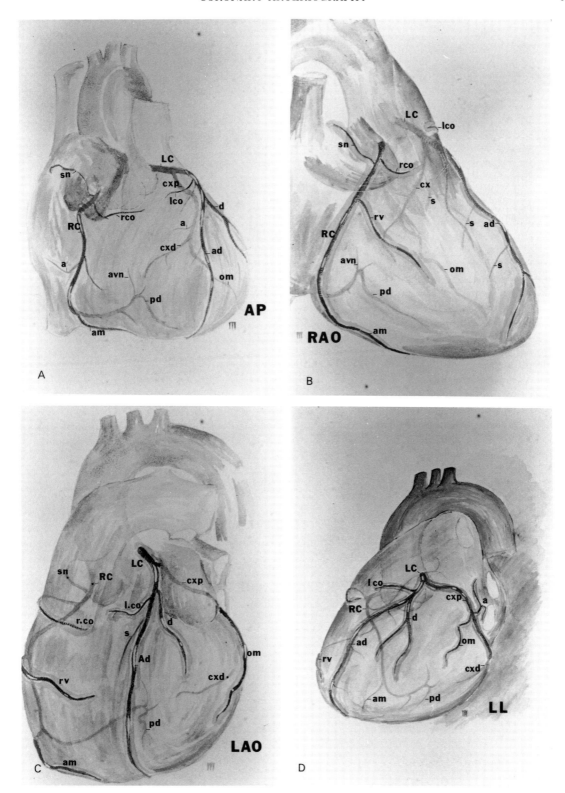

FIG. 370. A–D. SEE-THROUGH DIAGRAMS OF THE HEART

These illustrations show the coronary arteries as seen in four radiographic projections: AP, RAO, LAO, and LL views. The vessels on the cardiac surface closer to the observer are highlighted. The cardiac chambers, the aorta, pulmonary arteries, and the atrial appendages are outlined. Balanced type distribution.

coronary artery (anastomotic ring of Vieussens) (Figs. 377 and 405).

The septal branches of the anterior descending (Fig. 372) are variable in number and arise from the middle and distal thirds of the anterior descending, penetrate into the interventricular septum which they follow in a curvilinear course with convexity towards the right. The most constant is the first septal branch, the origin of which serves to mark the boundaries between the proximal and middle third of the anterior descending and it serves as an important intercoronary collateral pathway.

The left ventricular branches of the anterior descending also vary in size and number in an inverse relation with the number and size of left ventricular branches that arise from the circumflex. The most proximal or predominant branch to the left ventricle is called the diagonal branch. This branch occasionally can be as large as the anterior descending (Fig. 371) and may originate so proximally as to in fact appear as the third branch of the main left coronary artery. The diagonal branch follows a varied course along the epicardial surface of the free left ventricular wall. Several other left ventricular branches originating from the anterior descending also extend over the left ventricular surface; they may vary in number from two to six and their size is inversely proportional to the diagonal.

The left circumflex artery takes off at a rather sharp angle from the main left coronary artery and runs posteriorly, with a downward convexity, under the left atrial appendage (Figs. 371 and 372) into the left atrioventricular groove in a plane that is directed approximately 45° posterior to the frontal plane of the body. It may run a varied distance in the atrioventricular groove to reach in some instances (approximately 10%) the junction of the atrioventricular and the posterior interventricular grooves (the crux of the heart). In its course the circumflex gives off several anterior branches to the lateral surface of the left ventricle; the most prominent courses along or near the obtuse margin of the heart (the obtuse or left marginal branch) at an angle which depends entirely on its point of takeoff from the circumflex (Fig. 371). The circumflex can be divided into a proximal segment from its origin to the point at which it emerges from under the left atrial appendage near the obtuse margin of the heart and a distal segment from that point to its fullest reach in the atrioventricular groove (Fig. 372). Several other left ventricular branches may originate from both the proximal and distal segment of the circumflex; size varies in inverse proportion with the size of the obtuse marginal branch (Fig. 377).

The circumflex in its proximal and distal segments gives off branches that course posteriorly over the surface of the left atrium; they are named according to their origin as proximal and distal left atrial branches (Figs. 373 and 377). A recurrent branch of the proximal left atrial artery may course over the surface of the left atrium to cross between the root of the aorta and the superior vena cava and anastomose with its homologue, the atrial branch of the right coronary artery (Fig. 377). When the distal circumflex reaches the crux of the heart it may continue in a few cases to provide to a variable extent branches to the posteroinferior septum (Fig. 377).

In these cases the circumflex will provide the branch to the A-V node which penetrates the inferior portion of the interventricular septum in an upward directed course.

A small artery originally called by Kugel the arteria anastomotica auricularis magna, and now bearing his name, may be seen in coronary arteriograms of very good quality (Smith et al., 1973). It may arise from the proximal left circumflex or one of its branches and it courses in the lower portion of the atrial septum; it may anastomose either with the distal right coronary artery near the crux or with branches of the proximal right coronary artery. It constitutes the source of an infrequent collateral pathway.

The Right Coronary Artery. This artery originates from the right sinus of Valsalva on the anterior surface of the aorta and courses almost straight anteriorly and follows closely the anterior half of the sagittal plane of the body. It runs for a few millimeters ventrally and almost horizontally then courses more laterally under the right atrial appendage to enter the atrioventricular groove which it follows in its course around the lateral wall and then the inferior wall of the heart to reach the crux.

For descriptive purposes, three segments are recognized in the right coronary artery. The first segment extends from its origin to the point at or slightly after it emerges from under the right atrial appendage and changes to a downward course. The second segment extends from that point to the acute margin of the heart where a sudden change of direction occurs. The third segment begins at the acute margin of the heart and extends to the crux. At the crux of the heart the coronary artery takes a hairpin turn to enter the inferior interventricular groove where it becomes the posterior descending branch. The mode of termination of the distal right coronary artery is quite variable. The right coronary artery gives several branches. The first, originating in the proximal 2 cm, is the right conal branch

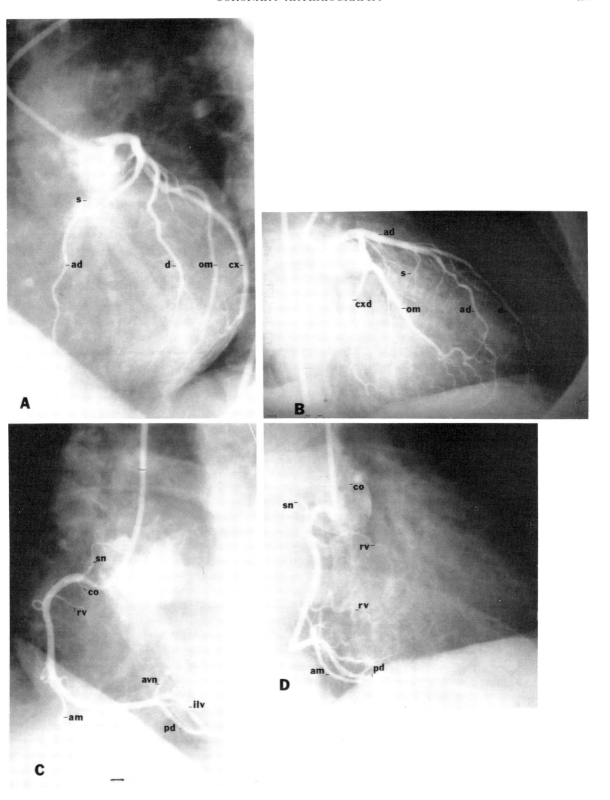

Fig. 371. Normal Coronary Arteriogram
(A) LCA, LAO. (B) LCA, RAO. (C) RCA, LAO. (D) RCA, RAO. The RCA is dominant but gives off only a moderate size inferior left ventricular branch. The distal circumflex is small but present distal to an early take-off of large obtuse marginal branch.

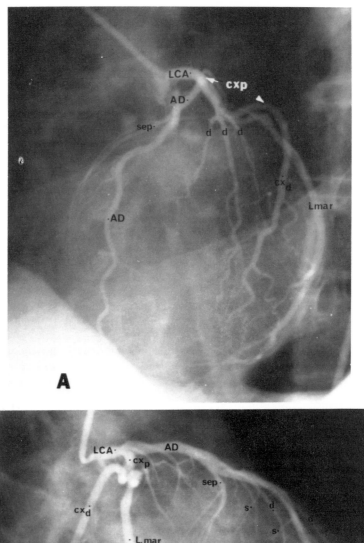

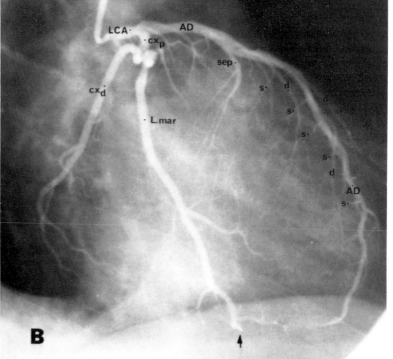

Fig. 372. Normal LCA

(A) LAO. (B) RAO. The septal branches are shown well. The diagonal branches are small. The obtuse (L. Mar.) is very large and enters the posterior interventricular sulcus replacing a segment of the PD (arrow).

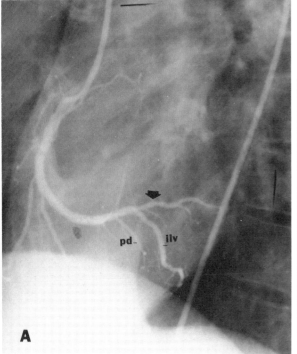

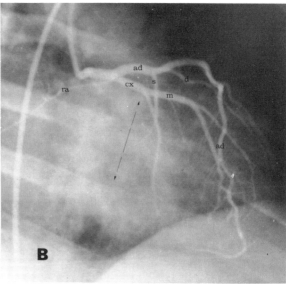

FIG. 373. DOMINANT RCA

The distal segment of the circumflex branch is absent and replaced by a large extension of the RCA (arrow) that gives off large inferior left ventricular branch. Line with arrows in B indicates the location of the left atrioventricular sulcus. The PD is small, and partly replaced by the AD. (A) RCA, LAO. (B) LCA, RAO.

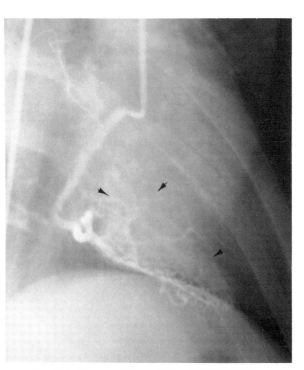

FIG. 374. NORMAL MYOCARDIAL BLUSH OF THE POSTERIOR INTERVENTRICULAR SEPTUM. RIGHT CORONARY ARTERY INJECTION RAO

which is directed anteriorly to encircle the right side of the outflow tract of the right ventricle where it anastomoses with its counterpart, the left conal branch of the left coronary artery (Figs. 402 and 405). The origin of this branch is quite variable and in 40–50% of the cases may originate as a separate vessel directly from the right sinus of Valsalva or from the aorta itself (Fig. 392).

The sinus node branch (Figs. 371 and 386) also originates from the initial portion of the right coronary, courses posteriorly and cranially below the right atrial appendage to reach the point where the superior vena cava enters the right atrium, to give off branches to the sinus node and occcasionally extending across the midline to variable length into the left atrium. In as many as 40% of cases the artery to the sinus node may originate from the proximal circumflex (Fig. 373). In the atrioventricular groove the right coronary artery gives origin to one or several anterior right ventricular branches distributed over the surface of the right ventricular wall. The number of these vessels is inversely related to their size. The most prominent and frequent of these branches is the so-called artery of the acute margin. Its origin is variable and may arise from either the first or second segment of the right coronary artery; the

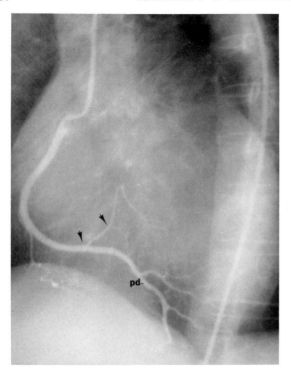

FIG. 375. THE DISTAL SEGMENT OF THE RCA
(BETWEEN ARROWS) IS HYPOPLASTIC

The RCA continues as a large inferior right ventricular
branch that enters the posterior interventricular groove
to become the posterior descending.

coronary distribution: the predominant right pattern, the predominant left pattern, and the balanced pattern. In each of these patterns there are certain consistencies which serve as valuable guides to anatomic and pathologic correlation. Bianchi (1904) and Smith (1962) have emphasized the fact that the fundamental variable is a reciprocal relationship of the length of the circumflex and of the right coronary artery.

Balanced Coronary Arterial Pattern. In this pattern, both the right and the left arteries terminate at the crux. The left coronary artery supplies the left ventricle and the anterior two-thirds of the interventricular septum, whereas the right coronary artery supplies the right ventricle and the posterior third of the interventricular septum.

Right Coronary Predominant Pattern. The circumflex branch of the left coronary artery does not extend into the distal atrioventricular groove and ends at the obtuse margin or by becoming the obtuse marginal artery itself. The right coronary artery here extends past the crux into the left atrioventricular groove from where it sends branches to the inferior surface of the left ventricle (Fig. 373).

Left Coronary Predominant Pattern. The left coronary artery extends beyond the crux into the inferior interventricular groove as a posterior

more proximal its origin the more oblique course it follows in the surface of the right ventricular wall. One or more inferior right ventricular branches are given off by the third segment of the right coronary artery to supply the inferior wall of the right ventricle. Its branches may reach the posterior interventricular groove to replace in part a segment of the posterior descending artery (Figs. 375 and 376).

From the second segment of the right coronary artery originates one or two right atrial branches of inconstant location. They supply the lateral and inferior walls of the right atrium.

At the crux, at the level of the U-shaped curve or slightly before it, originates the artery of the atrioventricular node (Fig. 371) which enters the posteroinferior septum and follows a fairly straight upward course to perfuse the region of the atrioventricular node.

It is very important to understand the reciprocal territorial interrelationships of both right and left coronary systems. The concept of dominance has been diversely defined by several authors.

In essence there are three basic patterns to the

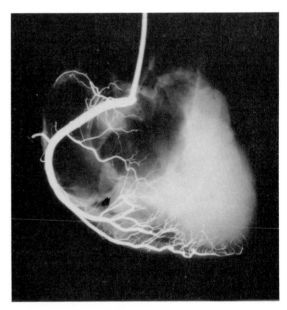

FIG. 376. INJECTED SPECIMEN

The RCA has been injected with a barium mixture, LAO view. The posterior descending has been replaced by numerous branches from the acute marginal and inferior right ventricular branches. As the case in Fig. 375, the same distal segment of the RC is hypoplastic (arrow).

descending and it may give branches to the inferior surface of the right ventricle. Reciprocally the right coronary artery may end at the acute margin of the heart or extend only a small distance into the right atrioventricular groove without reaching the crux (Fig. 377).

The reported frequencies with which each one of the patterns occur vary according to different authors and specifically according to their interpretations of the original definitions of dominance. Schlesinger (1940) divided coronary circulation into right, mixed, and left systems, depending upon the blood supply to the inferior wall of the left ventricle rather than to the origin of the posterior descending.

The relative frequency of each of these patterns was approximately 70, 20, and 10% for the right, mixed, and left, respectively.

It should again be emphasized that the predominance refers only to the reciprocal relationship of the right coronary artery and the circumflex in regard to the crux of the heart and not to the total mass of myocardium perfused. The left coronary artery perfuses most of the effective myocardial mass including the lateral and anterior walls of the left ventricle and the anterior two-thirds of the interventricular septum. The right coronary artery perfuses the smaller volume of the right ventricular wall and the posterior third of the interventricular septum. The right coronary artery is also responsible for the perfusion of the sinoatrial and atrioventricular nodes as well as the conducting system and in most instances the inferior papillary muscle.

Anatomy of the Coronary Vessels in the Angiographic Projections. The fundamental arteriographic principle that any vessel should be seen in at least two views at 90° angles from each other is essential in coronary angiography. The degrees of obliquity of the radiographic projections necessary to achieve this vary according to many factors: the size of the heart, the height of the diaphragm, the presence of right or left ventricular enlargement, common variations in the pattern of origin, branching, and distribution of the coronary vessels; therefore, selection must be made individually. Under most circumstances one left anterior oblique and two right anterior oblique views are sufficient for the left coronary and one left anterior and one right anterior oblique for the right coronary. In the evaluation of lesions of the main left coronary artery, and the proximal anterior descending and circumflex, additional views with a craniocaudal angulation are necessary and have been proven to be more reliable (Lesperance et al., 1974; Aldridge et al., 1975).

Left Coronary Artery. In the left anterior oblique projection, the ostium and the main left coronary artery are best seen. The first segment of the anterior descending, the proximal portions of the diagonal, the left ventricular branches of the circumflex, and the obtuse marginal artery are foreshortened. The proximal and distal segments of the circumflex are well displayed. The septal branches are a little foreshortened as they follow a curved branchless course with a slight convexity toward the right, slightly to the right, or overlapped by the undulating, anterior descending.

In the right anterior oblique projection the main left coronary artery is seen foreshortened as it courses perpendicularly away from the plane of the film. The first segment of the circumflex, which continues in the general direction of the main left coronary artery in this view, and as it courses under the left atrial appendage, is also markedly foreshortened. The middle segment of the circumflex as it rounds the obtuse margin is well seen, whereas the distal segment, coming toward the observer in the left atrioventricular groove, is also foreshortened. All of the segments of the anterior descending are displayed in this view. The anterior descending as it follows the anterior interventricular groove in this view, courses below the cardiac outline to a point at the beginning of its distal segment where it reaches the cardiac border to turn towards the apex of the heart. The anterior descending can be distinguished from the diagonal branch that in this projection runs along the border of the heart by the fact that it gives off numerous septal branches which arise almost perpendicular to its main course (Fig. 372). The well-displayed origin of the first septal branch in this view clearly helps to distinguish the proximal from the middle segment of the anterior descending. Some overlap is common, and the proximal few centimeters of the diagonal branch may be obscured by the anterior descending. The left ventricular branches of the circumflex along the lateral and inferior walls are well displayed without foreshortening. The atrial branches of the circumflex are seen coursing posteriorly into the lateral wall of the left atrium (Fig. 377) and the conal artery may be seen arising from the upper border of the proximal anterior descending. Directed upwards, it surrounds the outflow tract of the right ventricle (Fig. 396).

Right Coronary Artery. In the left anterior oblique projection the entire right coronary artery as it encircles the right atrioventricular groove is well displayed without any significant foreshortening, whereas its atrial and ventricular

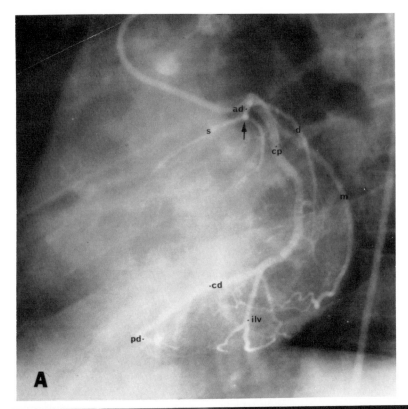

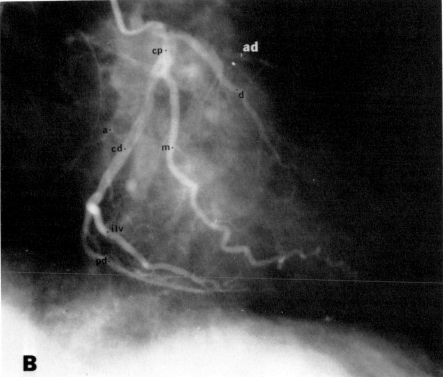

FIG. 377. DOMINANT LEFT CORONARY ARTERY

(A) LCA, LAO. (B) LCA, RAO. (C) RCA, LAO. The posterior descending is a branch of the circumflex. The anterior descending is completely occluded at the origin of the first septal branch (arrow). The RCA, distal to a right ventricular branch is very small and hypoplastic (open arrow). Right conal to the left conal anastomosis reconstitutes the anterior descending. Note a large left atrial branch of the distal circumflex (a).

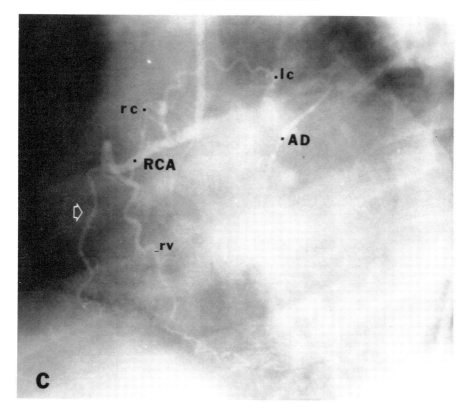

branches as well as the posterior descending are considerably foreshortened. Conversely, in the right anterior oblique projection, the right ventricular branches, the posterior descending, the atrial branches, and the second segment of the right coronary artery will be shown to better advantage. The first and third segments of the right coronary artery, because they are directed almost directly toward and away from the observer in this projection, cannot be well evaluated.

Late in the arterial phase and as the contrast substance disappears from the main branches (particularly with right coronary artery injections), a distinct, and sometimes intense stain appears in the interventricular septum (Fig. 374). This is particularly prominent in the presence of proximal stenosis or spasm and coincides in time with the maximum electrocardiographic effect produced by the injected contrast substance as it perfuses the conducting system of the heart and the atrioventricular node.

ANATOMICAL VARIATIONS, CONGENITAL ANOMALIES AND MALFORMATIONS

The classical anatomy of coronary vessels as described in the preceding section represents a composite of the most commonly encountered anatomical patterns. With this as a background, one should be aware of a certain number of variations in the origin, distribution, and interrelationships of the coronary vessels as well as the most frequently encountered congenital anomalies that can present a problem for the performance of the coronary arteriogram and its interpretation.

Anatomical variations or anomalies of origin, distribution, and territory, both inconsequential and of pathologic significance, can be encountered in normal individuals and in patients with congenital cardiovascular malformations.

A much-quoted classification of congenital anomalies of the coronary vessels (Edwards, 1958) divided the anomalies of the coronary vessels into those that had major or minor significance. Since then some of the anomalies of distribution of the coronary vessels that previously were considered inconsequential, have been recognized as the cause of serious and even fatal cardiac disease.

Since it is not possible to separate variations of frequent occurrence from congenital anomalies, for descriptive purposes, we propose the following classification.

I. Variations and Anomalies without Shunt

A. Not in association with congenital heart disease
1. Anomalies of the coronary ostia
   Ectopia
   Variations in number
2. Variations of origin
   Left coronary artery from right coronary sinus or right coronary artery
   Right coronary artery from left coronary sinus or left coronary artery
   Circumflex from right coronary sinus or right coronary artery
   Left anterior descending from right coronary artery
   Either coronary artery from noncoronary sinus
   Independent origin of branches from aorta or coronary sinus
3. Variations of distribution
   Distal segmental hypoplasia or underdevelopment of branches
   Marginal termination of circumflex
   Marginal termination of right coronary artery
   Marginal replacement of posterior descending
   Anterior descending replacement of posterior descending
   Duplication of branches
4. Single coronary artery
   Right coronary distribution
   Left coronary distribution
   Mixed distribution

B. In association with congenital heart disease
   Tetralogy of Fallot
   Complete transposition of the great vessels
   Corrected transposition of the great vessels
   Double outlet right ventricle
   Single ventricle
   Pulmonary atresia with intact septum
   Congenital aortic stenosis

II. Variations and anomalies with shunt

A. Origin of either or both coronary arteries from the pulmonary artery

B. Primary fistulas
With left to right shunt
With left to left shunt
   C. Secondary fistulas

III. Congenital Aneurysms and Ectasias

There are some variations and anomalies in origin, branching pattern, and distribution that are seen more frequently in patients with congenital cardiac malformations but are also seen in hearts that are otherwise normal.

The location of the coronary ostium in relation to its respective sinus may vary (Vlodaver *et al.*, 1972).

The ostia, as previously stated, in as many as 30% of hearts may be situated above the superior limits of the left cusp (the junctional line). The ostia can be found anywhere in the ascending aorta and in rare cases, quite high in location (Fig. 379).

Since any of the proximal or primary branches may originate directly from the corresponding cusps or the supravalvular aorta the number of ostia will vary accordingly. The most common branch that may arise independently is the conal, (Fig. 392) particularly the right, which according to classical descriptions (Bianchi, 1904) could be found in as many as 50% of the cases, receiving then the name "the third coronary artery." It may not be seen in a selective arteriogram.

In McAlpine's (1975) series, the right coronary orifice was single in 47%, 2 orifices were found in 48%, 3 in 4%, and 4 in 1%. The left orifice was single in all 100 hearts.

Similarly, an entire coronary artery or any of its primary branches may arise from the contralateral sinus or as a branch of the other coronary artery. The majority of these anomalies involve the left coronary artery.

Origin of the left circumflex branch from the right coronary sinus is the most frequent anomaly in this group (Engle *et al.*, 1975) and of itself is of no pathological significance. It is merely a potential source of diagnostic error since the lack of visualization of the circumflex from the left coronary artery injection may lead the observer to assume its occlusion. The vessel may arise directly from the right cusp (Fig. 408) or more commonly as a branch of the right coronary artery (Fig. 381), then course behind the great vessels to enter the atrioventricular groove under the left atrial appendage and continue in its usual distribution. The incidence of this variant in our experience has been one percent. Its existence

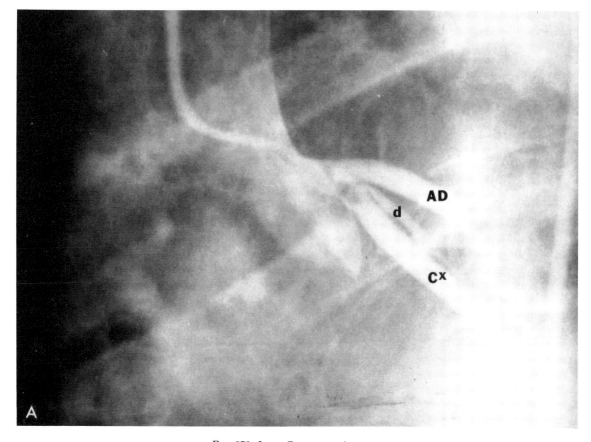

FIG. 378. LEFT CORONARY ARTERY

The main LCA is extremely short. The anterior descending, circumflex, and diagonal branches appear to arise from a common ostium. Close-up view of an injection in the left cusp.

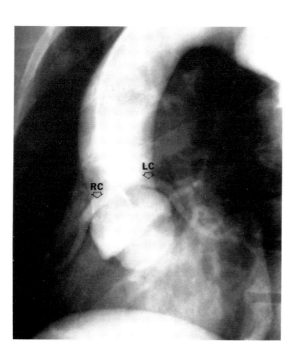

should be suspected when the absence of a vessel in the territory of circumflex, from a left coronary injection, is not accompanied by corresponding ventricular dysfunction.

Anomalous origin of the entire left coronary artery from the right coronary sinus was until recently considered a minor anatomical variation without significance. It appears from recent reports (Chaitman *et al.*, 1976; Cheitlin *et al.*, 1974) that sudden death from either massive myocardial infarction or arrhythmia during or immediately after some exertion may occur in 27% of cases of young men with this anatomical arrangement. In these individuals the left coronary artery arises from the right coronary sinus or as a part of a single coronary artery and forms a

FIG. 379. COMMON ORIGIN OF BOTH CORONARY ARTERIES FROM A SINGLE ECTOPIC OSTIUM LOCATED ABOVE THE SUPRAVALVULAR RIDGE IN A PATIENT WITH PSEUDOCOARCTATION OF THE AORTA. LAO.

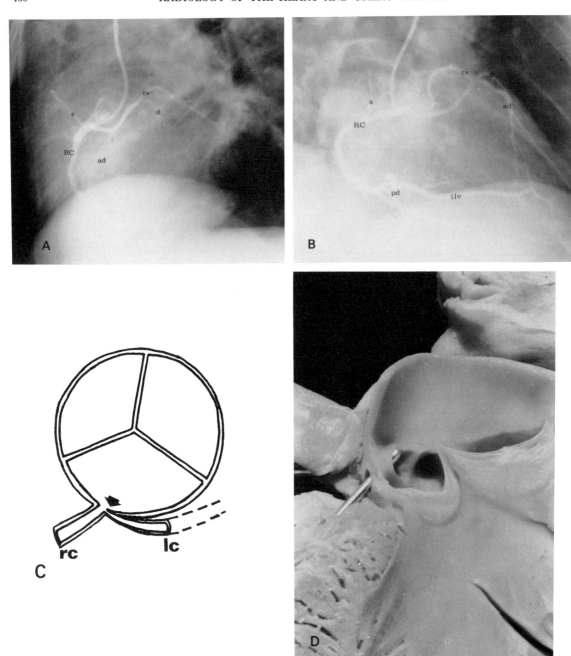

FIG. 380. ANOMALOUS ORIGIN OF THE ENTIRE LCA FROM THE RCA (SINGLE CORONARY ARTERY) IN A 30-YEAR-OLD
FEMALE WITH EXERTIONAL ANGINA

(A) LAO. (B) RAO. (C) Diagrammatic cross-section of aortic sinuses illustrating the relationships of the left coronary artery
(LC) to the anterior wall of the aorta, creating a valve-like opening (arrow). (D) Specimen of the aortic root of an 11-month-old
girl, with a similar anomaly, who died suddenly from an acute myocardial infarction. Note the slit-like configuration of the
proximal LC, which is included in the wall of the aorta (probe). (With permission, from Morettin, L. B., Coronary Arteriography,
Uncommon Observations. *Radiology Clinics of North America, 14:* 189–208, 1976.)

sharp acute angle as it courses leftwards between
the anterior wall of the aorta, into which it
sometimes is incorporated, and the pulmonary
artery (Fig. 380). The origin of the left coronary

artery then acquires a slit-like configuration.
With increased cardiac activity and expansion of
the pulmonary artery resulting from physical
exertion the left coronary artery is stretched and

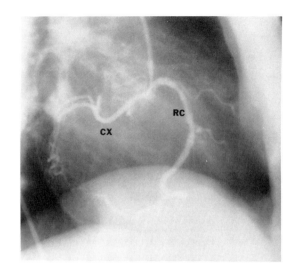

FIG. 381. ANOMALOUS ORIGIN OF LEFT CIRCUMFLEX FROM THE RIGHT CORONARY ARTERY

Anomalous origin of the left circumflex from the right coronary artery. Selective right coronary arteriogram, lateral view. The right coronary artery (RC) and the circumflex (CX) originate from a common ostium in the right coronary sinus. The circumflex courses around the aortic root posteriorly to its normal distribution in the left atrioventricular sulcus. (With permission, from Morettin, L. B., Coronary Arteriography. Uncommon Observations. *Radiologic Clinics of North America, 14:* 189–208, 1976.)

compressed, presumably resulting in the flap-like closure of the coronary artery near its orifice. The great majority of the reported deaths have been in very active young males in the second or third decades of life. We have seen an example of this situation in a 35-year-old female with angina, without infarction, and in a small infant dying of acute myocardial infarction (Fig. 380).

There is no evidence of increased incidence of sudden death or arrhythmia when the anomalous left coronary artery arising from the right sinus courses around and behind the aortic root. In fact, in this circumstance the left anterior descending could be considered a branch of an anomalous circumflex.

Both of these variants are indeed forms of a single coronary artery. When only the left anterior descending branch of the left coronary artery arises from the right coronary sinus it courses over the surface of the outflow tract of the right ventricle. This is much more common in congenital heart disease, particularly in the tetralogy of Fallot.

In addition to the conal branches other branches of the coronary artery may arise independently from the cusps or the aorta. This results when the main left coronary artery is absent and all branches appear to arise independently from the corresponding cusp (Fig. 378). This occurred in approximately 3% of our patients (Morettin, 1976).

Origin of either coronary artery from the posterior (noncoronary) cusp, in the absence of congenital heart disease, is extremely rare and has been reported only occurring with the right coronary artery.

A right coronary artery arising from the left coronary sinus was encountered only 3 times in 4,250 cases (Engle, 1975). Angina has been reported occurring when this anomalous right coronary artery courses between the aorta and the pulmonary artery. Sudden death has not been reported.

In the process of embryological development a reciprocal compensating relationship exists which determines that, when a branch of a coronary vessel does not develop in an area of the heart, a vessel from the contralateral system, or from the adjacent area will occupy its place. Consequently, when segmental hypoplasia or underdevelopment occurs in the distal circumflex, a branch of the right coronary artery distal to the crux (dominant) should occupy its place (Fig. 373). Similarly, when the right coronary artery is very small and does not extend into the right atrioventricular groove for more than a few centimeters, an extension of the left circumflex must take its place (Fig. 377). Congenital absence of the left circumflex, distal to the obtuse margin without compensatory development of the right coronary artery, has been observed in 89.5% of patients with the so-called systolic click syndrome (Gentzeler *et al.*, 1975). These patients exhibit marked reduction in the contraction of the mitral valvular ring and periannular myocardium accompanied by prolapse of the posterior mitral leaflet, causing a typical clicking sound followed by a late systolic murmur. Localized myocardial dysfunction with abnormal valvular closure is the proposed mechanism. It should be pointed out that a systolic click is known to occur in other circumstances such as inferior myocardial infarction, chest trauma, acute rheumatic fever, atrial septal defect, and hypertrophic subaortic stenosis.

Variations in the size and extent of distribution of the posterior descending are very frequent. In 18% of our cases one or more of the inferior right ventricular branches and/or the larger marginal branch could be seen entering the posterior interventricular groove to replace the entire or more frequently the most distal segments of the posterior descending. In these cases, the main right coronary tends to be very small distal to the origin of that branch (Figs. 375 and 376). When the entire posterior descending is replaced the usual hairpin turn of the right coronary at the crux is absent and, in this circumstance, the artery to the A-V node most frequently arises from the distal circumflex (Fig. 377). Similarly the anterior descending turning around the apex of the heart may occupy a sizable portion of the distal interventricular groove in a retrograde manner.

A considerable variation in the size of secondary branches of coronary arteries may occur. Particularly remarkable is the frequency of the presence of a large acute or obtuse marginal branch that may be even larger than the parent artery distal to its origin. A large obtuse marginal artery achieves considerable significance when it supplies both the lateral and inferior wall of the left ventricle, the distal circumflex being either very small or absent (Fig. 411). Similarly the acute marginal may replace the distal right coronary in the inferior wall of the right ventricle and inferior interventricular septum (Fig. 383).

Partial or complete duplication of either coronary artery or its main branches can be encountered in approximately 1% of cases (Morettin, 1976). In this variant, two vessels, generally of a smaller caliber than expected, run parallel courses very close to each other, to share a common territory (Figs. 382 and 383). Occlusion of one of these vessels may be easily overlooked.

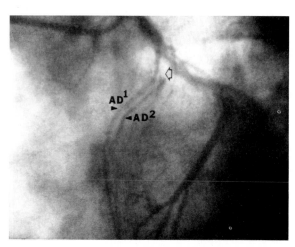

FIG. 382. DUPLICATION OF THE AD
Two separate arteries run next to each other in the anterior interventricular groove (AD₁ and AD₂). AD₂ is almost completely obstructed near its origin (open arrow). This vessel is not the first septal branch with which it may be confused. LAO view. Dominant left coronary artery. (With permission, from Morettin, L. B., Coronary Arteriography. Uncommon Observations. *Radiologic Clinics of North America, 14:* 189–208, 1976.)

This is more common in hearts with congenital deformities but can be encountered also in hearts that are otherwise normal. In order of frequency they involve the posterior descending branch, the anterior descending, and the right coronary artery.

Single coronary arteries of a right or left distribution may result when, through absence or insufficient development of the proximal segment of either vessel, the opposite artery running in a reverse direction in the atrioventricular groove occupies its territory. Consequently, only one ostium is present and a coronary artery originating from that ostium supplies the entire heart (Vlodaver *et al.*, 1975). This mechanism gives rise to the two most common types: a single artery of right or left distribution. The third type is a single coronary artery with a distribution and branching so atypical that it cannot be compared with the normal pattern of either right or left coronary. Single coronary arteries are found more frequently in association with other congenital anomalies of the heart than in normal hearts, particularly the third type. Single coronary arteries have been described in association with complete transposition of the great vessels, origin of both great vessels from the right ventricle, situs inversus, tetralogy of Fallot, and pulmonary atresia.

A single coronary artery results also when, as described above, the left coronary artery arises from the right coronary artery and after coursing either behind or in front of the aorta, reenters its normal distribution.

Anomalies and Variations in Association with Congenital Heart Disease

These have been extensively described by Elliott *et al.* (1966) and Vlodaver *et al.* (1975). Their descriptions are those we follow.

A large variety of anomalies of origin and distribution of the coronary vessels can be encountered in the tetralogy of Fallot. The most common (40% of the cases) is the presence of a very large conus artery arising from the right coronary sinus and distributed over a very large area of the right ventricle. A single coronary artery of right (most common) or left coronary distribution may be present. Next in frequency is the occurrence of an anomalous anterior descending that arises from the right coronary artery. In all these instances the anomalous vessel crosses over the anterior surface of the right ventricle and may be injured at the time of right ventriculotomy, leading to serious complications and even death (Hallman *et al.*, 1966). This circumstance is particularly dangerous when, as

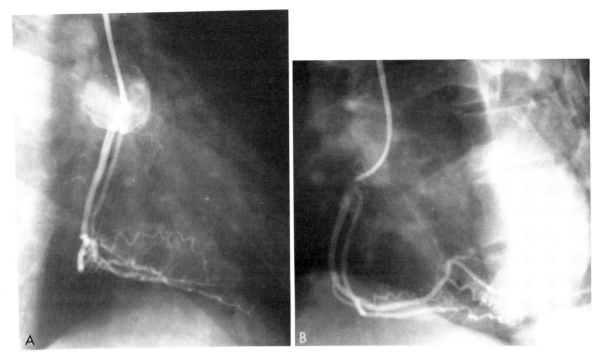

FIG. 383. RIGHT CORONARY ARTERIOGRAM

(A) Right anterior oblique. (B) Left anterior oblique. Unusual branching pattern resulting in actual duplication of the proximal right coronary artery. Occlusion of the smaller branch could be easily overlooked. (With permission, from Morettin, L. B., Coronary Arteriography. Uncommon Observations. *Radiologic Clinics of North America, 14:* 189–208, 1976.)

frequently occurs, the anomalous vessel is imbedded in the myocardium (mural artery). Other anomalies such as fistulous communications with the heart chambers and a bronchial artery and anomalous origin of the right coronary artery from the left sinus have been described, but they are very rare.

COMPLETE TRANSPOSITION OF THE GREAT VESSELS. In this case, the aorta, which gives origin to the coronary arteries, originates from the right ventricle, whereas the pulmonary trunk originates exclusively from the left ventricle. The connections of the systemic, pulmonary, and coronary veins are normal. In the great majority of cases, the anterior (right) is the noncoronary sinus with the right coronary artery arising from the posterior and the left coronary from the left coronary sinus. In the most common pattern of distribution the left coronary artery gives rise to both anterior descending and the left circumflex branch. This is found more frequently when there is an oblique relationship of the aorta to the pulmonary artery, with the aorta lying anterior and to the right of the pulmonary artery. The second most common pattern of distribution found in 20 of 60 cases of Elliott consisted of the anterior descending arising from the left coro-

nary sinus and the right coronary artery from the posterior sinus giving origin to a circumflex branch that coursed posterior to the great vessels. This pattern was more frequent in cases in which there was a side-to-side relationship of the aorta to the pulmonary artery, both situated almost in the same frontal plane.

CORRECTED TRANSPOSITION OF THE GREAT VESSELS. The two ventricles and atrioventricular valves are abnormally situated and with the exception of a possible ventricular septal defect, the ventricles are otherwise normal. The left-sided or arterial ventricle anatomically resembles a normal right ventricle and the right-sided or venous ventricle resembles a normal left ventricle. The aorta is located anteriorly and to the left and arises from the arterial ventricle. The pulmonary artery is located posteriorly and to the right, originating from the venous ventricle. In about one-third of the cases the aorta is directly anterior to the pulmonary artery. The anterior is the noncoronary cusp. The right coronary artery arises from the posterior sinus and gives origin to the anterior descending branch. The abnormal origin of the right coronary artery from the posterior sinus and its transverse direction, parallel to the frontal plane is quite characteristic. The left coronary artery in each case originates from the left aortic sinus and coursing in the left atrioventricular sulcus as a circumflex artery gives origin to the left ventricular and the posterior descending branches.

COMMON (SINGLE) CARDIAC VENTRICLE WITH TRANSPOSITION. In this entity, located anteriorly at the base of the heart is the infundibular chamber which is a small cavity separated from the main cardiac ventricular chamber by a rudimentary septum. The pulmonary artery arises from the common ventricular chamber whereas the aorta originates from the infundibular chamber. The atrioventricular valve or valves communicate with the main cardiac chamber only. Two types are distinguished according to the location of the infundibular chamber: (1) a single ventricle with noninverted infundibulum when the infundibular chamber is located on the right side of the base of the heart, and (2) a single ventricle with infundibular inversion when the chamber is located in the left side of the base of the heart. Coronary arterial patterns vary with each one of these subtypes (Elliott et al., 1966). When the infundibulum is in the noninverted position the origin and distribution of the coronary arteries is identical to that seen in complete transposition of the great vessels with an oblique relationship between the aorta and pulmonary artery.

When there is inversion of the infundibulum with the aorta situated anteriorly and to the left of the pulmonary artery, as in corrected transposition, the anterior is the noncoronary cusp and two patterns of coronary distribution may be encountered. In both the right coronary artery originates from the right cusp and the left coronary artery from the left cusp. But in the first and more common pattern, the anterior descending is a branch of the left coronary artery. This anatomical feature, when present, helps in distinguishing a single ventricle with infundibular inversion from corrected transposition. In the second and less frequent pattern of distribution, the anterior descending is, as in corrected transposition, a branch of the right coronary artery.

The origin and distribution of the coronary vessels can be, in some circumstances, of significant importance in helping to differentiate a single ventricle from transposition, and differentiation between complete transposition and origin of both great vessels from the right ventricle of the Taussig-Bing variety may be made from the study of the coronary arterial patterns. Specifically, when dealing with cases of suspected transposition, demonstration of a right coronary artery arising from a normal position rules out complete transposition, corrected transposition,

and common ventricle, and is in favor of origin of both great vessels from the right ventricle.

Determination of the site of origin of the anterior descending helps in the differentiation between corrected transposition and single ventricle with inversion of the infundibulum. In the presence of a case in which the position of the great vessels suggests corrected transposition or common ventricle, the demonstration of an anterior descending originating from the left coronary artery, which is characteristic of common ventricle with inverted infundibulum, rules out the presence of a corrected transposition. Conversely, the demonstration of a single anterior descending arising from the left cusp, and a circumflex as a branch of the right coronary artery, strongly favors the presence of a corrected transposition.

In cases of pulmonary atresia with intact interventricular septum and competent tricuspid valve, Williams et al. (1951) and Edwards et al. (1958) described an interesting anomaly of the coronary vessels. In such conditions, normally existing cardiac chamber-to-coronary artery anastomoses greatly expand in utero to form what in fact is an outflow to the obstructed ventricle. Blood then flows from the cardiac chamber via these connections into the coronary vessels and in a retrograde manner into the aorta, creating what is in fact a ventriculoaortic fistulous communication. A right ventricular angiocardiogram of a young infant with this abnormality (Fig. 384) clearly demonstrates large epicardial vascular structures in the distribution of the anterior descending and the right coronary arteries, leading to the aorta. This should not be confused with an intramyocardial injection that may result in opacification of the cardiac veins. The veins should drain posteriorly into the left atrium.

A significant difference has recently been observed (Higgins and Wexler, 1975) in the relative frequency in which the left coronary artery is the dominant vessel in patients with isolated congenital aortic stenosis and bicuspid aortic valve (36 and 56.8%, respectively). This clearly contrasts with 10–15% left dominance in the unselected population. This finding is consistent with our observation that variations of origin and distribution of the coronary arteries are more frequent in individuals with otherwise not significant and isolated anomalies of the aortic arch (Fig. 379).

Ostial stenosis may be encountered in association with supravalvular aortic stenosis (Vlodaver et al., 1976).

Anomalies with Shunt. In this group are included all of those anomalies and malformations that result in a direct communication of a

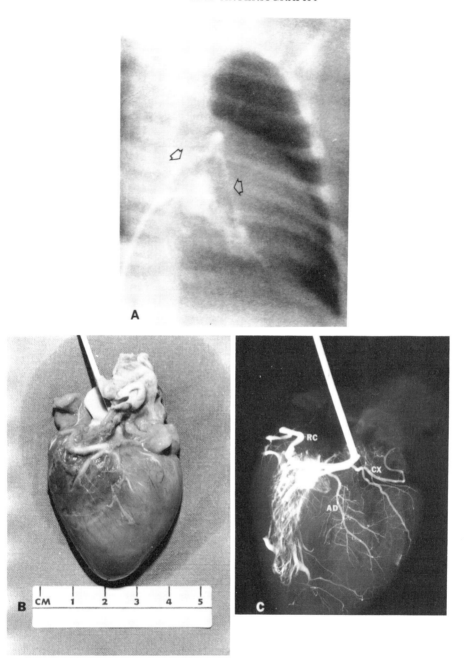

FIG. 384. PULMONARY ATRESIA WITH INTACT INTERVENTRICULAR SEPTUM AND COMPETENT TRICUSPID VALVE
(A) Right ventriculogram, AP view: Small right ventricular cavity and retrograde opacification of RCA and RV branches (arrows), draining into the aorta. This in fact represents a ventriculoaortic fistula. (B) Specimen with vessels injected with barium mixture showing a single coronary artery originating from the left sinus with large right ventricular branches that communicate with the RV cavity. (C) Radiograph of the specimen. Note the free communication of the coronary vessels with the RV cavity.

coronary artery and/or any of its branches with a cardiac chamber or extracardiac vessel resulting in a shunt of varying proportions.

Origin of both coronary arteries from the pulmonary artery is an extremely rare malformation of grave clinical significance. The entire myocardium is inadequately perfused by the low pulmonary pressure with desaturated blood. While relatively well compensated *in utero*, after birth, with a fall in the pulmonary artery pressure, rapid cardiac decompensation ensues. In rare cases this abnormality has occurred in association with tetralogy of Fallot or with large ventricular septal defects where severe pulmonary hypertension, under these circumstances, may result in improved myocardial perfusion.

Origin of the left coronary artery from the pulmonary artery is the most common anomaly of this group. The importance of its recognition resides in its early diagnosis and possible surgical correction. The evolution of the hemodynamic changes in this condition is related to the changes in pulmonary pressure that occur after birth. It is assumed that *in utero* the left ventricle is adequately perfused by the pulmonary artery with a pressure which at that time is equal to aortic pressure. With the fall in pulmonary pressure that occurs after birth, perfusion diminishes within the territory of the left coronary artery, leading to myocardial ischemia. Then, if the child survives, the reduction in left coronary artery pressure favors development of collaterals from the right to the left system through the ischemic myocardium and creates a fistula-like condition. The inconstant demonstration of flow into the pulmonary artery, in the newborn period and in young infants, indicates that shunting is an acquired phenomenon that develops some time after birth.

Cardiomegaly, sometimes massive, mostly left ventricular, is constant. Angina, congestive failure, and papillary muscle dysfunction leading to mitral insufficiency and left atrial enlargement, are frequently the presenting signs and symptoms. A continuous murmur of variable intensity appears some time in childhood and may progressively increase with the passage of years. Definite diagnosis is made by aortography or preferably by selective right coronary injection (Fig. 385). The right coronary artery arises normally from the right aortic cusps and is markedly dilated and through numerous intramyocardial connections communicates with branches of the left coronary artery in which the flow is reversed emptying into the pulmonary artery. When the shunt is sizable the pulmonary artery will be well opacified. Early diagnosis is essential because surgical ligation of the anomalous left coronary artery will improve myocardial perfusion. Other authors (Hallman *et al.*, 1966) recommend that ligation should be avoided or postponed until a later date when the child has grown and the vessels have achieved sufficient size to make vascular reconstruction feasible.

Origin of the right coronary artery from the pulmonary artery is a much rarer condition and

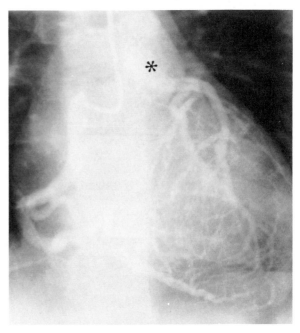

FIG. 385. ANOMALOUS ORIGIN OF THE ENTIRE LEFT CORONARY ARTERY FROM THE PULMONARY ARTERY
Selective right coronary arteriogram. The right coronary artery is markedly enlarged and tortuous. Its branches are increased in number and caliber, and through both epicardiac and intramural connections opacifies the very dilated branches of the left coronary artery and the pulmonary artery (*). (With permission, from Morettin, L. B., Coronary Arteriography. Uncommon Observations. *Radiologic Clinics of North America, 14:* 189–208, 1976.)

is considered to be a benign anomaly, found mostly at autopsy. It is thought that the pulmonary pressure is of sufficient magnitude to perfuse the right atrial and right ventricular walls that have lower intramural tension. This situation could suddenly be more serious when dealing with a dominant right coronary artery, or when obstructive lesions develop in the left coronary system necessitating right-to-left collaterals later in life. Anomalous origin of an accessory coronary artery, or one of its branches such as the conal, is very rare and mostly asymptomatic.

PRIMARY FISTULAS. These consist of a direct communication of the coronary artery or its branches with either right or left cardiac chambers or the great vessels. The reported incidence varies from 0.26–0.4%. They originate more commonly from the right coronary artery. Nearly 90% lead to the right side of the heart (in decreasing order of frequency) to the right ventricle, right atrium, pulmonary artery, and superior

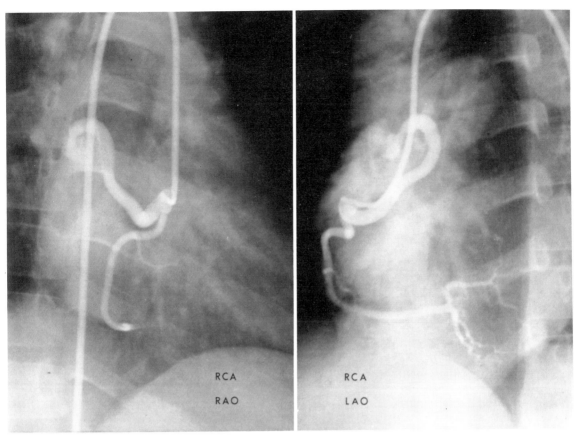

FIG. 386. CONGENITAL FISTULA

Right coronary arteriogram, right anterior oblique and left anterior oblique views. The sinoatrial branch is markedly enlarged and forms a direct fistulous communication between the right coronary artery and the superior vena cava. Note the opacification of the cavity of the right atrium. (With permission, from Morettin, L. B., Coronary Arteriography. Uncommon Observations. *Radiologic Clinics of North America, 14:* 189–208, 1976.)

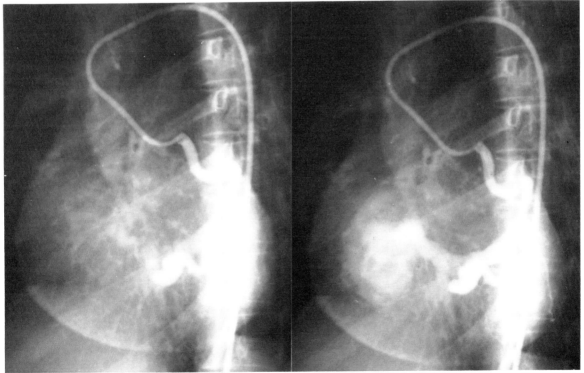

FIG. 387. CONGENITAL ARTERIOVENOUS FISTULA BETWEEN THE CIRCUMFLEX BRANCH AND THE CORONARY SINUS. LCA, LAO.

(Courtesy of Dr. Arnold Manske, Port Arthur, Texas.)

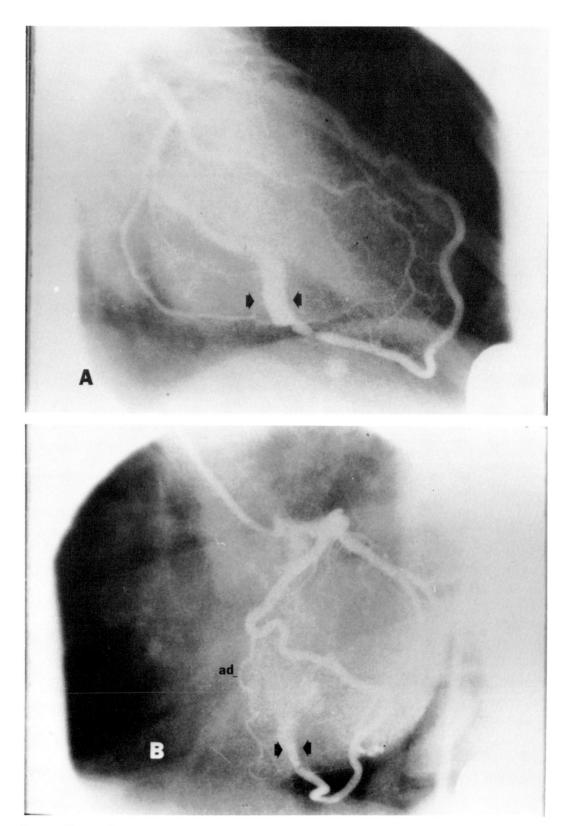

FIG. 388. FISTULA BETWEEN A DIAGONAL BRANCH OF THE ANTERIOR DESCENDING AND THE CAVITY OF THE LEFT
VENTRICLE (ARROWS)

(A) RAO diastole, a stream of contrast agent enters the LV cavity. (B) LAO systole; flow through the fistula is almost
completely stopped. The AD distal to the diagonal is small.

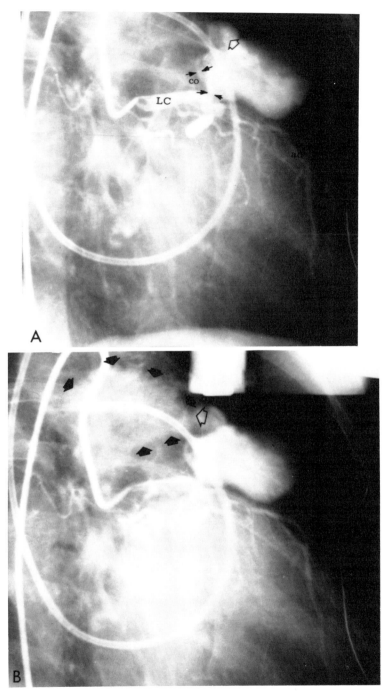

FIG. 389. CONGENITAL ANEURYSM-FISTULA

Left coronary arteriogram, right anterior oblique. The enlarged conal branch of the left coronary artery (A, small arrowheads, co) leads into a large aneurysm and through a connecting vessel (open arrow) opacifies the lumen of the pulmonary artery (B, solid arrows). LC, Left coronary artery. (With permission, from Morettin, L. B., Coronary Arteriography. Uncommon Observations. *Radiologic Clinics of North America, 14:* 189–208, 1976.)

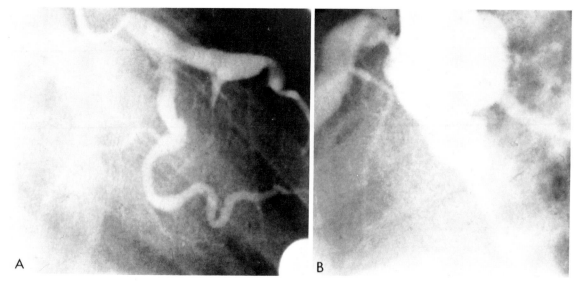

FIG. 390

(A) Left coronary arteriogram. (B) Aortogram in a 38-year-old male with Hurler's type mucopolysaccharide abnormality, multiple congenital stenotic valvular lesions, and aortic insufficiency. Both coronary arteries are markedly dilated. At autopsy the right coronary artery measured 2.5 cm in diameter. (With permission, from Morettin, L. B., Coronary Arteriography. Uncommon Observations. *Radiologic Clinics of North America, 14:* 189–208, 1976.)

vena cava (Fig. 386). When the left coronary artery is the source of the fistula, one of its branches may lead into the right ventricle, right atrium, (Fig. 387) left ventricle (Fig. 388) or pulmonary artery (Fig. 389).

The clinical picture varies across a wide spectrum according to the vessel involved, the magnitude of the shunt and the cavity or vessel in which it drains, and ranges from completely asymptomatic cases (the majority) to those with marked cardiomegaly and cardiac decompensation. Moderate cardiomegaly and some pulmonary enlargement are frequent. A continuous (postcardiac) murmur is generally present. When fistulas involve the left coronary artery, myocardial ischemia and ventricular dysfunction may develop if a sufficient amount of blood is diverted away from the left ventricular myocardium. Most of the fistulas with a communication between a branch of a coronary artery and the left ventricular cavity are asymptomatic and are found incidentally at coronary angiography. The shunt here, generally of small magnitude, occurs during diastole when the end diastolic ventricular pressure is lower than the aortic diastolic pressure (Fig. 388).

Secondary cardiac fistulas (Ogden, 1970) are those occurring in patients with severe stenosis or atresia of the pulmonary or aortic valve in association with competent tricuspid or mitral valve and intact interventricular septum. They have been described above in the subheading of those anomalies in association with congenital heart disease.

Congenital Aneurysms and Ectasia. Small saccular aneurysms have been described in association with branching anomalies (diverticula), most likely resulting from abortive branching; these can be found more commonly in patients with serious congenital anomalies of the heart such as transposition of the great vessels (Elliott *et al.*, 1966). Aneurysms are also frequent in fistulas of the coronary vessels (Fig. 389). In this situation it is likely that some of them are not primary aneurysms, but rather develop late in life as the consequence of increased flow through a structurally weak vessel. Most are asymptomatic and may be discovered when they develop calcifications in their walls. Daoud *et al.*, (1963), report that 17% of the aneurysms of the coronary arteries in their series were of congenital origin.

Localized aneurysms or diffuse aneurysmal ectasia of the coronary arteries are also frequently observed in patients with cystic medial necrosis in association with Marfan's syndrome and other disorders of mucopolysaccharide metabolism. We have seen massive diffuse aneurysmal dilatation of the coronary vessels in a 30-year-old man with Hurler's type mucopolysaccharide disturbance in association with multiple congenital valvular lesions (Fig. 390).

CORONARY ARTERIOGRAPHY AND VENTRICULOGRAPHY IN THE EVALUATION OF OCCLUSIVE CORONARY DISEASE

The irreplaceable role of coronary angiography in occlusive disease of the coronary vessels is the localization and quantitation of the obstructive lesions in the vessels of the heart. Arteriosclerosis, the most common disease of man, is responsible for the overwhelming majority of cases of ischemic coronary disease.

Early in the development of the arteriosclerotic process the degeneration of the elastic layer of the arterial wall produces no obvious arteriographic findings. Later, with early deposition of lipoid material, irregularity of the surface of the intimal layer causes irregularities in the lumen that may appear as minute, smooth elevations on the arteriogram. Localized intimal hyperplasia and the arteriosclerotic plaque are responsible for the obvious arteriographic changes. In addition, embolization, thrombosis, and dissection can account for rapid changes in the luminal configuration of a coronary vessel. An acutely occluded vessel may recanalize, even rapidly, accounting for some of the cases in which an arteriogram reveals no evidence of an arterial obstruction following a well-documented myocardial infarction. A fresh thrombus, unlike the gradual, funnel-like tapering lesion of mural sclerosis, appears frequently as an abrupt filling defect (Fig. 391).

As with narrowing of other arteries, there is no clear certainty as to what represents a "hemodynamically significant" lesion. What constitutes a critical stenosis depends not only on the actual reduction of the lumen of a vessel but on many other factors such as length of the lesion, its location, whether it is proximal or distal in a main vessel, its relation to side branches and their importance, the presence of spasm, the number of lesions, the size of the area perfused, and the collateral circulation from and to that vessel. In addition, general conditions such as arterial oxygen saturation, metabolic and hematologic abnormalities, etc., play an important role. The actual significance of a narrowed coronary segment depends, in the final analysis, on the consequences that that narrowing has on the function of the myocardial fiber and the left ventricle as a whole.

Purely from an angiographic point of view, numerous grading systems have been proposed to define and quantitate the stenosis (Gensini,

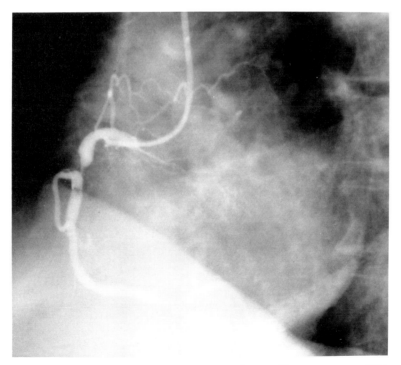

FIG. 391. SEVERE LOCALIZED STENOSIS AT THE SECOND SEGMENT OF THE RCA
LAO view. Note also polypoid defect distal to the area of stenosis, most likely a thrombus.

1975). This can be expressed in percentage of caliber reduction, descriptive terms, or numerical codes.

GRADING SYSTEMS TO EXPRESS THE MAGNITUDE OF NARROWING OF A CORONARY VESSEL

CODE	DESCRIPTIVE	% REDUCTION OF CALIBER
0	None	0
1	Minimal	0–25
2	Mild	25–50
3	Moderate	50–75
4	Severe	75–90
5	Very Severe	90–99
6	Complete	100

In an attempt to standardize the nomenclature and establish an acceptable method of quantitating coronary artery disease the Ad Hoc Committee for grading of coronary disease has recently published its guidelines (Austen *et al.*, 1975).

Most authors agree that a lesion is to be considered significant when a fixed narrowing of 50–75% can be demonstrated angiographically.

In addition to the magnitude of the stenosis a notation should be made of the length involved and distribution of the lesions. The velocity of flow, as estimated by the movement and the clearing of the contrast substance, gives additional evidence as to the significance of a stenosis. When there are multiple occlusive lesions and extensive collateral circulation one can observe abnormal, nonhomogenous, and sometimes dense myocardial staining representing delayed perfusion and a stagnation through ischemic myocardial sinusoids; this is best appreciated in the cinefluorogram.

The Incidence and Distribution of Coronary Lesions. From most of the reported series it appears that about 30% of the significant stenoses involve a single vessel (Gensini, 1975), 9% of the time at the level of the right coronary artery, 16% at the level of the anterior descending, and 5% at the level of the circumflex. In 30% of patients, two vessels are involved, and in the remaining 40%, significant stenosis of the 3 main vessels can be demonstrated (Fig. 392).

Of the complete occlusions 40% involve the right coronary artery, 32% the anterior descending, and 20% the circumflex. In only 5% of patients with complete occlusion of one artery, the other two major vessels were normal; in the remaining 95%, either one or both of the main vessels were involved by stenotic lesions.

Of the complete occlusions of the right coronary artery, 53% were located in the first segment, 38% in the middle segment, 10% in the distal segment, and 6.4% in the posterior descending or left ventricular branches (Fig. 393).

Of the occlusions of the anterior descending 39% are proximal to the first septal branch; 47% in the midsegment, most, just distal to the first septal branch; 5% involve the third or apical segment, and 25% involve the major diagonal branch. The majority of the occlusions of the circumflex were in the first few millimeters near its origin or in the region adjacent to the obtuse marginal branch (Fig. 394).

The right coronary artery tends to be more diffusely involved. In the anterior descending, the most frequently affected area is near the origin of its most prominent diagonal branch, or immediately distal to the origin of the first septal. Lesions of the circumflex appear more frequent and extensive in cases of dominant left coronary artery (Fig. 398).

In patients with a short main left coronary artery, the arteriosclerotic lesions in the anterior descending and proximal circumflex appear early, progress faster to a higher level of severity, and lead more frequently to myocardial infarctions than in patients with a long coronary artery trunk (Gazetopoulos *et al.*, 1976).

More than 75% of symptomatic patients have 90% or more stenosis of at least one vessel, and severe involvement of a single artery was more frequent in patients who had myocardial infarction without angina pectoris (Proudfitt *et al.*, 1967).

Localized dilatation, but much more frequently diffuse ectasia, is another manifestation of arteriosclerotic coronary disease (Figs. 398, 399). These result from loss of elasticity of the arterial wall. Turbulence of flow in association with a possible thrombogenic phenomenon may be responsible for the fact that the great majority of these patients are symptomatic and at autopsy reveal evidence of multiple small myocardial scars.

Arteries with pre-existing cystic medial necrosis, structural abnormalities, or other arterial diseases such as polyarteritis nodosa, collagen disorders, etc., are more susceptible to the development of arteriosclerotic disease.

Natural History of Coronary Artery Disease and the Prognostic Role of Coronary Angiography. In the presence of angina, the prognosis as to survival and progression to a complication, or a more serious manifestation, was shown by a recent report of the Framingham study, to be quite discouraging (Kannel and Fein-

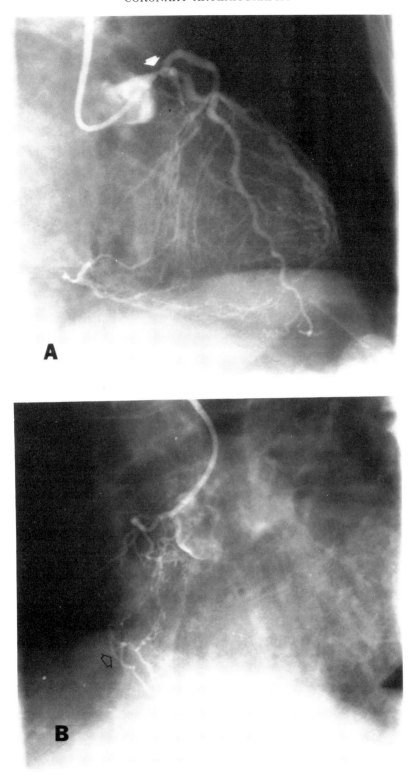

FIG. 392. SEVERE STENOSIS, MAIN LCA (WHITE ARROW)

(A) LC, RAO. Transeptal left to right collaterals to the posterior descending. The RC was obstructed at the ostium. (B) Injection in the right conal that originating directly from the right cusp, opacifies, through collaterals, a small segment of the occluded RC (open arrow).

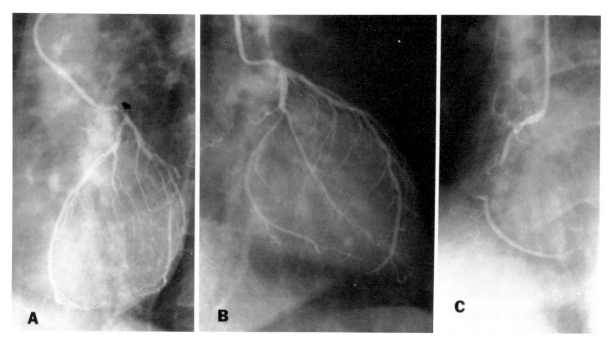

FIG. 393. SEVERE MAIN LC STENOSIS AND COMPLETE OBSTRUCTION OF SECOND SEGMENT OF RC WITH ADEQUATE DISTAL VESSELS

The severity of the LC stenosis could only be appreciated in the LAO (arrow). (A) LC, LAO. (B) LC, RAO. (C) RC, LAO.

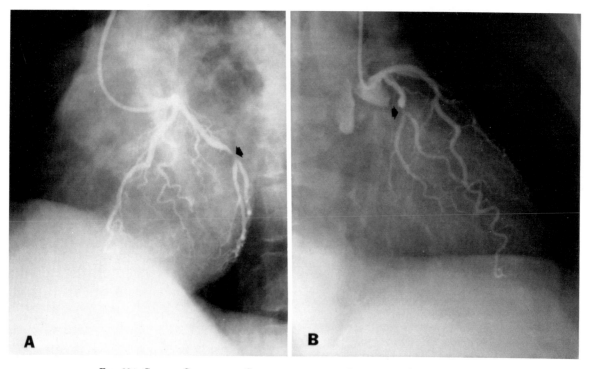

FIG. 394. SEVERE STENOSIS OF CIRCUMFLEX AT THE ORIGIN OF A SMALL MARGINAL

Slit-like lesion that in the RAO projection appears only as moderate stenosis. The LAO view shows 90% stenosis. (A) LC, LAO. (B) LC, RAO.

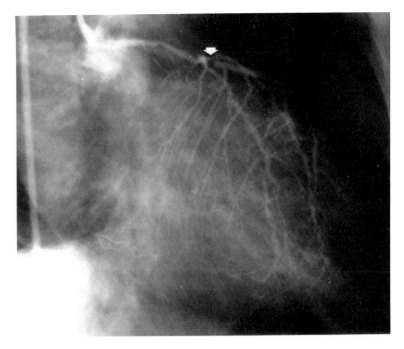

FIG. 395. DIFFUSE INVOLVEMENT OF THE LC MORE SEVERE THAN APPARENT

Long stenosis of main LC and localized lesions of its branches, particularly severe in the middle segment of AD just distal to the origin of 1st septal branch (arrow). This case illustrates the difficulties of quantitating the magnitude of stenosis; where a narrowed segment will, by necessity, be compared with another abnormal segment, resulting in underestimation of the severity of the lesion. The circumflex was occluded. LC, RAO.

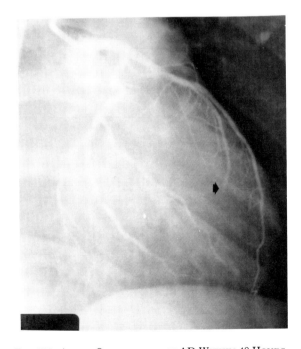

FIG. 396. ACUTE OBSTRUCTION OF AD WITHIN 48 HOURS OF ACUTE MYOCARDIAL INFARCTION DEMONSTRATES ABSENCE OF OPACIFICATION OF DISTAL AD WITH PROGRESSIVE DIMINUTION OF CONTRAST (ARROW)

The distal AD never opacified even after the administration of vasodilators. LC, RAO.

leib, 1972). One of every four men with angina will have a coronary attack within five years. The risk is half that for women. About 30% of all those over 55 with angina will die within eight years and 44% of the coronary deaths will be sudden. Reflecting the limitations of the clinical diagnosis, almost one in four myocardial infarctions were silent or unrecognized. Similarly, other studies (Fitzgibbon et al., 1971) have shown the unreliability of the Master's stress test when compared with the coronary and hemodynamic findings showing 16% false-positive responses in subjects without coronary disease and 33% false-negative results in patients with severe obstructions.

A number of studies have documented the importance of the location of the arterial stenosis or obstruction and the predictive prognostic value of coronary arteriography. Bruschke et al. (1973), studying patients with 50% or more stenosis of at least one major artery, in medically treated patients followed to nine years found a mortality of 34.4% for the entire population, 14.6% for patients with one vessel involvement, 37.8% in patients with two-vessel disease, 53.8% with three-vessel involvement, and 56.8% for those with main left coronary artery disease. Prognosis, as expected, was worse in those with

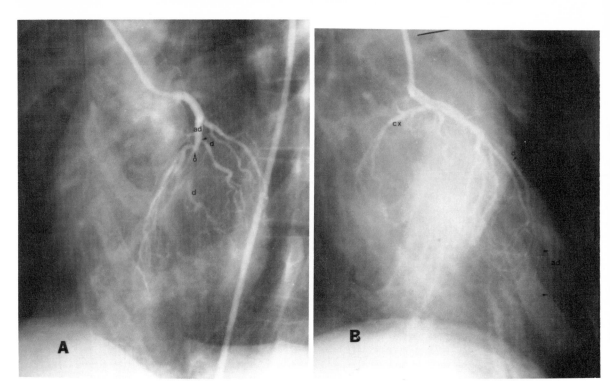

FIG. 397. COMPLETE OCCLUSION OF THE AD DISTAL TO THE ORIGIN OF A VERY LARGE 1ST SEPTAL BRANCH

One of the diagonal branches of the AD fills back to the obstruction at its origin, another more distal did not (underestimation). Only a small segment of the distal AD opacifies (LAO view, ad between arrows). This vessel was larger than would appear here. The involvement of a vessel distal to a complete obstruction tends to be overestimated. (A) LC, LAO. (B) LC, RAO.

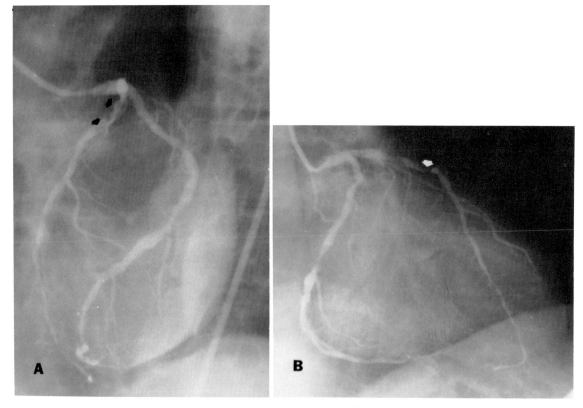

FIG. 398. DIFFUSE DISEASE WITH SEVERE PROXIMAL AND DISTAL NARROWING OF ANTERIOR DESCENDING AND DILATATION OF CIRCUMFLEX

Note also the sparcity of left ventricular branches suggesting that some may be completely obstructed at their origins and not filled through collaterals. (A) LC, LAO. (B) LC, RAO.

476

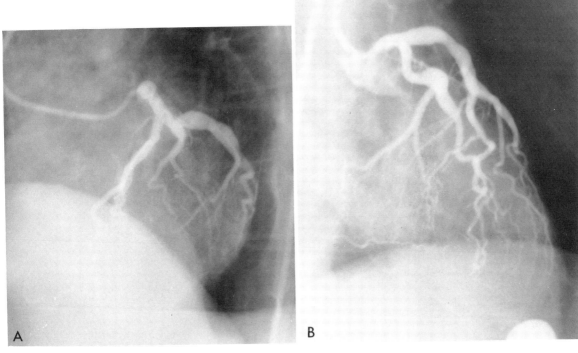

FIG. 399. LEFT CORONARY ARTERIOGRAM

(A) Left anterior oblique. (B) Right anterior oblique. Diffuse arteriosclerotic aneurysms without significant stenosis. The right coronary artery was completely occluded. (With permission, from Morettin, L. B., Coronary Arteriography. Uncommon Observations. *Radiologic Clinics of North America, 14*: 189–208, 1976.)

additional disease of distal vessels. Webster *et al.* (1974), studying 469 patients with 80–100% occlusive lesions of the proximal coronary tree, reported that those with isolated disease of the left anterior descending had an average 4% yearly attrition rate and a 6-year mortality rate of 25.5%. In isolated right coronary artery lesions, the yearly attrition rate was 2.3% and 14% 6-year mortality. In patients with double and triple vessel disease, the 6-year mortality was 41.5 and 63% respectively. The presence of prior myocardial infarction, the location of the lesion above or below the first septal branch in the anterior descending, in Webster's experience, did not alter the prognosis significantly. Others (Platia *et al.*, 1975) report a significant difference in the 8-year mortality of patients with greater than 70% stenosis of the anterior descending between those with obstruction proximal versus those with obstruction distal to the first septal branch (54 versus 22% respectively). Thus, the author thinks that this is an important consideration for the selection of those patients who are surgically suitable for bypass surgery. Other factors such as congestive heart failure and an abnormal left

ventricular function adversely affect the survival rates (Burggraf and Parker, 1975).

Coronary arteriography allows evaluation of the progression of the arteriosclerotic process. Recently, Rosch *et al.* (1976) encountered a statistically significant high rate of progression of lesions that appear as long tubular stenoses, contain ulcerating plaques, and as stenosis bridged by collateral circulation.

Bruschke *et al.*, (1973) studied the predictive value of the coronary arteriogram in patients with normal coronary arteries or narrowing of less than 50%. The minimal followup period was five years. Those with entirely normal coronary arteriograms had an incidence of 0.6% of presumed cardiac deaths and 0.9% myocardial infarctions within five years. These incidences are about half of the expected rates for the average unselected population matched by sex and age. In patients with less than 30% narrowing the prognosis was less good than the normal group but still better than the average population. In those with 30–50% narrowing, there was 5.3% cardiac deaths and 3.5% myocardial infarctions in five years, which reflects slightly higher incidences than the average population. The study confirms the major predictive value of the coronary arteriogram in that a normal arteriogram indicates an excellent prognosis regardless of other diagnostic parameters.

Brymer *et al.* (1974) confirmed the good prognostic value of the normal coronary arteriogram in evaluating patients with angina. The finding of a normal coronary arteriogram implies good prognosis regardless of the severity or variety of clinical symptoms.

"When the coronary arteries are proven to be free of obstructive lesions or irregularities in lumen diameter, coronary arteriosclerosis may be excluded as a cause of chest pain, abnormalities of the heart rhythm, electrocardiographic aberrations or myocardial insufficiency" (Sones, 1972).

Possible explanations for the presence of "angina pectoris" and "arteriographically normal coronary arteries" are (1) The nature of the symptoms is misinterpreted, probably the most common reason, where the chest pain is most likely atypical angina. (2) The arteriogram is technically inadequate, incomplete, or improperly interpreted. (3) The symptoms are caused by other myocardial or pericardial disease. (4) "Small-vessel disease" is responsible for myocardial ischemia, considered unlikely by most authors.

Shirey (1968), attempting to establish the significance of "small vessel disease" in angina pectoris, carried out a cine angiographic and pathologic study of the coronary microcirculation of 78 patients with primary myocardial disease. He concludes that arteriosclerotic small vessel disease does not exist and primary nonarteriosclerotic changes in the microcirculation are rare and do not constitute a cause of angina pectoris.

In recent years much attention has been given to a small group of patients with "myocardial infarction and angiographically normal coronary arteries". Arnett and Roberts (1976) emphasize that a normal coronary arterial tree has never been demonstrated by angiography *at the time* of acute myocardial infarction. An arteriogram performed after the acute infarction, and as early as 72 hours, may show no evidence of occlusion or even significant stenosis because of clot lysis, retraction, or recanalization of an obstruction which may then appear "angiographically normal" (Spring and Thomsen, 1973).

Considerable attention has been focused also on patients with stenosis of the left main coronary artery (Figs. 392 and 393). Patients with these lesions constitute a high-risk group both from the point of view of prognosis and of the

possible complications related to coronary arteriography. In Lim *et al.* series (1975), the 5-year mortality for patients with 50% or more stenosis of the main left coronary artery was 51%. Especially disturbing is the fact that 97% of those patients had additional lesions elsewhere in the coronary vessels. Another study (DeMots *et al.*, 1975) established that coexisting major disease of other vessels is an important determinant in the poor prognosis and prevented bypass surgery in 13% of the cases. Isolated left main artery disease is therefore uncommon, but because of its serious consequences, early diagnosis and revascularization surgery, even on emergency basis, seem justified (Cohen and Gorlin, 1975).

The Collateral Circulation. The nature and the significance of the collateral coronary circulation has been the subject of much debate. In the past few years a controversy has evolved and continues to divide opinions concerning the effectiveness of these vessels to maintain or restore ventricular function by compensating for the loss of flow caused by coronary occlusions.

Some authors have concluded that ventricular contractility does not appear to be improved, myocardial infarction is not prevented, and life is not prolonged significantly by the presence of angiographically demonstrable collaterals in patients with severe stenosis or occlusions of coronary arteries as compared with those who do not demonstrate collaterals (Lavine *et al.*, 1974). Others have shown completely opposite results with improved long-term prognosis and ventricular function (Levin, 1974; Hamby *et al.*, 1976). The problem of estimating the functional significance of the collaterals in any given patient is more complex than the simple demonstration of the presence or absence of collateral vessels. Many factors play an important role in their effectiveness, namely the rate with which the occlusion of the native circulation develops in relation to the speed with which mature collaterals form (James, 1970). Additional factors include the number and size of the anastomotic vessels, the mural tension in the area of myocardium through which they course, the transanastomotic pressure gradient, the viscosity of the blood, the cardiac rhythm, and the existence of functioning contracting myocardium distal to an occluded vessel to create the demand for the formation of new vessels. The exact contribution of each of these factors to the final effectiveness of the collateral circulation is as yet not completely known. That other extracardiac factors may play an important role in the rate of formation of collateral vessels is evidenced by the fact that patients with chronic hypoxia, resulting from chronic obstructive pulmonary disease, may be protected against myocardial infarction by the development of intercoronary or intracoronary collaterals.

We have noticed that the patients with proven chronic obstructive pulmonary disease reveal the presence of collateral vessels that are more numerous, larger, and more tortuous than a group of patients with comparable coronary occlusions without emphysema (Morettin, 1976) (Figs. 405 and 406). Under these circumstances, collaterals at the precapillary level develop before significant coronary artery disease, mature at a faster rate than that determined or induced by the rate of progression of the occlusive process of the native circulation, and by the time complete occlusion occurs, they are more numerous and carry a greater flow. The prophylactic effect of pre-existing anoxia in these patients is suggested by the presence of a larger number of silent coronary occlusions than in patients without chronic obstructive pulmonary disease (Nonkin et al., 1964).

It is agreed among most authors that severe stenosis (greater than 90%) is necessary to create the gradient of pressures that will stimulate the formation of angiographically visible collaterals (Levin, 1974). Hamby et al. (1976) observed that 83% of patients with complete obstruction of the dominant right coronary artery will have adequate visualization of the posterior descending via collaterals, but the frequency of myocardial infarction and inferior wall asynergy was not influenced by the presence of those collateral vessels. When the anterior descending was completely occluded, those patients without collateral vessels had a significantly greater frequency of heart failure, cardiomegaly, electrocardiographic evidence of anterior wall infarction, and angiographic findings of anterior wall asynergy.

It appears that the rate of progression from high degree stenosis to complete occlusion is faster in those individuals who have collateral circulation around the stenotic lesion than in those who do not (Rösch et al., 1976).

From an angiographic point of view, study of the collateral circulation is of important value in establishing the actual site of obstruction by careful evaluation of the reconstituted vessels distal to that obstruction and the direction of its

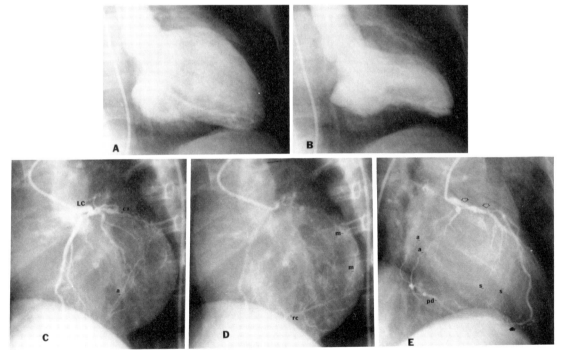

Fig. 400. Diffuse Left Ventricular Hypokinesia and Localized Apical and Posteroinferior Akinesia

(A) Left ventriculogram, RAO, Diastole. (B) Systole. Note the bulge of the posteroinferior surface of the left ventricle in the area supplied by a completely occluded large dominant RC, and diminished contraction of the apex, perfused by the AD with a severe proximal stenosis. (C and D) LC, LAO, early and late, respectively. Extensive severe stenosis of the CX. Reconstitution of the distal inferior left ventricular extension of the obstructed RC via collaterals from the left atrial, (a) and the marginal branch (m). (E) LC, RAO. Long severe stenosis of the proximal AD (open arrows). The 1st septal branch, obstructed at its origin, is not seen. Atrial (a), transseptal (s), and periapical (arrows) collaterals, reconstitute the PD.

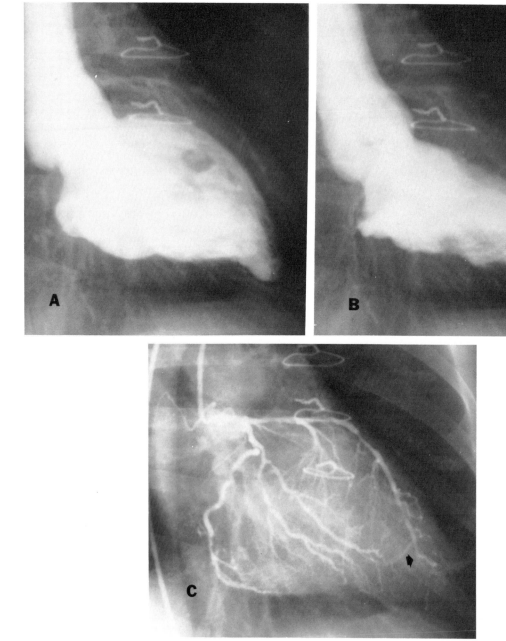

FIG. 401. MARKED DIFFUSE HYPOKINESIA WITH A PARADOXICAL SYSTOLIC BULGING OF THE APEX

The ventricular wall in this region was thin and the myocardium replaced by a fibrous scar resulting from an old infarction. Left Ventriculogram. (A) Diastole. (B) Systole. (C) LC, RAO, note segmental areas of moderate to severe stenosis and complete occlusion of distal AD (arrow) corresponding with the area of ventricular dysfunction.

flow. It also permits evaluation of the vessel distal to the obstruction and it's possible surgical suitability.

For descriptive purposes, collaterals can be classified as *intracoronary* (or *homocoronary*), and *intercoronary*. They may be *epicardiac* in location when they course over the surface of the heart, or *transmural* when they traverse myo-

cardial substance such as the ventricular walls or the interventricular septum; because of the mural tension in the area of myocardium through which they course, the latter, are less efficient (Fig. 403).

Innumerable collateral pathways result from a variety of obstructive lesions and anastomic variants in the pattern of distribution of the native

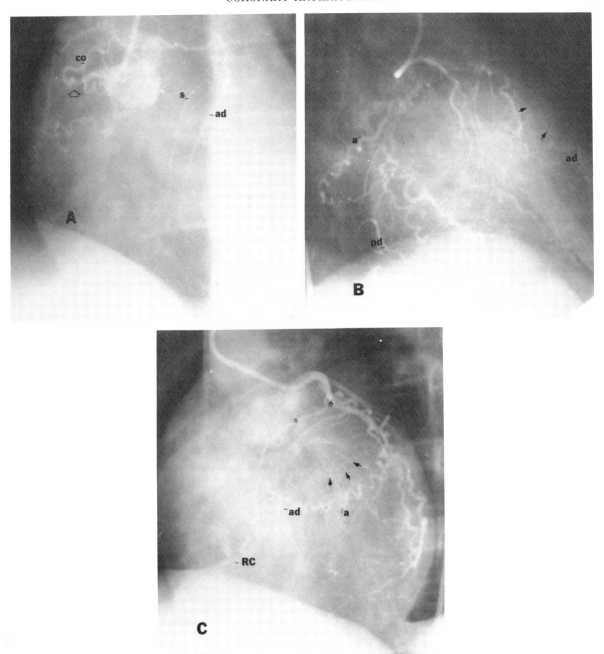

FIG. 402. INTERCORONARY COLLATERALS FROM RIGHT TO LEFT AND FROM LEFT TO RIGHT

The RC is obstructed at the beginning of the second segment (open arrow, A). The AD is obstructed at the origin (o). (A) Right to left conal collaterals, from RC to AD and large septal branch (s). (B and C) Left to right via left atrial branches (a) from circumflex to the distal RC, and intracoronary collaterals from diagonal to anterior descending (arrow points).

coronary circulation. The most common collateral pathways are shown in the accompanying illustrations. Most patients with severe, diffuse disease with multiple occlusions will exhibit one or more of these pathways and not infrequently the flow across collateral vessels can be bidirectional according to the coronary artery injected.

The most frequently encountered pathways are (1) left to right transseptal from the anterior descending to the posterior descending; (2) left to right, from the distal circumflex to the distal right coronary; (3) intracoronary collaterals around an obstruction of the second segment of the right coronary artery; (4) right to left inter-

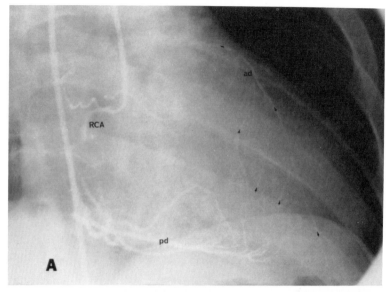

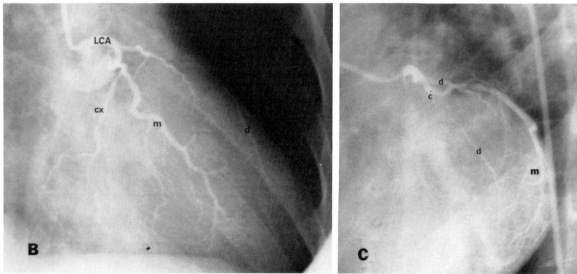

FIG. 403. COLLATERALS

Intercoronary right-to-left, transseptal collaterals, opacify in a retrograde manner (arrows in A); the AD that was completely occluded at its origin and did not fill with the LC injection. Also epicardiac collaterals from the obtuse marginal to an occluded diagonal. (A) RC, RAO. (B) LC, RAO. (C) LC, LAO.

conal; (5) right to left transseptal or periapical collaterals from posterior descending to the anterior descending; and (6) intracoronary collaterals between two or more branches of the left coronary artery. Numerous other pathways are found in decreasing order of frequency.

Collaterals may develop across pericardial adhesions but they are small and inadequate (Fig. 407).

LEFT VENTRICULOGRAPHY. Cine ventriculography, together with evaluation and recording of ventricular pressures performed at the time of

coronary angiography, is an essential part in the evaluation of patients with ischemic heart disease and in the planning of therapeutic alternatives. Ventriculography consists of the evaluation of the dimensions and sequential changes of shape and volume occurring during cardiac systole and diastole by means of an injection of radiopaque contrast substance in the left ventricle.

The majority of the investigators perform left ventriculography before injection in the coronary vessels and immediately after the recording of

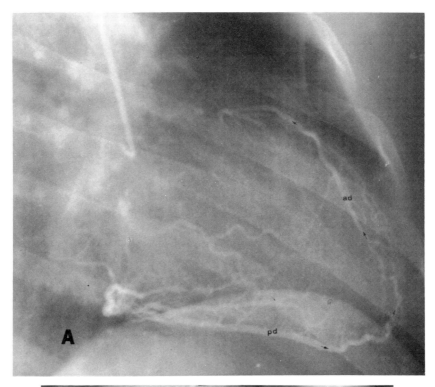

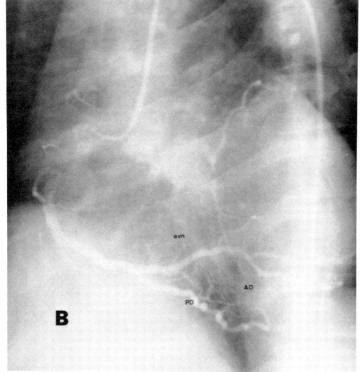

FIG. 404. COLLATERALS

Effective intercoronary right-to-left periapical collaterals from PD opacify the proximally obstructed AD and its branches. Ventricular function was normal. (A) RC injection, late, RAO. (B) RC, LAO.

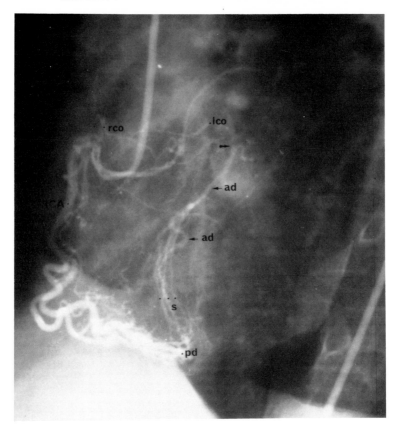

FIG. 405. 61-YEAR-OLD MAN WITH CHRONIC EMPHYSEMA

Right coronary arteriogram. Very tortuous vessels. Interconal (rco, lco) and transeptal (pd, s) collaterals from the right coronary artery to a proximally occluded, (double arrowhead), anterior descending (ad). There was no clinical or historical evidence of myocardial infarction. Left ventricular function was normal. (With permission, from Morettin, L. B., Coronary Arteriography. Uncommon Observations. *Radiologic Clinics of North America, 14:* 189–208, 1976.)

left ventricular pressures. Intraventricular and intracoronary injections of contrast substance produce transient changes in cardiac contractility with depression of the ejection fraction and slight increase in the end-diastolic volumes and pressures (Fig. 419) (Sos and Baltaxe, 1976).

Left ventriculography is usually performed in a 30° right anterior oblique projection. The degree of obliquity varies with the size and position of the heart. A left anterior oblique view is added when there is suspicion of involvement of the septal or posterolateral walls. An injection of 40–60 ml of a suitable water-soluble contrast agent is made and filming is obtained by means of a 35-mm cine at the rate of 60 frames/sec.

The normal contour of the left ventricular cavity in the right anterior oblique projection in diastole is an ellipsoid with its tip inclined downward at an angle of approximately 45° (Raphael and Allwork, 1974). During systole, the inward concentric motion of the anterior and posterior walls approximates the sides and the apex to-

wards the center without appreciable change in the dimension of its base, represented by the mitral valve ring. During systole the base-to-apex axis shortens approximately 20%. At the end of systole, the anterior and posterior walls approximate each other at the apex and the shadows of the anterior and posterior papillary muscles become more prominent.

The normal pattern of contraction becomes altered by the presence of premature ventricular beats, causing irregular contractions and followed by a prolonged postextrasystolic pause.

It can be observed that the left ventricular epicardial surface contracts in approximate symmetrical fashion with slight rotational movement along the long axis, most marked by the beginning and end of systole, while the surface of the left ventricular cavity appears less symmetrical because of the systolic increase in wall thickness, approximation of trabeculae and movements of the mitral valve (McDonald, 1970).

The ventricular mass can be divided into a

number of segments that in broad lines follow the distribution of the major arterial branches. Several classifications have been proposed. We follow the description of Gensini (1975) who di-

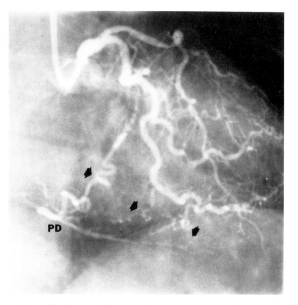

FIG. 406. LARGE MATURE INTERCORONARY LEFT-TO-RIGHT COLLATERALS (ARROWS) FROM DISTAL CIRCUMFLEX AND MARGINAL TO POSTERIOR DESCENDING IN A PATIENT WITH CHRONIC OBSTRUCTUVE PULMONARY DISEASE

(With permission, from Morettin, L. B., Coronary Arteriography. Uncommon Obstructions. *Radiologic Clinics of North America, 14:* 189–208, 1976.)

vides the ventricular wall into seven segments: (1) the anterior basal segment located near the base along the high anterolateral wall of the ventricle, usually supplied by the proximal branches of the left anterior descending, mostly high diagonals, and by proximal branches of the circumflex; (2) the anterolateral segment located inferior to the anterior basal and covering a large area of the anterolateral wall of the left ventricle, generally supplied by the midportion of the anterior descending and its diagonal branches; (3) the apical segment including the entire apex of the ventricle both in its anterior and posterior walls supplied by the anterior descending or when this is short by the posterior descending; (4) the diaphragmatic segment which includes most of the diaphragmatic surface of the left ventricle and is supplied by the posterior descending or inferior left ventricular branches; (5) the posterobasal segment located on the ventricular surface near the crux of the heart behind the diaphragmatic segment and near the posterior A-V cushion; (6) the septal segment, which can be divided into an anterior portion supplied by septal branches of the anterior descending (two-thirds) and the posterior portion supplied by branches of the posterior descending (one-third); and (7) the posterolateral segment encompassing a wedge of myocardium bounded superiorly by the left atrioventricular groove and extending to just above the shadow of the apex, being supplied most frequently by the obtuse marginal branch of the left coronary artery.

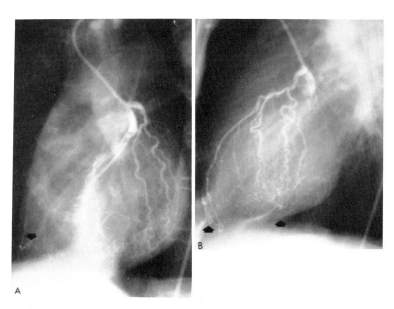

FIG. 407. PERICARDIAL ADHESIONS. LEFT CORONARY ARTERIOGRAM

(A) Left anterior oblique. (B) Left lateral. Several small, tortuous vessels (arrows) course through old adhesions bridging the pericardial space. The left circumflex was occluded at its origin. The RC was also completely occluded. These collaterals are not very effective.

Several specific terms are used to define the qualities of ventricular wall contraction and their alterations (Herman *et al.*, 1967).

A. *Synergy.*

May be defined as the cooperative and sequential contraction of the heart mass such as to produce maximum effective work at the minimal energy cost encompassing both temporal and spacial relations.

B. *Asynergy*

Defines the *localized* anomalies in the pattern of ventricular contraction and can be classified into four different types:

Dyskinesis

An abnormality of ventricular contraction consisting of paradoxic systolic expansion of a local portion of the left ventricle (Fig. 401). The bulge that is formed is caused by the inability of the area to build enough tension, creating a slack area that expands when other fibers contract.

Akinesis (Fig. 400)

This abnormality appears as an area with total lack of motion, rigid and nonmobile, that generates sufficient tension to prevent expansion in systole but without actual contraction.

Asyneresis

A localized area of "inadequate" ventricular motion that does not contribute to the stroke output.

Asynchrony

A disruption of the normal temporal sequence of contraction caused by delayed contraction of some fibers which causes alternating areas of contraction and expansion. Asynchrony may represent the most subtle expression of ventricular fibrillation.

C. *Hypokinesis* (Fig. 400)

A diffuse abnormality of contraction, characterized by generalized loss of strength of contraction, in which the ventricle appears sluggish or "quivering." Severe hypokinesis is also associated with massive increase in end-diastolic volume and elevated end-diastolic pressure.

Ventriculography permits a rough assessment of ventricular systolic and diastolic volumes. Mild increase in volumes are difficult to appreciate. Angiographic studies generally underestimate the true end-systolic volume.

Segmental early relaxation phenomenon (SERP) consists of a bulging or outward left ventricular wall motion occurring after the cessation of the systolic inward motion and before opening of the mitral valve, coinciding with the isovolumic relaxation period. Originally thought to be an abnormal type of movement related to ischemic myocardial disease it has been shown recently to be a normal variation of left ventricular relaxation (Altieri *et al.*, 1973).

The abnormalities of left ventricular wall motion related to ischemic coronary disease may be produced by fibrosis or by ischemia itself without fibrosis resulting from an intramyocardial coronary steal (Baltaxe *et al.*, 1974).

Abnormalities of left ventricular motion can be improved or changed in certain cases by the use of epinephrine infusion or nitroglycerin, suggesting the existence of residual contractile ability. This test may differentiate, then, between zones of potentially functional cardiac muscle and frank fibrosis (Horn *et al.*, 1974).

In assaying the significance of coronary artery disease as reflected by the changes in left ventriculography, it is important to remember that the performance of the left ventricular myocardium does not necessarily bear a consistent relation with the extent of coronary disease. Very advanced coronary artery lesions may be present with only minimal changes in ventricular volume and pattern or strength of contraction. When a sufficient number of fibers is not significantly affected, within a large mass of myocardium that is otherwise ischemic, both the electrocardiogram and the ventriculogram may be normal.

Filling defects. These may be demonstrated on left ventriculography. They are nearly always associated with a ventricular aneurysm or a severe or diffuse contraction abnormality and they represent thrombi adherent to the ventricular wall in areas with significant myocardial damage. Abnormal neovascularity may be present in the late phase of the coronary artery injection and it is presumably caused by the penetration of the organized thrombus by capillaries arising from the subendocardial vessels (Fig. 417).

The ventriculogram should be studied carefully for evidence of organic or functional valvular involvement. In the right anterior oblique the mitral valve plane is seen to better advantage. A small puff of contrast agent is frequently seen, particularly with the first systolic contraction following the onset of injection and especially following a premature ventricular contraction. This should not be considered an indication of mitral insufficiency. Mitral regurgitation can also be created by entrapment of the open mitral leaflets by the catheter. This can be recognized as artefactual by the fact that regurgitation stops with the end of injection. Ischemic disease can lead to mitral insufficiency by either means of damage to or dysfunction of the papillary muscles leading to shortening of the chordae tendineae or altered compliance or necrosis of the papillary muscles themselves. This is more frequently encountered with lesions of the right coronary artery and/or posterior descending involving the inferior papillary muscle.

Aortic stenosis is diagnosed by the demonstration of a pressure gradient and an alteration of the shape and motions of the aortic valve. Because aortic stenosis is accompanied by significant lesions of the coronary vessels in as much as 30–40% of the patients, evaluation of the aortic valve is essential in patients with angina.

Aneurysm of the ventricular septum, although uncommon, is one of the serious complications of coronary artery disease. Furthermore, rupture of a ventricular septal aneurysm is of extremely serious consequence with a mortality approaching 85%. The left anterior oblique projection is the most useful to evaluate this complication as ruptures are usually located in the muscular portion of the ventricular septum near the apex. The majority of cases are associated with marked diffuse hypokinesia, significant elevation of the end-diastolic pressure and mitral insufficiency.

PITFALLS, ERRORS, AND RELIABILITY OF THE CORONARY ARTERIOGRAM

The reliability and usefulness of coronary arteriography in the care and management of patients with ischemic coronary disease depend on many technical, anatomical, and human factors. Each of these potential sources of error should be considered separately.

1. **Technical**
   Inadequate equipment
   Insufficient projections
   Incomplete study
   Inadequate injection (volume, rate, site)
   Spasm
2. **Anatomical**
   Duplication of arteries or branches
   Replacement of one branch by others
   Hypoplasia of artery or segment
   Abnormal or ectopic origin of branch
   Collaterals from ectopic artery
   Muscular bridges
3. **Characteristics of Lesion(s)**
   Length
   Shape of lumen
   Location
   Status of the vessel distal to complete occlusion
   Recanalization of complete occlusion
   "Small vessel disease"
4. **Observer disagreement**

Technical causes

The quality of the coronary arteriogram is considered as the most important factor in limiting its accuracy in the management of ischemic heart disease. Inferior radiographic equipment that does not meet the minimal standards of performance and resolution, and an inexperienced or not sufficiently experienced investigator with insufficient volume of cases to maintain a high level of proficiency, are considered the two most common causes for examinations of less than acceptable diagnostic value and reliability.

Sufficient number of projections to allow each major vessel to be viewed isolated from other overlying vessels or structures in at least two projections at 90° from each other is absolutely essential. More recently, a higher level of accuracy has been demonstrated when additional views with craniocaudal angulation are added in the evaluation of lesions of the left coronary artery and its proximal branches (Lesperance *et al.,* 1974; Aldridge *et al.,* 1975).

A hesitant slow injection of inadequate volume and speed will cause insufficient, pulsating opacification of the vessels and poor anatomical detail.

Subselective injections into the proximal branches, particularly when the main left coronary artery is short, may lead to the erroneous assumption of occlusion of a branch proximal to the site of injection.

Spasm induced by the catheter tip could be a source of error, particularly in the proximal right coronary and in the left anterior descending. When spasm is recognized injection should be repeated after administration of a vasodilator (Fig. 409, 412).

Anatomical Causes

It is in the recognition of subtle degrees of anatomical variation that the experience of the angiographer plays an important role in distinguishing pathologic from normal conditions.

Complete duplication of a coronary artery or one of its branches may be encountered in approximately 1% of patients (Morettin, 1976). In this little-known variant, two vessels, generally of a smaller caliber than expected, run parallel courses very close to each other and share a common territory. It is easy to understand how occlusion of one of these vessels may be easily overlooked. In decreasing order of frequency they can be found in the posterior descending, anterior descending, and the entire right coronary artery (Figs. 382 and 383). Similarly the posterior descending may be replaced by two or more vessels, branches of either right or left inferior left ventricular arteries entering the posterior interventricular groove at various distances between the crux and the apex; obstruction of either of these vessels may easily go unnoticed. We have encountered this anatomical arrangement in 11% of our cases (Fig. 376).

Segmental hypoplasia occurring most frequently in the middle or distal segments of the right coronary artery and the distal circumflex (Figs. 373, 375, and 377) can lead to error. Failure to recognize the existence of subtle signs of territorial reciprocity with compensatory expansion of the circumflex, or the distal right coronary as the case may be, may lead to the erroneous assumption of the presence of an obstruction or serious stenosis.

Superimposition of two branches in a different territory in any given projection can be confusing. Particular attention should be paid in distinguishing the middle segment of the anterior descending from prominent diagonal branches, sometimes of equal size, in the right anterior oblique projection (Fig. 409). The angiographer should be suspicious of the presence of an undisputably normal left ventriculogram in the face of what appears to be a total occlusion of one of the two major coronary branches, particularly in the absence of any signs of attempted collateral circulation. Ectopic origin of a coronary branch should then be carefully sought. The most common anomaly causing these findings is the origin of the left circumflex from the right coronary sinus or right coronary artery (Fig. 408).

The right conal branch arising directly from the coronary sinus may be providing collaterals to a proximally obstructed but distally patent right coronary artery and overlooked unless selective injection in that vessel is performed (Fig. 392). This probably occurs more frequently than is realized, particularly in view of the fact that

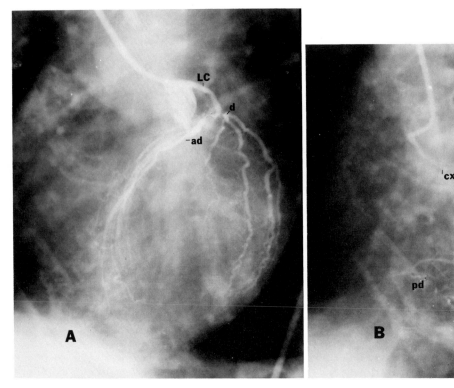

FIG. 408. ANOMALOUS ORIGIN OF THE CIRCUMFLEX FROM RIGHT CUSP. POSSIBLE SOURCE OF ERROR (OVERESTIMATION).

(A) LAO of LC injection reveals a small main LC. The circumflex branch is not seen. A moderately severe stenosis of the AD is present. A prominant diagonal (with 3 branches) has also a proximal area of stenosis. (B) The very large circumflex originates from the right coronary cusp and supplies a large portion of the left ventricular wall and numerous small collaterals to the posterior descending of an obstructed RC.

The resulting small main LC could have been considered abnormal (it was not), and the circumflex occluded. A deliberate search for a possible anomalous circumflex was made in this situation, because an apparent occlusion of the circumflex was not accompanied by a corresponding ventricular dysfunction.

the right conal may arise from the right sinus or aorta in as many as 50% of the patients.

Branches of the coronary arteries, most frequently the anterior descending, occasionally penetrate below the epicardial surface under small crossing bands of myocardial fibers. This may create the appearance of a stenotic lesion. It may be recognized angiographically (in the cine) by the transient nature of the narrowing that occurs during systole; the caliber in the area in question returns to normal during diastole (Vlodaver *et al.*, 1976).

Characteristics of Lesion(s)

The size, shape, and severity of a lesion also affects the reliability of the coronary arteriogram. Circumferential lesions involving a long segment of the lumen are a frequent source of error. This occurs because arteriography sees the vessel lumen but not its wall and the size of the lumen in areas adjacent to a lesion is most commonly used as a normal reference in determining residual luminal diameter. When the entire artery or several vessels are diseased these comparisons are misleading due to a lack of a true normal frame of reference (Fig. 411). Eccentric slit-like crescent shaped or fish-mouth shaped lesions account for some errors. When viewed from one angle, an eccentric lesion (Fig. 410) may appear normal, whereas, from a view that is at a slightly different angle its severity is greater (Gensini, 1975). A totally occluded vessel at its origin can be easily overlooked, particularly in the distribution of the diagonal branches of the anterior descending, the marginal branches, or the distal ventricular branches of the circumflex or right coronary artery (Fig. 411). When errors of diagnosis are made, they are usually underestimations of the degree of stenosis or obstruction. Conversely, in the presence of a severe proximal stenosis or a complete obstruction with reconstitution with collaterals, the degree of stenosis of the vessel distal to the stenosis tends to be overestimated. This is probably due to the fact that the distal vessel is incompletely distended and the pulse pressure is considerably reduced.

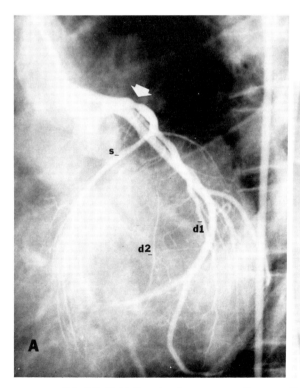
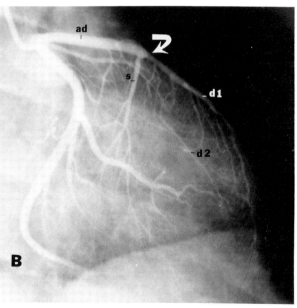

FIG. 409. THIS PATIENT ILLUSTRATES SEVERAL SITUATIONS THAT MAY LEAD TO DIAGNOSTIC ERRORS
(A) LCA, LAO. (B) LCA, RAO. 1. The main LC is very short. The catheter enters the AD causing a spasm at the tip (white arrow in A). Following vasodilator and repositioning of the catheter the AD is normal as shown in B. 2. The first septal branch is very large and could be mistaken in the LAO for the anterior descending that is completely occluded at the take-off of the first septal (curved arrow). 3. The larger of two diagonal branches (d_1) could be mistaken for the AD in the RAO; another small diagonal (d_2), completely occluded proximally, fills through collaterals. (A, with permission, from Morettin, L. B., Coronary Arteriography. Uncommon Observations. *Radiologic Clinics of North America, 14:* 189–208, 1976.)

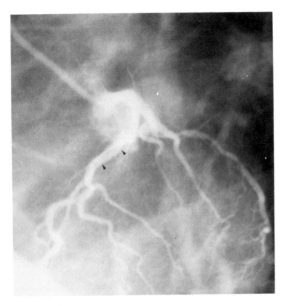

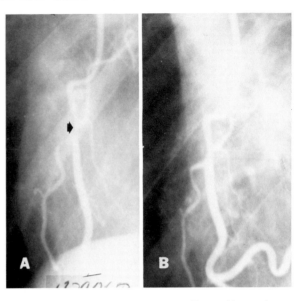

FIG. 410. ECCENTRIC STENOTIC PLAQUE, CREATING A
SUBTLE DEFECT IN THE PROXIMAL AD (ARROW POINTS)
AND LEAVING A CRESCENT- SHAPED STENOTIC LUMEN
MORE SEVERE THAN READILY APPARENT (LCA, LAO)

FIG. 412. TRANSIENT LOCALIZED SPASM (ARROW)
PRODUCED BY THE INJECTION, AT THE MIDDLE SEGMENT
OF THE RC; (A) BEFORE AND (B) AFTER VASODILATORS

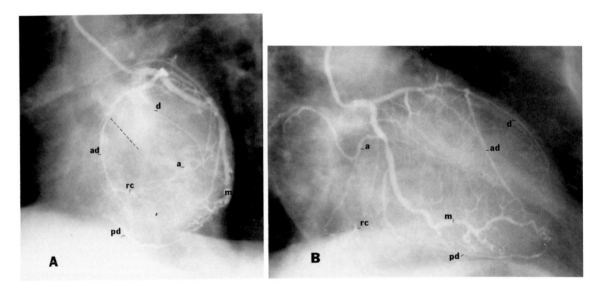

FIG. 411. HOW ACCURATE IS THE CORONARY ARTERIOGRAM?
1. Is the AD abnormal? 2. If so, how significant? 3. Are there any other occluded vessels? 4. Is the PD patent in its entirety?

The AD is small throughout its course due to diffuse (more severe than apparent) stenosis. Only a small diagonal branch (d) covers a large area of the anterolateral wall of the left ventricle. Another sizable branch to this area was completely occluded (course shown with line of dashes) leaving a bulging akinetic scar.

The posterior descending opacified from marginal collaterals appears interrupted proximally but was patent but not seen due to bidirectional flow. The distal RC fills from left atrial collaterals (a).

A myocardial scan, with injection in the LC revealed a sizable perfusion defect in the anterolateral wall of the left ventricle. (A) LC, LAO. (B) LC, RAO.

Schwartz *et al.* (1975) found, in a comparative angiographic postmortem study evaluating 225 stenotic arterial segments encountered at cine angiography, findings that were in good agreement with pathologic findings, showing less than 25% difference in estimation in 79% of the stenotic lesions examined. In 6% of the lesions, angiography overestimated, and in 15% it underestimated the degree of stenosis. This fact should be viewed with the understanding that autopsy studies do not evaluate the distended, pulsatile state of living coronary vessels.

Observer Disagreement

Analysis of inter- and intraobserver variability in the interpretation of the coronary arteriogram (Detre *et al.*, 1975) reveals that angiographic observations about which individual observers were more inconsistent from one reading to the other also had the largest interobserver disagreement. Areas of particular difficulty are the distal portions of the anterior descending and the circumflex branches. The areas of greater observer agreement are the main right coronary artery, collaterals, and the presence or absence of a ventricular aneurysm as judged by ventriculography. The use of more than one observer increases accuracy (Bjork *et al.*, 1975).

In assaying the reliability of coronary arteriography it must be kept in mind that although errors in diagnosis have been found to be real, they are not different from errors in other diagnostic or test methods where human judgment and interpretation must be expressed in quantitative terms (Detre *et al.*, 1975).

The significance of the normal coronary arteriogram in the presence of angina and myocardial infarction has been discussed in the preceding section.

COMPLICATIONS OF CORONARY ARTERIOGRAPHY

A frequently overlooked and probably the most significant complication of coronary arteriography is an incomplete or undiagnostic examination (Judkins, 1974). The quality of the patient's life is endangered by the serious consequences of an erroneous diagnosis and its very important prognostic and therapeutic implications. In the risk/benefit ratio, the benefit factor becomes of paramount importance.

Death associated with coronary arteriography can be due to either cardiac or noncardiac causes. Cardiac death may result from myocardial infarction complicating coronary artery injury or thrombosis, arrhythmias, or cardiogenic shock. Noncardiac causes of death include cerebral embolism and shock.

A report by Adams *et al.* (1973) supplied the statistics regarding the frequency of complications in a nationwide survey obtained during the years 1970 and 1971 encompassing 46,904 coronary arteriograms. Gensini (1975) reports on his experience in over 2,500 patients.

Table 11 shows the statistical frequency of the five major complications from both studies.

Several important conclusions can be made from those studies. Death or the serious nonfatal complications of myocardial infarction or cerebral embolus occur in 1.5% of all patients examined. If one considers the large number of coronary arteriograms performed yearly throughout the United States, as many as 1,000–1,500 patients may have died as a consequence of a diagnostic test. The mortality rate in institutions performing less than 100 examinations per year was eight times higher than in those institutions performing more than 400 examinations per year. Similarly the incidence of myocardial infarction, cerebral embolism, and serious arrhythmias was significantly higher when a smaller number of examinations were performed.

The higher incidence encountered with the percutaneous techniques in the report of Adams reflects the fact that 55% of laboratories using the femoral method do fewer than 50 cases per year. The most serious complications are the consequences of a thrombotic episode. From these reports the importance of two factors is clearly evident (Judkins, 1974): (1) The first factor is the operator and his ability to acquire and maintain skill and competence by performing a

TABLE 11
MAJOR COMPLICATIONS OF CORONARY ARTERIOGRAPHY

Complication	Gensini, 1975 Brachial	Adams et al., 1973	
		Brachial	Percutaneous
	%	%	
Death	0.05	0.13	0.78
Myocardial infarction	0.05	0.22	1.01
Cerebrovascular accident	0	0.03	0.43
Arterial damage	0.1	1.42	0.86
Ventricular fibrillation	0.75	1.15	1.41

sufficient number of examinations per year. The Report of the Intersociety Commission for Heart Disease Resources (1972) recommends that 500 cases per year are necessary to acquire and maintain adequate laboratory competence (2) The second factor is the length of the procedure and its influence on thrombogenicity; the longer the examination the greater the chances of serious complications. Takaro *et al.* (1973), in a cooperative study involving 18 hospitals over a four-year-period, encountered 0.3% fatalities with the brachial technique and 2.2% with the transfemoral, and explained the disparity by the mechanisms of coronary or cerebral arterial embolization from platelet deposits on the guide wires and catheters. In replacing the catheter after the performance of ventriculography, the very fine layer of fibrin and platelets that has been left on the surface of the wire is stripped by the second catheter when the guide wire is removed and it may become deposited or swept into a coronary artery or a brachiocephalic vessel. In those laboratories using systemic heparinization for the performance of percutaneous arteriography and performing more than 400 cases per year there is no significant difference in the rate of complications between each method (Adams and Abrams, 1975).

Other noncardiac complications include arterial lesions such as brachial artery obstruction and femoral embolization or thrombosis. Allergic reactions are exceedingly uncommon and reported to be more frequent with the brachial than with the percutaneous approach. This may reflect the fact that the catheters of Sones are not disposable but rather they are reused and what are in fact pyrogenic reactions may be misinterpreted as contrast agent reactions. The transfemoral approach uses preshaped disposable catheters. The incidences of allergic reactions are 0.25% for the brachial and 0.037% for the femoral techniques.

Predisposing Factors Causing Increased Risks.

The presence of left main coronary artery disease increases the risk of coronary arteriography. Fluoroscopic demonstration of calcification of the left main coronary artery is an important and reliable indicator of possible serious stenosis of that vessel. The possibility of this lesion should be kept in mind in patients with severe angina, angina at rest, or progressively increasing angina. Cohen and Gorlin (1975) report an average mortality of 13% for coronary arteriography in the presence of severe left main coronary artery disease. The mortality rate is greater with the per-

cutaneous femoral than with the brachial approach. The left coronary catheter of Judkins is stiffer, more resilient, and tends to penetrate deeper in the main left coronary artery; it may completely occlude it when it is severely stenotic or possibly dislodge a plaque or cause a dissection. Rösch *et al.* (1974) point out that with the use of a vasodilator, continuous monitoring of the catheter pressure, and careful technique, the percutaneous method can be used with safety and complications minimized.

We reported (Morettin, 1970) the uneventful perforation of a left coronary artery occurring during selective coronary arteriography by the percutaneous method of Judkins (Fig. 414). This occurred in a patient with severe aortic insufficiency, and it was possibly related to the force of the left coronary catheter augmented by prominent pulsations of the aorta and the wide pulse pressure.

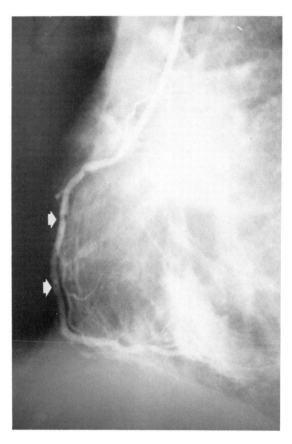

FIG. 413. SEVERAL SMALL AIR BUBBLES (AT AND BETWEEN ARROWS) ARE PRESENT IN THE RC

There were no adverse effects. Note also spasm at catheter tip and denser than usual stain of the posterior interventricular septum enhanced by the transient diminution of flow. RC, LAO.

The length of the examination and the catheter time is of considerable importance. Institutions reporting the lowest complication rates are those that do not combine arteriography with extensive physiological studies.

Air embolism (Fig. 413) may occur during coronary arteriography and unless of severe magnitude is not accompanied by serious complications. This results from faulty connectors, syringes and valves. This can be avoided by using, as we prefer, a closed system and a mechanical injector.

Metabolic conditions may increase the risk of complications, particularly hypokalemia. Low

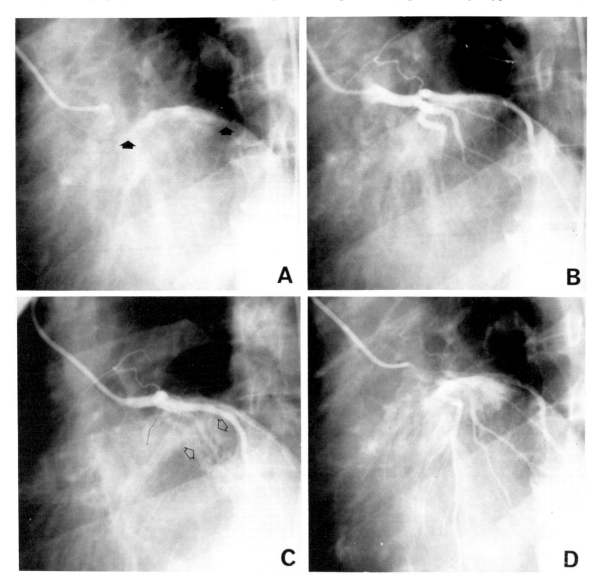

FIG. 414. UNEVENTFUL PERFORATION OF THE LEFT CORONARY ARTERY COMPLICATING ARTERIOGRAPHY
Roentgenograms of 4 different injections. Left anterior oblique projection. Left coronary artery. (A) Following the initial test dose the catheter tip has been removed from the left coronary artery and placed in the left coronary cusp. A crescent-shaped collection of contrast substance persists in the epicardiac surface of the heart (solid arrows). It is not in close proximity to the left aortic cusp. (B) A second injection shows its relation to the branches of the left coronary artery, which appear otherwise normal. (C) The walls of the diagonal branch are seen as a negative shadow outlined by the contrast substance outside (open arrows) and inside of the vessel. (D) The amount of extravascular contrast substance increased following the next injection.

There were no untoward effects. A small hematoma was found at surgery at the time of aortic valve replacement. (With permission, from *American Journal of Roentgenology, 100:* 185, 1970.)

potassium levels are common in patients treated with diuretics and should be corrected. Anoxia or hypoxia resulting from chronic pulmonary disease, or by even the moderate central respiratory depression caused by sedatives, increases myocardial irritability and the toxic effects of the contrast substance on the myocardium. Excessive sedation should be avoided.

Vasovagal reactions can be quite dangerous for two reasons: (1) A significant drop in arterial pressure causes decreased coronary perfusion that in patients with serious stenotic lesions of the coronary vessels may reach a critical level sufficient to produce arrhythmia or infarction. Similarly an acute cerebrovascular accident may occur in patients with already reduced cerebral flow. (2) The sluggish peripheral flow that accompanies vasovagal reactions increases the likelihood of arterial thrombosis.

Several anatomical situations increase the chances of complications. Injections in a dominant left coronary artery, particularly in the presence of severe disease in the right coronary artery, severe diffuse stenotic lesions, advanced cardiomegaly, and primary myocardial disease increase the possibility of serious arrhythmias. In 1970, one of the manufacturers of the water-soluble contrast substances used for coronary arteriography (Renografin 76, Squibb) removed most of the sodium from its formulation. This resulted in a higher incidence of ventricular fi-brillation. The present day Renografin 76 contains 0.19 *milliequivalents* of sodium/cm^3. The rate of ventricular fibrillation is the same with all contrast agents in common use today.

Prevention of Complications

In the prevention of complications the most important factors are (1) expeditious and meticulous technique; (2) systemic heparinization by the use of 4,000–6,000 units of heparin at the beginning of the procedure; (3) the acquisition and maintenance of an acceptable level of proficiency by the performance of at least 400 examinations per year.

Some authors (Judkins, 1974) believe that the angiographer should select one technique to the exclusion of others and become proficient with it. We disagree with this conclusion; there is no reason to think that anyone who has acquired experience in cardiac catheterization by other approaches cannot learn and practice percutaneous femoral arteriography provided that he deliberately maintains his skills by continuous use. We have practiced, and taught, both techniques by purposely using them, when feasible, on alternate patients. We have encountered situations in which the use of only one method would have resulted in an incomplete or less than ideal examination (a most important complication!), and the other method came to the rescue.

UNCOMMON OBSERVATIONS

In addition to arteriosclerosis there are other interesting aspects of coronary arteriography that, because of infrequent occurrence, are less well known. Angina may be the presenting symptoms of a number of abnormalities besides arteriosclerosis. The following, without intending to be complete, is a list of conditions that may cause coronary artery insufficiency and should be considered in the differential diagnosis of coronary occlusive disease (Morettin, 1976).

A. Inflammatory
Syphilis
Granulomatous arteritis
Sclerosing aortitis
Nonspecific infections
Lupus erythematosus
Polyarteritis nodosa
Rheumatoid arthritis
Ankylosing spondylitis

B. Traumatic
Closed chest trauma
Laceration
Traumatic fistulas
Iatrogenic injury
Radiation injury

C. Metabolic—Intimal Proliferation
Mucopolysaccharidosis
Homocystinuria
Fabry disease
Amyloidosis
Juvenile intimal sclerosis
Progeria
Pseudoxanthoma elasticum
Oral contraceptives and postpartum

D. Functional—Spasm
Prinzmetal angina
Iatrogenic (catheter)
Nitrate withdrawal

E. Embolic
Infective endocarditis
Prosthetic valve embolus
Myxoma
Atrial or ventricular thrombus
Iatrogenic

F. Miscellaneous

Aortic dissection
Cystic medial necrosis
Relapsing polychondritis
Syphilis
Papillary fibroelastoma of aortic-valve
Acquired aneurysms

Inflammatory Lesions

In the inflammatory conditions, specific diagnosis can be made only by clinical correlation and laboratory confirmation. A significant difficulty arises from the frequent impossibility to exclude, in most cases, concomitant or superimposed arteriosclerotic changes over a pre-existing abnormality of the arterial intima. The question of whether or not some lesions such as lupus erythematosus are predisposing factors for the development of severe arteriosclerotic changes remains to be answered (Gould *et al.*, 1968; Tsakraklides *et al.*, 1974). Arterial lesions have been observed in the coronary vessels in association with rheumatic fever (Cheitlin *et al.*, 1975). Rheumatoid disease, particularly the spondylitic form, may be associated with lesions of the proximal aorta, aortic valves, and proximal coronary vessels that resemble syphilis—consisting mostly of intimal sclerosis (Baggenstoss *et al.*, 1968; Sanerkin, 1968).

Polyarteritis nodosa of all the connective tissue disorders has been most frequently reported as involving the coronary vessels, even causing acute myocardial infarctions (Gould *et al.*, 1968).

It is quite likely that most of these patients will not come to coronary arteriography, because angina, in the absence of superimposed arteriosclerosis, must be exceedingly uncommon. The age of occurrence, the systemic symptoms, and the multiple organ involvement should help in the differentiation of the lesions associated with collagen disorders.

Syphilis deserves a special mention. Luetic aortitis characteristically affects the coronary ostia and the proximal main coronary arteries, which increases the risks of significant morbidity and mortality during coronary angiography. The coronary arteries should be evaluated very carefully before the repair of a syphilitic aneurysm of the aorta when utilizing extracorporeal circulation with coronary perfusion. Serious difficulties arise when unsuspected severe stenosis of the coronary ostia does not permit the passage of a perfusion cannula.

Granulomatous arteritis, or giant cell arteritis, is a progressive disease of unknown etiology characterized by destructive inflammatory changes of the elastic and muscular layers of medium sized arteries which may involve the coronary vessels, containing in its early stages abundant giant cells and granulomatous reaction. Later progressive stenosing fibrosis is the dominant feature (Gould *et al.*, 1968). Takayasu's disease is probably a related entity. It primarily affects young females and involves mostly the thoracic aorta and its branches. Patients experience visual disturbances, sometimes blindness, symptoms of cerebral ischemia, and progressive disappearance of pulses in the extremities.

Nonspecific coronary arteritis, presumably of viral origin, is known to produce marked acute inflammatory infiltration of the wall of the coronary vessels leading, in most cases, to ischemia and infarction (Cheitlin *et al.*, 1975).

Dego's syndrome is a cutaneosystemic disorder consisting of atrophic papular lesions of the skin and multiple ulcerations of the gastrointestinal tract, and diffuse occlusive arterial disease (Vlodaver *et al.*, 1972).

Trauma

Lacerations, thrombosis, and dissection have been occasionally described in penetrating or open injuries to the chest or as the result of inadvertent trauma at surgery (Danielson *et al.*, 1967; Fishman *et al.*, 1968) or coronary arteriography (see preceding section). Although there have been some reports of thrombosis following nonpenetrating chest trauma, only a few of them were well substantiated (Benray *et al.*, 1975; Jenkins *et al.*, 1975).

The anterior descending branch is always the site of thrombosis. The criteria necessary for the diagnosis include (1) evidence of recent localized thrombosis, (2) damaged myocardium in the area of distribution of the damaged vessel, and (3) absence of intrinsic disease in other vessels.

Figure 415 is the arteriogram of a 26-year-old man who developed an acute myocardial infarction following a severe nonpenetrating injury to the chest. Although it is impossible to determine how much of the myocardial damage is due to direct contusion of the heart and how much to acute thrombosis, cardiac contusion alone rarely leaves a clinically detectable abnormality (Benray *et al.*, 1975). In these cases the presence of a ventricular aneurysm or marked dysfunction may be explained by the demonstration of a coexisting localized coronary thrombosis. Penetrating wounds of the chest may result in acquired arteriovenous fistulas with direct communication between a coronary artery and vein

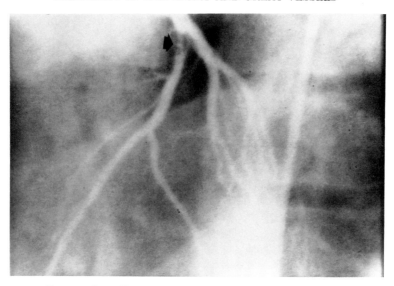

FIG. 415. LEFT CORONARY ARTERY, TRAUMATIC STENOSIS, LAO

The patient was a 26-year-old man who developed a large anterior myocardial infarction following nonpenetrating frontal chest trauma. Severe constricting lesion in the proximal anterior descending resulting from acute thrombosis (arrow). (With permission, from Morettin, L. B., Coronary Arteriography. Uncommon Observations. *Radiologic Clinics of North America,* *14:* 189–208, 1976.)

or cardiac chamber, or in localized traumatic aneurysms.

Constricting lesions of the epicardial vessels due to intimal fibrosis have resulted from radiation injury in patients receiving large doses to mediastinal fields for the treatment of a lymphoma. The critical dose has not been established. Pathologic features include abundant intimal proliferation and calcification (Tracy *et al.,* 1974).

Metabolic—Intimal Proliferation

Accumulation of an abnormal substance in some metabolic conditions may be responsible for coronary occlusions occurring in young individuals; mucopolysaccharides in Hurler's syndrome (Schiebler *et al.,* 1962), glycolipids in Fabry's disease (angiokeratoma corporis diffusum), and amyloid in primary and secondary amyloidosis (Cheitlin *et al.,* 1975).

Juvenile arterial sclerosis is a proliferative disease of the arterial wall which occurs in infancy and childhood, and is frequently accompanied by calcification that leads to early death (Witzleben, 1970). We have seen a case in a one-year-old child who died with extensive myocardial infarctions and calcified pulmonary arteries; the coronary arteries are the most frequently involved vessels. In pseudoxanthoma elasticum the elastic degeneration that affects the eyes, skin, and arteries is responsible for widespread vascular occlusions that may involve the coronary vessels.

Progeria is a rare idiopathic condition, characterized by growth retardation, baldness, premature closure of the epiphyses, loss of subcutaneous fat, and atherosclerotic and calcific lesions which may involve the coronary arteries early in childhood. Homocystinuria, an uncommon metabolic disorder, mostly affects the intramural branches; cases presenting with myocardial infarction have been reported.

Of particular interest is the increasing number of reports of young females who develop hyperplastic lesions of the intima of the coronary arteries while receiving oral steroids for contraception (Ivey and Norris, 1973). The exact nature of this problem awaits further elucidation. A similar mechanism may be responsible for the myocardial infarctions which complicate the postpartum of otherwise healthy young females.

Spasm

The role of spasm of the coronary artery in the so-called "variant" or Prinzmetal angina has recently received much attention (Higgins *et al.,* 1976). This type differs from classical angina in two important aspects: (1) the pain is not related to exercise, and (2) the electrocardiogram reveals transient S-T segment elevation rather than depression. Recent investigations reported the arteriographic demonstration of spasm which may occur in patients both with and without preexisting arteriosclerotic lesions (Donsky *et al.,* 1975). Spasm alone occurring in a normal artery is capable of producing the symptoms and electrocardiographic changes. To identify these individuals with a normal coronary arteriogram and variant angina, a provocative test has been proposed by Heupler *et al.* (1975). Patients with variant angina exhibit a positive response, consisting of the angiographic demonstration of severe segmental spasm with a greater than 90% narrowing, angina, and S-T elevation occurring within 10 minutes of the intravenous administration of 0.4 mg of ergonovine maleate. Spasm is not provoked in patients without Prinzmetal angina (Higgins *et al.*, 1976). Chahine *et al.* (1975) point out that the incidences of spontaneous spasm may be greater than can be documented during routine angiography and they recommend that vasodilators should be avoided when feasible until one complete set of coronary arteriograms is obtained. They point out that the angiographic contrast substance itself produces some coronary vasodilation which minimizes the opportunity for spasm.

Diffuse spasm has also been described and documented angiographically in individuals who develop anginal pains following removal from prolonged exposure to inhalation of nitrates, such as workers in ammunition factories or patients on large doses of nitroglycerin.

Embolic

Systemic embolization which may involve the coronary arteries occurs in situations that lead to the formation of cavitary thrombi such as rheumatic heart disease with mitral stenosis, endocarditis, cardiomyopathy, cardiac trauma, and left atrial myxoma. In patients with prosthetic valves, in addition to the possibility of embolism, fatal occlusion of the coronary ostia has been attributed to the development of abundant intimal hyperplasia surrounding the valve ring (Vlodaver *et al.*, 1972).

Miscellaneous

Aortic dissection which occurs in cystic medial necrosis of the aorta, arteriosclerosis, syphilis, trauma, and described in a few cases of relapsing polychondritis may extend to involve the origin of the coronary vessels, particularly when the ostia are situated above the supravalvular ring.

Papillary fibroelastoma of the aortic valve is a benign tumor-like growth which arises from the valve cusps and may extend to include the coronary orifices.

Although the existence of acquired aneurysms of the coronary arteries has been known for a long time (Bougon, 1812; Scott, 1948) it is only recently that their angiographic features became better known (Lipton *et al.*, 1975). Aneurysms of the coronary vessels have been described in patients with syphilitic aortitis, cystic medial necrosis, polyarteritis nodosa, and septic embolism, but in the majority of cases arteriosclerosis is responsible for both the localized and diffuse forms of arterial ectasia (Daoud *et al.*, 1963) (Fig. 399).

Bartel *et al.* (1974) found that in patients in whom calcification of the coronary vessels was identified at fluoroscopy, 97% had significant coronary disease with greater than 70% stenosis demonstrated angiographically. The angiographic severity of coronary artery disease increases with calcification of more than one vessel. Involvement of three of the major coronary branches occurred in 45%, 66%, and 82% of patients with one, two, and three vessel calcification respectively.

Abnormal Neovascularity

Abnormal neovascularity was reported by Grollman *et al.* (1974) to occur in a mural thrombus in a man with a history of myocardial infarction causing a left ventricular aneurysm. A prominent hypervascular blush was present in the anterolateral area of the left ventricle, presumably caused by penetration of the organized thrombus by capillaries arising from the subendocardial vessels.

We have encountered similar findings in a man with a cavitary filling defect on ventriculography without evidence of aneurysm (Fig. 417).

These abnormal blushes or accumulations of contrast agent are coarse, dense, irregular, and nonhomogeneous and should not be confused with the normally occurring staining of the myocardial wall or the dense areas of capillary staining demonstrated when the injection is made in a small coronary branch (Fig. 418). This stain represents stagnation of the contrast substance in the intramyocardial sinusoids. The sponge-like quality of the myocardial capillary bed is evidenced by the presence of this stain and the rapid filling of draining coronary veins.

I have been impressed by the intense and nonhomogeneous sinusoidal blush seen best in the cineflurograms in patients with rather diffuse coronary artery disease, particularly with severe proximal stenotic lesions, reflecting the presence of slow or stagnant flow.

Marshall *et al.* (1969) described a case of myxoma of the left atrium containing an abnormal collection of tumor-like vessels supplied by left atrial branches of the distal right coronary artery. Tumor-like vascularity in the left atrial wall, emptying directly in the left atrial cavity,

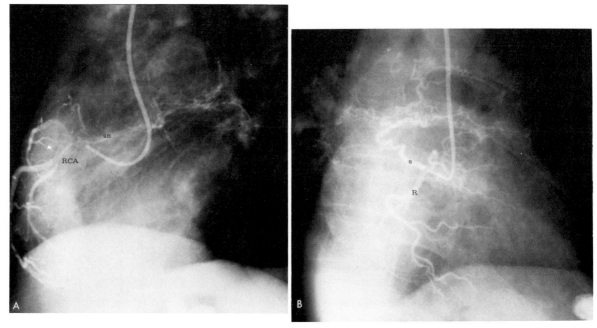

FIG. 416. RIGHT CORONARY ARTERIOGRAM IN A PATIENT WITH ADVANCED PULMONARY SILICOSIS
The sinoatrial artery (sn) is markedly enlarged and of almost the same caliber as the main right coronary artery (RCA) and gives origin to numerous large, tortuous vessels that supply mediastinal and hilar nodes. The atrial branches of the left circumflex were similarly enlarged. (A) Left anterior oblique. (B) Frontal view. (With permission, from Morettin, L. B., Coronary Arteriography. Uncommon Observations. *Radiologic Clinics of North America, 14:* 189–208, 1976.)

has also been reported in a patient with mitral valvular disease and a large left atrial thrombus (Standen, 1975).

Abnormal vessels may develop in adhesions across the pericardial cavity as the result of infarctions, hemorrhage or pericarditis (Fig. 407), and in pleuropericardial adhesions, the latter resulting frequently in communications between the bronchial and coronary circulations.

The existence of spontaneous bronchocoronary anastomosis has been well demonstrated (James, 1970), and although in some cases of obstructive coronary disease they may enlarge to provide some blood distal to obstructed coronary vessels, their value in adequately perfusing the myocardium remains doubtful. They occur around the base of the heart in the atrial walls. Conversely, the direction of flow may be reversed if the need for blood develops in the lung or hilar structures, and the coronary arteries become the suppliers rather than the receivers. Figure 416 illustrates such findings in a patient with advanced pulmonary silicosis in whom large and abundant newly formed vessels developed mostly from the atrial branches of both right and left coronaries to supply the hilar structures and anastomose with the bronchial arteries. In the absence of significant arteriosclerotic lesions or

desaturation it is tempting to theorize that the symptoms of typical angina in this patient may have been caused by a steal-like mechanism.

Physiological Effects of Coronary Arteriography and Ventriculography: Hemodynamic Changes

Measurement of ventricular pressures and the gradient across the aortic valve is performed routinely at the time of coronary arteriography and ventriculography.

Definite hemodynamic changes occur following the injection of contrast agent in the coronary arteries. Contrast substance decreases both the contractile force of the myocardial fiber and its compliance affecting both the ejection force of the myocardium and its relaxation during diastole.

Tracings obtained during coronary injections demonstrate both pressure and rhythm changes. The most constant findings are bradycardia and a drop in the peak systolic pressure that begin with the next systolic beat following the start of injection. These changes are transient and gradually return to the previous levels in the normal individual within 10–30 sec.

A transient elevation of the end-diastolic pressure also occurs lasting longer than the systolic

Electrocardiographic Changes (Fig. 420)

The electrocardiographic changes following injection of contrast substance in the coronary arteries consist of alterations of both conduction and depolarization. Although the quality and the intensity of the changes vary with the presence or absence of significant coronary artery disease, some patterns are constant in both groups.

Following injection into the left coronary artery, the ECG in the standard leads II and III shows a decrease in the amplitude of the P wave, a decrease in the R wave and/or an increase in the S wave. The most constant characteristic is a peaking of the T wave. The Q-T interval is prolonged and the heart rate is decreased.

Following injections in the right coronary artery, the sinus node is depressed resulting in bradycardia and even sinus block (Fig. 421). The PQ interval may be prolonged (Fig. 423) and there is a decrease in the amplitude of the Q-wave and the QRS complexes. The T wave in standard leads II and III show a progressive decrease in amplitude or inversion, becoming deep and peaked. The Q-T interval becomes prolonged.

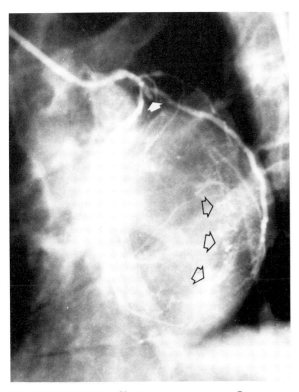

FIG. 417. ABNORMAL VASCULARITY IN AN ORGANIZED THROMBUS

A nonhomogeneous ripple-like stain and some globular dense collections of contrast (open arrows) are present along the lateral wall of the left ventricle. The ventriculogram revealed a sizable filling defect in the same region. A large diagonal branch (closed arrow) was completely occluded near its origin. (with permission, from Morettin, L. B., Coronary Arteriography. Uncommon Observations. *Radiologic Clinics of North America, 14:* 189–208, 1976.)

Marked bradycardia and transient periods of asystole (Fig. 424) occur more frequently with injections in the right coronary artery and at a time when a dense stain of the posterior interventricular septum is more apparent and reflecting depression of the sinus node and conduction system. This occurs particularly in patients with a dominant right coronary artery, or when there is spasm or significant stenosis of the proximal segments of the right coronary artery.

Several factors affect the magnitude and direction of the electrocardiographic changes following coronary artery injection. Injection in an occluded vessel frequently will show a little or no electrocardiographic response. When one coronary artery is occluded, injection in the opposite coronary artery will reveal the characteristic electrocardiographic changes expected with an injection of the occluded vessel (Fig. 420). For example, if the right coronary artery is proximally occluded and the distal right coronary artery is reconstituted through collaterals from the left coronary artery, an injection of the left coronary artery will produce an early elevation of the T-wave followed by a subsequent decrease and inversion. Similarly, injections in dominant vessels produce more pronounced electrocardiographic changes, and when the left coronary artery is dominant and the distal right coronary is hypoplastic, the changes following injection in the left coronary, will be identical to those expected from a normal right coronary (Fig. 422).

changes but gradually returning to the baseline values within the first minute in the normal individual. It is believed (Gensini, 1975) that the increase in the left ventricular end-systolic pressure is related to the amount of contrast material injected, which causes an increase in blood volume and consequently of the diastolic filling of the left ventricle. Another and equally as important mechanism is the diminution of left ventricular compliance, making the ventricles stiff and altering relaxation. Increase in left ventricular end-diastolic pressure is higher in patients with uncomplicated coronary disease (Fig. 419) and highest in those with coronary artery disease and left ventricular aneurysm. These findings closely correlate with ventricular function as assayed by cine ventriculography (Gensini, 1971) and may be used as an additional and useful test in evaluating the functional capacity of the left ventricle.

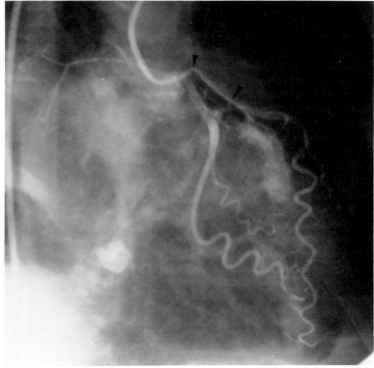

FIG. 418. MYOCARDIAL STAIN

Subselective injection in a small diagonal branch (arrow heads), results in a dense homogeneous myocardial blush. LC, RAO.

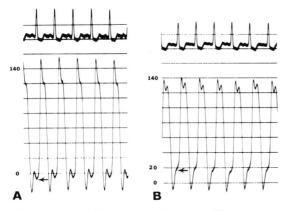

FIG. 419. LEFT VENTRICULAR PRESSURE TRACINGS

Before (A), and after (B), selective right and left coronary arteriography and left ventriculography, in a patient with moderate stenosis of the anterior descending and the right coronary arteries. The left ventriculogram was normal. Pressures in mm Hg. ECG, lead 2. Arrows indicate end-diastolic pressures.

The magnitude of the changes is related to the mass of myocardium perfused. This explains why normal individuals show a greater response than those with completely occluded vessels. Consequently when the myocardial mass is considerably increased such as in the presence of cardi-

omegaly particularly LVH, or myocardial disease, caution should be exercised, and the electrocardiographic changes closely observed in anticipation of the possibility of development of severe arrhythmias.

Myocardial Scanning

Coronary arteriography, while capable of demonstrating the anatomy and patency of the small coronary vessels, is limited in its ability to provide evaluation of the status of the myocardial sinusoidal bed and of the regional perfusion of the myocardium.

Ashburn *et al.* (1971) introduced the use of myocardial perfusion imaging by means of the selective injection in the coronary vessels of macroaggregated serum albumin particles labeled with 131-iodine and 99m Technetium. Radionuclide images thus obtained show the distribution of small (10–60 μ) biodegradable particles in the small vessels of the heart using a scintillation camera. The resulting images depict the relative distribution of blood flow throughout the myocardium.

By injecting a different isotope in each coronary artery, separate or complementary images of the relative small vessel perfusion via each vessel are obtained by electronic pulse-height

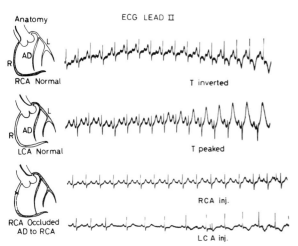

ECG LEAD II

Fig. 420. Lead II of Electrocardiogram Illustrating Changes Associated with Coronary Artery Opacification

Opacification of the normal right coronary artery is associated with inversion of the T wave, while opacification of the normal left coronary artery is associated with T-wave peaking. The last two strips of the electrocardiogram depict the changes seen in a patient with occlusion of the right coronary artery and filling of the distal branches of the right coronary by collateral vessels from the anterior descending. In this situation, right coronary injection is associated with T-wave peaking while left injection is followed by peaking and later inversion. Note that heart rate slows and that the T-wave vector moves away from the mass of myocardium being perfused with contrast material. (Courtesy of Drs. G. C. Friesinger and R. S. Ross, Departments of Medicine and Radiology of the Johns Hopkins University School of Medicine and the Johns Hopkins Hospital, Baltimore, Maryland.)

discrimination. This technique is remarkably free of complications. No significant S-T segment or T wave alterations or arrhythmias are noted during injection of the particles. Images of good quality are obtained. In the experience of Ashburn, all patients with stenosis of greater than 75% will have abnormal patterns. Abnormalities correlate very well with alterations of left ventricular wall motion demonstrated in ventriculography. In general, the underperfused regions are smaller than the areas with abnormal wall motion. This finding correlates well with the knowledge that in the fringes of an akinetic ventricular segment the myocardial fibers and sinusoids may be intact and that the abnormal function is caused by alterations of contraction and relaxation.

Generally myocardial perfusion scans can be done comfortably in 30 minutes. The particles are removed from the myocardial bed within 3–4 hours. This rate of clearance is similar to that of the same type of particles from the pulmonary capillary bed.

We have found myocardial perfusion imaging in conjunction with coronary arteriography quite useful in helping to differentiate, in some situations, discrepancies between the coronary arteriogram and the ventriculogram, specifically when a significant localized alteration of ventricular function is encountered, and the coronary arteriogram reveals normal or only slightly narrowed vessels in the area in question. In several cases (Figs. 397 and 411) an abnormal scan allowed us to suspect the complete occlusion of a branch at its origin without reconstitution, thus avoiding an error of underestimation.

Benchimol et al. (1968) described his observations on the findings on dye-dilution curves obtained following injection in a coronary artery at the time of arteriography. In normal patients with normal coronary arteries and in patients with evidence of coronary artery disease, 3.1 mg of Cardiogreen were used as the indicator and selectively injected in the ostium of the right or left coronary artery with continuous sampling from the main pulmonary artery.

Curves obtained in normal patients showed a fast appearance time, rapid build-up time, a tall peak concentration, and a rapid clearance and mean transient time. Significant obstructive lesions in one or more of the coronary arteries caused major alterations in the contour of the curves, resulting in prolonged appearance time, slurring, notches or a double hump in the ascending limb of the curve, slow build-up time, diminished peak amplitude, and prolonged mean transient and clearance time. Three factors play a role in the alteration of the dye-dilution curves, namely, delayed clearance of the indicator through an area of obstruction, the amount of the coronary flow and the extent of the collateral circulation.

This method has not encountered wide clinical application and more experience is needed to establish its value in the clinical setting.

Radiation Exposure and Dosimetry During Coronary Arteriography

A considerable concern has been expressed about the amount of radiation received by the operator, technicians, and patients during the performance of coronary arteriography. Wholey (1974) found that exposure to the hands of the operator was 1.1 mR/min for the Sones approach, versus 0.7 mR/min by the femoral technique. Exposure to the lens of the eye during fluoroscopy was 0.3 R/min. A technician posi-

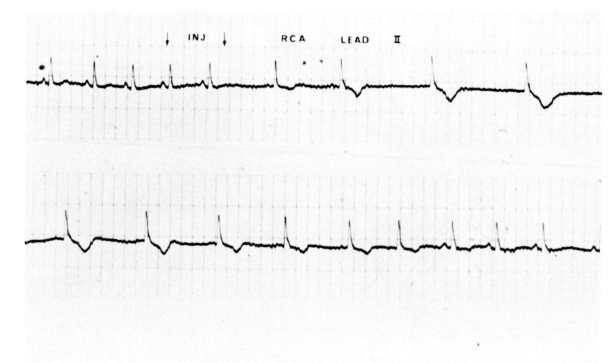

FIG. 421. FOLLOWING INJECTION (ARROWS) DEPRESSION OF THE SINUS NODE CAUSES TRANSIENT DISAPPEARANCE OF P WAVES, BRADYCARDIA, AND VENTRICULAR RHYTHM

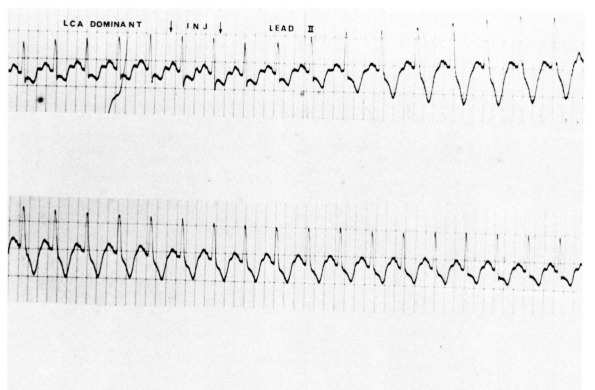

FIG. 422. T WAVE PROGRESSION FOLLOWING INJECTION OF A DOMINANT LC

T waves become deep and peaked. Changes reach maximum intensity 6–8 beats after end of injection and return to previous state 10–12 beats later. The right coronary was very small. Similar changes may be expected with an LC injection when the RC is obstructed, with left to right collaterals.

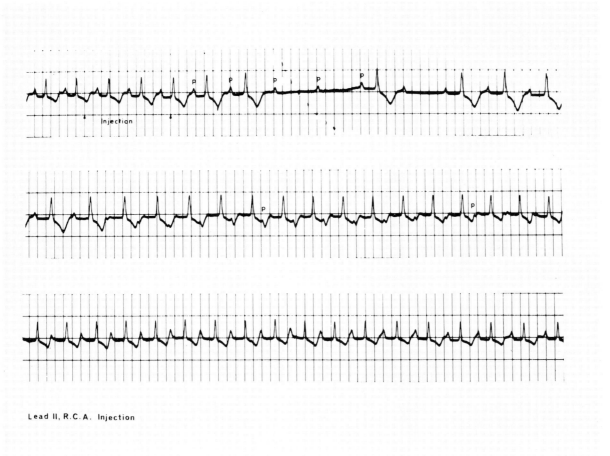

FIG. 423. A-V BLOCK

Following injection (arrow points) there is progressive prolongation of the P-Q segment and eventually, (at a time coinciding with maximum myocardial staining) complete A-V block, indicated by the presence of P waves without QRS complexes. Progressively the P-Q interval returns to normal. Dominant RC.

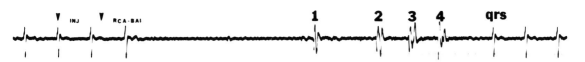

FIG. 424. COMPLETE ASYSTOLE BEGINNING ONE BEAT AFTER END OF INJECTION LASTING 8 SECONDS

The first "spontaneous" post-asystole beat (qrs) occurs after four blows (numbered) to the chest by an alert but overeager assistant. RC injection, balanced circulation.

tioned next to the patient's head receives 2 mR/min, or approximately 30 mR during 15 minutes of fluoroscopy. During the exposure of a 35-mm cine, the dose to the operator's hand was 11 mR/min with the brachial approach versus 4.5 mR/min with the femoral technique. The total dose accumulated during a coronary arteriogram can be as high as 43 mR per exam to the technician, 17 mR per exam to the radiologist's hands, and 10 mR/min to his lens. The techni-

cian positioned at the head of the unit to operate the cine controls and panning receives a dose greater than the maximal weekly permissible dose. Those participating in five examinations per day will get as much as 1,000 mR/week. Wholey (1974) strongly recommends that in those institutions where more than four examinations per day are performed, daily periodic rotation of both physicians and technical personnel should be practiced.

THE POST-OPERATIVE ARTERIOGRAM

Numerous surgical techniques have been used throughout the years with the purpose of increasing myocardial blood flow in an attempt to relieve the symptoms and complications of coronary artery obstructive lesions. The advent of direct coronary revascularization has determined the need of postoperative evaluation by means of angiographic studies of both the graft and the native circulation.

The earlier indirect attempts to promote increased collateral flow to the heart through extracardial anastomosis, by means of pericardial abrasions, partial ligation of the coronary sinus, ligation of the mammary artery, etc., have at the present time, only historical value.

Vineberg (1946) showed convincing evidence of increased coronary perfusion following implantation of the mammary arteries in the myocardium and that this was achieved through newly formed communications between the implanted vessel and the capillary-sinusoidal bed of the myocardium. This was predicated upon "a demand" created by the diminished pressure in the capillary bed distal to an area of significant stenosis. Depending on the extent of the disease, one or both mammary arteries were implanted in the myocardium. Sewell (1969) modified the preceding technique by the implantation of a mammary pedicle which consisted of the artery and the surrounding areolar tissue. The results were inconstant but in some patients symptomatic and even functional benefits were observed (Fig. 425).

Direct revascularization techniques originally included endarterectomy using several reaming techniques with or without the additional use of patch-graft reconstruction. The high frequency of complications and subsequent stenosis and thrombosis led to its loss of popularity.

Favaloro et al. (1970), in the Cleveland Clinic in 1967, performed for the first time a saphenous vein graft between the aorta and the coronary arteries. This proved to be a major advance in the surgical treatment of coronary artery disease.

An adequate segment of a saphenous vein is interposed, after ensuring incompetence of the venous system, between the aorta and a relatively nondiseased portion of the coronary artery distal to a stenosed or occluded segment. The graft is attached proximally to the lower portion of the ascending aorta. Distally it is anastomosed to the distal right coronary artery or the posterior descending near the crux of the heart on the right side or to the distal circumflex, anterior descending, or any of its larger branches as necessary.

In 1970, Green et al. reported their first experience with the coronary bypass using the internal mammary artery. The procedure is technically more demanding but it appears to have a higher patency rate than venous grafts.

Saphenous vein bypass grafts are indicated in patients suffering from angina with demonstrable

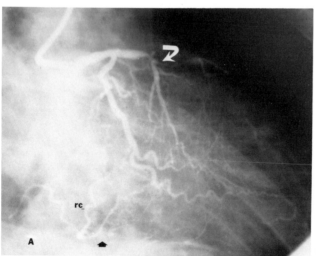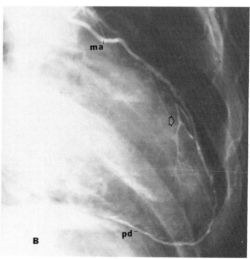

FIG. 425. FUNCTIONING MAMMARY ARTERY IMPLANT

(A) LC, RAO. The anterior descending is completely occluded proximally (curved arrow). The distal RC fills through collaterals and the posterior descending is obstructed (black arrow). (B) Selective left mammary arteriogram. RAO. The mammary artery has good flow and opacifies well, left ventricular (open arrow) and posterior descending branches. Ventricular function was minimally decreased.

segmental stenosis or complete occlusion of the proximal segments of the main three coronary branches with patent distal portions angiographically visualized directly or indirectly by collateral circulation and evidence of good distal run-off. The indications for coronary bypass surgery vary from institution to institution. Significant difference of opinion exists as to whether or not this should be performed in patients with acute myocardial infarction. Favaloro *et al.* (1971) state that when operations are performed within six hours of an acute myocardial infarction most of the heart muscle can be preserved or further myocardial damage prevented. Reul *et al.* (1976), reporting on their experience with 4,522 patients from one of the largest institutions in this country, conclude that coronary bypass can be recommended not only for patients with intractable angina, but also for patients with impaired ventricular function associated with angina, and in patients without angina who have a positive stress electrocardiogram.

The preoperative coronary arteriogram has been found useful in determining distal vessel suitability for bypass graft surgery. The accuracy diminishes when vessels distal to an obstruction are filled by insufficient collaterals.

Larger arteries with extensive peripheral vascular territories will show the higher rates of postoperative patency. Coronary calcifications should be sought carefully and reported; diffuse calcifications of the distal vessels often make bypass grafting technically impossible. The caliber of the vessel distal to an obstruction should be evaluated in light of the type of collateral circulation that contributes to its filling. Underdistention of a vessel distal to complete obstruction leads to underestimation of caliber. Furthermore, preoperative angiographic measurement of these partly distended vessels does not reveal the potential caliber that can be achieved following successful revascularization. Peripheral run-off capacity is an important factor in distal vessel suitability. If the run-off bed is small and of limited capacity, the resulting sluggish flow would predispose to thrombosis and graft failure (Rösch *et al.*, 1973). The condition of the myocardium to which the bypass is directed is very important. When the myocardium is normal the flow will be larger and will increase with time (Johnson *et al.*, 1970).

An intraoperative coronary arteriogram performed at the time of bypass may be of considerable value in assaying the actual caliber of a vessel distal to a complete obstruction when an accurate assessment of vessel diameter or potential distribution cannot be made from the preoperative examination (Kaplitt *et al.*, 1974).

Angiographic Technique

Postsurgical evaluation should include a repeat left ventriculogram and measurement of

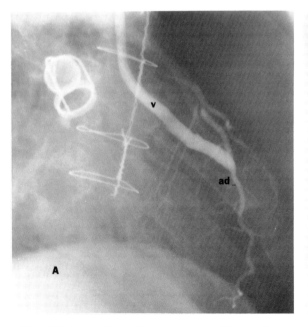 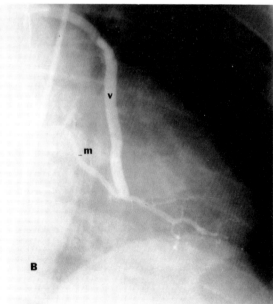

FIG. 426. AORTIC VALVE PROSTHESIS AND DOUBLE SAPHENOUS VEIN GRAFT (V) (ad) TO A LARGE LEFT MARGINAL (M) BRANCH IN A PATIENT WITH SEVERE STENOSIS OF THE MAIN LC AND ANGINA. GOOD ANASTOMOSIS

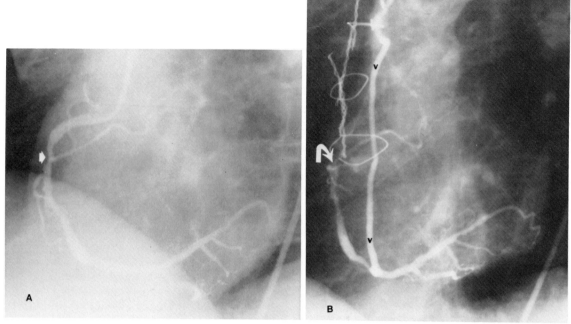

FIG. 427. THE AREA OF MODERATE STENOSIS (ARROW IN A) OF THIS LARGE DOMINANT RC WAS BYPASSED BY MEANS OF
A SAPHENOUS GRAFT

(A) RC, LAO. (B) Graft injection (v) 8 months following surgery reveals moderate stenosis of RC at the anastomosis and
progression of original stenosis to complete occlusion (curved arrow); good filling of distal branches.

ventricular pressures and gradients, then selective injection of all grafts, and finally selective right and left coronary injections. Ascending aortography becomes essential if any of the grafts cannot be catheterized. Most surgeons leave small metallic markers to indicate the site of the anastomosis of the graft to the aorta. Catheters specifically designed for the purpose are commercially available.

The origin and the course of the graft should be carefully examined for the presence of strictures, filling defects, kinking, etc. The distal anastomosis should be widely patent and at that point, generally, there is a slight dilatation of the coronary vessels. Stenosis occurs at the site of anastomosis either from the sutures themselves or intimal fibrosis or scarring (Fig. 428).

When the flow is normal (Fig. 426), injection in the graft will show a rapid filling of the native coronary circulation with complete washout of the contrast medium from the graft. Failure of visualization of the graft by means of an aortic injection does not necessarily mean that the graft is obstructed; when the flow is small, preferential layering posteriorly may prevent opacification of a graft directed anteriorly. Following injection in a graft, retrograde flow may be demonstrated in

the coronary artery back to site of proximal stenosis or occlusion (Fig. 427).

Occasionally, retrograde filling of a poorly functioning graft may be seen indicating lower pressure in the vein due to stenosis of a graft at its origin or in its distal anastomosis (Fig. 428).

Selective coronary injection may result in a lack of opacification of that coronary vessel at the site of previous stenosis or distal to the graft anastomosis. This may be caused by a good flow of nonopaque blood from the graft giving the erroneous impression that occlusion of the native coronary artery has occurred. This pseudo occlusion can usually be recognized by injecting the graft, though the area of stenosis may appear to be more severe due to the intermittent or incomplete opacification.

Previously demonstrated collaterals across an area of significant stenosis may regress following successful grafting. The regression may be more apparent than real and the collateral vessels do not obliterate but rather, because of the diminution of flow, are not opacified as well as they were preoperatively. The flow through a collateral vessel may reverse when a graft to a previously occluded vessel now provides blood flow to a diseased coronary artery that previously sup-

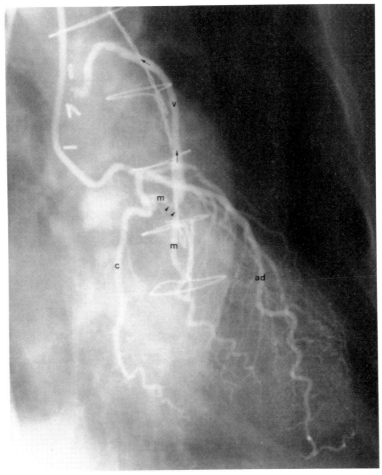

FIG. 428. POOR CHOICE OF GRAFT SITE

LAO view of injection in the LC. A venous graft (v) was made to a small marginal branch (m). An area of severe stenosis resulted at the anastomosis (arrow heads). Flow in the graft is poor and reversed by the injection (arrows).

plied the collateral vessel (Guthaner and Wexler, 1976).

Almost two-third of patients with patent grafts reveal evidence of normal or improved left ventricular contraction and decreased left ventricular end-diastolic pressure. Hypokineses show more improvement than localized akinetic areas.

Changes in the Graft and the Coronary Arteries. Their Evolution

Patency of the graft varies considerably between reported series, at rates between 72 and 85% at one year. Intraoperative flow measurements in vein grafts are considered to be of good prognostic value in predicting patency. If the graft flow is less than 20 ml/min, 50% of the grafts will be patent at one year. If the flow is between 20 and 40 ml/min, 79% of the grafts will be patent, and when the flow is greater than 40

ml/min, patency rate reaches 88% (Guthaner and Wexler, 1976).

The causes for immediate postoperative graft occlusion are related to faulty technique such as kinking of the graft or of the anastomosed artery, obstruction at the site of anastomosis, or traumatic injury of the graft or the coronary arteries. Some studies (Lespérance et al., 1973) suggest that early occlusion of the graft is secondary to thrombosis and it may be preventable by the use of systemic heparinization. Intimal fibroplasia begins to take place approximately one month following bypass surgery and accounts for the stenosis and occlusions that occur within the first year. This intimal fibrous hyperplasia seems to be a self-limited process that is not expected to progress after the first year following surgery. In that study there was no signfiicant difference in the amount of fibrous hyperplasia between the specimens obtained at one and at three years following bypass. Lawrie *et al.* (1976), in a similar study, confirm that moderate to marked intimal proliferation is an usual finding in long term grafts but is compatible with good graft patency.

Changes in the native coronary circulation both proximal and distal to the site of graft anastomosis have recently received a great deal of attention. A controversy exists regarding (1) whether or not coronary bypass surgery influences the rate of development of coronary artery disease and its complications, (2) whether or not coronary bypass surgery increases the incidence of new occlusions and, (3) whether the benefit of coronary bypass surgery is adversely affected by the development of new and unexpected lesions. Segal *et al.* (1973) observed that the competitive flow between the coronary artery and the bypass may result in actual progression of the proximal coronary arterial lesion. This is due to the fact that the coronary flow in the postoperative state is mostly through the bypass shunt and the reduced flow through the coronary artery may accelerate the progression of arteriosclerosis or thombosis or both in the proximal part of the vessel (Fig. 427). Consequently those patients who suffer delayed closure of the graft would be left in a disadvantageous situation. Similarly Maurer *et al.* (1974) noted that new total occlusions, new obstructive lesions, and progression of pre-existing stenoses were five times more frequent in grafted than in nongrafted arteries with comparable initial disease. The development of new and the progression of old lesions were encountered with the same frequency whether or not the graft remained patent or occluded. Occlusions occur more frequently in segments *proximal* than in those distal to the graft. In this series, 60% of the grafted arteries showed new total occlusions as opposed to only 2% of arteries that were not grafted. These facts should be kept in mind when evaluating a possible candidate for surgery particularly those with moderate degrees of stenosis.

Levine *et al.* (1975) established that the frequency of obstruction *distal* to the site of anastomosis is not significantly different from the progression of disease in nongrafted arteries and theorize that while proximal disease progression is probably a consequence of altered hydraulic factors, distal lesions seem to represent natural progression of arteriosclerotic disease.

Gensini *et al.* (1974), comparing patients that had coronary bypass surgery with a group of nonoperated patients, show differing results and conclude that coronary bypass surgery does not materially increase the incidence of new occlusions but it cannot be expected to arrest the natural progression of coronary arteriosclerosis. The answer to this question awaits longer follow up studies.

Particularly distressing are the reports that in as many as 63% of patients who have undergone coronary bypass surgery there is evidence of myocardial damage in the immediate postoperative period. These figures were reported in a recent study by Achuff *et al.* (1975). It is remarkable that in that study and in spite of the evidence of early myocardial damage, 88% of the late survivors report a significant symptomatic improvement. This author introduces the concept of "angina-producing" myocardial segment to explain the high rate of subjective improvement in angina, in spite of the occlusion of one or more bypass grafts and the frequent appearance of new total occlusions. A segment of myocardium can produce angina, only if it is viable and capable of some contraction. Dead tissue cannot cause pain as evidenced by the frequent improvement of angina following acute myocardial infarction in medically treated patients. It suggests that although the relief of angina pectoris can be accomplished in most patients by bypass surgery, the improvement in the symptoms is sometimes achieved by the conversion of ischemic to infarcted myocardium. It concludes that the relief of disabling angina is the major indication for surgery, but prevention of myocardial infarction and improvement of left ventricular function are less reliable objectives.

Acknowledgment—The very hard and diligent work of Peggy Smith, my secretary, is greatly appreciated.

General References

Baltaxe, H. A., Amplatz, K., and Levine, D. C.: Coronary Angiography. Springfield, Ill. Charles C Thomas, Publisher, 1973.

Gensini, G. G.: Coronary Arteriography. Mount Kisco, New York, Futura Publishing Company, Inc., 1975.

Guthaner, D. and Wexler, L.: The radiologic evaluation of patients with coronary bypass. Curr. Prob. Diag. Radiol. 6:6, 1976.

James, T. N.: Anatomy of the Coronary Arteries. New York, Paul B. Hoeber, Inc., 1961.

Morettin, L. B.: Coronary arteriography, uncommon observations. Rad. Clin. N.A. 14(2):189, 1976.

McAlpine, W. A.: Heart and Coronary Arteries—An Anatomical Atlas for Clinical Diagnosis, Radiological Investigation, and Surgical Treatment. Berlin, Heidelberg, New York, Springer-Verlag, 1975.

Vlodaver, D. P., Amplatz, M. H., Burchell, M. H., and Edwards, M. B.: Coronary Heart Disease, Clinical Angiographic and Pathologic Profiles, New York, Springer-Verlag, 1976.

Vlodaver, Z., Neufeld, H. N., and Edwards, J. E.: Coronary Arterial Variations in the Normal Heart and in Congenital Heart Disease, New York, Academic Press, Inc., 1975.

Paulin, Sven: Coronary Angiography, A Technical, Anatomic and Clinical Study, Acta Radiol. (Supp. 233), 1964.

15

The Cardiomyopathies

Cardiomyopathies refer to diseases of diverse etiology which primarily involve the myocardium rather than other portions of the cardiovascular system. An etiologic classification of the cardiomyopathies is shown in Table 12. In the handling of the individual patient the cardiomyopathies may be usefully classified according to the anatomical and functional changes (Goodwin, 1972). Congestive cardiomyopathy is the most common and is characterized by a weakened myocardium and poor systolic ejection fraction. Hypertrophic cardiomyopathy is characterized by irregular hypertrophy, impaired ventricular distensibility or compliance, and often some obstruction to the outflow tract of one or both ventricles. Obliterative cardiomyopathy is the rarest type, particularly in the United States, and is characterized by endocardial myofibrosis with stiffening of the myocardium, impaired ventricular filling and a small heart. It is usually a baffling diagnostic problem and may be difficult to differentiate from constrictive pericarditis. This type of cardiomyopathy is also known as constrictive myocarditis.

Positive identification of an etiologic agent is difficult and is often inferred. Chronic alcoholism frequently is indicted and seems quite authentic as either a predisposing or a direct etiologic agent (Tobin *et al.*, 1967). Cardiomyopathy can be associated with diseases due to malnutrition, such as beri-beri, or also to associated toxic agents, such as cobalt that is found in beer (Kesteloot *et al.*, 1968; Barlorik and Dusek, 1972).

Sarcoid is said to involve the heart in about 20% of cases studied at autopsy (Longcope and Freiman, 1952), and 5% may show clinical or electrocardiographic evidence of the disease (Lie *et al.*, 1974). The most common manifestations are arrhythmias and heart block, and sudden death has occurred with some frequency (Duvernoy and Garcia, 1971; Porter, 1960). The most common causes of congestive myocarditis are probably viral infections, such as Coxsackie B, mononucleosis, and varicella (Emanuel, 1970). An unusual and obscure type of cardiomyopathy is that associated with pregnancy. It is seen during the last antepartum month or more often during the first three months postpartum (Demakis and Rahintoola, 1971). In many cases and perhaps in the majority of those cases due to viral infection, the acute stages of the disease have occurred many years before the patient presents with the signs and symptoms of cardiomyopathy.

The pathologic features of cardiomyopathies are usually not specific and consist of interstitial fibrosis with consequent muscle replacement and an element of generalized myocardial hypertrophy. The left ventricle is characteristically the predominantly enlarged chamber, although all chambers are commonly affected. The aorta is usually normal in size. Involvement of the pericardium is not unusual, and there may be an associated pericardial effusion. Valvular abnormalities are not prominent, but some degree of insufficiency, particularly of the mitral valve, may develop with left ventricular dilatation. An obliterative myocarditis frequently involves either the tricuspid or mitral valve by a fibrotic process, and insufficiency of one or both of these valves may be a feature of this particular disease (Goodwin, 1972). A significant finding is the frequent occurrence of mural thrombi, particularly in the left ventricle. Peripheral emboli with or without infarction may be found in the lungs and in organs supplied by the systemic circulation. In the hypertrophic type the myocardial hypertrophy is occasionally localized to the interventricular septum and as has been described elsewhere may produce muscular subvalvular aortic stenosis. The pattern of the musculature of the myocardium in the hypertrophic type at times is highly suggestive of the diagnosis. Other microscopic findings depend on the specific etiology, such as round cell infiltration with myocarditis, and the specific histological appearances in car-

1. Infectious Myocarditis
   Bacteria, fungi, rickettsia, spirochetes, viruses, protozoa
2. Granulomatous Myocarditis
   Tuberculosis, sarcoidosis
3. Collagen Myocarditis
   Lupus erythematosus, periarteritis nodosa, rheumatoid arthritis, scleroderma
4. Fiedler's myocarditis
5. Infiltrative Diseases of Myocardium
   Amyloidosis, hemochromatosis, glycogen storage disease, tumor
6. Metabolic Diseases of Myocardium
   Thyrotoxicosis, myxedema, nutritional deficiency, gout, hypokalemia
7. Toxic Diseases of Myocardium
   Poisons, drugs, physical agents
8. Familial Diseases of Myocardium
   Friedreich's ataxia, muscular dystrophy, familial cardiomyopathy, glycogen storage disease
9. Idiopathic myocardial hypertrophy
   Idiopathic hypertrophic subaortic stenosis (sometimes familial)

TABLE 13
COMMON CAUSES OF HEART DISEASE

Arteriosclerotic heart disease
Acquired valvular heart disease
Congenital heart disease
Heart disease secondary to systemic hypertension
Heart disease secondary to hypertension of the pulmonary circulation

diac amyloidosis (Farrokh et al., 1964) and neoplasms.

The symptoms of cardiomyopathy are nondiagnostic. Weakness, fatigue, and exertional dyspnea are early manifestations, and dizziness and exertional syncope may occur. Sudden death is common, particularly in acute myocarditis and also with involvement due to sarcoid (Porter, 1960). Marked cardiomegaly may be asymptomatic for years until cardiac decompensation develops. Failure is often biventricular. Mural thrombi in the cardiac chambers may be the source of multiple pulmonary and systemic emboli and be productive of characteristic symptoms. Findings on physical examination depend upon the state of cardiac compensation. The patient may appear to be in good health or may show signs of intractable failure, with pallor and peripheral cyanosis, a rapid weak pulse, a low pulse pressure, diastolic gallop rhythm, functional murmurs, particularly those of mitral and tricuspid insufficiency, and ectopic rhythms and conduction defects. Cardiomegaly will be found in most cases and is predominantly left ventricular. The electrocardiogram is similarly nondiagnostic but is almost always abnormal. The most frequently seen pattern is that of left ventricular hypertrophy, low voltage, and nonspecific S-T wave changes. Arrhythmias are common, particularly atrial fibrillation and premature ventricular contractions. Second or third degree heart block has been seen associated with the Stokes-Adams syndrome (Duvernoy and Garcia, 1971).

Cardiac catheterization may show a low and relatively fixed cardiac output, increased arteriovenous oxygen difference, the absence of intra- and extracardiac shunts, and elevated end-diastolic pressures in the ventricles, particularly the left ventricle. In the obliterative or constrictive cardiomyopathies the left ventricular pressure curve may be highly suggestive in that it is a flat top and V type of curve indicating a sudden interruption of diastolic filling and delayed systolic ejection. In the hypertrophic type with localized hypertrophy of the interventricular septum there may be a variable subvalvular gradient between the main ventricular cavity and the immediate subvalvular area.

While certain features may suggest the diagnosis of primary myocardial disease, the diagnosis often depends upon the exclusion of the usual causes of heart disease (Table 13; Sanders, 1963). A thorough and exhaustive study is ordinarily required in order to make the diagnosis of primary myocardial disease with confidence.

RADIOLOGIC FINDINGS

The congestive type of cardiomyopathy is by far the most common. In this type the chest film usually shows diffuse cardiac enlargement, although there may be a predominance of the left ventricle. Fluoroscopy characteristically shows hypoactive and feeble pulsations. The right ventricle is often moderately dilated, and in the presence of relative or functional mitral and tricuspid insufficiency, the left and right atria may be moderately to greatly enlarged. In some cases, particularly those due to obliterative myocarditis, the valve structures may be actually distorted. The cardiac borders are usually sharply outlined due to the decreased pulsations of the weakened heart muscle. The aorta is of normal caliber and may appear relatively small in com-

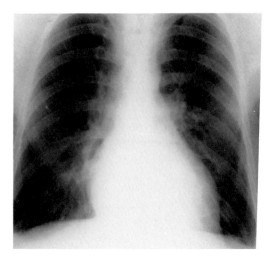

FIG. 429. PRIMARY MYOCARDIAL DISEASE

Thirty-seven-year-old white man who presented with edema of the lower extremities and genitalia of 1 month duration. Blood pressure was 128/48, pulse was 106 and regular. The only abnormal physical findings were the presence of a slightly enlarged liver and fixed splitting of the second pulmonary sound. A systolic murmur with maximal intensity midway between the left lower sternal border and the apex was heard. No diastolic murmurs were detected. Cardiac catheterization revealed normal pressures and showed no evidence of a shunt. The catheter passed easily to the right wall of the cardiac silhouette, demonstrating normal myocardial thickness here and militating strongly against the diagnosis of pericardial effusion. PA chest film shows mild

parison to the enlarged heart. The lungs are often quite clear, and the pulmonary blood vessels may be inconspicuous, particularly if the process involves both the right and left sides of the heart.

In the presence of congestive cardiac failure, the findings of moderate to great cardiomegaly may be accompanied by increase in size and decrease in clarity of the hilar vascular structures indicative of pulmonary congestion. The radiographic manifestations of pulmonary infarction may also be seen in all stages of development.

Venous or selective angiography of the congestive type of cardiomyopathy shows dilatation of the cardiac chambers with an increase in the circulation time and evidence of pooling of the contrast material on both sides of the heart. The left ventricular myocardium may be quite thick (Ruttenberg et al., 1964), and its internal surface may be thrown into coarse projections due to hypertrophy of the columnae carnae (Fig. 431C). This is in contrast to the usually smooth endocardial surface noted in endocardial fibroelastosis. When subvalvular muscular aortic stenosis is the predominant lesion, left ventriculography may show the characteristic funnel-shaped encroachment upon the left ventricular outflow tract that characterizes this condition.

left ventricular enlargement with a small pleural effusion on the right. The great vessels at the base of the heart are normal in appearance.

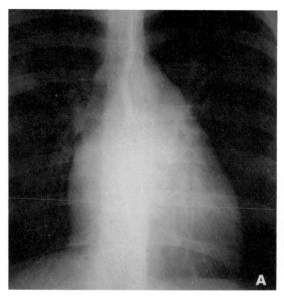
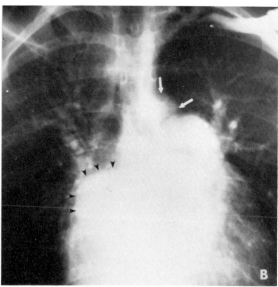

FIG. 430. IDIOPATHIC LEFT VENTRICULOPATHY (LEFT VENTRICULAR MYOCARDIAL INSUFFICIENCY) IN 26-YEAR-OLD WOMAN MIMICKING MITRAL STENOSIS

Repeated carefully performed left heart catheterizations showed no pressure gradient across the mitral valve. (A) Plain frontal film shows a prominent pulmonary trunk, small aorta, enlarged left atrial appendage, and steep left heart border giving the heart a "mitral" configuration. (B) Film from anteroposterior angiocardiogram. The upper lobe pulmonary vessels are dilated while the lower lobe channels are constricted. A sizeable left atrium (black arrowheads) and small aorta (white arrows) are shown.

DIFFERENTIAL DIAGNOSIS

The differential diagnosis includes all the other usual causes of cardiac disease. The most common of these, however, is the "burned out" hypertensive which may show great clinical similarity to the patient with a cardiomyopathy. In such cases, the roentgenographic demonstration of a normal-sized aortic knob, and the fluoroscopic observation of greatly diminished ventricular pulsations may be of some use in the differential diagnosis.

Fluoroscopy and films may be also of considerable value in excluding valvular and pericardial calcification. Pericardial calcification is said to be present in 55–70% of cases with constrictive pericarditis (Brigden, 1957), and in the small group of patients with obliterative endocarditis

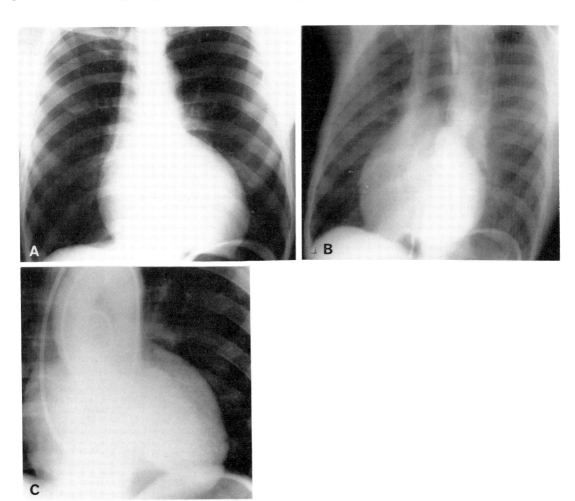

FIG. 431. PRIMARY MYOCARDIAL DISEASE

The patient is a 38-year-old black man. Cardiomegaly was first noted on a routine chest film, and careful questioning produced a history of shortness of breath after walking several blocks and some vague nocturnal chest pain. Physical examination revealed a blood pressure of 120/80. A Grade II systolic ejection murmur was heard along the left sternal border without radiation. No diastolic murmurs were heard. Cardiac catheterization showed slight elevation of the left ventricular end diastolic pressure and showed no systolic gradient across the aortic valve and no evidence of of intra- or extracardiac shunts. Repeat catheterization 1 week later showed normal pressures on both sides of the heart. Electrocardiogram showed left ventricular hypertrophy and some increase in the size of the P waves suggesting a right atrial abnormality. (A) Teleoroentgenogram of the chest shows mild cardiac enlargement, predominantly left ventricular. The aorta is normal in size. The left heart margin is unusually convex laterally, and the heart contour has a sharply defined "pencilled" outline. (B) Left anterior oblique view of the chest showing the prominent left ventricle and normal-sized aorta. (C) Left ventriculogram via a catheter introduced into the left ventricle across the aortic valve. The thickened left ventricular myocardium is well shown as well as the irregular inner surface of the left ventricle along the left heart border, thought to indicate considerable hypertrophy of the columnae carnae. No obstruction to left ventricular outflow was demonstrated.

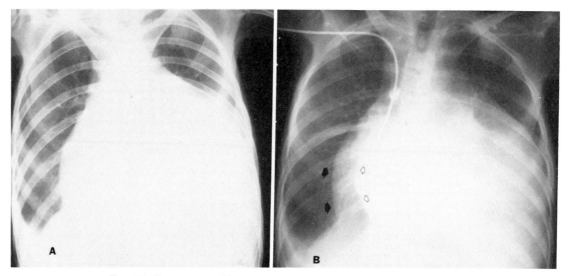

FIG. 432. POSTPARTUM MYOCARDIOPATHY WITH PERICARDIAL EFFUSION
Symptoms began 1 week postpartum. Present films were exposed 2 months later. (A) Marked cardiac enlargement with clear lungs. (B) Angiography shows a large pericardial effusion in addition to dilated heart.

and a normal-sized cardiac silhouette, the absence of such calcification may be helpful in the differential diagnosis. The presence of a large left atrium in association with a normal-sized left ventricle also is helpful in eliminating valvular disease, although this same finding may be seen with the constrictive type of cardiomyopathy.

Another differential consideration is pericardial effusion which may closely resemble the cardiovascular contour seen in primary myocardial disease. Cardiac pulsations may be greatly diminished in both abnormalities. Pericardial fluid can usually be detected by echocardiography, and this is the procedure of choice. Where this is not available, blood pool scanning should be considered as another noninvasive technique. Fluoroscopic detection of a thin fat line 5 mm below the cardiac contour is helpful but not always possible. Opaque angiocardiography is seldom necessary. The possible coexistence of myocardial disease and pericardial effusion must be borne in mind, however, and the mere demonstration of a thickened right cardiac-pericardial border does not eliminate the possibility of primary myocardial disease.

Other radiologic findings may occasionally be useful in determining the specific etiology of a cardiomyopathy. Intestinal and pulmonary changes in scleroderma may be helpful in diag-

nosis; plain films and angiography may, by demonstration of an irregular nodular cardiac contour or extension into the lumen, afford x-ray evidence of the presence of a cardiac neoplasm. Enlargement of the thyroid with deviation of adjacent organs may occasionally be seen in thyrotoxic heart disease, and roentgen changes in the extremities in progressive muscular dystrophy may suggest that the cardiac enlargement occasionally seen in that disease is due to myocardial involvement by the dystrophic process.

Other features helpful in differentiating the many causes of primary myocardial disease are chiefly clinical. Systemic signs of infection or toxicity suggest acute myocarditis. Blood chemical and complement fixation tests may cast additional light on the etiology. Myocardial biopsy, either by transthoracic needle puncture or removal of tissue by surgical exploration or by intraventricular catheter, may confirm the presence of a lesion in the myocardium and in some instances provide an etiological diagnosis (Mattingly, 1961). The disappearance of murmurs with return of cardiac compensation in primary myocardial disease is in striking contrast to the accentuation of such murmurs under similar circumstances in rheumatic valvular disease and provides a helpful clinical clue in distinguishing these broad groups.

THERAPY

Therapy consists of medical support of the myocardium, bed rest, and restriction of activity. At times specific therapy may be directed toward

the etiologic agent, as in diphtheria. Steroids, though harmful in acute infections, may be valuable in later stages and are frequently used in the management of cardiac disease associated with collagen disorders. Steroids may also be used in the treatment of sarcoid. Surgery, in the case of asymmetrical hypertrophy or tumor, may be curative. Chest films supply an important and useful means of detecting and following the response to therapy, chiefly by depicting changes in heart size and may aid in the diagnosis of embolic complications by demonstrating pulmonary infarction. The reader is referred to several reviews of primary myocardial disease for further information, particularly those of Mattingly (1961), Haskin et al. (1961), Brigden (1957), Saunders (1962, 1963), Sackner (1961), Bloomfield and Liebman (1963), Harris and Nghiem (1972), and Tobin et al. (1967).

IDIOPATHIC HYPERTROPHIC SUBAORTIC STENOSIS (IHSS)

Idiopathic hypertrophic subaortic stenosis is now, after some 15 years of investigation, a well documented and relatively clear-cut entity. Its origin and pathogenicity are still uncertain. In many, and perhaps all of the cases of IHSS, the myocardial abnormality is congenital, although obstruction in the outflow tract of the left ventricle may not appear for many years. In many, and perhaps the majority of cases, although there is a myocardial abnormality, outflow obstruction may never appear in which case the condition may be classified as a myocardiopathy. A considerable familial incidence has been observed, although many relatives may be asymptomatic and show no obvious clinical or hemodynamic findings. There is a preponderance of males to females of about 2:1 (Braunwald et al., 1960; 1964).

Brock (1959) was apparently the first to call attention to the possibility of the functional obstruction to the outflow tract of the left ventricle due to a localized hypertrophy of the myocardium. Bercu et al. (1958), Livesay et al. (1960), Menges et al. (1961), Nordenstrom and Ovenfors (1962), and Goodwin et al. (1960) all made important observations in small series of cases with muscular subaortic stenosis. Braunwald et al. (1964) reported on an extended series and documented in considerable detail the hemodynamic, clinical, and to a considerable extent the pathologic characteristics of this entity. Further contributions to the hemodynamic angiographic details were provided by Ross et al. (1966) and Criley et al. (1965). More recently, Simon et al. (1967) and Simon (1968) have described in considerable detail the angiographic characteristics of this condition.

The disease affects the ventricular myocardium, predominantly that of the left ventricle and interventricular septum. In patients with hemodynamically significant outflow obstruction, the upper part of the muscular septum is predominantly thickened, although the entire left ventricular myocardium is usually increased in thickness. Microscopic examination of the myocardium shows coarsening of the muscle bundles with bizarre and irregular arrangement and an abundant amount of collagenous tissue between the fibers. The histologic changes are sufficiently characteristic to permit a diagnosis to be made from biopsy of the interventricular septum via the right ventricle (Alexander and Gobel, 1974). The essential anatomic changes in those cases with outflow obstruction are (1) diffuse or irregular thickening of the left ventricular myocardium; (2) reduction in volume of the left ventricular cavity; (3) pronounced localized thickening of the interventricular septum, particularly the high ventricular septum; (4) enlargement and malalignment of the papillary muscles with resultant failure of proper closure of the mitral valve; and (5) elongation of the anterior leaflet of the mitral valve as has been documented in some cases (Fix et al., 1964), and this may be congenital or due to unusual stress over a number of years.

The age of onset of symptoms is quite variable. A few cases have been observed during the first year of life. The average age of onset in the series of Braunwald et al. (1964) was 22 years for males and 35 years for females. A number of cases have been observed in the fifth and sixth decades. In children, the symptoms are usually those of left ventricular failure. In adults, the symptoms are frequently those of dyspnea, angina, weakness, and syncope.

On physical examination, the heart may or may not be enlarged. A systolic murmur well localized to the left parasternal region is very common. Often an additional holosystolic murmur is found which is indicative of mitral insufficiency. The electrocardiogram is often abnormal, and about one-third of the cases show a left axis deviation and changes in the QRS complexes are very common. In many well documented instances, the heart was thought to have been normal on previous examination preceding by years the onset of symptoms.

The hemodynamic changes in IHSS are often characteristic and specific and are thus useful in diagnosis. The carotid pulse tracing shows a rapid upswing followed by a biphasic crest with a delayed second peak. This indicates a progressive increase in the severity of the obstruction reaching a maximum in late systole. Simultaneous tracings of the pressure curves obtained from the left ventricle and aorta or brachial artery have a number of unique characteristics that permit differentiation from other types of aortic stenosis. These pressure gradients and pulse contours were the source of considerable controversy (Criley *et al.*, 1965; Ross *et al.*, 1966), but most of these inconsistencies have been resolved or explained. The ventricular tracing is quite steep in its initial portion followed by a rounded crest which is different from that of fixed valvular or subvalvular stenosis. Any mechanism that increases the force of the ventricular contraction increases the severity of the outflow obstruction. This is commonly demonstrated by a tracing obtained during a premature ventricular contraction which is followed by a compensatory forcible ventricular contraction (Fig. 433). In patients with fixed stenosis, the pulse pressure in the peripheral arteries increases associated with the increased force of the compensatory ventricular contraction. In contrast in IHSS, the pulse pressure decreases due to the increased severity of the stenosis. A similar increase in the severity of the stenosis can be produced by the ionotropic agent, isoproterenol, and often by a well performed Valsalva manuever and other agents. In obtaining these tracings it is essential that the tip of the catheter be completely free in the sinus portion of the left ventricle. If the tip of the

catheter is wedged into the columnae carneae, the force of the contraction may produce variable and false increases in pressure recordings due to the contact of the catheter with the muscular wall of the left ventricle. General anesthesia di-

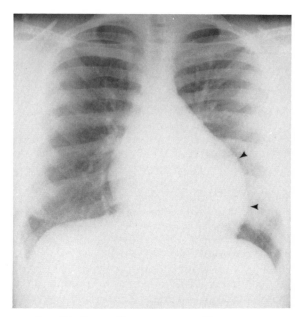

FIG. 434. SLIGHT FLATTENING AND NODULARITY (ARROWS) OF THE LEFT HEART BORDER IN A CASE OF IHSS

This seems to be an unusual manifestation of this condition.

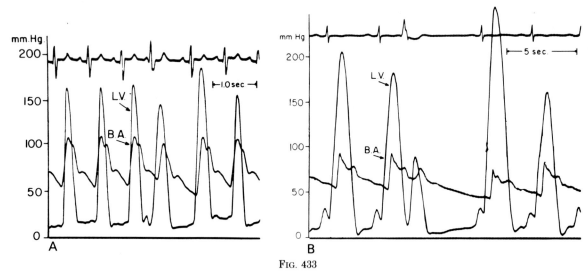

FIG. 433

(A) Simultaneous pressures recorded in the left ventricle (LV) and brachial artery (BA) of a patient with valvular aortic stenosis and aortic regurgitation. In the cycle following the premature contraction the pulse pressure in the brachial artery is greater than it is in the control beats. (B) Simultaneous pressures recorded in the left ventricle and brachial artery in a patient with IHSS. During the postpremature contraction beat the pulse pressure in the brachial artery is less than it is in the control beats.

(From Braunwald *et al.*, *Circulation*, *29–30:* (Suppl. 4), 1964; with permission, the American Heart Association, Inc.)

minishes the contractile force of the myocardium and may diminish or abolish the gradient. Consequently, observations at the operating table may be misleading and thus tended to confuse earlier observers. Variability in the gradient and the severity of the obstruction may be considerable, even during a single catheterization session and tends to support the diagnosis of IHSS.

Obstruction to the outflow tract of the right ventricle has been found in an appreciable num-ber of cases (Nghiem *et al.*, 1972). The hypertro-phied septum protrudes into the outflow tract and produces progressive obstruction during sys-tole. This can be demonstrated by pullback trac-ings and right ventricular angiography.

In patients with symptoms and signs of aortic stenosis and/or heart failure and where a ques-tion of surgical treatment has been raised, careful study by cardiac catheterization and ventriculog-raphy is indicated. Entrance into the left ventri-

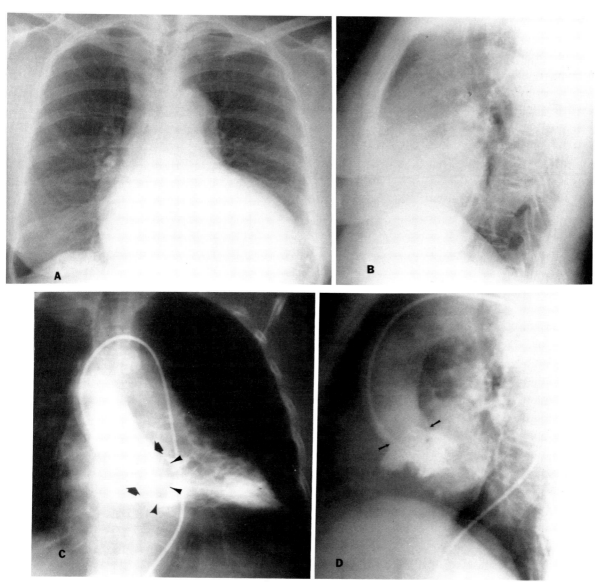

FIG. 435. IDIOPATHIC HYPERTROPHIC SUBAORTIC STENOSIS

(A and B) Heart is markedly enlarged with predominant enlargement of the left ventricle. Left atrium apparently not very large. (C and D) Frontal and lateral left ventriculograms. The frontal view exposed during systole shows the radiolucent area with sharp margin (arrowheads) due to anterior position of the anterior leaflet of the mitral valve. It partially obstructs the outflow tract of the left ventricle. In the lateral view the outflow tract is obscured due to the superimposed left ventricular cavity which occupies an abnormal horizontal position. Some reflux into the left atrium is seen in both projections. Arrows in D indicate aortic valve ring

cle is preferable by the transaortic route. Braunwald *et al.* (1964) state that there are 5 groups of
cases; those (1) with a gradient under all conditions, (2) with a gradient under basal conditions
that can be abolished with methoxamine or angiotensin, (3) with obstruction at certain times
only, (4) without obstruction in the basal state
but in whom an obstruction can be provoked by
nitroglycerin or the Valsalva maneuver, and (5)
with clear-cut clinical evidence of left ventricular
hypertrophy but no gradient under any circumstances. Many patients fall in the latter group.

Radiologic Findings

The conventional chest films are rarely helpful
or specific. The heart is enlarged in about one-
half of the patients with symptoms (Braunwald
et al., 1964). The left ventricle is always hypertrophied, and when the heart is enlarged, the left
border is rounded. The present authors have
observed one case in which the left border
showed a subtle but definite protrusion suggesting a localized or nodular area of thickening in
the left ventricle. This seems to be an isolated

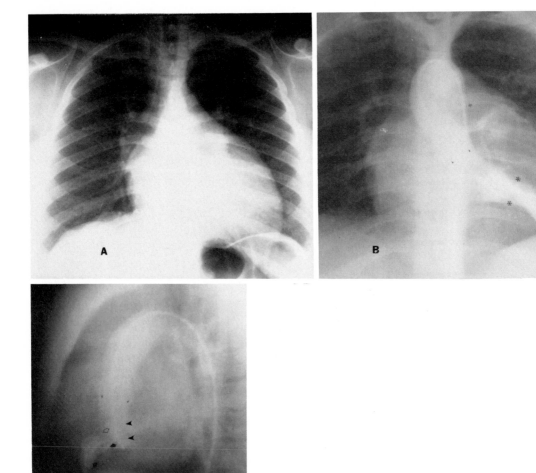

Fig. 436. Idiopathic Hypertrophic Subaortic Stenosis

(A) Marked cardiac enlargement, predominantly left ventricular. (B) Ventriculogram in systole. Small arrows indicate aortic
valve ring. Asterisks indicate impression on outflow tract of the anterior leaflet of the mitral valve. Note the marked thickening
of the ventricular myocardium. Faint mitral regurgitation is noted. (C) Lateral ventriculogram in systole. Small arrow indicates
aortic valve ring. Open arrow indicates hypertrophied and distorted interventricular septum. Entire posterior wall of left
ventricle is distorted and mal-aligned (closed arrows). The small arrowheads indicate anterior leaflet of mitral valve.

example, but its occurrence should suggest the possibility of this condition. Although the left ventricle is predominantly enlarged, the heart is more globular in contour than is usually seen with other forms of aortic stenosis. Left atrial enlargement secondary to mitral insufficiency is common and can be positively identified in over half of the patients with symptoms (Braunwald *et al.*, 1964). Right-sided enlargement occasionally occurs. When present, it suggests the possibility of pulmonary hypertension and/or left ventricular failure or is occasionally associated with an obstruction to the outflow tract of the right ventricle (Nghiem *et al.*, 1972). The size of the heart is not well correlated to the peak systolic gradient across the outflow tract of the left ventricle nor the functional classification of the patient. When the mitral insufficiency is sufficiently severe, pulmonary venous hypertension may be manifest by relative enlargement of the upper lobe blood vessels and other signs of left-sided heart failure. Calcium in any of the cardiac structures is rare.

Selective left ventriculography, preferably performed through the transoartic route, is often specific. Many authors have described various features of the ventriculogram (Nordenstrom and Ovenfors, 1962; Ross *et al.*, 1966; Braunwald *et al.*, 1964; Simon *et al.*, 1967; and Simon, 1969). The changes are best documented in the frontal and lateral projections using large films exposed at a rate of at least 4/sec so as to adequately delineate the ventricular cavity in both systole and diastole. Injection of the contrast substance should be made with the catheter tip free in the sinus portion of the left ventricle. The left ventricular wall is thickened, and the cavity is irregular in contour. In the lateral view in diastole, the hypertrophied septum impinges on the outflow tract as evidenced by a smooth curved indentation anteriorly below the aortic valve. The anterior leaflet of the mitral valve is in its usual position posteriorly in the outflow tract and together with the anterior septal muscle mass forms an inverted cone-shaped cavity below the aortic valve (Fig. 437). The ventricular cavity below the cone-shaped outflow tract is usually reduced in size, and often a sizeable localized indentation inferiorly also represents hypertrophied septal musculature. In the frontal projection in diastole, the inferior or diaphragmatic margin of the ventricle is often indented due to the wrapped around effect of the septal hypertrophy. The upper left lateral border may show a V-shaped indentation also due to the septum. The thin curved radiolucent line representing

the attachment of the posterior leaflet of the mitral valve is accentuated and is often wavy in appearance. This wavy linear shadow is due to the indentation posteriorly of the mitral valve and the thinning of the column of contrast substance in the outflow tract caused by the hypertrophied septum anteriorly. The ventricular cavity is reduced in volume and may have an irregular contour.

In systole in the lateral view, the impingement of the hypertrophied septum into the outflow tract is accentuated. The leaflets of the mitral valve, particularly the anterior leaflet, are tethered by the hypertrophied malaligned papillary muscles so that their leading edges are anterior and often in contact with the bulging septum anteriorly. The segment of narrowing or line of contact of the mitral leaflets with the septum correlates well with the site of change in pressure

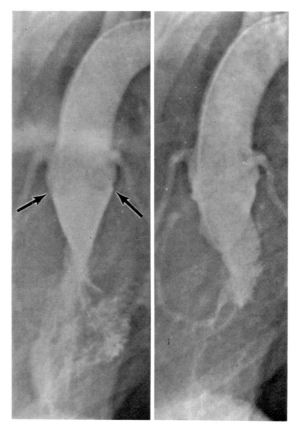

FIG. 437. HYPERTROPHIC MUSCULAR OBSTRUCTION OF LEFT VENTRICULAR INFUNDIBULUM

Catheter injection of contrast material into the left ventricle. Films exposed in lateral projection. A discrete, conical, subvalvular outflow tract chamber is shown (arrows point to normal appearing aortic valve). Pressures obtained at catheterization were as follows: left ventricle, 145/5; subvalvular chamber, 100/5; aorta, 100/72. (From Dotter *et al.* (1961).)

gradient found upon withdrawal of the catheter from the left ventricular sinus into the subvalvular region in the outflow tract. In the frontal view in systole, the usually thin edge of the mitral leaflets is seen outlining the subvalvular chamber and indicating their line of approximation to the bulging anterior septum. This line may be shaped like a V or a W. The indentation in the left upper margin of the ventricular cavity is due to the hypertrophied septum.

Mitral insufficiency is demonstrated in more than half of the cases with symptoms. Reflux of the contrast substance, best seen in the lateral or right anterior oblique projection, is seen to occur underneath the leading edge of the anterior leaflet. The left atrium is usually moderately enlarged.

The enlarged hypertrophied papillary muscles are easily identified and contribute to the distortion of the left ventricular cavity. In early and midsystole, the alignment of these structures is clearly abnormal with displacement towards the left in relation to the mitral ring. This results in an appearance of angulation and shortening of the line of attachment of the chordae tendineae (Fig. 436).

When the patient shows progressive symptoms and the gradient is persistent and supported by anatomic findings seen at angiography, operative treatment may be considered. A variety of operative attacks has been proposed (Morrow et al., 1964; Epstein et al., 1973). These involve partial removal or splitting of the hypertrophied ventricular muscles and/or replacement of the mitral valve.

CONNECTIVE TISSUE DISEASES INVOLVING THE HEART

Connective tissue or collagen diseases are often generalized and affect many organ systems, notably the lungs, heart, kidneys, gastrointestinal tract, and joints. The involvement of the pulmonary vascular system by collagen diseases is briefly discussed in the section devoted to that subject.

Connective tissue diseases may involve the heart directly or indirectly by several mechanisms: (1) pericarditis which may progress to pericardial effusion and even to tamponade and rarely to constrictive pericarditis; (2) direct involvement of the myocardium with edema, inflammation and/or fibrosis; (3) valvular disease with regurgitation or stenosis, and in the case of the aortic valve, this is often associated with aortitis (see section on Diseases of the Aorta); (4) involvement of the coronary arteries with obstruction and thrombosis followed by ischemia and infarction; (5) cor pulmonale secondary to involvement of the pulmonary vascular system; and (6) systemic hypertension secondary to renal involvement.

From clinical and pathological viewpoints, considerable overlap exists between the manifestations of the various connective tissue diseases, and this applies to involvement of the heart. However, each entity usually has some distinctive features.

Scleroderma

Congestive heart failure is seen with some frequency in scleroderma. Weiss et al. (1943) reported on 9 patients with similar clinical and electrocardiographic findings, and 3 of these were carefully studied at autopsy. A distinctive type of myocardial fibrosis was found that consisted of well defined scars 1–2 cm in length scattered throughout the myocardium. There was little if any evidence of coronary atherosclerosis or other cause for the fibrosis, and consequently it was considered to be an integral part and a fairly common accompaniment of scleroderma. The fibrosis at times affected the conduction system, but it had its most profound effect on left ventricular compliance and contractility. The pericardium was frequently involved with fibrosis and adhesions.

Sackner et al. (1966) in postmortem studies of 25 patients found only 3 in which myocardial fibrosis was a significant feature. Right ventricular hypertrophy and dilatation were found in about one-third of the cases usually associated with pulmonary atherosclerosis providing quite clear evidence of cor pulmonale. About one-third of the cases had extensive pulmonary fibrosis. Disease of the pericardium was found in 18 of the 25 cases. In several instances there was involvement of the kidney and associated hypertension.

James (1974) reported on 8 cases of scleroderma, 6 of whom died suddenly from cardiac arrhythmias. The large coronary arteries were open, but the small arteries (less than 1 mm) were extensively diseased with associated sclerosis of the conduction system.

Blakley et al. (1975) reported on a study of 52 patients at postmortem and found significant myocardial fibrosis in 26. In a number of cases a contraction band of fibrosis extended for a con-

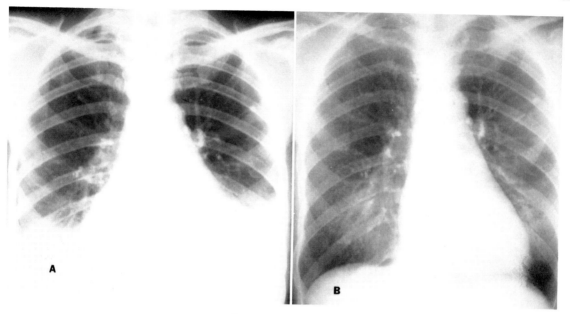

FIG. 438. SCLERODERMA
(A) Scleroderma with rapid onset of pancarditis and pleuritis with fluid. (B) After one month of therapy with steroids.

siderable distance through the myocardium and obviously affected the ventricular function. The pericardium was involved in approximately half of the cases, and in 10 patients this was attributed to the associated uremia.

The above studies suggest that scleroderma is a frequent cause of myocardial fibrosis and that heart failure is fairly common in this disease. The most frequent finding is pericarditis.

The heart as seen on conventional chest films is often enlarged due frequently to the presence of pericardial fluid. It has been described as triangular in shape (Weiss *et al.*, 1943). Pulmonary fibrosis and pleural fluid are quite common. The pulmonary trunk and pulmonary artery are often dilated, and this may be associated with distinctive enlargement of the right side of the heart. Heart failure may be due to myocardial fibrosis or cor pulmonale and rarely to pericarditis.

Lupus Erythematosus

Pericarditis is the most common manifestation of lupus erythematosus (Decker *et al.*, 1975). It is often manifest by a small to moderate collection of pericardial fluid that resolves under treatment with steroids. On the other hand, the pericarditis may advance to tamponade and rarely to constrictive pericarditis. Myocarditis is frequent and rarely leads to congestive heart failure.

Verrucous vegetations on the mitral valve (Libman-Sacks disease) are common and occur in about one-third of the cases but rarely lead to any hemodynamic consequences (Hejtmancik *et al.*, 1964). However, Bulkley and Roberts (1975) reported 3 cases with severe mitral regurgitation. They attributed this to the healing process following treatment with steroids. Reports by Bernhard *et al.* (1969) and Oh *et al.* (1974) indicate that the aortic valve may occasionally be involved. The valve tissue was thinned with retraction of the margins of the valve, and in the cases reported by Bernhard *et al.* (1969), there was perforation of one of the cusps producing pronounced aortic regurgitation and requiring replacement with a prosthetic valve. In the cases reported by Oh *et al.* (1974) the valve tissue was markedly thinned, and this was attributed to prolonged treatment by steroids.

The changes in the heart due to lupus erythematosus as seen on the conventional chest films depend on the type and extent of the cardiac involvement. Some enlargement of the heart due to pericardial fluid is the most common finding. Lesions of the mitral or aortic valve may be suspected if there is enlargement of the appropriate chambers similar to that found in association with rheumatic fever. There is no record that calcium is deposited in the valvular lesions of lupus erythematosus.

Dermatomyositis

Dermatomyositis often produces changes in the myocardium, but they are rarely extensive.

They may be a cause of tachycardia and arrhythmia but are seldom a conspicuous part of the symptomatology of the disease (Decker *et al.*, 1975).

Rheumatoid Arthritis, Ankylosing Spondylitis and Reiter Syndrome

All of these conditions occasionally produce an aortitis usually involving the root of the aorta (see section on Diseases of the Aorta). This is often accompanied by some dilatation of the valve ring and often some thickening and fibrosis of the valve cusps with retraction (Clark *et al.*, 1957; Weintraub and Zvaifler, 1963). This may progress to produce a clinically significant aortic regurgitation with associated left ventricular enlargement and heart failure. Lesions in the aorta and aortic valve were said to occur at a much later stage of the disease in ankylosing spondylitis as compared with rheumatoid arthritis. There is no evidence that these valvular lesions calcify.

PERIARTERITIS NODOSA

Periarteritis nodosa is a generalized disease, and the heart is one of the organs most frequently involved. Holsinger *et al.* (1962) found cardiac involvement in 51 of 66 cases, and congestive heart failure was the most frequent cause of death. The most severe manifestations are due to the involvement of the coronary arterial system by the necrotizing process. Coronary arteries of all sizes may be involved. Necrosis of the arterial wall may be followed by aneurysm formation or by thrombosis, obstruction and myocardial ischemia. Taubenhaus *et al.* (1955) reported an incidence of myocardial infarction of 17%, but Holsinger *et al.* (1962) found 41 out of 66 cases had a myocardial infarction. Askey (1950) reported a rupture of an anterior papillary muscle secondary to infarction following coronary arteritis. The disease can occur in infants and young children, and Sinclair and Nitsch (1949) reported a case with large aneurysms of the proximal coronary arteries with fatal rupture into the pericardium.

The kidneys are often involved with an ischemic process and hypertension. This increases the work of the left ventricle and may contribute to cardiac enlargement. Uremia was present in 9 of 66 cases reported by Holsinger *et al.* (1962). Pericarditis is common and may be secondary to uremia or a transmural myocardial infarction, or in some cases it is unexplained (Holsinger *et al.*, 1962).

Changes in the lungs are common with rapidly appearing pulmonary edema and at times frank hemorrhage (Fig. 83, page 136).

CARDIAC DISEASE ASSOCIATED WITH CARCINOID SYNDROME

Carcinoid tumors most commonly arise in the intestinal tract. They show a low grade of malignancy and frequently metastasize to the liver. A large majority of heart disease associated with the carcinoid syndrome have had hepatic metastases (Fowler, 1975). Carcinoid tumors are believed to elaborate 5-hydroxytryptamine (serotonin) (Mengel, 1966). If the carcinoid originates in the intestinal tract and particularly if it metastasizes to the liver, the serotonin may reach the right side of the heart where it has the unusual activity of inciting the formation of fibrous plaques in the endocardium. The plaques cause thickening of the atrial wall, the chordae tendineae and the papillary muscles in the right ventricle. The serotonin is inactivated by the lung so that the left side of the heart is rarely significantly affected. However, in the 9 patients studied by Roberts and Sjoerdsma (1964), one-third of the patients had some changes in the left side of the heart.

Roberts and Sjoerdsma (1964) reported that in their 9 patients there were no significant changes in the appearance of the heart as seen on the conventional chest films. Ardesty *et al.* (1966) reported on a patient with a 13-year history of a carcinoid originating in the ileum and metastasizing to the liver. The patient had hemodynamic and auscultatory signs of tricuspid stenosis and regurgitation and pulmonary stenosis. Angiocardiography showed thickening of both of these valves. The patient was improved by pulmonary valvotomy and replacement of the tricuspid valve by a prosthesis. Heart disease should be strongly suspected in a patient with a known history of a carcinoid tumor with probable metastases to the liver and the symptoms of attacks of flushing of the skin.

ENDOCARDIAL FIBROELASTOSIS

While the etiology of endocardial fibroelastosis is unknown, it is reasonable to believe that the disease is probably of a viral etiology and is a sequel to myocarditis or pancarditis. Such a conclusion was drawn by Schryer and Karnauchow (1974) after an extensive and detailed review of the world literature and the study of 106 cases of their own (1974). Numerous other theories have been propounded (Reddy et al., 1972). The disease is characterized by diffuse thickening of the endocardium associated with cardiac hypertrophy, the endocardial thickening being due to proliferation of collagen and elastic tissue. The endocardium may be as much as 15 times the thickness of the normal endocardium and presents as a whitish or grayish membrane. The left ventricle and left atrium are most frequently involved, and Denris et al. (1953) found the process to be limited to the left side of the heart in 82% of cases. Schryer and Karnauchow (1974), in a more recent review, found involvement of the left chambers of the heart only in 670 of 835 patients (1974). Valvular involvement was found in 51 percent of 131 cases reviewed by Dennis et al. (1953), the aortic and mitral valves being most frequently affected (contractures, thickening of leaflets, adhesions of leaflets). Cardiomegaly is an almost constant feature, and some degree of left ventricular enlargement is usually present.

Von Gronefeld and Hauke (1973) report an incidence of endocardial fibroelastosis of 1.5–2.0% of all cases of congenital heart disease. An incidence of primary endocardial fibroelastosis of 1 in 4000 in a study of 6000 total births was reported by Hunter and Keay (1973). The condition is apparently quite rare in the newborn.

Clinically the disease may be divided into three types (Dennis et al., 1953). In the fulminating type (about one-fourth of cases), symptoms begin before 6 weeks of age with the sudden onset of dyspnea and cyanosis leading to rapid death. Acute endocardial fibroelastosis occurs in about one-half the cases and has its onset between 6 weeks and 6 months of age. It is also characterized by dyspnea, cyanosis, and tachypnea; the average survival time from onset is about 15 days. In the chronic form (about one-fourth of cases), signs and symptoms develop slowly after 6 months of age and terminate in death months or years later. The usual symptoms and physical signs include paroxysmal dyspnea, cyanosis, coughing, anorexia, growth failure, irritability,

orthopnea, tachypnea, and tachycardia. With the development of cardiac failure rales, liver enlargement, and peripheral edema may occur. Murmurs may or may not be present. The electrocardiogram shows nonspecific changes but is almost always abnormal.

Endocardial fibroelastosis may be further classified into a "dilated" form, associated with marked left ventricular enlargement, low cardiac output and terminal heart failure; and a "contracted" form associated with normal or reduced ventricular volumes, markedly altered ventricular compliance, and secondary pulmonary hypertension. The contracted type probably accounts for no more than 5% of the reported cases (Sostre et al., 1974).

In about half of the reported cases some other cardiac abnormality was also found; the commonest associated condition is aortic stenosis (Still, 1961). In an analysis of 11,347 autopsies, McCormick (1958) found 15 cases of "primary" endocardial fibroelastosis and 9 cases in which the distinctive endocardial thickening occurred in association with interventricular septal defect, patent foramen ovale, patent ductus arteriosus, and coarctation of the aorta. In older persons and adults the abnormality occurs most often in association with other cardiac abnormalities, particularly left ventricular outflow obstructions. It may occur independently, however, as in the cases reported by McKusick (1952) and Thomas et al. (1954). In McKusick's case the signs and symptoms were those of chronic constrictive pericarditis, and in 1 of the 12 adult cases reported by Thomas and his associates the signs of constrictive pericarditis were sufficiently pronounced that exploratory thoracotomy (negative for pericarditis) was performed. In the case reported by Sostre et al. (1974) of the contracted form of endocardial fibroelastosis in an adult, the right ventricular angiographic pattern was indistinguishable from that of a primary cardiac neoplasm.

Catheterization studies in patients with this abnormality have shown markedly elevated left ventricular diastolic pressures. Lynfield et al. (1960), reporting 6 cases, found 3 with moderate and 3 with severe pulmonary hypertension. The increased pulmonary artery pressure was assumed to be due to the increased left ventricular diastolic pressure. In the cases with left ventricular dilatation, the dominant defect seemed to be impairment of systolic emptying resulting in a progressively larger residual volume and left ventricular dilatation. Impairment of ventricular distensibility appears to be the main difficulty in those with normal-sized left ventricles.

Radiologic Findings

The heart is moderately to greatly enlarged and may be globular, spherical, or oval in shape. Specific chamber enlargement is difficult to determine, though the left ventricle is usually predominantly involved. Left atrial enlargement may be a prominent feature in the presence of an associated lesion of the mitral valve or with the development of cardiac failure. According to Caffey (1961), endocardial fibroelastosis is probably the commonest cause of great cardiac enlargement in early infancy. The lungs are clear.

Ronderos (1960) observed a fluoroscopic sign in 2 autopsy-proved cases which may prove helpful. In the left anterior oblique projection no left ventricular pulsations were seen in contrast with normal contractility of the right ventricle.

Angiocardiography may occasionally be needed to distinguish endocardial fibroelastosis

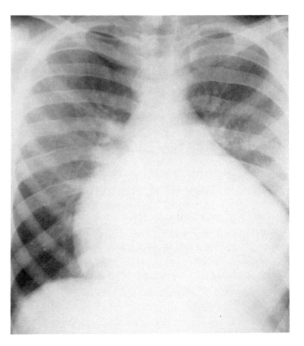

FIG. 440. ENDOCARDIAL FIBROELASTOSIS IN A 13-YEAR-OLD BOY WHO HAD HAD AN OPERATION FOR COARCTATION OF AORTA 10 YEARS BEFORE

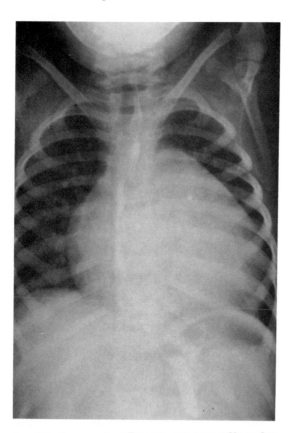

FIG. 439. ENDOCARDIAL FIBROELASTOSIS IN 2-YEAR-OLD CHILD (AUTOPSY CASE)
Film exposed shortly before death.

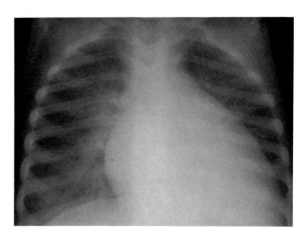

FIG. 441. ENDOCARDIAL FIBROELASTOSIS IN 17-MONTH-OLD BLACK GIRL

Congestive heart failure and cardiomegaly were noted first 1 month prior to death. No murmurs were heard, but a gallop rhythm was detected. ECG showed left ventricular hypertrophy. Improvement followed digitalization and diuresis. Cardiac decompensation recurred, however, and death due to cardiac arrest after lumbar puncture ensued. Autopsy showed endocardial fibroelastosis, marked dilatation and hypertrophy of the left ventricle, and pulmonary edema. Frontal film of the chest 1 month prior to death shows marked cardiomegaly, predominantly left ventricular, with moderate hilar vessel congestion and enlargement.

from surgically correctable cardiac anomalies. Following injection into a peripheral vein or selective introduction of the contrast material into one of the right heart chambers or pulmonary artery delayed and prolonged opacification of the left side of the heart is seen. Left ventricular contractility is greatly decreased. Linde *et al.* (1958) found no change in systolic and diastolic left ventricular volumes in consecutive cardiac cycles in 3 of 4 patients and prolonged retention of contrast material in an enlarged left ventricle in all. The present authors have measured left ventricular volumes in the range of 200–250 ml in brothers aged 5 and 9 years. These boys also showed incomplete systolic emptying and prolonged left ventricular opacification (decreased ejection fraction). Diastolic and systolic volumes were sufficiently different, however, so that a normal stroke volume was maintained. Moderate to severe mitral insufficiency was present in the older patient, a finding also reported by others (Johnsrude and Carey, 1965). Of the 6 patients

examined by Lynfield *et al.* (1960) 3 showed left ventricular dilatation, and 3 showed normal-sized or small left ventricles. Patients with the greatest left ventricular dilatation showed the smallest change in left ventricular chamber size during ventricular systole. All but one showed considerable systolic residual volume.

Differential diagnostic considerations include anomalous origin of the left coronary artery from the pulmonary artery, glycogen storage disease of the heart, beri-beri heart disease, cardiac tumors, and myocarditis (Eyler *et al.*, 1955). While some aid in differentiating these entities may come from specialized radiologic techniques, definitive diagnosis will more often depend on eliminating the other causes of cardiac enlargement.

Therapy is entirely medical and is directed for the most part toward the prevention and treatment of heart failure. Though occasional cases of survival to adulthood have been reported, the prognosis is generally poor, death frequently occurring by the end of the first year.

16

Syphilitic Heart Disease

Syphilitic heart disease is produced by gross pathologic changes in the root of the aorta with extension into the aortic valve, the aortic valve ring, and at times, involvement of the openings of the coronary arteries. An inflammatory reaction with scarring and fibrosis of the myocardium has been described by Hamman and Rich (1934), but its incidence is disputed. It must be quite rare. Heggtveit (1964), in a clinical, pathological, and autopsy study of 100 cases of syphilitic aortitis, found no case of syphilitic myocarditis.

SYPHILITIC AORTIC REGURGITATION

Involvement of the aortic valve is preceded by syphilitic aortitis and is due to an extension of the process into the region of the valve ring. The commissures between the valve cusps increase in width, and the attachment of the cusps may be separated by a distance as great as 1 cm. The cusps may be attacked. They become thickened and slightly to moderately retracted with rolling up of the free edges so that they no longer make accurate contact with each other. The thickening of the valve cusps does not produce aortic stenosis and calcification does not occur. The com-

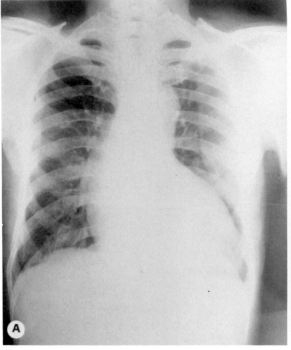 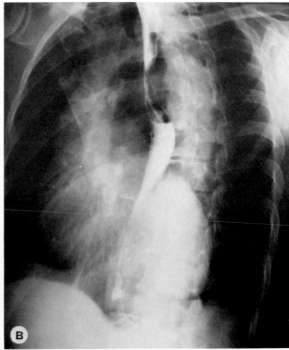

FIG. 442. AORTIC INSUFFICIENCY

Pulsations of the heart were quite violent, and the amplitude of pulsations of the left ventricle was increased. There was a history of a chancre, and the blood Wassermann was positive.

526

bination of shortened cusps and dilatation of the valve ring leads to severe aortic regurgitation. Other rare but very serious complications are (1) rupture and (2) eversion or retroversion of a cusp.

Another common and very important complication from a functional standpoint is an extension of the syphilitic aortitis into the region of the coronary ostia. The puckering and elevation of the aortic endothelium produce marked narrowing of the mouths of the coronary arteries with a corresponding decrease in the coronary blood flow. This coronary blood flow is further reduced by the decrease in diastolic pressure in the aorta so there may be severe myocardial ischemia and angina is a common symptom.

Syphilitic aortic regurgitation is different to a degree from other forms of aortic regurgitation in that it is the only valve involved, and is preceded by a significant degree of aortitis. The aortitis although causing considerable dilatation of the root of the aorta is difficult to detect unless there is a fine linear deposit of calcium in the aortic walls (Jackman and Lubert, 1945). Formerly, this was thought to be quite characteristic of syphilitic aortitis. Following the decline in the instance of syphilis during the past 30 years, calcium in the ascending aorta is no longer as suggestive of syphilis as formerly (see section on Diseases of the Aorta). Also, many other conditions may cause dilatation of the aortic root associated with aortic regurgitation namely rheumatoid arthritis, ankylosing spondylitis, the Marfan syndrome, cystic medial necrosis, etc.

Syphilitic aortic regurgitation produces the same changes in the hemodynamics of the left ventricle as other forms of regurgitation and these will not be discussed again in detail. After enlargement of the left ventricle occurs, the process is rapid, progressive, and severe especially when combined with decreased coronary flow and it may be rapidly fatal. In former years when it was more prevalent, some of the largest hearts were due to syphilitic aortic regurgitation (cor bovinum).

RUPTURE OR RETROVERSION OF AN AORTIC VALVE CUSP

In a study of 24 cases of nontraumatic aortic valve rupture, Caroll (1951) found 7 instances in which the condition was associated with leutic aortitis and some degree of aortic regurgitation. Rupture of a cusp of the aortic valve leads to a marked change in the circulatory dynamics. The patient may die suddenly. There is severe chest pain, cough, and a sense of suffocation. Consequently, the patient may be too ill to permit an immediate radiologic examination. The condition may be confusing, but an alert clinician may make the diagnosis mainly on the basis of the history and the loud murmurs heard over the precordium (Bean and Mohaupt, 1952). A chest film may show a contour suggestive of aortic regurgitation with an enlarged and a dilated left ventricle. Extensive pulmonary edema may appear secondary to left ventricular failure. The patient may die rapidly or may survive for some time and present some opportunity for correct diagnosis and surgical treatment.

In the present day setting a number of causes for rupture of an aortic cusp should be considered such as trauma, bacterial endocarditis, mucoid degeneration or mucopolysacharidosis, or rarely severe exertion.

Eversion or retroversion of a valve cusp also produces a severe regurgitation and this may follow syphilis of the aorta and the aortic valve or any other condition that changes the mechan-

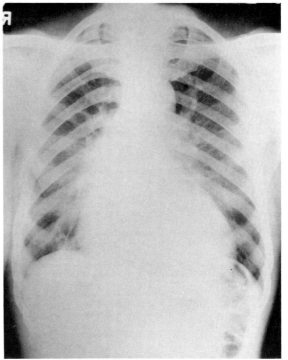

FIG. 443. AORTIC INSUFFICIENCY WITH POSSIBLE RUPTURE OR RETROVERSION OF AORTIC CUSP

There had been a sudden onset of severe dyspnea about 2 days before film was exposed. There was a quite loud cooing diastolic murmur over and just to the left of the sternum.

ical alignment of the valve ring and cusps. It is occasionally seen in association with a high membranous interventricular septal defect and in association with aneurysm of the sinus of Valsalva and a septal defect. The onset of retroversion may be more gradual than that associated with a ruptured cusp. The clinical and roentgen findings are similar. Supravalvular aortography will show the massive regurgitation but we know of no precise angiographic features that will make a precise diagnosis of retroversion of an aortic cusp.

17

Mucoid or Myxomatous Changes in the Cardiac Valves

Mucoid or myxomatous degeneration of the mitral valve produces a variety of structural changes accompanied by prolapse, billowing posteriorly or ballooning into the left atrium (Pomerance, 1969; Read *et al.*, 1965). The clinical findings associated with this change have been called "the floppy valve syndrome" (Read *et al.*, 1965). The reader is reminded that other causes may be associated with the billowing of the posterior leaflet of the mitral valve and can produce a similar syndrome (Pocock *et al.*, 1971). Some of these causes are rheumatic fever, ischemia of the papillary muscles and cardiomyopathies. Also, myxomatous change with degeneration is not limited to the mitral valve but may occur in all of the cardiac valves and at any age and can produce changes much more severe than the redundancy or prolapse of the cusps (O'Brien *et al.*, 1968; Read *et al.*, 1965; Shankar *et al.*, 1967; Fadell and Graziani, 1960).

Barlow and Bosman (1966) reported on four patients with a mid to late systolic murmur, a late systolic click and T wave inversions in leads II, III and AVF. Cineangiogram showed massive billowing or prolapse of the posterior leaflet of the mitral valve usually accompanied by mild to moderate mitral regurgitation. These patients had symptoms of chest pain, shortness of breath, and palpitation, and several kinships showed similar auscultatory findings, although they were asymptomatic.

Criley *et al.* (1966) reported on a similar group of five patients except one of the patients was 5 1/2 years of age, and one patient presented a rather typical Marfan syndrome with associated dilatation of the sinus of Valsalva and the ascending aorta. Several of the patients had had prior careful examinations of the heart without evidence of abnormality. It was assumed that the process had begun and progressed during the intervening period.

Read *et al.* (1965) reported on five cases of severe mitral insufficiency, two of which had had bacterial endocarditis. At operation the valve leaflets drooped into the ventricular cavity, and in one case the chordae tendineae were shortened, and in another the leaflets were described as diaphanous. The mitral valve leaflets in all cases showed partial replacement of the collagenous tissue by the myxomatous deposits accompanied by cystic areas, fibrosis, and destruction of the elastic tissue. The same authors have reported on three patients with moderate to severe aortic insufficiency in which the aortic cusps were redundant, floppy, and one or more had prolapsed into the outflow tract of the ventricle. One of these cases had cystic medial necrosis of the ascending aorta with aneurysm formation. Five other patients had a combination of pectus carinatum, or excavatum, blue sclera, and joint hypermobility. These authors suggested that the valvular abnormalities were a form fruste of the Marfan syndrome. It is well known (McKusick, 1972; Anderson *et al.*, 1968) that myxomatous deposits in the mitral valve with prolapse is an occasional accompaniment of the Marfan syndrome.

In a series of routine autopsies, Pomerance (1969) found an incidence of mucoid degeneration of the atrioventricular valves of approximately 1%. The mitral valve was involved in 35 instances, and in retrospect 16 of these were associated with signs and symptoms of heart disease during life. Grossly, the mitral valve leaflets were enlarged, redundant, often with thickened margins and loss of elasticity. The chordae tendineae were occasionally elongated or thickened, and in 3 cases a number of chordae tendineae were ruptured. In 2 cases there was evidence of a healed bacterial endocarditis. In no case was there calcification in the leaflets, although rarely, in an older person, there was calcification in the valve ring. Because of these changes the valve obviously would balloon and prolapse during ventricular systole and was often insufficient.

O'Brien et al. (1968) reported 2 cases of myxomatous degeneration of the aortic valve in which there was a rupture of one of the cusps producing an onset of a sudden severe aortic regurgitation. Shankar et al. (1967) reported severe congestive heart failure and death in a 5-month-old infant with the Marfan syndrome and myxomatous degeneration of both the mitral and tricuspid valves. Fadell and Graziani (1960) reported on 2 newborn infants who succumbed because of incomplete differentiation of the aortic valve accompanied by myxomatosis and aortic stenosis.

Read and Thal (1966) reported on the surgical management of similar cases and noted their marked propensity for postoperative dehiscence of the prosthetic valve attachments.

This brief review indicates that myxomatous or mucoid degeneration of the cardiac valves produces a wide spectrum of heart disease involving newborns, infants, children and adults. This is occasionally familial and has an association with the Marfan syndrome. The disease is often relatively benign but may produce severe disability and death. As indicated above, mucoid or myxomatous degeneration of the mitral valve has been most often a pathologic basis of the "floppy valve syndrome."

The "floppy valve syndrome," although applicable to all of the cardiac valves, has been most frequently applied to prolapse of the mitral valve and often to the posterior valve leaflet. The syndrome consists of a patient, usually an adult, with symptoms of chest pain, palpitations, shortness of breath and fatigue, and no history of rheumatic fever. There may be a history of bacterial endocarditis, and there is an increased susceptibility to this disease. Auscultation shows a mid to late systolic murmur accompanied by a late systolic click (Barlow and Bosman, 1966; Criley et al., 1966). The electrocardiogram typically shows T wave changes leads II-III and AVF and other changes which are occasionally accompanied by an arrhythmia. Although the syndrome is usually benign, when there are persistent electrocardiographic changes the prognosis is guarded (Barlow and Bosman, 1966). There is an increased incidence of bacterial endocarditis and also an increased incidence of sudden death in these patients. Trauma is often mentioned as a possible etiologic agent (Criley et al., 1966; Barlow and Bosman, 1966).

Radiologic Findings

Conventional chest films and fluoroscopy provide little significant information. The heart may be normal in size and contour or only minimally enlarged. The left atrium typically is only minimally enlarged and is rarely very large. Congestive changes in the lungs vary but are usually minimal depending on the severity of the associated mitral regurgitation. Some deformity of the thorax, such as kyphosis, scoliosis, and pectus excavatum, increases the possibility of the diagnosis. There is usually no evidence of calcium within the heart, although in some elderly people calcium may be deposited in the valve ring (Pomerance, 1969).

The prolapse of the posterior leaflet of the mitral valve is easily diagnosed by properly performed echocardiography (Feigenbaum, 1976), and this is one of the main uses of this procedure.

The most useful radiological procedure is left ventriculography with the catheter inserted by the transaortic route. Cinefluoroscopy is preferable because it is more likely to show the full range of motion of the valve structures and is more likely to show minor degrees of regurgitation. The RAO projection in about 30–35° of obliquity separates the left atrium from the ventricle and places the mitral valve in profile. A lateral and far LAO projections may provide additional important information, particularly when there is rupture of the chordae tendineae or marked posterior billowing of the posterior leaflet (Kittredge et al., 1970; Jeresaty, 1971). The angiographic appearance depends upon the extent of the changes in the valve which may vary from minimal prolapse of the posterior leaflet to ballooning of both leaflets to rupture of several chordae tendineae with a flail valve.

The posterior leaflet of the mitral valve has about one-third of the total surface area of the valve cusps and in the large majority of persons is divided into three scallops, the largest of which is the central one (Ranganathan et al., 1970). When the posterior leaflet of the mitral valve is normal, these scallops are scarcely visible during ventriculography. In prolapse of the posterior leaflet, these scallops may enlarge separately and prolapse producing a variety of contours. The posteromedial scallop projects downward and backward and is seen at the inferior margin of the valve. Dilatation and prolapse of all three scallops produce a triarcuate appearance during ventricular systole with a considerable collection of contrast substance trapped underneath the cusps. The regurgitation of contrast substance is usually minimal at this stage (Fig. 444). When both leaflets are involved, the entire valve presents as a rounded or ballooned-shaped structure protruding into the left atrium. The lateral or the far LAO position will show this prolapse or balloon effect to good advantage (Kittredge et al., 1970). A considerable amount of contrast substance stagnates underneath the leaflets of the balloon valve forming an oval shaped density. Jeresaty (1971) refers to this as a "doughnut," not only because of its exterior shape but because he identified a central radiolucency. At this stage mitral regurgitation may be moderate in degree associated with some dilatation of the left atrium. In some cases in which ballooning of the valve is not a prominent feature, thickening and irregularity of the valve margin may be noted (Anderson et al., 1968).

With rupture of one or more of the chordae tendineae a portion of the leaflet becomes partially or completely flail. The mitral regurgitation becomes more severe, and the rapid filling of the atrium with contrast substance obscures the valve contours. Typically with a prolapsed valve

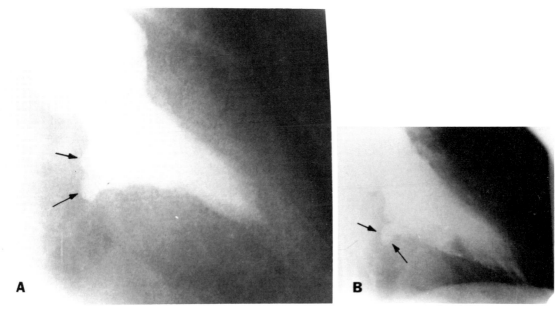

FIG. 444. TWO CASES OF MITRAL PROLAPSE

(A) Mild prolapse of two scallops of the posterior leaflet of the mitral valve. (B) Marked prolapse of a larger posterior scallop.

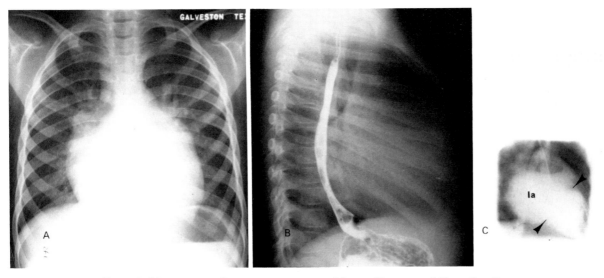

FIG. 445. MYXOMATOUS DEGENERATION OF THE MITRAL VALVE IN A 6-YEAR-OLD BOY

(A and B) Frontal and lateral chest films showing marked enlargement of left atrium and moderate enlargement of right atrium and right ventricle with some pulmonary congestion. (C) 16-mm cinefluorogram showing massive mitral regurgitation. la, left atrium, ➤ indicates mitral ring.

there is a jet effect representing the regurgitation of the contrast substance into the left atrium. The flail valve may be associated with a jet due to turbulence around the margin of the intact portion of the valve. The jet may give some clue as to the location of the involved leaflet. The distinctive features of the floppy or prolapsed posterior leaflet of the mitral valve may be modified or masked by marked regurgitation associated with the flail valve.

Associated dilatation of the sinuses of Valsalva and ascending aorta is frequent and suggests the presence of a cystic necrosis of the aorta. Dilatation of the ascending aorta was the most common associated finding in patients with the Marfan syndrome and a prolapsed mitral valve (Anderson et al., 1968).

Myxomatous changes or degeneration involving the aortic valve usually have a distinct gross appearance (Read and Thal, 1965) and are a cause of aortic regurgitation. However, it does not have any distinctive angiographic features which permit differentiation from other causes of aortic regurgitation.

Gooch et al. (1972) have studied cases with myxomatous degeneration of the tricuspid valve with prolapse. They recommend right ventriculography in the RAO projection with an injection into the outflow tract of the right ventricle. The valve may have a serrated contour or a distinct convex bulge into the right atrium.

The diagnosis of prolapse of the mitral valve is being made with increased frequency based predominantly on the findings of a late systolic murmur and click and confirmatory echocardiographic findings. Many of these patients are asymptomatic but are kept under observation. Those that are symptomatic often run a benign course, but a number progress to marked mitral regurgitation and require operative replacement of the mitral valve (Read and Thal, 1966).

18

Tumors of the Heart

Cardiac tumors may be primary in the heart or metastatic and secondary to disseminated malignant disease. The incidence of primary tumors as found in autopsy series varies from 1 in 1000 (0.1%; Davis *et al.*, 1969), 0.03% (Aldridge and Greenwood, 1960), 0.05% (White, 1951), to 0.0017% (Straus and Merliss, 1945). About 80% of primary tumors are benign (Griffiths, 1962), and the majority of these are myxomas. Other benign tumors are rhabdomyomas, hamartomas, hemangiomas, teratomas, and lymphangiomas, and these occur mainly in children. The most common primary malignant tumors are a variety of sarcomas, namely rhabdomyosarcoma, angiosarcoma, fibrosarcoma, and lymphosarcoma. The sarcomas occur in descending order of frequency in the right atrium, left atrium, right ventricle, and left ventricle (Abrams *et al.*, 1971; Scannell and Grillo, 1958).

MYXOMAS

Myxomas are the most common of the primary tumors and are particularly important because they are susceptible to diagnosis by radiologic means and can be excised and cured by surgical means. In the reported cases, 75% have been found in the left atrium, 25% in the right atrium, and a few have been attached inside one of the ventricles or to a valve leaflet (Griffiths, 1962; Harris and Adelson, 1965; Byron and Thompson, 1966). They are friable and jelly-like and tend to fragment and form systemic or less commonly pulmonary emboli. They are round, oval or more frequently polypoid (about 80%) with a pedicle attached to the interatrial septum in the region of the fossa ovalis. Small tumors usually produce no symptoms but may be a source of obscure and unexplained embolization. Large tumors obstruct the orifices of the valves, particularly the mitral valve. Since many of the tumors have a pedicle, they are mobile so that they may gyrate backward and forward through the valve orifices in phase with the heart cycle. About 10% of myxomas contain sufficient calcium to be recognized by fluoroscopy or films (Davis *et al.*, 1969), and a diagnosis has been made or confirmed by this observation in several cases (Smellie, 1962; Oliver and Missen, 1966). Buenger *et al.* (1956) described a spectacular case in which a pedunculated, peripherally calcified tumor was observed moving backward and forward through the tricuspid valve with each cardiac cycle. The tumor proved to be a rhabdomyoma rather than a myxoma. These tumors are moderately vascular, and pooled contrast substance has been identified in tumor vessels following coronary arteriography (Marshall *et al.*, 1969).

A patient with left atrial myxoma often presents with signs and symptoms which grossly resemble those of mitral stenosis. A detailed history, careful auscultation of the heart, and a high index of suspicion may lead one to suspect the correct diagnosis. Suggestive signs and symptoms are dizziness, syncope, dyspnea, and chest pain, with change in body position, presumably due to the intermittent obstruction of the mitral orifice (Van Buchem and Eerland, 1957); systemic arterial embolization in the absence of atrial fibrillation, due to fragmentation of the friable tumor (Scannell and Grillo, 1958); change in the character of the murmur with change in position of the patient (Jackson and Garber, 1958) and relentless progression of symptoms despite adequate therapy for cardiac failure (Aldridge and Greenwood, 1960). Unexplained fever and anemia are occasionally prominent features of the clinical picture (Greenwood, 1968). The presence of fever and evidence of multiple systemic or pulmonary emboli and failure to isolate a causative organism should suggest the possibility of an atrial myxoma.

When the myxoma is in the right atrium, it often obstructs the tricuspid valve and produces systemic venous obstruction. This produces edema of the feet and ankles, hepatic enlargement, ascites accompanied by weakness and shortness of breath, and occasionally some evidence of pulmonary emboli. A change in murmurs and symptoms with change in position may occur. Rarely a change in position may initiate a right-to-left shunt through a patent foramen ovale as reported by Coates and Drake (1958). Signs of isolated tricuspid stenosis, very rare in rheumatic heart disease, should suggest a right atrial tumor (Ashman et al., 1960). Constrictive pericarditis may occasionally present a similar clinical appearance.

Radiologic Findings

In symptomatic patients with left atrial myxoma, chest films, including oblique and lateral views, often resemble those of mitral stenosis. The left atrium is often moderately enlarged, and the left ventricle is normal or small. The right side of the heart may eventually enlarge secondary to pulmonary venous hypertension. The lungs often show a redistribution of blood flow and evidence of interstitial pulmonary edema is evidenced by indistinctness of the pulmonary blood vessels, hilar haze, and Kerley's septal B lines. Fluoroscopy adds little of importance unless calcium can be demonstrated in the tumor, and if the calcium indicates a gyrating motion with cardiac phase, the diagnosis can be suggested with considerable confidence, although angiography would still be indicated. Consequently we believe that fluoroscopy should be carried out in all cases of suspected left atrial myxoma.

Right atrial myxoma may cause some increase in prominence of the right heart border. It causes systemic venous obstruction and typically there is dilatation of the superior vena cava and azygos vein. The heart is usually small and often quite normal in appearance (Fig. 446).

The lung vasculature is usually diminished secondary to the obstruction in the right side of the heart.

Cardiac catheterization rarely provides decisive information and may be hazardous if the catheter is introduced into the chamber containing the myxoma. A portion may be easily dislodged producing an embolus (Davis et al., 1969). Winters et al. (1961) described a characteristic left atrial pressure curve which might support the diagnosis of a left atrial myxoma.

Angiography is the procedure of choice and when correctly performed has had a very satisfactory rate of success, although a number of false positive and false negative examinations have been reported (Wollenweber et al., 1968; Davis et al., 1969). A selective injection should be made upstream to the site of the suspected tumor. For the right atrium the injection should be in the superior vena cava, and for the left atrium the injection should be in the pulmonary artery. The myxoma is surrounded by the radiopaque blood and appears as a negative filling defect. It is often round or oval or polypoid. Cine recordings at 30–60 frames/sec are advantageous in showing motion of the tumor, and this is helpful in distinguishing it from immobile blood clots and spurious negative shadows due to streamlining of blood from the pulmonary veins or vena cava (Davis et al., 1969). A review of the pseudo tumors of the right heart which may resemble a myxoma is given by Wollenweber et al. (1968).

Facquet et al. (1949), using angiocardiography, demonstrated a bulging or convexity of the medial wall of the right atrium which could have been a myxoma, but there was no histologic proof. Goldberg et al. (1952) were the first to report the demonstration of a large mass in the left atrium of a 3 1/2-year-old child which was due to a myxoma, and the diagnosis was confirmed at operation and autopsy. Since this initial report many more confirmed cases of myxoma of the right and left atria have been reported, diagnosed preoperatively by angiocardiography (Steinberg and Dubilier, 1953; Van Buchem and Eerland, 1957; Belle, 1959; Ashman et al., 1960). One of us (R.N.C.) encountered in 1952 a large pedunculated myxoma of the right atrium in which the diagnosis was suspected from cardiac catheterization and confirmed by angiocardiography. The greater portion of the tumor was removed at surgery, but the patient survived less than 1 month (Bahnson and Newman, 1953).

Angiography should be seriously considered in any case of obscure obstruction of either the mitral or tricuspid valve in which the history and physical findings are bizarre and in which the patient is running a progressive downhill course. The occurrence of fever, anemia, and systemic embolization should likewise suggest the possibility of an atrial myxoma. Intracardiac surgery has now reached a status where an attack on such tumors has a good prospect of success and may thus cure the patient of an otherwise fatal disease.

Among the benign primary tumors, rhabdomyoma is probably the second most commonly

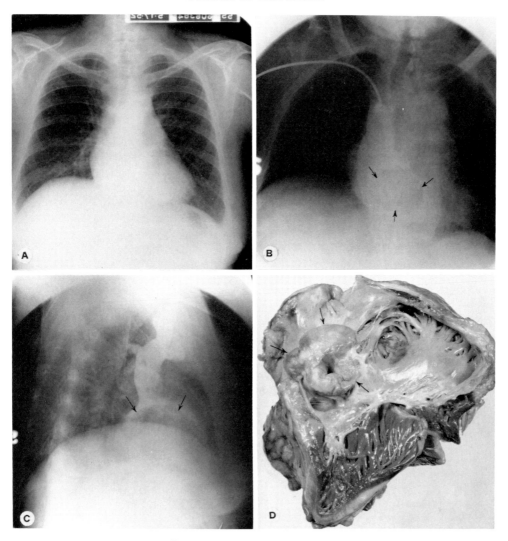

FIG. 446. MYXOMA OF RIGHT ATRIUM

(A) Conventional chest film of a 50-year-old patient who had had ascites and some shortness of breath for several years. The lungs are radiolucent. (B) Angiocardiogram in the AP projection showing large oval radiolucent shadow outlined by contrast substance in the right atrium. (C) Lateral view showing same radiolucent mass. (D) The heart at autopsy showing remnant of pedunculated tumor in right atrium. The greater portion of the tumor had been removed by previous surgery. (Case of Drs. E. V. Newman and H. T. Bahnson.)

encountered tumor. It is usually nodular and localized to the left ventricular wall (Nadas and Ellison, 1968). They have a considerable frequency of association with tuberous sclerosis, and the prognosis is poor. Fibromas are similar tumors and typically involve the myocardium but may protrude into the ventricle and often produce conduction defects and arrhythmias. Hamartomas and fibrolipomas belong to the same group of tumors. The important changes seen on a conventional chest film are changes in the cardiac contour often producing a bizarre shape with a localized hump or lump on the left ventricular contour; cardiac enlargement, partic-

ularly if there is outflow obstruction; calcification which occurs in about 20% of cases (Davis et al., 1969) and is highly suggestive of the diagnosis. Wilson et al. (1965) reported 2 cases of primary myocardial fibromas in children, each of which contained amorphous whorls of calcification within the ventricular silhouette on conventional chest films. Angiography may be used to better localize and determine the extent of the tumor and the degree of obstruction to blood flow. These tumors are susceptible to surgical removal (Castaneda and Varco, 1968).

About 20% of primary cardiac tumors are malignant and are mainly sarcomas. These fre-

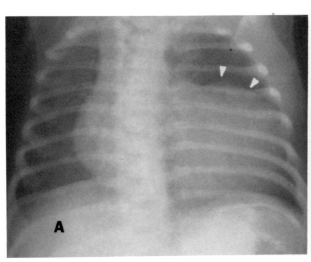
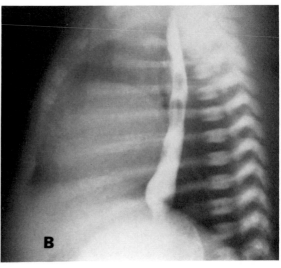

Fig. 447. Large Fibromyoma in the Left Ventricle in an Infant
(Courtesy of Radiology Department, Texas Children's Hospital, Houston, Texas.)

quently involve the pericardium and produce hemorrhagic effusions. They infiltrate the myocardium and may obstruct the blood flow by invading the ventricles or the great vessels at the base of the heart. Conventional chest films may show the heart to be considerably but nonspecifically enlarged, particularly if there is pericardial fluid. The contour may be distorted and bizarre. Most of these cases occur in an older age group of patients, and the heart with a hump should not be confused with a more common left ventricular aneurysm. Fluoroscopy is helpful in differentiating between the two. Angiography may confirm the presence of a pericardial effusion and will show the thickness and distortion of the myocardium. Pneumopericardium is also useful in delineating the true contour of the heart and the possible identification of nodules within the pericardium or on the cardiac surface. Displacement and distortion of the ventricular structures often with obstruction to outflow may be seen.

METASTATIC TUMORS

Metastatic tumors to the heart and pericardium are 20–40 times as common as primary tumors (Prichard, 1951). Cardiac metastases were found in 3.9% by Prichard (1951) and 3.8% by Abrams et al. (1956) of autopsies of patients with cancer. In the series of Abrams et al. (1956) when the pericardium was included along with the heart, the incidence of involvement was 16.3%. In both series the most frequent cancer to metastasize to the heart and pericardium was cancer of the breast followed closely by cancer of the lung. Other tumors in order of frequency were lymphoma, melanoma and carcinoma of the pancreas, stomach, and kidney.

The right side of the heart is involved more often than the left, and metastatic nodules may grow sufficiently to encroach on the cardiac chambers, although this is incommon. The tumor may invade the conduction system and produce an arrhythmia or heart block. The pericardium is involved more often than the myocardium, and the most frequent manifestation is a bloody pericardial effusion with an associated increase in the size of the heart. Hodgkin's disease involves the pericardium and produces an irregular enlargement of the heart (Abrams et al., 1971). Cardiac metastases may be suspected in a patient with cancer who develops a disturbance of cardiac rhythm. Radiation therapy, particularly in the case of lymphosarcoma, may decrease the pericardial effusion and cause the arrhythmia to disappear.

An unusual form of cardiac tumor metastases has been described by Wainwright (1938). In one case of sarcoma of the lung, an extensive thrombus-like mass of tumor extended along a pulmo-

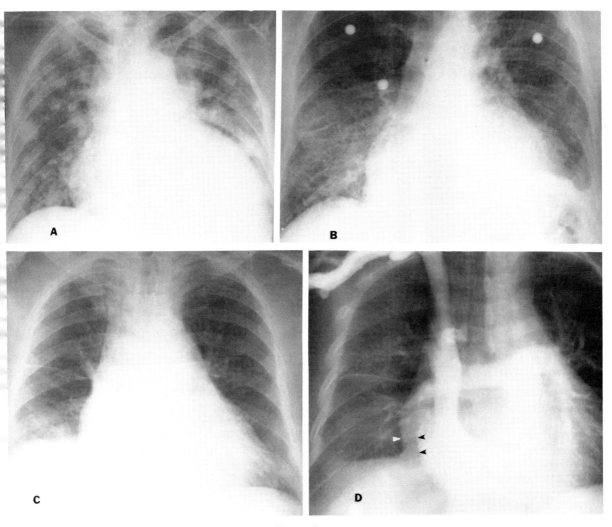

FIG. 448. THREE CASES OF METASTATIC TUMOR INVOLVING PERICARDIUM AND MYOCARDIUM

(A) Carcinoma of breast with metastasis to myocardium and pericardium. (B) Extension from occult cancer of the lung. (C and D) Extension from occult cancer of lung with cardiac tamponade.

nary vein into the left atrium. Here, the thrombus-like mass protruded through the mitral valve, producing the signs and symptoms of mitral valvular disease. In another case, there was a similar rod-like mass which originated in the pelvic veins and extended along the inferior vena cava to the right heart. There was evidence of tricuspid obstruction. Testicular tumors and hypernephromas are quite prone to enter the surrounding veins and continue by direct extension until they reach the right side of the heart. There they can cause some degree of valvular obstruction and enlargement of the right atrium.

19

The Heart in Systemic Disease

ENDOCRINE DISORDERS

Hyperthyroidism

Hyperthyroidism as a primary cause of heart disease is rather uncommon under modern conditions of medical practice since there is no doubt that proper treatment in the earlier stages of the disease greatly reduces the incidence of cardiac complications. Somewhat more common, however, are those cases of hypertensive or arteriosclerotic heart disease or rheumatic valvular disease in which thyrotoxicosis is a complicating factor. There has been some controversy as to whether or not hyperthyroidism alone can cause cardiac disability. What is important is that were thyroid function not increased, a considerable number of patients would not develop angina pectoris or cardiac failure (Silver *et al.,* 1962).

According to White (1951) there are several mechanisms which unfavorably affect the heart in thyrotoxicosis. The most important of these is an acceleration of the circulation associated with an increased cardiac output. Even under basal resting conditions, the increase may amount to as much as 50% of the average normal cardiac output. Furthermore, following ordinary activity or exercise, the increase in cardiac output is proportionately much greater than that which occurs in normal persons under similar circumstances. The increased output is accomplished by (1) tachycardia or increasing the number of beats per minute and (2) increasing the stroke volume. It is evident that in order to increase the volume of blood ejected with each beat, the ventricles must increase their capacity during diastole or dilate.

A second unfavorable factor is atrial fibrillation which occurs in about 20% (White, 1951) of all cases of thyrotoxicosis. It is rare in young individuals and is most common in older persons in whom congestive failure is either imminent or has actually occurred. The mechanism or cause for the fibrillation remains obscure.

Another factor which is frequently mentioned (White, 1951; Fishberg, 1966) is the effect of the thyrotoxic state on the myocardium. Both gross and microscopic changes have been observed in patients dying of myocardial exhaustion consisting of fatty infiltration, muscle necrosis and fibrosis and cellular infiltration (Goodposture, 1921). It is doubtful that these changes are found except in the most advanced cases of myocardial failure. On the other hand, it is probable that there is a functional disturbance in muscle metabolism, similar to that which occurs in skeletal muscle, which renders the myocardium less efficient and less able to cope with the increased demands for work. This may contribute to cardiac dilatation and heart failure.

Another probably minor factor is the large arteriovenous communications formed by the dilated thyroid vessels. These act in the same manner as any peripheral arteriovenous fistula by increasing the need for a larger cardiac output and thus increasing the burden on the heart.

In younger patients (20–40 years) with hyperthyroidism, the heart is rarely enlarged; the rhythm in most instances is regular. At fluoroscopy, the heart is seen to be exceedingly active and the ventricular pulsations are increased in amplitude. Often, there is a quite rapid, somewhat jerky or snappy inward excursion of the left ventricle during systole. This sort of movement is suggestive of thyrotoxicosis but is also often seen in PDA (Donovan *et al.,* 1943) or in any other condition in which there is an increased stroke volume associated with tachycardia. There is also increased activity of the pulmonary trunk and its major branches and the aorta. Thus, the pulmonary artery segment may be straightened or increased in convexity giving the heart a "mitralized" appearance. The left atrium is rarely significantly dilated in thyrotoxicosis, and this is important in differentiating between the thyrotoxic heart and either mitral valvular

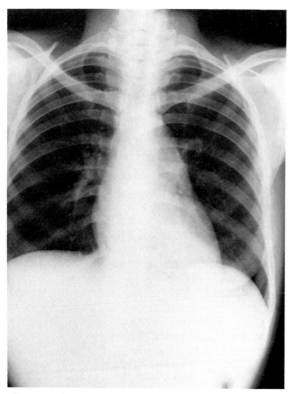

FIG. 449. CONVENTIONAL FILM OF 28-YEAR-OLD WOMAN
WITH DIFFUSE GOITER AND RAPID PULSE

There was an increased amplitude of pulsation of the cardiac borders.

ease, an incidence of less than 3% of the total number. In all 13 of these patients, left ventricular enlargement was demonstrated by a conspicuous increase in the transverse diameter of the heart in the posteroanterior projection and by posterior protrusion of the left ventricle in the left anterior oblique view. Enlargement of the pulmonary artery was present in 7, and enlargement of the aortic arch was present in 4. All were female. In all 13 patients with radiologic evidence of left ventricular enlargement there was electrocardiographic confirmation. These authors concluded that although thyrotoxicosis may not be the sole cause of the cardiac disability, in many patients with thyrotoxicosis and heart disease it is the predominant factor.

Following relief of the thyrotoxicosis either by surgery or medical treatment, there is usually a prompt decrease in pulse rate and cardiac activity. When the heart has been enlarged it may return to normal both in size and contour, but in none of the 13 patients discussed by Sandler and Wilson did the heart size revert to normal after I^{131} therapy. It appears that while milder changes in the heart may be reversible with therapy, the presence of both radiologic and electrocardiographic evidence of heart disease apparently represents a more severe and permanent form of cardiac damage.

Myxedema

In several respects, myxedema represents an opposite abnormal functional state to that seen in hyperthyroidism. In myxedema, the circulation is slowed, the cardiac output or minute volume of ejected blood is decreased, and the heart action is sluggish. In both myxedema and hyperthyroidism, however, there is probably some impairment of the ability of the myocardium to do work, and heart failure may appear in both conditions. The precise cause of the diminished cardiac activity in myxedema is not well understood.

At fluoroscopy, the cardiac pulsations are typically feeble and of low amplitude. The heart is usually symmetrically enlarged and globular in contour. It is probable that some of the enlargement is due to dilatation of the cardiac chambers following a general weakness or lack of tone of the myocardium (Edwards, 1961). Pericardial effusion is also quite common and is thought by some to be the predominant cause of cardiac enlargement (Kern et al., 1949). Significant pericardial effusion was demonstrated in 7 of 9 patients with myxedema heart disease by Kurtzman et al. (1965) utilizing carbon dioxide angiocardiography; in their experience pericardial ef-

disease or PDA. Also, there is rarely any evidence of pulmonary engorgement or edema unless the heart has begun to fail.

In patients over 40 and particularly in those in whom there is underlying hypertension or coronary arteriosclerosis or rheumatic valvular disease, the heart is much more likely to be enlarged. The enlargement is usually symmetrical although occasionally either the right or left ventricle is predominantly involved, depending somewhat on the nature of the underlying lesion. Also, in older individuals, atrial fibrillation is much more common. When the heart action is irregular and particularly when the rate is not too rapid, the amplitude of left ventricular pulsations is variable; many of the pulsations will show a marked excursion of the left ventricular wall, while others will be much smaller. Evaluation of cardiac activity under such circumstances is much more difficult than when the rhythm is normal.

Of 462 thyrotoxic patients studied by Sandler and Wilson (1959) 150 had cardiac involvement. Only 13 of these had cardiomegaly proved radiologically in the absence of atrial fibrillation, congestive heart failure, or associated heart dis-

fusion was the commonest cause for the apparent gross enlargement of the heart in myxedema heart disease. Certainly, the contour and activity of the heart are often compatible with the presence of a pericardial effusion, but this is not always so. A decrease in heart size and a change in contour occur quite rapidly following the administration of thyroid extract, and this confirms the diagnosis of myxedema. Also, the cardiac pulsations which formerly were quite sluggish become more vigorous and increase in amplitude so that there is a rapid return to normal of the cardiac status.

The heart changes ought to be regarded as part of the picture of myxedema and not as a separate cardiac entity. As such it has the favorable therapeutic and prognostic outlook of hypothyroidism. Patients with myxedema and findings suggestive of cardiac failure usually have hypertension and arteriosclerosis (Lerman et al., 1933).

Adrenal Disease

Adrenal medullary tumors (pheochromocytoma) may cause a paroxysmal type of hypertension, and this increases the work which the heart must perform. If the hypertension persists for a considerable period of time, the heart may respond in the same way that it does to hypertension due to any cause. After a long period of hypertension, irreversible changes occur, and at this stage, removal of the tumor will not relieve the hypertension (White, 1951).

Cushing's syndrome associated with either an adrenal tumor or a basophilic adenoma of the pituitary is often accompanied by a mild to moderate systemic hypertension. Consequently, a mild degree of left ventricular enlargement in this condition is commonly observed.

In Addison's disease, the heart is considerably smaller in weight and volume than normal. Chest films, therefore, often show a rather noticeable decrease in the size of the cardiac contour. Drug therapy may be followed by rapid and abnormal cardiac enlargement and even heart failure. Consequently, frequent teleoroentgenograms for the determination of heart size are quite helpful in regulating this form of treatment.

Acromegaly

Cardiac enlargement is common in acromegaly and may be part of the general splanchnomegaly which is present. The abnormal growth of other body organs and tissues probably imposes an increased work demand on the heart. Hypertrophy may be partially compensatory because of poor functioning of abnormally stimulated cardiac muscle cells. In 2 of 4 autopsied patients reported by Hejtmancik et al. (1951), conspicuous diffuse interstitial fibrous tissue proliferation was noted, and this proliferation may impair the function of the myocardium still further.

Heart disease in acromegaly appears to be rather common, being present in 13 of 21 patients reported by Hejtmancik et al. (1951) and in 18 of 24 patients discussed by Courville and Mason (1938). The heart may be quite large, and some patients with enormous hearts have been reported (up to 1300 gm). The enlargement is generalized and is associated microscopically with marked hypertrophy of myocardial fibers, with fragmentation of muscle fibers and loss of striations, and with diffuse interstitial fibrous tissue proliferation. In many acromegalics, cardiomegaly is associated with systemic hypertension, and there is an increased incidence of hypertension in acromegaly compared with the normal population (Balzer and McCullagh, 1959; Hamwi et al., 1960). It seems clear, however, that cardiomegaly and cardiac failure may develop in acromegaly in the absence of systemic hypertension.

The radiographic changes are those of generalized cardiomegaly which may be quite marked, associated with the hilar and pulmonary changes of congestion and edema when cardiac failure supervenes. Courville and Mason (1938) mention the possibility that cardiomegaly may be caused by a deformity of the spine and thoracic cage (kyphosis) often seen in acromegaly, but they point out that in the majority of cases of acromegaly in which cardiac hypertrophy and splanchnomegaly are present, the size of the heart is out of proportion to the size of the patient or to his muscular development, and they are of the opinion that the characteristic deformity of the chest, with upward displacement of the heart, plays a minor role in producing cardiac hypertrophy and failure.

ANEMIA

In anemia, there is a decrease in the oxygen carrying capacity of the blood. In order to compensate for this deficiency, there is an increase in the rate of blood flow through all of the body tissues. Just how this increased rate of flow is brought about is not completely clear, but an increased cardiac output is necessary in order to maintain this high rate of flow. Thus, the work of the heart is increased. Furthermore, because of the anemia, the myocardium receives a diminished supply of oxygen. This, in combination with the increased work demands, is instrumental in producing diffuse cardiac dilatation.

As seen on the conventional chest film, the heart is symmetrically enlarged. There is little if any congestion of the lungs. The pulsations of the heart are often rapid, jerky, and increased in amplitude. Unless there is accompanying hypertension or coronary arteriosclerosis, the heart returns to approximately its normal size and contour when the anemia is corrected, and this reversibility in the size of the heart is of considerable diagnostic weight. In some cases of chronic anemia there may be fatty infiltration of the muscle fibers of the myocardium producing irreversible change.

Enlargement is more pronounced and constant in the long standing chronic anemias. Of these, sickle cell anemia requires special comment not only because the anemia may be marked for many years but also because there are frequently changes in the small pulmonary arteries leading to thrombosis. Small infarct-like shadows are not uncommon in the lungs. When the vascular occlusions become sufficiently widespread, pulmonary hypertension and cor pulmonale may follow. The pulmonary trunk may dilate so that the cardiac contour may resemble that of mitral valvular disease. The important differential feature is that the left atrium is not significantly enlarged at fluoroscopy.

Cor pulmonale occurs only occasionally, however, in sickle cell anemia. In most cases, the heart is symmetrically enlarged. Murmurs are quite frequent and, when coupled with the fre-

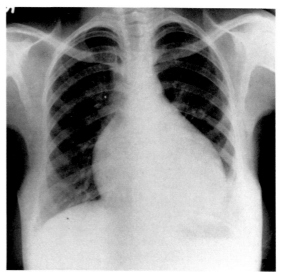

FIG. 450. SICKLE CELL ANEMIA IN 24-YEAR-OLD BLACK WOMAN
Loud systolic murmur and diffuse cardiac enlargement.

quent pain and swelling, the possibility of rheumatic heart disease is often considered. Actually, rheumatic heart disease has been uncommon in association with sickle cell anemia. Roentgen examination may be quite useful in that the usual signs of rheumatic valvular disease (left atrial enlargement, valvular calcification) are absent.

Other causes of chronic anemia in which the heart may be symmetrically enlarged are pernicious anemia, hookworm anemia, other chronic hemolytic anemias, and malaria. Sanghvi and Misra (1959) have reported the case of a young woman with severe congestive heart failure with loculated pleural effusion due to malaria.

NUTRITIONAL DEFICIENCY STATES

Starvation and Wasting

Simple starvation is said to cause (Keys *et al.*, 1950) a decrease in heart size, in the pulse rate, and the cardiac output. Consequently, in such cases a chest film might show a small cardiac silhouette which is in keeping with the patient's emaciation. The roentgenologist must be cautious in interpreting the significance of an apparent small frontal area of the heart, since the lower limits of the normal for this measurement have not been adequately investigated. Also, in hospital practice in the United States, severe degrees of starvation are rare. Marked bodily wasting is not uncommon in the late stages of malignant tumors and chronic infections, and it is the authors' impression that such patients

often show a relatively small cardiac silhouette. Studies of autopsy material (Hellerstein and Santiago-Stevenson, 1950) indicate that there is a definite incidence of cardiac atrophy (4.25% of all autopsied cases in their series) and that it is most common in the types of cases mentioned above.

Beriberi

It is well known that Oriental beriberi is often associated with a disturbance of cardiovascular function (Aalsmeer and Wenckebach, 1929). Also, there are a number of clinically similar states characterized predominantly by polyneuritis, gastrointestinal disturbances, and psychosis which are likewise associated with a deficient nutrition. Weiss and Wilkins (1937) in Boston studied the records of some 900 nutritionally deficient patients and found that 85 of these showed cardiovascular abnormalities which could not be attributed to usual or well recognized causes of heart disease such as hypertension, arteriosclerosis, or valvular disease. In an additional 35 patients of the same type they were able to make first hand observations. Circulatory signs and symptoms in these patients were remarkable. There were a rapid pulse, palpitation, dyspnea, venous engorgement, and frequently generalized peripheral edema, all of which indicated varying degrees of heart failure. Chest films usually showed a dilated or enlarged heart. Despite the evidence of heart failure, however, the circulation time (arm to tongue) was decreased, the extremities were warm and the skin was flushed, all indicating an increased velocity of peripheral blood flow and generalized arteriolar dilatation. The usual treatment for cardiac failure such as bed rest, digitalis, and diuretics did not bring about a significant betterment of these patients; however, after the daily administration of 20–50 mg of crystalline vitamin B_1 there was usually an immediate and striking improvement as evidenced by slowing of the pulse, decrease in dyspnea and palpitation, and a decreased venous pressure. A majority of their observed patients made a complete recovery.

Many of these patients were severe chronic alcoholics, some were "food cranks" or drug addicts, and in a few patients nutrition was poor due to the persistent nausea and vomiting of pregnancy. It was evident that there had been a marked decrease in vitamin B_1 intake for some time. Weiss and Wilkins suggested that this could well be a form of beriberi and proposed the term "Occidental beriberi."

More recently physiologic studies by Burwell and Dexter (1947) indicate that in beriberi heart disease there is a considerable increase in cardiac output, an elevation of the pulmonary artery pressure, an increased peripheral pulse pressure, and a high venous pressure. Thus, this is one of the few conditions in which there are signs of heart failure associated with an increased cardiac output. All of these hemodynamic changes revert to normal following the administration of vitamin B_1.

The clinical manifestations of Occidental beriberi heart disease may not be as dramatic as observed in the Orient (Jones, 1959). The commonest complaints are dyspnea, weakness, swelling of the ankles, and nonproductive nocturnal cough. Physical examination may disclose tachycardia, gallop rhythm, and murmurs which dis-

appear following treatment and relief of failure. Circulation time may be shortened but is usually moderately prolonged. Low voltage, T wave inversion, and QT interval prolongation are common electrocardiographic abnormalities. Significant arrhythmias are characteristically absent.

In the present authors' experience, disorders of the heart associated with beriberi have been rare or at least unrecognized, and this has been reported by others (Blankenhorn, 1951). The condition should be suspected whenever there is circulatory abnormality or failure which cannot be explained on the basis of the commoner causes of heart disease. Also, in all cases of clinical avitaminosis, latent disturbances of the circulation should be looked for. It is also possible that the commoner forms of heart disease may be complicated or aggravated by the effects of avitaminosis. Since the condition responds readily to proper treatment, early diagnosis is of considerable practical importance.

The authors have depended to a considerable extent on the description given by Sosman (1943). Fluoroscopy is the most important part of the roentgen examination. The heart is often enlarged, and this is due mainly to dilatation, although there may be some actual increase in weight. The heart rate is increased, and the heart is quite active with rapid, often jerky, movements of increased amplitude. A small pericardial effusion may tend to mask these movements, but the excursions of the aorta remain exaggerated. Either the right or left ventricle may be predominantly enlarged, although on the chest film and at fluoroscopy the heart appears to be symmetrically enlarged. The pulmonary artery segment on the left side of the heart may be increased in prominence and convexity, but this is rarely striking. There is often evidence of pulmonary edema and stasis, although this is variable and depends upon the extent of failure of either ventricle.

After the administration of thiamine hydrochloride, the roentgenograms may show a prompt decrease in the size of the heart, and within 3–4 weeks the silhouette may be entirely normal. This improvement substantiates the diagnosis, but in advanced cases cardiac enlargement may persist indefinitely (Jones, 1959).

Rickets and Scurvy

Some changes in the myocardium probably occur in severe cases of both rickets and scurvy. These are rarely an important factor in the course of either disease although it may contribute to a fatal collapse of the circulation in severe cases.

ABNORMALITIES OF RHYTHM

Abnormalities of cardiac rhythm can be studied by fluoroscopy and either roentgen or preferably electrokymography although these procedures are often inferior in reliability and exactness to clinical and electrocardiographic examinations.

Atrial Fibrillation

In atrial fibrillation, the abnormal or fibrillatory motion of the atrium is imperceptible; however, electrokymography shows that the normal atrial presystolic (atrial systole) curves disappear, whereas the waves accompanying ventricular systole persist. Ventricular pulsations can be studied by fluoroscopy. They are totally irregular and show considerable variation in the force and amplitude of the beats; some are forcible with an increased amplitude, whereas others are feeble with a just visible excursion of the ventricular border. These pulsations of variable force correspond with the pulse deficit which can be felt at the wrist and should always lead the fluoroscopist to suspect the presence of atrial fibrillation.

Paroxysmal Atrial Tachycardia

Paroxysmal atrial tachycardia may cause a slight decrease in size in a heart with a relatively healthy myocardium. On the other hand, if there is underlying coronary arteriosclerosis or hypertension, or, if the tachycardia persists for several hours to a day or so, definite cardiac enlargement may follow. Also, with the increased heart rate the amplitude of the pulsations is diminished and becomes progressively smaller as the heart dilates. Rarely, there may be evidence of left ventricular failure with pulmonary edema; more often there is right-sided failure with engorgement of the liver.

Bradycardia

Bradycardia due to any cause may bring about a considerable increase in the size of the heart as seen on a single chest film. This is because, with marked slowing of the heart, the stroke volume must increase if the cardiac output is to be maintained at a minimum level. Thus, the ventricles dilate in order to increase the amount of diastolic filling causing a moderate increase in the heart size. Also, there is a pronounced excursion of the ventricular margin with each beat. With complete heart block and a pulse rate of around 30/min, the excursions along the left border may be of the order of 10–12 mm and 6–8 mm along the right border. Thus, the difference in the transverse diameter and frontal area of the heart between systole and diastole is of considerable magnitude. A somewhat similar change may be seen in the well digitalized heart, particularly with atrial fibrillation where some of the beats are quite forceful. The excursions of the pulmonary trunk and aorta are likewise increased, corresponding to the forceful beats.

Ventricular Arrhythmias

The occurrence of premature ventricular contractions may be seen fluoroscopically as an intermittent irregularity in rhythm, and the forceful beat following the usual pause after a premature contraction may be quite pronounced and easily seen. Ventricular tachycardia shows only a rapid regular rhythm fluoroscopically. If failure supervenes, dilatation of the heart may occur, with pulmonary congestion and edema.

The selective injection of contrast material into a cardiac chamber or great vessel may, on occasion, precipitate an isolated premature ventricular contraction or even a short run of premature beats. Under such circumstances, the rise in ventricular pressure following a premature contraction may be insufficient to open the aortic (or pulmonary) valve, and the radiographic reflection of this delayed ventricular emptying may be confusing if note is not made of the temporary abnormal alteration in rhythm. Also, the occurrence of one or more premature contractions following injection of opaque material directly into a ventricle may allow a small puff of contrast material to regurgitate into the atrium (the atrioventricular valve may still be partially open), simulating mitral or tricuspid insufficiency when it is not present. Simultaneous film exposures and electrocardiographic tracings will allow the examiner to correlate film findings with the cardiac cycle and arrive at the correct interpretation.

20

Implantable Cardiac Pacemakers

Following the pioneering efforts of Zoll *et al.* (1954, 1956), Hunter *et al.* (1959), Furman *et al.* (1961), and Chardack *et al.* (1964), and others, implantable cardiac pacemakers are now available for routine use. In the United States and Canada, it is estimated as of 1973 that 90,000 units are in use (Parsonnet *et al.*—quoted from Green, 1975) or about one pacemaker for every 2,500 persons.

Pacemakers have three major components, all of which are visible to a considerable extent by radiologic means. These components are the pulse generator, the leads, and the electrodes. The generator contains 4–6 round mercury cells and a network of miniature electronic components which supply the appropriate electrical impulses to the positive $\oplus$ and negative $\ominus$ output terminals. The whole is mounted in a radiolucent epoxy base, although more recently electromagnetic shielding with titanium obscures the electronic components (Fig. 451). The entire generator is coated with impermeable silicone rubber.

TYPES OF GENERATORS

Four types of generators are available, namely, asynchronous, demand, ventricular synchronous, and atrial synchronous. The asynchronous generator is the simplest and delivers an electrical impulse of 4.7–7 volts lasting about 1 msec with a current flow of 5–20 mA. The pulses are delivered at a predetermined rate of 60–70 beats/min. These units are cheaper, require less current, and initially were more reliable than the other types. They work well in third degree heart block, but if there is a return to sinus rhythm or idioventricular rhythm, the pacemaker may compete with the cardiac impulses producing a disturbing arrhythmia.

The demand generators have a sensing circuit that detects spontaneous cardiac impulses and suppresses the impulses from the generator. If the spontaneous impulses fall below a certain rate or cease, the generator takes over at a predetermined rate and continues until spontaneous cardiac impulses return at a satisfactory rate, usually 60 beats/min or above. The circuitry of these generators is obviously more sophisticated than that of the asynchronous type. Also, the earlier models were easily inhibited by strong external electromagnetic radiation, such as might originate from microwave ovens, automobile ignition systems, elecrocautery units and airport metal detection devices. Later models are more heavily shielded and are programmed to switch to an asynchronous mode when affected by external radiation. Since these shortcomings have been largely eliminated, this type of generator is the most popular now in use.

Ventricular synchronous generators emit impulses continuously, but the timing is regulated by spontaneous cardiac impulses so that the generator impulses arrive during the absolute refractory stage of ventricular contraction and thus do not disturb the heart beat. If the spontaneous beat becomes too slow or stops, the continuous impulses from the generator take over the pacing. In a sense, these are demand pacemakers but differ in that it operates continuously and therefore has a larger drain on the batteries than the true demand type. On the other hand, it is much less sensitive to malfunction from exposure to external radiation than the earlier models of the demand type.

Atrial synchronous generators are still more sophisticated than the other types and require that an additional sensing electrode be placed in the atrium. This usually requires a thoracotomy or a mediastinoscopy. The generator produces pulses in phase with the atrial contractions so that the atria and ventricles function in something approaching a normal manner, and cardiac function is thereby improved. This type of generator has a limited use in persons in heart failure or in otherwise vigorous persons who may need a larger cardiac output for normal activities.

LEADS AND ELECTRODES

The pacemaker leads are composed of 47–70 fine strands of metallic alloys (stainless steel, braided steel, elgiloy or platinum iridium) coated with platinum with acceptable properties of flexibility, resistance to fatigue and satisfactory electrical conductivity. The leads (1 for unipolar and 2 for bipolar) are insulated by surrounding layers of rubberized silicone. The intracardiac leads are about 8 French in diameter.

The intracardiac electrodes are likewise platinum coated, rounded, and quite smooth and in the bipolar type are separated by a distance of about 3 cm. The unipolar electrode is about the same size and usually conducts negative current. When a unipolar electrode is used, the grounding electrode is usually attached to the case of the generator. The unipolar and bipolar electrodes each have their advantages, and it may suffice to say that bipolar electrodes are the most popular. The myocardial and epicardial electrodes have a corkscrew-like tip involving the distal 3–4 mm and are surrounded by a flange of silicone material for aid in fixation.

The implantable pulse generator is placed in the soft tissues of the upper abdomen or the transvenous pacemaker is often implanted underneath one of the pectoralis major muscles and in good alignment with the underlying ribs. The leads are placed subcutaneously with gradual curvatures so as to avoid undue angulation or stress with body movements. For the epicardial electrodes, the leads penetrate the thorax at about the level of the anterior 5th or 6th rib. The electrodes are preferably attached to the epicardium of the left ventricle about 3 cm apart. Where the electrodes are inserted through needles, they may be placed in the epicardium of the right ventricle. For the transvenous route, the leads are introduced preferably through the cephalic vein, or if this is unavailable, through the external or internal jugular vein. The electrodes are placed preferably in the apex of the right ventricle, although the pacemaker will work with the leads in the outflow tract or at other sites, such as the coronary sinus, but usually the action is less reliable or efficient.

The average life of present-day pacemakers is about 3 years (Green, 1975), although longer periods are occasionally observed. Exhaustion of the mercury batteries is a common cause of failure. Deterioration of the electronic components can occur, particularly if body fluid penetrates the plastic envelope. Occasionally the heart becomes more refractory to stimulation and thus requires a generator with a larger output. When it is necessary to exchange the pacemaker, the electrodes are usually left undisturbed. Experience has shown that properly placed endocardial electrodes, which have been in place for some time, are surrounded with fibrous tissue and are firmly attached to the endocardium. A fresh pulse generator may be successfully attached to the existing electrode.

RADIOLOGIC FINDINGS

The entire pacemaker is visible on properly exposed films of the chest or upper abdomen. Consequently, the radiologist may be of considerable help in determining the cause of pacemaker malfunction or failure. Fractured leads are reported to occur at a rate of 1.4–7.3% per year (Parsonnet *et al.,* 1973) and seem to be more common in the epicardial implants. Any sites at which the leads are bent or buckled, such as the site of entrance through the chest wall or the point of entrance into the myocardium, are suspect. Undue mobility of the generator in its pocket may cause torsion and predispose either to breakage of the leads or displacement of the electrodes (pacemaker twiddler's syndrome) (Tegtmeyer and Deignan, 1976). Undue motion of the generator has become less common since they have been implanted beneath the pectoral muscle. Various body motions of the patient may exert stress that is not appreciated when viewing a static film. The radiologist should search carefully for sites of disruption and should follow the leads all the way to the generator since breakage may be due to undue mobility of the generator. Failure to demonstrate breakage by radiologic means does not exclude this possibility. The ends of the metal leads may be in contact intermittently or slight motion may obscure fine detail.

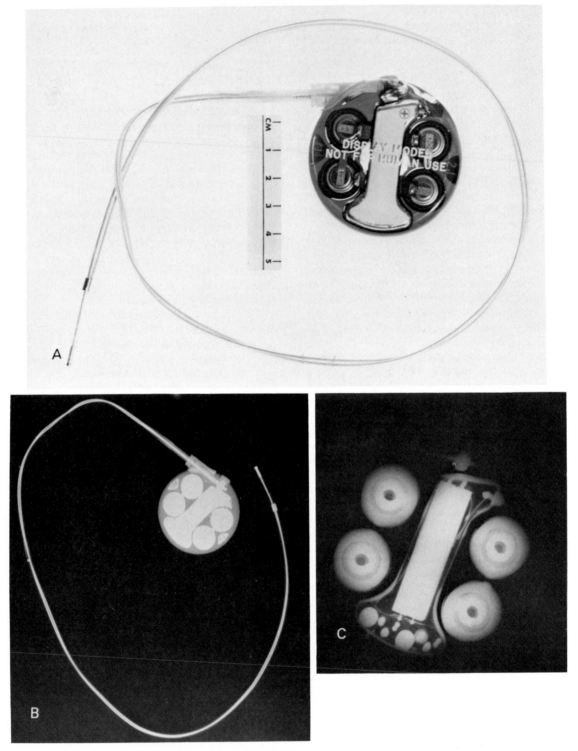

FIG. 451. MEDTRONICS DEMAND TYPE PACEMAKER COMPOSED OF POWER PACK LEADS AND ELECTRODES

(A) The central l-shaped metallic shield protects the vulnerable electronic circuits from externally generated electromagnetic waves. (B) Appearance with small x-ray exposure comparable to that used for chest film. (C) Heavy exposure to show appearance of fresh batteries.

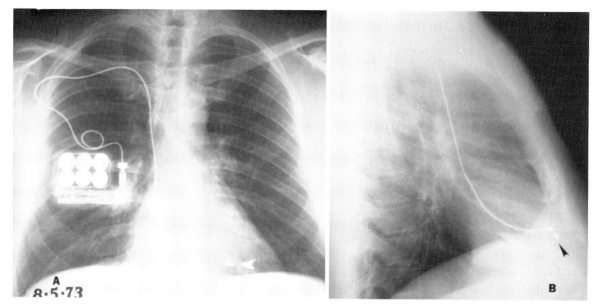

FIG. 452. GENERAL ELECTRIC DEMAND TYPE PACEMAKER SHOWING OPTIMUM POSITION OF THE LEADS IN THE APEX OF THE RIGHT VENTRICLE

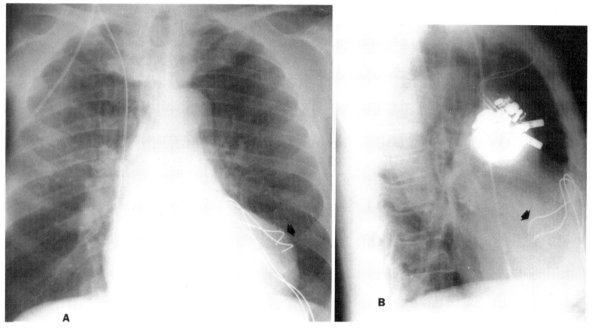

FIG. 453. SITE OF BREAKAGE OF A LEAD IMPLANTED IN THE LEFT VENTRICULAR MYOCARDIUM. A TRANSVENOUS PACEMAKER HAS BEEN INSERTED

Endocardial electrodes are correctly placed near the apex of the right ventricle, although the pacemaker may function with the leads in the outflow tract or occasionally in the coronary sinus. A lateral film is necessary to confirm that the leads are in the right ventricle rather than the coronary sinus as the appearance in the frontal view of these locations is often quite similar. Migration or displacement of the electrodes is most likely to occur in the first few days to weeks after implantation (Green, 1975; Hall and Rosenbaum, 1971). Interruption of pacemaker activity may or may not occur. If the migration is into the right atrium, the function is

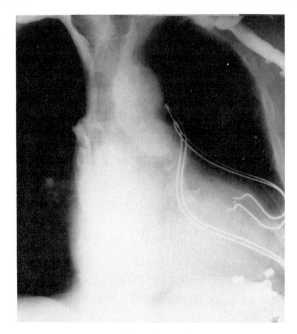

FIG. 454. BREAKS IN BOTH LEADS IMPLANTED IN THE
LEFT VENTRICULAR MYOCARDIUM

usually severely impaired. Perforation of the right ventricle or the coronary sinus has been reported with some frequency (Edmundowicz *et al.,* 1965; Nathan *et al.,* 1966; Hall and Rosenbaum, 1971). Attention may be directed to this complication by failure of the pacemaker, although this does not necessarily follow. Proximity of the electrodes to the diaphragm may cause hiccoughs and draw attention to this possibility (Hall and Rosenbaum, 1971). Hemorrhage into the pericardium with tamponade has been reported (Nathan *et al.,* 1966). Frontal and lateral films are useful in showing that the electrodes have penetrated beyond the margins of the right ventricle. Films in several projections or fluoroscopy may be necessary to confirm this. Gentle

and prolonged traction on the leads is probably justified as in some cases the electrodes can be replaced in the right ventricle by such a maneuver. Operation was necessary in one case reported by Nathan *et al.* (1966).

Infection is reported to occur in 0–43% of cases (quoted from Tegtmeyer *et al.,* 1974) and is more common in diabetics. Tegtmeyer *et al.* (1974) reported one case in which there was a draining fistula into the chest cavity that communicated with the bronchus. Common sites are around the generator or at the point of insertion of the leads through the chest wall. Occasionally, due to pressure or infection, a subcutaneous lead is extruded through the skin.

The fresh mercury batteries appear as target-like objects with a central radiolucent spot and a radiolucent band. As the mercury oxide is reduced to mercury, these radiolucent areas become progressively more opaque and are entirely obliterated in the exhausted cell. The state of the batteries can thus be roughly determined from a film that has been exposed properly to show the batteries. This requires proper positioning and considerable overexposure. Radiological examination is rarely used for this purpose but is frequently used to determine the state of the batteries in a malfunctioning pacemaker that has been removed.

MANUFACTURERS

At least 10 companies worldwide manufacture implantable pacemakers, and about 50 different models are available (Green, 1975). The American manufacturers are Medtronics, Inc., General Electric Company, Electrodyne Division of Becton, Dickinson and Company, Cordis Corporation, American Optical Company, and Phillips Medical Science Systems.

21

Calcification Within the Heart and Pericardium

The radiologist is concerned with (1) the detection of calcium within the heart and pericardium, (2) its location and extent, and (3) its significance. Careful studies, including x-ray examination of the hearts removed at autopsy in persons over 40 years of age show calcium in 83% (Blankenhorn and Stern, 1959). In more than 50% of these hearts, the deposit was 3 mm or larger in diameter and thus should be susceptible to radiologic demonstration. Although many of the small deposits were innocuous, most of the larger ones were associated with significant disease processes such as coronary atherosclerosis, valvular heart disease, and cardiac aneurysms. It is thus evident that the study of cardiac calcifications in patients is an important part of radiologic practice.

PROCEDURES FOR DETECTION

Fluoroscopy using the image amplifier is the basic procedure in detecting and identifying intracardiac calcifications (McGuire *et al.*, 1968; Oliver *et al.*, 1964). The technique proposed by Sosman (1943), although applied to conventional or nonamplified fluoroscopy, is still valid. The technique of fluoroscopy has already been discussed under fluoroscopy. Briefly, the examination is started with the patient in the frontal projection, and the shutters are opened sufficiently to encompass the entire cardiac contour. This is to enable the examiner to get his bearings and also to look for calcium in motion. The aperture is then quickly narrowed to an area of about 20–25 cm^2 and focused on the suspected calcium or on the most likely areas. The likely areas of calcification and their identity are shown in the diagrammatic drawings in Figures 455 and 456. With the suspected area of calcium under observation the patient is asked to take and hold a deep breath. These two maneuvers increase contrast and decrease motion in the surrounding lung. The same procedures are followed in both oblique and lateral projections. Prolonged study is rarely helpful, and experience is essential, particularly in detecting the smaller calcifications in the coronary arteries. McGuire *et al.* (1968) suggest that an experienced observer can complete the examination in an average of about 1 minute of fluoroscopic time. A majority of observers favor cinefluorography as the most sensitive method of detecting coronary calcifications (Lieber and Jorgens, 1961; Woodruff, 1962; Tampas and Soule, 1966), although obviously this accompanies fluoroscopy. The present authors prefer fluoroscopy alone because of its simplicity and decreased dose of radiation as compared with cinefluorography, although we regard the latter as a slightly more sensitive method. We have not had an opportunity to evaluate the use of tape recorders for this purpose but suspect that they may combine the advantages of fluoroscopy and cinerecordings.

Large films are much inferior to fluoroscopy in the demonstration of calcium. If filming is attempted for this purpose, the patient should be positioned at fluoroscopy and the exposure time should be quite short of the order of 0.01 sec. Tomography is recommended by Oliver *et al.* (1964) and is particularly useful in the demonstration of calcium in the left atrium (Gedgaudas *et al.*, 1968; Vickers *et al.*, 1959).

PERICARDIAL CALCIFICATIONS

The various causes of pericardial calcification have been classified by Freundlich and Lynn (1975) as follows:

I. Inflammation
  A. Infection
    1. Tuberculosis
    2. Histoplasmosis
    3. Syphilis
    4. Gonococcus
  B. Asbestosis (Talcosis)
  C. Autoimmune Diseases
    1. Rheumatic Heart Disease
    2. Systemic Heart Disease
    3. Rheumatoid Arthritis
II. Neoplasms
  A. Teratoma
  B. Pericardial Cyst
III. Hemopericardium
  A. Trauma
  B. Gaucher's Disease

In the authors' experience tuberculosis, histoplasmosis, rheumatic heart disease and trauma have been the etiologic agents in the vast majority of cases. The other causes listed above are quite rare and generally are the subject of individual case reports, and the interested reader is referred to the review by Freundlich and Lind (1975). Two other etiologic agents not mentioned above are chronic uremia and radiation. To date, calcification has not been reported secondary to either of these causes, but since they both can cause constrictive pericarditis, the possibility of calcium deposits should be kept in mind. In a sizeable group of patients the cause must be classified as idiopathic as the original injury apparently occurred many years before the appearance of the calcium.

Pericardial calcium may be laid down as a thin plaque or as a longer relatively thin linear curved layer which follows closely the cardiac contour.

The calcification may be minimal and confined to a single plaque or it may be so extensive that it encases almost the entire heart. It is commonly 2–3 mm in thickness but may become massive and reach a thickness of 1–2 cm. It is most commonly found in the lower and diaphragmatic portions of the pericardium and in the atrioventricular grooves. In this latter location, it may be associated with constriction of the mitral ring so as to produce a murmur and evidence of mild stenosis (White *et al.,* 1948). The incidence of calcification with constrictive pericarditis varies from 30 to about 70% of cases (Rigler *et al.,* 1941; Paul *et al.,* 1948; Chambers *et al.,* 1951; Evans and Jackson, 1952; Cornell and Rossi, 1968). It is an important sign of constrictive pericarditis but is not phathognomonic. Calcium may be present in the pericardium without any significant abnormality of the heart.

Radiologic Findings

Pericardial calcification is best detected and located by fluoroscopy in frontal, oblique, and lateral projections. The calcium can thus be viewed at its maximum thickness, and its peripheral location in the pericardium can be verified. Often pulsations associated with calcium are minimal, although occasionally they may reflect the normal pulsations of the heart. Particular attention should be given to the diaphragmatic surface of the heart and to the atrioventricular grooves. Filming is a much less sensitive procedure than fluoroscopy in the detection of pericardial calcification unless the calcium is massive. Overpenetrated Bucky films may occasionally show calcium on the diaphragmatic surface. Separation of myocardial from pericardial calcification is often difficult and requires completely tangential viewing of the calcium.

VALVULAR CALCIFICATIONS

The four main causes of valvular calcification are (1) rheumatic fever; (2) congenital deformities, such as bicuspid or unicommissural aortic valve; (3) previous inflammatory process or bacterial endocarditis; and (4) atherosclerosis.

Calcification of the mitral valve is due to preceding rheumatic fever in the overwhelming majority of cases, although bacterial endocarditis may be an uncommon cause. The incidence of calcium in the mitral valve in patients coming to surgical treatment has varied from 33% (McAfee

and Biondetti, 1957), to an average of 40% quoted from Bailey and Morse (1957), and an average of 40% as given by Wood (1954). In a select group of cases coming to surgery with predominant regurgitation, the incidence of calcium was 62% (Wood, 1954). A later series (Mitchell, 1960) showed 32 of 101 cases calcified with most having a combination of stenosis and insufficiency. In about half of the cases the calcium was described as heavy. The calcium was recognized preoperatively in only about 50–60% of the cases, although the thoroughness of the search among the various reported series apparently was quite variable. Heavy calcification is easily identified by image amplified fluoroscopy by an experienced observer. Massive calcification is a contraindication to valvotomy because of its frequent association with mitral insufficiency, the difficulty of obtaining a satisfactory cleavage of the mitral leaflets, and the fear of embolism. Its presence therefore is usually an indication for a valve replacement.

Combined calcification of both the aortic and mitral valve is almost always due to rheumatic heart disease. Its incidence is difficult to determine from the literature, but the incidence of combined aortic and mitral disease was given as 29% (Wallach and Angrist, 1958). Calcification in both the aortic and mitral valves might be expected in about 15% of cases with rheumatic valvular disease.

Roberts (1970, 1971) and Edwards (1962) have presented convincing evidence that isolated calcific aortic stenosis in the large majority of cases is secondary to a congenital deformity of the aortic valve. In about 70% of cases there is a bicuspid or unicommissural valve (Roberts, 1971). The disease is much more common in males than females, and the incidence increases with advancing age. In hemodynamically significant aortic stenosis, calcification is present in a very high proportion of cases. Schlant (1971) and Roberts *et al.* (1971) suggest that in elderly patients (above 65 years of age) calcium may be deposited in the aortic valve and ring by an atherosclerotic process. Often the annulus is involved, and the calcification may extend into the region of the annulus of the mitral valve. It is often associated with some degree of hypertension, and the stenosis is frequently not as severe or as progressive as that encountered in younger patients with calcific aortic stenosis presumably secondary to a congenital abnormality. Calcification is rarely seen in the aortic valve in patients under 30 years of age (Campbell and Kauntze, 1953).

Calcification in the pulmonic valve is quite rare. Rodriguez (1971) found 16 cases reported in the literature and added 2 of his own. All of the cases were associated with valvular pulmonic stenosis. Isolated calcification within the tricuspid valve is quite rare and limited to isolated case reports (Freundlich and Lind, 1975).

The amount of calcium deposited in the mitral valve is variable. It may consist of a few flattened plaques. In the more massive cases the entire valve appears calcified with some accentuation of the calcium toward one or other of the com-

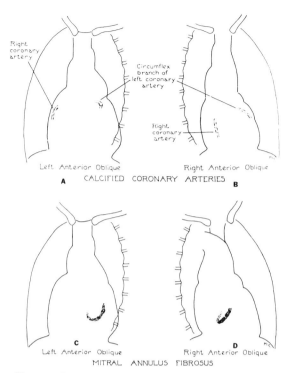

FIG. 455. DIAGRAMS SHOWING TYPICAL LOCATION OF CALCIUM IN MITRAL ANNULUS AND CORONARY ARTERIES
(After Sosman, M. C., and with permission, from the *American Journal of Roentgenology.*)

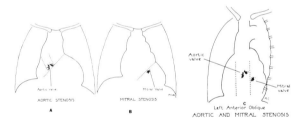

FIG. 456. DIAGRAMS SHOWING METHOD OF LOCALIZATION OF CALCIUM IN THE AORTIC AND MITRAL VALVES (SEE TEXT)
(After Sosman, M. C., and with permission, from the *American Journal of Roentgenology.*)

missures. Occasionally the calcium extends into the valve ring. Heavy calcification is rarely associated with pure mitral stenosis (Wood, 1954). It is more frequently associated with a combination of stenosis and insufficiency with insufficiency predominating.

In isolated aortic stenosis there is often a heavy deposit of calcium. The calcium extends into the valve ring. Some degree of regurgitation may be present, but this is usually minimal. Isolated or predominant aortic regurgitation rarely shows a significant amount of calcium in the aortic valve (Roberts, 1970). The common causes of aortic regurgitation are rheumatic fever, syphilis and

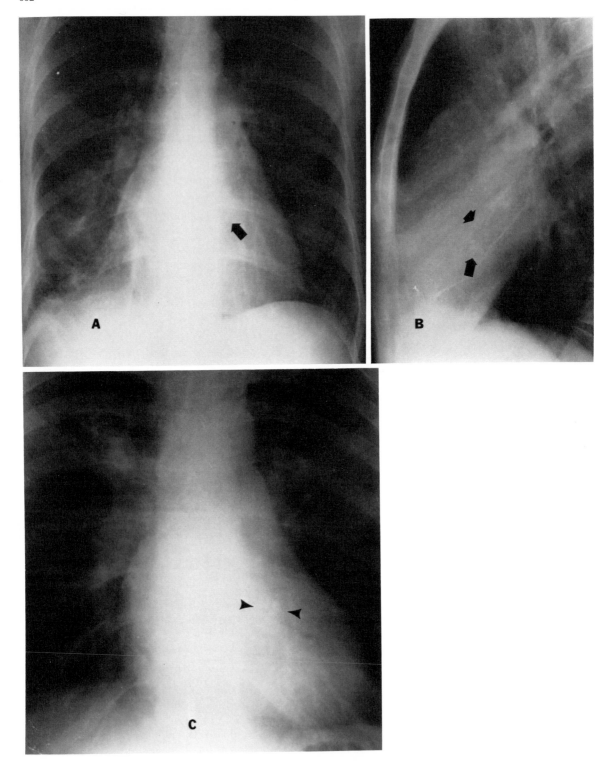

FIG. 457. TWO SEPARATE PATIENTS WITH CALCIUM IN MITRAL VALVE
(A and B) Calcium deposited in valve ring and leaflets (stenosis and insufficiency). (C) Frontal view only of another patient with mitral stenosis and insufficiency.

congenital deformities of the aortic valve. About 10% of congenital bicuspid valves will show predominant regurgitation (Roberts, 1970).

Radiologic Procedures and Findings

The procedure described by Sosman (1943) for locating the aortic and mitral valves is recommended. At fluoroscopy in the frontal projection the point of opposite pulsation or atrioventricular junction on the left heart border is located. From this point, an imaginary line is drawn obliquely downward across the cardiac contour at an angle of 45° with the vertical. The line is continued toward the right heart border. Both the aortic and mitral valves will be located close to this line (Fig. 456, A and B). By rotating the patient into a slight to moderate degree of left anterior obliquity, however, the valves are moved away from the vertebral column, and in general this is the optimum projection for detecting calcification (Fig. 456C).

The size and shape of the heart influence considerably the location of either the mitral or aortic valve. In mitral stenosis, the left atrium is enlarged whereas the left ventricle may be normal in size. Consequently, the mitral valve may lie farther toward the apex of the heart and closer to the diaphragm than is generally realized. In the frontal projection it lies just to the left of the vertebral column. With aortic stenosis, the left ventricle may hypertrophy, although the heart may have a relatively normal contour so the aortic valve is higher than the mitral, is more medially placed, and is often partially superimposed on the vertebral column in the frontal projection. If the oblique line mentioned above is again considered, it will be found that the aortic valve lies usually just above this line and the mitral valve just below.

Sosman (1943) recommended for further differentiation that the patient be rotated into about 45–50° of left anterior obliquity. The heart contour is then divided into three approximately equal parts by drawing two lines parallel to the spine (Fig. 456C). If the calcium is in the posterior third, it is in the mitral valve, and if in the middle third, it is in the aortic valve.

Movements of the two valves, when calcified, are quite similar. Intrinsic movements of the cusps or leaflets of the valve contribute very little to the observed motions since the cusps or leaflets are relatively fixed by the disease process. Most of the observed movement is due to the valve ring which is attached to the auriculoventricular septum. During systole the auriculoventricular septum moves downward toward the apex and in a reverse direction during diastole, and this is the major movement which is ob-

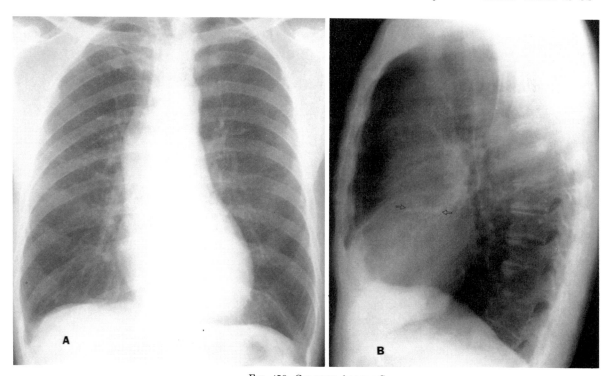

FIG. 458. CALCIFIC AORTIC STENOSIS
(A) Calcium lies over the spine in the frontal view and is obscurbed. It is easily seen in the lateral view (B).

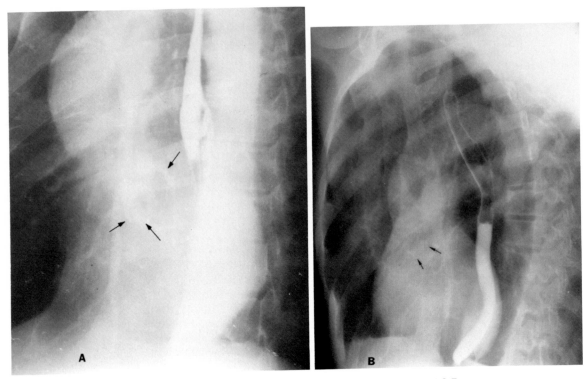

FIG. 459. TWO SEPARATE PATIENTS WITH CALCIFIC AORTIC STENOSIS, LAO PROJECTION

served at fluoroscopy. However, the motion is variable. It may be in a linear direction but more often is elliptical or oval in its course. The amplitude of the motion is often surprising, particularly when there is bradycardia, and it may exceed the range of left ventricular border motion. When both valves are calcified simultaneously, Sosman (1943) stated that there is a split second difference in the timing of their movements.

CALCIFICATION IN MITRAL AND AORTIC ANNULUS FIBROSUS

Calcification in the mitral annulus is rarely seen before the age of 60 years and is due to a degenerative process associated with aging. It is considerably more common in women (Korn *et al.*, 1962).

The mitral annulus is not a complete ring. Instead, it is shaped like a horseshoe and encircles the mitral orifice on three sides and is open in the area adjacent to the aorta. Consequently, calcification of the annulus is J-, H-, or C-shaped with the medial portion being free of calcium. The calcium is often extensive and has a homogeneous appearance, and this is in contrast with valvular calcification which is usually less massive and more irregular and nodular in appearance. Movements of the mitral annulus are similar to those of the calcified mitral valve. Calcification of the mitral annulus is usually of no clinical significance. However, if it is of massive proportions, it may deform the mitral orifice and produce serious cardiac impairment. Korn *et al.* (1962), analyzing 14 cases of massive noninflammatory calcification of the mitral annulus, found mitral insufficiency in all 14 and significant stenosis in 9. The lesion is therefore not entirely an innocuous one. It can give origin to a systolic or diastolic murmur.

The aortic annulus is rarely densely calcified unless there is an extension from massive calcification of the valve. As an isolated lesion it seems to be quite rare.

Between the right and left ventricular rings, there is a fibrous area known as the "trigona fibrosa." This fibrous mass is the basal thickening of the interventricular septum and is in close relationship to the bundle of His. Calcifications in this particular area are associated with heart block (Windholz and Grayson, 1947). The calcified area may be small and therefore not demonstrable by roentgen means. On the other hand, it

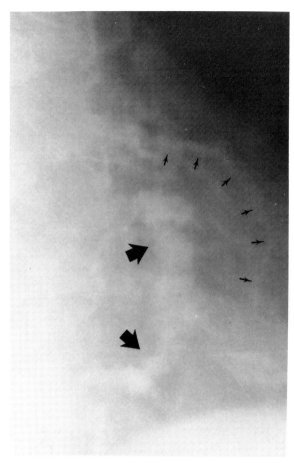

FIG. 460. CALCIFIED MITRAL ANNULUS

The two large arrows point to a densely calcified mitral annulus fibrosus in an 81-year-old woman. The smaller arrows point to a partly calcified left coronary artery (posteroanterior view of heart). The patient had a rasping systolic murmur at all valve areas, and the electrocardiogram showed anterior and posterior subendocardial injury and ischemia, left ventricular hypertrophy, and numerous premature ventricular contractions.

may extend for a considerable distance into the interventricular septum and also in the annulus fibrosus so as to be easily identified.

Left Atrial Calcification

Calcification in the left atrium is an uncommon manifestation of rheumatic mitral valvular disease. Its incidence has varied from 0.5–2.0% of

cases of rheumatic valvular disease (Seltzer et al., 1967; Gedgaudas et al., 1968). It may occur with mitral insufficiency but seems to be considerably more common with mitral stenosis (Seltzer et al., 1967; Vickers et al., 1959). The calcium is usually deposited in the endocardium and underlying muscle. Occasionally it has been found within mural thrombi, particularly in the atrial appendage (Vickers et al., 1959; Curry et al., 1953). The calcium is typically laid down in a sheet that follows the contour of the atrial wall. It is thus thin and often curvilinear and is more often located superiorly and posteriorly. Occasionally the calcium is shaggy or nodular (Gedgaudas et al., 1968), and this is suggestive of calcification in a mural thrombus. A forked or Y-shaped calcific configuration was noted in a thrombus in the atrial appendage (Vickers et al., 1959) and also occasionally appears as a dense homogeneous deposit. In some cases the calcium is so extensive that it encompasses almost the entire chamber. The left atrium is usually only slightly to moderately enlarged.

The presence of calcification is best detected and identified by image amplified fluoroscopy. If the calcium is of moderate extent, it may be identified on frontal chest films, particularly if they are overexposed. Bucky films are useful, and laminography is recommended by Gedgaudas et al. (1968). At fluoroscopy the lateral and oblique views are more likely to show the flat shell-like deposits in profile. The calcium must be differentiated from that deposited in the pericardium, valves, coronary arteries, root of aorta, tumors, hilar lymph nodes, and costal cartilages.

The identification of calcium in the left atrium is an important finding. It is diagnostic of rheumatic mitral valvular disease and most likely predominant stenosis. It poses a number of technical difficulties to surgical treatment. Entrance into the atrium may be difficult or impossible due to the resistant wall. Insertion of a catheter into the left atrium by the transseptal route may be impossible. Entrance through one of the pulmonary veins is seldom a satisfactory substitute for an attempt at valvotomy. The incidence of atrial thrombus considerably increases the risk of peripheral embolization. Also, the control of hemorrhage is complicated due to the stiffness of the atrial walls.

CALCIFICATION IN THE CORONARY ARTERIES

Using radiography Blankenhorn and Stern (1959) demonstrated calcium deposits in the coronary arteries of 80% of the hearts removed at

postmortem examination in patients over 40 years of age. More than half of these calcifications had a diameter exceeding 3 mm and would

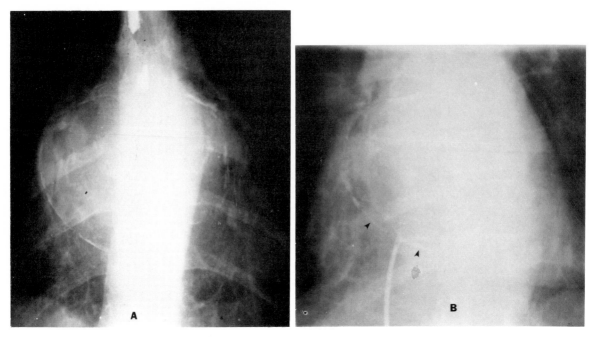

FIG. 461. Two Different Patients with Extensive Calcium in the Left Atrium
In B, the calcium has prevented the entrance of a trans-septal catheter into the left atrium.

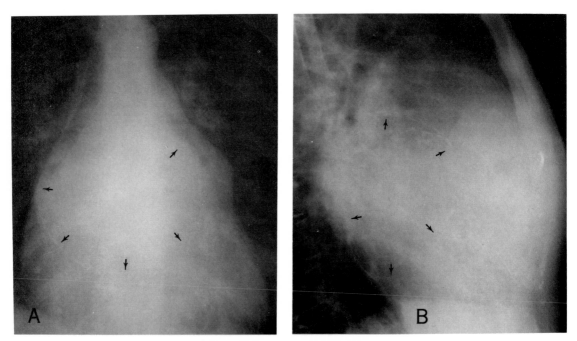

FIG. 462. Atrial Calcification
Calcified left atrium in a 51-year-old white woman with rheumatic mitral stenosis and atrial fibrillation. Calcification in the wall of the atrium was confirmed at the time of operation (mitral commissurotomy), and a large clot was found within the atrial chamber.

thus be susceptible to radiologic detection. In a somewhat similar study, Frink *et al.* (1970) found an incidence of calcification of 69%. In patients with myocardial infarction, the incidence was 93%, and with myocardial ischemia and infarction, there was a high incidence of heavy calcification. Small deposits of calcium were often inconsequential, but about 30–40% of the cases were associated with significant narrowing of the coronary arteries. Blankenhorn and Stern (1959) described four patterns of calcification, namely, punctate, blocky, double, and incomplete double. The block-like calcifications were more common in the left coronary system, specifically the proximal part of the left anterior descending artery. The double type, which was said to resemble a tramline, was most common in the right coronary artery. Both were associated with substantial narrowing of the artery. Calcifications were much more common in the proximal parts of the arterial system usually within 2 cm of the root of the aorta. It was most unusual to find calcium in the distal one-half of the coronary system without significant calcification in the proximal portion. In other words, the most significant calcification occurred within a few cms. of the origin of the coronary vessels from the aorta.

Tampas and Soule (1966) using cinefluorography examined routinely 1,087 patients over 40 years of age and found an incidence of coronary calcification in males of 19% and females of 12%. Thirty-six per cent of the group had substantial evidence of ischemic heart disease, and in this group 21% had calcium in the coronary arteries. Thus, 79% of patients with ischemic heart disease had no demonstrable calcium, and this method could not be used to exclude ischemic heart disease. However, in the 40–50 year age group, the incidence of calcium in patients with ischemic heart disease was 60% and was only 12% in those without evidence of ischemic heart disease. Also, in male patients with calcium demonstrated in a portion of both coronary arteries, the incidence of ischemic heart disease was 70%.

McGuire et al. (1968) using only image amplified fluoroscopy in patients in the age range of 15–90 years found an incidence of coronary calcification of 21% in males and 19% in females. In patients with well substantiated myocardial infarction or with significant findings on coronary arteriography, the incidence of calcium was 35% in males and 32% in females. The incidence of calcification increased progressively with age. When patients with calcification were matched with a similar group of controls and evaluated according to the presence of angina, myocardial infarction, hypertension, and diabetes, no significant differences could be detected. Only patients with hypercholesteremia showed a significant

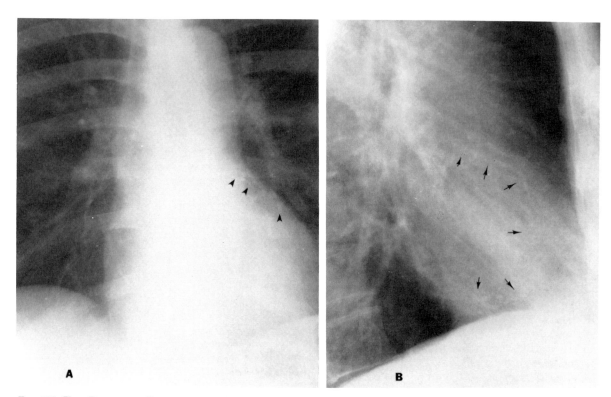

FIG. 463. TWO DIFFERENT PATIENTS WITH ANGINA AND CALCIUM IN THE CORONARY ARTERIES DEMONSTRATED ON CHEST FILMS

(A) Calcium like a railroad track in left main coronary artery and in circumflex branch (lower arrowhead). (B) Extensive calcification in right coronary artery (lateral projection).

difference of 41% with calcium vs. 23% without. The extent and the density of the calcification had an impressive correlation with the presence of angina or myocardial infarction. In patients with mild calcification, 25% had either angina or myocardial infarction. The prevalence increased to 48% when the calcification was moderate and to 83% when severe.

The literature concerning the incidence of calcification in the coronary arteries and its detection by radiologic means is extensive. The reader is referred to the contributions of Lieber and Jorgens (1961), Oliver et al. (1964), Shapiro et al.

(1963), Blankenhorn (1961), Beadenkopf et al. (1964), and the recent review by Freundlich and Lind (1975). The results of these contributions suggest that the radiologic examination for coronary calcification has a rather limited role in the detection and management of ischemic heart disease. The largest yield might come from an examination of a relatively young group of patients (35–50 years of age) in which the presence of substantial amounts of calcium, particularly in the proximal portions of the coronary arteries, would have considerable prognostic significance.

MYOCARDIAL CALCIFICATIONS

The causes of myocardial calcifications as presented by Freundlich and Lind (1975) are

I. Congenital
  A. Toxic degeneration
  B. Congenital syphilis
  C. Congenital aneurysm
II. Calcification following Myocardial Necrosis
  A. Postinfarction
    1. Without aneurysm
    2. With aneurysm
  B. Postmyocardial Infection
    1. Echinococcus cyst
    2. Tuberculosis
    3. Diphtheria
III. Idiopathic
IV. Metastatic (usually not visible by radiologic means)

Congenital aneurysms of the left ventricle are rare and most commonly involve the membranous interventricular septum, and these do not calcify. In the black race in Southern Africa, aneurysms in the subaortic and submitral segments of the left ventricle are seen in young individuals and are apparently of congenital origin (Chesler, 1972). Some of these have shown rim-like calcifications near the base of the heart.

Tuberculosis of the myocardium is quite rare and is usually due to direct invasion from an infection of the adjacent pericardium. Echinococcus involvement of the left ventricle is quite rare and is characterized by the formation of one or more cysts. These cysts typically have rim-like or circular rims of calcification that are highly suggestive (Zizmor and Szucs, 1945). The diagnosis should be supported by immunological tests for echinococcus. Dodek (1972) reported a single case in which there was a rounded tumor attached to the left ventricle, and this did not contain calcium.

Calcification due to congenital syphilis and following myocarditis due to diphtheria is ex-

ceedingly rare and is limited to a few case reports (Freundlich and Lind, 1975).

Metastatic calcification may be associated with hyperparathyroidism, hyper-vitaminosis D, and some metastatic tumors. These deposits are usually diffuse and of insufficient size to be detected by radiologic means. Trauma to the myocardium apparently can result in a sizeable scar with calcification (Grossman, 1974).

By far the most common cause of myocardial calcification is ischemic heart disease with myocardial infarction. Brean et al. (1950) reported on 14 cases, 9 of which were confirmed by autopsy examination. The incidence in one autopsy series

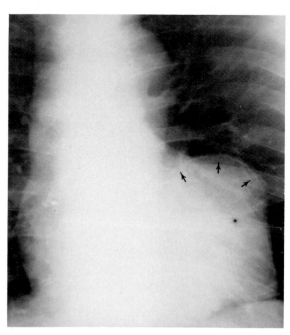

FIG. 464. CALCIFIED VENTRICULAR ANEURYSM IN 67-YEAR-OLD WHITE MAN

The ECG showed persistent ST segment elevation following myocardial infarction.

was 0.6%, and in 65 infarcts the incidence of calcification was 7.6% (Brean *et al.*, 1950). The most common site was the anterior wall of the left ventricle, but 2 cases were high posteriorly near the base of the heart, and 1 was in the interventricular septum. The infarcts were all quite extensive and larger than the calcium deposits, although these were often quite large and of the order of 6 × 6 cm in size. All of the patients were males. The calcium occasionally was curvilinear and was in the wall of an aneurysm, and aneurysm formation is quite common in association with calcification. Calcification in an aneurysm is compatible with a rather long period of

survival (Abrams *et al.*, 1963). Paradoxical pulsation of the calcium was noted in only 1 case in the series of Brean *et al.* (1950). In some cases, the calcium was massive, discoid or plate-like. The common characteristics and predisposing factors to myocardial calcification were (1) large infarct; (2) survival for at least 6 years; (3) most often involved the anterior surface or apex of the left ventricle; (4) often associated with angina but compatible with normal activity; (5) an increased risk of sudden death; and (6) usually associated with a preponderance of the right coronary circulation.

Freundlich and Lind (1975) have noted calci-

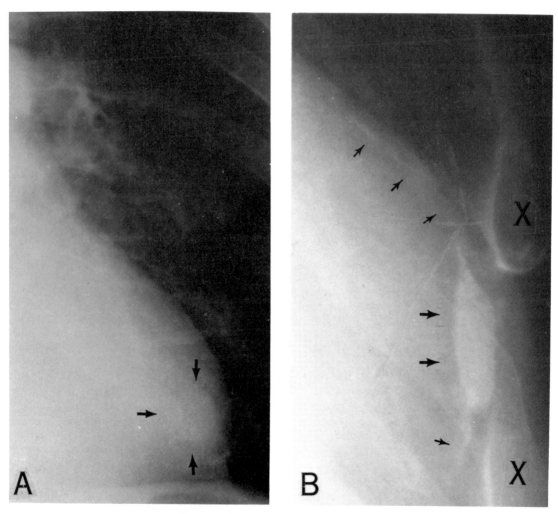

FIG. 465. CALCIFIED MYOCARDIAL INFARCT

Patient is a 61-year-old white male with symptoms of coronary insufficiency and electrocardiographic changes indicative of an old posterior myocardial scar and an anteroseptal infarction, age undetermined, with persistent subepicardial ischemia anteriorly. (A) Posteroanterior view of cardiac apex. Arrows point to rounded area of calcification. (B) Steep right anterior oblique view of cardiac apex. Large arrows point to calcium collection within the myocardium which pulsated with the heart at fluoroscopy. Smaller arrows point to superior and inferior strandlike extensions of the calcification. X's denote ribs seen on end.

fication in a right ventricular aneurysm secondary to surgery, and calcium in a papillary muscle has been described by Garfein *et al.* (1974).

The localization of myocardial calcification and its differentiation from pericardial calcification should be done by image-amplified fluoros-

copy. The localization of the calcium in the myocardium should be verified by fluoroscopy in several projections and the clear demonstration of at least 2 mm of soft tissue exterior to the calcium (representing the pericardium) should be demonstrated.

CALCIFICATION IN CARDIAC TUMORS

The most common primary tumor of the heart is a myxoma. About 10% of these calcify (Davis *et al.*, 1969) (Fig. 466). These are most commonly found in the left atrium. Other rare tumors that calcify are the benign fibromas and rhabdomyomas that are seen most frequently in infancy and childhood (Davis *et al.*, 1969). These tumors

have a high incidence of association with tuberous sclerosis. Other tumors that calcify are angiomas (Abrams *et al.*, 1971) and osteosarcomas.

Metastatic tumors are much more common than primary tumors, but these do not calcify sufficiently to be detected by radiologic means (Freundlich and Lind, 1975).

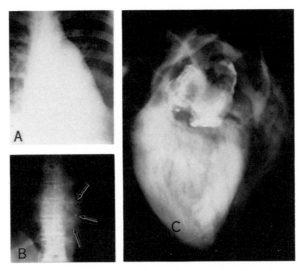

FIG. 466. CALCIFIED LEFT ATRIAL MYXOMA

The patient was a 52-year-old woman thought to have rheumatic heart disease since 1945. Exploratory cardiotomy in 1957 revealed only mild stenosis of the mitral valve, and valvulotomy was easily performed. Found at the time of surgery was a 6- × 4- × 4-cm tumor arising from the interatrial septum. Removal was not attempted. The patient died 5 years later in congestive cardiac failure. Autopsy showed a partly calcified left atrial myxoma and no evidence of mitral stenosis or previous rheumatic valvulitis. (A) Posteroanterior chest film. The pulmonary artery segment is prominent, the left heart border is straightened and steep, and the heart has a "mitral" configuration. (B) A heavily overpenetrated anteroposterior chest film shows irregular calcific deposits in the region of the left atrium. (C) Radiograph of autopsy specimen showing partly calcified left atrial tumor.

CALCIFICATION IN THE GREAT VESSELS

Calcification in the aorta has been discussed in the section devoted to diseases of the aorta (page 605). Calcification in a pulmonary artery has also been discussed in the section on diseases of the pulmonary vascular system. The most common cause is atherosclerotic plaques usually associated with pulmonary hypertension or increased blood flow.

Ductus arteriosus calcification may occasionally be detected radiographically. It appears in the shape of a curvilinear calcification with the

concavity upwards and is located just to the left of the midline between the aortic arch and the pulmonary artery. It must be differentiated chiefly from atheromatous calcification in the aorta (Shapiro *et al.*, 1963). Atheromatous calcifications commonly occur in the much older age group than that usually observed in cases of ductus calcification, and the size of the calcific arc is generally much larger in the aorta than within the ductus.

Calcification of the ductus arteriosus does not

necessarily indicate that the ductus is patent (Shapiro *et al.*, 1963), though most cases of calcification have been reported in adults with a patent rather than an obliterated ductus. Rarely, a ductus arteriosus aneurysm may calcify.

Apparently calcium deposited in the ligamentum botalli is much commoner than realized. Currarino and Jackson (1970) reported on 73 cases observed in patients between the age of 4 1/2 months to 16 years in which calcium was thought to be within the ligamentum botalli. The calcium in these instances consisted of a small dot-like deposit averaging about 1–3 mm in diameter or occasionally a streak a few millimeters in length just to the left of the vertebral column and near the tracheal bifurcation. It is best seen in frontal films. It is usually associated with a closed ductus and has no particular significance other than to realize that it is an innocuous finding.

22

Trauma to the Heart and Great Vessels

In the present milieu of automobile accidents, criminal violence, and warfare, the incidence of trauma to the heart is considerable and is probably increasing. A high proportion of severe injuries succumb before receiving medical attention and support. The lesser injuries, such as myocardial contusions, are often masked by more overt injuries to other organs, and often, unless there is a careful search, they may be overlooked. Also, permanent damage may go undetected for long periods and may be discovered long after the original injury has been forgotten.

CLASSIFICATION

I. Blunt Trauma—Chest or Abdomen
  A. Concussion
  B. Contusion
    (1) Myocardium
    (2) Coronary arteries
  C. Laceration of Myocardium
    (1) Atrial
    (2) Ventricular
  D. Rupture
    (1) Pericardium
    (2) Atrium
    (3) Ventricle
      a. Aneurysm
      b. Pseudoaneurysm
    (4) Interventricular septum
    (5) Papillary muscles
    (6) Chordae tendineae
    (7) Coronary arteries
    (8) Valves
II. Penetrating Injuries
  A. Gunshot
    (1) Laceration of pericardium, tamponade
    (2) Laceration of atrium, ventricle or septum
    (3) Foreign body embolism
  B. Sharp Instruments
    (1) Laceration of myocardium
    (2) Interventricular septal wounds and defects
  C. Intracardiac Catheters and Pacemaker Leads
    (1) Penetration of ventricular myocardium
    (2) Intracardiac injection of contrast substances
III. Unusual or Strenuous Exertion
  A. Rupture of Aortic Valve

Blunt Trauma

The heart has a modest mobility within the pericardial cavity. It is partially suspended by the attachment of the great vessels at its right side around the vena cava and at the base. It is subject to compression between the impacted sternum and thoracic spine. Fractures of the sternum and/or ribs should alert a search for cardiac injury. Sudden changes in intrathoracic pressure, such as occur with blast injuries or severe blows to the abdomen or sudden deceleration, change the pressure within the heart and great vessels drastically and may result in rupture of a chamber or the aortic valve.

Concussion

The borderline between concussion and contusion is indefinite, although contusion is accompanied by identifiable changes, such as hemorrhage and edema. The predominant manifestation of cardiac concussion is the onset of an arrhythmia (Parmley *et al.*, 1958). This is more likely in an already damaged heart. There are no significant radiographic changes.

Contusion

The myocardial muscle bundles may be ruptured or fragmented. Hemorrhage occurs between the muscle fibers, and there may be associated bleeding into the pericardium. These changes may resolve or heal by fibrosis (DeMuth and Zinsser, 1965; Parmley et al., 1958). Resemblance to myocardial infarction, both histologically and clinically, is close. The involved volume may vary from a few cubic millimeters to several cubic centimeters, and the left ventricle is most commonly affected. The common clinical signs are cardiac arrhythmias and associated changes in the ECG, such as deviations in the ST segment. Also, there is an elevation of the enzymes, CPK (creatinine phosphokinase), SGOT, and LDH (lactic dehydrogenase). Cardiac output is often profoundly decreased, depending on the extent of the injury. Chest films rarely show changes in cardiac size or contour.

Lacerations

Lacerations may involve the pericardium, the myocardium, or both. They are commonly associated with hemorrhage into the pericardium and tamponade. Associated arrhythmias and decreased cardiac output are common. Lacerations of the left ventricular myocardium may be followed by aneurysm formation even though they are initially repaired by surgical means. A contusion may result in aneurysm formation similar to that following infarction (Aronstam et al., 1970; Glancy et al., 1967). The late appearance of pseudoaneurysms which may offer quite a diagnostic problem is reported by Vix and Killen (1968). In 2 of their 3 cases, the aneurysm was mistaken for a mediastinal mass. These aneurysms may be the site of thrombosis and thus give rise to systemic embolization. The diagnosis is best established by angiocardiography or left ventriculography, although gated scanning using radioactive nuclides may supplement these procedures (Botvinick et al., 1976).

Rupture

The order of frequency of rupture of the cardiac chambers is the right ventricle, left ventricle, right atrium, and left atrium (Siderys and Strange, 1971). Rupture of either ventricle is followed by massive hemorrhage and death, and there are no recorded instances of survival. Four cases of rupture of the atria with repair and survival have been reported. The diagnosis can be suspected from the presence of pericardial hemorrhage and tamponade associated with a negative thoracic aortogram (Siderys and Strange, 1971). In a review, Parmley et al. (1958) found 14 of 66 cases of atrial rupture that survived for varying lengths of time, thus presenting an opportunity for diagnosis and repair.

Rupture of the interatrial septum was found to be uniformly fatal in the 25 cases reviewed by Parmley et al. (1958).

Rupture of the muscular interventricular septum can follow blunt trauma (9 of 22 cases of traumatic ventricular septal defect reported by Turneey et al., 1972). The appearance of the typical holosystolic murmur may be delayed for several days. The lungs may show engorgement. The most common site is the supracristal portion of the ventricular septum, and the openings vary from 1–3 cm with shunts varying from 1.2/1 to 3.4/1. A number of successful repairs have been reported using the technique of open heart surgery (Parmley et al., 1958; Turneey et al., 1972; Stinson et al., 1968). The appearance or detection of the ventricular septal defect may be delayed for several days to weeks.

Rupture of the papillary muscles of either the right or left ventricle may produce insufficiency of either the mitral or tricuspid valve (Mary et al., 1973; Parmley et al., 1958). Rupture can follow a severe contusion with resultant ischemia and necrosis (Hale and Martin, 1957; Halter, 1955). The resultant valvular insufficiency may be a cause of right or left atrial enlargement.

All of the heart valves are susceptible to damage from blunt trauma, although the aortic and tricuspid valves would seem to be the most frequently involved according to the scattered reports in the literature (Beasley, 1973; Bryant et al., 1973; Kissane et al., 1948; Shabetai et al., 1969; Tachovsky et al., 1970). An aortic valve damaged by disease may be more susceptible to partial rupture following blunt trauma. The predominant hemodynamic effect is some degree of insufficiency, although some degree of residual stenosis of the aortic valve is possible (Kissane et al., 1948).

The signs of valvular dysfunction may be obscured initially by the other effects of blunt trauma. One is impressed by the length of time between the injury and the diagnosis as recorded in a number of case reports. On the other hand, the symptoms of aortic insufficiency may appear suddenly and dominate the clinical picture. The physical findings are a loud murmur, and occasionally it is so loud as to be heard at a distance (Kissane et al., 1948; Bean and Mohaupt, 1952). The left ventricle may show rapid enlargement. In rupture of the aortic valve, the outlook is grave, and immediate replacement with a prosthetic valve is usually indicated. Supravalvular aortography may be useful in confirming the diagnosis and may be an emergency procedure.

In tricuspid insufficiency, the right side of the heart is often greatly enlarged with prominence and convexity of the right atrial border and dilatation of the superior vena cava and azygos vein. Right heart catheterization may show a marked increase in the A and V waves in the right atrium, and right atrial and ventricular angiography can confirm the diagnosis.

Prosthetic valves may suffer displacement or partial rupture of the tissues to which they are anchored following blunt trauma. In the case reported by Arditi et al. (1968), a diastolic murmur of mitral insufficiency appeared following trauma to the chest of a patient with a McGovern valve prosthesis.

Penetrating Wounds of the Heart

Gunshot

Lacerations. The most common injury is laceration of the pericardium and/or the myocardium with hemorrhage and cardiac tamponade. Bleeding into the pericardial sac sufficient to produce acute tamponade usually does not change the cardiac size or contour to a significant degree and may be unrecognized when viewed on a portable film. If leakage occurs into the pleura, it may become visible in the costophrenic angles or elsewhere. Aspiration of blood from the pericardium is the definitive diagnostic procedure and should be attempted if there are signs of tamponade. Aspiration of even a small amount of blood may have an immediate beneficial effect. Previously Blalock and Ravitch, 1943 recommended repeated aspirations as a form of treatment, but this is often ineffective since the blood tends to clot. If adequate surgical facilities are present, exploration of the pericardium and heart should be carried out immediately (Carrasquilla et al., 1972; Sugg et al., 1968).

Penetrating wounds of the cardiac chambers increase the gravity of the injury. Less than 2% of patients with penetrating wounds of the left ventricle reach the hospital alive (Sugg et al., 1968). Traumatic ventricular septal defect due either to blunt trauma or a penetrating wound may be overlooked initially. It is often followed by progressive cardiac enlargement, and the diagnosis is established by right heart catheterization and/or left ventriculography. Immediate surgical repair is indicated (Turneey et al., 1972; Desser et al., 1971).

Laceration of one of the coronary arteries is usually accompanied by other damage to the heart but increases the mortality because of an increased incidence of arrhythmias and cardiogenic shock. Injury to either main artery or their first branches is almost invariably fatal (Rea et al., 1969). Myocardial infarction, aneurysm or arteriovenous fistula may follow if the patient survives a sufficient length of time (Cheng and Adkins, 1973; Konecke et al., 1971). Immediate treatment with saphenous vein bypass graft has been carried out by Tector et al. (1973).

Rarely a bullet or a buckshot may be released inside a vein and be carried as an embolus into the right ventricle or pulmonary artery (Hilbert and Gregory, 1974). In an unusual case seen by one of the authors, a buckshot entered the venous system in the region of the left shoulder and was carried into the right ventricle where it lodged apparently among the chordae tendineae to the tricuspid valve.

Radiologic Procedures. Intracardiac catheters used for diagnostic purposes and central venous catheters used for monitoring may cause cardiac tamponade due to penetration of the myocardium with hemorrhage (Brandt et al., 1970; Bone et al., 1973). Care must be taken that monitoring catheters are soft and placed in one of the great veins rather than the cardiac chambers. Transvenous pacemaker leads may also penetrate the right ventricular myocardium. Since this process is a slow one, significant pericardial hemorrhage may not necessarily occur (see section on Pacemakers).

Intramyocardial injection of contrast substance via an intracardiac catheter occasionally occurs and has undoubtedly been observed by every experienced angiographer. It can be avoided by the use of a properly designed catheter and proper placement. An end hole is potentially more dangerous than a side hole catheter and care must be taken to see that the tip is free of the ventricular or atrial wall. However, the use of a side hole catheter will not guarantee that an intramyocardial injection will not occur. A side hole catheter if wedged cuts a space between the columnae carnae and may cause an extravasation. Fortunately, most extravasations are symptomless. The contrast substance is absorbed in 10–15 min without residual changes. In a few cases arrhythmias have developed.

Unusual or Strenuous Exertion

Ruptue of Aortic Valve

Following the report of Howard (1928) there is no doubt that rupture of a relatively normal aortic valve can occur due to unusual physical exertion or strain. In the case described by Howard (1928) the aortic intima in the region of the commissure between the right and posterior cusp was torn away causing a downward displacement of both cusps and producing a marked insufficiency that was followed by heart failure and death in a few months. Bean and Mohaupt (1952) described a similar case, although they did not have autopsy confirmation. Predisposing factors (Carroll, 1951) such as syphilis, bacterial endocarditis, atherosclerosis, and perhaps rheumatic fever might make the valve and adjacent aorta more susceptible to rupture following marked changes in aortic pressure associated with strain or exertion, but in the cases cited by Howard (1928) these diseases were not present to a significant extent. The murmur associated with a ruptured valve is often loud with a distinctive quality (Bean and Mohaupt, 1952) and should serve as an indication for angiographic studies to establish the diagnosis.

SIGNS AND SYMPTOMS OF TRAUMA TO THE GREAT VESSELS

The pulmonary artery and its branches are relatively short, and the intraluminal pressure is usually low so that lacerations and rupture are rarely immediately fatal. Intrapulmonary hemorrhage from such injuries is common and appears as homogeneous but ill-defined opacities as seen on the chest film. The large bronchial arteries such as occur in certain inflammatory and neoplastic conditions and bronchiectasis are susceptible to rupture and massive hemorrrhage and increase the risk of needle biopsy (McCartney, 1974).

The aorta because of its considerable length and higher intraluminal pressure and other anatomical peculiarities is quite susceptible to injury due to blunt trauma to the thorax. Greendyke (1966) found that approximately 1 in 6 fatal accidents were accompanied by rupture of the aorta. About 90–95% of the injuries due to blunt trauma involve the isthmus or that portion just beyond the left subclavian artery (Sanborn et al., 1970; Molnar and Pace, 1966; Pinet et al., 1973). The other 5–10% of injuries occur in the ascending aorta frequently inside the pericardial reflection. Multiple injuries at more than one site occasionally occur. Some disagreement exists as to which of the aortic segments is the most mobile, but there is considerable evidence that suggests that in blunt trauma the descending aorta is subject to considerable displacement, and there is no doubt that the maximum shearing force is centered around the isthmus (Parmley et al., 1958). The usual injury is a laceration of one or more of the aortic layers. The laceration is

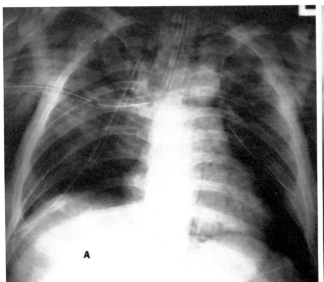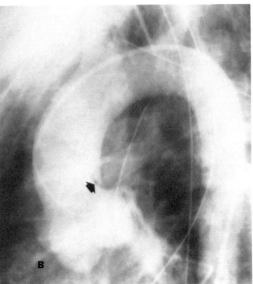

FIG. 467. TRACHEAL LACERATION

(A) Chest film exposed shortly after repair of a tracheal laceration and 24 hours following an automobile accident. Note widespread mediastinal and soft tissue emphysema. (B) Aortogram performed shortly thereafter. Arrow indicates a tear in the intima with possibly a short segment of dissection. At the ensuing operation several lacerations in the intima and media were found.

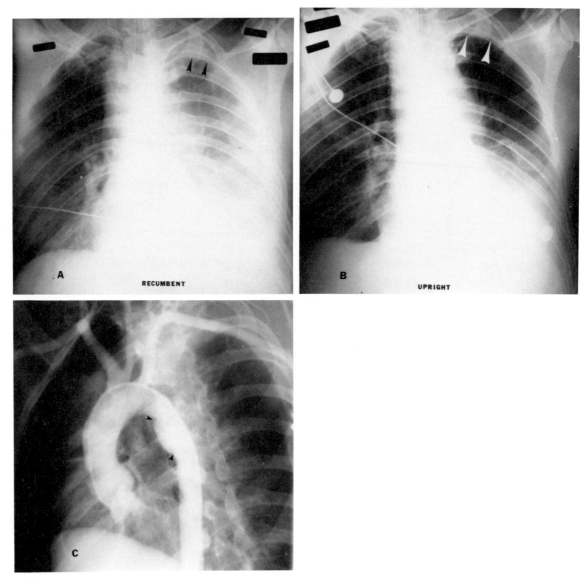

FIG. 468. AORTIC TEAR WITH FALSE ANEURYSM AT THE AORTIC ISTHMUS AND MEDIASTINAL HEMATOMA
(A) Recumbent film exposed about 3 hr after an automobile accident. Trachea is shifted slightly to right. Mediastinum is questionably widened toward the right. Haziness over lower portion of left lung could be due to pulmonary contusion and/or pleural fluid. No rib fracture. Opacity over apex of left lung is most important finding suggesting extrapleural seepage from a mediastinal hematoma. (B) Erect film. Some opacity remains at left base indicating pleural fluid. Apical opacity remains fixed indicating it is not free in pleural space. (C) Aortogram showing aneurysm in region of isthmus. The aorta was almost completely transected.

almost always transverse, and complete transection is surprisingly common (about 40% as observed by Alley *et al.,* 1966). The intima and a portion of the media are always torn, and this can produce the initimal flaps that are occasionally seen at aortography (Fig. 467). Frequently the laceration extends to the adventitia producing a false aneurysm which contains a hematoma. The partially torn adventitia may contain and limit the hematoma for varying periods of time or it may leak into the surrounding mediastinum and/or the left pleural space. If the laceration is in the ascending aorta, leakage may occur into the pericardium. Because of the restraining effects of the adventitia and other reasons, about 10–20% of patients will survive from a few hours to several weeks thus permitting time for diagnosis and treatment (Sanborn *et al.,* 1970; Freed *et al.,* 1968; Sutorius *et al.,* 1973; Griffin *et al.,* 1973). About 2% will survive for an indefinite period and may develop a chronic aneurysm which will be described below.

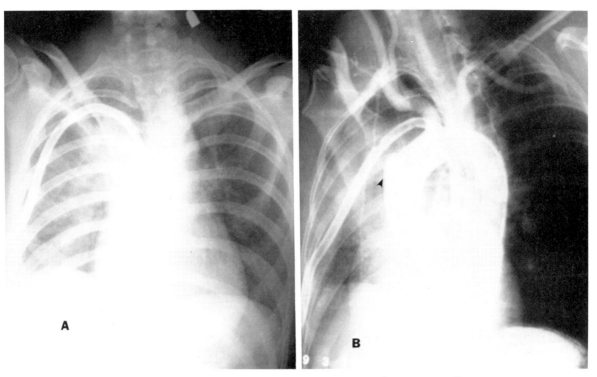

FIG. 469. "BLISTER-LIKE" ANEURYSM OF THE ASCENDING AORTA DUE TO GUNSHOT

(A) The bullet entered the upper part of the right thorax and penetrated upward to the root of the neck on the left side. Opacity in right lung is predominantly blood. (B) Aortogram performed a few hours later showed a blister-like protrusion which at operation was a localized aneurysm, although the intima was not lacerated.

Penetrating wounds may occur at any site due to bullets, stab wounds, and other foreign bodies, and also may be due to displaced fragments of fractured ribs, sternum, or clavicle. False aneurysm formation is much less common with penetrating injuries than with blunt trauma (Bennett and Cherry, 1967).

The innominate artery appears to be the most susceptible of the brachiocephalic vessels to avulsion, and the site is usually just beyond the point of origin (Eller and Ziter, 1970; Piwnica et al., 1961).

Signs and symptoms of aortic rupture are often overshadowed by injuries of other parts of the body. Major trauma to the thorax should always raise the possibility of aortic rupture. Severe chest pain, dysphagia and/or dyspnea are suggestive. Changes or differences in the blood pressure in the neck or arms should be looked for and are suggestive. Hypertension in the arms may be present (Laforet, 1965).

Radiologic Findings

One of the common radiologic findings of rupture of the thoracic aorta is widening of the mediastinum and change in the mediastinal contour as shown on conventional chest films. In the severely injured patient, these films are often exposed in the recumbent position and frequently with portable apparatus. Evaluation of the mediastinum is often perplexing and unreliable. Serial films in comparison with previous films, of course, are helpful. Close attention should be given to the paramediastinal lines which may be displaced laterally. The aortic margins may be irregular in contour or may be obliterated by surrounding hemorrhage. The trachea may be displaced to the right (Kirsh et al., 1970), and downward displacement of the left main stem bronchus with narrowing of the carinal angle is highly suggestive of a mediastinal hematoma (Sanborn et al., 1970). Hemorrhage may extend into the apex of the left thorax, and there may be clouding of the apex of the left lung. As pointed out by Simeone et al. (1975) the apical cap is due to extrapleural blood that extravasates from the mediastinum and seeps along the left subclavian artery. This remains fixed in the erect position and should not be confused with blood in the pleural space. Also it should not be confused with an apical cap or with hemorrhage from a fractured rib or clavicle. Hemothorax, most often on the left side, is common and is particularly suggestive when it accumulates in large volume.

Where there is a reasonable suspicion of aortic

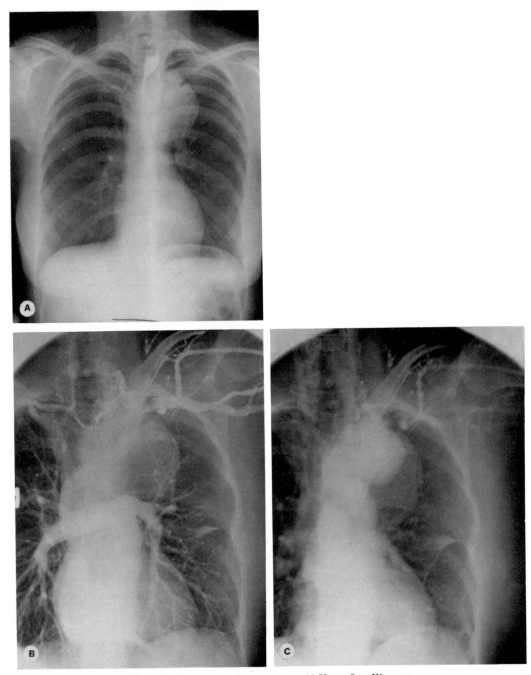

FIG. 470. TRAUMATIC ANEURYSM IN 38-YEAR-OLD WOMAN

Mass appeared adjacent to the left upper mediastinum a few weeks after an automobile accident in which there was trauma to the left upper thorax. The aneurysm was resected by Dr. H. T. Bahnson. The aneurysm arose from the aorta near the origin of the left subclavian artery. (A) Conventional film. (B) Angiocardiogram at 3 sec. (C) Angiocardiogram at 7 sec. The angiocardiogram was made after a previous attempt to treat the aneurysm by wrapping it with cellophane.

rupture, aortography should be performed immediately. The tip of the catheter should be placed in the ascending aorta. Some controversy centers about the appropriate route. Caution in the use of the transfemoral route seems justified

since the aorta may be transected and easily susceptible to further damage from the passage of the retrograde catheter. Molnar and Pace (1966) recommend the right axillary approach since most of the injuries are distal to the innom-

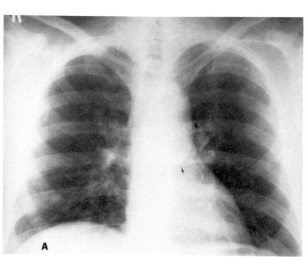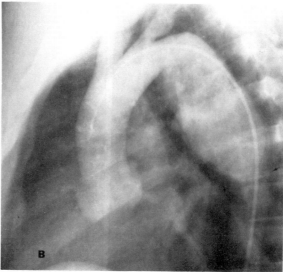

FIG. 471. CHRONIC TRAUMATIC ANEURYSM

Patient was a 24-year-old male who was in an automobile accident 7 years before. The aneurysm was producing no symptoms at the time of discovery.

inate artery. However, we believe that the femoral route can be used with safety if a soft pigtail type catheter is used with care. The right posterior oblique projection is used initially supplemented by a frontal projection if there is still doubt as to the presence or extent of the injury.

The aortogram may show an irregular eccentric false aneurysm or a fusiform widening usually with some irregularity of the contour. The contrast substance may penetrate into the ruptured adventitia producing an irregular shadow. Occasionally, only an intimal flap or radiolucent band in the aortic lumen is seen, although leakage has occurred into the mediastinum (Fig. 467). Technically satisfactory aortography is also valuable in *excluding* a laceration or rupture of the aorta, particularly in those cases where the mediastinum is widened due to other causes.

About 2% of patients with traumatic aortic rupture develop a chronic aneurysm (Bennett and Cherry, 1967; Steinberg, 1957). Steinberg (1957) reported on 5 patients who were asymptomatic for periods of from 5–27 years and recommended observation for stability rather than immediate attempts at repair or excision. Bennett and Cherry (1967), based on a review of the literature and their own experience, doubt that these traumatic aneurysms are ever stable and believe that they present a constant threat of rapid enlargement and rupture. Some produce pressure symptoms such as cough, dyspnea, and pain in the chest. Figure 471 shows a case in a 24-year-old male that was discovered during a routine work-up for a psychiatric condition.

23

Displacement of the Heart

There is considerable normal mobility of the heart; this has been discussed in the section on the normal heart. To summarize, the heart is restrained by (1) great vessels at its base, which are elastic and whose outer coats of fibrous tissue are continuous with the mediastinal fascia; and (2) the surrounding pericardium which in turn is loosely anchored to the diaphragm, sternum, and mediastinal fascia and is under restraining pressure from the surrounding lungs. The normal movements of the heart may be classified as either volumetric or positional in character. Positional changes are due to (1) changes in tension and lines of force inside the heart during systole and diastole; (2) effects of gravity (recumbent, erect, and lateral decubitus positions); (3) differences in pressure in the surrounding lung during respiratory activity; (4) height of the diaphragm; and (5) pressure from adjacent unyielding structures such as the sternum and ribs. Exaggeration of any of the last three factors mentioned above may produce an abnormal displacement of the heart.

Congenital displacements are most frequently due to diaphragmatic hernias, agenesis of one lung, and dextrocardia. Acquired displacements are due to deformities of the bony thorax, pneumothorax, massive unilateral pleural effusion, atelectasis, emphysema, pulmonary and pleural fibrosis, diaphragmatic hernias, defects in the pericardium (congenital or acquired), and eventration of the diaphragm. Dextrocardia has been considered in the section on congenital heart disease. Displacements of the heart due to either congenital or acquired causes are similar in the fundamental means of their production, and therefore will not be considered separately.

Displacement of the heart is of considerable practical importance because (1) displacement distorts the cardiac contour and thereby makes roentgen evaluation more difficult and (2) severe displacement is often accompanied by disturbances in the function of the heart and lungs which produce severe symptoms and shorten life.

DISPLACEMENT DUE TO THORACIC DEFORMITIES

These may be classified as (1) kyphosis, scoliosis, or, commonly, a combination of these two, namely, kyphoscoliosis; (2) pectus excavatum (funnel chest, trichterbrust); (3) pectus carinatum (pigeon breast); and (4) the straight back syndrome.

Kyphosis, Scoliosis, and Kyphoscoliosis

Thoracic kyphoscoliosis usually appears in early life, is progressive for a number of years and reaches its maximum and definitive deformity by the 20th year. Etiologic factors which are commonly mentioned are congenital, poliomyelitis, rickets, and tuberculous spondylitis. In many cases the cause is obscure. The primary curve is in the upper and midthoracic region and is much more frequently convex to the right than the left

(111 cases to right and 15 to left reported by Chapman *et al.* (1939)). Many patients with mild to moderate degrees of kyphoscoliosis are seen in daily practice and appear to be very little affected. Chest films of a right-sided kyphoscoliosis show the curve of the thoracic spine to the right. The right intercostal spaces are widened as the ribs follow the convexity of the vertebral curve and the volume of the right lung is often considerably larger than the left. There is always a less pronounced compensatory curve of the lower thoracic and upper lumbar spine to the opposite side so that the left side of the diaphragm is elevated and the left ribs are forced closer together. Consequently, the left lung is compressed and reduced in volume. The heart is displaced to the left to a variable degree depend-

570

ing upon the severity of the deformity. Its right border may be superimposed upon the vertebral column so that the exact outline is obscured; because of this superimposition, the heart may at first inspection appear enlarged. In the more severe cases, the heart is displaced far into the left chest and is no longer projected on the spine. Also, it is often rotated in a counterclockwise direction (as seen from above); consequently, when viewed in the PA projection, the contour is that of a slight to moderate degree of right anterior obliquity. Thus, the pulmonary trunk segment may appear more convex and prominent than usual. The aortic knob is variable in appearance; it is often increased in prominence due in part to elevation of the cardiac apex which tends to increase the redundancy of the aorta. The rotation of the heart may be partially compensated for by viewing the patient in a moderate degree of left anterior obliquity. The esophagus is also displaced and no longer holds its true relationships to the heart; evidence of left atrial enlargement as indicated by esophageal displacement is unreliable. The aortic impression may be less convex and longer and flatter.

The rarer left-sided kyphoscoliosis is more or less the reverse of the right-sided deformity. In the mild cases, however, the heart may not be significantly displaced and lies near the midline and retains its normal contour. The aorta, particularly if it is elongated and tortuous, tends to wander farther into the left thorax than usual and may produce a shadow lateral to the left heart border. With severe deformity, the heart is displaced into the right chest and is rotated in a clockwise direction (as seen from above). Thus, the contour in the PA projection may approach that seen with a normal heart in a moderate degree of left anterior obliquity, and this can be partially discounted by rotating the patient into a moderate degree of right anterior obliquity.

Severe degrees of kyphoscoliosis produce significant anatomic changes in the heart and lungs with severe symptoms which may lead to death. In a review of 69 fatal cases from the literature, Chapman *et al.* (1939) found 45 had right heart enlargement (hypertrophy and dilatation); also, there usually was an associated enlargement of the pulmonary artery. In a study of 12 additional cases, these same authors found that the vital capacity was reduced and the ratio of residual air to vital capacity was increased, thus producing a poor respiratory exchange. This is confirmed somewhat by fluoroscopy where the diaphragmatic movements are seen to be limited and the thoracic cage is fixed. At autopsy the lungs at times are small and light, indicating an actual loss of lung substance. Pulmonary infections such as pneumonia, chronic bronchitis, and bronchiectasis are quite common; also emphysema and atelectasis. A combination of these changes would seem sufficient to produce cor pulmonale, and this is a frequent occurrence, although there is no agreement that this is the cause of the severe symptoms which frequently are seen.

Chapman *et al.* (1939) use the term "pulmonocardiac failure" to describe the syndrome associated with severe kyphoscoliosis. It is characterized by dyspnea, palpitation, and cough; also, these patients are weak and may have episodes of fainting and asystole. Once severe symptoms appear, the average duration of life is a matter of months, and treatment is difficult. The patient may obtain some relief by lying in a position of dorsal hyperextension.

Radiologic Findings

The roentgen appearance of the far advanced cases is often confusing. In addition to the displacement and rotation of the heart, there are shadows due to inflammatory changes in the adjacent lungs and pleura which may partially obscure the heart borders. The heart often appears enlarged but the distortion of the cardiac contour and the frequent lack of contrast with the surrounding lung make a prediction of individual chamber enlargement hazardous. Also, some of these patients have associated valvular disease so that the right side of the heart is not always predominantly enlarged.

Dubilier *et al.* (1953) have described the angiocardiographic findings in kyphoscoliosis. In general the cardiac chambers were found to be tipped and rotated but not compressed. The distortion of the pulmonary arteries conformed to the misshapen lungs, and the aorta closely followed the deformed spine.

Thoracic kyphosis alone distorts the cardiac and mediastinal structures. The kyphosis may be secondary to a gibbus with a marked deformity of one or two vertebral bodies, or there may be a loss of height with anterior wedging of most of the thoracic segments. The ribs radiate out from the area of maximum kyphosis and are roughly bilaterally symmetrical. The lung apices appear to have an increased volume. The cardiac contour is in the midline and globular. The lower heart borders are submerged in the elevated diaphragmatic shadow and are therefore indistinct. The normal cardiac segments do not stand out, and since only the upper part of the cardiac contour is clearly visible, the heart may appear smaller than it actually is. On the other hand, the transverse width of the lower portion of the

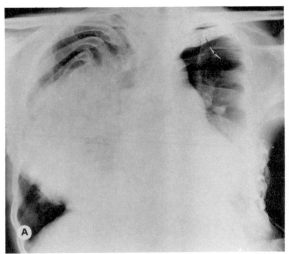 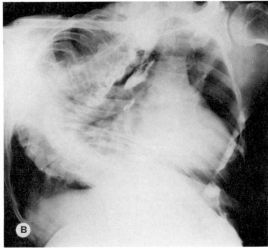

FIG. 472. MARKED RIGHT KYPHOSCOLIOSIS IN PATIENT WITH CONGESTIVE HEART FAILURE
There was no other evident cause for the heart failure. (A) Posteroanterior projection. (B) Right anterior oblique projection.

heart is increased due to the high diaphragm. In the lateral view, the AP diameter is considerably increased, and the heart has an oval or globular appearance.

Pectus Excavatum

Pectus excavatum is a thoracic deformity in which the lower portion of the sternum is depressed or displaced inward. As a result, the distance between the posterior surface of the sternum and the anterior surface of the vertebral bodies is decreased; in severe cases, this distance may be only a few centimeters or even less. The origin of the condition is obscure; it may be congenital or follow abnormal muscular changes during early life.

In the mild to moderately severe cases of this deformity, the heart is displaced almost invariably to the left, but there are no significant cardiac signs or symptoms. With severe or marked sternal depression in addition to cardiac displacement, however, there may be irregularities of rhythm, palpitation, and an elevation of right atrial and ventricular pressures (Ravitch, 1951).

Radiologic Findings

The diagnosis of pectus excavatum is easily made by palpation and inspection. In the lateral chest film, the linear shadow of the depressed lower one-third of the sternum can be recognized anteriorly. Furthermore, the cardiac contour is flattened so that the AP diameter is diminished. It is important for the rotentgenologist to recognize the evidence of the deformity as seen in the posteroanterior projection. The heart is displaced to the left and may appear slightly enlarged. Actually, the right border of the heart is obscured by the superimposed vertebral column; consequently, the precise frontal area or transverse diameter cannot be determined. Usually, the heart is not enlarged. The left border extends in a straight line obliquely downward from the inconspicuous aortic knob to the cardiac apex. The apex is rounded and slightly elevated. To the right of the vertebral column from about the level of the right main bronchus downward there is an ill-defined increase in density which extends laterally into the right lung for 3–4 cm. This is due to the oblique or almost lengthwise projection of the soft tissues of the right side of the sternal depression. The vascular markings in the lower portion of the lung are accentuated by the superimposed density so that the entire shadow may be wrongly attributed to pneumonitis or infiltration in the lower portion of the lung. The rib contours also may give another clue to the presence of the condition. The posterior ribs may be normal; the anterior ribs, particularly the second to sixth ribs, run obliquely downward at an increased angle; also, the third through the sixth anterior interspaces are relatively narrower than normal.

In the severe cases, the distance between the posterior surface of the sternum and anterior surface of the vertebral bodies may be incredibly small. In the case reported by Ravitch (1951), the distance was about 3 cm (compare fig. 473). Severe cardiac embarrassment may follow due to (1) direct pressure on the heart, with restric-

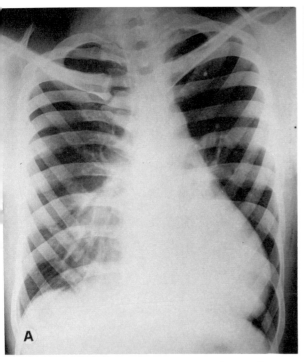
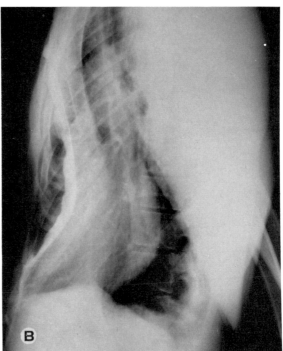

FIG. 473. WELL-MARKED PECTUS EXCAVATUM WITH SOME CARDIAC DISPLACEMENT

Barium was placed over the sternum in the laterval view in order to demonstrate more clearly the degree of depression. The patient had auricular fibrillation.

tion of expansion; (2) cardiac rotation, with twisting or angulation of the great veins, impeding the return of blood to the right heart; (3) cardiac arrhythmias secondary to atrial impingement; and (4) a decrease in respiratory reserve (Wachtel *et al.*, 1956). In such cases, division of the costosternal cartilages with elevation of the sternum may relieve the cardiac embarrassment.

Pectus Carinatum

Deformities of the thorax are common in congenital heart disease. In many instances, they are due to pressure on the soft, yielding, bony structures of early life by a large heart. The chest is frequently asymmetrical, and one side is more full or more convex than the other. Often the left anterior chest is protuberant, and the right side is flat. Occasionally, the deformity may be symmetrical and resemble a true pigeon breast. These deformities are best evaluated by palpation when the patient is fluoroscoped. They are often associated with minor cardiac displacement.

The Straight Back Syndrome

The straight back syndrome was first described by Rawlings (1960, 1961) as a new cause

of "pseudo heart disease." Its main importance is that it is usually a benign condition and may be easily confused with more serious organic heart disease. Most of the patients reported by Rawlings (1960, 1961); Daty *et al.* (1964); DeLeon *et al.* (1965) and Twigg *et al.* (1967) were seen because of a heart murmur. Rarely the patients had mild symptoms of palpitation and dyspnea which usually could be attributed to other causes. Their murmurs were described as ejection type or late systolic murmurs and rarely accompanied by a thrill (Daty *et al.*, 1964). Careful physical examination showed a lack of normal thoracic kyphosis. There is rarely any change or depression in the sternum.

Radiologic Findings

The frontal chest film may be normal but infrequently the heart appears enlarged and "pancake" in appearance. This occurs in more extreme cases. In the lateral view, the thoracic spine is straight and as a consequence the distance between the posterior surface of the sternum and the anterior surfaces of the mid thoracic vertebrae is reduced to 10 cm or less on average (Twigg *et al.*, 1967). The area of the heart in contact with the sternum anteriorly is usually

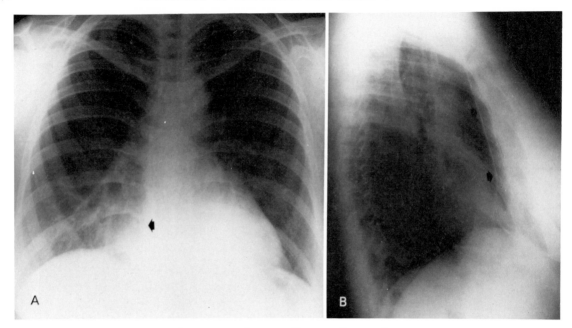

FIG. 474. FRONTAL AND LATERAL VIEWS OF PECTUS EXCAVATUM

The frontal view (A) shows slight displacement of heart to the left and soft tissue density to right of spine (arrow). In the lateral view (B), arrows show depression of sternum.

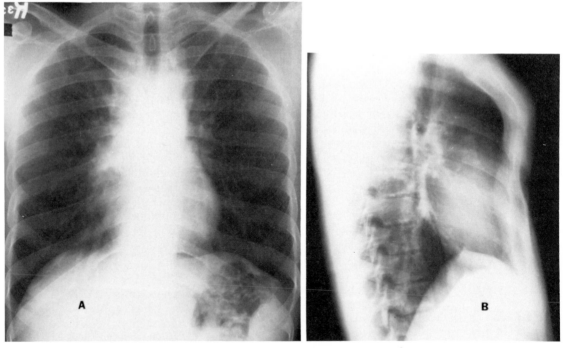

FIG. 475. PECTUS CARINATUM WITH THE APPEARANCE OF WIDENING OF THE MEDIASTINUM

increased, and it is probable that some pressure is exerted on the heart. Because of this, the heart may be rotated creating a minor torsion of the great vessels which in turn could produce tur-

bulence and a murmur. The right ventricular outflow tract and pulmonary artery are brought into close contact with the anterior chest wall so that any turbulence is easily transmitted to the

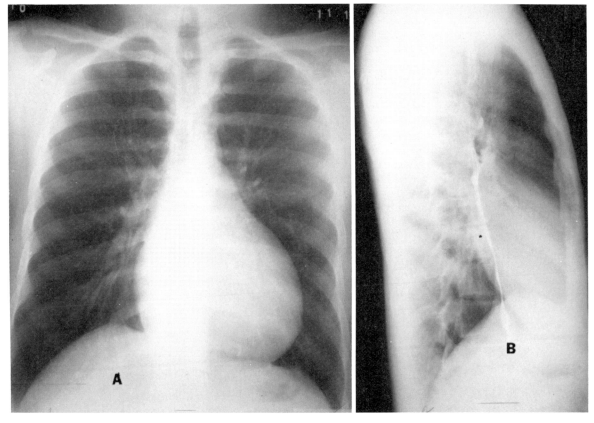

FIG. 476. STRAIGHT BACK SYNDROME IN A YOUNG MALE

The thoracic spine is quite straight, and the distance between the posterior surface of the sternum and anterior surface of vertebral colum is diminished. The heart is flattened in its A-P dimension and appears enlarged and slightly deformed. The patient had a prolapse of the mitral valve but only minor symptoms.

chest wall.

When the heart is deformed, it is usually the midportion of the heart that is flattened with suggestive enlargement of the pulmonary artery, although occasionally the ventricles will be flattened and the entire heart will appear enlarged as seen in the frontal view (Fig. 476).

The diagnosis is easily made by inspection of a properly exposed lateral chest film. The straight thoracic spine and decreased distance between the posterior surface of the sternum and the spine is evident from inspection, but measurements can be made. Twigg et al. (1967) used a horizontal line from the posterior surface of the sternum to the anterior surface of the 8th thoracic vertebra (APT). In normal males and females, this averaged 14.2 cm and 11.96 cm, respectively. In patients with the straight back syndrome, the average distance in males and females was 10.65 and 9.81, respectively. For details of other measurements conducted on the

thorax concerning the transverse diameter of the heart and of the chest, the reader is referred to the articles by Twigg et al. (1967) and Tampas and Lurie (1968). Further support to the legitimacy of the straight back syndrome is given by the paper of Tampas and Lurie (1968). These authors found that in children and infants the incidence of functional murmurs was related to the ratio of the AP diameter to the transverse diameter of the chest, and the patients with the lower ratio had an increased incidence of heart murmurs and a large heart as measured by the transverse diameter.

The importance of the condition is not to confuse it with some serious cardiac disorder. The appearance of the heart and the presence of a murmur and at times a thrill could suggest a diagnosis of ASD, VSD, AS, or PS. Although the abnormalities of the chest comprising the straight back syndrome are present, they cannot be used to rule out a minor defect with certainty.

The presence of a straight thoracic spine greatly decreases the importance of the auscultatory findings. In many of the reported cases cardiac catheterization was carried out with normal findings.

DISPLACEMENT DUE TO PULMONARY AND PLEURAL DISEASE

Displacement of the heart in these conditions is due to (1) traction, (2) pressure, or (3) a combination of these two. Traction is exerted by fibrous adhesions between the pericardium and a fibrotic lung or extensive pleural fibrosis. Normally, the pressure of the two lungs on the exterior of the pericardium is equal. When this relationship is upset, the heart may be displaced.

Traction displacement to a minor degree is common in chronic pulmonary infections with fibrosis. A scar in either apex may elevate the pulmonary artery and other hilar structures. A large area of fibrosis involving an entire lobe may shift the entire heart toward the involved side, partially due to traction and partially due to chronic atelectasis and loss of volume of the involved lobe.

Atelectasis of a sizeable volume of the lung causes the surrounding elastic structures to alter their shape in order to compensate for the loss in volume. The heart shifts to the involved side. The shift is more pronounced with lower than with upper lobe collapse. A left lower lobe collapse may cause some rotation of the heart (counterclockwise as seen from above) and a change in the left border contour. Massive atelectasis of an entire lung is followed by a pronounced shift of the heart and mediastinal structures to the involved side. The degree of cardiac embarrassment caused by such a shift is difficult to evaluate because of the accompanying lung changes. The rapidity with which the displacement occurs is influential in the degree of embarrassment which follows. When the displacement takes place slowly, it may become quite pronounced without significant symptoms.

A sizeable accumulation of pleural fluid displaces the heart towards the opposite side; this is more pronounced with left-sided effusions. If a large effusion is present without a shift of the heart, one should suspect malignant fixation, although, rarely, a chronic infectious process will produce the same result. A rapid accumulation of fluid may produce severe symptoms of dyspnea and shortness of breath; slower accumulation may give comparatively few symptoms.

Spontaneous pneumothorax may cause an almost complete collapse of one lung with displacement of the heart to the opposite side; if there are pleuropericardial adhesions, there may be some rotation of the heart also. Fluoroscopy of a large pneumothorax shows a diminished motion of the diaphragm on the involved side. There may be a slight shift away from the involved side during inspiration.

Induced or therapeutic pneumothorax also displaces the heart; it is much better tolerated than a spontaneous pneumothorax because of its slower accumulation. When the pneumothorax is allowed to absorb, the heart may return to its normal position, or adhesions, thickening, and fibrosis of the mediastinal pleura may keep it permanently displaced.

Following a pneumonectomy, the hemithorax on the operated side fills with fluid which eventually organizes and is replaced by fibrous tissue. The heart commonly shifts to the operated side to a slight to moderate degree, providing there has not been previous fixation of the mediastinal structures.

DISPLACEMENT DUE TO CHANGES IN THE DIAPHRAGM

Changes in the cardiac contour due to normal variations in the height of the diaphragm have been described in the section on the normal heart. In certain conditions such as pregnancy or ascites, the diaphragm is elevated for considerable periods of time. The major change in the cardiac contour in pregnancy may be due to the elevated diaphragm, but there is an increase in cardiac output, plasma volume, and blood volume which may be associated with an increase in cardiac volume. According to Kjellberg et al.

(1949) there may be a 30–35% increase in cardiac volume, about 10% of which occurs in the first half of pregnancy. With elevation of the diaphragm, the left border of the heart moves toward the left. The transverse diameter of the heart is thus increased. Also, the heart is displaced slightly posteriorly as is shown by a curved posterior displacement of the barium-filled esophagus. The length of the curve is longer than that seen with left atrial enlargement. The aorta is deviated by the elevation of the heart, and the knob increases in prominence. The pulmonary artery segment is often prominent during the latter months of pregnancy, and there may be some actual enlargement of the right ventricle and pulmonary artery due to the increased cardiac output.

In chronic emphysema, the diaphragm is depressed and has a small range of motion. The transverse diameter of the heart is decreased and the long diameter becomes much more vertical. Thus, a transverse heart may approach the vertical type.

Diaphragmatic hernias are either congenital or acquired. Left-sided far outnumber right-sided hernias. Many of the congenital hernias are due to a failure of development of a portion of the diaphragm and are quite large. These are occasionally seen in newborns and infants. The symptoms of cyanosis and difficult respiration are quite alarming, and immediate operative treatment is often necessary. It is wise to determine the length of the esophagus and organs involved in the hernia before repair is attempted.

Acquired left-sided hernias also displace the heart and mediastinum toward the right. Occasionally, a hiatus hernia may be of sufficient size to exert pressure on the heart posteriorly. Anterior hernias through the foramen of Morgagni often appear as small, rounded masses in the right cardiophrenic angle and do not displace the heart. Larger hernias may be present on either side; when they are left-sided, they displace the heart toward the right.

Eventration of the left diaphragm, elevation due to massive pleural adhesions or left phrenic paralysis also elevates the apex of the heart and displaces it to the right and slightly posterior.

24

Diseases of the Pericardium

GENERAL CONSIDERATIONS

The pericardium is a fibroserous sac which completely surrounds the heart and extends for short but variable distances along the aorta, the pulmonary trunk, the venae cavae, and the pulmonary veins. The outer layer or pericardium is mainly fibrous tissue and is continuous with the inner epicardium which is closely applied to the heart surface. The interior or apposing surfaces of these two layers are lined with a smooth serous membrane; between these two layers is the pericardial cavity. *Gray's Anatomy* (1942) states that the cavity is a potential space although it normally contains a small amount of clear fluid which has lubricating qualities. It is unlikely that the pericardium is everywhere closely approximated to the heart, else the activity of the heart would be hampered. Arendt (1948) indicates that "the diaphragmatic surface of the pericardium is considerably larger than the corresponding surface area of the heart which rests and moves about within it." This would suggest that there is some redundancy of at least the basilar portions, and this would be necessary if diaphragmatic movements are to take place without undue traction on the heart.

Two redundancies or potential recesses exist that may be of importance as sites for collection of small amounts of pericardial fluid. These are the oblique sinus posteriorly around the pulmonary veins and vena cava and the transverse sinus more anteriorly around the aorta and pulmonary artery.

The actual and potential pericardial cavity normally is not large. Torrance (1953) found at autopsy that only 200–300 ml of water could be injected into the pericardial space of a normal heart using a hand syringe, and this amount tightly distended the pericardium. If the heart was enlarged, as little as 80–100 ml would cause a marked tenseness of the pericardial sac. Furthermore, the pericardium was relatively unyielding and inelastic and when tightly distended brought the injection to an abrupt stop. These observations are of considerable importance in connection with the clinical course of acute pericardial effusion.

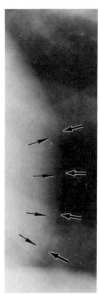

FIG. 477. NORMAL PERICARDIAL FAT LINE
Enlargement of a posteroanterior view of the cardiac apex and adjacent hemidiaphragm from the chest film of a healthy 19-year-old girl. The film was exposed at 1/60 sec. The curvilinear radiolucent line (arrows on left) 2 mm deep to the lateral heart margin (arrows on right) represents epicardial fat, and the intervening thin soft tissue band represents the normal pericardium. This is seldom seen in normal subjects, in part perhaps because of the longer exposure times commonly used in chest radiography.

The pericardium covers the ascending aorta for approximately one-half the distance from the aortic valve to the origin of the innominate artery (2–3 cm). The pulmonary trunk is covered to a point just below its bifurcation. The investments

578

of the venae cavae, particularly the inferior vena cava, and the pulmonary veins are relatively quite short.

Exteriorly, the fibrous coat of the pericardium is continuous with the external coat of the great vessels and the mediastinal pleura. The lower portion or base is in close contact with the diaphragm, and over a small area in the region of the central tendon the diaphragm and pericardium are completely fused. Near the cardiac apex the outer layer of the pericardium is separated from the mediastinal pleura by the pericardial fat pad; a similar collection of fat is often present on the right side anterior to the inferior vena cava.

In addition to fusing with the external coats of the great vessels, the pericardium is continuous with the pretracheal fascia. Superior and inferior ligaments are present anteriorly between the pericardium and the sternum. All of these connections tend to stabilize the pericardium within the mediastinum; nevertheless, a considerable range of mobility exists.

The normal pericardium cannot ordinarily be recognized as such by conventional roentgen examination. Its density is almost the same as that of the heart; it is thin and is applied so closely to the exterior of the heart that under normal circumstances it is considered roentgenologically as an intrinsic part of the heart. It is visible only when (1) calcified, (2) separated from the heart by presence of air in the pericardial cavity, and (3) separated from the heart by a layer of fat in the epicardium (Kremens, 1955) (Fig. 477). Angiocardiography permits a close appraisal of the thickness of the pericardium in the area adjacent to the right atrium. The soft tissue here is composed of the endocardium of the right atrium, the myocardium, the epicardium, the pericardium and the parietal and visceral pleura. It should not exceed 4 mm in thickness (Figley and Bagshaw, 1957).

Changes in the pericardium are manifested radiologically by (1) changes in the cardiac contour, such as smoothing out of the normal curves, bulging posteriorly or anteriorly, etc.; (2) changes in pulsation; (3) changes in mobility with changes in posture, e.g., fixation; and (4) calcification. These changes are due to (1) collections of fluid in the pericardial sac; (2) extensive fibrosis and/or calcification of the pericardium with thickening and hardening and/or adhesions to surrounding structures and compression of the heart; (3) partial or complete absence of the pericardium; and (4) tumors, cysts, and diverticula of the pericardium.

ETIOLOGIC AGENTS AND OTHER CONDITIONS AFFECTING THE PERICARDIUM

I. Infection
  A. Tuberculosis
  B. Pyogenic—pneumococcus, streptococcus
  C. Virus
  D. Histoplasmosis
  E. Amebiasis (Faerber et al., 1974)
II. Metabolic
  A. Myxedema
  B. Uremia
III. Autoimmune Diseases
  A. Scleroderma
  B. Lupus erythematosus
  C. Rheumatic fever
IV. Physical Agents
  A. Radiation
  B. Asbestosis (Freundlich and Lind, 1975)

V. Neoplasms
  A. Cysts
  B. Primary malignant
  C. Metastatic
VI. Postoperative
  A. Hemorrhage
    (1) Heparin therapy
  B. Post-pericardiotomy syndrome
VII. Trauma (see Chapter 22)
VIII. Circulatory
  A. Congestive heart failure
IX. Rupture of the Heart and Aorta
  A. Dissecting aneurysm
  B. Myocardial infarction
X. Idiopathic
  A. Secondary to cardiomyopathies

PERICARDIAL FLUID

Pericardial fluid may be a transudate, an exudate or blood. Specific diseases are often associated with a typical fluid. In congestive heart failure the fluid is usually serous with low specific gravity; with myxedema the fluid may contain a considerable amount of cholesterol. Tuberculosis is often associated with a sanguineous effusion, and uremia and metastatic tumor almost always produce a bloody effusion. Pyogenic infections usually produce a purulent effusion.

Acute Pericardial Effusion

Of major importance is the rapidity with which fluid collects in the pericardium. Since the pericardium is predominantly a fibrous structure, it is not particularly elastic, and the rapid accumulation of a relatively small amount of fluid may be sufficient to produce some degree of cardiac tamponade. Much depends upon the elasticity of the pericardium. Cardiac tamponade is manifest clinically by a drop in blood pressure, hypotension, small pulse pressure and pulsus paradoxus, and a striking increase in systemic venous pressure.

Radiologic Findings. The accumulation of small amounts of fluid (probably less than 200 cc) is difficult to detect on conventional chest films. A change in the size of the heart may be minor, and careful comparison of previous chest films or a series of films exposed at daily intervals may be helpful in determining minor changes in size and contour of the heart. Some of the normal minor curvatures may become effaced. The left border may become straightened. Dilatation of the superior vena cava and azygos vein is suggestive of cardiac tamponade, but this may be difficult to evaluate. The lungs are often clear unless there is associated pulmonary disease such as pneumonia or injury or a previous operative procedure.

Fluoroscopy is potentially helpful in demonstrating diminished pulsations. In the authors' experience this has not been too reliable because there was no previous baseline fluoroscopy, and significant pulsations may persist in the presence of a small amount of pericardial fluid. Furthermore, patients may be too ill to cooperate properly for the examination.

Echocardiography properly performed can detect pericardial fluid in amounts of 20 cc (Horowitz *et al.*, 1974), although Fiegenbaum (1976) does not give such a precise figure. Furthermore, the apparatus can be brought to the patient and carried out with minimum disturbance. Recent echocardiographic studies (D'Cruz *et al.*, 1975) of cardiac tamponade have shown an increase in filling of the right and a decreased filling of the left ventricle accompanied by motion of the anterior leaflet of the mitral valve with inspiration which they took as further confirmatory evidence of cardiac tamponade. Also, echocardiography can be used to follow the course of the effusion.

Angiocardiography (using either contrast substance or CO_2) and blood pool isotope scanning may be used in the diagnosis of pericardial effusion (see below). Their use would be indicated only where echocardiography was not available. Angiocardiography besides its invasive and complex nature has not established its reliability in the detection of small effusions (less than 200

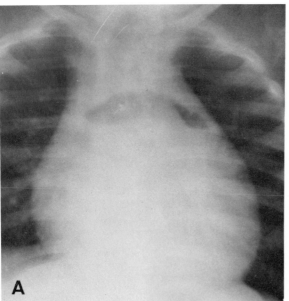 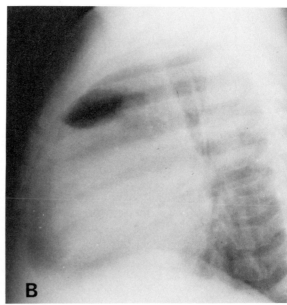

FIG. 478. PERICARDIAL EFFUSION

Chest film on an 18-month-old male infant being treated for pneumonia revealed cardiac enlargement. The liver was also enlarged, and there was ECG evidence of pericarditis. Fluid removed by pericardial tap was a transudate and was sterile. The etiology of the effusion is unknown. Erect posteroanterior and lateral films of the chest (A and B) show air in the pericardial sac following paracentesis. The air fills and outlines the anterior-superior pericardial recess, which is quite spacious and rises to surround the bases of the great vessels, demonstrating the superior extension of the pericardial attachment.

cc). Blood pool scanning (Kriss, 1969) may be used as a noninvasive technique but has a low sensitivity to small effusions (Strauss *et al.*, 1974; Christensen and Bonte, 1968).

The radiologist should be alert to small changes in heart size and contour, particularly in the appropriate clinical setting such as suspected dissecting aneurysm, uremia, and postoperative cardiac cases.

Subacute and Chronic Pericardial Effusion

When pericardial fluid accumulates slowly (a few days or a week or longer) distention and dilatation of the pericardium occur. Under these circumstances a large collection is possible without severe symptoms. Changes in the cardiac contour may therefore be pronounced and depend upon the amount of fluid present. Resiliency of the pericardium depends to a considerable extent on the nature of the process causing the fluid. If the process is inflammatory after a period of time the pericardium thickens, becomes fibrotic and unyielding. This limits the size of the effusion and may precipitate cardiac tamponade with only a moderate-sized effusion. With effusions in excess of 500 ml there are significant changes. The heart is enlarged. One is usually impressed by its symmetrical appearance although it continues to extend farther to the left than to the right. Its contour has been described as globular, spherical, onion-like, triangular, and like a water bottle. The transverse diameter increases, whereas the vertical length remains constant. The base of the heart is narrow, and the length of the vascular pedicle in relation to the remainder of the heart contour is decreased. There is straightening of the upper borders, particularly on the left side where fluid distends the pericardium around the roots of the great vessels. With a large effusion the esophagus is displaced posteriorly. The curvature of the displaced segment is longer than that due to an enlarged left atrium and begins at the level of the carina and extends to the diaphragm.

In a relaxed pericardium the position of the fluid is influenced considerably by gravity, and in the erect or recumbent position, it tends to collect inferiorly and laterally. As the size of the effusion increases the fluid tends to collect anteriorly and in the retrosternal area as well as in the infracardiac and lateral recesses (Steinberg *et al.*, 1958; Steinberg, 1958; Golden, 1950). This produces posterior displacement of the heart contour as well as filling in of the retrosternal space. Mellins *et al.* (1959) experimentally produced opaque pericardial effusions in dogs and showed that the pericardial fluid collected ante-

riorly, superiorly, and, to a lesser degree, inferiorly, with almost no posterior localization. Changes in position of the animals were found to have little or no effect on the location of the fluid. This is evidently due to the fixation of the posterior heart surface to the soft tissues of the posterior mediastinum by the six sizeable veins which enter the heart posteriorly. Kymographic studies showed that the pulsations of the anterior pericardial surface were dampened while the barium-filled esophagus posteriorly showed good transmitted cardiac pulsations without evidence of an intervening fluid collection. This differential dampening of the cardiac pulsations is thought to be a dependable radiologic sign of pericardial effusion. Image amplified fluoroscopy and cinefluorography may be adequate to demonstrate this sign though the present authors have had no experience with their use.

In large chronic effusions there is an increase in the width of the base of the heart in the recumbent as compared with the erect position. This sign is rarely very helpful. It should be remembered that the base of the normal heart widens with recumbency. Also, since recumbent films are often exposed in the anteroposterior projection they must not be compared with erect films made in the same projection at a greater distance.

A review of serial films exposed at frequent intervals is helpful. In acute effusion there may be a rapid return to normal as the fluid resolves. Any sudden change in heart size should raise the suspicion of pericardial fluid.

Differential Diagnosis and Radiologic Findings. The differential diagnosis between diffuse cardiac enlargement and pericardial effusion by conventional radiologic means is difficult. Pulsations may be diminished in both conditions; they are rarely completely absent with myocarditis or cardiac enlargement secondary to decompensation. Diminished pulsations anteriorly with normal posterior cardiac border pulsations favor the diagnosis of pericardial effusion. The lungs are clear, and the superior vena cava is widened in both pericardial effusion and myocarditis; congestive heart failure is commonly accompanied by signs of lung stasis. Both an effusion and myocarditis may coexist as in rheumatic fever, and in congestive heart failure there may be an associated hydropericardium which further increases the heart size. Even when enlarged, however, the heart responds to changes in intrathoracic pressure by changes in contour. This is brought out by filming or fluoroscopy during the Valsalva and Mueller maneuvers; with an effusion, there is minimal or no change in cardiac contour in response to these tests (Ar-

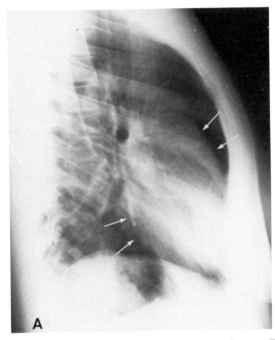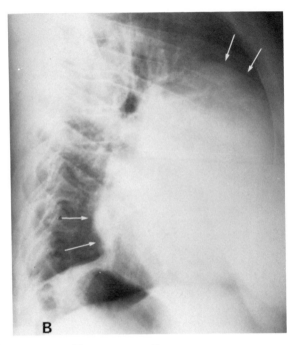

FIG. 479. PERICARDIAL EFFUSION DUE TO FIBROSARCOMA, METASTATIC TO PERICARDIUM

(A) Lateral chest film exposed in December 1947. No abnormality is seen. Arrows point to the anterosuperior and posteroinferior aspects of the cardiovascular shadow. (B) Lateral chest film exposed in January, 1949. Pericardial effusion has produced massive enlargement of the cardiac-pericardial shadow, the bulk of the fluid having collected anterosuperiorly and posteroinferiorly (arrows). (Courtesy of Dr. Ross Golden.)

endt, 1948). Unfortunately, many patients are too sick or uncomfortable to carry out effectively these breathing exercises, and in the authors' experience this procedure has not been helpful.

The diagnosis of pericardial effusion may be established with certainty and its differentiation from generalized cardiac enlargement established if any of the several normally occurring collections of subepicardial fat can be seen more than 2 mm deep to the external contour of the pericardial shadow. Jorgens et al. (1962) described several epicardial fat deposits and demonstrated their radiographic appearance in various positions. Cinefluorography was used to demonstrate a decreased amplitude of pulsation of the pleuropericardial border and an increase in the distance between the epicardial fat lines and this border. The present authors have used this method with success and, particularly in the presence of massive effusion, have clearly visualized a heart of normal size, outlined at one or more points by radiolucent epicardial fat, pulsating within an enlarged and immobile pericardial sac distended with fluid. Failure to demonstrate a fat line does not exclude the presence of a pericardial effusion.

Angiocardiography will give highly suggestive evidence of increased width of the pericardial cavity and is thus a reliable method for demonstrating pericardial fluid (Williams and Steinberg, 1949). The crucial interface is the space between the right atrial cavity and the adjacent right lung. This provides a soft tissue band that is visible between the right atrial cavity (outlined by contrast substance) and the air-containing right lung. This band follows the contour of the right atrium and normally should not exceed 4 mm in thickness. A greater width suggests pericardial disease. It does not follow that this increased width is always due to fluid. It may be due to fibrosis or thick exudate or hemorrhage or rarely to extrinsic pleural fluid (McKusick, 1952; Turner et al., 1966; Figley and Bagshaw, 1957). It is highly suggestive of pericardial disease, and if the band is greater than 1 cm in thickness, it is quite likely due to fluid (Figley and Bagshaw, 1957).

Angiocardiography may be performed using opaque contrast material or carbon dioxide. In the average adult, 50–100 ml of carbon dioxide are injected rapidly into a peripheral vein (ordinarily the left antecubital vein) with the patient lying on the left side. Immediately following the completion of the injection 6 films, using a film changer, are exposed over a period of 12 seconds. With the patient in the left-side-down decubitus position, the gas rises and outlines the internal aspect of the right atrial cavity. This permits one to evaluate the soft tissue band adjacent to the right atrium.

Turner *et al.* (1966) advocated the use of cinefluorography because of the importance of certain dynamic changes in contour of the soft tissue band that can only be demonstrated by this method. Although the soft tissue band was greater than 5 mm in thickness, the presence of

fluid waves visible within the band by cinefluorography was a highly predictive sign of pericardial fluid. In the absence of fluid waves the thickened band was due to a variety of conditions which caused pericardial thickening, such as constrictive pericarditis, invasion by Hodgkin's disease and chronic pericarditis due to uremia. Flattening and asymmetry of the band with absence of fluid waves were highly suggestive of thickening of the pericardium. Several cases were

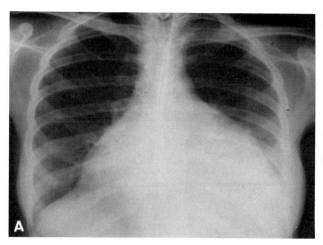
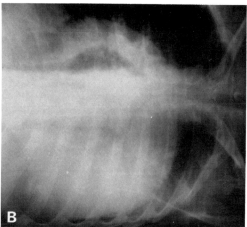

FIG. 480. PERICARDIAL EFFUSION

Eighteen-year-old dyspneic black woman with systemic lupus erythematosus. Blood pressure was 90/60. A paradoxical pulse was noted. Electrocardiogram showed low voltage and ischemic changes anterolaterally. Chest film (A) showed marked globular cardiomegaly. Intravenous carbon dioxide injection with the patient lying on her left side (B) showed a wide band of water density between the gas in the right atrium and the air in the right lung. Pericardial effusion was thought to be present and was confirmed by pericardial tap.

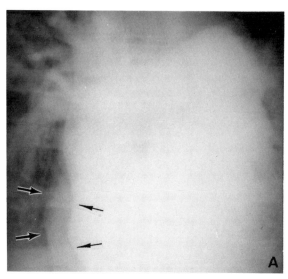
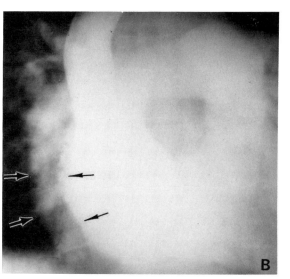

FIG. 481. PERICARDIAL EFFUSION

Opacification of the right side of the heart by venous angiocardiography in two different patients (A and B) in whom pericardial effusion was suspected. In each case the lateral-most portion of the right atrium (arrows on right) is 1–2 cm deep to the right heart margin (arrows on left), indicating the presence of pericardial disease, usually effusion.

observed of initial trapping of the gas under the crista terminalis with incomplete filling of the right atrium. This could also give an appearance of a thickened soft tissue band. Complete filling of the lateral wall of the right atrium could best be demonstrated by the cinefluorographic method.

Carbon dioxide angiography is simple and has few contraindications. It possibly should not be employed in patients with intracardiac right to left shunts because of the danger of gas embolization to the brain or coronary arteries should the gas reach the left side of the circulation (Phillips, 1961). Turner et al. (1966) think that the only contraindication is severe pulmonary disease in which carbon dioxide retention can cause acidosis and narcosis.

Patients with pericardial effusion have tolerated opaque angiography quite well. One injection of contrast substance usually suffices, and this may be less than the usual amount since good visualization of the right atrium is often all that is necessary to make the diagnosis (Holman and Steinberg, 1958; Soloff and Zatuchni, 1957). The demonstration of a thickened soft tissue band has the same significance and limitations that have been discussed with carbon dioxide angiography. Angiocardiography with an opaque contrast material may also demonstrate pericardial thickening or effusion in areas other than the right heart border, and demonstration of all of the cardiac chambers is desirable such as in cases of suspected constrictive pericarditis. The present authors prefer opaque angiocardiography when angiocardiography is required because of the occasional false negative studies using carbon dioxide.

Pericardial effusion or thickening may be determined during the progress of a right heart catheterization. The catheter tip can be placed against the lateral wall of the right atrium and an estimate of the thickness of the soft tissue band can be obtained (Connolly et al., 1959).

All of the radiologic procedures just described are usually unnecessary where satisfactory echocardiography is available. The reader is referred to articles by Fiegenbaum (1970, 1976), Gramiak and Shaw (1971) and Horowitz et al. (1974).

Blood pool scanning for the detection of pericardial effusion is a noninvasive technique that may also be used when echocardiography is not available. It consists of scanning the heart, lungs, and liver following the injection of ^{99}mTcO$_4$ bound to serum albumin. The radioactive material is trapped in the lung and liver but also enters the blood sufficiently to outline the cardiac chambers. A halo between the cardiac chambers and the adjacent lungs and liver constitutes evidence of a pericardial effusion (Kreiss, 1969). The experiments of Christensen and Bonte (1968) suggest that the method is less sensitive than either carbon dioxide or opaque angiography or echocardiography.

Aspiration of the pericardium is a common procedure and may establish the diagnosis of fluid and also its etiology. The fluid may be replaced with air so that the pericardium remains distended and is seen as a curved shadow extending from the base of the heart downward to the area where fluid remains (Maurer and Mendez, 1960). The pericardial wall is usually thin but may be thickened, particularly in tuberculous pericarditis or invasion by tumor. A width of 3–4 mm suggests thickening and therefore may have some diagnostic significance, although it should be remembered that the projected width varies somewhat with the curvature in relation to the x-ray beam. Irregular areas of thickening, of course, are significant. In the erect position there is a fluid level; it may be bilateral, or when small in amount, it may be on one side only. Varying positions of the heart contour are made visible by the surrounding air; frequently all of the contour can be seen by filming in both lateral decubitus positions. A remarkable feature is the freedom of motion of the heart within the air-containing pericardium. The amplitude of pulsations is increased, and both systolic and diastolic movements are quick. Left border motion as shown by roentgenkymography may be as much as 1.5 cm, or 3 times the normal. Furthermore, the normal pendulum motion and positional changes which occur during the various phases of the cardiac cycle are exaggerated, and this excess movement indicates the restraining effect of the surrounding normal pericardium and lungs. The pericardial fluid is constantly agitated by the heart beat so that small rapid waves cross the surface continuously.

The rate at which air disappears must vary somewhat with the condition of the pericardial cavity. This has not been carefully studied. Certainly a considerable amount will disappear within 1–2 days, and a large amount will be entirely gone within a week.

Pneumopericardium

Pneumopericardium of any extent can hardly be confused with any other condition. At times, however, it may resemble a number of lesions such as (1) an abscess or fluid-containing cyst in the adjacent portions of the lower lung, particularly on the left side; (2) achalasia of the esophagus with a fluid level; and (3) diaphragmatic

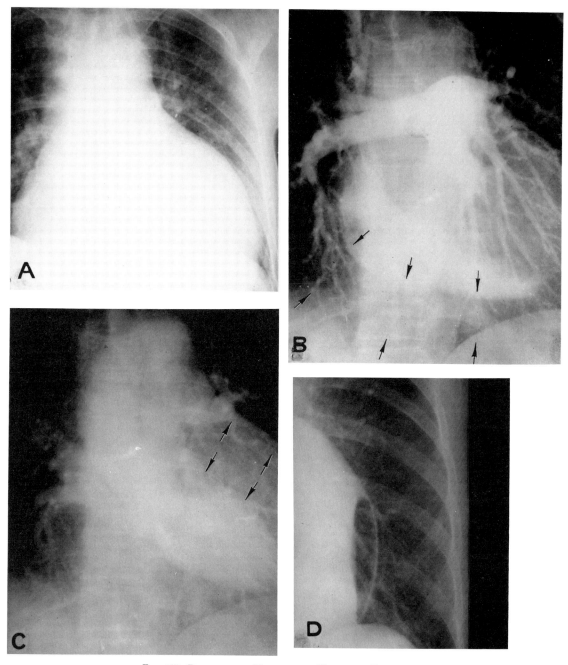

FIG. 482. PERICARDIAL EFFUSION OF UNKNOWN ETIOLOGY

Fifty-three-year-old white woman with no complaints referable to the heart. Globular cardiac enlargement (A) was noted on a routine chest film. Pericardial effusion was suspected, and image-amplified fluoroscopy and cinefluorography in the frontal projection were performed. During fluoroscopy a curvilinear epicardial fat line along the left heart border was seen to pulsate vigorously several centimeters deep to the external cardiac-pericardial shadow. The outer contour was motionless. On the basis of this finding, a large pericardial effusion was thought to be present, and venous angiocardiography was performed for confirmation. Contrast material in the right atrium and ventricle was seen to be widely separated from the right lateral heart margin and from the diaphragm (B). Later in the angiographic series the left ventricular cavity became opacified, and its outer margin was clearly shown to be several centimeters deep to the left lateral aspect of the silhouette of the heart (C). Following these procedures pericardial tap was performed with confirmation of the diagnosis of pericardial effusion. A small amount of air was introduced into the pericardial sac, and a film exposed in the right lateral decubitus position showed the air outlining a normally thin and smooth parietal pericardium (D). Examination of the fluid revealed it to be a transudate, and no cause for the patient's pericardial effusion was discovered.

hernia with fluid in the stomach or bowel. Fluoroscopy and barium studies of the esophagus and intestines usually eliminate these possibilities. A small amount of air is much more difficult to locate; it often localizes along the left border in the region of the pulmonary artery segment and may be confused with mediastinal emphysema. With mediastinal emphysema, however, there

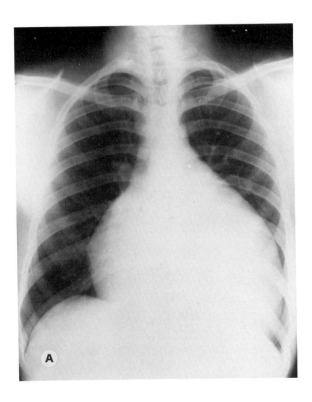

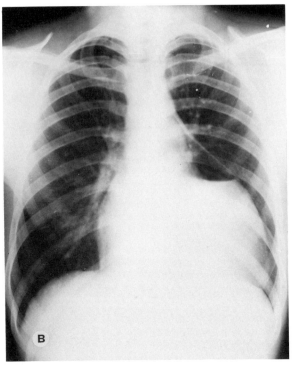

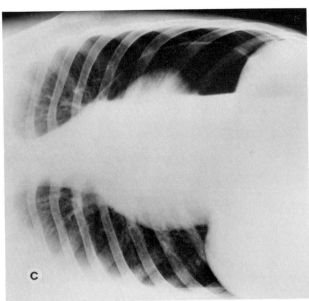

FIG. 483. MASSIVE PERICARDIAL EFFUSION IN YOUNG MAN; ETIOLOGY UNDETERMINED, POSSIBLY TUBERCULOUS
(A) Marked enlargement of cardiac contour although the base of the heart remains narrow. The lungs show no signs of congestion. (B) After removal of some fluid and replacement of about 150 cc of air. (C) Right lateral decubitus film showing a thin pericardium and evidence of a small heart.

may be a number of blebs along the lateral heart borders and around the great vessels, some of which are clearly outside the pericardium.

The etiology and treatment of pericardial fluid are influential in determining its duration. A single or repeated aspiration (Blalock and Ravitch, 1943) is recommended for control of hemopericardium secondary to trauma. Present day surgical consensus is in favor of exploration of the heart and pericardium (see section on Trauma to the Heart). Acute suppurative pericarditis usually requires open drainage, and this may be an emergency procedure.

Some degree of pericardial effusion is exceedingly common with acute rheumatic myocarditis; it may be the principal cause of cardiac enlargement in this condition. The fluid may accumulate within a day or so; rarely is the effusion sufficiently acute or extensive as to require treatment per se. It may continue for several weeks or resolve quickly depending somewhat on the clinical course of the patient, and it is prone to recur with each exacerbation of the disease. In the majority of cases it leaves no significant residual changes, but it is thought to be an uncommon cause of constrictive pericarditis and pericardial calcification.

Tuberculous effusions may exist for some time before they are diagnosed and typically run a course of many months. They are treated by aspiration, induced pneumopericardium and an-

tibiotics. The effusion may be bloody. Residual changes, such as thickening of the pericardium and calcification, are common. Tuberculosis was formerly thought to be the single most common cause of constrictive pericarditis (McKusick, 1952; Paul et al., 1948; Chambers et al., 1951). Hydropericardium is common in congestive heart failure and contributes to the roentgen picture of cardiac enlargement. It is thought by Kerley (1951) that a rapid reduction in heart size following medical treatment of this condition is due to resolution of the fluid. It seems likely that the fluid would add to the cardiac embarrassment, but this is rarely sufficient to demand specific treatment.

Malignant Tumors

Metastatic malignant tumors, such as carcinoma of the breast, lymphosarcoma and Hodgkin's disease, may produce a bloody effusion by invading the pericardium or myocardium. Radiation therapy may be followed by a complete but usually temporary resolution of the fluid.

In a considerable number of cases no adequate cause for the effusion is found. It may run a benign course and disappear without residual changes.

A pericardial effusion of slight to moderate extent is a frequent finding in myxedema. Certainly, the size, shape and activity of the heart are often typical of an effusion, although there

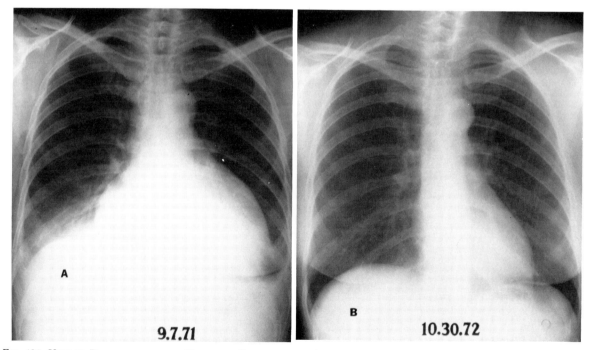

FIG. 484. UREMIC PERICARDITIS THAT RESOLVED FOLLOWING AN ACTIVE DIALYSIS PROGRAM AND MEDICAL MANAGEMENT

may be changes in the myocardium. The effusion disappears rapidly following thyroid medication.

Uremic Pericarditis

Formerly uremic pericarditis was part of a terminal illness and did not require specific diagnosis and treatment. Following an extensive use of hemodialysis, during which the patient may survive for many years, uremic pericarditis has become an increasingly important problem. Goldberg (1976) gives the incidence in patients on prolonged hemodialysis as 15%. Bailey et al. (1968) reporting on 83 patients found 33 (41%) had pericarditis at some time during the illness as evidenced by a friction rub. Most of these occurred prior to hemodialysis, but 11 episodes occurred during treatment. The cause of the pericarditis is not clearly understood, and the interested reader is referred to the extensive literature (Guild et al., 1957; Alfrey et al., 1968; Comty et al., 1971; Wray and Stone, 1976). The pericardial fluid is always bloody. Rapid and better control of dialysis is often beneficial, but some cases are progressive despite treatment and result in pericardial thickening and cardiac tamponade (Baldwin and Edwards, 1976; Singh et al., 1974; Moraski and Bousnaios, 1969). Pericardial aspiration may be helpful and at times lifesaving as the fluid can collect with amazing rapidity and can produce fatal tamponade. Some cases come to pericardiectomy because of constrictive pericarditis.

In the initial stages the heart contour increases in size (Bailey et al., 1968) and accompanying pleural effusions are common. Consequently, the radiologist should be sensitive and alert to an increase in heart size in a patient on hemodialysis. Following treatment the heart may return to normal, but if the signs of pleural fluid and heart failure persist, the possibility of constrictive pericarditis should be considered.

RADIATION INJURY TO THE HEART

The heart and pericardium are considered as relatively resistant to radiation. Following the use of moderately high doses (4400 rads in 4–5 weeks) such as is common with the mantle technique for the treatment of Hodgkin's disease and carcinoma of the breast, cardiac disease has been observed with some frequency (Stewart et al., 1967; Stewart and Fajardo, 1971; Martin et al., 1975; Byhardt et al., 1975; Ruckdeschel et al., 1975). Changes due to the radiation have been found in the valves, endocardium, myocardium, including myocardial infarcts, and most commonly the pericardium. With a dose of 4000 rads in 4 weeks, Ruckdeschel et al. (1975) found a 20% incidence of pericarditis. Byhardt et al. (1975) found 24 patients with pericarditis out of 83 treated to a pericardial dose of 5325 rads or 1823 rets. Ten of these were asymptomatic, and the main evidence of pericarditis was an increase in the transverse diameter of the heart of 1.5 cm or more. In the majority of cases the fluid resolved after a period of months to years, but in a few the process progressed to thickening of the pericardium producing constrictive pericarditis and requiring pericardiectomy (McCleod et al., 1969; Ruckdeschel et al., 1975). Retreatment of the mediastinum to a high dose is particulary hazardous and may carry an incidence of pericarditis of 40% (Stewart and Fajardo, 1971).

CONSTRICTIVE AND ADHESIVE PERICARDITIS

Small areas of thickening and fibrosis of both the epicardium and pericardium are commonly seen at autopsy. Adhesions between the pericardial layers or between the exterior of the pericardium and the surrounding pleural surfaces are not unusual; a sizeable area of the pericardial cavity may be obliterated, yet produce no symptoms and be an incidental finding at autopsy.

When fibrosis of the pericardium is more extensive and particularly when the scar is dense and unyielding or calcified, the heart may be partially or completely enclosed in a rigid case (concretio cordis). Also, external adhesions may extend anteriorly to the sternum and chest wall and/or to the lung, lung hilus, and mediastinum laterally and posteriorly. When these adhesions are massive or rigid and particularly when they extend to a bony structure, they restrict the heart action (accretio cordis). Constriction of the heart and adhesions to surrounding structures often coexist, and both may contribute to the clinical and roentgen picture in any one patient. Physiologically the constrictive effects are most important and probably more common and may give rise to a well established clinical entity, namely "chronic constrictive pericarditis."

Tuberculosis was proven as the etiologic agent in 25–33% of several older series of cases of constrictive pericarditis (McKusick, 1952; Paul *et al.,* 1948; Chambliss *et al.,* 1951). Recently chronic uremia with hemodialysis and radiation therapy using the mantle technique have become increasingly important etiologic agents. Other proven agents are histoplasmosis and Coxsackie B (Steinberg and Hagstrom, 1968), trauma, pyogenic infections, rheumatic fever and malignant tumors (White, 1948). In a sizeable proportion of cases the etiologic agent has disappeared and the cause is unknown.

Chronic constrictive pericarditis has received considerable attention since 1928, due in part to the fact that it is often amenable to surgical treatment. Undiagnosed and untreated, this condition commonly produces chronic invalidism and eventually death, although mild cases are seen. The diagnosis is not an easy one. It should be suspected in a patient with Beck's (1935) triad of a quiet heart, increased venous pressure and ascites out of proportion to dependent edema. Other signs and symptoms are shortness of breath and increased systemic venous pressure. It has been a cause of protein-losing enteropathy (Plauth *et al.,* 1964) and nephrotic syndrome (Pastor and Cohn, 1960) and associated with the syndrome of mulibrey nanism (Voorhees, 1976). The diagnosis is usually established by a combination of clinical, radiologic and physiologic studies.

In a study of six cases, Sawyer *et al.,* (1952) demonstrated that the basic disturbance in constrictive pericarditis was an inability of the ventricles to dilate sufficiently during diastole to maintain an adequate stroke volume and cardiac output. They found no evidence that one ventricle was selectively more constricted or that a constriction of the atria or narrowing of the vena cava were important factors. Also they noted that a long postoperative convalescence was usual before the heart function and dynamics returned to normal levels. In most of the patients the heart did not become entirely normal in its response to exercise and these investigators attributed this to atrophy of the myocardium. Summerville (1968) however suggests a more likely reason was the failure to obtain a complete removal of the adherent pericardium. Sawyer *et al.* (1952) found that pressures were significantly elevated in the right atrium, right ventricle, pulmonary artery and in the pulmonary capillary wedge position. These changes were compatible with pulmonary congestion which is a common finding on the chest film in constrictive pericarditis (Heinz and Abrams, 1957; Cornell and Rossi, 1968). The elevated wedge pressure indicated an elevated pressure in the left atrium and was attributed to involvement of the left ventricle by the constrictive process.

As seen on conventional chest films the heart in constrictive pericarditis is normal in size in about one-half of the cases (45% of 53 cases, Paul *et al.,* 1948; 50% of 16 cases, Heinz and Abrams, 1957). Consequently it should be emphasized that in only 40–45% of the cases the heart is slight to moderately enlarged and in a few cases it is markedly enlarged (Chambliss *et al.,* 1951). Cardiac enlargement when present is due mainly to thickening of the pericardium. Pleural fluid, pleural, and pleuro pericardial adhesions and an

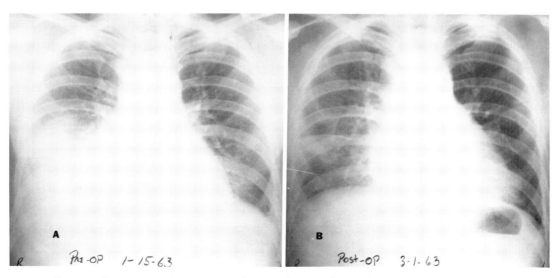

FIG. 485. CONSTRICTIVE PERICARDITIS BEFORE (A) AND 6 WEEKS AFTER PERICARDIECTOMY (B).

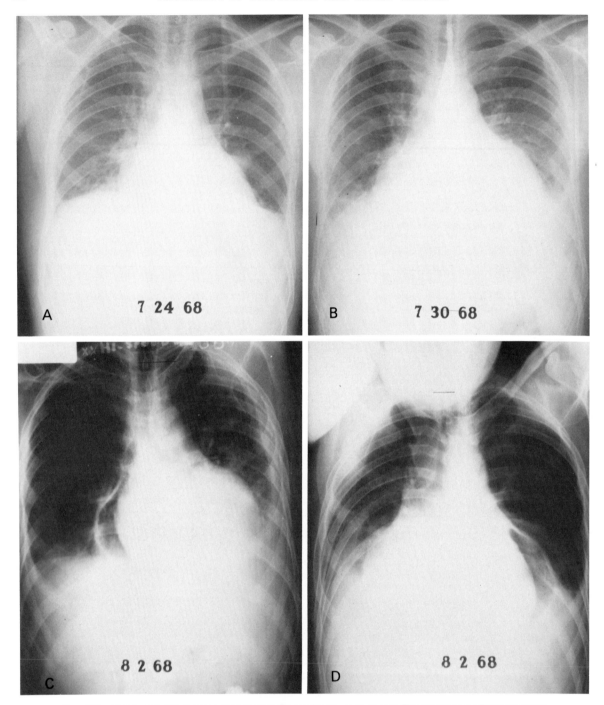

FIG. 486. TUBERCULOUS PERICARDITIS WITH RAPID PROGRESSION AND THICKENING OF PERICARDIUM
C and D show air injected after aspiration of fluid. Constrictive pericarditis developed requiring pericardiectomy.

elevated diaphragm are quite common with constrictive pericarditis and may partially obscure the cardiac contour. The cardiac contour is rarely normal. The usual indentation at the junction of the superior vena cava with the right atrium may be obliterated. A rigid right atrial border which

has lost its normal outward convexity is emphasized by Zatuchi *et al.* (1961) as a finding indicative of structural abnormality of the pericardium but does not necessarily signify hemodynamic abnormality. The aortic knob is usually small or normal in size. Enlargement of individual chambers is difficult to determine with certainty. The right ventricle is often enlarged (81%, Cornell and Rossi, 1968, and 3 of 17 cases, Heinz and Abrams, 1957). Pulmonary congestion is present in about one-half of the cases and the pulmonary artery is enlarged in the majority of cases. Pulmonary edema is an unusual finding (Sawyer *et al.*, 1952). Enlargement of the left atrium has been variable in different series—76% in the series of Cornell and Rossi (1968) and 3 of 21 cases in the series of Heinz and Abrams, (1957). The superior vena cava and azygous vein are frequently dilated giving an increased width to the upper mediastinum.

Calcification in the Pericardium

Calcification in the pericardium is a sign of considerable importance and occurs in 30–60% of cases of constrictive pericarditis (Rigler, 1941; Powell *et al.*, 1948; Chambliss *et al.*, 1951; Evans and Jackson, 1952; Cornell and Rossi, 1968). It is not pathognomonic of constriction, however, and may produce no symptoms (Mathewson, 1955). On the other hand, when associated with definite clinical and radiologic signs, it may strongly support the diagnosis. It may be elusive and is best demonstrated by careful fluoroscopy or over penetrated films using a high speed bucky diaphragm. The calcium may be found over any part of the heart, but the most frequent sites are the diaphragmatic and anterior surfaces. Dense deposits are frequent in the atrial-ventricular sulci; these may compress the heart sufficiently over a localized area to produce stenosis at the valve ring. White *et al.* (1948) report a case in which left atrial enlargement was due to mitral stenosis secondary to external compression on the lateral aspect of the mitral valve by fibrous scarring in the pericardium. The apex is often free of calcium. At times the entire heart is encased in a calcific shell. The calcium may be thin like an egg-shell or it may be dense, massive and reach a centimeter in thickness. Occasionally the calcium extends into the myocardium and is extensive; it is frequently molded close to the heart contour and often appears to be holding or supporting the heart.

Pulsations of the heart have been variable in the authors' experience and rarely provide decisive information. Typically they should be diminished or absent over some portion or other of the cardiac contour but this is not always so. Pulsations were normal in 8 of 53 cases reported by Paul *et al.* (1948) and in 33% of 24 cases reported by Heinz and Abrams (1957) and only 5% of 21 cases reported by Cornell and Rossi (1968).

Roentgen kymographic studies of constrictive pericarditis were reported by Rigler *et al.* (1941)

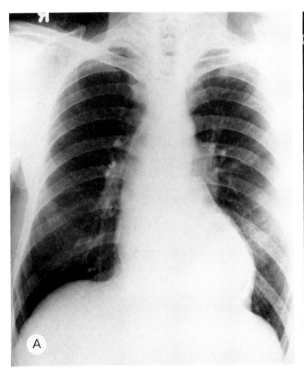
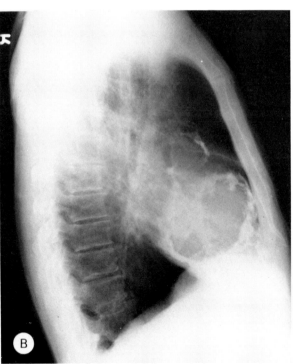

FIG. 487. CONSTRICTIVE PERICARDITIS WITH EXTENSIVE PLATE-LIKE CALCIFICATION IN PERICARDIUM

and electrokymographic studies by Gillick and Reynolds (1950) and McKusick (1952). The kymographic curves particularly of ventricular pulsations are distinctive and are mentioned here because they represent the fundamental nature of the disorder. The systolic limb as seen on the electrokymograph is steep and rather straight. The diastolic limb is almost equally as steep and terminates abruptly in a flat top which persists for the remainder of diastole. There are no minor secondary positional or rotational waves which usually occur at the beginning of systole and diastole. The period during which the heart is motionless is relatively increased and such a change is occasionally perceptible to the eye at fluoroscopy. These curves have been called "The flat-top and V pattern" (see Fig. 488B). They have their counterparts in the pressure curves taken from the right and left ventricles in constrictive pericarditis (Plauth *et al.*, 1964; Sawyer *et al.*, 1952). These curves are described as showing the early diastolic dip and plateau curve and indicate that there is a rapid filling of the ventricles during early diastole following by an abrupt stop to ventricular filling with a high end diastolic pressure. The diastolic pressure curve is often as steep in descent as the systolic curve is steep in ascent. This type of pressure tracing taken from the ventricles is of considerable di-

agnostic importance. Desilets *et al.* (1966) using cineangiography in cases of constrictive pericarditis, demonstrated the abrupt stop to both atrial and ventricular filling that would be the counterpart of the pressure curves.

Dotter and Steinberg (1951), Figley and Bagshaw (1957), and Steinberg and Hagstrom (1968) have reported on the angiographic features of constrictive pericarditis. These are as follows: (1) increased width of the soft tissue band between the right atrial cavity filled with contrast substance and the adjacent air containing lung. In the normal heart this should not exceed 4 mm. In constrictive pericarditis it was 6–9 mm in thickness and in pericardial effusion it was often 1 cm. more in thickness (Figley and Bagshaw, 1957). The authors caution against confusing pleural fluid with thickening of the right atrial wall. (2) The right atrial border lacked its usual normal convexity. It was often straight or concave. (3) No change in contour of the right atrium was demonstrated from film to film. (4) Dilatation of the superior vena cava was often present and where there was reflux the inferior vena cava was also dilated. (5) In diastole the ventricles were normal or reduced in size. This is of value in excluding most cardiomyopathies and other conditions that cause chronic heart failure. (6) Occasional evidence of right atrial and left atrial

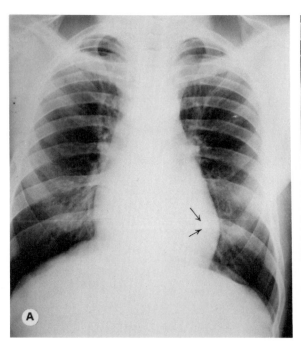 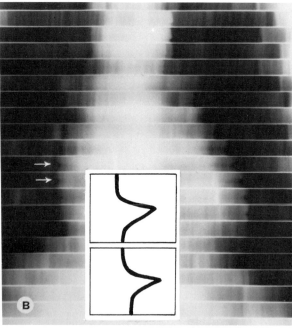

FIG. 488. CONSTRICTIVE PERICARDITIS (OPERATIVE CASE) SECONDARY TO BULLET WOUND IN 19YEAR-OLD BLACK MALE PATIENT

(A) Conventional film showing a bullet in the neighborhood of the pericardium. The film was exposed more than a year after the initial injury. (B) Roentgenkymogram showing flat top and V controus particularly along the right lower border.

enlargement that is quite compatible with the diagnosis of constrictive pericarditis.

In the authors' experience the diagnosis of constrictive pericarditis is made from a combination of clinical, angiographic, and hemodynamic studies. Cardiac catheterization is essential in ruling out other forms of cardiac disease and the ventricular pressure curves (diastolic dip and plateau pattern) are highly suggestive of constriction. Conditions that can mimic constrictive pericarditis are primary amyloid of the heart (Gunnar et al., 1955) and certain types of constrictive cardiomyopathies (McKusick, 1952). The radiologist is reminded that an enlarged heart with normal pulsations and radiologic evidence of pulmonary congestion is quite compatible with the diagnosis of constrictive pericarditis.

CONGENITAL ANOMALIES

Congenital defects in the pericardium are rare. Hipona and Crummy (1964) found 108 recorded cases and added 3 of their own. About 75% of the defects are on the left side (Ellis et al., 1959), and about 75% are incomplete or partial (Hipona and Crummy, 1964). Moene et al. (1973) and Ellis et al. (1959) suggest that the defect is the result of a faulty development of the primitive pleuropericardial canal. The development of the left canal is more complicated and therefore more subject to anomalous development.

Associated congenital anomalies occurred in about 30% of reported cases and include atrial septal defect, patent ductus arteriosus, bicuspid aortic valve, bronchogenic cysts, pulmonary sequestration, and hiatus hernia (Tabakin et al., 1965).

Most patients are asymptomatic, and the condition is compatible with a normal life span. Chest pain has been reported in several instances (Fisher and Ehrenhaft, 1964). Pain could be due to a number of mechanisms, such as undue torsion or strain on the great vessels which serve as the only anchor for a ptotic heart; lack of a

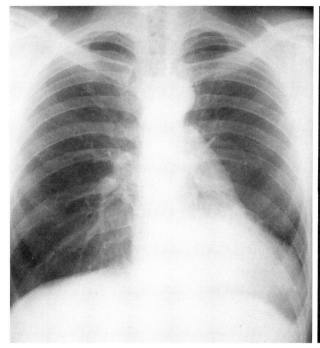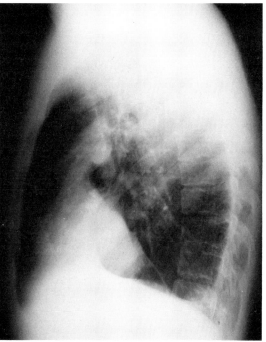

FIG. 489. CONGENITAL ABSENCE OF PERICARDIUM (COMPLETE)

Patient is 39-year-old white man with frequent colds and productive cough. On physical examination there were no murmurs or other abnormal cardiac findings. Posteroanterior and lateral chest films, above, show prominence of the pulmonary trunk with increased length of its arc. The pulmonary artery is unusually well defined on both frontal and lateral films. The heart appears to be unrestrained and to "sag" toward the left, its shape conforming to that of the left hemidiaphragm. The lingula of the left upper lobe is partly and irregularly consolidated. At operation complete absence of the pericardium was found. The heart was shifted toward the left and covered a large part of the left hemidiaphragm. Adhesions between the lingula and the heart had produced distortion of the left upper lobe bronchus, with atelectasis of the lingula.

cushioning effect of the pericardium, allowing the heart to pound freely on the overlying lung or chest wall; tension on pleuropericardial adhesions which form in the absence of a parietal pericardium; or impingement of the rim of the defect on the coronary arteries. Both the left and right atrial appendages are susceptible to herniation and may produce severe symptoms (Chang and Leigh, 1961; Duffie *et al.*, 1962; Dimond *et al.*, 1960). Right-sided defects may have a reverse herniation of the lung into the pericardium (Moene *et al.*, 1973; Hipona and Crummy, 1964). One case was reported in which a 28-year-old woman died suddenly following herniation of the heart through a large left pericardial foramen (Kavanheh-Gray *et al.*, 1961).

Radiologic Findings. The appearance of partial defects of the pericardium as seen on conventional chest films is variable depending on whether or not there is associated herniation of the heart or lung. If the heart is herniated, it appears as a mass projecting from the cardiac border. In the frontal projection, the pericardial sac extends ordinarily between the level of the third and seventh ribs in their anterior aspects, and the mass should be located within this level. The size and shape of the herniated mass are

dependent upon the size of the foramen and the herniated part. The left atrial appendage is the most common portion of the heart that is liable to herniation. The appendage may appear as a wedge-shaped density interposed between the pulmonary trunk above and the left ventricle below. In 2 cases of partial right-sided defects, the right lung herniated into the pericardium around the base of the heart (Moene *et al.*, 1973; Hipona and Crummy, 1964). This produced a radiolucent shadow that surrounded the aorta as seen in the lateral view and was suggestive of a pneumopericardium. In one case (Moene *et al.*, 1973), the herniation exerted pressure on the superior vena cava producing a minor degree of obstruction.

With complete left-sided pericardial defect one may see a shift of the heart to the left and an unusual cardiac silhouette in the frontal projection. The left heart border may be flattened as the heart stretches out over the left dome of the diaphragm (Fig. 489). Three convexities are seen along the left heart border, the aortic knob, a long prominent and sharply demarcated pulmonary artery segment, and a distinct left ventricular contour. These findings presumably result from the more intimate contact between the left

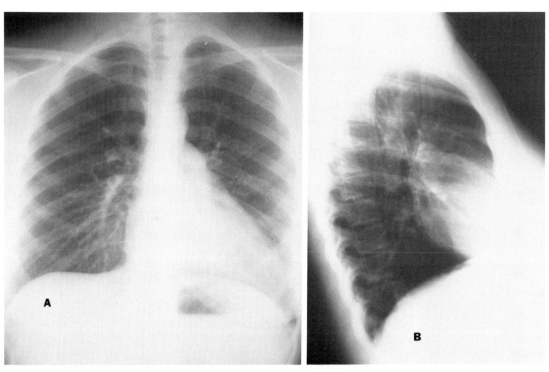

FIG. 490. PARTIAL ABSENCE OF THE LEFT SIDE OF PERICARDIUM

(A and B) Frontal and lateral chest films of an asymptomatic young woman. The pulsations of the pulmonary artery segment were exaggerated and cardiac contour in the upper portion of left side is quite sharply defined as well as over the posterior surface of the heart.

lung and the heart and great vessels (Fisher and Ehrenhaft, 1964). Frequently the radiolucent lung may extend underneath the heart contour separating it for a variable distance from the diaphragm.

Diagnostic pneumothorax is an important method of investigation when congenital pericardial defect is suspected. The demonstration of pneumopericardium following induction of an artificial pneumothorax is diagnostic. The absence of pneumopericardium following pneumothorax does not necessarily rule out the presence of a pericardial defect, however, since in some cases adhesions might prevent the accumulation of air in the pericardial sac. Such cases are unusual, however. In the case of a small defect, considerable maneuvering of the patient may be necessary to permit air to enter the pericardium.

Angiocardiography may help to rule out other cardiac abnormalities and will give positive information concerning the anatomic location of the herniated part in the case of a partial pericardial defect (Hering *et al.*, 1960; Dimond *et al.*, 1960). Chang and Amory (1965) report a case of partial right pericardial defect through which the right atrial appendage had herniated. The diagnosis was established by angiocardiography.

A supine lateral chest film utilizing a horizontally directed beam may reveal the ability of the heart to fall away from the anterior chest wall and diaphragm in the complete absence of the left pericardium (Ellis *et al.*, 1959). Payvandi and Kerber (1976) advocate both the right and left lateral decubiti with filming in the frontal projection to show abnormal movement of the heart. They also employed echocardiography to show abnormal movement of the ventricular septum which suggests abnormal mobility of the heart. Failure to demonstrate the pericardium in its usual position posterior to the heart or elsewhere

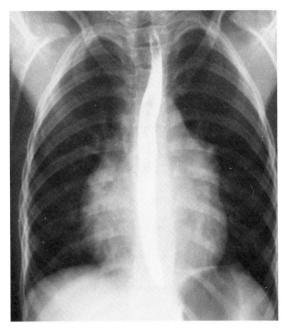

FIG. 491. PARTIAL ABSENCE OF LEFT UPPER PERICARDIUM WITH HERNIATION OF ATRIAL APPENDAGE CONFIRMED AT OPERATION FOR PATIENT DUCTUS ARTERIOSUS
The lateral border of the pulmonary artery is clearly inside of the localized convexity.

by echocardiography is unreliable.

In the case of partial pericardial defect with herniation of a portion of the heart, ordinarily the left atrial appendage, differential diagnosis includes aneurysm of the heart, dilatation of the pulmonary artery, and bronchogenic or mediastinal neoplasm. In the absence of symptoms, surgical repair is not indicated. In the presence of symptoms, surgical closure of the defect, perhaps combined with amputation of the herniated atrial appendage, may be undertaken (Dimond *et al.*, 1960).

CYSTS AND DIVERTICULA

Cysts and diverticula of the pericardium may be congenital or acquired. Congenital cysts are presumably due to a deviation in the development of the pericardial cavity. In the early embryo the forerunner of the pericardium is a series of mesothelial lacunae. These fuse to form the large definitive pericardial cavity. In rare instances a lacuna fails to fuse properly; it may remain separate from but communicates with the pericardium through a small opening and thus represents a diverticulum. More frequently there may be no communication, the resulting cyst being attached to the pericardium by a

pedicle and receiving its blood supply by the same route. These are known as "pericardial celomic cysts." Both cysts and diverticula contain a thin watery fluid. The cysts may be multilocular.

Acquired cysts or diverticula may be due to a number of mechanisms. A hydropericardium may produce a herniation of a weakened segment of the pericardium, and this may become encysted or remain as a diverticulum (Kerley, 1951). Maier (1958) suggests that this is the more common cause since pericardial diverticula have not been reported in infants. Inflammatory proc-

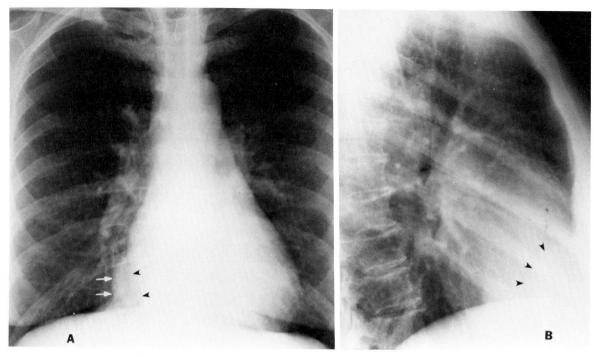

FIG. 492. PERICARDIAL CYST IN THE RIGHT CARDIOPHRENIC ANGLE.
THIS IS THE MOST COMMON LOCATION FOR THESE CYSTS

esses in the pericardium can produce fluid which may herniate through the pericardium and produce a cystic structure (Loehr, 1952). Bronchial cysts may be embedded in the heart (Dabbs *et al.*, 1957), and teratomas may be attached to the heart. Certain tumors, such as lymphangiomas, are cystic, but these are exceedingly rare. Pericardial cysts were classified by Loehr (1952) as follows:

True Cysts
    Congenital
        Pericardial celomic cyst
        Cystic lymphangioma
        Bronchial cyst
        Teratoma
    Acquired
        Cystic hematoma
        Neoplastic cyst
        Parasitic cyst
Pseudocysts
    Pericardial diverticulum
    Encapsulated pericardial exudate

The majority of pericardial cysts produce no symptoms and are an incidental finding as seen on a conventional chest film. If they reach a large size, they may produce chest pain. It is not unusual to note that they have appeared over a period of a few years (Klatte and Yune, 1972). Under observation they grow very slowly or more often are stationary in size over a considerable period of time. They are most commonly encountered during middle age.

Radiologic Findings. As seen on conventional chest films the cyst or diverticulum is a smooth, rounded or elliptical structure that presents along one of the heart borders. They are more frequently found near the cardiophrenic angle and more often on the right side. They are seldom seen around the base of the heart (Klatte and Yune, 1972). Pericardial cysts rarely calcify, and it is probable that the celomic variety does not calcify. If calcium is found, an inflammatory origin is suggested (Loehr, 1952). The calcium is usually thin like an eggshell and peripheral and may actually be in the pericardium adjacent to the inflammatory cyst. The presence of calcium also suggests the possibility of a teratoma or a bronchogenic cyst (Dabbs *et al.*, 1957). Echinococcus cysts calcify, but the calcium is typically quite heavy (Zigmor and Scuzs, 1945). Frequently a pericardial cyst will show an acute angle at its junction with the pericardium. This suggests that in some cases the mass is connected with the pericardium by a broad pedicle. Pericardial cysts and diverticula have a density similar to that of the heart. However, in certain projections the cyst may appear slightly less dense, and this could be of some diagnostic significance (Loehr, 1952).

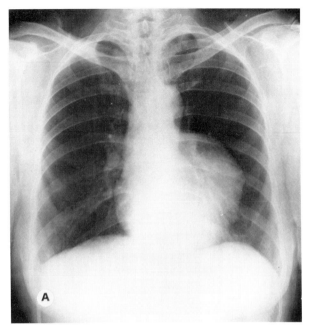

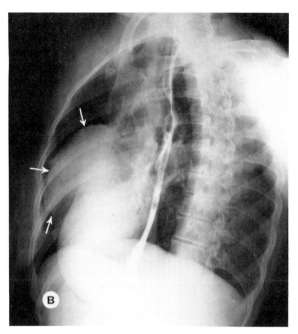

FIG. 493. PERICARDIAL CYST ATTACHED HIGH ON LEFT HEART BORDER
(A) Posteroanterior projection. (B) Left anterior oblique projection. Arrows indicate the anterior outline of the cyst. The patient had very minor symptoms.

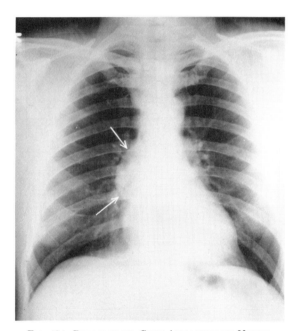

FIG. 494. PERICARDIAL CYST ATTACHED TO UPPER
PORTION OF PERICARDIUM ON RIGHT
The patient was completely asymptomatic. Transmitted pulsations of the lateral wall of the cyst (arrows) were minimal.

The cyst typically changes in contour with respiration. It usually elongates with inspiration and becomes shorter and wider with expiration. This change in contour is a sign of some diag-

nostic significance and tends to exclude a solid tumor.

Diverticula tend to become smaller in certain positions due to the drainage of the fluid from the cyst into the pericardial cavity. The patient should be placed in a suitable decubitus position, and the size and contour of the cyst should be observed (Fell *et al.*, 1959). A cyst may show pulsations, but these are transmitted (Fell *et al.*, 1959). Angiocardiography may be used to exclude a cardiac aneurysm, a cardiac tumor or abnormal chamber enlargement. It is not diagnostic.

Formerly definitive diagnosis could be established only by thoracotomy. Klatte and Yune (1972) advocate aspiration of the cyst and injection of water soluble contrast substance. In the typical celomic cyst the fluid is thin and watery. The fluid, of course, can be examined for inflammatory cells, bacteria and tumor cells. The interior of the cyst should be smooth in all projections. The contrast substance is withdrawn. In 2 cases in which this procedure was carried out, the cyst collapsed and did not reappear over a 3 year period of follow-up. This procedure is recommended in lieu of a thoracotomy provided the benignity of the cyst is established by examination of the withdrawn fluid and the contour of the cyst wall.

Computed tomography is now the recommended procedure in that diagnosis of pericardial cyst.

The differential diagnosis includes diaphragmatic hernia through the foramen of Morgagni, mediastinal teratomas and other neoplasms, cardiac chamber enlargement, aneurysm of the heart, ascending aorta or sinuses of Valsalva, pericardial fat pad (Nahon, 1955), pericarditis, anterior mediastinal pleuritis, and occasionally bronchogenic carcinoma and solitary metastatic pulmonary nodules.

TUMORS

Primary tumors of the pericardium are rare. The ratio of benign to malignant tumor is about one-to-one (Abrams *et al.*, 1971). Yater (1931) found fibromas and sarcomas arising from the fibrous tissue of the pericardium, also mesotheliomas, neurofibromas and teratomas. Vascular tumors, such as hemangiomas, lymphangiomas, and lymphangioendotheliomas, are uncommon and are often incidental findings (Abrams *et al.*, 1971). DeCarlo and Lindquist (1950) described a hemangiosarcoma of the pericardium in which the cardiac silhouette was greatly enlarged and angiocardiography showed an obstruction of the superior vena cava and displacement of both the atrium and vena cava due to a large tumor mass in the right side of the pericardium. In intrapericardial masses, conventional chest films are of little aid in diagnosis, but angiocardiography may show characteristic rotation of the heart by the intrapericardial mass (Steinberg, 1960). Angiocardiography may also demonstrate associated pericardial effusion. The exclusion of heart disease by angiocardiography when there is a massive cardiac silhouette will hasten surgical exploration of the mediastinum and pericardium and permit definitive diagnosis and appropriate therapy. Waldhausen *et al.* (1959) report the case of a 23-year-old man in whom a primary mesothelioma of the pericardium compressed the pulmonary artery and produced the physical findings of obstruction to right ventricular outflow. A selective right ventricular angiogram demonstrated the extrinsic character of the obstruction and its anatomic relations. The tumor was successfully excised.

Primary pericardial tumors may produce only a localized bulge in the cardiac contour. The diagnosis should be considered whenever a bizarre cardiac silhouette is encountered.

Metastatic or secondary tumors of the pericardium are much more common than primary tumors. The most common is carcinoma of the lung which usually reaches the pericardium by direct extension (Hanfling, 1968). Other common metastases are from the breast, lymphoma and leukemia, and malignant melanoma. The pericardial metastases usually do not cause symptoms (Hanfling, 1968) but may produce a serous or bloody effusion. Metastatic carcinoma may also contribute to a constrictive pericarditis (Sla-

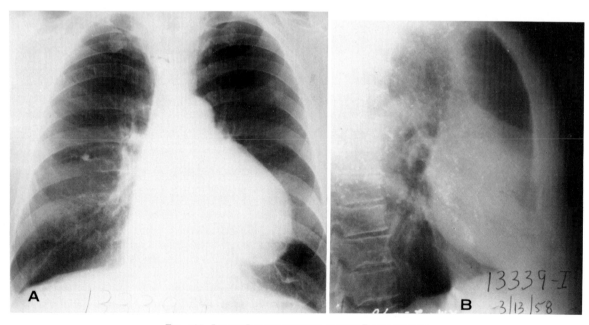

FIG. 495. LARGE LYMPHANGIOMA OF THE PERICARDIUM

ter *et al.*, 1952). The possibility of pericardial metastases should be considered when the heart enlarges in a patient with known disseminated malignant disease.

POSTPERICARDIOTOMY SYNDROME

The clinical profile of patients with this syndrome consists of an abrupt onset of chest pain which may radiate to the shoulder, fever, cough and often physical signs of pleuritis or pericarditis. It is most commonly seen in patients who have had open heart surgery or in any operation in which the pericardium has been opened. A similar picture may follow myocardial infarction (Dressler's Syndrome, Dressler, 1956; Arnold, 1963), blunt or penetrating trauma to the chest and implantation of a transvenous pacemaker (Kaye *et al.*, 1975). The incidence following open heart surgery was estimated at 20–30%, but this seems too high in the authors' experience (McCabe *et al.*, 1974). Adequate postoperative drainage from the thoracic and mediastinal cav-

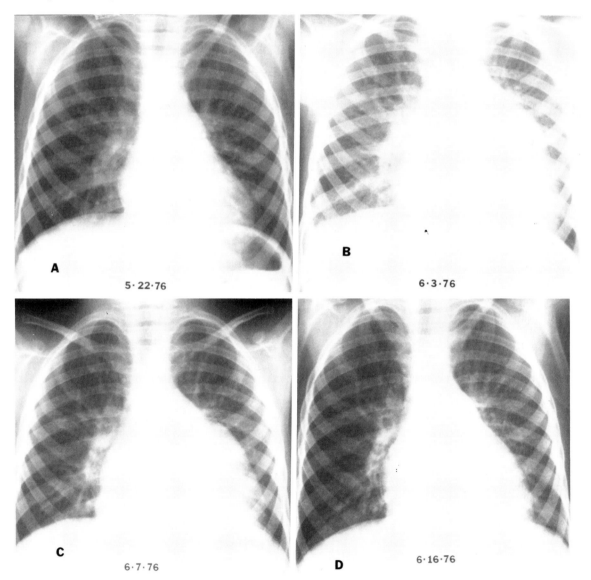

FIG. 496. POSTPERICARDIECTOMY SYNDROME IN A 2-YEAR-OLD

(A) Three days postoperative following repair of ASD. (B) Patient returned with mild elevation of temperature, pulse 150/min and vomiting. Treated with digitalis and later with aspirin. C and D represent gradual response and patient was discharged.

ities seems to be helpful in preventing the syndrome (Cunningham *et al.*, 1975). Serologic tests using autologous pericardium and myocardium indicate that the syndrome is due to hypersensitivity (Engle *et al.*, 1974, 1975).

There may be no radiologic changes, but when they occur they are suggestive although not specific. The syndrome is most frequent in the first 2–3 weeks, although it may occur as long as 14 months postoperatively. Rapid enlargement of the heart is suggestive, particularly when accompanied by fever, dampening of the heart sounds, and ECG evidence of pericardial reaction. Echocardiographic evidence of pericardial fluid is helpful in diagnosis. A small amount of pleural fluid and rarely pulmonary opacities are seen. Rapid regression in heart size, particularly following the use of steroids, is also suggestive. Rarely a pericardiectomy may be necessary to control the recurrent pericardial effusion (McCabe *et al.*, 1974). The condition at times may be confused with recurrent rheumatic fever.

25

Diseases of the Thoracic Aorta and Its Branches

ANATOMICAL CONSIDERATIONS

The aorta originates at the aortic valve which lies slightly to the left of but near the midline and roughly at the level of the eighth to ninth thoracic vertebrae. In its first or intracardiac portion the ascending aorta extends toward the right and upward and soon crosses the midline where it lies just anterior to the superior vena cava. After crossing the midline, the aorta curves so as to extend upward and parallel to the vertebral column, and its medial part normally overlays the vertebral column. After a short distance the aorta again crosses the midline at about the level of the fifth thoracic vertebra and by arching obliquely posteriorly forms the aortic knob as seen in the posteroanterior projection of the chest. The first part of the descending aorta is posterior to and in close relationship with the left pulmonary artery and then the left main bronchus. Usually the descending aorta deviates slightly medialward and descends within the mediastinum to the diaphragmatic hiatus which lies at the level of the eleventh or twelfth thoracic vertebra. The aorta is anchored or fixed to a degree at two points, namely (1) at its origin at the aortic valve and (2) at the diaphragmatic hiatus, whereas the remainder of the aorta is supported by rather loose mediastinal connective tissue which permits a considerable degree of motion and redundancy. Some support of the aortic arch is also provided by the large brachiocephalic branches, and some degree of fixation is provided by the intercostal arteries.

The aortic valve is deep within the cardiac silhouette, and the first 3 cm of the ascending aorta cannot be demonstrated except by the use of angiography. Even after the aorta emerges from the heart contour its shadow is superimposed on that of the superior vena cava, and it can be seen by conventional x-ray means only where the margins are brought into contrast with some other structure of different density such as the air-containing lung or trachea or barium within the esophagus. Often the entire width of the upper part of the ascending portion and arch of the aorta in persons of slender or medium build may be seen on good quality films exposed in the left anterior oblique projection. Also, in the region of the aortic knob in the posteroanterior projection an approximate transverse section of the arch is outlined by the contrast with the lung on one side and the barium-filled esophagus on the other.

In the posteroanterior projection the lateral margin of the descending aorta is frequently visible through the cardiac silhouette, although the medial border is obscured by the overlying vertebral column and heart. In the lateral view the descending aorta often casts a faint shadow anterior to the thoracic spine.

DISEASE PROCESSES THAT AFFECT THE AORTA

Disease processes that affect the aorta sufficiently to produce radiologic findings are quite numerous. Congenital abnormalities of the aorta (aneurysm of the sinuses of Valsalva, coarctation, PDA, etc.) are considered in the section on congenital heart disease. Also, conditions due to inherited abnormalities of connective tissue, such as the Marfan syndrome and homocystinuria, are treated in a special section. Trauma to the aorta is treated in Chapter 22.

The most common disease process in the thoracic aorta is atherosclerosis, and it has gross and microscopic characteristics that allow it to be positively identified in most instances. Atherosclerosis is a ubiquitous process and is often superimposed on many other diseases of the aorta and may be so extensive as to obscure the underlying original cause of an aortitis.

Until the past three decades, syphilis was a common cause of changes in the ascending aorta and the adjacent valve cusps and ring. With the advent of treatment by penicillin, a drastic decline in the incidence of late syphilis of the cardiovascular system has been noted. It was formerly believed that the gross and microscopic changes of syphilitic aortitis were specific and recognizable by gross and microscopic examination. The disease process begins and is predominantly confined to the aortic media with some later involvement of the adventitia. The medial coat is partially or completely replaced by fibrous tissue with weakening of the wall. Probably due to changes in thickness and elasticity of the underlying media the intima shows longitudinal ridges and also transverse striations giving a "tree-bark" appearance that grossly is highly suggestive of syphilis. In addition to these changes in the aortic root and ascending aorta, the adjacent valve ring and cusps are often involved. The valve ring is usually dilated. The valve cusps are often fibrotic and shortened. The dilatation of the valve ring leads to separation of the commissures, and the entire process results in some degree of aortic regurgitation. A pulsatile blood flow against the weakened aortic wall frequently causes dilatation, usually localized, and in many cases there is a formation of an aneurysm. It is now known that similar changes are associated with a sizeable number of other diseases, and these have become increasingly important. The more common of these along with important contributions to the literature are aortitis associated with rheumatoid arthritis (Mallory, 1936; Clark et al., 1957), ankylosing spondylitis (Zvaifler and Weintraub, 1963), the Reiter syndrome (Paulus et al., 1972), scleroderma (Roth and Kissane, 1964), rheumatic fever (Paptenheimer and Von Glahn, 1924), giant cell arteritis (Zumbrow et al., 1975; Austin et al., 1965), tuberous sclerosis (Dutton and Singleton, 1975), relapsing polychondritis (Haimer et al., 1969), and in a number of cases the origin has been obscure and designated as idiopathic (Marquis et al., 1968).

Bacterial infections may attack the aorta at any point but are most common just above the aortic valve usually secondary to bacterial endocarditis, or distal to some point of obstruction such as a coarctation. The inflammatory process may progress to the formation of a mycotic aneurysm (Osler, 1885; Osler and McCray, 1908, Pg. 454). Mycotic aneurysms may be primary and "not associated with any demonstrable intravascular inflammatory focus" (Crane, 1937) or secondary to some other inflammatory process such as endocarditis or infection in the surrounding lung or mediastinum.

Takayasu's arteritis, although having some of the characteristics of the other types of aortitis, grossly is different in that it produces marked thickening of the aortic wall with proliferation of the intima and narrowing or occlusion of the aorta or one of its major branches. It is proposed by Lande (1976) that it is the major cause of coarctation at unusual sites including those in the abdominal aorta. It may be a cause of aneurysm formation (Lande and Berkman, 1976; Deutsch et al., 1974). The distribution of Takayasu's arteritis is different from the other common types of aortitis in that it has a predilection for the arch, descending and abdominal aorta and frequently involves one or more of the major branches. It is a cause of the aortic arch syndrome (Ross and McKusick, 1953). It also may involve the pulmonary arteries producing narrowing or occlusion (Lande and Beckman, 1976).

Cystic medial necrosis may have several causes. It occurs frequently in the Marfan syndrome and is described as an abiotrophy of the connective tissue in the media of the aorta (McKusick, 1972). It also may appear as a reaction to increased stress or turbulence secondary to aortic stenosis (McKusick et al., 1957). It is the cause of dilatation of the ascending aorta and aneurysm formation and predisposes to a dissecting hematoma.

Hypertension causes dilatation of the thoracic aorta most pronounced in its ascending portion. It is a more important factor when it is associated with aortitis and associated weakening of the aortic wall.

Gross changes in the aorta which are susceptible to demonstration by radiologic means may be classified as follows:
1. Elongation (tortuosity)
2. Dilatation
   (a) Localized
   (b) Generalized
3. Increased amplitude of pulsation
4. Increase in density
   (a) Fine, linear calcification in aortic wall
   (b) Irregular, lumpy calcification in aortic wall
5. Irregularities in aortic contour

6. Irregularities in contour of lumen (lack of parallelism of walls)
7. Aneurysm formation
    (a) Fusiform
    (b) Saccular
    (c) Dissecting
    (d) False and mycotic
8. Obstruction
    (a) Coarctation at unusual sites

Atherosclerosis

Atherosclerosis is so commonly seen with advancing years that it is considered to be a part of the aging process. Its onset is variable; however, when atherosclerosis of the aorta is pronounced or when it is detectable before the age of 40, it should be considered abnormal.

Atherosclerosis produces elongation of the aorta. Since the aorta is fixed to a degree at its origin from the heart and at the diaphragmatic hiatus, elongation must bring on a more devious course between these two points. On conventional posteroanterior roentgenograms elongation is manifested by deviation of the ascending aortic contour toward the right. The aortic shadow extends lateralward beyond the shadow of the superior vena cava. The aortic knob is increased in prominence; also, the knob may be elevated and be just below the left sternoclavicular joint. The tortuous descending aorta can be followed through the superimposed cardiac contour or the tortuosity may be so great that the descending aorta extends beyond the left heart border or is distinguished only with difficulty from the left heart border. As the aorta approaches the diaphragm, it swings toward the midline; occasionally the tortuosity of the aorta is so great that a knuckle-like projection is visible beyond the left heart border.

Associated with the atherosclerotic change, there is an increase in aortic density. The aortic wall is actually thickened, and there may be deposits of calcium which are too small to be individually visible but are sufficient to give a general increase in aortic density. Calcified plaques which are easily visible by roentgen means are common. These are crescent or sickle shaped and are most frequently seen in the region of the aortic knob. Isolated deposits of gross calcium due to atherosclerosis alone are rarely seen in the root and ascending portion of the aorta but are occasionally associated with calcium in the arch. Calcium due to atherosclerosis is usually irregular and lumpy and is to be distinguished from fine, linear sharply defined calcium which is occasionally seen in the ascending aorta associated with aortitis such as syphilis. How-

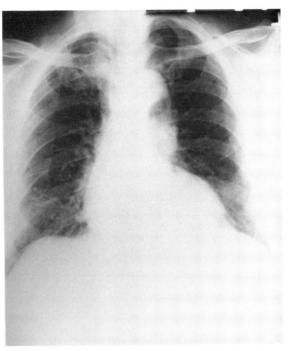

Fig. 497. Hypertensive and Arteriosclerotic Changes in Aorta in 70-Year-Old Man

The aorta is elongated and tortuous, particularly in its descending portion.

ever, atherosclerosis may be superimposed upon the dystrophic calcification due to aortitis and obscure it. Higgins and Reinke (1974) believe that even distinct linear calcification in the ascending aorta is no longer commonly due to syphilis and is more likely due to atherosclerosis.

The normal aortic root lies deep within the cardiac mass and is not visible on the frontal films of the chest. In the oblique view, it is partially obscured by the superior vena cava. In the far LAO or lateral view and films of good quality, the greater part of the thoracic aorta is visible. In atherosclerosis the arch is unfolded, and the descending aorta may be deviated posteriorly so as to be superimposed upon the thoracic spine. As it approaches the diaphragm the aorta may slant forward in order to pass through the hiatus just posterior to the esophagus.

With atherosclerosis the diameter of the ascending aorta may be increased, and this can sometimes be determined from films of good contrast in the far left oblique projection. An aortic diameter greater than 3.8 cm in an adult is suggestive of dilatation (Steinberg et al., 1949). The dilatation is rarely very great due to atherosclerosis alone, and if the diameter is greater than 4 cm without allowances for magnification, the possibility of aortitis or hypertension or an aneurysm must be suspected.

The tortuous course of the aorta causes a considerable deviation in the course of the barium-filled esophagus. The depth of the aortic indentation may be increased, and the lateral border of the aortic knob may extend farther to the left of the midline than usual. Thus, with barium in the esophagus an estimate of the aortic diameter may indicate considerable dilatation. Such an estimate, however, may be unreliable due to a more oblique course of the elongated aorta. A more accurate measurement can be with the patient rotated into about 10–15° of right anterior obliquity.

The tortuous descending aorta carries the esophagus in a somewhat irregular course to the left and posterior (Fig. 498). Just above the diaphragm the esophagus lies in front of the aorta, and this causes a large posterior impression on the esophagus which is best seen in the extreme left oblique or lateral view. Occasionally the dilated and tortuous aorta may compress the lower esophagus just above the diaphragm sufficiently to produce dysphagia. This should not be confused with an intrinsic lesion of the esophagus. Because of the devious course of the esophagus, associated with the wandering tortuous aorta, its

relationship to the posterior surface of the heart and the left atrium is disturbed. Consequently, in such instances the degree of posterior deviation of the esophagus cannot be relied upon in estimating the size of the left atrium.

Pulsations of an atherosclerotic aorta are not remarkable unless there is a considerable degree of hypertension or aortic insufficiency.

Differentiation of an elongated and tortuous aorta from an aneurysm by conventional roentgen means is not always possible. A degree of dilatation of the aorta does occur with atherosclerosis and advancing years; however, if the ascending aorta is definitely visible in the left anterior oblique view and measures in excess of 4.0 cm, dilatation due to some cause other than atherosclerosis should be suspected. At times, angiography, either forward angiography or preferably retrograde aortography, may be necessary in delineating the anatomy of a tortuous aorta and differentiating it from an aneurysm.

Syphilitic Aortitis

Syphilis typically involves the aortic root and adjacent portions of the ascending aorta and more rarely other portions of the thoracic aorta.

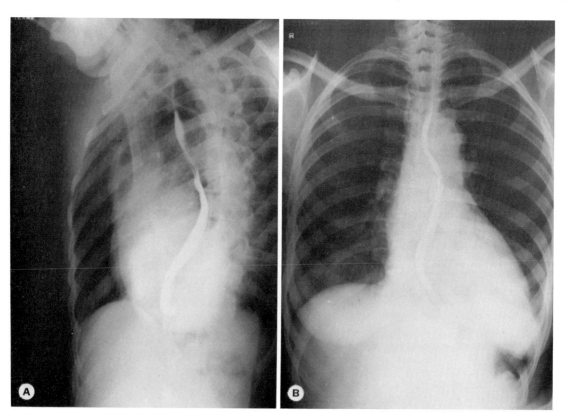

FIG. 498. DEVIATION OF BARIUM-FILLED ESOPHAGUS DUE TO ELONGATED TORTUOUS AORTA
(A) Left anterior oblique projection. (B) Posteroanterior projection.

It is quite rate in the abdominal aorta. The aortic wall in the region of the sinuses of Valsalva and the first 3–4 cm beyond is weakened due to invasion of the medial coat and replacement by fibrous tissue. The intima may become thickened and calcified at times, and this process may encroach upon the orifices of the coronary arteries. The syphilitic process often involves the valve ring and produces dilatation. Also, the valve cusps are frequently involved, and their change is characterized by some shortening and rolling of the margins; associated with the dilated valve ring there is some widening of the commissures between the valve cusps. Consequently, some degree of aortic regurgitation may complicate syphilitic aortitis. Also, involvement of the ostia of the coronary arteries may produce some degree of ischemia. The combined effects of aortic regurgitation and decreased coronary flow produce angina in a significant number of patients with luetic aortitis. Another complication is aneurysm formation which is due to weakening and replacement of the muscle and elastic tissue in the aortic wall by fibrous tissue. This may progress to aneurysm formation. Thus, uncomplicated syphilitic aortitis occurs in a minority of cases, and it is usually one or more of the complications mentioned above that produce the symptomatology which brings the patient to the physician. Changes of interest to the radiologist in syphilitic aortitis are dilatation of the root and adjacent portions of the ascending aorta and the deposition of linear, thin eggshell-like calcification in the involved aortic segment. When dilatation with calcification is associated with a positive serology and other evidence of syphilis, the presumption of syphilitic aortitis is very strong. Also, when there is evidence of aortic regurgitation or evidence of myocardial ischemia associated with dilatation of the aortic root, the presumption of aortitis is very strong but again the type will depend somewhat upon the associated findings, particularly the serology.

The aortic root because of its deep position in the cardiac contour as has been described above is not easily susceptible to demonstration by conventional chest films, and the diagnosis of aortitis is impossible by this method unless there is calcification. Calcification in the aortic root is best detected in the far left oblique or lateral view using a short exposure time and some overpenetration of the films or by fluoroscopy. The frequency of calcification in luetic aortitis is uncertain, and its absence has no diagnostic significance. Jackman and Lubert (1945) found radiologic evidence of calcium in 15 of 66 cases of syphilitic aortitis in which the diagnosis was confirmed by autopsy. Wolkins (1954) found calcium

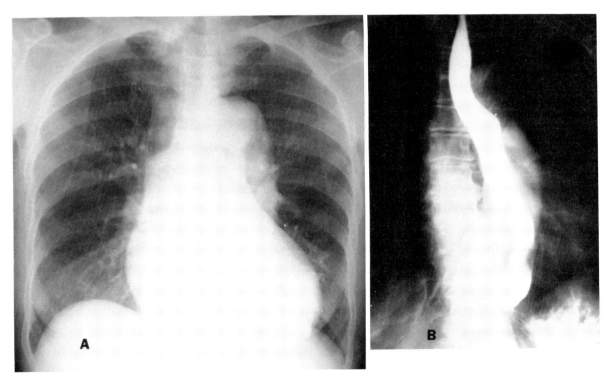

FIG. 499. ELONGATED AND TORTUOUS AORTA COMPRESSING LOWER ESOPHAGUS AND PRODUCING MILD DYSPHAGIA

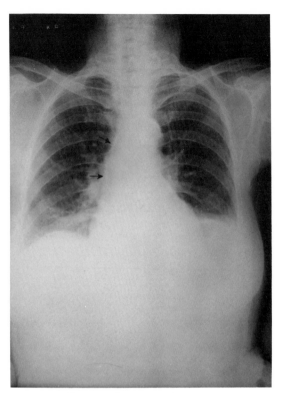

FIG. 500. SYPHILITIC AORTITIS

Rimlike deposit of calcium (arrows) seen in the ascending aorta in a 50-year-old black man with a positive blood serologic test for syphilis.

in the ascending aorta in 54 of 95 patients diagnosed as syphilitic aortitis. In 43 of these, calcium was also demonstrated in the transverse and descending aorta, and in only 11 was it limited to the ascending aorta. Rich and Webster (1952) found calcium in the ascending aorta in only 2 instances among 141 patients diagnosed as syphilitic aortitis by "clinical and x-ray means" and a considerable period of follow-up observation. Higgins and Reinke (1974) applied a delicate serological test to 20 patients with distinct linear calcification in the ascending aorta and found only 5 with evidence of syphilis. In 3 of these, the calcium was not limited to the ascending aorta. Other differences between the two groups (syphilitic and nonsyphilitic) were looked for such as lack of parallelism and irregularity of the aortic margins, elongation and aneurysm formation, but no significant differences were found. In the non-syphilitic group, calcium was found in association with calcific aortic stenosis and rheumatic aortic regurgitation. It is probable that the incidence of syphilitic aortitis has markedly decreased during the past 25 years and that calcium in the aortic root and even localized to the aortic

root and ascending aorta is more often due to atherosclerosis or to some other cause of aortitis.

Radiologic Findings

Angiography, preferably retrograde aortography, is the most reliable radiologic procedure in making the diagnosis of syphilitic aortitis (Steinberg et al., 1949; Rich and Webster, 1952). Steinberg et al. (1949) found that a diameter of the ascending aorta in excess of 3.8 cm as seen in the far anterior oblique projection and in the absence of marked hypertension was highly suggestive of aortitis. Associated thickening of the aortic wall with lack of parallelism of the walls and roughening of the lumen strengthen the diagnosis. Documentation of associated aortic regurgitation at the same time strengthened the diagnosis. Uncomplicated aortitis (without aortic regurgitation or coronary insufficiency) rarely produces symptoms sufficiently severe as to warrant the use of aortography.

Aortitis associated with other systemic diseases is being reported with increasing frequency. The reader is referred to the recent review by Lande and Berkman (1976).

Rheumatoid Arthritis and Ankylosing Spondylitis

Rheumatoid arthritis and ankylosing spondylitis produce lesions in the heart with a predilection for the aortic valve and aortic root (Mallory, 1936; Clark et al., 1957). The changes in the aorta are similar to those due to syphilis. Aortic valvular lesions associated with these two diseases are said to be a cause of about 5 percent of those patients needing a prosthetic replacement of the aortic valve (Zvaifler et al., 1963). Valvular lesions associated with ankylosing spondylitis seem to be more severe than those with rheumatoid arthritis.

Giant Cell Arteritis

Giant cell aortitis is a rare manifestation of a more generalized arteritis which commonly affects the large and medium-sized arteries, such as the carotids, subclavian, vertebral, coronary, and superior mesenteric. A specific syndrome, "temporal arteritis," is due to the same process. When the aorta is affected it may lead to aneurysm formation. It is characteristically a disease of elderly persons but has been associated with aneurysm formation in a child of 8 and an adult of 30 years of age (Zumbro et al., 1975; Austin et al., 1965). Giant cell arteritis is thought to be due to an autoimmune mechanism and often responds to steroid therapy.

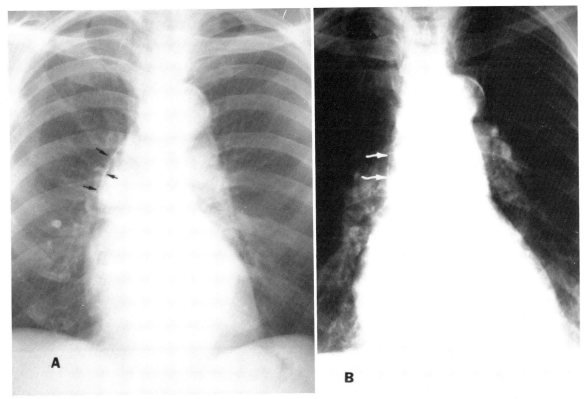

FIG. 501. TWO SEPARATE PATIENTS WITH FINE PENCILLED TYPE CALCIFICATION IN ASCENDING AORTA
(A) Ascending aorta is prominent and probably dilated and patient had a positive serologic test for syphilis. (B) Aorta is not prominent and probably not dilated. Sensitive serologic tests for syphilis were repeatedly negative. Calcium assumed to be due to atherosclerosis alone.

Relapsing Polychondritis

Relapsing polychondritis (Pearson *et al.*, 1960) is a systemic inflammatory disease which affects multiple cartilaginous structures, such as the external ear, nose, bronchial and costal cartilages, and interarticular surfaces of the joints and the sacroiliac joints. About 10% of cases have evidence of aortitis (Lande and Berkman, 1976). The disease affects the elastic tissue in the aorta, and the process of dilatation and aneurysm formation is the same as in other types of aortitis. Haimer and Hamilton (1969) reported a case with a dissecting aneurysm of the aorta.

The Reiter Syndrome

The Reiter syndrome consists of a nonspecific urethritis, conjunctivitis and arthritis. About 2–5% of patients will have dilatation of the aortic ring, an aortitis of the ascending aorta and aortic regurgitation (Lande and Berkman, 1976). Paulus *et al.* (1972) found that signs of aortic and cardiac involvement appeared on an average 15 years after the initial onset of the disease. The changes in the aorta are similar to those seen in association with rheumatoid arthritis.

Takayasu's Arteritis

As first described (Takayasu, 1908—quoted from Lande and Berkman, 1976) this disease affected the carotid arteries producing narrowing or occlusion and visual symptoms. A more detailed study (Shimizu and Sano, 1952) delineated a clinical profile of young Japanese females with discrepancies in the pulses of the upper part of the body and with symptoms of ischemia of the head and arms. The ischemia produced a variety of symptoms, such as vertigo, loss of consciousness, headache, visual difficulties and blindness. A synonym was adopted (Shimizu and Sano, 1952) of "pulseless disease," and this unusual condition is one of the causes of "aortic arch syndrome" so well described by Ross and Mc-Kusick (1953).

Further experience has shown that the disease frequently involves the descending thoracic and abdominal aorta and its major branches, particularly the renal arteries (Nakao *et al.*, 1967). Inada *et al.* (1962) and Lande (1976) proposed on good evidence that most of the coarctations at unusual sites in the thoracic or abdominal aorta (atypical coarctation) are the end results of this form of aortitis.

This disease is more common in Japan and the oriental countries and seems clearly to have an ethnic distribution (Deutsch *et al.*, 1974). It occurs infrequently in males and is rare in the United States, although the disease may have been unrecognized, particularly as related to the cases of atypical coarctation. In the majority of cases the onset is characterized by fever, weakness, arthritis and pains in various parts of the body. The occlusive and ischemic phase appears after the systemic symptoms subside. An autoimmune inflammatory process with connective tissue reaction has been proposed as the mechanism of this disease, but the evidence is inconclusive (Nakao *et al.*, 1967).

Although the disease process is common in the brachiocephalic arteries, it rarely involves the ascending portion and arch of the aorta. Occasionally it produces dilatation and aneurysm formation, and the aneurysm may contain linear calcium (Deutsch *et al.*, 1974). The aortic ring may be dilated causing aortic insufficiency, and the heart was enlarged in one-half of the patients described by Deutsch *et al.* (1974). Corticosteroid therapy is recommended and may cause a remission in a majority of patients (Nakao *et al.*, 1967).

Retrograde aortography, and where necessary selective injection into the potentially involved arteries, is the radiological procedure of choice. The obstructed areas, particularly those in the aorta, are variable but usually are relatively smooth and often concentric in appearance. Long or short areas of the descending aorta may be involved. The disease attacks the pulmonary arteries and produces occlusions (Lande and Berkman, 1976). Pulmonary angiography is indicated in evaluating these patients. The heart is enlarged in the majority of the patients, and this may be associated with hypertension or aortic regurgitation. Involvement of the aorta may lead to narrowing of the ostia of the coronary arteries and myocardial ischemia.

THE AORTIC ARCH SYNDROMES

The aortic arch syndromes (Ross and McKusick, 1953) refer to a collection of disorders of the aortic arch and brachiocephalic vessels that are manifest by "pulsus differens," a diminution or absence of the pulse in one or more of the major arterial systems arising from the aortic arch. In some cases the pulses in the upper extremities and the blood pressure are less than in the lower extremities. These cases were labelled as "reversed" or "paradoxical" coarctation. Ross and McKusick (1953) listed at least 10 documented causes for the syndromes. The most common in their opinion was syphilitic aortitis with or without aneurysm formation. Atherosclerosis usually contributed to the obstruction or obliterative process. Other proven causes were chronic aortic dissections, thrombophilia, congenital anomalies and nonsyphilitic arteritis. A number of cases were collected before aortography was a popular procedure, and the precise anatomy and cause were unexplained.

Symptoms due to these syndromes are very variable, the most common of which are vertigo, loss of consciousness, headache, impairment of memory and vision and trophic changes in the extremities and claudication. Careful physical examination will show that some manifestation of these syndromes is a rather common finding. In the authors' experience atherosclerosis has played an important part. Radiological investigation, and specifically aortography, is the optimum means for diagnosis.

Aneurysms of the Thoracic Aorta

Aneurysms of the thoracic aorta may be classified according to: (1) their location or point of origin, *e.g.*, those of the sinus of Valsalva, ascending portion, arch or descending aorta; (2) their etiology (congenital, arteriosclerotic, luetic, etc.); and (3) their anatomy (saccular, fusiform, or dissecting). Dissecting aneurysms are treated as a separate section.

In older reviews (Brindley and Stembridge, 1956; Kampmeier, 1938) saccular aneurysms in the ascending aorta due to syphilis were the most frequent type. Fomon *et al.* (1967) in a study of 110 cases at autopsy found a distribution as follows: ascending aorta, 55; arch, 29; descending aorta, 19; and thoracoabdominal (partly below the diaphragm), 7. In more recent years in dealing with clinical material, atherosclerosis is the most common etiologic agent, and there has been an increase in the relative number of aneurysms of the descending aorta (DeBakey and Noon, 1976; Higgins *et al.*, 1975). Atherosclerotic aneurysms in contrast to those due to syphilis are more often fusiform than saccular. All of the etiologic agents mentioned in the discussion of aortitis may be a cause of aneurysm formation.

Aneurysms of the sinuses of Valsalva may be

sis or rarely to atherosclerosis (Reinke *et al.*, 1974).

Acquired aneurysms may be discreet and involve only a single sinus or diffuse. The Marfan syndrome and cystic medial necrosis are frequent causes of diffuse dilatation of the sinuses. These aneurysms, whatever their cause, often become quite large and displace or intrude upon adjacent structures, such as the pulmonary artery, left atrium, right ventricle, or adjacent lung. They may rupture into the pericardial cavity, the right ventricle (Harris, 1956) or into the pulmonary artery (Shipp *et al.*, 1955). When the aneurysm ruptures into the right ventricle or pulmonary artery, it produces evidence of a left to right shunt, often a continuous murmur and engorgement of the lungs. Calcification in the walls of the aneurysm is common (Harris, 1956; Shipp *et al.*, 1955; Schneider and Spitz, 1968) and when fine and linear is usually attributed to syphilis. Fine eggshell-like calcification has been reported in nonsyphilitic aneurysms (Reinke *et al.*, 1974) (Fig. 504). Acquired aneurysms may interfere with the coronary circulation and by distorting the aortic valve or ring may produce regurgitation.

Acquired aneurysms are usually symptomless until they reach a considerable size unless they are associated with some complication as interference with the coronary circulation or pronounced aortic regurgitation. Since they are deep in the cardiac silhouette, they are not demonstrable by chest films or fluoroscopy unless they contain calcium or until they reach a size sufficient to distort the cardiac contour. As they enlarge they may displace the pulmonary artery segment causing an apparent fullness. They may intrude into the left atrium (Shipp *et al.*, 1955) suggesting enlargement of that chamber. At times they form a large mass at the base of the heart that must be differentiated from a cystic teratoma or some other extracardiac tumor.

Radiologic Findings

Retrograde aortography with injection of the contrast substance into the root of the aorta will demonstrate the aneurysm, although rarely the extent of the aneurysm may not be shown because of contained thrombus.

The ascending aorta is a common site of aneurysm formation. A fusiform aneurysm may extend from the aortic valve to the origin of the innominate artery or in some cases it may involve the entire thoracic aorta. In such cases, there is often in the frontal projection an obvious widening of the aorta to the right, and the aortic knob is grossly dilated. In the left anterior oblique or

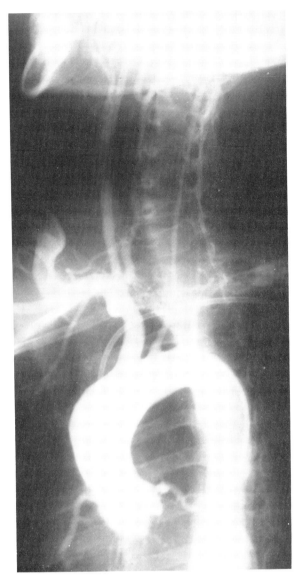

FIG. 502. "PULSELESS DISEASE" (ARTERITIS OF BRACHIOCEPHALIC VESSELS COMPATIBLE WITH TAKAYASU'S ARTERITIS)
Patient was 15-year-old white girl with physical findings of weakness, decreased pulse, and decreased blood pressure in the left upper extremity. Retrograde femoral arch aortogram shows irregular but smooth and marked narrowing of the left common carotid and left subclavian arteries just distal to their origin from the aorta. The normal caliber of the carotid artery appears to be restored at the level of its bifurcation into internal and external branches.

congenital or acquired. The congenital aneurysms are discussed in a separate section. Acquired aneurysms may be due to syphilis, the Marfan syndrome (discussed in a separate section), bacterial endocarditis, cystic medial necro-

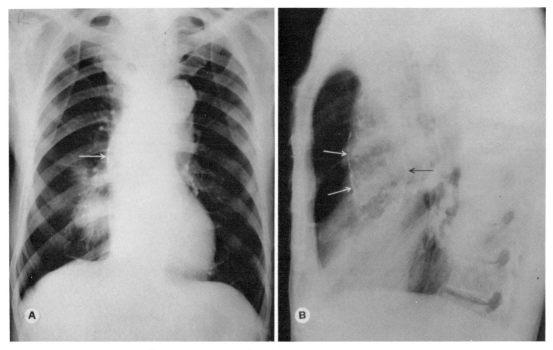

FIG. 503. FUSIFORM ANEURYSM OF ASCENDING AORTA

The dilated segment (arrows) is partially outlined by calcium deposited in its walls. The rounded shadow in the right lower lung adjacent to the heart was a primary bronchogenic carcinoma.

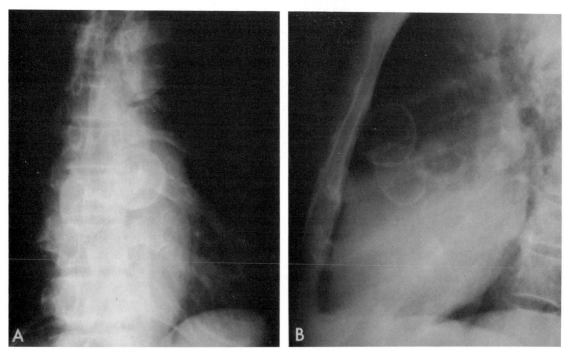

FIG. 504. CALCIFIED ANEURYSMS OF AORTIC SINUSES OF VALSALVA

A 70-year-old black male patient had clinical evidence of aortic stenosis and insufficiency. Serologic tests for syphilis were repeatedly negative, and his heart disease is presumed to be arteriosclerotic in origin. Blood pressure is 170/70; ECG shows left ventricular hypertrophy and strain. The patient takes maintenance doses of digitalis regularly and is asymptomatic. Frontal (A) and lateral (B) chest films show three rounded, peripherally calcified lesions at the root of the aorta, just anterior to a partly calcified aortic annulus. The two views at right angles to one another establish the location of the lesions within the heart and in intimate relation with the aortic root.

lateral projection, the diameter of the aorta is increased. Linear deposits of calcium may aid in the recognition of the aortic walls. A combination of saccular and fusiform aneurysms may be present as in Figure 506 in which the entire aorta was dilated and there is a saccular aneurysm in the descending aorta.

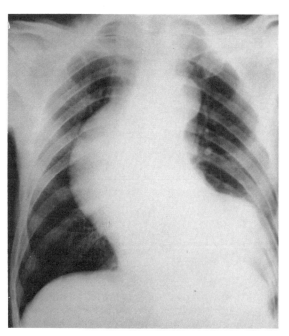

FIG. 505. LARGE FUSIFORM ANEURYSM OF ASCENDING PORTION AND ARCH OF AORTA
Some degree of aortic insufficiency was present.

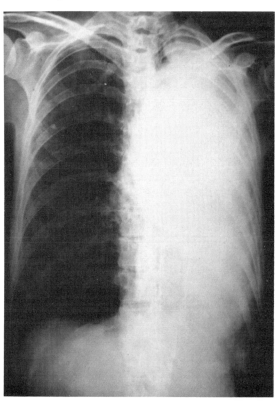

FIG. 507. MASSIVE ATELECTASIS OF LEFT LUNG DUE TO COMPRESSION FROM LARGE ANEURYSM OF ARCH AND DESCENDING AORTA

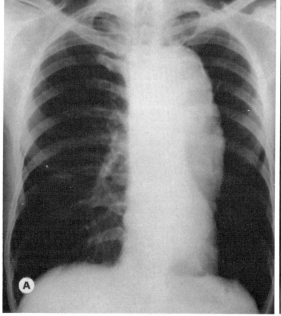

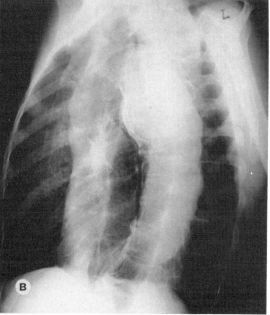

FIG. 506. FUSIFORM ANEURYSM OF ASCENDING PORTION AND SACCULAR ANEURYSM OF ARCH OF AORTA
Calcium is visible in the ascending aorta and in the aneurysm.

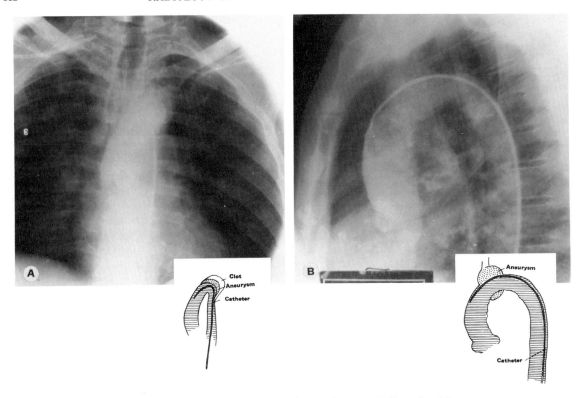

FIG. 508. SACCULAR ANEURYSM OF AORTIC ARCH IN 62-YEAR-OLD MAN

The patient suffered from attacks of dizziness and fainting spells. There was no pulse in either carotid or brachial arteries, and the blood pressure in the arms was unobtainable. In the thighs the BP was 150/90. A catheter inserted into the right brachial artery met an obstruction near the bifurcation of the innominate artery. (A) A catheter inserted into the aorta through the femoral artery follows the upper margin of the aortic arch, yet contrast substance has entered a rounded structure which protrudes above the aortic arch. (B) Lateral view showing a saccular aneurysm of the aortic arch which undoubtedly impinges on the openings of the brachiocephalic vessels. The aneurysm was invisible on the conventional chest film.

Saccular aneurysms of the ascending aorta usually produce rounded or oval-shaped shadows which frequently present to the right of the midline and which are continuous with the central mediastinal or aortic shadow. Pressure on a bronchus is common and atelectatic lung surrounding or adjacent to an aneurysm may produce a bizarre-shaped shadow. Infection may occur in the lung distal to an obstruction, and this may tend to obscure or draw attention away from the underlying condition. The aneurysm may impinge on and erode the sternum producing a rounded bony defect. This is best seen in oblique views of the sternum but is a very uncommon finding under the circumstances of modern medical practice. Occasionally, a saccular aneurysm of the ascending aorta may present to the left of the midline and in the region of the left lung. Obviously, in such a case the aneurysm must extend across the midline in the region of the anterior mediastinum.

The shadow of a saccular aneurysm is of medium density and usually of slightly greater density than the aorta because its diameter is often greater. A thin rim of calcium may be seen anywhere within the aneurysmal mass, although it is most frequent near the outer margin. Typically, in all projections the shadow of the aneurysm cannot be separated or projected away from contact with the aortic shadow. Pulsations are variable and depend to a considerable extent upon the amount of laminated clot within the aneurysmal sac. Fluoroscopy of suspected aneurysms generally is not useful since the information obtained cannot be substituted for aortography If expansile pulsations are present, the chances of any given mediastinal mass being an aneurysm are slightly improved. The differentiation by fluoroscopy or kymogrpahy between intrinsic expansile pulsations and pulsations transmitted from the aorta to a solid mass is difficult and unreliable.

Aneurysms of the aortic arch may present either to the right or left of the midline; they may project anteriorly and eventually erode the sternum or they may project posteriorly and erode the vertebral bodies. Aneurysms in this location characteristically displace the trachea,

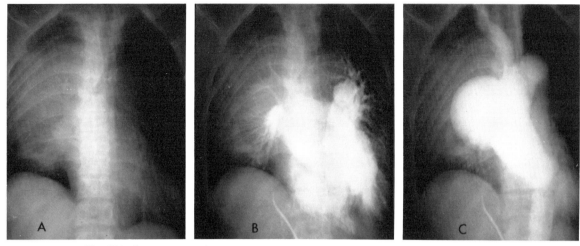

FIG. 509. ANEURYSM OF ASCENDING AORTA DEMONSTRATED BY VENOUS ANGIOGRAPHY

(A) Preliminary film shows a large mass in the right hemithorax inseparable from the cardiovascular silhouette. (B) A catheter was placed into the inferior vena cava, and contrast material was injected. This film shows the right side of the cardiopulmonary circulation, demonstrating marked displacement of the cardiac chambers and pulmonary artery toward the left. (C) A later film in this series shows opacification of the ascending aorta, the brachiocephalic vessels, and the descending thoracic aorta. A huge aneurysm arises from the lateral aspect of the ascending aorta. The opacified lumen of the aneurysm is much smaller than the size of the entire structure due to the presence of a large amount of laminated thrombus within it.

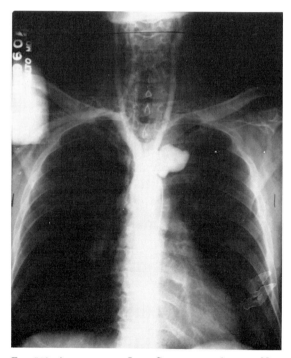

FIG. 510. ANEURYSM OF LEFT SUBCLAVIAN ARTERY NEAR ITS ORIGIN FROM AORTA

The polyethylene tube was inserted percutaneously through a cannula into the femoral artery and threaded into the arch of the aorta. (Courtesy Dr. E. C. Pierce, II.)

esophagus or both, and this is easily demonstrated by conventional chest films and barium swallow. Aneurysms originating near the origin of the innominate artery typically displace the trachea to the right and the esophagus posteriorly and to the right. Aneurysms in this location may be so small that they are not visible at fluoroscopy or on conventional films. On the other hand, they may be large enough to compress the great veins and seriously interfere with blood flow from the head and arms.

Aneurysms of the descending aorta present as irregular rounded or fusiform shadows in the left posterior thorax. They characteristically produce various degrees of atelectasis of the left lung either by direct pressure or bronchial obstruction. Rarely they erode the bodies of the thoracic vertebrae. The erosion takes place on the anterior or left lateral surface; the midportion of the vertebral bodies characteristically shows the deepest or most pronounced erosion whereas the adjacent intervertebral disc area is less markedly involved. Bony erosion is a very rare occurrence in modern day medical practice. The differentiation of an aneurysm, either saccular or fusiform, from a tortuous descending aorta is difficult and usually requires aortography.

Aneurysms of the major branches of the aorta may be saccular or fusiform and vary in appearance according to their location. Some of these aneurysms are quite small and are not demonstrable by conventional chest films and fluoroscopy. These aneurysms may be a cause of the aortic arch syndrome. Some widening of the innominate and subclavian arteries with advancing years is common. An aneurysm should not be confused with tortuosity (buckling of the innominate artery) (see page 407).

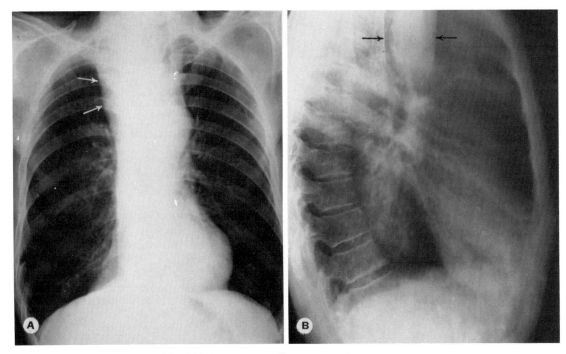

FIG. 511. ANEURYSM OF INNOMINATE ARTERY

MYCOTIC ANEURYSMS

Only about 2.5% of all aneurysms are of mycotic origin (Weintraub and Abrams, 1968), but these aneurysms deserve special consideration because of their often rapid progress and poor outcome if not properly treated. Osler (1895, 1908) applied the word "mycotic" to those aneurysms produced by bacteria, fungi, or other infectious agents. The medium-sized arteries in the mesentery, brain, spleen, and extremities are most frequently involved. Aortic mycotic aneurysms are more often secondary to septicemia and particularly bacterial endocarditis of the aortic valve and are thus most common in the ascending aorta. The much rarer primary mycotic aneurysms are lesions that develop without any other demonstrable intravascular source of infection and without any inflammatory process in the surrounding tissues (Crane, 1937). Mycotic aneurysms of the aorta, in addition to direct extension from an endocarditis, may be due to lodgement of bacteria in an atherosclerotic plaque, lymphatic extension, lodgement of bacteria in the vasa vasorum of the aortic wall or direct extension from an infectious process in the surrounding lung or mediastinum. Coarctation of the aorta or any condition that increases the turbulence or stress on the aortic intima may be a predisposing factor. A large variety of bacteria have been isolated from the aneurysms among which there are salmonella (Yanoff et al., 1965;

Weintraub and Abrams, 1968), streptococcus, staphylococcus, and in infants cytomegalic inclusion disease has been incriminated (quoted from Wood et al., 1973). Tuberculosis is a rare cause and may originate from a previous miliary tuberculosis (Kline and Durant, 1961; Ferrucci et al., 1975) on direct extension from adjacent tuberculosis in the lung, hilar lymph nodes, or vertebral column (Felson et al., 1977). Intravenous drug abuse may be a predisposing factor (Jaffe and Koschman, 1970; Jaffe and Condor, 1975), particularly in producing a mycotic aneurysm of the pulmonary artery.

Mycotic aneurysms are often associated with unexplained fever. They typically appear relatively suddenly and increase rapidly in size and are prone to early rupture and death. An aortic mycotic aneurysm should be suspected in any patient who has a mass that cannot be separated from the aorta by using multiple conventional films and which is associated with a persistent elevation of temperature or evidence of septicemia. It should be suspected in all cases of bacterial endocarditis.

Radiologic Findings

The diagnosis is established usually by retrograde aortography. Care should be exercised in manipulating the catheter in the region of the aneurysm in order that it does not enter the sac

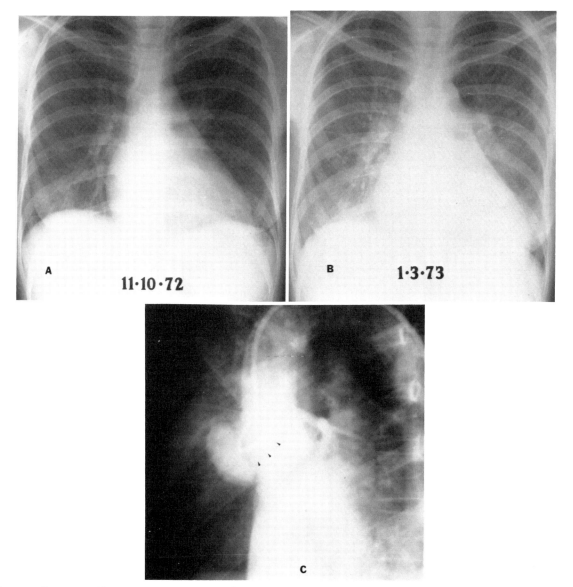

FIG. 512. BACTERIAL ENDOCARDITIS OF MITRAL VALVE WITH MYCOTIC ANEURYSM AND AORTIC REGURGITATION. PATIENT WAS A HEROIN ADDICT

(A) Patient had had fever, chills, and weakness for 2 weeks. Staphylococcus aureus cultured from blood. Patient placed on antibiotics and organisms disappeared from blood. (B) Several weeks later. Heart is larger with evidence of left ventricular failure. (C) Supravalvular aortogram showing massive regurgitation and a mycotic aneurysm. Small arrowheads indicate site of deformed aortic cusp.

or contribute to dislodgement of infectious material or rupture. An injection into the pulmonary artery may demonstrate the aorta satisfactorily and is a substitute procedure.

The most reliable means of establishing the diagnosis of aneurysm of the thoracic aorta at any site is by retrograde aortography. In most circumstances it is desirable to see the entire aorta, and the contrast substance should be injected in the ascending portion of the aorta. Filming is preferably carried out in two projec-

tions, but always the right posterior oblique projection is used. Where there is redundancy of the aorta, two projections are mandatory. The examination should be sufficient to show the origin of the brachiocephalic vessels and several cms. of their length. Rarely, it is technically impossible to insert a catheter in a retrograde direction into the thoracic aorta, particularly in patients with widespread atherosclerosis. In these cases, an injection into the right side of the heart or preferably into the pulmonary artery may be a

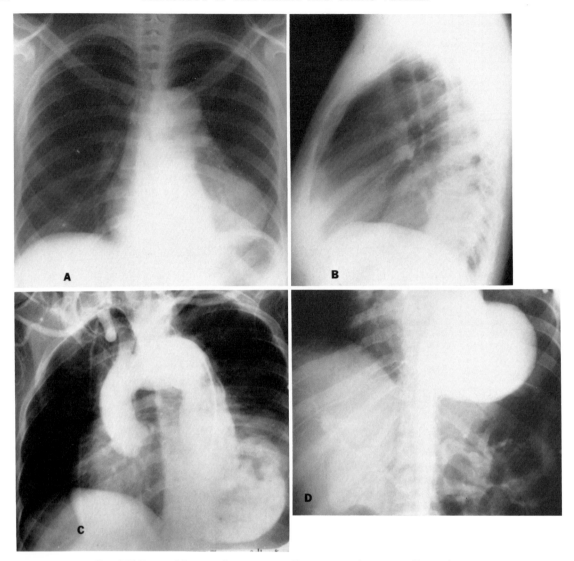

FIG. 513. LARGE MYCOTIC ANEURYSM OF DESCENDING AORTA IN A DRUG ADDICT

Patient had fever and chills for 10 days and pain in back. (A and B) Chest films show mass in lower thorax behind the heart and dilatation of aortic knob. (C and D) Aortogram shows large aneurysmal sac attached to descending aorta but aneurysm involves aortic arch also.

Resected aneurysm showed acute inflammatory process with degeneration of elastic tissue.

satisfactory substitute. Visualization of the right side of the heart using forward angiocardiography at times may be advantageous in indicating involvement of the great veins or pressure on the pulmonary artery. Forward angiocardiography is rarely completely satisfactory in demonstrating the anatomy of an aortic aneurysm. In some cases, a direct left ventricular injection is necessary. Visualization of the thoracic aorta is a necessary prerequisite to surgical treatment. Surgical treatment of aneurysms of the thoracic aorta and its branches is commonly used in most medical centers. A precise diagnosis is an essential preliminary to surgical attack, and contrast visualization studies provide the maximum preoperative information regarding size, structure, location and relation of the aneurysm to the surrounding structures.

Associated diseases of the cardiovascular system commonly accompany an aneurysm of the thoracic aorta and should be evaluated before surgical treatment is attempted. Joyce *et al.* (1964) found that 47% of 107 cases had hypertension, 16 percent had symptomatic coronary atherosclerosis and 13% had atherosclerosis of the peripheral arteries.

Tortuosity (Buckling) of Innominate Artery

Atherosclerosis of the thoracic aorta, with commonly associated dilatation, elongation and uncoiling of the aortic arch, is often associated with tortuosity or buckling of the innominate artery. Atherosclerotic elongation and dilatation of the innominate artery itself further accentuates the prominence of this vessel. On posteroanterior films of the chest the tortuous innominate artery may simulate an aneurysm or a tumor of the lung or mediastinum, and in 1 case of which we are aware thoracotomy was performed for suspected neoplasm (Fig. 514). If the index of suspicion is high, it should be possible to make the correct diagnosis of innominate artery buckling in most cases.

Clinically there may be evidence of generalized arteriosclerosis, systemic hypertension, or other cardiac disease, and a small pulsating mass may be palpated in the right supraclavicular fossa or lower cervical area. Film findings include contiguity of the mass with the aortic arch in all projections, a smooth lateral border, occasional linear or curvilinear calcifications on the lateral margin of the soft tissue opacity, prominence of the left superior mediastinum above the aortic knob (suggesting a similar process in the left subclavian artery), and evidence of atherosclerosis of the thoracic aorta (Schneider and Felson, 1961). Fluoroscopy is apt to be of limited value in the differential diagnosis.

The definitive diagnosis can be made in one of several ways. Catheter aortography will produce excellent contrast and good definition of the brachiocephalic vessels and is an entirely satisfactory means of establishing the diagnosis. Intravenous angiocardiography has much to recommend it as well, for in some cases the buckled and tortuous innominate artery may displace the right innominate vein to the right, and the lateral margin of the right superior paramediastinal mass may in fact be produced by the innominate vein rather than the innominate artery. Early filming following intravenous injection will define the location of the mediastinal veins, and late filming will establish the location and the size of the innominate artery. Intravenous angiocardiography is apt to be less than entirely satisfactory when the circulation time is prolonged or when intra- or extracardiac shunts from left to right are present.

Tortuosity or buckling of the innominate artery bears implications no more serious than the arteriosclerosis which is responsible; establishment of the correct diagnosis by angiography will help to avoid unnecessary surgical intervention.

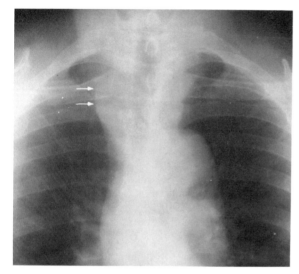

FIG. 514. TORTUOUS INNOMINATE ARTERY
Posteroanterior chest film of a 67-year-old black male patient showing a smoothly circumscribed laterally rounded right superior paramediastinal soft tissue opacity. The patient had no complaints referable to the lesion, and there were no abnormal physical signs in the area. Neoplasm and aneurysm were suspected. Exploratory thoracotomy revealed only a tortuous and somewhat dilated innominate artery in the region of the soft tissue opacity seen on the chest film.

DISSECTING ANEURYSM (HEMATOMA)

The term "dissecting aneurysm" is widely used, although it is inaccurate in that the aortic lumen in this condition is usually not dilated. "Dissecting hematoma" more accurately describes this entity.

This condition is relatively uncommon with an incidence of about 1 in 380 adult autopsies, and large medical centers see about 3–10 cases per year (Erb and Tullis, 1960).

Dissecting hematoma develops because of defects or deterioration in the smooth muscle and/or elastic tissue of the aortic media. The exact cause of these defects is often uncertain (Hirst and Gore, 1976). Arteriosclerosis with thickening and changes in the vasa vasorum leading to ischemia and atrophy of the smooth muscle is one probable cause. A loss of elastic tissue accompanied by cyst-like areas filled with ground substance (cystic medial necrosis of Erdheim) may be another mechanism. Hypertension is often a contributing cause by tending to extend the original localized tear in the media.

At any rate, some disease process in the media is a necessary prerequisite. The process usually produces a tear in the intima, and it is not entirely clear whether an intimal tear always precedes the splitting of the media or not. The conditions that predispose to aortic dissection are hypertension, atherosclerosis, pregnancy, coarctation of the aorta, Marfan's syndrome, and valvular aortic stenosis (Fukuda *et al.*, 1976). This condition is about twice as common in males as in females and is quite uncommon under the age of 30 years, although it has been encountered in infancy.

The classification of DeBakey *et al.* (1955) into Groups I, II, and III is quite important because of the differences in prognosis and treatment between the three groups (Grondin *et al.*, 1967; Daily *et al.*, 1970). Group I comprises those cases in which the dissection originates in the ascending aorta and extends beyond the left subclavian artery into the descending and often into the abdominal aorta. Group II has a similar origin but does not extend beyond the left subclavian artery. Group III comprises those cases in which the dissection originates beyond the left subclavian artery and extends into the descending aorta and beyond. In Type I and III cases, the dissection may extend into the lower thoracic and abdominal aorta and into any of the major branches and may involve any or all of the brachiocephalic vessels. However, the dissection tends to follow a pattern (Siegelman *et al.*, 1970; Hayashi *et al.*, 1974). In the ascending aorta the lateral wall is usually involved. In the arch the

dissection tends to be superior and posterior, and in the descending aorta it is lateral and somewhat posterior. In the abdomen the dissection is much more common posteriorly and to the left with a frequent extension into the left renal artery (Siegelman *et al.*, 1970). The left renal artery may be involved in at least half of the cases, and this can be a contributing factor to continuing hypertension. Type I and II dissections (originating in the ascending aorta) are about twice as frequent as the Type III cases (Hirst and Barbour, 1958). In those cases originating in the ascending aorta the prognosis, whether treated or not, is considerably worse than in those originating in the descending aorta (Grondin *et al.*, 1967; Daily *et al.*, 1970; Dinsmore *et al.*, 1972). The most frequent cause of death is external rupture of the hematoma. In those originating in the ascending aorta the most frequent cause of death is rupture into the pericardium (Beachley *et al.*, 1974). Another important factor in prognosis is duration of the symptoms. In several series the percentage of chronic dissections varied from 16–28% (Daily *et al.*, 1970; Grondin *et al.*, 1967). Many of these chronic cases survived for extended periods of time. Shennan (1932) in a review found 79 cases of healed dissecting aneurysm among a total of 300 cases, and Levinson *et al.* (1950) found 28% of 58 cases lived 3 months or longer. Symptom-free or chronic cases are occasionally encountered as incidental findings. Aortic insufficiency is a common accompaniment of dissections in the ascending aorta.

The role of medical and surgical therapy depends to a considerable extent on the origin and extent of the aneurysm, whether there is severe aortic insufficiency, duration of symptoms, and the presence of associated conditions, such as congestive heart failure and diabetes (Fukuda *et al.*, 1976). The surgical treatment of dissection of the aorta is given considerable impetus by the report of DeBakey *et al.* (1955), and the medical treatment in recent years has been popularized by Wheat and Palmer (1968).

The role of the radiologist, besides establishing the diagnosis, is also to determine the site of the intimal tear and presumably the site of origin, the extension of the hematoma, and the extent and degree of blockage of the major arterial branches.

Radiologic Findings

Conventional Chest Films. The findings on the frontal chest film that are suggestive of aortic dissection are (1) about 70% show widening of the mediastinum, but this is nonspecific. This may be quite difficult to evaluate on a recumbent

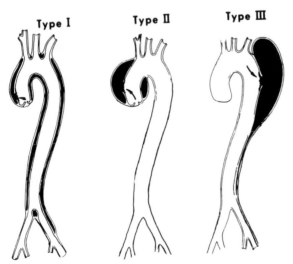

FIG. 515. THREE TYPES OF AORTIC DISSECTION (AFTER DEBAKEY)
(With permission, from Hayashi, Meaney, Zelch, and Taras, and the *American Journal of Roentgenology*.)

portable chest film which so often is the only film available; (2) prominence of the ascending aorta, particularly the lateral border as seen in Types I and II dissections; (3) enlargement of the aortic knob; (4) haziness of the aortic knob; (5) irregularities or angular jagged contour of the ascending aorta and aortic knob; (6) displacement of the trachea to the right; (7) enlargement

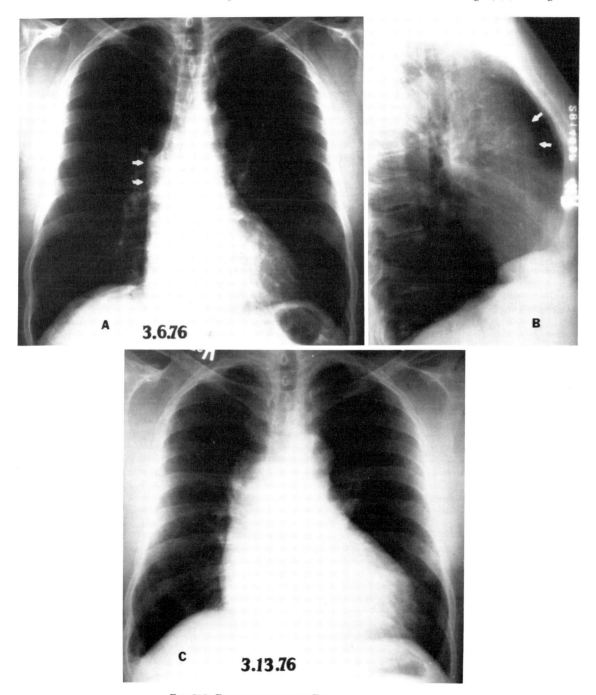

FIG. 516. DEVELOPMENT OF A DISSECTING ANEURYSM

(A and B) On first visit (3/6/76) patient complained of dizziness and abdominal pain. Chest film was reported as normal. In retrospect a localized convexity is seen on the lateral wall of ascending aorta (arrows) and a "blister"-like localized bump on the anterior surface of ascending aorta in the lateral view. (C) One week later, patient now complaining of severe chest pain. Entire aorta is larger and the heart has increased considerably in size. Echocardiography showed pericardial effusion. Patient died within a few hours from rupture of the hematoma into pericardium with tamponade.

of the descending aorta; (8) widening of the mediastinal stripe as seen in the lower thoracic region on the left side; and (9) thickening of the aortic wall as indicated by soft tissue density 1 cm or greater in thickness outside of the calcification of the intima as seen in the aortic knob (Wyman, 1957). Oblique and lateral films may show the thoracic aorta in contour and show localized bulges and/or irregular soft tissue densities that may not be seen on the frontal films (Fig. 517, B and C). Comparison with previous films if available should always be attempted and is quite helpful and will permit a more confident evaluation of the small deviations in the aortic contour.

Leakage of the hematoma into the mediastinum may cause widening of the mediastinal stripe as indicated or there may be leakage into the pleural space most often on the left side. Consequently, a left pleural effusion tends to support the diagnosis in combination with the other findings.

Acute cardiac tamponade does not usually cause a dramatic change in the size of the heart. However, a cardiac contour suggestive of pericardial effusion or the presence of pericardial fluid as determined by echocardiography or other means may support a suspected diagnosis of dissecting hematoma. Conventional films, including oblique and lateral projections, will show some abnormality in most cases, but the findings although suggestive are rarely specific. Where the changes develop under observation and in a matter of hours or a few days the diagnosis becomes more certain. However, angiography is necessary for diagnosis.

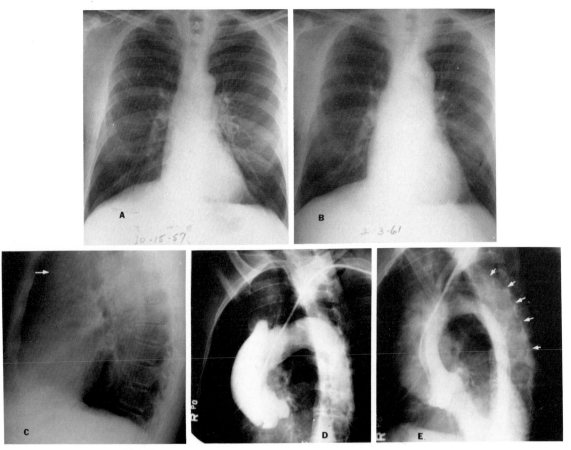

FIG. 517. TYPE I DISSECTING ANEURYSM (HEMATOMA) WITH ORIGIN IN THE ASCENDING AORTA

(A) Chest 3½ years prior to onset of dissection. (B) Chest film exposed about 24 hr after onset of severe chest pain. Note change in ascending aorta and aortic knob. In some cases these borders have an irregular crenated appearance. (C) Lateral view suggests unusual protrusion into retrosternal space. (D) Injection unintentionally in false passage. Note extension into innominate artery and deformity of sinuses of Valsalva. No untoward results of this injection were apparent. (E) Injection into lumen. Note normal appearing sinuses of Valsalva and marked aortic regurgitation. A large hematoma is seen in aortic wall (arrowhead) and the lumen of the aorta is narrowed.

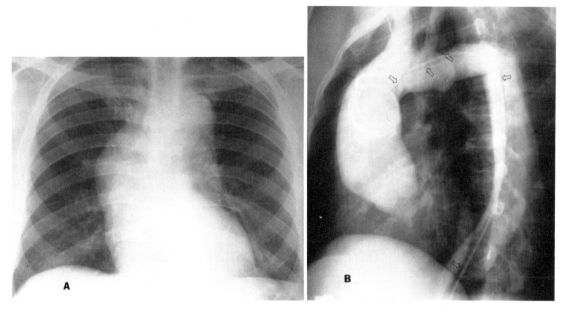

FIG. 518. PROBABLE TYPE I DISSECTION ORIGINATING IN THE ASCENDING AORTA,
PROBABLY NEAR PROXIMAL ARROW IN B

Several radiolucent internal flaps are seen in the transverse arch which is elongated. A large periaortic soft tissue shadow representing hematoma is seen. The dissection extends into the abdominal aorta (lower arrow). Abdominal aortography should be performed in order to determine the extent of the dissection. (Courtesy of Dr. Luis B. Morettin.)

Angiography. Satisfactory visualization of the aorta occasionally can be obtained by forward angiography with injection intravenously, or into the right atrium, or preferably into the pulmonary artery. Hart *et al.* (1963) suggested these routes as preferable to aortography because of the hazards of injection of the false channels of the aneurysm. Krouzon *et al.* (1975) recommended a transseptal approach to the left atrium with injection as a desirable alternate route if there was any technical difficulty with aortography. However, complete and satisfactory visualization is much less certain with these routes than with retrograde aortography. Frequent causes for failure of forward angiography are decreased cardiac output (heart failure) and aortic insufficiency. The majority of recent investigators recommend the retrograde route most often using the femoral and less often the axillary or brachial arteries (Beachley *et al.*, 1974; Hayashi *et al.*, 1974; Dinsmore *et al.*, 1972). Using the retrograde route the catheter may enter the false channel and a pressure injection conceivably could cause an extension of the dissection. Usually there is little difficulty in determining if the catheter is in the false channel. The position of the catheter is carefully monitored under image amplification using small hand injections of contrast substance. When the catheter is in the false channel, the injected contrast substance is slow to clear, the pressure is substantially less than systemic, and if the injection is made in the region of the arch of the aorta the sinuses of Valsalva will not be visualized. Also, the usual snapping movement of the aorta with the heart beat is greatly reduced when the catheter is in the false channel. An injection into the false channel is not necessarily disastrous and may be informative. The injection should be carried out by hand pressure. This should be followed by an attempt to place the catheter in the true lumen, and at times it may be necessary to select a second puncture site. The femoral route is preferable because it gives easier access to the abdominal aorta and its branches. These arteries must be examined in all cases in which the dissection extends below the diaphragm.

In the thorax biplane AP and lateral projections are recommended occasionally supplemented by a right posterior oblique projection. In the abdomen frontal and oblique projections are useful with particular reference to the aortic branches.

The flow of contrast substance into a double aortic lumen is positive evidence of a dissecting hematoma. However, the demonstration of a false lumen may be uncertain unless a central radiolucent septum is seen dividing the false and

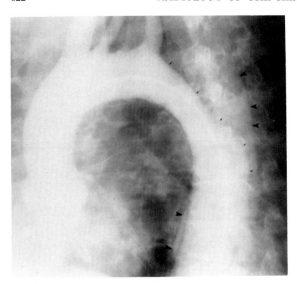

FIG. 519. TYPE II DISSECTION WITH A LARGE SOFT TISSUE
COMPONENT, AT LEAST 3 CM IN THICKNESS
(ARROWHEADS) AND SLIGHT NARROWING OF AORTIC
LUMEN

Lower arrows show contrast substance in false passage
outside of aorta.

true channels or unless there is a markedly differential rate of filling and emptying. Delayed films may be helpful.

The true channel usually has a rapid flow, but this may be slowed by aortic insufficiency. The true channel is often compressed or flattened on one side. In those cases in which the false channel does not fill, a soft tissue swelling indicates a false passage which in the arch and descending aorta is often superior and lateral to the true lumen. The soft tissue density should be at least 1 cm in thickness as lesser densities may be due to other causes, such as atherosclerotic thickening of the aortic wall, aortitis, true aneurysm with laminated thrombus, or neoplasia (Shuford et al., 1969; Kanick et al., 1964). The interior of the true channel often is irregular with a bump or ulcer-like protrusion. Small amounts of contrast substance may extravasate slowly into the false channel and stagnate. The proximal margin of the soft tissue mass representing either a thrombosed or closed false lumen is usually very near the origin or most proximal portion of the aneurysm. However, in a sizeable number of cases the dissection extends in a retrograde di-

rection all the way to the aortic valve ring. The detection of an intimal flap inside the true lumen is also helpful in determining the site of origin of the aneurysm. An important observation is sometimes possible during the injection of contrast substance with the tip of the catheter in the ascending aorta. The catheter rebounds against the upper and outer margin of the aorta. This facilitates the detection of an extrinsic soft tissue thickening representing the false channel.

Brachiocephalic and abdominal branches of the aorta may be occluded by the dissection, and it is the obligation of the radiologist to detect these. At times these vessels may opacify entirely from the false channel, and this may suffice to maintain the function of the organ and this is important in determining treatment. Attempts to locate a re-entry site of the false channel, if such is not readily apparent, are usually not justified. A free flow of contrast substance in the false channel suggests that there is a re-entry site, and stagnation suggests that there is no functioning re-entry site. Dinsmore et al. (1972) believe the absence of a demonstrable false channel in which there is active blood flow suggests a better prognosis and increases the probability of containment of the hematoma.

The diagnosis of dissecting aneurysm by retrograde aortography in many instances is quite easy. On the other hand, there are a number of pitfalls (Shuford et al., 1969; Kanick et al., 1964). Since treatment and particularly surgical treatment depends on a diagnosis and precise localization of the site of origin, a false positive or negative diagnosis is fraught with considerable risk to the patient. A negative diagnosis should not be given until the entire aorta is seen in profile, and occasionally a third projection (other than AP and lateral) may show a finding of importance. Special care must be taken in the interpretation of soft tissue thickening as due to a false channel. In the ascending aorta in the oblique position the shadow of the right atrium and vena cava may appear as a soft tissue mass. The soft tissue thickening in the arch and descending aorta should be at least 1 cm thick as indicated above. Small flattened seeming extravasations should be viewed with caution as they are more likely due to atherosclerotic plaque formation in the aortic intima.

CARDIOVASCULAR DISEASE ASSOCIATED WITH THE MARFAN SYNDROME

The Marfan syndrome is designated by Mc-Kusick (1972) as an abiotrophy of connective tissue rather than a congenital anomaly. The syndrome is often familial and is due to a muta-

tion in an autosomal dominant gene or genes. The principal abnormalities are manifested in the skeletal system, the eye, and the cardiovascular system. The more striking changes in the skeletal system are excessive length of the limbs, loose jointedness, scoliosis, kyphosis, pectus carinatum and excavatum, and typically arachnodactyly. In the eye the characteristic change is an ectopia of the lens, but there is often a high degree of myopia and retinal detachment.

Significant involvement of the cardiovascular system occurs in 30–60% of cases (Murdoch et al., 1971) and presents the most common threat to life and health. A frequent basic defect is found in the tunica media of the ascending aorta. The elastic fibers are defective. After a variable period of time, associated with the pulsating pressure in the aorta, the elastic tissue breaks and fragments. Cystic areas filled with mucoid material appear, and the wall of the aorta is weakened. Similar changes are found less frequently in the proximal portions of the pulmonary artery and its branches. The mitral valve cusps and chordae tendineae also may show mucoid degeneration with lengthening and some degree of deformity. Similar changes rarely occur in the tricuspid valve, and McKusick (1972) believes that the aortic valve cusps per se rarely are involved.

The earliest gross anatomical changes usually occur at the valve ring and in the adjacent sinuses of Valsalva. The aortic valve ring dilates, and the dilatation extends into the sinuses of Valsalva and they may become aneurysmal. All of the sinuses are usually involved in contrast to the congenital aneurysms of the sinuses of Valsalva which typically involve only one sinus. Also, the aneurysms of the sinuses of Valsalva associated with the Marfan syndrome rarely if ever rupture into the right atrium or right ventricle (McKusick, 1972). The orifices of the coronary arteries are frequently high and above the sinuses of Valsalva. The dilatation of the sinuses frequently leads to a distortion of the orifices and undoubtedly interferes with coronary blood flow. As the process continues the adjacent ascending aorta also dilates forming a large aneurysm. The dilatation rarely extends beyond the origin of the innominate artery.

Because of the dilatation of the valve ring, the aortic cusps become insufficient, and aortic regurgitation ensues. If the regurgitation becomes severe, left ventricular hypertrophy, then dilatation and enlargement occur. Patients may present with anginal-like chest pain, and the physical signs of aortic regurgitation are often seen.

Involvement of the mitral valve is one of the causes of the "billowing" or "floppy" valve syndrome (Read et al., 1965). This may progress to severe mitral insufficiency, left ventricular failure, and death.

The pulmonary artery, particularly its proximal portion, may have a weakened media and also become dilated. This may be one of the causes of the so-called "idiopathic dilatation of the pulmonary artery" (Castellanos et al., 1957).

The histologic changes in the media of the ascending aorta are similar or identical to those of cystic medial necrosis described by Erdheim (Baer et al., 1943). The media is therefore susceptible to disruption and dissecting aneurysm is a fairly frequent occurrence. The dissection typically begins in the ascending aorta and may become an additional cause of aortic regurgitation or it may leak or rupture into the pericardium. In patients under 40 years of age with dissecting aneurysm, 16% were found to have the Marfan syndrome (Hirst et al., 1958).

The causes of death due to cardiovascular disease in the Marfan syndrome in order of frequency are dilatation of the ascending aorta with aortic regurgitation, rupture, dissection and surgical deaths following attempts to repair the dilated aorta or one of its complications (Murdoch et al., 1972). Other rare causes are bacterial endocarditis, usually involving the mitral valve (McKusick, 1972; Soman et al., 1974) and cor pulmonale secondary to chest deformity (Wanderman et al., 1975).

Coarctation of the aorta has an increased frequency with the Marfan syndrome but is rarely hemodynamically significant. The aortic knob and descending aorta may show changes suggestive of coarctation or pseudocoarctation, but notching of the ribs is unusual. Originally it was thought that atrial septal defect was a common associated congenital anomaly, but this has not been borne out by a review of the larger series of cases. Ventricular septal defect seems to be quite uncommon in association with the Marfan syndrome (McKusick et al., 1972).

Radiologic Findings

Conventional chest films may show evidence of pectus carinatum or excavatum. Prominence of the ascending aorta and some minor degree of enlargement of the left ventricle are the earliest changes detected on the conventional chest film. The prominence of the aorta may be better detected in the left oblique or lateral view. Since the dilatation of the aorta begins at the valve ring and the sinuses of Valsalva, it is remarkable the extent of dilatation that may occur before this becomes noticeable on the conventional chest film. This is due to the fact that the first part of the aorta is inside the pericardium and does not form an interface with the lung. In the more advanced cases, the ascending aorta and the left ventricle are definitely enlarged, and the ascending aorta may show increased pulsations.

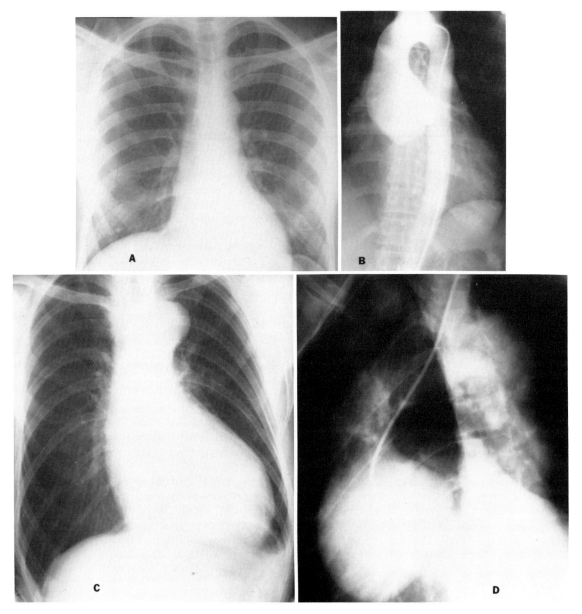

FIG. 520. TWO SEPARATE CASES OF THE MARFAN SYNDROME WITH ANEURYSMAL DILATATION OF THE ASCENDING AORTA
Note that the frontal contour of heart shows almost no evidence of the dilatation of this portion of the aorta.

At this stage, the disease is usually rapidly progressive. Occasionally, the other stigmata of the Marfan syndrome may be incompletely developed or overlooked, and consequently rheumatic or syphilitic disease of the aorta and aortic valve may be considered. With involvement of the mitral valve (the "floppy" valve syndrome), the left atrium is enlarged, and in the later stages there may be congestive changes in the lungs.

Retrograde aortography with selective injection into the ascending aorta is the procedure of choice. In the earlier cases, the sinuses of Val-

salva may be individually dilated (Steinberg and Geller, 1955). The dilatation may involve only the valve ring. As the process progresses, the adjacent portion of the ascending aorta distends and become quite large with associated aortic regurgitation (Fig. 521B). The extent of the aortic regurgitation can be grossly quantitated.

The patient may first appear because of a dissection which begins in the dilated and often aneurysmal ascending aorta. A selective aortogram will show the dissection (see page 620). At times aortography may show a linear radiolucent

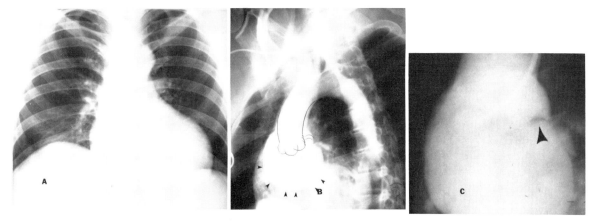

FIG. 521. THE MARFAN SYNDROME WITH ANEURYSM OF AORTIC ROOT AND AN INTIMAL FLAP, BUT NO EVIDENCE OF A
DISSECTING HEMATOMA
(A) No evidence of dilated aortic root. (B) Large aneurysm with some aortic regurgitation and enlargement of valve ring.
(C) Internal flap just above origin of left coronary artery. (Courtesy of Dr. Luis B. Morettin.)

rim or line representing the avulsed intima and portion of the media and thus indicate the origin of the dissection.

In cases with involvement of the mitral valve and mitral insufficiency, left ventriculography is the procedure of choice. Reflux into the left atrium will indicate in a gross way the severity of the insufficiency and often shows the redundant and billowing cusps that are typical of the diagnosis.

The cardiovascular manifestations of the Marfan syndrome must be differentiated from rheumatic aortic and mitral valvular disease, syphilis of the aorta and aortic valve, and the cardiovascular involvement associated with homocystinuria.

Surgical treatment (Nasrallah *et al.,* 1975; Symbas *et al.,* 1970) consists of replacement of the aortic valve with a prosthesis. This is often accompanied by inserting a graft inside the redundant aorta or less often by primary plastic procedures. In those cases of the "floppy" valve syndrome, the valve is replaced by a prosthesis. The operative mortality for the aorta and aortic valve is high and has varied from 20–30%.

Homocystinuria

Homocystinuria is an inborn error of metabolism due to the marked reduction or absence of the enzyme, cystathionine synthetase (Mc-

Kusick, 1972; Smith, 1967). Homocystinuria is mentioned here because of its frequent confusion in the past with the Marfan syndrome. Differentiation by clinical and radiologic observations is usually possible. In contrast to the Marfan syndrome, patients with homocystinuria show a considerable frequency of mental retardation, frequent generalized osteoporosis and localized enlargements of the ends of the long bones with some stiffness of the joints.

The cardiovascular manifestations in the two diseases are quite different. In homocystinuria the basic changes occur in the intima of the large and medium-sized arteries and veins, and this is often followed by localized thrombosis. The thoracic aorta is rarely obstructed by thrombosis and is rarely dilated unless there is associated hypertension (McKusick, 1972). The medium-sized arteries, such as the carotids, renals, iliacs and coronaries, are subject to thrombosis with recanalization and permanent narrowing. Ischemic heart disease with myocardial infarction at a young age may occur. Surgery and arteriography are quite hazardous because of the risk of localized thrombosis in contrast to the Marfan syndrome. Aortic aneurysms and dissecting aneurysms are quite rare.

The diagnosis is confirmed by the demonstration of homocystine in the urine by the use of the cyanide nitroprusside test or by high-voltage paper electrophoresis.

26

Valve Replacements

The mitral, aortic, and tricuspid valves have been excised and replaced by so-called "biologic valves" or by prostheses. The biologic valves may be homografts, xenografts, or fascial transplants (Ross, 1972). The biologic valves, except the circular supporting metal ring, are invisible to the radiologist unless they calcify. Calcification unfortunately is common after 2–3 years (Ross, 1972). Also, these valves tend to become insufficient, and Ross (1972) reported that approximately 16% had to be replaced due to degenerative changes. The biologic valves are singularly free from thromboembolic phenomena and do not require continuous anticoagulant treatment.

Since the initial reports of Harken *et al.* (1960) and Starr and Edwards (1961), prosthetic valves have been used on an increasing scale. All or part of these devices are visible to the radiologist who has a substantial role in detecting local malfunction and other complications. Visualization of the valve and its range of motion are determined by fluoroscopy or cinefluorography. Chun and Nelson (1977) have recently published a useful table of   currently available prostheses (Table 14) along with their x-ray appearance.

Prosthetic valves are of four basic designs. These are (1) a ball and cage arrangement as exemplified by the Starr-Edwards, Mcgovern, Braunwald-Cutter, and the Smeloff-Cutter prostheses; (2) the tilting disc type as exemplified by the Bjork-Shiley and the Lillehei-Kaster prostheses; (3) the moving disc type as exemplified

by the Beall mitral prosthesis; and (4) the leaflet type as exemplified by the Gott-Daggett type. All of these valves have a rigid ring composed of radiopaque stellite or titanium covered by a Dacron velour or Teflon plus polypropylene or some other similar substance. The major exception is the Gott-Daggett valve, the ring of which is composed of a polycarbonate housing with two hinged Teflon leaflets that are supported by fine metallic struts. The base is relatively radiolucent, but the leaflets when seen end-on are faintly visible (Wilson *et al.*, 1967).

The struts for the ball and cage type prostheses are made of stellite and are three in number except certain series of the Starr-Edwards valve has four struts, and these are easily visible by image amplified fluoroscopy, cinefluorography, and usually by conventional films. The Starr-Edwards valve has a closed cage whereas in the other three mentioned above, the cage is open at the apex. The two supporting struts of the Beall valve were originally of titanium but later changed to non-ferrous metal coated with pyrolite carbon, but these are likewise easily visible by radiologic means. The Bjork-Shiley valve has a single strut that limits the tilt of the disc to 60°, and the Lillehei-Kaster valve has two struts, low in profile, that limit the tilt to 80° from the vertical in relation to the valve ring. The base of the prosthesis or valve ring is covered with slightly redundant Teflon or Dacron which acts as a sewing-ring. The base is shaped specifically to fit either the aortic or the mitral orifices.

SPECIFIC FEATURES OF PROSTHESES

The Starr-Edwards prostheses come in four sizes and with basal rings adaptable to either aortic or mitral implantation. The ball or poppet originally was composed of silastic rubber (Dow Chemical Company) with a specific gravity of approximately 1.14 (Wilson *et al.*, 1967; Hipona *et al.*, 1971). The usual specific gravity of blood

is 1.056 which provides a sufficient contrast to permit visualization with image amplified fluoroscopy. Two percent barium impregnated balls were introduced in 1962 (Hylen *et al.*, 1969), and these were replaced by a stellite poppet in 1967 (Bonchek and Starr, 1975). Originally the struts and seating studs were bare metal. In newer models the struts were covered by two layers of Teflon, and more recently an outer layer of polypropylene has been added. The cloth cover has been added to provide an acceptable surface for the ingrowth of fibrin and platelets and an ultimate covering of endothelium which would prevent thrombus formation. This also deadened the noise produced by the stellite poppet which occured in those valves where the metal cage was bare. The Starr-Edwards valve produces a small gradient usually less than 10 mm Hg, depending on the orifice size and the volume of blood flow (Kirklin, 1973).

The Magovern prosthesis is quite similar to the Starr-Edwards design except that it has an open end cage, three struts, and the cloth ring is sutureless and fixed by pins and hooks (Magovern, 1963). Its use is contraindicated in patients with extensive scar tissue, cystic medial necrosis or with large and redundant annuluses.

The Braunwald-Cutter valve uses a specially cured silastic rubber ball, an open ended cage, and is completely covered with polypropylene and Dacron mesh (Braunwald et al., 1971). It may have a lesser tendency to thrombus formation (Brawley et al., 1975).

The Smeloff-Cutter prosthesis has a double cage design with the shorter cage protruding in a retrograde position into the atrium or ventricle as the case may be. This design permits a larger effective orifice and a lower gradient at the expense of a small amount of regurgitation. The forward portion of the valve has a lower profile than the Starr-Edwards valve and therefore may be useful in patients with small ventricles. The ball is made of a specially cured silicone rubber material.

The Bjork-Shiley prosthesis (Bjork, 1969) initially had a tilting disc of Delrin, and later this was replaced by a pyrolytic carbon disc which withstands autoclaving and has better wear characteristics. The Bjork-Shiley valve has a low profile and is thus desirable for mitral replacements in patients with small ventricles. It provides less gradient than most of the ball and cage type valves (quoted from Brawley et al., 1975).

The Lillehei-Kaster valve is also of the disc type with a pyrolite disc that tilts to 80° with the plane of the valve ring. It has a low profile and the same advantages as the Bjork-Shiley prosthesis.

The Beall valve was designed for mitral valve replacement (Beall et al., 1973). Its base is covered with Dacron velour, and the struts are covered with Teflon. This prosthesis has a low profile and a minimum gradient. The disc occluder was initially made of a specially treated Teflon but was later replaced by a much more wear resistant disc of pyrolite. It has had a good performance in the prevention of thromboembolism (quoted from Brawley et al., 1975). Strut fracture with release of the disc occluder has been reported (Nathan, 1973).

At least ten other prosthetic valves are available but have seen limited use. The interested reader is referred to the review articles by Hipona et al. (1971) and Chun and Nelson (1977).

COMPLICATIONS OF PROSTHETIC VALVE REPLACEMENT

Operative or hospital mortality initially was of the order of 15%, but following a more extended experience and averaged over a period of several years the mortality stated for the mitral valve is about 5 percent and slightly higher for the aortic valve (Bonchek and Starr, 1975). Other authors give higher figures (quoted from Hipona et al., 1971).

Later results in a relatively large series of cases reported by Bonchek and Starr (1975) show that about 78% of patients who survived the operative procedure for the mitral valve were alive at 8 years. Of those who survived the aortic valve replacement, 72% were alive at 8 years (Bonchek and Starr, 1975). In those patients who survive operation the heart often decreases in size. The change in size is least in those with the larger hearts (Braun et al., 1973), and those with the larger hearts preoperatively have the poorest survival.

The immediate complications other than those associated with any type of major surgery are infection and heart failure. Infectious endocarditis occurs in 1–10% of cases and may have a high mortality (Kloster, 1975), although many cases may be controlled by antibiotics. Occasionally an ingrowth of granulation tissue secondary to the endocarditis may interfere with valve function or disturb the anchoring component. Radiologic examination at this time may show undue tilting or rocking of the valve base. Lansing (1967) and Stinson et al. (1968) diagnosed a loose valve base and undue motion by prolonged exposure chest films. Since this is a rather innocuous procedure and can be brought to the patient's bedside, it should be thought of when this complication is suspected.

Long-term complications are due to thrombus formation on the prosthesis, thromboembolism, infection, persistent hemolysis with anemia, and

BALL VALVES

VALVE	SHAPE	X-RAY	X-RAY OUTLINE	MITRAL TRICUSPID	AORTIC	IDENTIFYING FEATURES	COMPLICATIONS
Starr-Edwards 6000	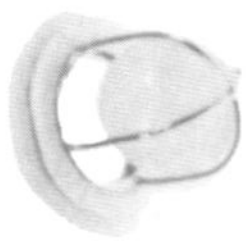	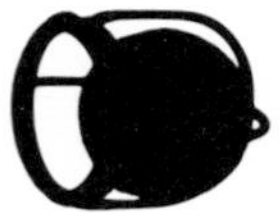	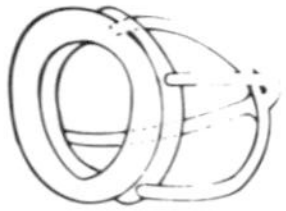	●		1. double donut 2. 4 thick struts joined at apex 3. radiolucent poppet (some with barium)	1. thromboemboli 2. ball variance 3. left ventricular incorporation of cage
6300	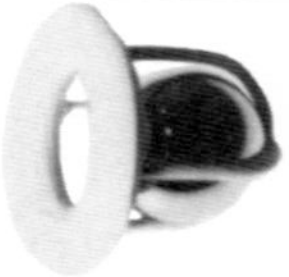	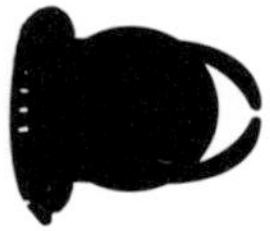	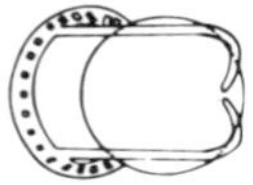	●		1. concave perforations 2. 4 thin struts not joined at apex 3. radiopaque poppet (in systole sits far from equator)	1. thromboemboli 2. bacterial endocarditis
1000	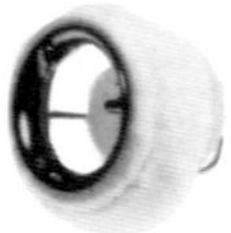	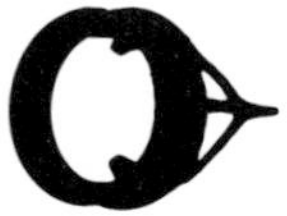	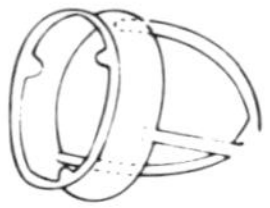		●	1. conical valve with 3 feet in orifice 2. 3 thin struts joined at apex 3. radiolucent poppet	1. thromboemboli 2. ball variance
1200	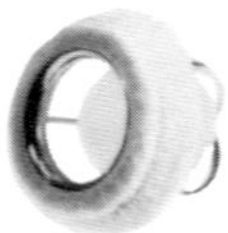	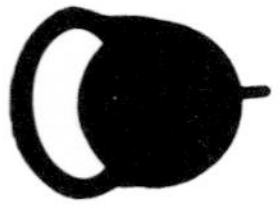	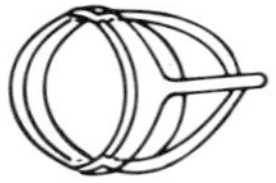		●	1. tapered support at each strut junction 2. 3 thin struts fused at apex 3. some barium poppets	1. thromboemboli 2. ball variance
2310	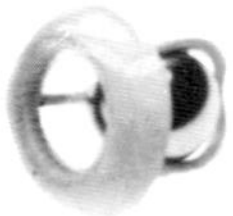	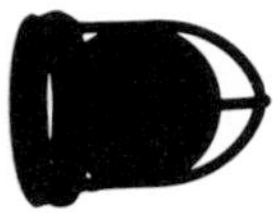	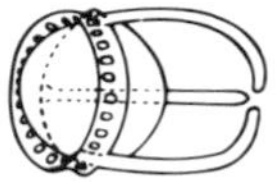		●	1. perforated concave valve base 2. 3 thin struts joined at apex after 12/69 3. radiopaque poppet (diastole sits close to equator)	1. close clearance model with poppet impacted in open position*
Braunwald-Cutter	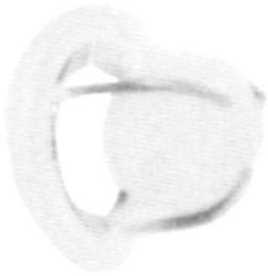	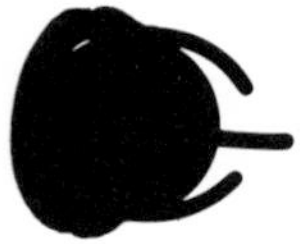	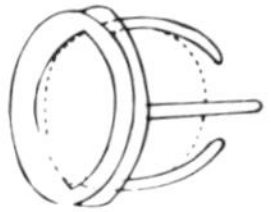	●	●	1. open-ended cage 2. radiolucent poppet	1. thromboemboli 2. ball variance 3. hemolysis 4. cloth wear at apex 5. peri-valvular leaks
Smeloff-Cutter	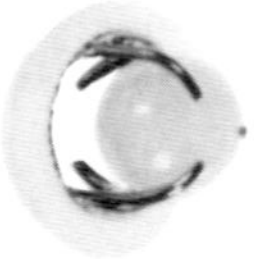	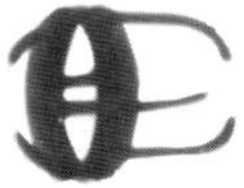	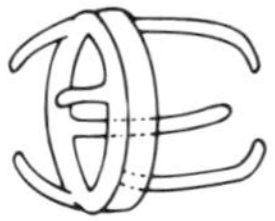	●	●	1. open-ended cage 2. 3 struts 3. full-flow orifice ball valve 4. radiolucent poppet	1. thromboemboli 2. hemolysis 3. ball variance 4. open top buried in ventricular septum*

TABLE 14

RADIOLOGIC IDENTIFICATION OF COMMON CARDIAC PROSTHETIC VALVES AND THEIR ASSOCIATED COMPLICATIONS

* Characteristic for sub-

VALVE	SHAPE	X-RAY	X-RAY OUTLINE	MITRAL/TRICUSPID	AORTIC	IDENTIFYING FEATURES	COMPLICATIONS
MaGovern-Cromie				●	●	1. sutureless mechanical fixation prosthesis 2. open-ended cage 3. 3 struts 4. vertical fixation pins 5. radiopaque poppet	1. thromboemboli 2. hemolysis 3. ball variance
DeBakey-Surgitool					●	1. closed-ended cage 2. 3 struts 3. serrated ring 4. radiolucent poppet	
LOW PROFILE VALVES A. DISC VALVES							
6520				●		1. low profile cage 2. cross struts 3. radiopaque poppet 4. concave perforations	
Starr-Edwards 6500				●		1. low profile cage 2. cross struts 3. radiolucent poppet with radiopaque ring in poppet	1. thromboemboli 2. cocking of disc
Kay-Shiley				●		1. single or double muscle guard 2. 4 parallel struts 3. radiolucent poppet	1. thromboemboli 2. sudden, unexpected, unexplained death 3. grooving and disc wear 4. restenosis with disc ingrowth· 5. perivalvular leaks 6. disc cocking, variance
Kay-Suzuki				●	●	1. close-ended cage 2. 4 struts 3. 4 short open base struts 4. double ring valve base 5. radiolucent poppet	1. thromboemboli 2. disc variance
Cross-Jones				●		1. open-ended cage 2. radiolucent poppet with radiopaque ring in poppet	1. thromboemboli 2. cocking of disc 3. disc variance

DISC VALVES continued

VALVE	SHAPE	X-RAY	X-RAY OUTLINE	MITRAL/ TRICUSPID	AORTIC	IDENTIFYING FEATURES	COMPLICATIONS
Beall				●		1. 2 parallel indented struts 2. radiopaque poppet	1. obstruction of prosthesis orifice by thrombus 2. cocking of disc 3. hemolysis 4. disc variance 5. gallstones
Harken				●	●	1. thin cross struts 2. radiopaque poppet	1. thromboemboli 2. disc variance
Cooley-Bloodwell-Cutter						1. discoid valve 2. open-ended cage 3. 4 struts 4. radiolucent poppet	1. thromboemboli 2. prosthetic leaks 3. thrombotic valve occlusion
LOW PROFILE VALVES B. HINGED-LEAFLET VALVE							
Gott-Daggett					●	1. central cross strut 2. multiple projecting prongs from ring 3. radiolucent leaflets	1. thromboemboli 2. hemolysis 3. gallstones
LOW PROFILE VALVES C. CENTRAL FLOW ECCENTRIC MONOCUSP VALVES							
Lillehei-Kaster				●	●	1. 2 teardrop-shaped pivots 2. 2 lateral disc guide-shields 3. radiolucent poppet	1. thromboemboli
Wada-Cutter				●	●	1. base ring with 2 notches 2. disc with 2 notches 3. radiolucent poppet	1. early disc wear 2. total valve thrombosis 3. thromboemboli 4. peri-basilar leaks with significant regurgitation
Bjork-Shiley				●	●	1. 2 eccentrically located support struts 2. radiolucent poppet	1. thromboemboli

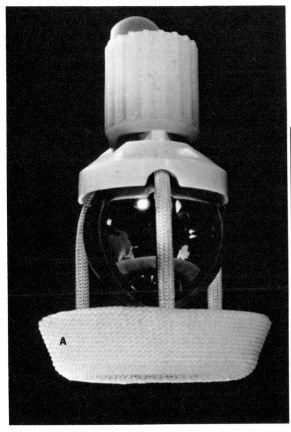
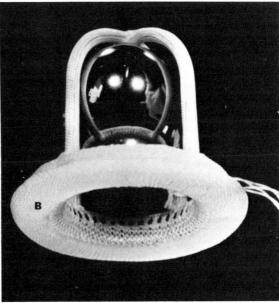

FIG. 522. RECENT MODELS OF THE STARR-EDWARDS CLOTH-COVERED AORTIC (A) AND MITRAL (B) PROSTHETIC HEART VALVES
The fluted device at the top of the aortic valve is used for handling.

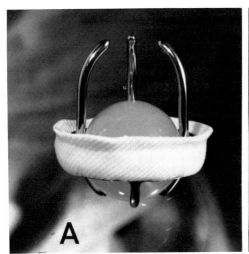
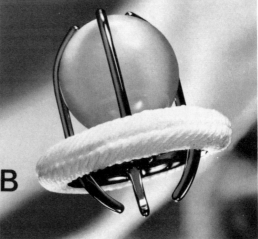

FIG. 523. THE SMELOFF®-CUTTER AORTIC (A) AND MITRAL (B) PROSTHETIC HEART VALVES
(Courtesy of Cutter Laboratories, Inc., Berkeley, California 94710.)

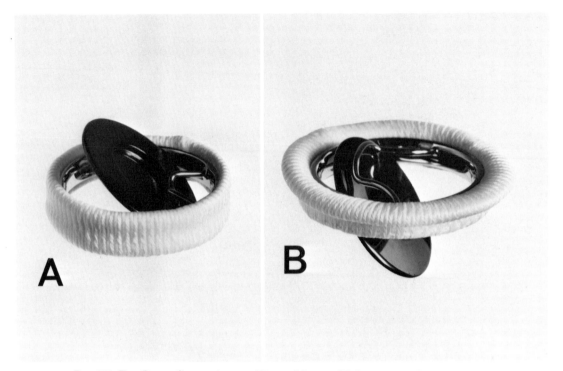

FIG. 524. THE BJORK-SHILEY AORTIC (A) AND MITRAL (B) PROSTHETIC HEART VALVES

The prosthesis is available in two other suture ring configurations. (Courtesy of Shiley Laboratories, Inc., Santa Ana, California 92705.)

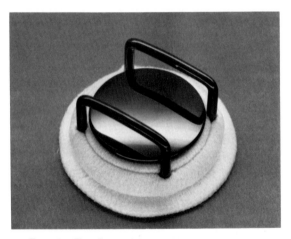

FIG. 525. THE BEALL MITRAL VALVE PROSTHESIS, MODEL 106

(Courtesy of Surgitool Travenol Laboratories, Pittsburgh, Pennsylvania 15234.)

mechanical failure of the prosthesis. Rarely coronary ostial stenosis may occur (Yates *et al.*, 1974; Bonchek and Starr, 1975; Hipona *et al.*, 1971). The radiologist may have a role to play in each of these complications.

Thromboembolism which is the commonest

long term complication is due to thrombus formation usually at the junction of the metal portions of the prosthesis with the surrounding tissue, but may occur on the struts and particularly at the non-contact space at the apex of the older Starr-Edwards prosthesis (Garamella *et al.*, 1964; Spencer *et al.*, 1965). Cloth covering of the metal surfaces has greatly reduced the incidence of thrombus formation (Braunwald, 1971; Bonchek and Starr, 1975). The thrombus material may become so extensive as to inhibit the motion of the poppet. Auscultation and phonocardiography may show a change in the relative intensities of the opening and closing sounds. However, cinefluorography may show a decreased or abnormal excursion (Wilson *et al.*, 1967; Feist and Magovern, 1967). A left ventriculogram in the case of a mitral prosthesis showed a radiolucent defect at the base of the valve (Pfeifer *et al.*, 1972) due to a mound of thrombus material. Chronic fibrous obstruction due to organization of the thrombus material may produce the same effect (Seyfer *et al.*, 1974).

Although covering of the metallic portion of the cage with Teflon mesh has reduced the incidence of thrombus formation and thromboembolism, anticoagulants on a long term basis are usually necessary (Bonchek and Starr, 1975). Also, the cloth tends to fray and split providing an irregular surface that produces excessive hemolysis, and this may necessitate valve replacement (Santinga *et al.*, 1974; Bonchek and Starr, 1975). A later type of the Starr-Edwards prosthesis has inside tracks for contact with the ball which tend to overcome this difficulty. The other common cause of excess hemolysis is regurgitation around the base of the valve, and this is best detected by supravalvular aortography or left ventriculography as indicated (Fig. 526).

The tilting disc Bjork-Shiley valve is subject to thrombus formation, and this may restrict the motion of the disc (Ben-Zvi *et al.*, 1974). Angiography is helpful in demonstrating regurgitation and treatment should be instituted immediately.

Aortic ball variance was a troublesome defect in the earlier Starr-Edwards prosthesis. In an early series, 25% of the cases were documented as showing ball variance, and in 9 cases the variance was a cause of death. The silicone rubber ball absorbs lipids from the blood, often becomes discolored, may shrink in diameter and may become cracked, grooved or contain lakes of fluid. The ball may decrease in size to such an extent that it escapes either momentarily or permanently from the cage (Newman *et al.*, 1967; Kunstadt *et al.*, 1976). In the case reported by Ridolfi and Hutchins (1974), the poppet fragmented and embolized into the portal triads of the liver. The usual signs of improper motion of the poppet are changes in the opening and closing sounds as seen on the phonocardiogram. Ball variance such as cracks or fissures can occur without changes in the valve sounds (Hylen *et al.*, 1969). Fissures, clefts, changes in ball motion and unusual vibrations may be detected by cinefluorography (Wilson *et al.*, 1967; Feist and Magovern, 1967) and by serial radiography using a rapid film changer (Hylen *et al.*, 1969). In those prostheses that are subject to ball variance such as the older Starr-Edwards prosthesis, constant radiologic monitoring is probably indicated (Hylen *et al.*, 1969). The threat of ball variance as a complication has been alleviated by the use of the stellite poppet introduced in 1967. Also, bet-

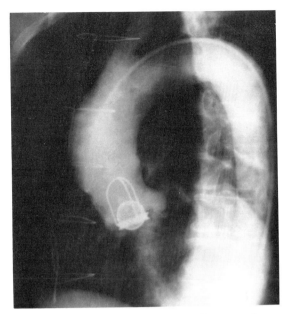

FIG. 526. REGURGITATION AROUND THE BASE OF A STARR-EDWARDS PROSTHESIS ASSOCIATED WITH EXCESSIVE HEMOLYSIS AND ANEMIA

ter curing of the silicone rubber has improved the situation in the use of the Braunwald-Cutter and Smeloff-Cutter valves.

An uncommon complication of aortic valve replacement is stenosis of one or both of the coronary ostia. Yates *et al.* (1974) reported 8 of 292 patients who underwent aortic valve replacement developed stenosis of one or both coronary ostia. Typically angina appeared within 2–6 months following what was thought to be a satisfactory replacement procedure. A number of causes were suspected such as excessive trauma during coronary perfusion, turbulence in the proximal aorta secondary to flow from the prosthetic valve, and tissue overgrowth arising from the base of the implanted valve. When coronary arteriography is attempted in such cases, a preliminary cusp injection should precede attempts to catheterize the artery. Ostial stenosis is otherwise difficult to document. Ostial stenosis may require a coronary bypass procedure.

Bibliography

Aalsmeer, W. C. and Wenckenbach, K. F.: Herz und Kreislauf bei der Beri-beri Krankheit. Wien Arch. Inn. Med. *16:*193, 1929.

Abbott, M. E.: Clinical and developmental study of a case of ruptured aneurysm of the right anterior sinus of Valsalva. Contributions to Medical and Biological Research (Osler Memorial) *2:*899, 1919.

Abbott, M. E.: Atlas of Congenital Cardiac Disease. New York, American Heart Association, 1936.

Abdulla, H. M., Demany, M. A., and Zimmerman, H. A.: Cor triatriatum: preoperative diagnosis in an adult patient. Am. J. Cardiol. *26:*310, 1970.

Abrams, D. L., Edelist, A., Luria, M. H., and Miller, A. J.: Ventricular aneurysm: reappraisal based on a study of 65 consecutive autopsied cases. Circulation *27:*164, 1963.

Abrams, H. L.: Radiologic aspects of operable heart disease. III. The hazards of retrograde thoracic aortography. A survey. Radiology *68:*812, 1957.

Abrams, H. L.: Persistence of fetal ductus function after birth: the ductus arteriosus as an avenue of escape. Circulation *18:*206, 1958.

Abrams, H. L.: The opaque media: physiologic effects and systemic reactions. *In* Angiography, 2nd ed., Vol. 1, pp. 15–35, Little, Brown & Co., Boston, Mass., 1971.

Abrams, H. L., Adams, D. F., and Grant, H. A.: Radiology of tumors of the heart. Radiol. Clin. N.A. *9:*299, 1971.

Abrams, H. L., Adelstein, S. J., Elliott, L. P., Ellis, K., Greenspan, R. H., Judkins, M. P., and Viamonte, M.: Optimal radiologic facilities for examination of the chest and cardiovascular system. Circulation *43:*A-135, 1971.

Abrams, H. L. and Kaplan, H. S.: Angiographic Interpretation in Congenital Heart Disease, pp. 160–162, Springfield, Ill., Charles C Thomas, 1956.

Abrams, H. L., Spiro, R., and Goldstein, N.: Metastases in carcinoma. Analysis of 1000 autopsied cases. Cancer *3:*74, 1956.

Achuff, S. C., Griffith, L. S. C., Conti, C. R., Humpries, J. O., Brawley, R. K., Gott, V. L., and Ross, R. S.: The "angina-producing" myocardial segment: an approach to the interpretation of results of coronary bypass surgery. Am. J. Cardiol. *36:*723, 1975.

Adams, D. F. and Abrams, H. L.: The Complications of Coronary Arteriography, Presented at the Radiological Society of North America Meeting, Chicago, Illinois, 1975.

Adams, D. F., Fraser, D. B., and Abrams, H. L: The complications of coronary arteriography. Circulation *48:*609, 1973.

Adams, J. C. L. and Hudson, R.: A case of Ebstein's anomaly surviving to the age of 79. Brit. Heart J. *18:*129, 1956.

Adams, W. E.: Bilateral resection for arteriovenous fistulae of lung. Proc. Inst. Med. Chicago *18:*294, 1951.

Adams, W. E., Thornton, T. F., Jr., and Eichelberger, L.: Cavernous hemangioma of lung (arteriovenous fistula). Arch. Surg. *49:*51, 1944.

Agarwala, B., Doyle, E. F., Danilowicz, D., Spencer, F. C., and Mills, N. M.: Double outlet right ventricle with pulmonic stenosis and anteriorly positioned aorta (Taussig-Bing variant). Report of a case and surgical correction. Am. J. Cardiol. *32:*850, 1973.

Agustsson, M. H., Gasul, B. M., Fell, E. H., Graettinger, J. S., Bicoff, J. P., and Waterman, D. F.: Anomalous origin of left coronary artery from pulmonary artery. Diagnosis and treatment of infantile and adult types. J.A.M.A. *180:*15, 1962.

Albers, W. H., Hugenholz, P. G., and Nadas, A. S.: Significance of left ventricular volumes in constrictive pericarditis and myocarditis. Circulation *35 & 36:*II-50, 1967.

Aldridge, H. E. and Greenwood, W. F.: Myxoma of the left atrium. Brit. Heart J. *22:*189, 1960.

Aldridge, H. E., McLouglin, M. J., and Taylor, K. W.: Improved diagnosis in coronary cinearteriography with routine use of 110° oblique views and cranial and caudal angulations. Am. J. Cardiol. *36:*468, 1975.

Alexander, C. S. and Gobel, F. L.: Diagnosis of idiopathic hypertrophic subaortic stenosis by right ventricular septal biopsy. Am. J. Cardiol. *34:*142, 1974.

Alfrey, A. C., Goss, J. E., Ogden, D. A., Vogel, J. H. K., and Holmes, J. H.: Uremic hemopericardium. Am. J. Med. *45:*391, 1968.

Alley, R. D., Van Mierop, L. H. S., Li, E. Y., Jagdish, K. R., Kausel, Ho W., and Stranahan, A.: Traumatic aortic aneurysm. Four cases of graftless excision and anastomosis. Ann. Thoracic Surg. *2:*514, 1966.

Alpert, B. S., Mellits, E. D., and Rowe, R. D.: Spontaneous closure of small ventricular septal defects, probability rates in the first five years of life. Am. J. Dis. Child. *125:*194, 1973.

Althaus, U., Kaufmann, M., and Gertsch, M.: Surgical closure of atrial septal defects. J. Cardiovasc. Surg. *15:*300, 1974.

Altieri, P. I., Sharon, M. W., and Leighton, R. F.: Left ventricular wall motion during the isovolumic relaxation period. Circulation *48:*499, 1973.

Amundsen, P.: The diagnostic value of conventional radiological examination of the heart in adults. Acta Radiol., Suppl. 181, 1959.

Amplatz, K., Ernst, R., Lester, R. G., Lillehei, C. W., and Lillie, A.: Retrograde left cardioangiography as a test of valvular competence. Radiology *72:*268, 1959.

Amplatz, K., Lester, R. G., Schiebler, G. L., Adams, P., Jr., and Anderson, R. C.: The roentgenologic features of Ebstein's anomaly of the tricuspid valve. Am. J. Roentgenol. *81:*788, 1959.

Anderson, R. C., Obata, W., and Lillehei, C. W.: Truncus arteriosus (clinical study of fourteen cases). Circulation *16:*586, 1957.

Anderson, R. C., Lillehei, C. W., and Lester, R. G.: A review of corrected transposition of the great vessels of the heart: 17 cases. Pediatrics *20:*626, 1957.

Anderson, R. E., Grondin, C., and Amplatz, K.: The mitral valve in Marfan's syndrome. Radiology *91:*910, 1968.

Anselmi, G., Munoz, S., Blanco, P., Carbonell, L., and Puigbo, J. J.: Anomalous coronary artery communicating with the right ventricle associated with pulmonary stenosis and atrial septal defect. Am. Heart J. *62:*406, 1961.

Apley, J., Horton, R. E., and Wilson, M. G.: The possible role of surgery in the treatment of anomalous left coronary artery. Thorax *12:*28, 1957.

Ardesty, J. M., DeWeese, J. A., Hoffman, M. J., and Yu, P. N.: Carcinoid heart disease: successful repair of the valvular lesions under cardiopulmonary bypass. Circulation *34:*105, 1966.

Arditi, L. I., Holswade, G. R., and Steinberg, I.: Aortic regurgitation following trauma in a patient with a Magovern valve prosthesis. Am. J. Roentgenol. *104*:420, 1968.

Arendt, J.: Radiological differentiation between pericardial effusion and cardiac dilatation. Radiology *50*:44, 1948.

Armer, R. M., Schumacker, H. B., Jr., and Klatte, E. C.: Origin of the right pulmonary artery from the ascending aorta. Report of a surgically corrected case. Circulation *24*:662, 1961.

Arnett, E. N. and Roberts, W. C.: Acute myocardial infarction and angiographically normal coronary arteries. Circulation *53*:395, 1976.

Arnold, H. R.: Postmyocardial infarction syndrome. Am. J. Roentgenol. *90*:628, 1963.

Aronstam, E. M., Strader, B. D., Geiger, J. P., and Gomez, A. C.: Traumatic left ventricular aneurysms. J. Thoracic Cardiovasc. Surg. *59*:239, 1970.

Arnulf, G. and Buffard, P.: L'arteriographie des coronaries grace a l'acetylcholine. Ann. Radiol. (Paris)*2*:685, 1959.

Arvidsson, H., Carlsson, E., Hartmann, A., Jr., Tsifutis, A., and Crawford, C.: Supravalvular stenoses of the pulmonary arteries. Acta Radiol. *56*:466, 1961.

Ashburn, W. L., Braunwald, E., Simon, A. L., Peterson, J. L., and Gault, J. H.: Myocardial perfusion imaging with radio-active-labeled particles injected directly into the coronary circulation of patients with coronary artery disease. Circulation *44*:851, 1971.

Ashcraft, W., Nghiem, Q. X., Nishimura, A., and Padula, R. T.: Double chambered right ventricle. Ann. Thoracic Surg. *16*:273, 1973.

Ashman, H., Zaroff, L. I., and Baronofsky, I.: Right atrial myxoma. Am. J. Med. *28*:487, 1960.

Askey, J. M.: Spontaneous rupture of a papillary muscle of the heart. Review with eight additional cases. Am. J. Med. *9*:528, 1950.

Astley, R., Oldham, J. S., and Parsons, C.: Congenital tricuspid atresia. Brit. Heart J. *15*:287, 1953.

Astley, R. and Parsons, C.: Complete transposition of the great vessels. Brit. Heart. J. *14*:13, 1952.

Atlas, P., Deutsch, V., Lieberman, Y., and Neufeld, H. N.: False aneurysm of the left atrium after closed mitral commissurotomy: diagnosis by cineangiocardiography. Report of one case treated surgically. J. Cardiovasc. Surg. *17*:170, 1976.

Austen, W. G. and Blennerhassett, J. B.: Giant cell aortitis causing an aneurysm of the ascending aorta and aortic insufficiency. New England J. Med. *272*:80, 1965.

Austen, W. G., Edwards, J. E., Frye, R. L., Gensini, G. G., Gott, V. L., Griffith, L. S. C., McGoon, D. W., Murphy, M. L., and Roe, B. B.: AHA Committee Report: A reporting system on patients evaluated for coronary artery disease. Circulation *51*:7, 1975.

Austen, W. G., Sanders, C. A., Averill, J. H., and Friedlich, A. L.: Ruptured papillary muscle. Report of case with successful mitral valve replacement. Circulation *32*:597, 1965.

Austen, W. G., Sokol, V. M., DeSanctis, R. W., and Sanders, C. A.: Surgical treatment of papillary muscle rupture complicating myocardial infarction. N. Engl. J. Med. *278*:113, 1968.

Baer, R. W., Taussig, H. B., and Oppenheimer, E. H.: Congenital aneurysmal dilatation of the aorta associated with arachnodactyly. Bull. Johns Hopkins Hosp. *72*:309, 1943.

Baer, S., Behrend, A., and Goldburgh, H. L.: Arteriovenous fistulas of lung. Circulation *1*:602, 1950.

Baggenstoss, A. H. and Titus, J. L.: Rheumatic and collagen disorders of the heart. *In* Gould, S. E. (ed.): Pathology of the Heart and Great Vessels, Springfield, Charles C Thomas, 1968, pp. 699.

Bahn, R. C., Edwards, J. E., and DuShane, J. W.: Coarctation of the aorta as a cause of death in early infancy. Pediatrics *8*:192, 1951.

Bahnson, H. T., Bauersfeld, S. R., and Smith, J. W.: Pathological anatomy and surgical correction of Ebstein's anomaly. Circulation *31*:I-3, I-8, Suppl. #1, 1965.

Bahnson, H. T., Cooley, R. N., and Sloan, R. D.: Coarctation of the aorta at unusual sites. Am. Heart J. *38*:905, 1949.

Bahnson, H. T. and Newman, E. V.: Diagnosis and surgical removal of intracavitary myxoma of right atrium. Bull. Johns Hopkins Hosp. *93*:150, 1953.

Bahnson, H. T., Spencer, F. C., and Neill, C. A.: Surgical treatment of thirty-five cases of drainage of pulmonary veins to the right side of the heart. J. Thoracic Surg. *36*:777, 1958.

Bailey, C. P., Lemmon, W. M., and Musser, B. G.: Experiences with coarctation of the aorta. Am. J. Cardiol. *4*:775, 1959.

Bailey, C. P. and Morse, D. P.: Mitral commissurotomy performed from the right side. J. Thoracic Surg. *33*:427, 1957.

Bailey, G. L., Hampers, C. L., Hager, E. B., and Merrill, J. P.: Uremic pericarditis. Clinical features and management. Circulation *38*:582, 1968.

Baker, C. G., Benson, P. F., Joseph, M. C., and Ross, D. N.: Congenital mitral stenosis. Brit. Heart J. *24*:498, 1962.

Baker, C. and Trounce, J. R.: Arteriovenous aneurysm of lung. Brit. Heart J. *11*:109, 1949.

Baldwin, J. J. and Edwards, J. E.: Uremic pericarditis as a cause of cardiac tamponade. Circulation *53*:896, 1976.

Balkoura-Christopoulus, M. H., and Kittle, C. F.: Post superior vena cava—right pulmonary artery shunt; total surgical correction of Ebstein's anomaly with Starr-Edwards prosthesis. Chest *63*:120, 1973.

Baltaxe, H. A.: The current uses of coronary angiography. Radiol. Clin. N.A. *9*:597, 1971.

Baltaxe, H. A., Alonso, D. R., Lee, J. G., Prat, J., Husted, J. W., and Stakes, J. W.: Impaired left ventricular contractility in ischemic heart disease: angiographic and histopathologic correlations. Radiology *113*:581, 1974.

Balzer, R. and McCullagh, E. P.: Hypertension in acromegaly. Am. J. Med. Sci. *237*:449, 1959.

Banas, J. S., Meister, S. G., Gazzaniga, A. B., O'Connor, N. E., Haynes, F. W., and Dalen, J. E.: A simple technique for detecting small defects of the atrial septum. Am. J. Cardiol. *28*:467, 1971.

Barcia, A., Kincaid, O. W., Davis, G. D., Kirklin, J. W., and Ongley, P. A.: Transposition of the great arteries: an angiocardiographic study. Am. J. Roentgenol. *100*:249, 1967.

Bardeen, C. R.: Determination of the size of the heart by means of the x-rays. Am. J. Anat. *23*:423, 1918.

Barden, R. P.: Reflections of disease in the pulmonary medulla. Radiology *75*:454, 1960.

Barden, R. P.: Pulmonary edema: correlation of roentgenologic appearance and abnormal physiology. Am. J. Roentgenol. *92*:495, 1964.

Barker, N. W., Nygaard, K. K., Watlers, W., and Priestley, J. T.: Statistical study of post-operative venous thrombosis and pulmonary embolism. III—Time of occurrence during the preoperative period. Proc. Staff. Meet. Mayo Clin. *16*:17, 1941.

Barlorik, M. and Diesek, J.: Cardiomyopathy accompanying industrial Cobalt exposure. Brit. Heart J. *34*:113, 1972.

Barlow, J. B. and Bosman, C. K.: Aneurysmal protrusion of the posterior leaflet of the mitral valve. An auscultatory-electrocardiographic syndrome. Am. Heart J. *71*:166, 1966.

Barnard, C. N. and Schrire, V.: Surgical correction of Ebstein's malformation with prosthetic tricuspid valve. Surgery *54*:302, 1963.

Barnhard, H. J. and Barnhard, F. M.: The emergency treatment of reactions to contrast media. Radiol. Clin. N.A. *3*:51, 1965.

Baron, M. G.: Endocardial cushion defects. Radiol. Clin. N.A.

6:343, 1968.

Baron, M. G.: Post-infarction aneurysm of the left ventricle. Circulation 43:762, 1971.

Baron, M. G.: Radiologic notes in cardiology. Angiographic differentiation between tetralogy of Fallot and double-outlet right ventricle. Relationship of the mitral and aortic valves. Circulation 43:451, 1971.

Baron, M. G.: Abnormalities of the mitral valve in endocardial cushion defects. Circulation 45:672, 1972.

Baron, M. G., Wolf, B. S., Steinfeld, L., and Gordon, A. J.: Left ventricular angiocardiogram in the study of ventricular septal defect. Radiology 81:223, 1963.

Baron, M. G., Wolf, B. S., Steinfeld, L., and Van Mierop, L. H. S.: Endocardial cushion defects: specific diagnosis by angiocardiography. Am. J. Cardiol. 13:162, 1964.

Baronofsky, I. D., Gordon, A. J., Grishman, A., Steinfeld, L., and Kreel, I.: Aorticopulmonary septal defect. Diagnosis and report of case successfully treated. Am. J. Cardiol. 5:273, 1960.

Barratt-Boyes, B. G., Nicholls, T. T., Brandt, P. W. T., and Neutze, J. M.: Aortic arch interruption associated with patent ductus arteriosus, ventricular septal defect, and total anomalous pulmonary venous connection. Total correction in an 8-day-old infant by means of profound hypothermia and limited cardiopulmonary bypass. J. Thoracic Cardiovasc. Surg. 63:367, 1972.

Bartel, A. G., Chen, J. T., Peter, R. H., Behar, V. S., Kong, Y., and Lester, R. G.: The significance of coronary calcification detected by fluoroscopy. Circulation 49:1247, 1974.

Bauersfield, S. R., Adkins, P. C., and Kent, E. M.: Patent ductus arteriosus in infancy. J. Thoracic Surg. 33:123, 1957.

Bayley, R. H. and Holoubek, J. E.: Coarctation of the aorta at or above the origin of the left subclavian artery. Brit. Heart J. 2:208, 1940.

Beachley, M. C., Ranniger, K., and Roth, F. J.: Roentgenographic evaluation of dissecting aneurysms of the aorta. Am. J. Roentgenol. 121:617, 1974.

Beadenkopf, W. G., Daoud, A. S., and Love, B. M.: Calcification in the coronary arteries and its relationship to arteriosclerosis and myocardial infarction. Am. J. Roentgenol. 92:865, 1964.

Beall, A. C., Morris, G. C., Noon, G. P., Guinn, G. A., Raul, G. R., Lefrak, E. A., and Greenberg, S. D.: An improved mitral valve prosthesis. Ann. Thoracicc Surg. 15:25, 1973.

Bean, W. B. and Mohaupt, F. X.: Rupture of the aortic valve. J.A.M.A. 150:92, 1952.

Beasley, K.: Traumatic tricuspid insufficiency. Texas Med. 69:71, 1973.

Beck, W., Schrire, V., Vogelpoel, L., Nellen, M., and Swanepoel, A.: Corrected transposition of the great vessels. Brit. Heart J. 23:497, 1961.

Becker, A. E., Becker, M. J., and Edwards, J. E.: Malposition of pulmonary arteries (crossed pulmonary arteries) in persistent truncus arteriosus. Am. J. Roentgenol. 110:509, 1970.

Becu, L. M., Swan, H. J. C., DuShane, J. W., and Edwards, J. E.: Ebstein's malformation of the left atrioventricular valve in corrected transposition of the great vessels with ventricular septal defect. Proc. Staff Meet. Mayo Clin. 30:483, 1955.

Belle, M. S.: Right atrial myxoma. Circulation 19:910, 1959.

Bellon, E. M., Borkat, G., Whitman, V., and Perrin, E. G.: Unusual catheter course in aortic arch atresia associated with aortopulmonary window. Brit. J. Radiol. 47:144, 1974.

Benchimol, A., Maia, I. G., and Maroko, P. R.: Selective coronary dye dilution curves in normal subjects and in patients with coronary disease. Amer. J. Cardiol. 22:844, 1968.

Benry, J. Price, E. C., Massin, E. K., Bowers, J. C., and Cooley, D. A.: Coronary occlusion secondary to nonpene-trating chest trauma. Texas Medicine, 71:60, 1975.

Bennett, D. E. and Cherry, J. K.: The natural history of traumatic aneurysms of the aorta. Surgery 61:516, 1967.

Ben-Zvi, J., Hildner, F. J., Chandraratna, P. A., and Samet, P.: Thrombosis on Bjork-Shiley aortic valve prosthesis: clinical, arteriographic, echocardiographic and therapeutic observations in seven cases. Am. J. Cardiol. 34:538, 1974.

Bercu, B. A., Diettert, G. A., Danforth, W. H., Pund, E. E., Jr., Ahlvin, R. C., and Belliveau, R. R.: Pseudoaortic stenosis produced by ventricular hypertrophy. Am. J. Med. 25:814, 1958.

Berg, N. O., Idbohrn, H., and Wendeberg, B.: Investigation of the tolerance of the rabbit's kidney to the newer contrast media in renal angiography. Acta Radiol. 50:285, 1958.

Bernhard, G. C., Lange, R. L., and Hensley, G. T.: Aortic disease with valvular insufficiency as the principal manifestation of systemic lupus erythematosus. Ann. Int. Med. 71:81, 1969.

Bernhard, W. F., Keane, J. F., Fellows, K. E., Lotwin, S. B., and Gross, R. E.: Progress and problems in the surgical management of congenital aortic stenosis. J. Thoracic Cardiovasc. Surg. 66:404, 1973.

Bernheim, H.: De l'asytole veineuse dans l'hypertrophie du coeur gouche par stenose comcomitante du ventricule droit. Rev. Med. 30:785, 1910.

Bernstein, J., Nolke, A. C., and Reed, J. O.: Extrapulmonic stenosis of the pulmonary veins. Circulation 19:891, 1959.

Berthrong, M. and Sabiston, D. C.: Cerebral lesions in congenital heart disease. A review of autopsies on 162 cases. Bull. Johns Hopkins Hosp. 89:384, 1951.

Bertrand, C. A. and Cooley, R. N.: Congenital aneurysm of the left ventricle. A case report. Ann. Int. Med. 43:426, 1955.

Best, P. V. and Heath, D.: The right ventricle and small pulmonary arteries in aneurysmal dilatation of the left atrium. Brit. Heart J. 26:312, 1964.

Betriu, A., Wigle, E. D., Felderhof, C. H., and McLoughlin, M. J.: Prolapse of the posterior leaflet of the mitral valve associated with secundum atrial septal defect. Am. J. Cardiol. 35:363, 1975.

Beuren, A.: Differential diagnosis of the Taussig-Bing heart from complete transposition of the great vessels with a posteriorly overriding pulmonary artery. Circulation 21:1071, 1960.

Beuren, A. J., Apitz, J., and Harmjanz, D.: Supravalvular aortic stenosis in association with mental retardation and certain facial appearance. Circulation 26:1235, 1962.

Bhariti, S. and Lev, M.: Congenital polyvalvular disease. Circulation 47:575, 1973.

Bhariti, S., McAllister, H. A., Rosenquist, G. C., Miller, R. A., Tatooles, C. J., and Lev, M.: The surgical anatomy of truncus arteriosus communis. J. Thoracic Cardiovasc. Surg. 67:501, 1974.

Bialostozky, D., Horwitz, S., and Espino-Vela, J.: Ebstein's malformation of the tricuspid valve. A review of 65 cases. Am. J. Cardiol. 29:826, 1972.

Bianchi, A.: Morfologia delle arterie coronariae cordis. Arch. Ital. Anat. Embriol. 3:87, 1904.

Bindelglass, I. L. and Trubowitz, S.: Pulmonary vein obstruction: an uncommon sequel to chronic fibrous mediastinitis. Ann. Int. Med. 48:876, 1958.

Bing, R. J., Vandam, L. D., and Gray, F. D., Jr.: Physiological studies in congenital heart disease. I. Procedures. II. Results of preoperative studies in patients with tetralogy of Fallot. III. Results obtained in five cases of Eisenmenger's complex. Bull. Johns Hopkins Hosp. 80:107, 121, 323, 1947.

Biorck, G. and Crafoord, C.: Arteriovenous aneurysm of the pulmonary artery simulating patent ductus arteriosus botale. Thorax 2:65, 1947.

Bjork, L. and Lodin, H.: The heart and blood vessels: angiographic determination of left atrial and left ventricular volumes in normal children and adults. Acta Radiol. *3:*577, 1965.

Bjork, L., Spindola-Franco, H., Van Houten, F. X., Cohn, P. F., and Douglass, F. A.: Comparison of observer performance with 16mm cinefluorography and 70mm camera fluorography in coronary arteriography. Am. J. Cardiol. *36:*474, 1975.

Bjork, V. O.: Ventricular aneurysm. Thorax *19:*162, 1964.

Bjork, V. O.: A new tilting disc valve prosthesis. Scan. J. Thorac. Cardiovasc. Surg. *3:*1, 1969.

Black, J. A. and Bonham-Carter, R. E.: Association between aortic stenosis and facies of severe infantile hypercalcemia. Lancet *2:*745, 1963.

Blake, H. A., Manion, W. C., Mattingly, T. W., and Baroldi, G.: Coronary artery anomalies. Circulation *30:*927, 1964.

Blake, H. A., Manion, W. C., and Spencer, F. C.: Atresia or absence of the aortic isthmus. J. Thoracic Cardiovasc. Surg. *43:*607, 1962.

Blakley, B. H., Ridolfi, R. L., Salyer, W. R., and Hutchins, D. M.: Myocardial lesions of progressive systemic sclerosis. The cause of cardiac dysfunction. Circulation *53:*483, 1976.

Blalock, A. and Hanlon, C. R.: The surgical treatment of complete transposition of the aorta and pulmonary artery. Surg. Gynecol. Obstet. *90:*1, 1950.

Blalock, A. and Ravitch, M. M.: A consideration of the nonoperative treatment of cardiac tamponade resulting from wounds of the heart. Surgery *14:*157, 1943.

Blalock, A. and Taussig, H. B.: The surgical treatment of malformations of the heart in which there is pulmonary stenosis or pulmonary atresia. J.A.M.A. *128:*189, 1945.

Blankenhorn, D. H.: Coronary arterial calcification. A review. Am. J. Med. Sci. *242:*1, 1961.

Blankenhorn, D. H. and Stern, D.: Calcification of coronary arteries. Am. J. Roentgenol. *81:*772, 1959.

Blankenhorn, M. A.: The heart in vitamin deficiencies. *In* Disorders of the Heart and Circulation. Edited by R. L. Levy. Chap. XIX. Baltimore, The Williams & Wilkins Co., 1951.

Blieden, L. C., Randall, P. A., Castaneda, A. R., Lucas, R. V., Jr., and Edwards, J. E.: The "gooseneck" of the endocardial cushion defect: anatomic basis. Chest *65:*13, 1974.

Bloomfield, D. K., and Liebman, J.: Idiopathic cardiomyopathy in children. Circulation *27:*1071, 1963.

Bloor, B. M., Wrenn, F. R., and Margolis, G.: An experimental evaluation of certain contrast media for cerebral angiography: electroencephalographic and histopathological correlations. J. Neurosurg. *8:*585, 1951.

Blount, S. G., Jr., Vigoda, P. S., and Swan, H.: Isolated infundibular stenosis. Am. Heart J. *57:*684, 1959.

Bonchek, L., Anderson, R., and Rosch, J.: Should coronary arteriograms be performed routinely prior to valve replacement? Circulation *56:*II-133, 1972.

Bonchek, L. I. and Starr, A.: Ball valve prostheses: current appraisal of late results. Am. J. Cardiol. *35:*843, 1975.

Bonchek, L. I., Sunderland, C. O., and Starr, A. K.: Spontaneous closure of ventricular septal defect following pulmonary artery banding. Chest *63:*453, 1973.

Bone, D. K., Maddrey, W. C., Eagan, J., and Cameron, J. L.: Cardiac tamponade. Arch. Surg. *106:*868, 1973.

Bonte, F. J., Parkey, R. W., Graham, K. D., Moore, J., and Stokely, E. M.: A new method for radionuclide imaging of myocardial infarcts. Radiology *110:*473, 1974.

Bookstein, J. J. and Sigmann, J. M.: Intramural deposition of contrast agent during selective angiocardiography. Radiology *81:*932, 1963.

Boone, M. L., Swenson, B. E., and Felson, B.: Rib notching: its many causes. Am. J. Roentgenol. *91:*1075, 1964.

Bose, J. S., Levin, D. C., Goldstein, S., and Laster, W.: Congenital absence of the pulmonary valve associated with congenital aplasia of the thymus (DiGeorge's syndrome). Am. J. Roentgenol. *122:*97, 1974.

Bosher, L. H., Jr. and McCue, C. M.: Diagnosis and surgical treatment of aortopulmonary fenestration. Circulation *25:*456, 1962.

Bosniak, M. A.: An analysis of some anatomic roentgenologic aspects of the brachiocephalic vessels. Am. J. Roentgenol. *91:*1222, 1964.

Bothwell, T. H., Van Lingen, B., Whidborne, J., Kaye, J., McGregor, M., and Elliot, G. A.: Patent ductus arteriosus with partial reversal of the shunt. Am. Heart J. *44:*360, 1852.

Botvnick, E. H., Shames, D., Hutchinson, J. C., Roe, B. B., and Fitzpatrick, M.: Noninvasive diagnosis of a false left ventricular aneurysm with radioisotope gated cardiac blood pool imaging. Differentiation from true aneurysm. Am. J. Cardiol. *37:*1089, 1976.

Bougon, M.: Observations sur un anevrisme d'une des arteres coronaires ou cardiaques. Bib. Med. *37:*85 and *37:*183, 1812.

Bourassa, M. G., Lesperance, J., and Campeau, L.: Selective coronary arteriography by the percutaneous femoral artery approach. Am. J. Roentgenol. *107:*377, 1969.

Boyden, E. A.: A synthesis of the prevailing patterns of the bronchopulmonary segments in the light of their variations. Dis. Chest *15:*657, 1949.

Brandt, R. L., Foley, W. L., and Fink, G. H.: Mechanism of perforation of the heart with production of hydropericardium by a venous catheter and its prevention. Am. J. Surg. *119:*311, 1970.

Brantigan, O. C.: Anomalies of the pulmonary veins. Surg. Gynecol. Obstet. *84:*653, 1947.

Braun, K.: Pulmonary artery dilatation as a cause of chest pain. Am. Heart J. *62:*715, 1961.

Braun, L. O., Kincaid, O. W., and McGoon, D. C.: Prognosis of aortic valve replacement in relation to the preoperative heart size. J. Thoracic Cardiovasc. Surg. *65:*381, 1973.

Braunwald, E. and Gorlin, R.: Cooperative study on cardiac catheterization. Total population studied, procedures employed, and incidence of complications. Circulation *37* (Supp. 3):8, 1968.

Braunwald, E., Lambrew, C. T., Rockoff, S. D., Ross, J., Jr., and Morrow, A. G.: Idiopathic hypertrophic subaortic stenosis. Circulation *30* (Supp. 4):3, 1964.

Braunwald, E. and Morrow, A. G.: Left ventriculo-right atrial communication: diagnosis by clinical, hemodynamic and angiographic methods. Am. J. Med. *28:*913, 1960.

Braunwald, E., Morrow, A. G., Cornell, W. P., Aygen, M. M., and Hilbish, T. F.: Idiopathic hypertrophic subaortic stenosis: clinical, hemodynamic and angiographic manifestations. Am. J. Med. *29:*924, 1960.

Braunwald, N. S., Tatooles, C., and Turina, M.: New development in the design of fabric-covered prosthetic heart valves. J. Thoracic Cardiovasc. Surg. *62:*673, 1971.

Bravo, A. J., McIntosh, C. L., and Morrow, A. G.: A correlation of chest roentgenograms and hemodynamic findings following operative treatment of congenital cardiac valvular lesions. Radiol. Clin. N.A. *9:*219, 1971.

Brawley, R. K., Donahoo, J. S., and Gott, V. L.: Current status of the Beall, Bjork-Shiley, Braunwald-Cutter, Lillehei-Kaster and Smeloff-Cutter cardiac valve prosthesis. Am. J. Cardiol. *35:*855, 1975.

Brean, H. P., Marks, J. H., Sosman, M. C., and Schlesinger, M. J.: Massive calcification in infarcted myocardium. Radiology *54:*33, 1950.

Breckenridge, I. M., Stark, J., Waterston, D. J., and Bonaham-Carter, R. E.: Multiple ventricular septal defects. Ann. Thoracic Surg. *13:*128, 1972.

Brenner, O.: Pathology of the vessels of the pulmonary circulation. Arch. Int. Med. *56:*(Part I) 211, (Part II) 457, (Part III) 724, (Part IV) 976, (Part V) 1189, 1935.

Brettner, A., Heitzman, E. R., Woodin, W. G.: Pulmonary complications of drug therapy. Radiology 96:31, 1970.

Brigden, W.: Uncommon myocardial diseases. The non-coronary cardiomyopathies. Lancet 2:1243, 1957.

Brindley, P. and Stembridge, V. A.: Aneurysms of the aorta: a clinicopathologic study of 369 necropsy cases. Am. J. Path. 32:67, 1956.

Brink, A. J.: Telangiectasis of lung, with two case reports of hereditary haemorrhagic telangiectasia with cyanosis. Quart. J. Med. 19:239, 1951.

Brock, R.: Functional obstruction of the left ventricle (acquired aortic subvalvular stenosis). Guy's Hosp. Rep. 108:126, 1959.

Brockenbrough, E. C. and Braunwald, E.: New technic for left ventricular angiography and transseptal left heart catheterization. Am. J. Cardiol. 6:1062, 1960.

Broden, B., Jonsson, G., and Karnell, J.: Thoracic aortography. Observations on technical problems connected with the method and various risks involved in its use. Acta Radiol. 32:498, 1949.

Brodey, P. A., Doppman, J. L., and Bisaccia, L. J.: An unusual complication of aortography with the pigtail catheter. Radiology 110:711, 1974.

Brody, H.: Drainage of the pulmonary veins into the right side of the heart. Arch. Path. 33:221, 1942.

Broman, T. and Olsson, O.: Experimental study of contrast media for cerebral angiography with reference to possible injurious effects on the cerebral blood vessels. Acta Radiol. 31:321, 1949.

Bruno, F. P., Cobb, F. R., and Rivas, F.: Evaluation of 99m technetium stannous pyrophosphate as an imaging agent in acute myocardial infarction. Circulation 54:71, 1976.

Bruschke, A. V. G.: Progress study of 590 consecutive non-surgical cases of coronary disease followed five to nine years. I. Arteriographic correlations. J.A.M.A. 225:1012, 1973.

Bruschke, A. V. G., Proudfitt, W. L., and Sones, F. M.: Clinical course of patients with normal and slightly or moderately abnormal coronary arteriograms. Circulation 47:936, 1973.

Brust, A. A., Howard, J. M., Bryant, M. R., and Goodwin, J. T.: Coarctation of the abdominal aorta with stenosis of the renal arteries and hypertension. Clinical and pathologic study of two cases and review of the literature. Am. J. Med. 27:793, 1959.

Bruwer, A. and Pugh, D. G.: A neglected roentgenologic sign of coarctation of the aorta. Proc. Staff Meet. Mayo Clin. 27:377, 1952.

Bruwer, A. J., Ellis, F. H., and Kirklin, J. W.: Costophrenic septal lines in pulmonary venous hypertension. Circulation 12:807, 1955.

Bryant, L. R., Mobin-Uddin, K., Dillon, M. L., Hinshaw, M. A., and Utley, J. R.: Cardiac valve injury with major chest trauma. Arch. Surg. 107:279, 1973.

Brymer, J. F., Buter, T. H., Walton, J. A., Jr., and Willis, P. W., III.: A natural history study of the prognostic role of coronary arteriography. Am. Heart J. 88:2, 1974.

Buckley, M. J., Mundth, E. D., Daggett, W. M., DeSanctis, R. W., Sanders, C. A., and Austen, W. G.: Surgical therapy for early complications of myocardial infarction. Surgery 70:814, 1971.

Buckley, M. J., Mason, D. T., Ross, J., Jr., and Braunwald, E.: Reversed differential cyanosis with equal desaturation of the upper limbs. Syndrome of complete transposition of the great vessels with complete interruption of the aortic arch. Am. J. Cardiol. 15:111, 1965.

Buenger, R. E., Paul, O., and Fell, E. H.: Calcified polyp of the heart. Radiology 67:531, 1956.

Bulkley, D. H. and Roberts, W. C.: Systemic lupus erythe-matosus as a cause of severe mitral regurgitation. New problem in an old disease. Am. J. Cardiol. 35:305, 1975.

Burggraf, G. W. and Parker, J. O.: Prognosis in coronary artery disease. Circulation 51:146, 1975.

Burroughs, J. T. and Edwards, J. E.: Total anomalous pulmonary venous connection. Am. Heart J. 59:913, 1960.

Burroughs, J. T. and Kirklin, J. W.: Complete surgical correction of total anomalous pulmonary venous connection: report of three cases. Proc. Staff Meet. Mayo Clin. 31:182, 1956.

Burwell, C. S. and Dexter, L.: Beri-beri heart disease. Trans. Assoc. Am. Physicians 60:59, 1947.

Burwell, C. S., Eppinger, E. C., and Gross, R. E.: The effects of patency of the ductus arteriosus on the circulation. J. Clin. Invest. 19:774, 1940.

Byhardt, R., Brace, K., Ruckdeschel, J., Chang, P., Martin, R., and Wiesnik, P.: Dose and treatment factors in radiation-related pericardial effusion associated with mantle techniques for Hodgkin's disease. Cancer 35:795, 1975.

Byron, F. and Thompson, W.: Myxoma of the right ventricle. Ann. Thoracic Surg. 2:424, 1966.

Caffey, J.: Pediatric X-ray Diagnosis, ed. 4, p. 461. Chicago, Year Book Medical Publishers Inc., 1961.

Caldicott, W. J. H., Hollenberg, N. K., and Abrams, H. L.: Characteristics of response of renal vascular bed to contrast media. Evidence for vasoconstriction induced by renin angiotensin system. Invest. Radiol. 5:539, 1970.

Calenoff, L.: Multiple mycotic pulmonary artery aneurysms. Am. J. Roentgenol. 91:379, 1964.

Campbell, M. and Deuchar, D. C.: The left-sided superior vena cava. Brit. Heart J. 16:423, 1954.

Campbell, M. and Deuchar, D. C.: Absent inferior vena cava, symmetrical liver, splenic agenesis, and situs inversus, and their embryology. Brit. Heart J. 29:268, 1967.

Campbell, M. and Forgacs, P.: Laevocardia with transposition of the abdominal viscera. Brit. Heart J. 15:401, 1953.

Campbell, M. and Gardner, F.: Radiological features of enlarged bronchial arteries. Brit. Heart J. 12:183, 1950.

Campbell, M. and Kauntze, R.: Congenital aortic valvular stenosis. Brit. Heart J. 15:179, 1953.

Capp, M. P., Levin, A. R., Jarmakani, M. M., Canent, R. V., Jr., Graham, T. P., and Lester, R. G.: New concepts of isolated ventricular septal defect. Radiol. Clin. N.A. 6:327, 1968.

Carey, L. S. and Edwards, J. E.: Roentgenographic features in cases with origin of both great vessels from the right ventricle without pulmonary stenosis. Am. J. Roentgenol. 93:269, 1965.

Carey, L. S., Sellers, R. D., and Shone, J. D.: Radiologic findings in the developmental complex of parachute mitral valve, supravalvular ring of left atrium, subaortic stenosis, and coarctation of aorta. Radiology 82:1, 1964.

Carlsson, E. S.: The cardiovascular system, in the A.U.R. Symposium, "Quantitative Data from Radiological Images". Invest. Radiol. 7:293, 1972.

Carlsson, E. S., Keene, R. J., Lee, P., and Goerke, R. J.: Angiocardiographic stroke volume correlation of the two cardiac ventricles in man. Invest. Radiol. 6:44, 1971.

Carmichael, J. H. E., Julian, D. G., Jones, G. P., and Wren, E. M.: Radiological signs in pulmonary hypertension. The significance of lines B of Kerley. Brit. J. Radiol. 27:393, 1954.

Carney, E. K., Braunwald, E., Roberts, W. C., Aygen, M., and Morrow, A. H.: Congenital mitral regurgitation: clinical, hemodynamic and angiocardiographic findings in nine patients. Am. J. Med. 33:223, 1962.

Carrasquilla, C., Wilson, R. F., Walt, A. J., and Arbulu, A.: Gunshot wounds of the heart. Ann. Thoracic Surg. 13:208, 1972.

Carroll, D.: Non-Traumatic aortic valve rupture. Bull. Johns Hopkins Hosp. *89*:309, 1951.

Cascade, T. N., Kantrowitz, A., Wajszczuk, W. J., and Rubinfar, E. M.: The chest x-ray in acute left ventricular power failure: an aid to determining prognosis of patients supported by intra-aortic balloon pumping. Am. J. Roentgenol. *126*:1147, 1976.

Case, R. B., Hurley, H. W., and Keating, P.: Detection and measurement of circulatory shunts by use of a radioactive gas. Prog. Cardiovascular Dis. *2*:186, 1959.

Castaneda, A. R., Sade, R. M., Lamberti, J., and Nicoloff, D. M.: Reoperation for residual defects after repair of tetralogy of Fallot. Surgery *76*:1010, 1974.

Casteneda, A. R. and Varco, R. L.: Tumors of the heart. Surgical considerations. Am. J. Cardiol. *21*:357, 1968.

Castellanos, A. and Hernandez, F. A.: Angiocardiographic determination of the size of the left ventricular cavity in congenital aortic disease. Am. J. Roentgenol. *100*:299, 1967.

Castellanos, A., Jr., Ugarriza, R., de Cardenas, A., and Cano, L. A.: Sindrome de Marfan: reporte de seis casos en una misma familia. Arch. Hosp. Univ. (Habana) *9*:353, 1957.

Castellanos, A., Pereiras, R., and Garcia, A.: La angiocardiographia radio opaca. Arch. Soc. Estud. Clin. Habana *31*:523, 1937.

Cavalcanti, I. D. L., Tompson, G., DeSouza, N., and Barbosa, F. S.: Pulmonary hypertension in schistosomiasis. Brit. Heart J. *24*:363, 1962.

Cayler, C. G.: Spontaneous functional closure of symptomatic atrial septal defects. N. Engl. J. Med. *276*:65, 1967.

Cayler, C. G., Smeloff, E. H., and Miller, G. E., Jr.: Surgical palliation of hypoplastic left heart. N. Engl. J. Med. *282*:780, 1970.

Celoria, G. C. and Patton, R. B.: Congenital absence of aortic arch. Am. Heart J. *58*:407, 1959.

Chahine, R. A., Raizner, A. E., Ishimori, T., Luchi, R. J., and McIntosh, H. D.: The incidence and clinical implications of coronary artery spasm. Circulation *52*:972, 1975.

Chait, A., Cohen, H. E., Meltzer, L. E., and Vandurme, J. P.: The bedside chest radiograph in the evaluation of incipient heart disease. Radiology *105*:563, 1972.

Chait, A., Summers, D., Krasnow, N., and Wechsler, B. M.: Observations on the fate of large pulmonary emboli. Am. J. Roentgenol. *100*:364, 1967.

Chaitman, B. R., Lesperance, J., Saltiel, J., and Bourassa, M. G.: Clinical, angiographic, and hemodynamic findings in patients with anomalous origin of the coronary arteries. Circulation *53*:122, 1976.

Challis, T. W. and May, J. E.: Isolated dilatation of the main pulmonary artery: a report of three cases and a review of the literature. J. Assn. Canad. Radiol. *10*:180, 1969.

Chambers, A. A.: Traumatic aortic rupture. J.A.M.A. *229*:463, 1974.

Chambliss, J. R., Jaruszewski, E. J., Brofman, B. L., Martin, J. F., and Feil, H.: Chronic cardiac compression (chronic constrictive pericarditis) A critical study of 61 operated cases with follow-up. Circulation *4*:816, 1951.

Chang, C. H.: The normal roentgenographic measurement of the right descending pulmonary artery in 1,085 cases. Am. J. Roentgenol. *87*:929, 1962.

Chang, C. H. and Amory, H. I.: Congenital partial right pericardial defect associated with herniation of the right atrial appendage. Radiology *84*:660, 1965.

Chang, C. H. and Leigh, T. F.: Congenital partial defect of the pericardium associated with herniation of the left atrial appendage. Am. J. Roentgenol. *86*:517, 1961.

Chapman, C. B., Baker, O., Mitchell, J. H., and Collier, R. G.: Experience with a cinefluorographic method for measuring ventricular volume. Am. J. Cardiol. *18*:25, 1966.

Chapman, C. B. and Robbins, S. L.: Patent ductus arteriosus with pulmonary vascular sclerosis and cyanosis. Ann. Int. Med. *12*:312, 1944.

Chapman, E. M., Dill, D. B., and Graybeil, A.: The decrease in functional capacity of the lungs and heart resulting from deformities of the chest. Medicine *18*:167, 1939.

Chardack, W. M., Gage, A. H., Federico, A. J., Schimert, G., and Greatbach, W.: Clinical experience with an implantable pacemaker. Ann. N. Y. Acad. Sci. *111*:1075, 1964.

Chavez, I., Dorbecker, N., and Celis, A.: Direct intracardiac angiocardiography: its diagnostic value. Am. Heart J. *33*:560, 1947.

Cheitlin, M. D., de Castro, C. M., and McAllister, H. A.: Sudden death as a complication of anomalous left coronary origin from the anterior sinus of Valsalva, a not-so-minor congenital anomaly. Circulation *50*:787, 1974.

Cheitlin, M. D., McAllister, H. A., and de Castro, C. M.: Myocardial infarction without atherosclerosis. J.A.M.A. *231*:951, 1975.

Cheng, T. O.: Incidence of ventricular aneurysm in coronary artery disease: an angiographic appraisal. Am. J. Med. *50*:340, 1971.

Cheng, T. O. and Adkins, P. C.: Traumatic aneurysm of left anterior descending coronary artery with fistulous opening into left ventricle and left ventricular aneurysm after stab wound of chest. Report of case with successful surgical repair. Am. J. Cardiol. *31*:384, 1973.

Chesler, E.: Aneurysms of the left ventricle. Cardiovascular Clin. *4*:187, 1972.

Chesler, E., Beck, W., and Schrire, V.: Selective catheterization of pulmonary or bronchial arteries in the preoperative assessment of pseudotruncus arteriosus and truncus arteriosus type IV. Am. J. Cardiol. *26*:20, 1970.

Childe, A. E. and Mackenzie, E. R.: Calicification in the ductus arteriosus. Am. J. Roentgenol. *54*:370, 1945.

Chiechi, M. A.: Incomplete transposition of the great vessels with biventricular origin of the pulmonary artery (Taussig-Bing complex): report of 4 cases and a review of the literature. Am. J. Med. *22*:234, 1957.

Christensen, E. E. and Bonte, F. J.: The relative accuracy of echocardiography, intravenous CO2 studies, and blood-pool scanning in detecting pericardial effusion in dogs. Radiology *91*:265, 1968.

Christensen, E. E., Curry, T. S., III, and Nunnally, J.: An Introduction to the Physics of Diagnostic Radiology, pp. 172–186, Lea & Febiger, Philadelphia, 1972.

Chun, P. K. C. and Nelson, W. P.: Common cardiac prosthetic valves. Radiologic identification and associated complications. J.A.M.A. *238*:401, 1977.

Chung, K. J., Alexson, C. G., Manning, J. A., and Gramiak, R.: Echocardiography in truncus arteriosus. Circulation *58*:281, 1973.

Civins, W. H. and Edwards, J. E.: The postnatal structural changes in the intrapulmonary arterioles. Arch. Pathol. *51*:192, 1951.

Clagett, A. H., Jr.: Cardiac roentgenology. The value of exact cardiac measurements. Am. J. Roentgenol. *46*:794, 1941.

Clark, W. S., Kulka, J. P., and Bower, W.: Rheumatoid aortitis with aortic regurgitation: an unusual manifestation of rheumatoid arthritis including spondylitis. Am. J. Med. *22*:580, 1957.

Clarkson, P. M., Barratt-Bores, B. G., Neutze, J. M., and Lowe, J. B.: Results over a ten year period of palliation followed by corrective surgery for complete transposition of the great arteries. Circulation *45*:1251, 1972.

Coates, E. O., Jr. and Drake, E. H.: Myxoma of the right atrium, with variable right-to-left shunt. N. Engl. J. Med. *259*:165, 1958.

Cohen, L. S., Friedman, W. F., and Braunwald, E.: Natural history of mild congenital aortic stenosis elucidated by serial hemodynamic studies. Am. J. Cardiol. *30:*1, 1972.

Cohen, L. S., Kokko, J. P., and Williams, W. H.: Hemolysis and hemoglobinuria following angiography. Radiology *92:*329, 1969.

Cohen, M. V. and Gorlin, R.: Main left coronary artery disease: clinical experience from 1964–1974. Circulation *52:*275, 1975.

Cokkinos, D. V., Plessas, S. T., Tolis, G., and Voridis, E. M.: Tricuspid atresia with dextroversion. A not very rare combination. J. Thoracic Cardiovasc. Surg. *68:*268, 1974.

Coleman, E. N., Reid, J. M., Barclay, R. S., and Stevenson, J. G.: Ventricular septal defect repair after pulmonary artery banding. Brit. Heart J. *34:*134, 1972.

Collett, R. W. and Edwards, J. E.: Persistent truncus arteriosus. A classification according to anatomic types. Surg. Clin. N.A. *29:*1245, 1949.

Comty, C. M., Cohen, S. L., and Shapiro, F. L.: Pericarditis in chronic uremia and its sequels. Ann. Int. Med. *75:*173, 1971.

Connolly, D. C., Dry, T. J., Good, C. A., Clagett, O. T., and Burchell, H. B.: Chronic idiopathic pericardial effusion without tamponade. Circulation *20:*1095, 1959.

Conte, E. and Costa, A.: Angiopneumography. Radiology *21:*461, 1933.

Conti, C. R.: Coronary arteriography. Circulation *55:*227, 1977.

Contis, G., Fung, R. H., Vawter, G. F., and Nadas, A. S.: Stenosis and obstruction of the pulmonary veins associated with pulmonary artery hypertension. Am. J. Cardiol. *20:*718, 1967.

Cooley, D. A. and Beall, A. C., Jr.: Progress in cardiovascular surgery: surgical treatment of acute massive pulmonary embolism using temporary cardiopulmonary bypass. Dis. Chest *41:*102, 1962.

Cooley, D. A., Belamonte, B. A., Zeis, L. B., and Schnur, S.: Surgical repair of ruptured interventricular septum following acute myocardial infarction. Surgery *41:*930, 1957.

Cooley, D. A., Hallman, G. L., and Leachman, R. D.: Total anomalous pulmonary venous drainage. J. Thoracic Cardiovasc. Surg. *51:*88, 1966.

Cooley, D. A., Henly, W. S., Amad, K. H., and Chapman, D. W.: Ventricular aneurysm following myocardial infarction—results of surgical treatment. Ann. Surg. *150:*595, 1959.

Cooley, D. A. and McNamara, D. G.: Pulmonary telangiectasis: report of a case proved by pulmonary biopsy. J. Thoracic Surg. *27:*614, 1954.

Cooley, D. A., McNamara, D. G., and Latson, J. R.: Aorticopulmonary septal defect: diagnosis and surgical treatment. Surgery *42:*101, 1957.

Cooley, D. A., Wukasch, D. C., and Hallman, G. L.: Acute dissecting aortic aneurysm resulting from coronary arteriography: successful surgical treatment. Chest *61:*317, 1972.

Cooley, R. N., Bahnson, H. T., and Hanlon, C. R.: Angiocardiography in congenital heart disease of cyanotic type with pulmonic stenosis or atresia. I. Observations on the tetralogy of Fallot and "pseudotruncus arteriosus". Radiology *52:*329, 1949.

Cooley, R. N., Harris, L. C., and Rodin, A. E.: Abnormal communication between the aorta and left ventricle. Aortico-left ventricular tunnel. Circulation *31:*564, 1965.

Cooley, R. N., Schreiber, M. H., and Brown, R. W.: Effects of transaortic catheter injection of Renografin, Urokon, Hypaque and Miokon into the superior mesenteric arteries of dogs. Angiology *15:*107, 1964.

Cooley, R. N., Sloan, R. D., Hanlon, C. R., and Bahnson, H. T.: Angiocardiography in congenital heart disease of cyanotic type. II. Observations on tricuspid stenosis or atresia

with hypoplasia of the right ventricle. Radiology *54:*848, 1950.

Coon, W. W. and Coller, F. A.: Clinicopathologic correlation in thromboembolism. Surg. Gynecol. Obstet. *109:*259, 1959.

Cordell, A. R., McKone, R. C., and Bhatti, M. A.: Pulmonary-artery debanding. Ann. Thoracic Surg. *14:*24, 1972.

Cornell, S. H.: Angiocardiography in endocardial cushion defects. Radiology *84:*907, 1965.

Cornell, S. H. and Rossi, N. P.: Roentgenographic findings in constrictive pericarditis. An analysis of 21 cases. Am. J. Roentgenol. *102:*301, 1968.

Cote, M., Davignon, A. and Fouron, J.: Congenital hypoplasia of right ventricular myocardium (Uhl's anomaly) associated with pulmonary atresia in a newborn. Am. J. Cardiol. *31:*658, 1973.

Cournand, A., Motely, H. L., Hummelstein, A., Dresdale, D., and Baldwin, J. S.: Recording of blood pressure from the left auricle and the pulmonary veins in human subjects with interauricular septal defects. Am. J. Physiol. *150:*267, 1947.

Cournand, A. and Ranges, H. M.: Catheterization of the right auricle in man. Proc. Soc. Exp. Biol. Med. *46:*462, 1941.

Courville, C. and Mason, V. R.: The heart in acromegaly. Arch. Int. Med. *61:*704, 1938.

Coussement, A. M., Gooding, C. A., and Carlsson, E.: Left atrial volume, shape, and movement in total anomalous pulmonary venous return. Radiology *107:*139, 1973.

Cramer, R., Moore, R., and Amplatz, K.: Reduction of the surgical complication rate by the use of a hypothrombogenic catheter coating. Radiology *109:*585, 1973.

Crane, A. R.: Primary multiocular mycotic aneurysms of the aorta. Arch. Path. *24:*634, 1937.

Crane, P., Lerner, H. H., and Lawrence, E. A.: Syndrome of arteriovenous fistula of the lung. Am. J. Roentgenol. *62:*418, 1949.

Criely, J. M., Lewis, K. B., Humphries, J. O., and Ross, R. S.: Prolapse of the mitral valve; clinical and cine-angiographic findings. Brit. Heart J. *28:*488, 1966.

Criley, J. M., Lewis, K. B., Lewis, R. I., and Ross, R. S.: Pressure gradients without obstruction: a new concept of hypertrophic subaortic stenosis. Circulation *32:*71, 1965.

Cross, F. S. and Mowlem, A.: A survey of the current status of pulmonary embolectomy for massive pulmonary embolism. Circulation (Supp. I) *35 & 36:*86, 1967.

Cunningham, J. N., Jr., Spencer, F. C., Zeff, R., Williams, C. D., Cukingnan, R., and Mullin, M.: Influence of primary closure of the pericardium after open-heart surgery on the frequency of tamponade, postcardiotomy syndrome, and pulmonary complications. J. Thoracic Cardiovasc. Surg. *70:*119, 1975.

Currarino, G. and Jackson, J. H.: Calcification of the ductus arteriosus and ligamentum botalli. Radiology *94:*139, 1970.

Currarino, G., Willis, K. W., Johnson, A. F., Jr., and Miller, W. W.: Pulmonary telangiectasia. Am. J. Roentgenol. *127:*775, 1976.

Curry, J. L., Lehman, J. S., and Schmidt, E. C. H.: Left atrial calcification. Report of eight cases verified at surgery for relief of mitral stenosis. Radiology *60:*559, 1953.

Dabbs, C. H., Peirce, E. C. II, and Rawson, F. L.: Cyst of the pericardium or bronchogenic cyst. N. Engl. J. Med. *256:*541, 1957.

Dack, S., Paley, D. H., and Susman, M. L.: A comparison of electrokymography and roentgenkymography in the study of myocardial infarction. Circulation *1:*551, 1950.

Daily, P. O., Trueblood, H. W., Stinson, E. B., Wuesflein, R. D., and Shumway, T. E.: Management of acute aortic dissections. Ann. Thoracic Surg. *10:*237, 1970.

Dalen, J. E. and Dexter, L.: Pulmonary embolism. J.A.M.A.

207:1505, 1969.

Dalinka, M. K., Rubinstein, B. M., and Lopez, F.: The roentgen findings in truncus arteriosus. J. Canad. Assoc. Rad. 21:85, 1970.

Dalith, F. and Neufeld, H. N.: Radiological diagnosis of anomalous venous connection: a tomographic study. Radiology 74:1, 1960.

d'Allaines, F., Donzelot, E., Dubost, Ch., Durand, N., Metianu, G. et Heim de Balzac.: Aneurysmes arterioveineaux pulmonaires. Diagnostic par angiocardiographie. Interventions. Mem. Acad. Cir. 76:713, 1950.

Dammann, J. F., Berthrong, M., and Bing, R. J.: Reverse ductus: a presentation of the syndrome of patency of the ductus arteriosus with pulmonary hypertension and a shunting of blood from pulmonary artery to aorta. Bull. Johns Hopkins Hosp. 92:128, 1953.

Dammann, J. F., and Sell, C. G.: Patent ductus arteriosus in the absence of a continuous murmur. Circulation 6:110, 1952.

Dammann, J. F., Thompson, W. M., Jr., Sosa, O., and Christlieb, I.: Anatomy, physiology and natural history of simple ventricular septal defects. Am. J. Cardiol. 5:136, 1960.

Danielson, G. K., Cooper, E., and Tweeddale, D. N.: Circumflex coronary artery injury during mitral valve replacement. Ann. Thoracic Surg. 4:53, 1967.

Daoud, G., Kaplan, S., Perrin, E. V., Dorst, J. P., and Edwards, F. K.: Congenital mitral stenosis. Circulation 27:185, 1963.

Daoud, A. S., Pankin, D., Tulgan, H., and Florentin, R. A.: Aneurysms of the coronary artery: report of ten cases and review of the literature. Am. J. Cardiol. 11:228, 1963.

Darling, R. C., Rothney, W. B., and Craig, J. M.: Total pulmonary venous drainage into the right side of the heart. Lab. Invest. 6:44, 1957.

Daty, K. K., Deshmukh, M. M., Engineer, S. D., and Dalvi, C. P.: Straight back syndrome. Brit. Heart J. 26:614, 1964.

Davachi, F., Moller, J. H., and Edwards, J. E.: Diseases of the mitral valve in infancy. An anatomic analysis of 55 cases. Circulation 43:565, 1971.

Davies, L. G., Goodwin, J. F., Steiner, R. E., and Van Leuven, B. A.: The clinical and radiological assessment of the pulmonary arterial pressure in mitral stenosis. Brit. Heart J. 15:393, 1953.

Davignon, A. L., DuShane, J. W. Kincaid, O. W., and Swan, H. J. C.: Pulmonary atresia with intact ventricular septum: report of 2 cases studied by selective angiocardiography and right heart catheterization. Am. Heart J. 62:690, 1961.

Davis, G. D., Kincaid, O. W., and Hallermann, F. J.: Roentgen aspects of cardiac tumors. Sem. Roentgenol. IV:4:384, 1969.

Davis, R. H., Schuster, B., Knoebel, S. B., and Fisch, C.: Myxomatous degeneration of the mitral valve. Am. J. Cardiol. 28:449, 1971.

Davis, W. C.: Immediate diagnosis of pulmonary embolus. Am. Surgeon 30:291, 1964.

Davis, W. H., Jordaan, F. R., and Snyman, H. W.: Persistent left superior vena cava draining into the left atrium as an isolated anomaly. Am. Heart J. 57:616, 1959.

D'Cruz, I. A. and Ascilla, R. A.: Anomalous venous drainage of the left lung into the inferior vena cava. Am. Heart J. 67:539, 1964.

D'Cruz, I. A., Cohen, H. C., and Prabhu, R.: Diagnosis of cardiac tamponade by echocardiography: changes in mitral valve motion and ventricular dimensions with special reference to paradoxical pulse. Circulation 52:460, 1975.

De Bakey, M. E., Cooley, D. A., and Creech, O. Jr.: Surgical considerations of dissecting aneurysm of the aorta. Ann.

Surg. 142:586, 1955.

De Bakey, M. E. and Noon, G. P.: Aneurysms of the thoracic aorta. Mod. Concepts Cardiovasc. Dis. 44:53, 1975.

Decker, J. L., Steinberg, A. D., Gershwin, M. E., Seaman, W. B., Kippel, J. H., Plotz, P. H., and Paget, S. A.: Systemic lupus erythematosus. Contrast and comparisons. Ann. Int. Med. 82:391, 1975.

Dekker, A., Mehrizi, A., and Vengsarkar, A. S.: Corrected transposition of great vessels with Ebstein malformation of left atrioventricular valve. Circulation 31:119, 1965.

de la Cruz, M. V., Polansky, B. J., and Navarro-Lopez, F.: Diagnosis of corrected transposition of great vessels. Brit. Heart J. 24:483, 1962.

DeLeon, A. C., Perloff, J. K., Twigg, H., and Majd, M.: The straight back syndrome. Clinical cardiovascular manifestations. Circulation 32:193, 1965.

Demakis, J. E., Rahimtoola, S. H.: Peripartum cardiomyopathy. Circulation 44:964, 1971.

De Meules, J. E., Cramer, G., and Perry, J. F. Jr.: Rupture of aorta and great vessels due to blunt thoracic trauma. J. Thoracic & Cardiovascular Surg. 61:438, 1961.

De Mots, H., Boncheck, L. I., Rosch, J., Anderson, R. P., Starr, A., and Rahimtolla, S. H.: Left main coronary artery disease. Am. J. Cardiol. 36:136, 1975.

De Muth, W. E., and Zinsser, H. F.: Myocardial contusion. Arch. Int. Med. 115:434, 1965.

Dennis, J. L., Hansen, A. E., and Corpening, T. N.: Endocardial fibroelastosis. Pediatrics 12:130, 1953.

De Sanctis, R. W., Dean, D. C., and Bland, E. F.: Extreme left atrial enlargement: some characteristic features. Circulation 29:14, 1964.

Deshmukh, M., Guvene, S., Bentivaglio, L., and Goldberg, H.: Idiopathic dilatation of the pulmonary artery. Circulation 21:710, 1960.

Desilets, D. T., and Beckenbach, E. S.: Myocardial function from cineangiocardiograms with a digital computer. Radiology 99:319, 1971.

Desilets, D. T., and Hoffman, R.: A new method of percutaneous catheterization. Radiology 85:147, 1965.

Desser, K. B., Benchimol, A., Cornell, W. P., and Nelson, A. R.: Traumatic ventricular septal defect, aortic insufficiency, and sinus aneurysm. J. Thoracic Cardiovasc. Surg. 62:830, 1971.

Deterling, R. A., Jr., and Clagett, O. T.: Aneurysms of the pulmonary artery: review of the literature and report of a case. Am. Heart J. 34:471, 1947.

Detre, K. M., Wright, E., Murphy, M. L., and Takaro, T.: Observer agreement in evaluating coronary angiograms. Circulation 52:979, 1975.

Deutsch, V., Shen-Tov, A., Yakini, J. H., and Neufeld, H. N.: Sub-aortic stenosis (discrete form). Classification and angiographic features. Radiology 101:275, 1971.

Deutsch, V., Yahini, J. H., Shen-Tov, A., and Neufeld, H. N.: The parachute mitral valve complex: angiographic observations. Chest 65:262, 1974.

Dexter, L., Dow, J. W., Haynes, F. W., Wittenberger, J. L., Ferris, B. G., Goodale, W. T., and Hellems, H. K.: Studies of the pulmonary circulation in man at rest. Normal variations and the interrelations between increased pulmonary blood flow, elevated pulmonary arterial pressure and high pulmonary "capillary" pressures. J. Clin. Invest. 29:602, 1950.

Dexter, L., Haynes, F. W., Burwell, C. S., Eppinger, E. G., Siebel, R. E., and Evans, J. M.: Studies of congenital heart disease. I. Technique of venous catheterization as a diagnostic procedure. J. Clin. Invest. 26:547, 1947.

Dhanavaravibul, S., Nora, J. J., and McNamara, D. G.: Pulmonary valvular atresia with intact ventricular septum:

problems in diagnosis and results of treatment. J. Pediat. 77:1010, 1970.

DiChiro, G.: Unintentional spinal cord arteriography: a warning. Radiology 112:231, 1974.

Dick, M., Fyler, D. C. and Nadas, A. S.: Tricuspid atresia: clinical course in 101 patients. Am. J. Cardiol. 36:327, 1975.

Dickie, K., de Groot, W., Cooley, R. N., Guest, M. M. and Bond. T.: Urokinase in pulmonary thromboembolic disease: a preliminary report. Tex. Rep. Biol. Med. 25:613, 1967.

DiGuglielmo, L., and Guttadauro, M.: Roentgenologic study of coronary arteries in living. Acta Radiol. Supp. 97, 1952.

Dimisch, I., Steinfeld, L., and Park, S. C.: Symptomatic atrial septal defect in infants. Am. Heart J. 85:601, 1973.

Dimond, E. G., Kittle, C. F. and Youth, D. W.: Extreme hypertrophy of the left atrial appendage. The case of the giant dog ear. Am. J. Cardiol. 5:122, 1960.

Dinsmore, R. E., Willerson, J. T. and Burkley, M. J.: Dissecting aneurysm of the aorta. Aortographic features affecting prognosis. Radiology 105:567, 1972.

Dische, M. R., Tsai, M., and Baltaxe, H. A.: Solitary interruption of the arch of the aorta. Clinico-pathologic review of eight cases. Am. J. Cardiol. 35:271, 1975.

Dobell, A. R. C., Henry, J. N., and Murphy, D. A.: Surgical experience with recurrent ventricular septal defect. Ann. Thorac. Surg. 14:405, 1972.

Dodek, A.: Cardiac mass in a young woman. Chest 62:317, 1972.

Dodge, H. T., Sandler, H., Baxley, W. A., and Hawley, R. R.: Usefulness and limitations of radiographic methods for determining left ventricular volume. Am. J. Cardiol. 18:10, 1966.

Donahoo, J. S., Brawley, R. K., Haller, J. A., Elkins, R. C., Bender, H. W. Jr., and Gott, V. L.: Correction of tetralogy of Fallot in patients with one pulmonary artery in continuity with the right ventricular outflow tract. Surgery 74(6):887, 1973.

Donaldson, G. A., Williams, C., Scannel, J. G. and Shaw, R. S.: A reappraisal of the application of the Trendelenburg operation to massive fatal embolism. Report of a successful pulmonary artery thrombectomy using a cardiopulmonary bypass. N. Engl. J. Med. 268:171, 1963.

Donovan, M. S., Neuhauser, E. B. D., and Sosman, M. C.: The roentgen signs of patent ductus arteriosus: a summary of 50 surgically verified cases. Am. J. Roentgenol. 50:293, 1943.

Donsky, M. S., Harris, J. D., Curry, G. C., Blomqvist, G., Willerson, J. T., and Mullins, C. B.: Variant angina pectoris: a clinical and coronary arteriographic spectrum. Am. Heart J. 89:571, 1975.

Dotter, C. T.: Left ventricular and systemic arterial catheterization: a simple percutaneous method using a spring guide. Am. J. Roentgenol. 83:969, 1960.

Dotter, C. T.: The normal pulmonary angiogram, In Angiography. Edited by H. L. Abrams, ed. 2, pp. 451–463, Boston, Little, Brown, & Co., 1971.

Dotter, C. T., and Frische, L. H.: Visualization of the coronary circulation by occlusion aortography: a practical method. Radiology 76:502, 1958.

Dotter, C. T., Hardisty, N. M., and Steinberg, I.: Anomalous right pulmonary vein entering the inferior vena cava: two cases diagnosed during life by angiocardiography and cardiac catheterization. Am. J. Med. Sci. 218:31, 1949.

Dotter, C. T., and Jackson, F. S.: Death following angiocardiography. Radiology 54:527, 1950.

Dotter, C. T., Lukas, D. S., and Steinberg, I.: Tricuspid insufficiency: observations based on angiocardiography and cardiac catheterization in twelve patients. Am. J. Roentgenol. 70:786, 1953.

Dotter, C. T., and Steinberg, I.: Angiocardiography. Annals of Roentgenology, vol. II. New York, Paul B. Hoeber, Inc., 1951.

Doub, H. P., Goodrich, B. E., and Gish, J. R.: The pulmonary aspects of polyarteritis (periarteritis) nodosa. Am. J. Roentgenol. 71:785, 1954.

Dow, J. W., Levine, H. D., Elkin, M., Hayes, F. W., Hellems, H. K., Whittenberger, J. W., Ferris, B. G., Goodale, W. T., Harvey, W. P., Eppinger, E. C., and Dexter, L.: Studies of congenital heart disease. IV. Uncomplicated pulmonic stenosis. Circulation 1:267, 1950.

Doyle, A. E., Goodwin, J. F., Harrison, C. V., and Steiner, R. E.: Pulmonary vascular patterns in pulmonary hypertension. Brit. Heart J. 19:353, 1957.

Dressler, W.: Post-myocardial-infarction syndrome. J.A.M.A. 160:1379, 1956.

Drexler, C. J., Stewart, J. R., and Kincaid, O. W.: Diagnostic implications of rib notching. Am. J. Roentgenol. 91:1064, 1964.

Dubilier, W., Steinberg, I., and Dotter, C. T.: Kyphoscoliosis: angiocardiographic findings. Radiology 61:56, 1953.

Duffie, E. R., Jr., Moss, A. J., and Maloney, J. V., Jr.: Congenital pericardial defects with herniation of the heart into the pleural space. Pediatrics 30:746, 1962.

DuShane, J. W., Weidman, W. H., Ongley, P. A., Swan, H. J. C., Kirklin, J. W., Edwards, J. E., and Schmutzler, H.: Clinical-pathologic conference. Am. Heart. J. 59:782, 1960.

DuShane, J. W., Weidman, W. H., Bradenburg, R. O., and Kirklin, J. W.: Differentiation of interatrial communications by clinical methods: ostium secundum, ostium primum, common atrium and total anomalous pulmonary venous connection. Circulation 21:363, 1960.

Dutton, R. V. and Singleton, E. B.: Tuberous sclerosis: a case report with aortic aneurysm and unusual rib changes. Pediatric Radiology 3(3):184, 1975.

DuVernoy, W. F. C., and Garcia, R.: Sarcoidosis of the heart presenting with ventricular tachycardia and atrio-ventricular block. Am. J. Cardiol. 28:348, 1971.

Dye, C. L., Genovese, P. D., Daly, W. J., and Behnke, R. H.: Primary myocardial disease - Part II. Hemodynamic alterations. Ann. Internal Med. 58:442, 1963.

Dye, C. L., Rosenbaum. D., Lowe, J. C., Behnke, R. H., and Genovese, P. D.: Primary myocardial disease - Part I. Clinical features. Ann. Internal Med. 58:426, 1963.

Dworkin, H. J., Smith, J. R., and Bull, F.: A reaction following administration of macroaggregated albumin (MAA) for a lung scan. Am. J. Roentgenol. 98:427, 1966.

Eaton, S. B., James, A. E., Potsaid, M. S., and Fleischner, F. G.: Scintigraphic findings in pulmonary microembolism. Am. J. Roentgenol. 106:778, 1969.

Ebstein, W.: Uber einen sehr seltenen Fall von Insufficienz der Valvula tricuspidalis, bedingt durch eine angeborene hochgradige Missbildung derselben. Arch. Anat. Physiol. 33:238, 1866.

Edie, R. N., Ellis, K., Gersony, W. M., Krongrad, E., Bowman, F. O., Jr., and Malm, J. R.: Surgical repair of single ventricle. J. Thoracic & Cardiovascular Surg. 66:350, 1973.

Edmundowicz, A. C., Morgan, D. A., and Marshall, R. J.: Perforation of the right ventricle: A complication of transvenous endocardiac catheter pacemaking. Circulation 32(Supp. 2):80, 1965.

Edwards, J. E.: Congenital Malformations of the Heart and Great Vessels. In Gould, S. E., Pathology of the Heart. Springfield, Ill., Charles C Thomas, 1953.

Edwards, J. E.: Functional pathology of the pulmonary vascular tree in congenital cardiac disease. Circulation 15:164, 1957.

Edwards, J. E.: Anomalous coronary arteries with special reference to arteriovenous-like communications. Circulation 17:1001, 1958.

Edwards, J. E.: The congenital bicuspid aortic valve. Circulation 23:485, 1961.

Edwards, J. E.: An Atlas of Acquired Diseases of the Heart and Great Vessels, vol. 2, Philadelphia, W. B. Saunders Co., 1961.

Edwards, J. E.: Pathology of left ventricular outflow tract obstruction. Circulation 31:586, 1965.

Edwards, J. E. and Burchell, H. B.: The pathological anatomy of deficiencies between the aortic root and the heart, including aortic sinus aneurysms. Thorax 12:125, 1957.

Edwards, J. E., Carey, L. S., Neufeld, H. N., and Lester, R. G.: Congenital Heart Disease, Correlation of Pathologic Anatomy and Angiocardiography, vol. 1. Philadelphia, W. B. Saunders Co., 1965.

Edmunds, L. H., Gregory, G. A., Heymann, M. A., Kitterman, J. A., Rudolph, A. M., and Tooley, W. H.: Surgical closure of the ductus arteriosus in premature infants. Circulation 48:856, 1973.

Eiseman, B. and Rainer, W. G.: Clinical management of post-traumatic rupture of the thoracic aorta. J. Thoracic Surg. 35:347, 1958.

Eisenmenger, V.: Die angeborenen Defect der Kammerscheidewand des Herzens. Klin. Med. 32:1, 1897.

Eller, J. L. and Zieter, F. M. H.: Avulsion of the innominate artery from the aortic arch. An evaluation of roentgenographic findings. Radiology 94:75, 1970.

Ellis, K., Malm, J. R., Bowman, F. O., Jr., and King, D. L.: Roentgenographic findings after pericardial surgery. Radiol. Clin. N.A. 9:327, 1971.

Elliott, L. P., Adams, P., Jr., and Edwards, J. E.: Pulmonary atresia with intact ventricular septum. Brit. Heart J. 25:489, 1963.

Elliott, L. P., Amplatz, K., Anderson, R. C., and Edwards, J. E.: Cor triloculare biatriatum with pulmonary stenosis and normally related great vessels. Am. J. Cardiol. 11:469, 1963.

Elliott, L. P., Amplatz, K., and Edwards, J. E.: Coronary arterial patterns in transposition complexes. Am. J. Cardiol. 17:362, 1966.

Elliott, L. P., Anderson, R. C., and Edwards, J. E.: The common cardiac ventricle with transposition of the great vessels: association of pulmonary stenosis and atresia of the atrioventricular valves. Brit. Heart J. 26:289, 1964.

Elliott, L. P. and Gedgaudas, E.: Roentgenologic findings in common ventricle with transposition of the great vessels. Radiology 82:850, 1964.

Elliott, L. P., Jue, K. L., and Amplatz, K.: A roentgen classification of cardiac malpositions. Invest. Radiol. 1:17, 1966.

Elliott, L. P. and Morgan, A. D.: Common ventricles. Heart Disease in Infants, Children, and Adolescents. Chap. 28, pp. 589–601, Baltimore, Williams & Wilkins Co., 1968.

Elliott, L. P., Ruttenberg, H. D., Eliot, R. S., and Anderson, R. C.: Vectorial analysis of the electrocardiogram in common ventricle. Brit. Heart J. 26:302, 1964.

Elliott, L. P., Van Mierop, L. H. S., Gleason, D. C., and Schiebler, G. L.: The roentgenology of tricuspid atresia. Sem. Roentgenol. 3:399, 1968.

Ellis, E., Griffiths, S. P., Burris, J. O., Ramsay, C. G., and Fleming, R. J.: Ebstein's anomaly of the tricuspid valve. Angiocardiographic considerations. Am. J. Roentgenol. 92:1338, 1964.

Ellis, F. H. and Kirklin, J. W.: Congenital valvular aortic stenosis: anatomic findings and surgical technique. J. Thoracic & Cardiovascular Surg. 43:199, 1962.

Ellis, F. H., Ongly, P. A., and Kirklin, J. W.: Ventricular septal defect with aortic valvular incompetence. Surgical considerations. Circulation 27:789, 1963.

Ellis, K., Casarella, W. J., Hayes, C. J., Gersony, W. M., Bowman, F. O., Jr., and Malm, J. R.: Pulmonary atresia

with intact ventricular septum. New developments in diagnosis and treatment. Am. J. Roentgenol. 116:501, 1972.

Ellis, K., Griffiths, S. P., Jesse, M. J., and Jameson, A. G.: Cor triatriatum. Angiocardiographic demonstration of the obstructing left atrial membrane. Am. J. Roentgenol. 92:669, 1964.

Ellis, K., Leeds, N. E., and Himmelstein, A.: Congenital deficiencies in the parietal pericardium. A review with 2 new cases including successful diagnosis by plain roentgenography. Am. J. Roentgenol. 82:125, 1959.

Ellis, K., Morgan, B. C., Blumenthal, S., and Anderson, D. H.: Congenitally corrected transposition of the great vessels. Radiology 79:35, 1962.

Ellis, L. B. and Harken, D. E.: Clinical results in first 500 patients with mitral stenosis undergoing valvuloplasty. Circulation 11:637, 1955.

El-Said, G., Galioto, F. M., Mullins, C. E., and McNamara, D. G.: Natural hemodynamic history of congenital aortic stenosis in childhood. Am. J. Cardiol. 30:6, 1972.

El-Said, G., Mullins, C. E., and McNamara, D. G.: Management of total anomalous pulmonary venous return. Circulation 45:1240, 1972.

Emanuel, R.: A classification for the cardiomyopathies. Am. J. Cardiol. 26:438, 1970.

Emslie-Smith, D., Hill, I. G. W., and Lowe, K. G.: Unilateral membranous pulmonary venous occlusion, pulmonary hypertension, and patent ductus arteriosus. Brit. Heart J. 17:79, 1955.

Engel, H. J., Torres, C., and Page, H. L.: Major variations in anatomical origin of the coronary arteries. Cath. & Cardiovascular Diag. 1:157, 1975.

Engle, M. A.: Ventricular septal defect: status report from the 70's. Cardiovascular Clin. 4:282, 1972.

Engle, M. A., Goldsmith, E. I., Holswade, G. R., Goldberg, H. P., and Glenn, F.: Congenital coronary arteriovenous fistula. Diagnostic evaluation and surgical correction. N. Engl. J. Med. 264:856, 1961.

Engle, M. A., McCabe, J. C., Ebert, P. A., and Zabriskie, J.: The postpericardiotomy syndrome and antiheart antibodies. Circulation 49:401, 1974.

Engle, M. A., Zabriskie, J. B., Senterfit, L. B., and Ebert, P. A.: Postpericardiotomy syndrome. A new look at an old condition. Mod. Concepts. Cardiovascular Dis. 44:59, 1975.

Epstein, S. E., Morrow, A. G., Henry, W. L., and Clark, C. E.: The role of operative treatment in patients with idiopathic hypertrophic subaortic stenosis. Circulation 48:677, 1973.

Erb, B. D. and Tullis, I. F.: Dissecting aneurysm of the aorta. The clinical features of thirty autopsied cases. Circulation 22:315, 1960.

Espino-Vela, J.: Rheumatic heart disease associated with atrial septal defect. Clinical and pathologic study of 12 cases of Lutembacher's syndrome. Am. Heart J. 57:185, 1959.

Esposito, M. J.: Focal pulmonary hemosiderosis in rheumatic heart disease. Am. J. Roentgenol. 73:351, 1955.

Evans, J. R., Rowe, R. D., and Keith, J. D.: Spontaneous closure of ventricular septal defects. Circulation 22:1044, 1960.

Evans, W.: The less common forms of pulmonary hypertension. Brit. Heart J. 21:197, 1959.

Evans, W. and Jackson, F.: Constrictive pericarditis. Brit. Heart J. 14:53, 1952.

Evans, W., Short, D. S., and Bedford, D. E.: Solitary pulmonary hypertension. Brit. Heart J. 19:93, 1957.

Everts-Suarez, E. A. and Carson, C. P.: Triad of congenital absence of aortic arch (isthmus aortae), patent ductus arteriosus and interventricular septal defect-trilogy. Ann. Surg. 150:153, 1959.

Eyler, W. R., Ziegler, R. F., Shea, J. J., and Knabe, G. W.:

Endocardial fibroelastosis: Roentgen appearance. Radiology 64:797–809, 1955.

Facquet, J., Durant, M., Hyatt, P. Y., and Piequet, J.: Gros coeur solitaire. Diagnostic angiocardiographique. Tumeur du coeur. Cardiologia 15:313, 1949–50.

Fadell, E. J. and Graziani, L. J.: Incomplete differentiation of the aortic valve (myxomatosis). A cause of myocardial infarction in the neonate. J. Pediatrics 57:892, 1960.

Faesber, E. N., Segal, F., and Sischy, N. L.: Amoebic pericarditis. Brit. J. Radiol. 47:816, 1974.

Falicov, P. E., and Cooney, D. F.: Takayasu's arteritis and rheumatoid arthritis. Arch. Int. Med. 114:594, 1964.

Falkenbach, K. H., Zheutlin, N., Dowdy, A. H., and O'Loughlin, B. J.: Pulmonary hypertension due to pulmonary arterial coarctation. Radiology 73:575, 1959.

Farrar, J. F., Reye, R. D. K., and Stuckey, D.: Primary pulmonary hypertension in childhood. Brit. Heart J. 23:605, 1961.

Farrokh, A., Walsh, T. J., and Massie, E.: Amyloid heart disease. Am. J. Cardiol. 13:750, 1964.

Favaloro, R. G., Effler, D. B., Groves, L. K. Westcott, R. N., Saurez, E., Lozoda, J.: Ventricular aneurysm. Clinical experience. Am. J. Thoracic Surg. 6:227, 1968.

Favaloro, R. G., Effler, D. B., Cheanvechai, C., Quint, R. A., Sones, F. M., Jr.: Acute coronary insufficiency (impending myocardial infarction and myocardial infarction). Am. J. Cardiol. 28:598, 1971.

Favaloro, R. G., Effler, D. R., Groves, L. K., Sheldon, W. C., Shirey, E. K., and Sones, F. M.: Severe segmental obstruction of the left main coronary artery and its divisions. Surgical treatment by the saphenous vein graft technique. J. Thoracic Cardiovasc. Surg. 60:469, 1970.

Feigenbaum, H.: Echocardiographic diagnosis of pericardial effusion. Am. J. Cardiol. 26:475, 1970.

Feigenbaum, H.: Echocardiography. Philadelphia, Lea & Febiger, 1976.

Feist, J. H. and Magovern, G. J.: In vivo behavior of artificial aortic and mitral valve prosthesis: preliminary observations. Radiology 88:791, 1967.

Fell, S. C., Schein, C. J., Bloomberg, A. E., and Rubinstein, B. M.: Congenital diverticula of the pericardium. Ann. Surg. 194:117, 1959.

Fellows, K. E., Martin, E. C., and Rosenthal, A.: Angiocardiography of obstructing muscular bands of the right ventricle. Am. J. Roentgenol. 128:249, 1977.

Felson, B., Akers, P. V., Hall, G. S., Schreiber, J. T., Greene, R. E., and Pedrosa, C. S.: Mycotic tuberculous aneurysm of the thoracic aorta. J.A.M.A. 237:1104, 1977.

Felson, B. and Palayew, M. J.: The two types of right aortic arch. Radiology 81:745, 1963.

Ferencz, C., Johnson, A. L., and Wiglesworth, F. W.: Congenital mitral stenosis. Circulation 9:161, 1954.

Ferris, E. J., Stanzler, R. M., Rourke, J. A., Blumenthal, J., and Messar, J. V.: Pulmonary angiography in pulmonary embolic disease. Am. J. Roentgenol. 100:355, 1967.

Ferrucci, J. T., Rubin, R. H., and Scully, R. E.: Case records of the Massachusetts General Hospital, N. Engl. J. Med. 292:579, 1975.

Figley, M. M.: Accessory roentgen signs of coarctation of the aorta. Radiology 62:671, 1954.

Figley, M. M.: Angiocardiography in valvular heart disease: morphological and volumetric considerations. Rad. Clin. N.A. 2:409, 1964.

Figley, M. M., and Bagshaw, M. A.: Angiographic aspects of constrictive pericarditis. Radiology 69:46, 1957.

Figley, M. M., Gerdes, A. J., and Ricketts, H. J.: Radiographic aspects of pulmonary embolism. Sem. Roentgenol. 2(4):389, 1967.

Figley, M. M., Nordenstrom, B., Stern, A., and Sloan, H.:

Angiocardiographic mixing defects as indicators of left to right shunts. Acta Radiol. 45:1956.

Findlay, C. W., Jr. and Maier, H. C.: Anomalies of the pulmonary vessels and their surgical significance. With a review of literature. Surgery 29:604, 1951.

Fischer, H. W.: Hemodynamic reactions to angiographic media. A survey and commentary. Radiology 91:66, 1968.

Fischer, H. W. and Doust, V. L.: An evaluation of pretesting in the problem of serious and fatal reactions to excretory urography. Radiology 103:497, 1972.

Fischer, H. W. and Eckstein, J. W.: Comparison of cerebral angiographic contrast media by their circulatory effects. An experimental study. Am. J. Roentgenol. 86:166, 1961.

Fisher, C. H., James, A. E., Humphries, J. O., Foster, J., and White, R. I.: Radiographic findings in anomalous muscle bundles of the right ventricle.: an analysis of 15 cases. Radiology 101:35, 1971.

Fisher, F. D. and Ehrenhalft, J. L.: Congenital pericardial defect. J.A.M.A. 188:78, 1964.

Fisher, R. D., Brawley, R. K., Neill, C. A., Donahoo, J. S., Haller, J. A., Rowe, R. D., and Gott, V. L.: Severe tricuspid regurgitation after repair of ventricular septal defect. J. Thoracic Cardiovasc. Surg. 65:702, 1973.

Fishman, N. H., Youker, J. E., and Roe, B. B.: Mechanical injury to the coronary arteries during operative cannulation. Am. Heart J. 75:26, 1968.

Fitzgibbon, G. M., et al.: Double Master's two-step test: clinical, angiographic and hemodynamic correlations. Ann. Int. Med. 74:509, 1971.

Fix, P., Moberg, A., Soderberg, H., and Karnell, J.: Muscular subvalvular aortic stenosis: abnormal anterior mitral leaflet possibly the primary factor. Acta Radiol. (Diagn.) 2:177, 1964.

Fleischner, F. G.: Occurrence and diagnosis of dilatation of the aorta distal to the area of coarctation. Am. J. Roentgenol. 61:199, 1949.

Fleischner, F. G.: Pulmonary embolism. Clin. Radiol. 13:169, 1962.

Fleischner, F. G.: Observations on the radiologic changes in pulmonary embolism. In Sasahara, A. A., and Stein, M. (eds.), Pulmonary Embolic Disease, pp. 206–213. New York, Grune and Stratton, 1965.

Fleischner, F. G.: Angiographic diagnosis of pulmonary embolism in the "mitral lung." Radiology 87:705, 1966.

Fleischner, F., Hampton, A. O., and Castleman, B.: Linear shadows in the lung (interlobar pleuritis, atelectasis, and healed infarction). Am. J. Roentgenol. 46:610, 1941.

Fleischner, F. G. and Sagall, E. L.: Pulmonary arterial oligemia in mitral stenosis as revealed on the plain roentgenogram. Radiology 65:857, 1955.

Fleming, J. S. and Gibson, R. V.: Absent right superior vena cava as an isolated anomaly. Brit. J. Radiol. 37:696, 1964.

Fleming, P. R. and Simon, M.: The hemodynamic significance of intrapulmonary septal lymphatic lines (lines B of Kerley). J. Fac. Radiologists 9:33, 1958.

Fletcher, G., DuShane, J. W., Kirklin, J. W., and Wood, E. H.: Aortic-pulmonary septal defect: report of a case with surgical division along with successful resuscitation from ventricular fibrillation. Proc. Staff Meet. Mayo Clin. 29:285, 1954.

Fomon, J. J., Kurzweg, F. T., and Broadaway, R. K.: Aneurysm of the aorta: a review. Ann. Surg. 165:557, 1967.

Fontan, F. and Baudet, E.: Surgical repair of tricuspid atresia. Thorax 26:240, 1971.

Forssman, W.: Die sondierung des rechten herzen. Klin. Wchnshr. 8:2085, 1929.

Fouche, R. F., Beck, W., and Schrire, V.: The roentgenologic assessment of the degree of left-to-right shunt in secundum type atrial septal defect. Am. J. Roentgenol. 89:254, 1963.

Fowler, N. O.: Congenital defect of the pericardium. Its resemblance to pulmonary artery enlargement. Circulation 26:114, 1962.

Fowler, N. O., Black-Schaffer, B., Scott, R. C., and Gueron, M.: Idiopathic and thromboembolic pulmonary hypertension. Am. J. Med. 40:331, 1966.

Fraser, R. S., Dvorkin, J., Rossall, R. E., and Eidem, R.: Left superior vena cava. Am. J. Med. 31:711, 1961.

Fray, W. W.: The roentgenologic diagnosis of coarctation of the aorta (adult type). Am. J. Roentgenol. 24:349, 1930.

Fred, H. L., Axelrad, M. A., Lewis, J. M., and Alexander, J. K.: Rapid lysis of pulmonary thromboemboli in man: an angiographic study. Clin. Res. 13:25, 1965.

Fred, H. L., Burdine, J. A., Jr., Gonzalez, D. A., Lockhart, R. W., Peabody, C. A., and Alexander, J. K.: Arteriographic assessment of lung scanning in the diagnosis of pulmonary thromboembolism. N. Engl. J. Med. 275:1025, 1966.

Freed, M. D., Keane, J. F., and Rosenthal, A.: The use of heparinization to prevent arterial thrombosis after percutaneous cardiac catheterization in children. Circulation 50:565, 1974.

Freed, T. A., Neal, M. P., and Vinik, M.: Roentgenographic findings in extracardiac injury secondary to blunt chest automobile trauma. Am. J. Roentgenol. 104:424, 1968.

Freeman, E., Ziskin, M. C., Bone, A. A., Gimenez, J. L., and Lynch, P. R.: Cineradiographic frame rate selection for left ventricular volumetry. Radiology 96:587, 1970.

Freiman, D. G., Suyemoto, J., and Wessler, S.: Frequency of pulmonary thromboembolism in man. N. Engl. J. Med. 272:1278, 1965.

Freis, E. D.: Effects of treatment on morbidity in hypertension. II. Results in patients with diastolic blood pressure averaging 90 through 114 mm. Hg. Veterans Administration cooperative study group on antihypertensive agents. J.A.M.A. 213:1143, 1970.

Freundlich, I. M. and Lind, T. A.: Calcification of the heart and great vessels. CRC Crit. Rev. Clin. Radiol. Nuc. Med. 6:171, 1975.

Friedberg, Charles K.: Pulmonary hypertension with special reference to its occurrence in congenital heart disease. Prog. Cardiovasc. Dis. 1:356, 1959.

Friedberg, C. K.: Diseases of the Heart. Vols. I & II. 3rd Ed., Philadelphia, W. B. Saunders, Co., 1966.

Friedenberg, M. J., Hartmann, A. F., Jr., Silverman, J. L., and Burford, T. H.: Opacification from the pulmonary artery of an anomalous left coronary artery. Radiology 80:806, 1963.

Friedenberg, M. J., Carlsson, E., Hartmann, A. F., Jr., and Behrer, M. R.: Evaluation of the degree of aortic valve stenosis by direct roentgenologic measurement of the ostium. Am. J. Roentgenol. 91:1347, 1964.

Friedli, B., Kidd, B. S. L., Mustard, W. T., and Keith, J. D.: Ventricular septal defect with increased pulmonary vascular resistance. Am. J. Cardiol. 33:403, 1974.

Friedlich, A., Bing, R. J., and Blount, S. G., Jr.: Physiological studies in congenital heart disease. IX. Circulatory dynamics in the anomalies of venous return to the heart including pulmonary arteriovenous fistula. Bull. Johns Hopkins Hosp. 86:20, 1950.

Friedman, C. E. In Proceedings of the Swedish Society for Cardiology: Symposium on Roentgenologic Heart Volume Determinations. Cardiologia 14:368, 1949.

Friesinger, G. C., Schaefer, J., Criley, J. M., Gaertner, R. A., and Ross, R. S.: Hemodynamic consequences of the injection of radiopaque material. Circulation 31:730, 1965.

Frink, R. J., Achor, R. W. P., Brown, A. L., Jr., Kincaid, O. W., and Bradenburg, R. O.: Significance of calcification of the coronary arteries. Am. J. Cardiol. 26:241, 1970.

Fukuda, T., Tadavarthy, M., and Edwards, J. E.: Dissecting aneurysm of aorta complicating aortic valvular stenosis. Circulation 53:169, 1976.

Furby, N., Evans, J. A., and Steinberg, I.: Reactions from intravenous organic iodide compounds. Radiology 71:15, 1958.

Furman, S. and Schwedel, J. B.: An intracardiac pacemaker for Stokes-Adams seizures. N. Engl. J. Med. 261:943, 1959.

Furman, S., Schwedel, J. B., Robinson, G., and Hurwitt, E. S.: Use of an intracardiac pacemaker in the control of heart-block. Surgery 49:98, 1961.

Galioto, F. M., Jr., Cooley, D. A., El-Said, G., Mullins, C. E., and Sandiford, S. M.: Closure of ventricular septal defect through the aortic valve. Chest 64:683, 1973.

Garamella, J. J., Lynch, M. F., Schmidt, W. R., and Jensen, N. K.: Fatal clotting of the Starr-Edwards mitral ball valve nineteen months postoperatively. J. Thoracic Cardiovasc. Surg. 47:673, 1964.

Garbode, F. and Carr, I.: Defects of the atrial septum. Cardiovasc. Clin. 3:130, 1971.

Garland, L. H. and Sisson, M. A.: Roentgen findings in the "collagen" diseases. Am. J. Roentgenol. 71:581, 1954.

Garvin, C. F.: Tricuspid stenosis; incidence and diagnosis. Arch. Int. Med. 72:104, 1943.

Gasul, B. M., Arcilla, R. A., Fell, E. H., Lynfield, J., Bicoff, J. P., and Luan, L. L.: Congenital coronary arteriovenous fistula. Pediatrics 25:531, 1960.

Gasul, B. M., Dillon, R. F., Vrla, V., and Hait, G.: Ventricular septal defects; their natural transformation into those with infundibular stenosis or into the cyanotic or noncyanotic type of tetralogy of Fallot. J.A.M.A. 164:847, 1957.

Gasul, B. M., Fell, E. H., and Casas, R.: The diagnosis of aortic septal defect by retrograde aortography. Report of a case. Circulation 4:251, 1951.

Gates, G. F., Sette, R. S., and Cope, J. A.: Acute cardiac herniation following pneumonectomy. Radiology 94:561, 1970.

Gay, B. B., Jr. and Franck, R. H.: Pulsations in the pulmonary arteries as observed with roentgenoscopic image amplification; observations in patients with isolated pulmonary valvular stenosis. Am. J. Roentgenol. 83:335, 1960.

Gay, B. B., Jr., Franck, R. H., Shuford, W. H., and Rogers, J. V.: Roentgenologic features of single and multiple coarctations of the pulmonary artery and branches. Am. J. Roentgenol. 90:599, 1963.

Gay, W. A., Jr. and Ebert, P. A.: Aorta-to-right pulmonary artery anastomosis causing obstruction of the right pulmonary artery. Management during correction of tetralogy of Fallot. Ann. Thoracic Surg. 16:402, 1973.

Gazetopoulos, N., Ioannidis, P. J., Karydis, C., Lolas, C., Kiriakou, K., and Tountas, C.: Short left coronary artery trunk as a risk factor in development of coronary atherosclerosis: pathologic study. Br. Heart J. 38:1160, 1976.

Gedgaudas, E., Kieffer, S. A., and Erickson, C.: Left atrial calcification. Am. J. Roentgenol. 102:293, 1968.

Gensini, G. G., Buonanno, C., and Palacio, A.: Anatomy of the coronary circulation in living man. Dis. Chest. 52:125, 1967.

Gensini, G. G., Dubiel, J., Huntington, P. P., and Kelly, A. E.: Left ventricular end-diastolic pressure before and after coronary arteriography; the value of coronary arteriography as a stress test. Am. J. Cardiol. 27:453, 1971.

Gensini, G. G. and DiGiorgi, S.: Myocardial toxicity of contrast agents used in angiography. Radiology 82:24, 1964.

Gensini, G. F., Esente, P., and Kelly, A.: Natural history of coronary disease in patients with and without coronary bypass graft surgery. Circulation (Supp. II) 49 & 50:11, 1974.

Gentzler, R. D., II, Gault, J. G., Liedtke, A. J., McCann, W. D., and Mann, R. H., and Hunter, A. S.: Congenital absence of the left circumflex coronary artery in the systolic click syndrome. Circulation 52:490, 1975.

Gerald, B. and Dungan, W. T.: Cor pulmonale and pulmonary edema in children secondary to chronic upper airway obstruction. Radiology 90:679, 1968.

Gerbode, F., Hultgren, H., Melrose, D., and Osborn, J.: Syndrome of left ventricular-right atrial shunt: successful surgical repair of defect in five cases, with observation of bradycardia on closure. Ann. Surg. 148:433, 1958.

Gersony, W. M., Bowman, F. O., Jr., Steeg, C. N., Hayes, C. J., Jesse, M. H., and Malm, J. R.: Management of total anomalous pulmonary venous drainage in early infancy. Circulation 43 & 44:I-19-I-24 (Supp. I), 1971.

Gibbon, J. H., Hopkinson, M., and Churchill, E. D.: Changes in the circulation produced by gradual occlusion of the pulmonary artery. J. Clin. Invest. 11:543, 1932.

Gibson, R. and Wood, E.: Diagnosis of tricuspud stenosis. Brit. Heart J. 17:552, 1955.

Gilbert, J. W., Morrow, A. G., and Talbert, J. L.: The surgical significance of hypertrophic infundibular obstruction accompanying valvular pulmonic stenosis. J. Thoracic Cardiovasc. Surg. 46:457, 1963.

Gillick, F. G. and Reynolds, W. F.: Electrokymographic observations in constrictive pericarditis. Radiology 55:77, 1950.

Girod, D. A., Hurwitz, R. A., King, H., and Jolly, W.: Recent results of two stage surgical treatment of large ventricular septal defect. Circulation 50 (Supp. II):9, 1974.

Girod, D., Raghib, G., Wang, Y., Adams, P., Jr., and Amplatz, K.: Angiocardiographic characteristics of persistent common atrioventricular canal. Radiology 85:442, 1965.

Glancy, D. L., Yarnell, P., and Roberts, W. C.: Traumatic left ventricular aneurysm. Cardiac thrombosis following aneurysmectomy. Am. J. Cardiol. 20:428, 1967.

Glenn, W. W. L. and Patino, J. F.: Circulatory bypass of right heart. J. Biol. Med. 27:147, 1954.

Goerke, R. J. and Carlsson, E.: Calculation of right and left cardiac ventricular volumes. Methods using standard computer equipment and biplane angiocardiograms. Invest. Radiol. 2:360, 1967.

Goetz, R. H.: A new angiographic sign of patent ductus arteriosus. Brit. Heart J. 13:242, 1951.

Gokcebay, T. M., Batillas, J., and Pinck, R. L.: Complete interruption of the aorta at the arch. Am. J. Roentgenol. 114:362, 1972.

Goldberg, H. P., Glenn, F., Dotter, C. T., and Steinberg, I.: Myxoma of the left atrium. Diagnosis made during life with operative and postmortem findings. Circulation 6:762, 1952.

Goldberg, M.: Uremic pericarditis: a review. Military Med. 141:606, 1973.

Golden, R.: Remarks before the annual meeting of the American Roentgen Ray Society, St. Louis, September, 1950.

Goldenberg, D. L., Leff, G., and Grayzel, A. I.: Pericardial tamponade in systemic lupus erythematosus; with absent hemolytic complement activity in pericardial fluid. N.Y. State J. Med. 75:910, 1975.

Goldsmith, M., Farina, M. A., and Shaher, R. M.: Tetralogy of Fallot with atresia of the left pulmonary artery: surgical repair using a homograft aortic valve. J. Thoracic Cardiovasc. Surg. 69:458, 1975.

Gomes, M. M. R., Feldt, R. H., McGoon, D. C., and Danielson, G. K.: Total anomalous pulmonary venous connection. J. Thoracic Cardiovasc. Surg. 60:116, 1970.

Gomes, M. M. R., Weidman, W. H., McGoon, D. C., and Danielson, G. K.: Double-outlet right ventricle with pulmonic stenosis. Surgical considerations and results of operation. Circulation 43:889, 1971.

Gonzalez-Cerna, J. L. and Lillehei, C. W.: Patent ductus with pulmonary hypertension simulating ventricular septal defect. Circulation 18:871, 1958.

Gooch, A. S., Maranhao, V., Scampordonis, G., Cha, S. D., and Yang, S. S.: Prolapse of both mitral and tricuspid leaflets in systolic murmur-click syndrome. N. Engl. J. Med. 287:1218, 1972.

Goodpasture, E. W.: Significance of certain pulmonary lesions in relation to etiology of influenza. Am. J. Med. Sci. 158:863, 1919.

Goodwin, J. F.: The nature of pulmonary hypertension. Brit. J. Radiol. 31:174, 1958.

Goodwin, J. F.: Cardiomyopathies. Mod. Concepts Cardiovasc. Dis. No. 9: 41, 1976.

Goodwin, J. F., Harrison, C. V., and Wilcken, D. E.: Obliterative pulmonary hypertension and thromboembolism. Brit. Med. J. 1:701 and 777, 1963.

Goodwin, J. F., Hollman, A., Cleland, W. P., and Teare, D.: Obstructive cardiomyopathy simulating aortic stenosis. Brit. Heart J. 22:403, 1960.

Goodwin, J. F., Rab, S. M., Sinha, A. K., and Zoob, M.: Rheumatic tricuspid stenosis. Brit. Med. J. 2:1383, 1957.

Goor, D. A. and Lillehei, C. W.: Congenital Malformations of the Heart, pp. 388, New York, Grune & Stratton, 1975.

Gorfein, O. B., Mau, R. D., and Shimonmura, S.: Cineradiographic recognition of papillary muscle calcification. Chest 66:207, 1974.

Gorham, L. W.: A study of pulmonary embolism. I. A clinicopathologic investigation of 100 cases of massive embolism of the pulmonary artery; diagnosis by physical signs and differentiation from acute myocardial infarction. Arch. Int. Med. 108:8, 1961.

Gorham, L. W.: A study of pulmonary embolism. II. The mechanism of death; based on a clinicopathological investigation of 100 cases of massive and 285 cases of minor embolism of the pulmonary artery. Arch. Int. Med. 108:189, 1961.

Gorlin, R., Klein, M.D., and Sullivan, J. M.: Prospective correlative study of ventricular aneurysm. Mechanistic concept and clinical recognition. Am. J. Med. 42:512, 1967.

Gotsman, M. S., Beck, W., and Schrire, V.: Selective angiography in arteritis of the aorta and its major branches. Radiology 88:232, 1967.

Gough, J.: Correlation of radiological and pathological changes in some diseases of the lung. Lancet 1:161, 1955.

Gould, D. M. and Torrance, D. J.: Pulmonary edema. Am. J. Roentgenol. 73:366, 1955.

Gould, L., Guttman, B., and Larrasco, J.: Partial absence of the right ventricular musculature. Am. J. Med. 42:636, 1967.

Gould, S. E. and Ionnides, G.: Disease of the coronary vessels. In Gould, S. E. (ed.). Pathology of the heart and great vessels, pp. 545–600. Springfield, Ill., Charles C Thomas, 1968.

Gouley, B. A.: Anomalous left coronary artery arising from pulmonary artery (adult type). Am. Heart J. 40:630, 1950.

Grace, R. R., Angelini, P., and Cooley, D. A.: Aortic implantation of anomalous left coronary artery arising from pulmonary artery. Am. J. Cardiol. 39:608, 1977.

Graham, E. A.: Aneurysm of the ductus arteriosus, with a consideration of its importance to the thoracic surgeon. Report of two cases. Arch. Surg. 41:324, 1940.

Grainger, R. G.: Interstitial pulmonary edema and its radiological diagnosis. A sign of pulmonary venous and capillary hypertension. Brit. J. Radiol. 31:201, 1958.

Grainger, R. G. and Hearn, J. B.: Intrapulmonary septal lymphatic lines (B lines of Kerley): their significance and their prognostic evaluation before mitral valvotomy. J. Fac. Radiol. 7:66, 1955.

Gramiak, R., Chung, J. K., Nanda, N., and Manning, J.: Echocardiographic diagnosis of transposition of the great vessels. Radiology 106:187, 1973.

Grant, R. P.: The morphogenesis of corrected transposition and other anomalies of cardiac polarity. Circulation 29:71, 1964.

Grant, R. P., Sanders, R. J., Morrow, A. G., and Braunwald, E.: Symposium on diagnostic methods in the study of left-to-right shunts. Circulation 16:791, 1957.

Gray, H.: Anatomy of the Human Body. Edited by W. H. Lewis, ed. 24, p. 550. Philadelphia, Lea & Febiger, 1942.

Gray, H.: Anatomy of the Human Body. Edited by C. M. Goss, ed. 28, p. 545. Philadelphia, Lea & Febiger, 1966.

Grayson, T., Margulis, A. R., Heinbecker, P., and Saltzstein, S. L.: Effects of intra-arterial injection of Miokon, Hypaque, and Renografin in the small intestine of the dog. Radiology 77:776, 1961.

Green, G. D.: The Assessment and Performance of Implanted Cardiac Pacemakers. Butterworths & Co., London, 1975.

Green, G. E., Spencer, F. C., Tice, D. A., and Stertzer, S. H.: Arterial and venous microsurgical bypass grafts for coronary artery disease. J. Thoracic Cardiovasc. Surg. 60:491, 1970.

Greendyke, R. M.: Traumatic rupture of the aorta: special reference to automobile accidents. J.A.M.A. 195:527, 1966.

Greene, D. G., Baldwin, E. F., Baldwin, J. S., Himmelstein, A., Roh, C. E., and Cournand, A.: Pure congenital stenosis and idiopathic congenital dilatation of the pulmonary artery. Am. J. Med. 6:24, 1949.

Greene, D. G. and Bunnell, I. L.: Left ventricular volumes from one-plane cine frames in the right anterior oblique projection in adult human subjects. Presentation to the North American Society for Cardiac Radiology, New Orleans, March, 1974.

Greene, D. G., Carlisle, R., Grant, C., and Bunnell, I. L.: Estimation of left ventricular volume by one-plane cineangiography. Circulation 35:61, 1967.

Greenfield, L. D. and Bennett, L. R.: Detection of intracardiac shunts with radionuclide imaging. Sem. Nuc. Med. 3:139, 1973.

Greenspan, R. H. and Steiner, R.: The Radiologic Diagnosis of Pulmonary Thromboembolism. In Simon, M., Potchen, E. J., and LeMay, M. (eds.). Frontiers of Pulmonary Radiology, pp. 222–245, New York, Grune & Stratton, 1969.

Greenwold, W. E., DuShane, J. W., Burchell, H. B., Bruwer, A., and Edwards, J. E.: Congenital pulmonary atresia with intact interventricular septum: two anatomic types. Circulation 14:945, 1956.

Greenwood, W. F.: Profile of atrial myxoma. Am. J. Cardiol. 21:367, 1968.

Griepp, E., French, J. W., Shumway, N. E., and Baum, D.: Is pulmonary artery banding for ventricular septal defects obsolete? Circulation 50(Supp II):14, 1974.

Griffin, J. F.: Congenital kinking of the aorta (pseudocoarctation). N. Engl. J. Med. 271:726, 1964.

Griffin, J. S., Ochsner, J. L., and Bower, P. J.: Posttraumatic coarctation of the aorta. Am. J. Cardiol. 31:391, 1973.

Griffiths, G. C.: Primary tumours of the heart. Clin. Radiol. 13:183, 1962.

Griffiths, G. C. and Varol, I. L.: Polyarteritis nodosa: a correlation of clinical and post-mortem findings in 17 cases. Circulation 3:481, 1951.

Griffiths, S. P., Levine, O. R., and Andersen, D. H.: Aortic origin of the right pulmonary artery. Circulation 25:73, 1962.

Grishma, A., Sussman, M. L., and Steinberg, M. F.: Angiocardiographic analysis of the cardiac configuration in rheumatic mitral disease. Am. J. Roentgenol. 51:33, 1944.

Griswold, H. E., Jr. and Young, M. D.: Double aortic arch: report of 2 cases and review of the literature. Pediatrics 4:751, 1949.

Grollman, J. H., Gray, R. K. Spiegler, P. Moler, C., MacAlpin, R., and Eber, L.: 105 mm. serial photofluorography of the coronary arteries. Radiology 108:577, 1973.

Grollman, J. H., Jr., Hoffman, R. B., Price, J. E., Jr., O'Reilly, R. J., Lilley, J. M., and Herman, N. P.: Abnormal vascularity in left ventricular mural thrombus demonstrated by selective coronary arteriography. Radiology 113:591, 1974.

Grollman, J. H., Jr. and Horns, J. W.: The collateral circulation in coarctation of the aorta with a distal subclavian artery. Radiology 83:622, 1964.

Grondin, C., David, P. R., Goor, D. A., Edwards, J. E., and Lillehei, C. W.: Dissecting aneurysms of the thoracic aorta: review of 52 cases with consideration of factors influencing prognosis. Ann. Thoracic Surg. 4:29, 1967.

Grondin, C., Leonard, A. S., Anderson, R. C., Amplatz, K. A., Edwards, J. E., and Varco, R. L.: The heart and blood vessels. Cor triatriatum: a diagnostic surgical enigma. J. Thoracic Cardiovasc. Surg. 48:527, 1964.

Gross, R. E.: Surgical closure of an aortic septal defect. Circulation 5:858,1952.

Gross, R. E.: Vascular Anomalies in the Thorax Producing Compression of the Trachea or Esophagus in Surgery of Infancy and Childhood, pp. 913–935. Philadelphia, W. B. Saunders Co., 1953.

Gross, R. E. and Hubbard, J. P.: Surgical ligation of a patent ductus arteriosus: report of first successful case. J.A.M.A. 112:729, 1939.

Gross, R. E. and Longino, L. A.: The patent ductus arteriosus: observations from 412 surgically treated cases. Circulation 3:125, 1951.

Grossman, C. M.: Posttraumatic ossification of the myocardium. J. Trauma 14:85, 1974.

Guerin, R., Soto, B., Karp, R. B., Kirklin, J. W., and Barcia, A. Transposition of the great arteries: determination of the position of the great arteries in conventional chest roentgenograms. Am. J. Roentgenol. 110:747, 1970.

Guild, W. R., Bray, G., and Merrill, J. P.: Hemopericardium with cardiac tamponade in chronic uremia. N. Engl. J. Med. 257:230, 1957.

Gulotta, S. J.: Coronary arteriography 1976 - for whom? Am. J. Cardiol. 38:537, 1976.

Gunnar, R. M., Dillon, R. F., Wallyn, R. J., and Elsberg, E. I.: The physiologic and clinical similarity between primary amyloid of the heart and constrictive pericarditis. Circulation 12:827, 1955.

Gutgesell, H. P. and McNamara, D. G.: Transposition of the great arteries: results of treatment with early palliation and later intracardiac repair. Circulation 51:32, 1975.

Hainer, J. W. and Hamilton, G. W.: Aortic abnormalities in relapsing polychondritis. N. Engl. J. Med. 280:1166, 1969.

Hairston, P., Parker, C. F., Arrants, J. E., Bradham, R. R., and Lee, W. H. Jr.: The adult atrial septal defect: results of surgical repair. Ann. Surg. 179:799, 1974.

Halasz, N. A., Halloran, K. H., and Liebow, A. A.: Bronchial and arterial anomalies with drainage of the right lung into the inferior vena cava. Circulation 14:826, 1956.

Hale, H. W., Jr. and Martin, J. W.: Myocardial contusion. Am. J. Surg. 93:558, 1957.

Hall, R. M. and Margolin, F. R.: Oxygen alveolopathy in adults. Clinical Radiology 23:11, 1972.

Hall, W. M. and Rosenbaum, H. D.: The radiology of cardiac pacemakers. Rad. Clin. N.A. 9(2):343, 1971.

Hallermann, F. J., Davis, G. D., Ritter, D. G., and Kincaid, O. W.: Roentgenographic features of common ventricle. Radiology 87:409, 1966.

Hallerman, F. J., Kincaid, O. W., Tsakiris, A. G., Ritter, D. G., and Titus, J. L.: Persistent truncus arteriosus: a radiographic and angiocardiographic study. Am. J. Roentgenol. 107:827, 1969.

Hallman, G. L., Cooley, D. A., and Singer, D. B.: Congenital anomalies of the coronary arteries: anatomy, pathology, and surgical treatment. Surgery 59:133, 1966.

Halpern, M.: Percutaneous transfemoral arteriography. An analysis of the complications in 1000 consecutive cases. Am. J. Roentgenol. 92:918, 1964.

Halter, B. L.: Nonpenetrating trauma to the heart. Am. J. Surg. 90:237, 1955.

Hamby, R. I., Aintablian, A., and Schwartz, A.: Reappraisal of the functional significance of the coronary collateral circulation. Am. J. Cardiol. 38:305, 1976.

Hamilton, W. F. and Abbott, M. F.: Coarctation of the aorta of the adult type. Am. Heart J. 3:381, 574, 1928.

Hamman, L. and Rich, A. R.: A case of syphilitic myocarditis. Intern. Clinics, 4:221, 1934.

Hampton, A. O. and Castleman, J.: Correlation of postmortem chest teleoroentgenograms with autopsy findings: with special reference to pulmonary embolism and infarction. Am. J. Roentgenol. 43:305, 1940.

Hamwi, G. J., Skillman, T. G., and Tufts, K. C., Jr.: Acromegaly. Am. J. Med. 29:690, 1960.

Hanenson, I. B.: Curable forms of systemic hypertension. In Cardiac Diagnosis and Treatment, p. 727. New York, Harper and Row, 1976.

Hanfling, S.: Metastatic cancer to the heart: review of the literature and report of 127 cases. Circulation 22:474, 1968.

Hansen, J. F. and Wennevold, A.: The diagnosis of Ebstein's disease of the heart. Acta Med. Scand. 189:515, 1971.

Hanson, D. J. and Rosenbaum, H. D.: Posterior cardiac prominence in Ebstein's anomaly simulating mitral disease. Am. J. Roentgenol. 92:1131, 1964.

Hardin, N. J., Wilson, J. M., III, Gray, G. F., and Gay, W. A., Jr.: Experience with primary tumors of the heart—clinical and pathological study of seventeen cases. Johns Hopkins Med. J. 134:141, 1974.

Harken, D. E., Soroff, H. S., and Taylor, W. J.: Partial and complete prosthesis in aortic insufficiency. J. Thoracic Cardiovasc. Surg. 40:744, 1960.

Harley, H. R. S.: The radiological changes in pulmonary venous hypertension, with special reference to the root shadows and lobular pattern. Brit. Heart J. 23:75, 1961.

Harrell, J. E. and Manion, W. C.: Sclerosing aortitis and arteritis. Sem. Roentgenol. 5:260, 1970.

Harris, E. J.: Aneurysms of the sinus of Valsalva. Am. J. Roentgenol. 76:767, 1956.

Harris, L. C., Nghiem, Q. X., Schreiber, M. H., and Wallace, J. M.: Severe pulsus alternans associated with primary myocardial disease in children. Circulation 34:948, 1966.

Harris, L. C. and Nghiem, Q. X.: Cardiomyopathies in infants and children. Prog. Cardiovasc. Dis. 15(3):255, 1972.

Harris, L. S. and Adelson, L.: Fatal coronary embolism from myxomatous tumor of aortic valve. Am. J. Clin. Pathol. 43:61, 1965.

Harrison, C. V.: The pathology of the pulmonary vessels in pulmonary hypertension. Brit. J. Radiol. 31:217, 1958.

Harrison, M. D., Coute, P. M., and Heitzman, E. R.: Radiological detection of clinically occult cardiac failure following myocardial infarction. Brit. J. Radiol. 44:265–272, 1971.

Hart, K.: Uber das aneurysma des rechten sinus valsalvae der aorta und seine beziehungen zum oberen ventrikelseptum. Virchows Arch. Path. Anat. 182:167, 1905.

Hart, W. L., Berman, E. J., and LaCom, R. J.: Hazard of retrograde aortography in dissecting aneurysm. Circulation 27:1140, 1963.

Hartman, A. F., Goldring, D., and Carlsson, E.: Development of right ventricular obstruction by aberrant muscular bands. Circulation 30:679, 1964.

Hartmann, A. F., Jr., Tsifutis, A. A., Arvidsson, H., and Goldring, D.: The two-chambered right ventricle. Report

of nine cases. Circulation 26:279, 1962.

Haskin, M. E., Kricheff, I. I., Sackner, M. A., and Widmann, B. P.: Idiopathic myocardial hypertrophy. Am. J. Roentgenol. 86:1073, 1961.

Hawkins, I. F., Jr. and Kelley, M. J.: Benzalkonium-Heparin-Coated angiographic catheters. Radiology 109:589, 1973.

Hawley, R. R., Dodge, H. T., and Graham, T. P.: Left atrial volume and its changes in heart disease. Circulation 34:989, 1966.

Hayashi, K., Meaney, T. F., Zelch, J. V., and Tasas, R.: Aortographic analysis of aortic dissection. Am. J. Roentgenol. 122:775, 1974.

Healey, J. E., Jr.: An anatomic survey of anomalous pulmonary veins: their clinical significance. J. Thoracic Surg. 23:433, 1952.

Healey, R. F., Dexter, L., Elkin, M., and Sosman, M. C.: Roentgenographic changes in pulmonic stenosis: a report of 9 cases. Am. J. Roentgenol. 63:813, 1950.

Heath, D. and Whitaker, W.: The pulmonary vessels in mitral stenosis. J. Pathol. Bacteriol 70:291, 1955.

Heggtveit, H. A.: Syphilitic aortitis. A clinicopathologic autopsy study of 100 cases, 1950 to 1960. Circulation 29:346, 1964.

Heinz, R. and Abrams, H. L.: Radiologic aspects of operable heart disease. IV. Constrictive pericarditis. Radiology 69:54, 1957.

Heitzman, E. R., Markarian, B., and Dailey, E. T.: Pulmonary thromboembolic disease. A lobular concept. Radiology 103:529, 1972.

Hejtmancik, M. R., Bradfield, J. Y., Jr., and Hermann, G. R.: Acromegaly and the heart: a clinical and pathologic study. Ann. Int. Med. 34:1145, 1951.

Hejtmancik, M. R., Wright, J. C., Quint, R., and Jennings, F. L.: The cardiovascular manifestations of systemic lupus erythermatosus. Am. Heart J. 68:119, 1964.

Hellerstein, H. K. and Santiago-Stevenson, D.: Atrophy of the heart: a correlative study of 85 proved cases. Circulation 1:93, 1950.

Helmsworth, J. A., McGuire, J., and Felson, B.: Arteriography of the aorta by means of the polyethylene catheter. Am. J. Roentgenol. 64:196, 1950.

Henry, J., Kaplan, S., Helmsworth, J. A., and Schreiber, J. T.: Management of infants with large ventricular septal defects. Ann. Thoracic Surg. 15:109, 1973.

Henry, J. N., Devloo, R. A. E., Ritter, D. G., Mair, D. D., Davis, G. D., and Danielson, G. K.: Tricuspid atresia—successful surgical "correction" in two patients using porcine xenograft valves. Mayo Clin. Proc. 49:803, 1974.

Henry, M., Hoeffel, J. C., and Pernot, C.: Congenital localized stenosis of the pulmonary veins. Pediatric Radiology 4:49, 1975.

Hepburn, J. and Dauphinee, J. A.: Successful removal of hemangioma of the lung, followed by disappearance of polycythemia. Am. J. Med. Sci. 204:681, 1942.

Hering, A. C., Wilson, J. S., and Ball, R. E., Jr.: Congenital deficiency of the pericardium. J. Thoracic Cardiovasc. Surg. 40:49, 1960.

Herman, M. V., Heinle, R. A., Klein, M. D., and Gorlin, R.: Localized disorders in myocardial contraction. N. Engl. J. Med. 277:222, 1967.

Hernandez, F. A., Rochkind, R., and Cooper, H. R.: The intracavitary electrocardiogram in the diagnosis of Ebstein's anomaly. Am. J. Cardiol. 1:181, 1958.

Herr, R. H., Starr, A., Pierie, W. R., Wood, J. A., and Bigelow, J. C.: Aortic valve replacement: a review of six years experience with ball valve prosthesis. Ann. Thoracic Surg. 6:199, 1968.

Herrnheiser, G., and Hinson, K. F. W.: An anatomical explanation of the formation of butterfly shadows. Thorax 9:198, 1954.

Heupler, F., Proudfit, W., Siegel, W., Shirey, E., Razavi, M., and Sones, F. M.: The ergonovine maleate test for the diagnosis of coronary artery spasm. Circulation 51 and 52 (Supp. II):1975.

Hiebert, C. A. and Gregory, F. J.: Bullet embolism from the head to the heart. J.A.M.A. 229:442, 1974.

Higashino, S. M., Shaw, G. G., May, I. A., and Ecker, R. R.: Total anomalous pulmonary venous drainage below the diaphragm. J. Thoracic Cardiovasc. Surg. 68:711, 1974.

Higgins, C. B. and Reinke, R. T.: Nonsyphilitic etiology of linear calcification of the ascending aorta. Radiology 113:609, 1974.

Higgins, C. B., Silverman, N. R., Harris, R. D., and Albertson, K. W.: Localized aneurysms of the descending thoracic aorta. Clinical Radiology 26:475, 1975.

Higgins, C. B. and Wexler, L.: Reversal of dominance of the coronary arterial system in isolated aortic stenosis and bicuspid aortic valve. Circulation 52:292, 1975.

Higgins, C. B. and Wexler, L.: Clinical and angiographic features of pulmonary arteriovenous fistulas in children. Radiology 119:171, 1976.

Higgins, C. B., Wexler, L., Silverman, J. F., Hayden, W. G., Anderson, W. L., and Schroeder, J. H.: Spontaneously and pharmacologically provoked coronary arterial spasm in Prinzmetal variant angina. Radiology 119:521, 1976.

Hightower, B. M., Barcia, A., Bargeron, L. M., and Kirklin, J. W.: Double-outlet right ventricle with transposed great arteries and subpulmonary ventricular septal defect. The Taussig-Bing malformation. Circulation (Supp. 1), 39:49, 1969.

Hilal, S. K.: Hemodynamic changes associated with intraarterial injection of contrast media: new toxicity test and a new experimental contrast medium. Radiology 86:615, 1966.

Hilbish, T. F. and Cooley, R. N.: Congenital mitral stenosis. Roentgen study of its manifestations. Am. J. Roentgenol. 76:743, 1956.

Hilbish, T. F. and Morgan, R. H.: Cardiac mensuration by roentgenologic methods. Am. J. Med. Sci. 224:586, 1952.

Hill, M. C., Muto, C. N., Mani, J. R., and Dozier, W. E.: The value of pneumoperitoneum in diagnosis of sequestered lung. Am. J. Roentgenol. 91:291, 1964.

Hiller, H. G. and McClean, A. D.: Pulmonary artery ring. Acta Radiol. 48:434, 1957.

Hills, T. H. and Stanford, R. W.: The problem of excessive radiation during routine investigations of the heart. Brit. Heart J. 12:45, 1950.

Hipona, F. A. and Crummy, A. B.: Congenital pericardial defect associated with tetralogy of Fallot. Herniation of normal lung into the pericardial cavity. Circulation 29:132, 1964.

Hipona, F. A. and Jamshidi, A.: Observations of the natural history of varicosity of pulmonary veins. Circulation 35:471, 1967.

Hipona, F. A., Lerona, P. T., and Paredes, S.: Radiologic diagnosis of late complications associated with cardiac valve surgery in acquired heart disease. Radiol. Clin. N.A. 9:265, 1971.

Hirst, A. E. and Barbour, B. H.: Dissecting aneurysm with hemopericardium. Report of a case with healing. N. Engl. J. Med. 258:116, 1958.

Hirst, A. E. and Gore, I.: Is cystic medionecrosis the cause of dissecting aortic aneurysm? Circulation 53:915, 1976.

Hirst, A. E., Jr., Johns, V. J., Jr., and Kima, S. W., Jr.: Dissecting aneurysm of the aorta: a review of 505 cases. Medicine 37:217, 1958.

Ho, C. S., Krovetz, L. J., Strise, J. L., Brawley, R. K., and

Rowe, R. D.: Postoperative assessment of residual defects following cardiac surgery in infants and children. II. Ventricular septal defect. Johns Hopkins Med. J. 133:278, 1973.

Hodges, P. C.: Heart size from routine chest films. Radiology 47:355, 1946.

Hodges, P. C. and Eyster, J. A. E.: Estimation of cardiac area in man. Am. J. Roentgenol. 12:252, 1924.

Hoffman, J. I. E.: Natural history of congenital heart disease. Problems in its assessment with special reference to ventricular septal defects. Circulation 37:97, 1968.

Hoffman, J. I. E.: Treatment of ventricular septal defect. Western J. Med. 120:315, 1974.

Hoffman, J. I. E. and Rudolph, A. M.: Natural history of ventricular septal defect in infancy. Abstract. Circulation 28:737, 1963.

Hoffman, J. I. E., Rudolph, A. M., Nadas, A. S., and Gross, R.E.: Pulmonic stenosis, ventricular septal defect, and right ventricular pressure above systemic level. Circulation 22:405, 1960.

Holman, B. L.: Radionuclide methods in the evaluation of myocardial ischemia and infarction. Circulation 53 (Supp. 1):112, 1976.

Holman, C. W. and Steinberg, I.: The role of angiocardiography in the surgical treatment of massive pericardial effusions. Surg. Gynecol. Obstet. 107:639, 1958.

Holman, E. and Beck, C. S.: The physiological response of the circulatory system to experimental alterations. III. The effect of aortic and pulmonary stenosis. J. Clin. Invest. 3:283, 1926.

Holsinger, D. R., Osmundson, P. J., and Edwards, J. E.: The heart in periarteritis nodosa. Circulation 25:610, 1962.

Hopps, H. C. and Wissler, R. W.: Uremic pneumonitis. Am. J. Pathol. 31:261, 1955.

Horn, H. R., Teichholz, L. E., Cohn, P. F., Herman, M. V., and Gorlin, R.: Augmentation of left ventricular contraction pattern in coronary artery disease by an inotropic catecholamine. Circulation 49:1063, 1974.

Horowitz, M. S., Schultz, C. S., Stinson, E. B., Harrison, D. C., and Popp, R. L.: Sensitivity and specificity of echocardiographic diagnosis of pericardial effusion. Circulation 50:239, 1974.

Howard, R. J., Moller, J., Castaneda, A. R., Varco, R. L., and Nicoloff, B. M.: Surgical correction of sinus of Valsalva aneurysm. J. Thoracic Cardiovasc. Surg. 66:420, 1973.

Hoyos, J. M. and Campo, C. G.: Angiography of the thoracic aorta and coronary vessels with direct injection of an opaque solution into the aorta. Radiology 50:211, 1948.

Hudson, R.: The normal and abnormal inter-atrial septum. Brit. Heart J. 17:489, 1955.

Hughes, C. W. and Rumore, P. C.: Anomalous pulmonary veins. Arch. Pathol. 37:364, 1944.

Humblet, L., Stainier, L., Joris, H., Collignon, P., Kulbertus, H., and Delvigne, J.: Observations cliniques la stenose mitrale congenitale. Acta Cardiol. 26:500, 1971.

Hung, J. S., Ritter, D. G., Seldt, R. H., and Kincaid, O. W.: Electrocardiographic and angiographic features of common atrium. Chest 63:970, 1973.

Hunt, C. E. and Lucas, R. B.: Symptomatic atrial septal defect in infancy. Circulation 47:1042, 1973.

Hunter, A. S. and Keay, A. J.: Primary endocardial fibroelastosis. An inherited condition. Arch. Dis. Childhood 48:66, 1973.

Hunter, S. W., Roth, N. A., Bernardez, D., and Noble, J. H.: A bipolar myocardial electrode for complete heart block. Lancet 79:506, 1959.

Hurley, P. J., Cooper, M., Reba, R. C., Poggenbing, K. J., and Wagner, H. J., Jr.: ^{43}KCL: A new radiopharmaceutical for imaging the heart. J. Nucl. Med. 12:516–519, 1971.

Husson, G. S., Blackman, M. S., Riemenschneider, P., and

Berne, A. S.: Isolated congenital mitral insufficiency. J. Pediat. 64:248, 1964.

Hylen, J. C., Judkins, M. P., Herr, R. H., and Starr, A.: Radiologic diagnosis of aortic-ball variance. J.A.M.A. 207:1120, 1969.

Idbohrn, H. and Berg, N.: On the tolerance of the rabbit's kidney to contrast media in renal angiography - a roentgenologic and histologic investigation. Acta Radiol. 42:121, 1954.

Idriss, F. S., Aubert, J., Paul, M., Nikaidoh, H., Lev, H., and Newfield, E. A.: Transposition of the great vessels with ventricular septal defect: surgical and anatomic considerations. J. Thoracic Cardiovasc. Surg. 68:732, 1974.

Imai, Y., Nishiya, Y., Morikawa, T., Kurosawa, H., and Konno, S.: Total correction of tetralogy of Fallot associated with an anomalous left pulmonary artery arising from the aortic arch. J. Thoracic Cardiovasc. Surg. 68(1):51, 1974.

Inada, K., Shimizu, H., Kobayashi, T., Ishiai, S., and Kawamoto, S.: Pulseless disease and atypical coarctation of the aorta. Arch. Surg. 84:306, 1962.

Ionescu, M. I., Macartney, F. J., and Wooler, G. H.: Intracardiac repair of single ventricle with pulmonary stenosis. J. Thoracic Cardiovasc. Surg. 65:602, 1973.

Israel, H. L. and Patchefsky, A. S.: Wegener's granulomatosis of lung: diagnosis and treatment—experience with 12 cases. Ann. Int. Med. 74:881, 1971.

Ivemark, B. J.: Implications of agenesis of spleen in pathogenesis of conotruncus anomalies in childhood. Acta Paediat. 44(Supp. 104):590, 1955.

Ivey, N. S. and Norris, H. J.: Intimal vascular lesions associated with female reproductive steroids. Arch. Pathol. 96:227, 1973.

Jackman, J. and Lubert, M.: Significance of calcification in the ascending aorta as observed roentgenographically. Am. J. Roentgenol. 53:432, 1945.

Jackson, A. and Garber, P. E.: Myxoma of the left atrium: report of 3 cases. Am. Heart J. 55:591, 1958.

Jacobson, G., Cosby, R. S., Griffith, G. C. and Meyer, B. W.: Valvular stenosis as a cause of death in surgically treated coarctation of the aorta. Am. Heart J. 45:889, 1953.

Jacobson, G., Turner, A. F., Balchum. O. J., and Jung, R.: Vascular changes in pulmonary emphysema. The radiologic evaluation by selective and peripheral pulmonary wedge angiography. Am. J. Roentgenol. 100:374, 1967.

Jacobson, G. and Weidner, W.: Dilatation of the left auricular appendage by the Valsalva maneuver: an aid in the diagnosis of mitral valve disease. Radiology 79:274, 1962.

Jaffee, R. B.: Complete interruption of the aortic arch. I. Characteristic radiographic findings in 21 patients. Circulation 52:714, 1975.

Jaffe, R. B. and Condon, V. R.: Mycotic aneurysms of the pulmonary artery and aorta. Radiology 116:291, 1975.

Jaffe, R. B. and Figley, M. M.: Roentgenographic evaluation of bronchial size following pulmonary embolization. Radiology 88:245, 1967.

Jaffe, R. B. and Koschmann, E. B.: Intravenous drug abuse. Pulmonary, cardiac, and vascular complications. Am. J. Roentgenol. 109:107, 1970.

Jager, B. V. and Wollenman, O. J. Jr.: Anatomical study of closure of ductus arteriosus. Am. J. Pathol. 18:595, 1942.

Jahnke, E. J. Jr., Fisher, G. W., and Jones, R. C.: Acute traumatic rupture of the thoracic aorta. Report of six consecutive cases of successful early repair. J. Thoracic Cardiovasc. Surg. 48:63, 1964.

James, A. E. Jr., Conway, J. J., Chang, C. H., Cooper, M., White, R. I., and Strauss, H. W.: The fissure sign: its multiple causes. Am. J. Roentgenol. 111:492, 1971.

James, T. N.: The delivery and distribution of coronary collateral circulation. Chest 58(3):183, 1970.

James, T. N.: DeSubitaneis Mortibus. VIII. Coronary arteries and conduction system in scleroderma heart disease. Circulation 50:844, 1974.

Jeffery, R. F., Moller, J. H., and Amplatz, K.: The dysplastic pulmonary valve: a new roentgenographic entity. With a discussion of the anatomy and radiology of other types of valvular pulmonary stenosis. Am. J. Roentgenol. 114:322, 1972.

Jegier, W., Gibbons, J. E., and Wiglesworth, F. W.: Cor triatriatum: clinical, hemodynamic and pathological studies: surgical correction in early life. Pediatrics 31:255, 1963.

Jenkins, J. L. and Nishimura, A.: Coronary artery obstruction and myocardial infarction resulting from nonpenetrating chest trauma. Texas Med. 71:78, 1975.

Jensen, J. B. and Blount, S. G. Jr.: Total anomalous pulmonary venous return Am. Heart J. 82:387, 1971.

Jeresaty, R. M.: Ballooning of the mitral valve leaflets. Angiographic study of 24 patients. Radiology 100:45, 1971.

Joffe, N.: Roentgenologic findings in post-shock and post-operative pulmonary insufficiency. Radiology 94:369, 1970.

Johns, T. N. P., Williams, G. R., and Blalock, A.: The anatomy of pulmonary stenosis and atresia with comments on surgical therapy. Surgery 33:161, 1953.

Johnson, L. W., Grossman, W., Dalen, J. E., and Dexter, L.: Pulmonic stenosis in the adult. Long-term follow-up results. N. Engl. J. Med. 287:1159, 1972.

Johnson, P. M., Wood, E. H., Pasternack, B. S., and Jones, M. A.: Roentgen evaluation of pulmonary arterial pressure in mitral stenosis. Radiology 76:541, 1961.

Johnson, W. D., Flemma, R. J., and Lepley, D.: Determinants of blood flow in aortic-coronary saphenous vein bypass grafts. Arch. Surg. 101:806, 1970.

Johnsrude, I. S. and Carey, L. S.: Roentgenographic manifestations of endocardial fibroelastosis. Am. J. Roentgenol. 94:109, 1965.

Jones, E. L., Conti, C. R., Neill, C. A., Gott, V. L., Brawley, R. K., and Haller, J. A., Jr.: Long-term evaluation of tetralogy patients with pulmonary valvular insufficiency resulting from outflow-patch correction across the pulmonic annulus. Circulation 48(Supp. 3):11, 1973.

Jones, J. C. and Thompson, W. P.: Arteriovenous fistula of lung. J. Thoracic Surg. 13:357, 1944.

Jones, R. H., Jr.: Beriberi heart disease. Circulation 19:275, 1959.

Jönsson, G.: Thoracic aortography by means of a cannula inserted percutaneously into the common carotid artery. Acta Radiol. 31:376, 1949.

Jönsson, G., Broden, B., and Karnell, J.: Thoracic aortography with special reference to its value in patent ductus arteriosus and coarctation of the aorta. Acta Radiol. (Supp. #89), 1951.

Jönsson, G. and Saltzman, G. F.: Infundibulum of patent ductus arteriosus. A diagnostic sign in conventional roentgenograms. Acta Radiol. (Stockholm) 38:8, 1952.

Jorgens, J., Kundel, R., and Lieber, A.: The cinefluorographic approach to the diagnosis of pericardial effusion. Am. J. Roentgenol. 87:911, 1962.

Joyce, J. W., Fairbairn, J. F. II, Kincaid, O. W., and Juergens, J. L.: Aneurysms of the thoracic aorta. A clinical study with special reference to prognosis. Circulation 29:176, 1964.

Judkins, M. P.: Selective coronary arteriography—Part I: A percutaneous transfemoral technic. Radiology 89:815, 1967.

Judkins, M. P.: Percutaneous transfemoral selective coronary arteriography. Rad. Clin. N. A. (VI)3:467, 1968.

Judkins, M. P., Abrams, H. L., Bristow, J. D., Carlsson, E., Criley, J. M. Elliott, L. P., Ellis, K. B., Freisinger, G. C., Greenspan, R. H., and Viamonte, M., Jr.: Report of the Intersociety Commission for Heart Disease Resources. Optimal resources for examination of the chest and cardiovascular system. A hospital planning and resource guideline. Radiologic facilities for conventional x-ray examination of the heart and lungs. Catheterization angiographic laboratories. Radiologic resources for cardiovascular surgical operating rooms and intensive care units. Circulation *53*:A1, 1976.

Judkins, M. P. and Gander, M. P.: Prevention of complications of coronary arteriography. Circulation *49(4)*:599, 1974.

Jue, K. L., Amplatz, K., Adams, P. A., and Anderson, R.: Anomalies of great vessels associated with lung hypoplasia: the scimitar syndrome. Am. J. Dis. Child. *111*:35, 1966.

Kahlstorf, A.: Ueber eine orthodiagraphische Herzvolumenbestimmung. Fortschr. Gebiete Roentgenstrahlen *45*:123, 1932.

Kalke, B. R., Carlson, R. G., Ferlic, R. M., Sellers, R. D., and Lillehei, C. W.: Partial anomalous pulmonary venous connections. Am. J. Cardiol. *20*:91, 1967.

Kampmeier, R. H.: Saccular aneurysms of the thoracic aorta: a clinical study of 633 cases. Ann. Int. Med. *12*:624, 1938.

Kanick, V., Hemley, S. D., Kittredge, R. D., and Finby, N.: Some problems in the angiographic diagnosis of dissecting aneurysms of the thoracic aorta. Am. J. Roentgenol. *91*:1283, 1964.

Kannel, W. B. and Feinleib, M.: Natural history of angina pectoris in the Framingham study. Am. J. Cardiol. *29*:154, 1972.

Kaplan, B. M., Schlichter, J. G., Graham, G., and Miller, G.: Idiopathic congenital dilatation of the pulmonary artery. J. Lab. Clin. Med. *41*:697, 1953.

Kaplitt, M. J., Frantz, S. L., Beil, A. R., Stein, H. L., and Gulotta, S. J.: Analysis of intraoperative coronary angiography in aortocoronary bypass grafts. Circulation (Supp. II)*49 and 50*:II-141, II-148, 1974.

Kardjiev, V., Symeonov, A., and Chankov, I.: Etiology, pathogenesis and prevention of spinal cord lesions in selective angiography of the bronchial and intercostal arteries. Radiology *112*:81, 1974.

Kartagener, M.: Zur Pathogenese der Bronchiektasien; Bronchiektasien bei situs viscerum inversum. Beitr. Klin. Tuberk. *83*:489, 1933.

Kasser, I. and Kennedy, J. W.: The measurement of left ventricular volumes from single plane cineangiocardiography. Clin. Res. *14*:110, 1968.

Kauff, M. K., Bloch, J., and Baltaxe, H. A.: Complete interruption of the aortic arch in adults. Radiology *106*:53, 1973.

Kavanheh-Gray, D., Musgrove, E., and Stanwood, D.: Congenital pericardial defects: report of a case. N. Engl. J. Med. *265*:692, 1961.

Kawashima, Y., Ueda, T., Naito, Y., Morikawa, E., and Manabe, H.: Stenosis of pulmonary veins: report of a patient corrected surgically. Ann. Thoracic Surg. *12*:196, 1971.

Kaye, D., Frankl, W., and Arditi, L. I.: Probable postcardiotomy syndrome following implantation of a transvenous pacemaker: report of the first case. Am. Heart J. *90*:627, 1975.

Keane, J. F., Maltz, D., Bernhard, W. F., Corwin, R. D., and Nadas, A. S.: Anomalous origin of one pulmonary artery from the ascending aorta: diagnostic, physiological, and surgical considerations. Circulation *50*:588, 1974.

Keats, T. E. and Enge, I. P.: Cardiac mensuration by the cardiac volume method. Radiology *85*:850, 1965.

Keats, T. E. and Martt, J. M.: Acyanotic tetralogy of Fallot. Am. J. Roentgenol. *82*:417, 1959.

Keats, T. E. and Martt, J. M.: False paradoxic movement of the posterior wall of the left ventricle simulating myocardial aneurysm. Radiology *78*:381, 1962.

Keats, T. E. and Martt, J. M.: Selective dilatation of the right

atrium in pregnancy. Am. J. Roentgenol. *91*:307, 1964.

Keats, T. E. and Steinbach, H. L.: Patent ductus arteriosus: a critical evaluation of its roentgen signs. Radiology *64*:528, 1955.

Keck, E. W. O., Ongley, P. A., Kincaid, O. W., and Swan, H. J. C.: Ventricular septal defect with aortic insufficiency: a clinical and hemodynamic study of 18 proved cases. Circulation *27*:203, 1963.

Keith, J. D., Neill, C. A., Vlad, P., Rowe, R. D., and Chute, A. L.: Transposition of the great vessels. Circulation *7*:830, 1953.

Keith, J. D., Rowe, R. P., and Vlad, P.: Heart Disease in Infancy and Childhood. New York, The Macmillan Co., 1958.

Keith, J. D., Rowe, R. P., and Vlad, P.: Heart Disease in Infancy and Childhood, 2nd ed. New York, The Macmillan Co., 1967.

Kelly, D. P., Wullsberg, E., and Rowe, R. D.: Discrete subaortic stenosis. Circulation *46*:309, 1972.

Keneidel, J. H.: A case of aneurysm of ductus arteriosus with postmortem and roentgenologic study after instillation of barium paste. Am. J. Roentgenol. *62*:223, 1949.

Kerley, P.: Radiology in heart disease. Brit. Med. J. *2*:594, 1933.

Kerley, P.: The cardiovascular system. *In* A Text Book of X-ray Diagnosis, Vol. 2, Shanks, S. C., and Kerley, P. (eds.). Philadelphia, W. B. Saunders Co., 1951.

Kern, R. A., Soloff, W. A., Snape, W. J., and Bellow, C. T.: Pericardial effusion: a constant, early and major factor in the cardiac syndrome of hypothyroidism (myxedema heart). Am. J. Med. Sci. *217*:609, 1949.

Kesteloot, H., Roelandt, J., Willems, J., Claes, J. H., and Joossens, J. V.: An enquiry into the role of cobalt in the heart disease of chronic beer drinkers. Circulation *37*:854, 1968.

Keys, A., Brozek, J., Henschel, A., Mickelsen, O., and Taylor, H. L.: The Biology of Human Starvation, vol. 1, pp. 198–208, Minneapolis, University of Minnesota Press, 1950.

Keys, A. and Shapiro, M. J.: Patency of the ductus arteriosus in adults. Am. Heart J. *25*:158, 1943.

Kezdi, P. and Wennemark, J.: Ebstein's malformation (clinical findings and hemodynamic alterations). Am. J. Cardiol. *2*:200, 1958.

Kidd, B. S. L., Tyrell, M. J., and Pickering, D.: Transposition 1969. *In* The Natural History and Progress in Treatment of Congenital Heart Defects, Kidd, B. S. L., and Keith, J. D. (eds.), pp. 127–137. Springfield, Ill., Charles C Thomas, 1971.

Kieffer, S. A., Amplatz, K., Anderson, R. C., and Lillehei, C. W.: Proximal interruption of a pulmonary artery: roentgen features and surgical correction. Am. J. Roentgenol. *95*:592, 1965.

Kieffer, S. A. and Carey, L. S.: Roentgen evaluation of pulmonary atresia with intact ventricular septum. Am. J. Roentgenol. *89*:999, 1963.

Kiely, B., Filler, J., Stone, S., and Doyle, E. F.: Syndrome of anomalous venous drainage of the right lung to the inferior vena cava. Am. J. Cardiol. *20*:102, 1967.

King, D. L., Steeg, C. N., and Ellis, K.: Demonstration of transposition of the great arteries by cardiac ultrasonography. Radiology *107*:181, 1973.

King, T. D. and Mills, N. L.: Non-operative closure of atrial septal defects. Surgery *75*:383, 1974.

Kinsley, R. H., McGoon, D. C., Danielson, G. K., Wallace, R. B., and Mair, D. D.: Pulmonary arterial hypertension after repair of tetralogy of Fallot. J. Thoracic & Cardiovascular Surg. *67*:110, 1974.

Kirklin, J. W.: Advances in Cardiovascular Surgery, New York, Grune & Stratton, 1973.

Kirklin, J. W., Connolly, D. C., Ellis, F. H., Burchell, H. B., Edwards, J. E., and Wood, E. H.: Problems in the diagnosis and surgical treatment of pulmonic stenosis with intact ventricular septum. Circulation 8:849, 1953.

Kirklin, J. W., DuShane, J. W., Patrick, R. T., Donald, D. E., Hetzel, P. S., Harshbarger, H. G., and Wood, E. H.: Intracardiac surgery with the aid of a mechanical pump-oxygenator system (Gibbon type): report of eight cases. Proc. Staff Meet. Mayo Clin. 30:201, 1955.

Kirklin, J. W. and Karp, R. B.: The Tetralogy of Fallot from a Surgical Viewpoint. Philadelphia, W. B. Saunders Co., 1970.

Kirsh, M. M., Crane, J. D., Redman, H., Bookstein, J. J., and Sloan, H. Roentgenographic evaluation of traumatic rupture of the aorta. Surg., Gynecol. Obstet. 131:900, 1970.

Kissane, R. W.: Traumatic heart disease, especially myocardial contusion. Postgrad. Med. 15:114, 1954.

Kistin, A. D., Evans, J. M., and Brigulio, A. E.: Ebstein's anomaly of the tricuspid valve: angiocardiographic diagnosis. Am. Heart J. 50:634, 1955.

Kittredge, R. D. and Cameron, A.: Abnormalities of left ventricular wall motion and aneurysm formation. Am. J. Roentgenol. 116:110, 1972.

Kittredge, R. D., Gamboa, D., and Kemp, H. D.: Radiographic visualization of left ventricular aneurysms on lateral chest film. Am. J. Roentgenol. 126:1140, 1976.

Kittredge, R. D., Shimomura, Cameron, A., and Bell, A. L. L.: Prolapsing mitral valve leaflets; cineangiographic demonstration. Am. J. Roentgenol. 109:84, 1970.

Kjellberg, S. R., Lonroth, H., and Rudhe, U.: The effects of various factors on the roentgenological determination of the cardiac volume. Acta Radiol. 35:413, 1951.

Kjellberg, S. R., Mannheimer, E., Rudhe, U., and Jönsson, B.: Diagnosis of Congenital Heart Disease, ed. 2., New York, Year Book Publishers, Inc., 1958.

Kjellberg, S. R., Rudhe, U., and Sjostrand, T.: The condition of the cardiac volume during pregnancy. Acta Radiol. 31:123, 1949.

Klatte, E. C., Tampas, J. P., Campbell, J. A., and Lurie, P. R.: The roentgenographic manifestations of aortic stenosis and aortic valvular insufficiency. Am. J. Roentgenol. 88:57, 1962.

Klatte, E. C. and Yune, H. Y.: Diagnosis and treatment of pericardial cysts. Radiology 104:541, 1972.

Kline, J. L. and Durant, J.: Surgical resection of a tuberculous aneurysm of the ascending aorta: report of a case. N. Engl. J. Med. 265:1185, 1961.

Kloster, F. E.: Diagnosis and management of complications of prosthetic heart valves. Am. J. Cardiol. 35:872, 1975.

Knight, M. and Lennox, S.: Results of surgery for atrial septal defect in patients of 40 years and over. Thorax 27:577, 1972.

Koch, W. and Silva, A.: Anomalous drainage of pulmonary veins into the inferior vena cava. Radiology 75:592, 1960.

Kohout, F. W., Silber, E. N., Schlichter, J. G., and Katz, L. N.: The dynamics of the Eisenmenger complex. Am. Heart J. 50:337, 1955.

Konecke, L. S., Spitzer, S., Mason, D., Kasparian, H., and James, P. M.: Traumatic aneurysm of the left coronary artery. Am. J. Cardiol. 27:221, 1971.

Korn, D., DeSanctis, R. W., and Sell, S.: Massive calcification of the mitral annulus. N. Engl. J. Med. 267:900, 1962.

Korn, D., Gore, I., Blenke, A., and Collins, D. P.: Pulmonary arterial bands and webs: unrecognized manifestation of organized pulmonary emboli. Am. J. Pathol. 40:129, 1962.

Kozuka, T., Sato, K., Fujino, M., Kawashima, Y., and Nosaki, T.: Roentgenographic diagnosis of single ventricle. Analysis of forty-two cases. Am. J. Roentgenol. 119:512, 1973.

Kramer, R. A. and Abrams, H. L.: Radiologic aspects of operable heart disease. VII. Left ventricular-right atrial shunts. Radiology 78:171, 1962.

Kravath, R. E., Scarpelli, E. M., and Bernstein, J.: Hepatogenic cyanosis: arteriovenous shunts in chronic active hepatitis. J. Pediat. 78:238, 1971.

Kremens, V.: Demonstration of the pericardial shadow on the routine chest roentgenogram: a new roentgen finding: preliminary report. Radiology 64:72, 1955.

Kruetzer, G., Galindez, E., Bono, H., de Palma, C., and Laura, J. P.: An operation for the correction of tricuspid atresia. J. Thoracic Cardiovasc. Surg. 66:613, 1973.

Kriss, J. P., Enright, L. P., Hayden, W. G., Wexler, L., and Shumway, N. E.: Radioisotopic angiocardiography: findings in congenital heart disease. J. Nuc. Med. 13:31, 1972.

Krongrad, E., Ritter, D. G., and Kincaid, O. W.: Aorticopulmonary tunnel: angiographic recognition of pulmonary atresia and coronary artery-to-pulmonary artery fistula. Am. J. Roentgenol. 119:498, 1973.

Kronzon, I., Deutsch, P. G., Lefleur, R., and Glassman, E.: Diagnosis of dissecting aortic aneurysm by left atrial angiography. Am. J. Roentgenol. 124:458, 1975.

Krovetz, L. J.: Hemodynamics of left-to-right shunts. Radiol. Clin. N.A. 6:319, 1968.

Kundstadt, D., Adeboyo, A., and Clauss, R. H.: Aortic insufficiency: a result of intermittent migration of aortic valve prosthesis poppet. J.A.M.A. 235:2847, 1976.

Kupic, E. A. and Abrams, H. L.: Supravalvular aortic stenosis. Am. J. Roentgenol. 98:822, 1966.

Kurlander, G. J., Petry, E. L., Taybi, H., Lurie, P. R., and Campbell, J. A.: Supravalvular aortic stenosis: the roentgen analysis of 27 cases. Am. J. Roentgenol. 98:782, 1966.

Kurtzman, R. S., Otto, D. L., and Chepey, J. J.: Myxedema heart disease. Radiology 84:624, 1965.

Laforet, E. G.: Acute hypertension as a diagnostic clue in traumatic rupture of the aorta. Am. J. Surg. 110:948, 1965.

Lam, C. R., Gale, H., and Drake, E.: Surgical treatment of left ventricular aneurysms. J.A.M.A. 187:1, 1964.

Lam, C. R., Green, E., and Drake, E.: Diagnosis and surgical correction of two types of triatrial heart. Surgery 51:127, 1962.

Lande, A.: Takayasu's arteritis and congenital coarctation of the descending thoracic and abdominal aorta: a critical review. Am. J. Roentgenol. 127:227, 1976.

Lande, A. and Berkmen, Y. M.: Aortitis. Pathologic, clinical and arteriographic review. Rad. Clin. N.A. 14:219, 1976.

Lande, A. and Rossi, P.: The value of total aortography in the diagnosis of Takayasu's arteritis. Radiology 114:287, 1975.

Landing, B. H.: Syndromes of congenital heart disease with tracheobronchial anomalies. Edward B. D. Neuhauser Lecture, 1974. Am. J. Roentgenol. 123:679, 1974.

Lang, E. K.: A survey of the complications of percutaneous retrograde arteriography. Seldinger technique. Radiology 81:257, 1963.

Lansing, A. M.: Unusual radiologic sign of loose mitral valve prosthesis. Radiology 88:789, 1967.

Larsson, H. and Kjellberg, S. R.: Roentgenological heart volume determination with special regard to pulse rate and the position of the body. Acta Radiol. 29:159, 1948.

Lasser, E. C.: Basic mechanisms of contrast media reactions: theoretical and experimental considerations. Radiology 91:63, 1968.

Lasser, E. C., Walters, A., Reuter, S. R., and Lang, L.: Histamine release by contrast media. Radiology 100:683, 1971.

Laubry, C. H., Cottenot, P., Routier, D., and Heim de Balsac, R.: Radiologie Clinique du Coeur et des Gros Vaisseaux, Paris, Masson et Cie, Editeurs, 1939.

Lauer, R. N. DuShane, J. W. and Edwards, J. E.: Obstruction

of the left ventricular outlet in association with ventricular septal defect. Circulation *18*:110, 1960.

Lavine, P., Zbigniew, F., Moosa, N., Demetrios, K., Segal, B. E., and Linhart, J. W.: Clinical and hemodynamic evaluation of coronary collateral vessels in coronary artery disease. Am. Heart J. *87*:3:343, 1974.

Lawrence, E. A. and Rumel, W. R.: Arteriovenous fistula of lung. J. Thoracic Surg. *20*:142, 1950.

Lawrie, G. M., Lie, J. T., Morris, G. C., and Beazley, H. L.: Vein graft patency and intimal proliferation after aortocoronary bypass: early and long-term angiopathologic correlations. Am. J. Cardiol. *38*:856, 1976.

Lees, M. H.: Commentary. Patent ductus arteriosus in premature infants—a diagnostic and therapeutic dilemma. J. Pediat. *132*:34, 1975.

Lehman, J. S., Boyer, R. A., and Winter, F. S.: Coronary arteriogram. Am. J. Roentgenol. *81*:749, 1959.

Lehman, J. S., Boyle, J. J. Jr., and Debbas, J. N.: Quantitation of aortic valvular insufficiency by catheter thoracic aortography. Radiology *709*:361, 1962.

Lehman, J. S., Musser, B. G., and Lykens, H. D.: Cardiac ventriculography. Am. J. Roentgenol. *77*:207, 1957.

Lehman, J. S. and Debbas, J. N.: An evaluation of cardiovascular contrast media. Radiology *76*:548, 1961.

Lenkei, S. C., Swan, H. J. C., and DuShane, J. W.: Transposition of the great vessels with atrial septal defect: a hemodynamic study in 2 cases. Circulation *20*:842, 1959.

Lequime, J., et al: Aneurysmes arterioveineux pulmonaires et angiomatose generalizee. Acta Cardiol. *5*:63, 1950.

Lerman, J., Clark, R. J., and Means, J. H.: The heart in myxedema. Electrocardiograms and roentgen-ray measurements. Ann. Int. Med. *6*:1251, 1933.

Lesage, C. H., Vogel, G. H. K., and Blount, S. G., Jr.: Iatrogenic coronary occlusive disease in patients with prosthetic heart valves. Am. J. Cardiol. *26*:123, 1970.

Lesperance, J., Bourassa, M. G., Saltiel, J., Campeau, L., and Grondin, C. M.: Angiographic changes in aortocoronary vein grafts: lack of progression beyond the first year. Circulation *48*:633, 1973.

Lesperance, J., Saltiel, J., Petitclerc, R., and Bourassa, M. G.: Angulated views in the sagittal plane for improved accuracy of cinecoronary angiography. Am. J. Roentgenol. *121(3)*:565, 1974.

Lester, R. G., Anderson, R. C., Amplatz, K., and Adams, P.: Roentgenologic diagnosis of congenitally corrected transposition of the great vessels. Am. J. Roentgenol. *83*:985, 1960.

Lester, R. G., Mauck, H. P., and Grubb, W. L.: Anomalous pulmonary venous return to the right side of the heart. Sem. Roentgen. *1*:102, 1966.

Lester, R. G., Osteen, R. T., and Robinson, A. E.: Infundibular obstruction secondary to pulmonary valvular stenosis. Am. J. Roentgenol. *94*:78, 1965.

Lev, M.: Pathologic anatomy and interrelationships of hypoplasia of the aortic tract complexes. Lab. Invest. *1*:61, 1952.

Levin, D. C.: Pulmonary abnormalities in the necrotizing vasculitides and their rapid response to steroids. Radiology *97*:521, 1970.

Levin, D. C.: Pathways and functional significance of the coronary collateral circulation. Circulation *50*:831, 1974.

Levin, D. C., Baltaxe, H. A., Goldberg, H. P., Engle, M. A., Ebert, P. A., Sos, T. A., and Levin, A. R.: The importance of selective angiography of systemic arterial supply to the lungs in planning surgical correction of pseudotruncus arteriosus. Am. J. Roentgenol. *121*:606, 1974.

Levin, D. C., Baltaxe, H. A., Lee, J. G., and Sos, T. A.: Potential sources of error in coronary arteriogram. I. In performance of the study. Am. J. Roentgenol. *124(3)*:378, 1975.

Levin, D. C., Baltaxe, H. A., and Sos, T. A.: Potential sources of error in coronary arteriography. II. In interpretation of the study. Am. J. Roentgenol. *124(3)*:386, 1975.

Levine, J. A., Bechtel, D. J., Gorlin, R., Cohn, P. F., Herman, M. V., Cohn, L. H., and Collins, J. J., Jr.: Coronary artery anatomy before and after direct revascularization surgery: clinical and cinearteriographic studies in 67 selected patients. Am. Heart J. *89(5)*:561, 1975.

Levinson, D. C., Edmeades, D. T., and Griffith, G. C.: Dissecting aneurysm of aorta: its clinical, electrocardiographic and laboratory features: report of 38 autopsy cases. Circulation *1*:360, 1950.

Levy, A. M.: Hypertrophied adenoids causing pulmonary hypertension and severe congestive heart failure. N. Engl. J. Med. *277*:506, 1967.

Levy, M. J., Lillehei, C. W., Anderson, R. C., Amplatz, K., and Edwards, J. E.: Aortico-left ventricular tunnel. Circulation *27*:841, 1963.

Lew, E. A.: High blood pressure, other risk factors and longevity: the insurance viewpoint. Am. J. Med. *55*:281, 1973.

Lewis, F. J., Taufic, M., Varco, R. L., and Niazi, S.: The surgical anatomy of atrial septal defects: experiences with repair under direct vision. Ann. Surg. *142*:401, 1955.

Lewis, R. P., Bristow, J. D., and Griswold, H. E.: Radiographic heart size and left ventricular volume in aortic valve disease. Am. J. Cardiol. *27*:250, 1971.

Lie, J. T., Hunt, D., and Valentine, P. A.: Sudden death from cardiac sarcoidosis with involvement of conduction system. Am. J. Med. Sci. *267*:123, 1974.

Lieber, A. and Jorgens, J.: Cinefluorography of coronary artery calcification. Correlation with clinical arteriosclerotic heart disease and autopsy findings. Am. J. Roentgenol. *86*:1063, 1961.

Liebow, A. A., Moser, K. M., and Southgate, M. T.: Rapidly progressive dyspnea in a teenage boy. J.A.M.A. *223*:1243, 1973.

Liese, G. J., Brainard, S. C., and Goto, U: Giant blood cyst of the pulmonary valve. Report of a case. N. Engl. J. Med. *269*:465, 1963.

Lillehei, C. W., Cohen, M., Warden, H. E., Read, R. C., Aust, J. B., DeWall, R. A., and Varco, R. L.: Direct vision intracardiac surgical correction of the tetralogy of Fallot, pentalogy of Fallot, and pulmonary atresia defects—report of first ten cases. Ann. Surg. *142*:418, 1955.

Lillehei, C. W., and Gannon, P. G.: Ebstein's malformation of the tricuspid valve—method of surgical correction utilizing a ball-valve prosthesis and delayed closure of atrial septal defect. Circulation *31*:I-9, I-18, Supp. No. 1, 1965.

Lillehei, C. W., Levy, M. J., DeWall, R. A., and Warden, H. E.: Resection of myocardial aneurysms after infarction during temporary cardiopulmonary bypass. Circulation *26*:206, 1962.

Lim, J. S., Proudfit, W. L., and Sones, F. M.: Left main coronary arterial obstruction: long-term follow-up of 141 nonsurgical cases. Am. J. Cardiol. *36*:2:131, 1975.

Linbert, M. C. F. and Correll, H. L.: Rupture of pulmonary aneurysm accompanying patent ductus arteriosus. Occurrence in a 67 year old woman. J.A.M.A. *143*:888, 1950.

Lind, J. and Wegelius, C.: Atrial septal defects in children: an angiocardiographic study. Circulation *7*:819, 1953.

Lind, J.: Heart volume in normal infants: a roentgenological study. Acta Radiol. (Supp. #82), 1950.

Liljestrand, G., Lysholm, E., Nylin, G., and Zachrisson, C. G.: The normal heart volume in man. Am. Heart J. *17*:406, 1939.

Linde, L. M., Adams, F. H., and O'Loughlin, B. J.: Endocardial fibroelastosis (angiocardiographic studies). Circulation

17:40, 1958.

Lindgren, P.: Hemodynamic responses to contrast media. Invest. Rad. 5:424, 1970.

Lindskog, G. E., Liebow, A., Kausel, H., and Janzen, A.: Pulmonary arteriovenous aneurysms. Ann. Surg. 132:591, 1950.

Lipchik, E. O. and Robinson, K. E.: Acute traumatic rupture of the thoracic aorta. Am. J. Roentgenol. 104:408, 1968.

Lipton, M. J., Pfeifer, J. F., Lopes, M. J., and Hultgren, H. N.: Aneurysms of the coronary arteries in the adult: clinical and angiographic features. Radiology 117:11, 1975.

Little, J. B., Lavender, J. P., and De Sanctis, R. W.: Narrow infundibulum in pulmonary valvular stenosis: its preoperative diagnosis by angiocardiography. Circulation 28:182, 1963.

Livesay, W. R., Wagner, E. L., and Armburst, C. A. Jr.: Functional subaortic stenosis due to cardiomyopathy of unknown origin. Am. Heart J. 60:955, 1960.

Loehr, W. M.: Pericardial cysts. Am. J. Roentgenol. 68:584, 1952.

Longcope, W. T. and Freeman, D. G.: Study of sarcoidosis; based on combined investigations of 160 cases including 30 autopsies from Johns Hopkins Hospital and Massachusetts General Hospital. Medicine 31:1, 1952.

Lopez-Majano, V., Tow, D. E., and Wagner, H. N., Jr.: Regional distribution of pulmonary arterial blood flow in emphysema. J.A.M.A. 197:81, 1966.

Lucas, R. V. Jr., Adams, P., Jr., Anderson, R. C., Meyne, N. G., Lillehei, C. W., and Varco, R. L.: The natural history of isolated ventricular septal defect. A serial physiologic study. Circulation 24:1372, 1961.

Lucas, R. V., Jr. and Schmidt, R. E.: Cor Triatriatum. In Heart Disease In Infants, Children and Adolescents. Moss, A. J. and Adams, F. H. (eds.), pp 702–707. Baltimore, Williams & Wilkins Co., 1968.

Lucas, R. V. and Schmidt, R. E.: Anomalies Of The Systemic Venous System. In Heart Disease In Infants, Children and Adolescents, pp 713–727. Moss, A. J., and Adams, F. H. (eds.), Baltimore, Williams & Wilkins Co., 1968.

Lucas, R. V., Jr., Varco, R. L., Lillehei, C. W., Adams, P., Jr., Anderson, R. C., and Edwards, J. E.: Anomalous muscle bundle of the right ventricle. Hemodynamic consequences and surgical considerations. Circulation 25:443, 1962.

Lundquist, C. B., and Amplatz, K.: The subvalvular aortic jet. Radiology 85:635, 1965.

Lundquist, C. and Amplatz, K.: Anomalous origin of the left coronary artery from the pulmonary artery. Am. J. Roentgenol. 95:611, 1965.

Lundstrom: N.: Echocardiography in the diagnosis of Ebstein's anomaly of the tricuspid valve. Circulation 47:597, 1973.

Lynfield, J., Gasul, B. M., Luan, L. L., and Dillon, R. F.: Right and left heart catheterization and angiocardiographic findings in idiopathic cardiac hypertrophy with endocardial fibroelastosis. Circulation 21:386, 1960.

Macafee, C. A. J. and Patterson, G. C.: Congenital tricuspid atresia with transposition of the great vessels. Brit. Heart J. 23:308, 1961.

Macartney, F. J., Scott, O., Ionescu, I., and Deverall, P. B.: Diagnosis and management of parachute mitral valve and supravalvular mitral ring. Brit. Heart J. 36:641, 1973.

Maddison, F. E., Wright, R. R., and Tooley, W. H.: Chest radiography following unilateral pulmonary artery occlusion. An experimental study. Radiology 88:435, 1967.

Magovern, G. J., Kent, E. M., and Cromie, H. W.: Sutureless artificial heart valves. Circulation 27:784, 1963.

Maier, H. C.: Diverticulum of the pericardium with observations on mode of development. Circulation 16:1040, 1957.

Maier, H. C., Himmelstein, A., Riley, R. L., and Bunin, J. J.: Arteriovenous fistula of the lung. J. Thoracic Surg. 17:13, 1948.

Mair, D. D., Ritter, D. G., Davis, G. D., Wallace, R. B., Danielson, G. K., and McGoon, D. C.: Selection of patients with truncus arteriosus for surgical correction. Circulation 59:144, 1974.

Mair, D. D., Ritter, D. G. Ongley, P. A., and Helmholz, H. F.: Hemodynamics and evaluation for surgery of patients with complete transposition of the great arteries and ventricular septal defect. Am. J. Cardiol. 28:632, 1971.

Mallory, T. B.: Case records of the Massachusetts General Hospital. Case 22141 & 42. N. Engl. J. Med. 214:690, 1936.

Mann, M. R.: The pharmacology of contrast media. Proc. Roy. Soc. Med. 54:473, 1961.

Mannix, E. P. and Berroya, R. B.: Prosthetic replacement of the tricuspid valve for Ebstein's anomaly. J. Cardiovasc. Surg. 12:355, 1971.

Marchand, E. J., Marcial-Rojas, R. A., Rodriguez, R., Polanco, G., and Diaz-Rivera, R. S.: The pulmonary obstruction syndrome in schistosoma Mansoni pulmonary endarteritis: report of 5 cases. Arch. Internal Med. 100:965, 1957.

Margolis, G., Tindall, G. T., Phillips, R. L., Kenan, P. D., and Grimson, K. S.: Evaluation of roentgen contrast agents used in cerebral angiography. I. A simple screening method. J. Neurosurg. 15:30, 1958.

Margulis, A. R., Figley, M. M., and Stern, A. M.: Unusual roentgen manifestations of patent ductus arteriosus. Radiology 63:334, 1954.

Marin-Garcia, J., Tandon, R., Moller, J. H., and Edwards, J. E.: Common (single) ventricle with normally related great vessels. Circulation 49:565, 1974.

Marin-Garcia, J., Tandon, R., Moller, J. H., and Edwards, J. E.: Single ventricle with transposition. Circulation 49:994, 1974.

Marin-Garcia, J., Tandon, R., Lucas, R. V., and Edwards, J. E.: Cor triatriatum: study of 20 cases. Am. J. Cardiol. 35:59, 1975.

Marquis, R. M.: Ventricular septal defect in early childhood. Brit. Heart J. 12:265, 1950.

Marquis, Y., Richardson, J. B., Ritchie, A. C., and Wigle, E. D.: Idiopathic medial aortopathy and arteriopathy. Am. J. Med. 44:939, 1968.

Marr, K., Giargiana, F. A., Jr., and White, R. I., Jr.: The radiographic diagnosis of pulmonary hypertension following Blalock-Taussig shunts in patients with tetralogy of fallot. Am. J. Roentgenol. 122(1):125, 1974.

Marshall, R.: The physiology and pharmacology of the pulmonary circulation. Prog. Cardiovasc. Dis. 1:341, 1959.

Marshall, W. H., Steiner, R. M., and Wexler, L.: "Tumor vascularity" in left atrial myxoma. Radiology 93:815, 1969.

Martin, R. G., Ruckdeschel, J. C., Chang, P., Byhart, R., Bouchard, R. J., and Wiernik, P. H.: Radiation-related pericarditis. Am. J. Cardiol. 35:216, 1975.

Mascarenhas, E., Javier, R. P., and Samet, P.: Partial anomalous pulmonary venous connection and drainage. Am. J. Cardiol. 31:512, 1973.

Mattingly, T. W.: Clinical features and diagnosis of primary myocardial disease (II). Mod. Concepts Cardiovasc. Dis. 30:683, 1961.

Mauer, B. J., Oberman, A., Holt, J. H., Kouchoukos, N. T., Jones, W. B., Russell, R. O., and Reeves, T. J.: Changes in grafted and nongrafted coronary arteries following saphenous vein bypass grafting. Circulation 50:293, 1974.

Maurer, E. R. and Mendez, F. L., Jr.: Diagnostic pneumopericardium: its clinical application. Dis. Chest 37:13, 1960.

Marvel, R. J. and Genovese, P. D.: Cardiovascular disease in Marfan's syndrome. Am. Heart J. 42:814, 1951.

McAfee, J. G.: A survey of complications of abdominal aortography. Radiology 68:825, 1957.

McAfee, J. G. and Biondetti, P.: Roentgenologic follow-up on 150 consecutive mitral commissurotomy patients. Am. J. Roentgenol. 78:213, 1957.

McAlister, W. H. and Blatt, E.: Calcified pulmonary artery thrombus. Am. J. Roentgenol. 87:908, 1962.

McAlpine, W. A.: Heart and Coronary Arteries. Springer-Verlag, New York, 1975.

McCabe, J. C., Engle, M. A., and Ebert, P. A.: Chronic pericardial effusion requiring pericardiectomy in the post-pericardiotomy syndrome. J. Thoracic Cardiovasc. Surg. 67:814, 1974.

McCartney, R. L.: Hemorrhage following percutaneous lung biopsy. Radiology 112:305, 1974.

McCleod, C. A., Schwarz, H., and Linton, D. B.: Constrictive pericarditis following irradiation therapy. J.A.M.A. 207:2281, 1969.

McConnell, T. H.: Bony and cartilaginous tumors of the heart and great vessels. Cancer 25:611, 1970.

McClure, C. W. F. and Butler, E. G.: The development of the vena cava inferior in man. Am. J. Anat. 35:331, 1925.

McCue, C. M., et al.: Persistent truncus arteriosus: clinical correlation with the pathological anatomy. Dis. Chest 46:507, 1964.

McDonald, I.G.: The shape and movements of the human left ventricle during systole. Am. J. Cardiol. 26:221, 1970.

McGoon, D. C., McMullan, M. H., Mair, D. D., and Danielson, G. K.: Correction of complete atrioventricular canal in infants. Mayo Clin. Proc. 48:769, 1973.

McGoon, D. C., Rastelli, G. C., and Ongley, P. A.: An operation for the correction of truncus arteriosus. J.A.M.A. 205:59, 1968.

McGuire, J., Schneider, H. J., and Chore, T.: Clinical significance of coronary artery calcification seen fluoroscopically with the image intensifier. Circulation 37:82, 1968.

McHugh, T. J., Forrester, J. S., Adler, L., Zion, D., and Swan, H. J.: Pulmonary vascular congestion in acute myocardial infarction: hemodynamic and radiologic correlations. Ann. Int. Med. 76:29, 1972.

McKusick, V. A.: Chronic constrictive pericarditis. I. Some clinical and laboratory observations. Bull. Johns Hopkins Hosp. 90:3, 1952.

McKusick, V. A.: Chronic constrictive pericarditis. II. Electrokymographic studies and correlations with roentgenkymography, phonokymography, and right ventricular pressure curves, Bull. Johns Hopkins Hosp. 90:27, 1952.

McKusick, V. A.: The cardiovascular aspects of Marfan's syndrome: a heritable disorder of connective tissue. Circulation 11:321, 1955.

McKusick, V. A. and Cochran, T. H.: Constrictive endocarditis. Report of a case. Bull. Johns Hopkins Hosp. 90:90, 1952.

McKusick, V. A.: Heritable Disorders of Connective Tissue, ed. 4, St. Louis, C. V. Mosby Co., 1972.

McKusick, V. A. and Cooley, R. N.: Drainage of right pulmonary vein into inferior vena cava—report of a case with a radiologic analysis of the principal types of anomalous venous return from the lung. N. Engl. J. Med. 252:426, 1955.

McKusick, V. A., Logue, R. B., and Bahnson, H. T.: Association of aortic valvular disease and cystic medial necrosis of the ascending aorta. Report of 4 instances. Circulation 16:188, 1957.

McMullan, M. H., McGoon, D. C., Wallace, R. B., Danielson, G. K., and Weidman, W. H.: Surgical treatment of partial atrioventricular canal. Arch. Surg. 107:705, 1973.

McMyn, J. K.: Radiological appearances of pulmonary hypertension. J. Coll. Radiol. Australasia 4:21, 1960.

McNamara, D. G. and Sommerville, R. J.: Aortic-pulmonary window. In Heart Disease in Infants, Children and Adolescents, Moss, A. J., and Adams, F. H. (eds.) Baltimore, Williams & Wilkins Co., 1968.

McWhorter, J. E. and LeRoy, E. C.: Pericardial disease in scleroderma (systemic sclerosis). Am. J. Med. 57:566, 1974.

Meadows, W. R. and Sharp, J. T.: Persistent left superior vena cava draining into the left atrium without arterial oxygen unsaturation. Am. J. Cardiol. 16:273, 1965.

Meckel, J. F.: Verschliessung der aorta am vierten Brustwirbel. Arch. Anat. u. Physiol. 345–354 (Table V; Fig. 1), 1827.

Mehrizi, A. and Taussig, H. B.: Acyanotic transposition of the great vessels. Circulation 20:740, 1959.

Mellins, H. Z., Kottmeier, T., and Kiely, B.: Radiologic signs of pericardial effusion; an experimental study. Radiology 73:9, 1959.

Mengel, C. E.: Carcinoid and the heart. Mod. Concepts Cardiovasc. Dis. 35:75, 1966.

Menges, H., Jr., Brandenburg, R. O., and Brown, A. L., Jr.: Clinical, hemodynamic and pathologic diagnosis of muscular subvalvular aortic stenosis. Circulation 24:1126, 1961.

Mesko, Z. G., Jones, J. E., and Nadas, A. S.: Diminution and closure of large ventricular septal defects after pulmonary artery banding. Circulation 48(1):847, 1973.

Meszaros, W. T.: Cardiac Roentgenology, pp. 506–513. Springfield, Ill., Charles C Thomas, 1969.

Meyers, G. S., Scannell, J. G., Wyman, S. M., Dimond, E. G., and Hurst, J. W.: Atypical patent ductus arteriosus with absence of the usual aortic pulmonary pressure gradient and the characteristic murmur. Am. Heart J. 41:819, 1951.

Meyers, R. A. and Kaplan, S.: Echocardiography in the diagnosis of hypoplasia of the left or right ventricle in the neonate. Circulation 46:55, 1972.

Miller, G. A. H., Ongley, P. A., Anderson, M. W., Kincaid, O. W., and Swan, H. J. C.: Cor triatriatum: hemodynamic and angiocardiographic diagnosis. Am. Heart J. 68:298, 1964.

Miller, R. A., Lev, M., and Paul, M. H.: Congenital absence of pulmonary valve: clinical syndrome of tetralogy of Fallot with pulmonary regurgitation. Circulation 26:266, 1962.

Milne, E. N. C.: Physiological interpretation of the plain radiograph in mitral stenosis, including a review of criteria for the radiological estimation of pulmonary arterial and venous pressure. Brit. J. Radiol. 36:902, 1963.

Mirowski, M., Mehrizi, A., and Shah, K. D.: Right ventricular aneurysm: a complication of transventricular pulmonary valvulotomy. Am. Heart J. 68:799, 1964.

Mirowski, M., Shah, K. D., Neill, C. A., and Taussig, H. B.: Long term (10 to 13 years) follow up study after transventricular pulmonary valvulotomy for pulmonary stenosis with intact ventricular septum. Circulation 28:906, 1963.

Mitchell, G.: Calcified mitral stenosis and mitral valvotomy. Brit. J. Med. 1:687, 1960.

Moller, J. H. and Edwards, J. E.: Interruption of aortic arch. Anatomic patterns and associated cardiac malformations. Am. J. Roentgenol. 95:557, 1965.

Molnar, W. and Pace, W. G.: Traumatic rupture of the thoracic aorta. Radiol. Clin. N.A. 4:403, 1966.

Moniz, E., DeCarvalho, L., and Lima, A.: Angiopneumographie. Presse Med. 39:996, 1931.

Morales, R. A., Garcia, F., Grover, F. L., and Trinkle, J. K.: Aneurysm of the left ventricle after repair of a penetrating injury. J. Thoracic Cardiovasc. Surg. 66:632, 1973.

Moraski, R. E. and Bousnaios, G.: Constrictive pericarditis due to chronic uremia. N. Engl. J. Med. 281:542, 1969.

Morettin, L. B. and Wallace, J. M.: Uneventful perforation of a coronary artery during selective arteriography. A case report. Am. J. Roentgol. 110:184, 1970.

Moore, C. B., Kraus, W. L., Dock, D. S., Woodward, D. E., and Dexter, L.: The relationship between pulmonary arterial pressure and roentgenographic appearance in mitral stenosis. Am. Heart J. 58:576, 1959.

Morgan, J. R., Forker, A. D., Fosburg, R. G., Neugebauer, M. K., Rogers, A. K., and Bemiller, C. R.: Interruption of the aortic arch without a patent ductus arteriosus. Circulation 42:961, 1970.

Morgan, J. R., Rogers, A. K., and Fosbus, R. G.: Ruptured aneurysms of sinus of Valsalva. Chest 61:640, 1972.

Morrow, A. G., Baker, R. R., Hanson, H. E., and Mattingly, T. W.: Successful surgical repair of a ruptured aneurysm of the sinus of Valsalva. Circulation 16:533, 1957.

Morrow, A. G., Greenfield, L. J., and Braunwald, E.: Congenital aortopulmonary septal defect: clinical and hemodynamic findings, surgical technic, and results of operative correction. Circulation 25:463, 1962.

Morrow, A. G., Lambrew, C. T., and Braunwald, E.: Idiopathic hypertrophic subaortic stenosis. II. Operative treatment and the results of pre- and postoperative hemodynamic evaluations. Circulation 30 (Suppl. #4), 1964.

Morrow, A. G., Sharp, E. H., and Braunwald, E.: Congenital aortic stenosis. Circulation 18:1091, 1958.

Morrow, A. G., Waldhausen, J. A., Peters, R. L., Bloodwell, R. D., and Braunwald, E.: Supravalvular aortic stenosis—clinical, hemodynamic and pathologic observations. Circulation 20:1003, 1959.

Moss, A. J.: Conquest of the ventricular septal defect—a period of uncertainty. Am. J. Cardiol. 25:457, 1970.

Moss, A. J. and Siassi, B.: The small atrial septal defect—operate or procrastinate? J. Pediat. 79:854, 1971.

Motley, H. L., Cournand, A., Werko, L., Himmelstein, A., and Dresdale, D.: The influence of short periods of induced acute anoxia upon pulmonary artery pressures in man. Am. J. Physiol. 150:315, 1947.

Moyer, J. H. and Ackerman, A. J.: Hereditary hemorrhagic telangiectases associated with pulmonary arteriovenous fistula in two members of a family. Ann. Internal Med. 29:775, 1948.

Moyer, J. H., Glantz, G., and Brest, A. N.: Pulmonary arteriovenous fistulas: physiologic and clinical considerations. Am. J. Med. 32:417, 1962.

Mudd, J. G., Willman, V. L., and Riberi, A.: Origin of one pulmonary artery from the aorta. Am. Rev. Resp. Dis. 89:255, 1964.

Muller, W. H., Littlefield, J. B., and Beckwith, J. R.: Surgical treatment of Lutembacher's syndrome. J. Thoracic Cardiovasc. Surg. 51:66, 1966.

Mundth, E. D., Buckley, M. J., Daggett, W. M., Sanders, C. A., and Austen, W. G.: Surgery for complications of acute myocardial infarction. Circulation 45:1279, 1972.

Murdoch, J. L., Walker, B. A., Halpern, B. L., Kuzma, J. W., and McKusick, V. A.: Life expectancy and causes of death in the Marfan syndrome. N. Engl. J. Med. 286:804, 1972.

Muroff, L. R. and Freedman, G. S.: Radionuclide angiography. Sem. Nuc. Med. 2:217, 1976.

Murphy, D. A. Collins, G., and Dobell, A. R. C.: Surgical correction of type A congenital aortic arch interruption. Ann. Thoracic Surg. 11:593, 1971.

Murray, J. A.: Quantitative angiocardiography. II. Normal left atrial volume in man. Circulation 37:800, 1968.

Mustard, W. T.: Successful two-stage correction of transposition of the great vessels. Surgery 55:469, 1964.

Muster, A. J., Paul, M. H., and Nikaidoh, H.: Tetralogy of Fallot associated with total anomalous pulmonary venous drainage. Chest 64;323, 1973.

Nadas, A. S.: Pulmonic stenosis: indications for surgery in children and adults. N. Engl. J. Med. 287:1196, 1972.

Nadas, A. S. and Alimurung, M. M.: Apical diastolic murmurs in congenital heart disease. Am. Heart J. 43:69, 1952.

Nadas, A. S. and Ellison, R. C.: Cardiac tumors in infancy. Am. J. Cardiol. 21:363, 1968.

Nadas, A. S. and Eyler, D. C.: Pediatric Cardiology, ed. 3, pp. 438–443. Philadelphia, W. B. Saunders Co., 1972.

Nadas, A. S., Gamboa, R., and Hugenholtz, P. G.: Anomalous left coronary artery originating from the pulmonary artery: report of two surgically treated cases with a proposal of hemodynamic and therapeutic classification. Circulation 29:167, 1964.

Nadas, A. S., Rosenbaum, H. D., Wittenborg, M. H., and Rudolph, A. M.: Tetralogy of Fallot with unilateral pulmonary atresia; a clinically diagnosable and surgically significant variant. Circulation 8:328, 1953.

Nadas, A. S., Scott, L. P., Hauck, A. J., and Rudolph, A. M.: Spontaneous functional closing of ventricular septal defects. N. Engl. J. Med. 264:309, 1961.

Nadas, A. S., Thilenius, O. G., LaFarge, C. G., and Hauck, A. J.: Ventricular septal defect with aortic regurgitation: medical and pathologic aspects. Circulation 29:862, 1964.

Nadas, A. S., Van der Hauwaert, L., Hauck, A. J., and Gross, R. E.: Combined aortic and pulmonic stenosis. Circulation 25:346, 1962.

Nadel, J. A., Colebatch, J. H., and Olsen, C. R.: Location and mechanism of airway constriction after barium sulfate microembolism. J. Appl. Physiol. 19:387, 1964.

Naeim, F., De La Maza, L., and Robbins, S. L.: Cardiac rupture during myocardial infarction. Circulation 45:1231, 1972.

Nagao, G. I., Daoud, G. K., McAdams, A. J., Schwartz, D. C., and Kaplan, S.: Cardiovascular anomalies associated with tetralogy of Fallot. Am. J. Cardiol. 20:206, 1967.

Nahon, J. R.: Roentgenologic characteristics of the epipericardial fat pad, with a case report. Radiology 65:745, 1955.

Nakao, K., Ikeda, M., Kimata, S., Niitani, S., Miyahara, M., Ishimi, Z., Hashiba, K., Takeda, Y., Ozawa, T., Matsushita, S., and Kuramochi, M.: Takayasu's arteritis: clinical report of eighty-four cases and immunological studies of seven cases. Circulation 35:1141, 1967.

Nakib, A., Moller, J. H., Kanjuh, V. T., and Edwards, J. E.: Anomalies of the pulmonary veins. Am. J. Cardiol. 20:77, 1967.

Nasrallah, A. T., Cooley, D. A., Goussous, Y., Hallman, G., Lufschanowski, R., and Leachman, R. D.: Surgical experience in patients with Marfan's syndrome, ascending aortic aneurysm and aortic regurgitation. Am. J. Cardiol. 36:338, 1975.

Nathan, D. A., Center, S., Pina, R. E., Medow, A., and Keller, W., Jr.: Perforation during indwelling catheter pacing. Circulation 33:128, 1966.

Nathan, M.: Strut fracture: a late complication of Beall mitral valve replacement. Ann. Thoracic Surg. 16:610, 1973.

Neal, W. M., Bessinger, F. B., Jr., and Hunt, C. E.: Patent ductus arteriosus complicating respiratory distress syndrome. J. Pediat. 86:127, 1975.

Neches, W. H., Park, S. C., Lenox, C. C., Zuberbuhler, J. R., and Bahnson, H. T.: Tricuspid atresia with transposition of the great arteries and closing ventricular septal defect. Successful palliation by banding of the pulmonary artery and creation of an aorticopulmonary window. J. Thoracic Cardiovasc. Surg. 65:538, 1973.

Neill, C. A., Ferencz, C., Sabiston, D. C., and Sheldon, H.: The familial occurrence of hypoplastic right lung with systemic arterial supply and venous drainage. "Scimitar syndrome." Bull. Johns Hopkins Hosp. 107:1, 1960.

Neufeld, H. N., DuShane, J. W., Wood, E. H., Kirklin, J. W., and Edwards, J. E.: Origin of both great vessels from the right ventricle. I. Without pulmonary stenosis. Circulation 23:399, 1961.

Neufeld, H. N., DuShane, J. W., and Edwards, J. E.: Origin of both great vessels from the right ventricle. II. With pulmonary stenosis. Circulation 23:603, 1961.

Neufeld, H. N., Lester, R. G., Adams, P., Anderson, R. C., Lillehei, C. W., and Edwards, J. E.: Congenital communication of a coronary artery with a cardiac chamber or the pulmonary trunk ("coronary artery fistula"). Circulation 24:171, 1961.

Neufeld, H. N., Lester, R. G., Adams, P., Anderson, R. C., Lillehei, C. W., and Edwards, J. E.: Aorticopulmonary septal defect. Am. J. Cardiol. 9:12, 1962.

Neufeld, H. N., Lucas, R. V., Jr., Lester, R. G., Adams, P., Jr., Anderson, R. C., and Edwards, J. E.: Origin of both great vessels from the right venticle without pulmonary stenosis. Brit. Heart J. 24:393, 1962.

Neufeld, H. N., McGoon, B. C., DuShane, J. W., and Edwards, J. E.: Tetralogy of Fallot with anomalous tricuspid valve simulating pulmonary stenosis with intact septum. Circulation 22:1083, 1960.

Neufeld, H. N., Ongley, P. A., and Edwards, J. E.: Combined congenital subaortic stenosis and infundibular pulmonary stenosis. Brit. Heart J. 22:686, 1960.

Neuhauser, E. B. D.: Roentgen diagnosis of double aortic arch and other anomalies of the great vessels. Am. J. Roentgenol. 56:1, 1946.

Newcombe, C. P., Ongley, P. A., Edwards, J. E., and Wood, E. H.: Clinical, pathologic and hemodynamic considerations in coarctation of the aorta associated with ventricular septal defect. Circulation 24:1356, 1961.

Newman, M. M., Hoffman, M. S., and Gesink, M. H.: Mechanical failure of Starr-Edwards aortic prosthesis due to ball fracture. J. Thoracic Cardiovasc. Surg. 53:398, 1967.

Newton, T. H. and Preger, L.: Selective bronchial arteriography. Radiology 84:1043, 1966.

Nghiem, Q. X., Schreiber, M. H., and Harris, L. C.: Cardiac volume in normal children and adolescents. Circulation 35:509, 1967.

Ngheim, Q. X., Toledo, J., Schreiber, M. H., Harris, L. C., Lockhart, L. L., and Tyson, K. R. T.: Congenital idiopathic hypertrophic subaortic stenosis associated with a phenotypic Turner's syndrome. Am. J. Cardiol. 30:683, 1972.

Nickey, W. A., Chinitz, J. L., Flynn, J. J., Adam, A., Kim, K. E., Schwartz, A. B., Onesti, G., and Swartz, C. D.: Surgical correction of uremic constrictive pericarditis. Ann. Int. Med. 75:227, 1971.

Nicoloff, D. M., Zamora, R., Castaneda, A. R., Moller, J. H., Hunt, C. E., and Lucas, R. V.: Transatrial closure of high pressure, high resistance ventricular septal defects. J. Pediat. Surg. 6:650, 1971.

Nielsen, P. B.: Intralobar bronchopulmonary sequestration: review of the literature and report of 2 cases. Am. J. Roentgenol. 92:547, 1964.

Niwayama, G.: Cor triatriatum. Am. Heart J. 59:291, 1960.

Nonkin, P. M., Dick, M. M., and Baum, G. L.: Myocardial infarction in respiratory insufficiency. Arch. Int. Med. 113:92, 1964.

Noonan, C. D., Margulis, A. R., and Wright, R.: Bronchial arterial patterns in pulmonary metastasis. Radiology 84:1033, 1965.

Noonan, J. A.: Hypoplastic left ventricle. In Heart Disease in Infants, Children and Adolescents, Chap. 31, pp. 660–671, Moss, A. J., and Adams, F. H. (eds.). Baltimore, The Williams & Wilkins Co., 1968.

Noonan, J. A. and Nadas, A. S.: Hypoplastic left heart syndrome. Pediat. Clin. N.A. 5:1029, 1958.

Noonan, J. A., Nadas, A. S., Rudolph, A. M., and Harris, G. B. C.: Transposition of the great arteries. N. Engl. J. Med. 263:592, 637, 684, 739, 1960.

Nordenstrom, B. and Ovenfors, C. O.: Septal defect between the left ventricle and right atrium, diagnosed by cineangiography. Acta Radiol. 54:393, 1960.

Nordenstrom, B. and Ovenfors, C. R.: Low subvalvular aortic and pulmonic stenosis with hypertrophy and abnormal arrangement of the muscle bundles of the myocardium. Acta Radiol. 57:321, 1962.

Nuvoli, I.: Arteriografia dell'aorta toracica mediante puntura dell'aorta ascendente o del ventricolo S. Policlinico Sez. Prat., 227–237, 1936. Abstracted in Zentralblatt Gesamte Radiol. 22:382, 1936.

OBrien, K. P., Hitchcock, G. C., Barratt-Boyes, B. G., and Love, J. B.: Spontaneous aortic cusp rupture associated with valvular myxomatous transformation. Circulation 37:273, 1968.

Oderr, C. P., Pizzolato, P., and Ziskind, J.: Emphysema studied by microradiology. Radiology 71:236, 1958.

Ödman, P.: The appearance of the internal mammary arteries in coarctation of the aorta. Acta Radiol. 39:47, 1953.

Ödman, R., and Philipson, J.: Aortic valvular diseases studied by percutaneous thoracic aortography. Acta Radiol. (Supp. #172), 1958.

O'Donovan, T. G., Schrire, V., and Barnard, C. N.: Surgical closure of ventricular septal defect in infancy. South African Med. J. 46:883, 1972.

Ogden, J. A.: Congenital anomalies of the coronary arteries. Am. J. Cardiol. 25:474, 1970.

Oh, W. M. C., Taylor, R. P., and Olsen, E. G. J.: Aortic regurgitation in systemic lupus erythematosus requiring aortic valve replacement. Brit. Heart J. 36:413, 1974.

Oliver, C. G., and Messen, G. A. K.: A heavily calcified right atrial myxoma. Guy's Hosp. Reports 115:37, 1961.

Oliver, M. F., Samuel, E., Morley, P., Young, G. B., and Kapur, P. L.: Detection of coronary artery calcification during life. Lancet 1:891, 1964.

Olsson, O.: Antihistaminic drugs for inhibiting untoward reactions of injections to contrast medium. Acta Radiol. 35:65, 1951.

Ongley, P. A., Titus, J. L., Khoury, G. H., Rahinetoola, S. H., Marshall, H. J., and Edwards, J. E.: Anomalous connection of pulmonary veins to right atrium associated with anomalous inferior vena cava, situs inversus and multiple spleens—a developmental complex. Mayo Clinic Proc. 40:609, 1965.

O'Rielly, J. R. and Grollman, J. H., Jr.: The lateral chest film as an unreliable indicator of azygos continuation of the inferior vena cava. Circulation 53:891, 1976.

Osler, W.: The Gulstonian lectures. Lecture I. Malignant Endocarditis. Br. Med. J. 1:467, 1885.

Osler, W. and McCrae, T.: Modern Medicine: Its Theory and Practice, vol. 4, Philadelphia, Lea & Febiger, 1908.

Otto, J. F., Hutcheson, J. M., Jr., Abelman, W. H., Harken, D. E., Gary, J. E., and Ellis, L. B.: Clinical observations before and after mitral valvuloplasty. N. Engl. J. Med. 253:995, 1955.

Ovitt, T. W., Durst, S., Moore, R., and Amplatz, K.: Guide wire thrombogenicity and its reduction. Radiology 111:43, 1974.

Pacifico, A. D., Kirklin, J. W., Bargeron, L. M., Jr., and Soto, B.: Surgical treatment of common arterial trunk with pseudotruncus arteriosus. Circulation 50(2):20 (Suppl #2), 1974.

Packard, G. B. and Waring, J. J.: Arteriovenous fistula of lung treated by ligation of pulmonary artery. Arch. Surg. 56:725, 1948.

Pacofsky, K. B. and Wolfel, D. A.: Azygos continuation of the inferior vena cava. Am. J. Roentgenol. 113:362, 1971.

Pansegrau, D. G., Kioshos, J. M., Durnin, R. E., and Kroetz, F. W.: Supravalvular aortic stenosis in adults. Am. J. Cardiol. 31:635, 1973.

Pappenheimer, M. A. and Von Glahn, C. W.: Lesions of the aorta associated with acute rheumatic fever, and with chronic cardiac disease of rheumatic origin. J. Med. Res. 44:489, 1924.

Paraskos, J. A., Adelstein, S. J., Smith, R. E., Rickman, F. D., Grossman, W., Dexter, L., and Dalen, J. E.: Late prognosis of acute pulmonary embolism. N. Engl. J. Med. 289:55, 1973.

Pariser, S., Zuckner, J., Taylor, H. K., and Messinger, W. J.:

Mitral stenosis without clinically demonstrable left auricular enlargement. Am. J. Med. Sci. 221:431, 1951.

Parker, F., Jr. and Weiss, S.: The nature and significance of the structural changes in the lungs in mitral stenosis. Am. J. Pathol. 12:573, 1936.

Parkey, R. W., Bonte, F. J., Meyer, S. L., Atkins, J. M., Curry, G. L., Stokely, E. M., and Willerson, J. T.: A new method for radionuclide imaging of acute mycardial infarction in humans. Circulation 50:540–46, 1974.

Parkhurst, G. F. and Decker, J. P.: Bacterial aortitis and mycotic aneurysm of aorta. Am. J. Pathol. 31:821, 1955.

Parmley, L. F., Manion, W. C., and Mattingly, T. W.: Nonpenetrating traumatic injury of the heart. Circulation 18:371, 1958.

Parmley, L. F., Mattingly, T. W., Manion, W. C., and Jahnke, E. J., Jr.: Non-penetrating traumatic injury of the aorta. Circulation 17:1086, 1958.

Parsonnet, V., Gilbert, L., and Zucker, I. R.: The natural history of pacemaker wires. J. Thoracic Cardiovasc. Surg. 65:315, 1973.

Pastor, B. H. and Cahn, M.: Reversible nephrotic syndrome resulting from constrictive pericarditis. N. Engl. J. Med. 262:872, 1960.

Patel, R. G., Ihenacho, H. N. C., Abrams, L. D., Astley, R., Parsons, C. G., Roberts, K. D., and Singh, S. P.: Pulmonary-artery banding and subsequent repair in ventricular septal defect. Brit. Heart J. 35:651, 1973.

Pattinson, J. N. and Grainger, R. G.: Congenital kinking of the aortic arch. Brit. Heart J. 21:555, 1959.

Paul, M. H., Van Praagh, S., and Van Praagh, R.: Transposition of the great arteries, In Pediatric Cardiology, Watson, H. (ed.), p. 576. St. Louis, C. V. Mosby Company, 1968.

Paul, O., Castleman, B., and White, P. D.: Chronic constrictive pericarditis: a study of 53 cases. Am. J. Med. Sci. 216:361, 1948.

Paul, R. E., Dusant, T. M., Oppenheimer, M. J., and Stauffer, H. M.: Intravenous carbon dioxide for intracardiac gas contrast in the roentgen diagnosis of pericardial effusion and thickening. Am. J. Roentgenol 78:224, 1957.

Paul, R. N.: A new anomaly of the aorta: left aortic arch with right descending aorta. J. Pediat. 32:19, 1948.

Paulus, H. E., Pearson, C. M., and Pitts, W.: Aortic insufficiency in 5 patients with Reiter's syndrome. Am. J. Med. 53:464, 1972.

Payvandi, M. N. and Kerber, R. E.: Echocardiography in congenital and acquired absence of the pericardium. An echocardiographic mimic of right ventricular volume overload. Circulation 53:86, 1976.

Pearson, C. M., Kline, H. M., and Newcomer, V. D.: Relapsing polychondritis. N. Engl. J. Med. 263:51, 1960.

Peirce, E. C., II: Percutaneous femoral artery catheterization in man with special reference to aortography. Surg. Gynecol. Obstet. 93:56, 1951.

Peirce, E. C., II, and Ramey, W. P.: Renal arteriography: report of percutaneous methods using femoral artery approach and disposable catheters. J. Urol. 69:578, 1953.

Pendergrass, E. P., Hodes, P. J., Tondreau, R. L., Powell, C. C., and Burdick, E. D.: Further consideration of deaths and unfavorable sequelae following the administration of contrast media in urography in the United States. Am. J. Roentgenol. 74:262, 1955.

Pendergrass, H. P., Tondreau, R. L., Pendergrass, E. P., Ritchie, D. J., Hildreth, E. A., and Askovitz, S. I.: Reactions associated with intravenous urography: historical and statistical review. Radiology 71:1, 1958.

Perry, E. L., Burchell, H. B., and Edwards, J. E.: Congenital communication between the left ventricle and the right atrium: co-existing ventricular septal defect and double tricuspid orifice. Proc. Staff Meet. Mayo Clin. 24:198, 1949.

Perry, T. M.: Brucellosis and heart disease. IV. Etiology of calcific aortic stenosis. J.A.M.A. 166:1123, 1958.

Pfeifer, J., Goldschlager, N., Sweatman, T., Gerbode, F., and Selzer, A.: Malfunction of mitral ball valve prosthesis due to thrombus: report of 2 cases with notes on early clinical diagnosis. Am. J. Cardiol. 29:95, 1972.

Phillips, J. H., Jr., Burch, G. E., and Hellinger, R.: The use of intracardiac carbon dioxide in the diagnosis of pericardial disease. Am. Heart J.61:748, 1961.

Pichard, A.: Coronary Arteriography for everyone? Am. J. Cardiol. 38:533, 1976.

Pieroni, D. R., Strife, J. L., Donahoo, J. S., and Krovetz, L. J.: Postoperative assessment of residual defects following cardiac surgery in infants and children. III. Atrial septal defects. Johns Hopkins Med. J. 133:287, 1973.

Pillsbury, R. C., Lower, R. R., and Shumway, N. E.: Atresia of aortic arch. Circulation 30:749, 1964.

Pinet, F., Michaud, P., Amiel, M., Chassignole, J., Rubet, A., Dalloz, C., Froment, J. C., and Kadi, A.: Aortography of traumatic aneurysms of the thoracic aorta: a study of 10 cases. Ann. Radiol. 16:11, 1973.

Piwnica, A. H., Chetochine, F., Soyer, R., and Winckler, C.: Traumatic rupture of the aortic arch with disinsertion of the innominate artery. Report of a case with successful treatment. J. Thoracic Cardiovasc. Surg. 61:246, 1961.

Plaeith, W. H., Jr., Waldmann, T. A., Wackner, R. A., Braunwald, N., and Braunwald, E.: Protein-losing enteropathy secondary to constricting pericarditis in children. Pediatrics 34:636, 1964.

Platia, E., Griffith, L., and Humphries, O. J.: Location and severity of coronary artery narrowings as predictors of survival. Circulation (Supp. II) 51 and 52: 1975.

Pocock, W. A. and Barlow, J. B.: Etiology and electrocardiographic features of the billowing posterior mitral leaflet syndrome. Analysis of a further 130 patients with a late systolic murmur or nonejection systolic click. Am. J. Med. 51:731, 1971.

Poe, N. D., Dore, E. K., Swanson, L. A., and Taplin, G. V.: Fatal pulmonary embolism. J. Nucl. Med. 10:28, 1969.

Pomerance, A.: Ballooning deformity (mucoid degeneration) of atrioventricular valves. Brit. Heart J. 31:343, 1969.

Ponsdomenech, E. R. and Nunez, V. B.: Heart puncture in man for Diodrast visualization of the ventricular chambers and great arteries. I. Its experimental and anatomophysiological basis and technique. Am. Heart J. 41:643, 1951.

Pool, P. E., Vogel, J. H. K., and Blount, S. G., Jr.: Congenital unilateral absence of pulmonary artery: importance of flow in pulmonary hypertension. Am. J. Cardiol. 10:706, 1962.

Popp, R. L. and Harrison D. C.: Ultrasound for the diagnosis of atrial tumor. Ann. Int. Med. 71:785, 1969.

Porter, G. H.: Sarcoid heart disease. N. Engl. J. Med. 263:1350, 1960.

Potts, W. J., Holinger, P. H., and Rosenblum, A. H.: Anomalous left pulmonary artery causing obstruction to right main bronchus: report of a case. J.A.M.A. 155:1409, 1954.

Potts, W. J., Smith, S., and Gibson, S.: Anastomosis of the aorta to a pulmonary artery for certain types of congenital heart disease. J.A.M.A. 132:627, 1946.

Prado, S., Levy, M., and Varco, R.: Successful replacement of "parachute" mitral valve in a child. Circulation 32:130, 1965.

Price, A. C., Lee, D. A., Kagan, K. E., and Baker, W. P.: Aortic dysplasia in infancy simulating anomalous origin of the left coronary artery. Circulation 48:434, 1973.

Price, J. D., Isabel, J., Muldr, D. G., and Gyepes, M. T.: The radiographic diagnosis of complications of the Mustard procedure. Am. J. Roentgenol. 112:52, 1971.

Prichard, R. W.: Tumors of the heart: review of the subject and report of one hundred and fifty cases. Arch. Pathol.

51:98, 1951.

Prioton, J. B., Thevenet, A., Pelissier, M., Puech, P., Latour, H., and Pourquier, J.: Cardiographie ventriculaire gauche par catheterisme retrograde percutane femoral: technique et premiers resultats. Presse Med. *65*:1948, 1957.

Proudfit, W. L., Shirey, E. K., and Sones, F. M., Jr.: Distribution of arterial lesions demonstrated by selective cinecoronary arteriography. Circulation *36*:54, 1967.

Pryce, D. M., Sellors, T. H., and Blair, L. B.: Intralobar sequestration of lung associated with an abnormal pulmonary artery. Brit. J. Surg. *35*:18, 1947–48.

Radner, S.: An attempt at the roentgenologic visualization of the coronary blood vessels in man. Acta Radiol. *26*:497, 1945.

Radner, S.: Thoracal aortography by catheterization from the radial artery. Acta Radiol. *29*:178, 1948.

Railsback, O. C. and Dock, W.: Erosion of the ribs due to stenosis of the isthmus (coarctation of the aorta). Radiology *12*:58, 1929.

Randall, P. A., Goodman, D. J., and Schroeder, J. S.: Left ventricular angiographic anatomy of ostium primum defect in the adult. Am. J. Roentgenol. *121*:597, 1974.

Ranganathan, N., Lam, J. H. C., and Wigle, E. D.: Morphology of the human mitral valve. II. The valve leaflets. Circulation *41*:459, 1970.

Ranniger, K. and Valvassori, G. E.: Angiographic diagnosis of intralobar pulmonary sequestration. Am. J. Roentgenol. *92*:540, 1964.

Rao, B. N. and Edwards, J. E.: Conditions simulating the tetralogy of Fallot. Circulation *49(1)*:173, 1974.

Raphael, M. J. and Allwork, S. P.: Angiographic anatomy of the left ventricle. Clin. Radiol. *25*:95, 1974.

Rashkind, W. J.: Balloon atrioseptostomy. Adv. Cardiol. *11*:2, 1974.

Rashkind, W. J. and Miller, W. W.: Creation of an atrial septal defect without thoracotomy. J.A.M.A. *196*:173, 1966.

Rastelli, G. C., McGoon, D. C., Ongley, P. A., Mankin, H. T., and Kirklin, J. W.: Surgical treatment of supravalvular aortic stenosis. J. Thoracic Cardiovasc. Surg. *51*:873, 1966.

Ravitch, M. M.: Pectus excavatum and heart failure. Surgery *30(1)*:178, 1951.

Rawlings, M. S.: The "straight back" syndrome. A new cause of pseudo heart disease. Am. J. Cardiol. *5*:333, 1960.

Rawlings, M. S.: The straight back syndrome: a new heart disease. Dis. Chest *39*:435, 1961.

Rea, W. J., Sugg, W. L., Wilson, L. C., Webb, W. R., and Ecker, R. R.: Coronary artery lacerations. Ann. Thoracic Surg. *7*:518, 1969.

Read, R. C. and Thal, A. P.: Surgical experience with symptomatic myxomatous valvular transformation (the floppy valve syndrome). Surgery *59*:173, 1966.

Read, R. C., Thal, A. P., and Wendt, V. E.: Symptomatic valvular myxomatous transformation (the floppy valve syndrome): a possible forme fruste of the Marfan syndrome. Circulation *32*:897, 1965.

Reddy, C. R. R. M., Sudareshwar, B., and Rajakumari, K.: Congenital endocardial fibroelastosis. Indian J. Pediat. *39*:293, 1972.

Rees, J. R., Goor, D. A., Holswade, G. R., and Lillehei, C. W.: Closure of atrial septal defects in adults. Rocky Mountain Med. J. *70*:46, 1973.

Reid, J. M., Coleman, E. N., Barclay, R. S., and Stevenson, J. G.: Blalock-Taussig anastomosis in 126 patients with Fallot's tetralogy. Thorax *28*:269, 1973.

Reid, R. C., Johnson, J. A., Vick, J. A., and Meyers, M. W.: Vascular effects of hypertonic solutions. Cir. Res. *8*:538, 1960.

Reifenstein, G. H., Levine, S. A., and Gross, R. E.: Coarctation of the aorta: a review of 104 cases of the "adult type," 2

years of age or older. Am. Heart J. *33*:146, 1947.

Reinke, R. T., Coel, M. N., and Higgins, C. B.: Calcified nonsyphilitic aneurysms of the sinuses of Valsalva. Am. J. Roentgenol. *122*:783, 1974.

Reul, G. J., Jr., Cooley, D. A., Sandiford, F. M., Kyger, E. R., III, Wukasch, D. C., and Hallman, G. L.: Aortocoronary artery bypass—present indications and risk factors. Arch. Surgery *111*:414, 1976.

Revell, S. T. R.: Primary mycotic aneurysm. Ann. Int. Med. *22*:431, 1945.

Rich, C. and Webster, B.: The natural history of uncomplicated syphilitic aortitis. Am. Heart J. *43*:321, 1952.

Ricketts, H. J. and Abrams, H. L.: Percutaneous selective coronary cine arteriography. J.A.M.A. *181*:620, 1962.

Ridolfi, R. L. and Hutchins, G. M.: Detection of ball variance in prosthetic heart valves by liver biopsy. Johns Hopkins Med. J. *134*:131, 1974.

Rigler, L. G., Wangensteen, O. H., and Friedell, H. L.: Roentgen kymography in constrictive pericarditis. Am. J. Roentgenol. *46*:765, 1941.

Rizk, G., Cueto, L., and Amplatz, K.: Rebound enlargement of the thymus after successful corrective surgery for transposition of the great vessels. Am. J. Roentgenol. *116*:528, 1972.

Rizk, G., Moller, J. H., and Amplatz, K.: The angiographic appearance of the heart following the Mustard procedure. Radiology *106*:269, 1973.

Robb, G. H.: Management of atrial septal defect in middle age. Am. Heart J. *85*:837, 1973.

Robb, G. P. and Gottlieb, C.: Report of case of pulmonary arteriovenous fistula in left lower pulmonary field. Exp. Med. Surg. *9*:431, 1951.

Robb, G. P. and Steinberg, I.: Visualization of the chambers of the heart, the pulmonary circulation and the great blood vessels in man. Am. J. Roentgenol. *41*:1, 1939.

Robbins, S. L.: Pathology, ed. 3, p. 743. Philadelphia, W. B. Saunders Co., 1967.

Roberts, N., and Moes, C. A. F.: Supravalvular pulmonary stenosis. J. Pediat. *82*:838, 1973.

Roberts, W. C.: Anatomically isolated aortic valvular disease. The case against it being of rheumatic etiology. Am. J. Med. *49*:151, 1970.

Roberts, W. C.: Congenitally bicuspid aortic valve. A study of 85 autopsy cases. Am. J. Cardiol. *26*:72, 1970.

Roberts, W. C. and Elliott, L. P.: Lesions complicating the congenitally bicuspid aortic valve. Radiol. Clin. N.A. *6*:409, 1968.

Roberts, W. C., Mason, D. T., and Braunwald, E.: Survival to adulthood in a patient with complete transposition of the great vessels: including a note on the association of endocrine tumors with heart disease. Ann. Int. Med. *57*:834, 1962.

Roberts, W. C., Perloff, J. K., and Costantino, T.: Severe valvular aortic stenosis in patients over 65 years of age. Am. J. Cardiol. *27*:487, 1971.

Roberts, W. C., Perry, L. W., Chandra, R. S., Meyers, G. E., Shapiro, S. R., and Scott, L. P.: Aortic valve atresia: a new classification based on necropsy study of 73 cases. Am. J. Cardiol. *37*:753, 1976.

Roberts, W. C. and Sjoerdsma, A.: The cardiac disease associated with the carcinoid syndrome (carcinoid heart disease). Am. J. Med. *36*:5, 1964.

Robin, E. Silberberg, B., Ganguly, S. N., and Magnisalis, K.: Aortic origin of the left pulmonary artery. Variant of tetralogy of Fallot. Am. J. Cardiol. *35(2)*:324, 1975.

Robinson, A. S.: Acute pancreatitis following translumbar aortography: case report with autopsy findings 7 weeks following aortogram. Arch. Surg. *72*:290, 1956.

Rockoff, S. D., Braasch, R., Kuhn, C., and Chraplyvy, M.:

Contrast media as histamine liberators. I. Mast cell histamine release in vitro by sodium salts of contrast media. Invest. Radiol. 5:503, 1970.

Rockoff, S. D. and Aker, U. T.: Contrast media as histamine liberators. VI. Arterial plasma histamine and hemodynamic responses following angiocardiography in man with 75% Hypaque. Invest. Radiol. 7:403, 1972.

Rodriquez-Alvarez, A. and Rodriquez, G. M.: Injection of radiopaque material in technique of selective angiocardiography: influence of viscosity upon flow rates through catheter. Monograph on therapy. Squibb Inst. Med. Res. 2:279, 1957.

Rodriguez, G. R.: Calcification of the pulmonary valves. Chest 59:160, 1971.

Roesler, H.: Beitrage zur Lehre von den Angenborenen Herzfehlern: Untersuchungen an Zwei Fallen von Isthmusstenose der Aorta. Wien. Arch. Inn. Med. 15:521, 1928.

Roesler, H.: Interatrial septal defect. Arch. Internal Med. 54:339, 1934.

Roesler, H.: Clinical Roentgenology of the Cardiovascular System. Springfield, Ill., Charles C Thomas, 1946.

Rogers, H. M. and Edwards, J. E.: Incomplete division of the atrioventricular canal with patent interatrial foramen primum (persistent common atrioventricular ostium): report of 5 cases and review of the literature. Am. Heart J. 36:28, 1948.

Rohrer, F.: Volumbestimmung von Korpenhohlen und Organen auf orthodiagraphischem Wege. Fortschr. Gebiete Roentgenstrahlen 24:285, 1916–17.

Ronderos, A.: Endocardial fibroelastosis. Am. J. Roentgenol. 84:442, 1960.

Rösch, J., Antonovic, R., Trenouth, R. S., Shebudin, H., Rahimtoola, M. B., Sim, D. N., and Dotter, C. T.: The natural history of coronary artery stenosis. A longitudinal angiographic assessment. Radiology 119:513, 1976.

Rösch, J., DeMots, H., Antonovic, R., Rahimtolla, S. H., Judkins, M. P., and Dotter, C. T.: Coronary arteriography in left main coronary artery disease. Am. J. Cardiol 36:136, 1975.

Rösch, J., Dotter, C. T., Antonovic, R., Bonchek, L., and Starr, A.: Angiographic appraisal of distal vessel suitability for aortocoronary bypass graft surgery. Circulation 48:202, 1973.

Rosenbaum, H. D.: Roentgen demonstration of broken cardiac pacemaker wires. Radiology 84:933, 1965.

Rosenbaum, H. D., Pellegrino, E. D., and Treciokas, L. J.: Acyanotic levocardia. Circulation 26:60, 1962.

Rosenberg, S. A.: A Study of the etiological basis of primary pulmonary hypertension. Am. Heart J. 68:484, 1964.

Rosengart, R., Jarmakani, J. M., and Emmanouilides, G. C.: Single film retrograde umbilical aortography in the diagnosis of hypoplastic left heart syndrome with aortic atresia. Circulation 54(2):345, 1976.

Rosenow, E. C., III: The spectrum of drug induced pulmonary disease. Ann. Int. Med. 77:977, 1972.

Rosenquist, G. C.: Congenital mitral valve disease associated with coarctation of the aorta: a spectrum that includes parachute deformity of the mitral valve. Circulation 49:985, 1974.

Rosenquist, G. C., Stark, J., and Taylor, J. F. N.: Congenital mitral valve disease in transposition of the great arteries. Circulation 51:731, 1975.

Rosenquist, G. C., Taylor, J. F. N., and Stark, J.: Aortopulmonary fenestration and aortic atresia. Report of an infant with ventricular septal defect, persistent ductus arteriosus, and interrupted aortic arch. Brit. Heart J. 36:1146, 1974.

Rosenthall, L. and Mercer, E. N.: Intravenous radionuclide cardiography for the detection of cardiovascular shunts. Radiology 106:601, 1973.

Ross, D. N.: The sinus venosus type of atrial septal defect. Guy's Hosp. Rep. 105:376, 1956.

Ross, D. N.: Replacement of the aortic and mitral valves with a pulmonary autograft. Lancet 2:956, 1967.

Ross, D. N.: Biologic valves: their performance and prospects. Circulation 45:1259, 1972.

Ross, D. N. and Somerville, J.: Surgical correction of tricuspid atresia. Lancet 1:845, 1973.

Ross, J., Jr.: Catheterization of the left heart through the interatrial septum: a new technique and its experimental evaluation. Surg. Forum 9:297, 1959.

Ross, J., Jr., Braunwald, E., Gault, J. H., Mason, D. T., and Morrow, A. G.: The mechanism of the intraventricular pressure gradient in idiopathic hypertrophic subaortic stenosis. Circulation 34:558, 1966.

Ross, J., Jr., Gault, J. H., Mason, D. T.: On the question of obstruction in idiopathic hypertrophic subaortic stenosis. Ann. Int. Med. 65:859, 1966.

Ross, R. S. and Criley, J. M.: Contrast radiography in mitral regurgitation. Prog. Cardiovasc. Dis. 5:195, 1962.

Ross, R. S., Feder, F. P., and Spencer, F. C.: Aneurysm of the previously ligated patent ductus arteriosus. Circulation 23:350, 1962.

Ross, S. R. and McKusick, A. V.: Aortic arch syndrome. Arch. Int. Med. 92:701, 1953.

Rossall, R. E. and Gunning, A. J.: Basal horizontal lines on chest radiographs: significance. Lancet 1:604, 1956.

Roth, L. M. and Kessane, J. M.: Panaortitis and aortic valvulitis in progressive systemic sclerosis. Am. J. Clin. Pathol. 41:287, 1964.

Rousthoi, P.: Uber angiokardiographie. Vorlaufige mitteilung. Acta Radiol. 14:419, 1933.

Rowe, R. D.: Maternal rubella and pulmonary artery stenosis: report of eleven cases. Pediatrics 32:180, 1963.

Rowe, R. and Macdonald, D.: Partial absence of right ventricular musculature: partial parchment heart. Am. J. Cardiol. 14:415–419, 1964.

Ruckdeschel, J. C., Chang, P., Martin, R. E., Byhardtir, W., O'Connell, M. J., Sutherland, J. C., and Wiernik, P. H.: Radiation-related pericardial effusion in patients with Hodgkin's disease. Medicine 54:245, 1975.

Rudolph, A. M.: Congenital Diseases of the Heart, pp. 527–545. Chicago, Year Book Medical Publisher, 1974.

Ruel, G. J., Cooley, D. A., Sandiford, F. M., and Hallman, G. L.: Complications following contoured dacron baffle in correction of transposition of the great arteries. Surgery 76:946, 1974.

Ruskin, H. and Samuel, E.: Calcification in the patent ductus arteriosus. Brit. J. Radiol. 23:710, 1950.

Ruttenberg, H. D.: Congenital absence of the pulmonary valve. In Heart Disease in Infants, Children, and Adolescents. Moss, A. J., and Adams, F. H. (eds.), pp. 487–491. Baltimore, Williams & Wilkins Co. 1968.

Ruttenberg, H. D.: Corrected transposition of the great vessels. In Heart Disease In Infants, Children, and Adolescents. Moss, A. J., and Adams, F. H. (eds.), p. 553. Baltimore, Williams & Wilkins Co., 1968.

Ruttenberg, H. D., Carey, L. S., Adams, P., Jr., and Edwards, J. E.: Absence of the pulmonary valve in the tetralogy of Fallot. Am. J. Roentgenol. 91:500, 1964.

Ruttenberg, H. D., Steidl, R. M., Carey, L. S., and Edwards, J. E.: Glycogen-storage disease of the heart. Hemodynamic and angiocardiographic features in 2 cases. Am. Heart J. 67:469, 1964.

Ruzyllo, W., Nihill, M. R., Mullins, C. E., and McNamara, D. G.: Hemodynamic evaluation of 221 patients after intracardiac repair of tetralogy of Fallot. Am. J. Cardiol. 34(5):565, 1974.

Sabiston, D. C., Jr., Neill, C. A., and Taussig, H. B.: The

direction of blood flow in anomalous left coronary artery arising from the pulmonary artery. Circulation 22:591, 1960.

Sackner, M. A., Heinz, E. R., and Steinberg, A. J.: The heart in scleroderma. Am. J. Cardiol. 17:542, 1966.

Sackner, M. A., Lewis, D. H., Robinson, M. J., and Bellet, S.: Idiopathic myocardial hypertrophy. Am. J. Cardiol. 7:714, 1961.

Sakakibara, S. and Konno, S.: Congenital aneurysm of the sinus of Valsalva: anatomy and classification. Am. Heart J. 63:405, 1962.

Sakakibara, S. and Konno, S.: Congenital aneurysms of sinus of Valsalva: a clinical study. Am. Heart J. 63:708, 1962.

Salvioni, D. and Goldin, R. R.: Intralobular pulmonary sequestration. Dis. Chest 37:122, 1960.

Samaan, H. A.: Congenital pulmonary valve stenosis with intact ventricular septum and interatrial communication. J. Cardiovasc. Surg. 13:554, 1972.

Samarrai, A. A. R., McCloy, R., and Ablett, M. B.: Biloculate false aneurysm of the right ventricle after cardiac surgery. Brit. Heart J. 38:297, 1976.

Sanborn, J. C., Heitzman, E. R., and Markarian, B.: Traumatic rupture of the thoracic aorta: roentgen-pathological correlations. Radiology 95:293, 1970.

Sanders, J. M.: Bilateral superior vena cavae. Anat. Rec. 94:657, 1946.

Sanders, J. S. and Martt, J. M.: Multiple small pulmonary arteriovenous fistulas: diagnosis by cardiac catheterization. Circulation 25:383, 1962.

Sanders, V.: Idiopathic disease of the myocardium. Arch. Int. Med. 112:661, 1963.

Sandler, G. and Wilson, G. M.: The nature and prognosis of heart disease in thyrotoxicosis. Quart. J. Med. 28:347, 1959.

Sandler, H.: Use of single-plane angiocardiogram for calculation of left ventricular volume in man. Am. Heart J. 75:325, 1968.

Sanerkin, N. G.: Extracardiac anastomosis in coronary ostial occlusion. Brit. Heart J. 30:440, 1968.

Sanfelippo, P. M., DuShane, J. W., McGoon, D. C., and Danielson, G. K.: Ventricular septal defect and aortic insufficiency. Ann. Thoracic Surg. 17:213, 1974.

Sanford, W., Armstrong, R. G., Cline, R. E., and King, T. D.: Right atrium-pulmonary artery allograft for correction of tricuspid atresia. J. Thoracic Cardiovasc. Surg. 66:105, 1973.

Sanghvi, L. M. and Misra, S. N.: Loculated pleural effusion in congestive heart failure due to severe anemia: report of a case. Am. Heart J. 55:421, 1958.

Santinga, J. T., Flora, J. D., Batsakis, J., and Kirsh, M. M.: Hemolysis in patients with the cloth-covered aortic valve prosthesis: changing severity of hemolysis and prediction of anemia. Am. J. Cardiol. 34:533, 1974.

Saric, S., Vuletic, V., Gvozcanocic, V., and Mark, B.: Case of kinking of the aortic arch. Circulation 21:1147, 1960.

Sasahara, A. A., Nadas, A. S., Rudolph, A. M., Wittenborg, M. H., and Gross, R. E.: Ventricular septal defect with patent ductus arteriosus: a clinical and hemodynamic study. Circulation 22:254, 1960.

Sawyer, E. G., Burwell, C. S., Dexter, L., Eppinger, E. C., Goodale, W. T., Gorlin, R., Harkins, D. E., and Haynes, F. W.: Chronic constrictive pericarditis: further considerations of the pathologic physiology of the disease. Am. Heart J. 44:207, 1952.

Scannell, J. G. and Grillo, H. C.: Primary tumors of the heart. J. Thoracic Surg. 35:23, 1958.

Scatliff, J. H., Kummer, A. J., and Janzen, A. H.: The diagnosis of pericardial effusion with intracardiac carbon dioxide. Radiology 73:871, 1959.

Schachner, A., Varsano, I., and Levy, M. J.: The parachute mitral valve complex: case report and review of the literature. J. Thoracic Cardiovasc. Surg. 70:451, 1975.

Scheinin, T. M., Inberg, M. V., and Kallio, V.: Supravalvular aortic stenosis and multiple aneurysms of the ascending aorta. Scand. J. Thoracic Cardiovasc. Surg. 3:107, 1969.

Schiebler, G. L., Adams, P., Jr., Anderson, R. C., Amplatz, K., and Lester, R. G.: Clinical study of twenty-three cases of Ebstein's anomaly of the tricuspid valve. Circulation 19:165, 1959.

Schiebler, G. L., Loring, A. E., and Brogdon, B. G.: Cardiovascular manifestations of Hurler's syndrome. Circulation 26:782, 1962.

Schieken, R. M., Friedman, S., and Pierce, W. S.: Severe congenital pulmonary stenosis with pulmonary valvular dysplasia syndrome. Ann. Thoracic Surg. 15:570, 1973.

Schlant, R. C.: Acute rheumatic fever. The Heart Arteries and Veins, 2nd ed. Hurst, J. W. and Logue, R. N. (eds.), pp. 752–53. McGraw-Hill Book Company, 1970.

Schlant, R. C.: Calcific aortic stenosis. Am. J. Cardiol. 27:581, 1971.

Schlesinger, M. J.: Relation of anatomic pattern to pathologic conditions of the coronary arteries. Arch. Pathol. 30:403, 1940.

Schneider, H. J. and Felson, B.: Buckling of the innominate artery simulating aneurysm and tumor. Am. J. Roentgenol. 85:1106, 1961.

Schneider, H. J. and Spitz, H. B.: Unruptured aortic sinus aneurysm: plain film diagnosis. Dis. Chest 53:340, 1968.

Schoonmaker, F. W. and King, S. B.: Coronary arteriography by the single catheter percutaneous femoral technique. Circulation 50:735, 1974.

Schreiber, M. H.: The volume of the heart—a roentgenographic determination. Arizona Med. 21:551, 1964.

Schreiber, M. H.: Resemblence of normal pulmonary veins to pulmonary lesions on lateral chest films. Am. Rev. Resp. Dis. 91:434, 1965.

Schuster, S. R. and Gross, R. E.: Surgery for coarctation of the aorta. A review of 500 cases. J. Thoracic Cardiovasc. Surg. 43:54, 1962.

Schwedel, J. B., Escher, D. W., Aaron, R. S., and Young, D.: The roentgenologic diagnosis of pulmonary hypertension in mitral stenosis. Am. Heart J. 53:163, 1957.

Schwarz, G. S.: Determination of frontal plane area from the product of the long and short diameters of the cardiac silhouette. Radiology 47:360, 1946.

Schwartz, J. N., Kong, Y., Hackel, D. B., and Bartel, A. G.: Comparison of angiographic and postmortem findings in patients with coronary artery disease. Am. J. Cardiol. 36:174, 1975.

Schryer, M. J. P. and Karnauchow, P. N.: Endocardial fibroelastosis. Etiologic and pathogenetic considerations in children. Am. Heart J. 88:557, 1974.

Scott, D. H.: Aneurysm of the coronary arteries. Am. Heart J. 36:403, 1948.

Scott, H. W., Jr. and Sabiston, D. C., Jr.: Surgical treatment for congenital aortico-pulmonary fistula. J. Thoracic Surg. 25:26, 1953.

Scott, L. P., Dempsey, J. J., Timmis, H. H., and McClenathan, J. E.: A surgical approach to Ebstein's disease. Circulation 27:574, 1963.

Scott, L. P., Hauck, A. J., and Nadas, A. S.: Endocardial cushion defect with pulmonic stenosis. Circulation 25:653, 1962.

Seckelj, P. and Bensey, B. G.: Historical landmarks: Ebstein's anomaly of the tricuspid valve. Am. Heart J. 88:108, 1974.

Segal, B. L., Likoff, W., Broek, H. Vanden, Kimbiris, D., Najmi, M., and Linhart, J. W.: Saphenous vein bypass surgery for impending myocardial infarction: critical evaluation and current concepts. J.A.M.A. 223:767, 1973.

Segers, M., Regnier, M., and Denolin, H.: Tumeur pulmonaire pulsatile avec shunt arterioveineux. Acta Cardiol. *5:*156, 1950.

Seldinger, S. I.: Catheter replacement of the needle in percutaneous arteriography. Acta Radiol. *39:*368, 1953.

Seltzer, R. A., Harthorne, J. W., and Austen, W. G.: Appearance and significance of left atrial calcification. Am. J. Roentgenol. *100:*307, 1967.

Sewell, W. H.: Coronary disease management. *In* Coronary Arteriography, Nitrates, and the Triple Pedicle Operation. St. Louis, Warren H. Green, Inc., 1969.

Selzer, A.: Pulmonary hypertension and its relation to congenital heart disease. Dis. Chest *25:*253, 1954.

Seyfer, A. E., Heydorn, W. H., Nelson, W. P., Spicer, M. J., and Strevey, T. E.: Starr-Edwards mitral valve failure ten years after replacement surgery: chronic fibrous obstruction of the prosthesis frustrum area: report of a case. Circulation *50:*372, 1974.

Shabetai, R., Aravindakshan, V., Danielson, G., and Bryant, L.: Traumatic hemopericardium with tricuspid incompetence. J. Thoracic Cardiovasc. Surg. *57:*294, 1969.

Shabetai, R., Fowler, N. O., and Gunthoroth, W. G.: The hemodynamics of cardiac tamponade and constrictive pericarditis. Am. J. Cardiol. *26:*480, 1970.

Shaffer, A. B. and Silber, E. N.: Rheumatic fever and rheumatic heart disease, *In* Heart Disease, Silber, E. N. and Katz, L. N. (eds.), p. 699. Macmillan Co., Inc., 1975.

Shaher, R. M., Moes, C. A. F., and Khoury, G.: Radiologic and angiocardiographic findings in complete transposition of the great vessels with left ventricular outflow tract obstruction. Radiology *88:*1092, 1967.

Shapiro, J. H., Jacobson, H. G., Rubinstein, B. M., Poppel, M. H., and Schwedel, J. B.: Calcifications of the Heart. Springfield, Ill., Charles C Thomas, 1963.

Shauker, K. R., Hultgren, M. K., Lauer, R. M., and Diehl, A. M.: Lethal tricuspid and mitral regurgitation in Marfan's syndrome. Am. J. Cardiol. *20:*122, 1967.

Shariatzadeh, A. N., King, H., Girod, D., and Shumaker, H. B. J.: Discrete subaortic stenosis. A report of 20 cases. J. Thoracic & Cardiovascular Surg. *63:*258, 1972.

Shennan, T.: Completely healed dissecting aneurysm of aorta with obliteration of sac. J. Pathol. Bacteriol. *35:*161, 1932.

Sherman, F. E., Stengel, W. F., and Bauersfeld, S. R.: Congenital stenosis of pulmonary veins at their atrial junctions. Am. Heart J. *56:*908, 1958.

Shernick, D. W., Kincaid, O. W., and DuShane, J. W.: Agenesis of main branch of pulmonary artery. Am. J. Roentgenol. *87:*917, 1962.

Shimizu, K. and Sano, K.: Pulseless diasese. J. Neuropathol. Clin. Neurol. *1:*37, 1951.

Shipp, J. C., Crowley, L. V., and Wigh, B.: Aortic sinus aneurysm: Production of intracardiac calcification and pulmonary artery fistula. Am. J. Med. *18:*160, 1955.

Shirey, E. K.: Correlative pathologic study of the coronary microcirculation with coronary arteriography. Circulation (Supp. VI) *38:*179, 1968.

Shone, J. D., Amplatz, K., Anderson, R. C., Adams, P., and Edwards, J. E.: Congenital stenosis of individual pulmonary veins. Circulation *26:*574, 1962.

Shone, J. D., Sellers, R. D., Anderson, R. C., Adams, P., Jr., Lillehei, C. W., and Edwards, J. E.: The developmental complex of "parachute mitral valve," supravalvular ring of left atrium, subaortic stenosis, and coarctation of aorta. Am. J. Cardiol. *11:*714, 1963.

Short, D. S.: Post-mortem pulmonary arteriography with special reference to the study of pulmonary hypertension. J. Fac. Radiol. *8:*118, 1956.

Shuford, W. H., Sybers, R. G., and Edwards, F. K.: The three types of right aortic arch. Am. J. Roentgenol. *109(1):*67, 1970.

Shuford, W. H., Sybers, R. G., Milledge, R. D., and Brinsfield, D.: The cervical aortic arch. Am. J. Roentgenol. *116:*519, 1972.

Shuford, W. H., Sybers, R. G., and Schlant, R. C.: Right Aortic arch with isolation of the left subclavian artery. Am. J. Roentgenol. *109(1):*75, 1970.

Shuford, W. H., Sybers, R. G., and Weens, H. S.: Problems in the aortographic diagnosis of dissecting aneurysm of the aorta. N. Engl. J. Med. *280:*225, 1969.

Shuford, W. H., Sybers, R. G., and Weens, H. S.: The angiographic features of double aortic arch. Am. J. Roentgenol. *116:*125, 1972.

Shuford, W. H., and Weens, H. S.: Azygos vein dilatation simulating mediastinal tumor. Am. J. Roentgenol. *80:*225, 1958.

Siderys, H. and Strange, P. S.: Rupture of the heart due to blunt trauma. J. Thoracic Cardiovasc. Surg. *62:*84, 1971.

Siegelman, S. S., Caplan, L. H., and Annes, G. P.: Complications of catheter angiography. Study with oscillometry "pullout" angiograms. Radiology *91:*251, 1968.

Siegelman, S. S., Sprayregen, S., Strasberg, Z., Attai, L. A., and Robinson, G.: Aortic dissection and the left renal artery. Radiology *95:*73, 1970.

Sievers, J.: Cardiac rupture and acute myocardial infarction. Geriatrics *21:*125, 1966.

Silver, S., Delit, C., and Eller, M.: The treatment of thyrocardiac disease with radioactive iodine. Prog. Cardiovasc. Dis. *5:*64, 1962.

Silverman, J. J. and Scheinesson, G. P.: Persistent truncus arteriosus in a 43-year-old man. Am. J. Cardiol. *17:*94, 1966.

Simeone, J. F., Minagi, H., and Putman, C. E.: Traumatic disruption of the thoracic aorta: significance of the left apical extrapleural cap. Radiology *117:*265, 1975.

Simon, A. L.: Angiographic diagnosis of idiopathic hypertrophic subaortic stenosis. Rad. Clin. N.A. *6(3):*423, 1968.

Simon, A. L., Friedman, W. F., and Roberts, W. C.: The angiographic features of a case of parachute mitral valve. Am. Heart J. *77:*809, 1969.

Simon, A. L., and Reis, R. L.: The angiographic features of bicuspid and unicommissural aortic stenosis. Am. J. Cardiol. *28:*353, 1971.

Simon, A. L., Ross, J., Jr., and Gault, J. H.: Angiographic anatomy of the left ventricle and mitral valve in idiopathic hypertrophic subaortic stenosis. Circulation *36:*852, 1967.

Simopoulos, A. P., Rosenblum, D. J., Mazumdar, H., and Kiely, B.: Intralobar bronchopulmonary sequestration in children: diagnosis by intrathoracic aortography. J. Dis. Child. *97:*796, 1959.

Sinclair, W. and Nitsch, E.: Polyarteritis nodosa of the coronary arteries. Report of a case in an infant with rupture of an aneurysm and intrapericardial hemorrhage. Am. Heart J. *38:*898, 1949.

Sirgh, R., McGuire, L. B., Carpenter, M., and Dammann, J. F.: Mitral stenosis with partial anomalous pulmonary venous return (with intact atrial septum). Am. J. Cardiol. *28:*226, 1971.

Singh, S., Newmark, K., Ishikawa, I., Mitral, S., and Berman, L. B.: Pericardiectomy in uremia. The treatment of choice for cardiac tamponade in chronic renal failure. J.A.M.A. *228:*1132, 1974.

Singh, R., Nolan, S. P., and Schrank, J. P.: Traumatic left ventricular aneurysm. Two cases with normal coronary angiograms. J.A.M.A. *234:*412, 1975.

Singleton, E. B., Dutton, R. V., and Wagner, M. L.: Pulmonary isomerism. Rad. Clin. N.A. *10(2):*343, 1972.

Singleton, E. V., McNamara, D. G., Leachman, R. D., Cooley, D. A., and Chau, P. M.: Radiological evaluation of isolated ventricular septal defects before and after surgical closure. Radiology *73:*37, 1959.

Singshinsuk, S., Hartmann, A., Elliot, L.: Stenosis of individual pulmonary veins. A rare cause of pulmonary hypertension. Radiology 87:514, 1966.

Sinha, K. P., Uricchio, J. F., and Goldberg, H.: Ebstein's syndrome. Brit. Heart J. 22:94, 1960.

Sissman, N. J. and Abrams, H. L.: Bidirectional shunting in a coronary artery–right ventricular fistula associated with pulmonary atresia and an intact ventricular septum. Circulation 32:582, 1965.

Skinner, J. F. and Burroughs, J. T.: Intracardiac knotting of the catheter during right heart catheterization. Circulation 23:81, 1961.

Slater, S. R., Kroop, I. G., and Zuckerman, S.: Constrictive pericarditis caused by solitary metastatic carcinosis of pericardium and complicated by radiation fibrosis of mediastinum. Am. Heart J. 43:401, 1952.

Slezak, P., Steinhart, L., Prochizka, J., Endrys, J., and Jusin, I.: The angiographic appearance of subvalvular aortic stenosis. Brit. J. Radiol. 38:350, 1965.

Sloan, R. D. and Cooley, R. N.: Coarctation of the aorta: the roentgenologic aspects of 125 surgically confirmed cases. Radiology 61:701, 1953.

Sloan, R. D. and Cooley, R. N.: Congenital pulmonary arteriovenous aneurysm. Am. J. Roentgenol. 70:183, 1953.

Smellis, H.: Myxoma of the left atrium. Proc. Roy. Soc. Med. 55:226, 1962.

Smith, C. and Amplatz, K.: Angiographic demonstration of Kugel's artery (arteria anastomotica auricularis magna). Radiology 106:113, 1973.

Smith, D. E. and Matthews, M. B.: Aortic valvular stenosis with coarctation of the aorta: with special reference to the development of aortic stenosis upon congenital bicuspid valve. Brit. Heart J. 17:198, 1955.

Smith, G. T., Dammin, G. J., and Dexter, L.: Post-mortem arteriographic studies of the human lung in pulmonary embolism. J.A.M.A. 188:143, 1964.

Smith, G. W. and Muller, W. H., Jr.: The evolution and current concepts of the surgical treatment of constrictive pericarditis. Prog. Cardiovasc. Dis. 4:346, 1961.

Smith, G. T.: The anatomy of the coronary circulation. Am. J. Cardiol. 9:327, 1962.

Smith, H. L. and Horton, B. T.: Arteriovenous fistula of lung associated with polycythemia vera. Report of case in which diagnosis was made clinically. Am. Heart J. 18:589, 1939.

Smith, R. A.: A theory of the origin of intralobar sequestration of lung. Thorax 11:10, 1956.

Smith, S. W.: Roentgen findings in homocystinuria. Am. J. Roentgenol. 100:147, 1967.

Soloff, L. A. and Zatuchni, J.: The definitive diagnosis of effusive or constrictive pericarditis. Am. J. Med. Sci. 234:687, 1967.

Soloff, L. A., Stauffer, H. M., and Zatuchni, J.: Ebstein's disease: report of the first case diagnosed during life. Am. J. Med. Sci. 222:554, 1951.

Soloff, L. A., Zatuchni, J., Mark, G. E., Jr., and Stauffer, H. M.: Size of the pulmonary artery in rheumatic heart disease with mitral stenosis and its significance. Circulation 16:940, 1957.

Soman, V. R., Breton, G., Hershkowitz, M., and Mark, H.: Bacterial endocarditis of mitral valve in the Marfan syndrome. Brit. Heart J. 36:1247, 1974.

Somerville, W.: Constrictive pericarditis with special reference to change in natural history brought about by surgical intervention. Circulation 38(Supp. 5):102, 1968.

Sones, F. M.: Indications and value of coronary arteriography. Circulation 45:6, 1155, 1972.

Sones, F. M., Jr., and Shirey, E. K.: Cine coronary arteriography. Mod. Concepts Cardiovasc. Dis. 31:735, 1962.

Sones, F. M., Shirey, E. K., Proudfit, W. C., and Westcott, R. N.: Cine arteriography. In abstracts of 32nd Scientific Sessions of American Heart Association. Circulation

20:773, 1959.

Sos, T. A., and Baltaxe, H. A.: The importance of coronary angiography in the evaluation of patients with aortic valvular disease. Am. J. Roentgenol. 122(4):793, 1974.

Sos, T. A., and Baltaxe, H. A.: Comparison of left ventricular ejection fraction and regional contractility fraction pre and post-coronary angiography. Invest. Radiol. 2:138, 1976.

Sos, T. A., Tay, D., Levin, A. R., Levin, D. C., and Baltaxe, H. A.: Angiographic demonstration of the absence of an atrial septal defect in the presence of partial anomalous pulmonary venous connection. Am. J. Roentgenol. 121:591, 1974.

Sosman, M. C.: Subclinical mitral stenosis. J.A.M.A. 115:1061, 1940.

Sosman, M. C.: X-ray in curable heart disease. Radiology 41:351, 1943.

Sosman, M. C.: The technique for locating and identifying pericardial and intracardiac calcifications. Am. J. Roentgenol. 50:461, 1943.

Sostre, S., Hurley, E. J., and Zaret, B. L.: The contracted form of endocardial fibroelastosis in an adult: hemodynamic and angiographic observations. Chest 65:544, 1974.

Sounders, C. R., Pearson, C. M., and Adams, H. D.: Aortic deformity simulating mediastinal tumor: subclinical form of coarctation. Dis. Chest 20:35, 1951.

Spencer, F., Trinkle, K., and Reeves, J. T.: Successful replacement of a thrombosed mitral ball-valve prosthesis. J.A.M.A. 194:1249, 1965.

Spencer, F. C., Bahnson, H. T., and Neill, C. A.: The treatment of aortic regurgitation associated with a ventricular septal defect. J. Thoracic Cardiovasc. Surg. 43:222, 1962.

Spencer, F. C., Neill, C. A., Sank, L., and Bahnson, H. T.: Anatomical variations in 46 patients with congenital aortic stenosis. Am. Surg. 26:204, 1960.

Sprague, H. B., Ernlund, C. H., and Albright, F.: Clinical aspects of persistent right aortic root. N. Engl. J. Med. 209:679, 1933.

Spring, D. A., and Thomsen, J. H.: Recanalization in a coronary artery thrombus. J.A.M.A. 224:1152, 1973.

Standen, J. R.: "Tumor vascularity" in left atrial thrombus demonstrated by selective coronary arteriography. Radiology 116:549, 1975.

Stahlman, M., Kaplan, S., Helmsworth, J. A., Clark, L. C., and Scott, H. H., Jr.: Syndrome of left ventricular-right atrial shunt resulting from high interventricular septal defect associated with defective septal leaflet of the tricuspid valve. Circulation 12:813, 1955.

Stannard, M., Sloman, J. G., Hare, W. S. C., and Goble, A. J.: Prolapse of the posterior leaflet of the mitral valve: a clinical, familial, and cineangiographic study. Brit. Med. J. 3:71, 1967.

Stark, J., Silove, E. D., Taylor, J. F. N., and Graham, G. R.: Obstruction to systemic venous return following the Mustard operation for transposition of the great arteries. J. Thoracic Cardiovasc. Surg. 68:742, 1974.

Starr, A., and Edwards, M. L.: Mitral replacement: clinical experience with a ball valve prosthesis. Ann. Surg. 154:726, 1961.

Stauffer, H. M., and Pote, H. H.: Anomalous right subclavian artery originating on the left as the last branch of the aortic arch. Report of a probable case diagnosed roentgenographically. Am. J. Roentgenol. 56:13, 1946.

Stecher, W. R.: Cardiac mensuration aided by horizontal orthodiagraphy. Am. J. Roentgenol. 42:264, 1939.

Steeg, C. N., Ellis, K., and Gersony, W. M.: Total anomalous pulmonary venous drainage with ventricular septal defect. Am. Heart J. 86:341, 1973.

Stein, G. N., Chen, J. T., Goldstein, F., Israel, H. L., and Finkelstein, A.: The importance of chest roentgenography in the diagnosis of pulmonary embolism. Am. J. Roentgenol. *81:*255, 1959.

Steinberg, I: Angiocardiography in the differential diagnosis of pericardial and mediastinal tumors. Am. J. Roentgenol. *84:*409, 1960.

Steinberg, I., Dubilier, W., and Lucus, D.: Persistence of left superior vena cava. Dis. Chest *24:*479, 1953.

Steinberg, I.: Chronic traumatic aneurysm of the thoracic aorta. N. Engl. J. Med. *257:*913, 1957.

Steinberg, I.: Diagnosis of arteriosclerotic aneurysms of the thoracic aorta: report of 6 cases. Ann. Int. Med. *46:*218, 1957.

Steinberg, I.: Diagnosis and surgical treatment of pulmonary arteriovenous fistula. Report of three new and review of nineteen consecutive cases. Surg. Clin. N.A. *41:*523, 1961.

Steinberg, I.: Pericarditis with effusion: new observations with a note on Ewart's sign. Ann. Int. Med. *48:*428, 1958.

Steinberg, I.: Bilateral simultaneous intravenous angiocardiography. Am. J. Roentgenol. *88:*38, 1962.

Steinberg, I., Dotter C., Peabody, G., Reader, G., Heimoff, L., and Webster, B.: The angiocardiographic diagnosis of syphilitic aortitis. Am. J. Roentgenol. *62:*655, 1949.

Steinberg, I., and Dubilier, W., Jr.: Myxoma of the atrium. Roentgen diagnosis during life. Exhibit, 54th Annual Meeting of the American Roentgen Ray Society. Cincinnati, Ohio, September, 1953.

Steinberg, I., and Engle, M. A.: Angiocardiographic diagnosis of both great vessels originating from right ventricle. Am. J. Roentgenol. *94:*45, 1965.

Steinberg, I., and Finby, N.: Clinical manifestation of unperforated sinus aneurysm. Circulation *14:*115, 1956.

Steinberg, I., and Gelles, W.: Aneurysmal dilatation of aortic sinuses in arachnodactyly: diagnosis during life in three cases. Ann. Int. Med. *43:*120, 1955.

Steinberg, I., and Hagstrom, J. W. C.: Congenital aortic valvular stenosis and pseudocoarctation ("kinking, buckling") of the arch of the aorta. Report of four cases including an autopsy study on one case with parietal endocardial fibrosis and fibroelastosis. Circulation *25:*545, 1962.

Steinberg, I., and Hagstrom, J. W. C.: Angiocardiography in diagnosis of effusive-restrictive pericarditis. Am. J. Roentgenol. *102:*305, 1968.

Steinberg, I., Miscall, L., Redo, S. F., and Goldberg, H. P.: Angiocardiography in diagnosis of cardiac tumors. Am. J. Roentgenol. *91:*364, 1964.

Steinberg, I., and Stein, H. L.: Intravenous angiocardiography, abdominal aortography, and peripheral arteriography with single arm pressure injection. Am. J. Roentgenol. *92:*893, 1964.

Steinberg, I., Tillotson, P. M., and Halpern, M.: Roentgenography of systemic (congenital and traumatic) arteriovenous fistulas. Am. J. Roentgenol. *89:*343, 1963.

Steinberg, I., von Gal, H. V., and Finby, N.: Roentgen diagnosis of pericardial effusion: new angiocardiographic observations. Am. J. Roentgenol. *79:*321, 1958.

Steinberg, M. F., Greshman, A., and Sussman, M. L.: Angiography in congenital heart disease—III patent ductus arteriosus. Am. J. Roentgenol. *50:*306, 1943.

Steiner, R. E.: Radiologic aspects of cardiac tumors. Am. J. Cardiol. *21:*344, 1968.

Steiner, R. E.: A physiological approach to radiology. Radiology *100:*497, 1971.

Steiner, R. M., Bull, M. I., Kumpel, F., Wexler, L., and Kriss, J. P.: The diagnosis of intracardiac metastasis of colon carcinoma by radioisotopic and roentgenographic studies. Am. J. Cardiol. *26:*300, 1970.

Steinfeld, L., Dimich, I., Park, S. C., and Baron, M. G.: Clinical diagnosis of isolated subpulmonic (supracristal) ventricular septal defect. Am. J. Cardiol. *30:*19, 1972.

Stevens, G. M.: Buckling of the aortic arch (pseudocoarctation, kinking): a roentgenographic entity. Radiology *70:*67, 1958.

Stewart, J. R., Cohn, K. E., Fajurdo, L. F., Handcock, E. W., and Kaplan, H. S.: Radiation-induced heart disease. A study of twenty-five patients. Radiology *89:*302, 1967.

Stewart, J. R., and Fajardo, L. F.: Dose response to human and experimental radiation-induced heart disease. Application of the nominal standard dose (NSD) concept. Radiology *99:*403, 1971.

Stewart, J. R., Kincaid, O. W., and Edwards, J. E.: An Atlas of Vascular Rings and Related Malformations of the Aortic Arch System. Springfield, Ill., Charles C Thomas, Publisher, 1964.

St. Geme, J. W., Davis, C. W., and Noren, G. R.: An overview of primary endocardial fibroelastosis and chronic viral cardiomyopathy. Perspect. Biol. Med., 495–505, Summer, 1974.

Still, W. J. S.: Endocardial fibroelastosis. Am. Heart J. *61:*579, 1961.

Stinson, E. B., Rowles, D. F., and Shumway, N. E.: Repair of right ventricular aneurysm and ventricular septal defect caused by non-penetrating cardiac trauma. Surgery *64:*1022, 1968.

Stinson, E. V., Castellino, R. A., and Shumway, N. E.: Radiologic signs in endocarditis following prosthetic valve replacement. J. Thoracic Cardiovasc. Surg. *56:*554, 1968.

Stork, W. J.: Pulmonary arteriovenous fistulas. Am. J. Roentgenol. *74:*441, 1955.

Straus, R., and Merliss, S. R.: Primary tumors of the heart. Arch. Pathol. *39:*74, 1945.

Strauss, P., Abrams, H. L., and Robinson, S.: Radiologic aspects of operable heart disease. VI. Changes following surgical closure of patent ductus arteriosus. Circulation *17:*1047, 1958.

Strauss, H. W., Pitt, B., and James, A. E., Jr.: Cardiovascular Nuclear Medicine. St. Louis, C. V. Mosby, Co., 1974.

Sugg, W. L., Rea, W. J., Ecker, R. R., Webb, W. R., Rose, E. F., and Shaw, R. R.: Penetrating wounds of the heart. J. Thoracic Cardiovasc. Surg. *56:*531, 1968.

Sukumar, I. P., Prabhu, S., Bakthaviziam, A., Munsi, S. C., McArthur, J. D., Krishnaswami, J. S., and Cherian, G.: The diagnosis of origin of both great vessels from the right ventricle. J. Assoc. Phys. India *20:*557, 1972.

Sukumar, I. P., Sarvotham, S. G., Bhaktaviziam, A., John, S., Krishnaswami, S., McArthur, J. D., and Cherian, G.: Total anomalous pulmonary venous connection. Indian Heart J. *25:*328, 1973.

Sundararajan, V., Mich, E., and Molthan, M. E.: Truncus arteriosus (type II) associated with interruption of the aortic arch (type B). Am. J. Dis. Child. *123:*494, 1972.

Sussman, M. L., Dack, S., and Master, A. M.: The roentgenkymogram in myocardial infarction. I. Abnormalities in left ventricular contraction. Am. Heart J. *19:*453, 1940.

Sutorius, D. J., Schreiber, J. T., and Helmsworth, J. A.: Traumatic disruption of the thoracic aorta. J. Trauma *13:*583, 1973.

Swan, H. J. C.: Indicator-dilution methods in the diagnosis of congenital heart disease. Prog. Cardiovasc. Dis. *2:*143, 1959.

Swan, H. J. C., Forrester, J. S., Diamond, G., Chattesjce, K., and Parmley, W. W.: Hemodynamic spectrum of myocardial infarction and cardiogenic shock. Circulation *45:*1097, 1972.

Swan, H. J. C., Hetzel, P. S., Burchell, H. B., and Wood, E. H.: Differential diagnosis at cardiac catheterization of anomalous pulmonary venous drainage to atrial septal defects or abnormal venous connections. Mayo Clinic Proc. *28:*452, 1953.

Swan, H. J. C., Zapata-Diaz, J., Burchell, H. B., and Wood, E. H.: Pulmonary hypertension in congenital heart disease.

Am. J. Med. *16:*12, 1954.

Syhers, R. G., Syhers, J. L., Dickie, H. A., and Paul, L. W.: Roentgenographic aspects of hemorrhagic pulmonary-renal disease (Goodpasture's syndrome). Am. J. Roentgenol. *94:*674, 1965.

Symbas, P. N., et al: Rupture of aorta. Ann. Thoracic Surg. *15:*405, 1973.

Symbas, P. N., Baldwin, B. J., Silverman, M. E., and Galambos, J. T.: Marfan's syndrome with aneurysm of the ascending aorta and aortic regurgitation. Am. J.Cardiol. *25:*483, 1970.

Symbas, T. N., and Sehdeva, J. S.: Penetrating wounds of the thoracic aorta. Ann. Surg. *171:*441, 1970.

Szweda, J. A., and Drake, E. H.: Ruptured congenital aneurysms of the sinuses of Valsalva. A report of two cases treated surgically. Circulation *25:*559, 1962.

Tabakin, B. S., Hanson, J. S., Tampas, J. P., and Caldwell, E. J.: Congenital absence of the left pericardium. Am. J. Roentgenol. *94:*122, 1965.

Tachovsky, T. J., Giuliani, E. R., and Ellis, F. H.: Prosthetic valve replacement for traumatic tricuspid insufficiency: report of a case originally diagnosed as Ebstein's malformation. Am. J. Cardiol. *26:*196, 1970.

Takaro, T., Hultgren, H. N., Littmann, D., Wright, E. C., and Oteen, N. C.: An analysis of deaths occurring in association with coronary arteriography. Am. Heart J. *86:*587, 1973.

Takekawa, S. D., Kincaid, O. W., Titus, J. L., and DuShane, J. W.: Congenital aortic stenosis. Am. J. Roentgenol. *98:*800, 1966.

Talner, N. S., Stern, A. M., and Sloan, H. E., Jr.: Congenital mitral insufficiency. Circulation *23:*339, 1961.

Tampas, J. P., and Lurie, P. R.: The roentgenographic appearance of the chest in children with functional murmurs. Am. J. Roentgenol. *103:*78, 1968.

Tampas, J. P., and Soule, A. B.: Coronary artery calcification: incidence and significance in patients over 40 years of age. Am. J. Roentgenol. *97:*369, 1966.

Tandon, R., and Edwards, J. E.: Tricuspid atresia: a re-evaluation and classification. J. Thoracic Cardiovasc. Surg. *67:*530, 1974.

Tandon, R., Manchanda, S. C., and Roy, S. B.: Mitral stenosis with left-to-right shunt at the atrial level. Brit. Heart J. *33:*773, 1971.

Tandon, R., Marin-Garcia, J., Moller, J. H., and Edwards, J. E.: Tricuspid atresia with l-transposition. Am. Heart J. *88:*417, 1974.

Tasaka, S., Yoshikoshi, Y., Seki, K., Koide, K., Ogata, E., and Nakamura, K.: Congenital aneurysm of the right coronary sinus of Valsalva with rupture into the left ventricle. Jap. Heart J. *1:*106, 1960.

Taubenhaus, M., Eisenstein, B., and Pick, A.: Cardiovascular manifestations of collagen disease. Circulation *12:*903, 1955.

Taubman, J. O., Goodman, D. J., and Steiner, R. E.: The value of contrast studies in the investigation of aortic valve disease. Clin. Radiol. *17:*23, 1966.

Taussig, H.: Congenital Malformations of the Heart. II. Specific Malformations. Cambridge, The Harvard University Press, 1960.

Taussig, H. B. and Bing, R. J.: Complete transposition of the aorta and a levoposition of the pulmonary artery: clinical, physiological and pathological findings. Am. Heart J. *37:*551, 1949.

Taussig, H. B., Keinonen, R., Momberger, N., and Kirk, H.: Long-time observations on the Blalock-Taussig operation. IV. Tricuspid atresia. Johns Hopkins Med. J. *132:*135, 1973.

Taussig, H. B., Momberger, N., and Kirk, H.: Long-time observations on the Blalock-Taussig operation. VI. Truncus arteriosus, type IV. Johns Hopkins Med. J. *133:*123, 1973.

Tector, A. J., Reuben, C. F., Hoffman, J. F., Gelfand, E. T., Keelan, M., and Worman, L.: Coronary artery wounds treated with saphenous vein bypass grafts. J.A.M.A. *225:*282, 1973.

Tegtmeyer, C. J., and Deignan, J. M.: The cardiac pacemaker: a different twist. Am. J. Roentgenol. *126:*1017, 1976.

Tegtmeyer, C. J., Hunter, J. G., Jr., and Keats, T. E.: Bronchocutaneous fistula as a late complication of permanent epicardial pacing. Am. J. Roentgenol. *121:*614, 1974.

Teplick, J. G., Haskin, M. E., and Steinberg, S. B.: Changes in the main pulmonary artery segment following pulmonary embolism. Am. J. Roentgenol. *92:*557, 1964.

Thibeault, D. W., Emmanouilides, C. G., Nelson, R. J., Lackman, R. S., Rosengart, R. M., and Oh, W.: Patent ductus arteriosus complicating the respiratory distress syndrome in preterm infants. J. Pediat. *86:*120, 1975.

Thilenius, O. C., Bharati, S., and Lev, M.: Subdivided left atrium: an expanded concept of cor triatriatum sinistrum. Am. J. Cardiol. *37:*743, 1976.

Thomas, W. A., Randall, R. V., Bland, E. F., and Castleman, B.: Endocardial fibroelastosis: a factor in heart disease of obscure etiology. N. Engl. J. Med. *251:*327, 1954.

Thompson, S. I., Vieweg, W. V. R., Alpert, J. S., and Hagan, A. D.: Anomalous origin of the right coronary artery from the left sinus of valsalva with associated chest pain: report of two cases. Cath. Cardiovasc. Diag. *2:*397, 1976.

Tobin, J. R., Jr., Driscoll, J. F., Lim, M. T., Satton, G. C., Szanto, P. B., and Gunnar, R. M.: Primary myocardial disease and alcoholism: the clinical manifestations and course of the disease in a selected population of patients observed for three or more years. Circulation *35:*754, 1967.

Toledo, J., Nghiem, Q., and Harris, L.: Newborn emergency: pulmonary atresia or severe pulmonic stenosis with intact ventricular septum. Texas Med. *67:*78, 1971.

Torrance, D.: Personal communication. November, 1953.

Torrance, D. J., Jr.: Roentgenographic signs of pulmonary artery occlusion. Am. J. Med. Sci. *237:*651, 1959.

Tow, D. E. and Wagner, H. N., Jr.: Recovery of pulmonary flow in patients with pulmonary embolism. N. Engl. J. Med. *276:*1053, 1967.

Tracy, G. P., Brown, D. E., Johnson, L. W., and Gottlieb, A. J.: Radiation-induced coronary artery disease. J.A.M.A. *228:*1660, 1974.

Trent, J. K., Adelman, A. G., Wigle, E. D., and Silver, M. D.: Morphology of a prolapsed posterior mitral valve leaflet. Am. Heart J. *79:*539, 1970.

Trusler, G. A., Moes, C. A. S., and Kidd, D. S. L.: Repair of ventricular septal defect with aortic insufficiency. J. Thoracic Cardiovasc. Surg. *66:*394, 1973.

Tsakraklides, V. G., Blieden, L. C., and Edwards, J. E.: Coronary atherosclerosis and myocardial infarction in association with lupus erythematosus. Am. Heart J. *87:*637, 1974.

Tsioulias, T.: Calibre variations in the left ventricular outflow tract. Acta Radiol. *3:*209, 1965.

Turneey, S. Z., Mathai, J., Singleton, R., and Cowley, R. A.: Traumatic ventricular septal defect. Ann. Thoracic Surg. *13:*36, 1972.

Turner, A. F., Lau, F. Y. K., and Jacobson, G.: A method for the estimation of pulmonary venous and arterial pressures from the routine chest roentgenogram. Am. J. Roentgenol. *116:*97, 1972.

Turner, A. F., Meyers, H. I., Jacobson, G., and Lo, W.: Carbon dioxide cineangiocardiography in the diagnosis of pericardial disease. Am. J. Roentgenol. *97:*342, 1966.

Twigg, H. L., DeLeon, A. C., Perloff, J. K., and Majd, M.: The straight-back syndrome. Radiographic manifestations. Radiology *88:*274, 1967.

Tynan, M.: Survival of infants with transposition of the great arteries after balloon atrial septostomy. Lancet 1:621, 1971.

Tyson, K. R. T., Harris, L. C., and Nghiem, Q. X.: Repair of aortic arch interruption in the neonate. Surgery 67:1006, 1970.

Uhl, H. S.: Previously undescribed congenital malformation of the heart: almost total absence of the myocardium of the right ventricle. Bull. Johns Hopkins Hosp. 91:197, 1952.

Ungerleider, H. E. and Gubner, R.: Evaluation of heart size measurements. Am. Heart J. 24:494, 1942.

Upshaw, C. B.: Congenital coronary arteriovenous fistula: report of a case with an analysis of 73 reported cases. Am. Heart J. 63:390, 1962.

Urokinase Pulmonary Embolism Trial. Phase 1 results: a cooperative study. J.A.M.A. 214:2163, 1970.

Urokinase Pulmonary Embolism Trial. Circulation 47(Supp. 2):II-1, 1973.

Utley, J. R.: Hemodynamic determinants of risk in pulmonary artery banding. Am. J. Surg. 126:30, 1973.

Vacca, J. B., Bussmann, D. W., and Mudd, J. G.: Ebstein's anomaly: complete review of 108 cases. Am. J. Cardiol. 2:210, 1958.

Van Buchem, F. S. P. and Eerland, L. D.: Myxoma cordis. Dis. Chest 31:61, 1957.

Van Buchem, F. S. P., Nieveen, J., Marring, W., and Van Der Slikke, L. B.: Idiopathic dilatation of the pulmonary artery. Dis. Chest 28:326, 1955.

Vanderhoeft, P. J.: Broncho-pulmonary circuits: a synoptic appraisal. Thorax 19:537, 1964.

Van Epps, E. F.: Primary pulmonary hypertension in brothers. Am. J. Roentgenol. 78:471, 1957.

Van Mierop, L. H. S.: Cyanotic congenital heart disease. Cardiovasc. Clin. 5:1, 1973.

Van Mierop, L. H. S., Alley, R. D., Kausel, H. W., and Stranahan, A.: Ebstein's malformation of the left atrioventricular valve in corrected transposition, with subpulmonary stenosis and ventricular septal defect. Am. J. Cardiol. 8:270, 1961.

Van Mierop, L. H. S., Alley, R. D., Kausel, H. W., and Stranahan, A.: The anatomy and embryology of endocardial cushion defects. J. Thoracic Cardiovasc. Surg. 43:72, 1962.

Van Praagh, R.: Malpositions of the heart, In Heart Disease in Infants, Children and Adolescents. Edited by Moss, A. J., and Adams, F. H. (eds.), Chap. 29. Baltimore, The Williams & Wilkins Co., 1968.

Van Praagh, R.: What is the Taussig-Bing Malformation? Editorial. Circulation 38:445, 1968.

Van Praagh, R., Bernhard, W. F., Rosenthal, A., Parisi, L. F., and Eyler, D. C.: Interrupted aortic arch: surgical treatment. Am. J. Cardiol. 27:200, 1971.

Van Praagh, R., Ongley, P. A., and Swan, H. J. C.: Anatomic types of single or common ventricle in man: morphologic and geometric aspects of 60 necropsied cases. Am. J. Cardiol. 13:367, 1964.

Van Praagh, R., Van Praagh, S., Nebesar, R. A., Muster, A. J., Sinha, S. N., and Paul, M. H.: Tetralogy of Fallot: underdevelopment of the pulmonary infundibulum and its sequelae. Am. J. Cardiol. 26:25, 1970.

Van Praagh, R., Van Praagh, S., Vlad, P., and Keith, J. D.: Diagnosis of the anatomic types of congenital dextrocardia. Am. J. Cardiol. 15:234, 1954.

Van Praagh, R., Van Praagh, S., Vlad, P., and Keith, J. D.: Diagnosis of the anatomic types of single or common ventricle. Am. J. Cardiol. 15:345, 1965.

Van Tassel, R. A. and Edwards, J. E.: Rupture of the heart complicating myocardial infarction: analysis of 40 cases including nine examples of left ventricular false aneurysm. Chest 61:104, 1972.

Venables, A. W. and Hiller, H. G.: Complications of cardiac

investigation. Brit. Heart J. 25:334, 1963.

Viamonte, M., Jr.: Selective bronchial arteriography in man; preliminary report. Radiology 83:830, 1964.

Viamonte, M., Jr., Parks, R. E., and Barrera, F.: Roentgenographic prediction of pulmonary hypertension in mitral stenosis. Am. J. Roentgenol. 87:936, 1962.

Vickers, C. W., Kincaid, O. W., Ellis, F. H., and Bruwer, A. J.: Left atrial calcification. Radiology 72:569, 1959.

Victorica, B. E. and Elliott, L. P.: The roentgenologic findings and approach to persistent truncus arteriosus in infancy. Am. J. Roentgenol. 104:440, 1968.

Victorica, B. E., Krovetz, L. J., Elliott, L. P., Van Mierop, L. H. S., Bartley, T. D., Gessner, I. H., and Schiebler, G. L.: Persistent truncus arteriosus in infancy. Am. Heart J. 77:13, 1969.

Vieweg, W. V. R., Alpert, J. S., and Hagan, A. D.: Caliber and distribution of normal coronary arterial anatomy. Cath. Cardiovasc. Diag. 2:269, 1976.

Vineberg, A. M.: Development of an anastomosis between coronary vessels and a transplanted internal mammary artery. Canad. Med. Assoc. J. 55:117, 1946.

Vix, V. A. and Killen, D. A.: Traumatic pseudoaneurysm of the left ventricle. Am. J. Roentgenol. 104:413, 1968.

Vlodaver, Z., Neufeld, H. N., and Edwards, J. E.: Pathology of coronary disease. Sem. Roentgenol. 7:376, 1972.

Von Gronefeld, V. and Hauke, H.: Endocardial fibroelastosis: Radiological and angiocardiographic signs. Ann. Radiol. 17:405, 1973.

Voorhess, M. L., Husson, G. S., and Blackman, M. S.: Growth failure with pericardial constriction: the syndrome of Mulibrey nanism. Am. J. Dis. Child. 130:1146, 1976.

Wachtel, F. W., Ravitch, M. M., and Grisham, A.: The relation of pectus excavatum to heart disease. Am. Heart J. 52:121, 1956.

Wagenvoort, C. A., Neufeld, H. N., Birge, R. F., Caffrey, J. A., and Edwards, J. E.: Origin of right pulmonary artery from ascending aorta. Circulation 23:84, 1961.

Wagenvoort, C. A., Neufeld, H. N., DuShane, J. W., and Edwards, J. E.: The pulmonary arterial tree in ventricular septal defect: a quantitative study of anatomic features in fetuses, infants and children. Circulation 23:740, 1961.

Wagner, H. N., Jr., Sabiston, D. C., Jr., Iio, M., McAfee, J. G., Meyer, J. K., and Langan, J. K.: Regional pulmonary blood flow in man by radioisotope scanning. J.A.M.A. 187:601, 1964.

Wagner, H. N., Jr., Sabiston, D. C., Jr., McAfee, J. G., Tow, D., and Stern, H. S.: Diagnosis of massive pulmonary embolism in man by radioisotope scanning. N. Engl. J. Med. 271:377, 1964.

Wagner, H. N., Jr. and Tow, D. E.: Radioisotope scanning in the study of pulmonary circulation. Prog. Cardiovasc. Dis. 9:382, 1967.

Wagner, H. R. and Vlad, P.: Sudden unexpected death in cardiovascular disease in children: a cooperative international study. Am. J. Cardiol. 34:89, 1974.

Wainwright, C. W.: Intracardiac tumor producing the signs of valvular heart disease. Bull. Johns Hopkins Hosp. 63:187, 1938.

Wakai, C. S., Swan, H. J. C., and Wood, E. H.: Hemodynamic data and findings of diagnostic value in nine proved cases of persistent common atrioventricular canal. Proc. Staff Meet. Mayo Clin. 31:500, 1956.

Waldhausen, J. A., Lombardo, C. R., and Morrow, A. G.: Pulmonic stenosis due to compression of the pulmonary artery by an intrapericardial tumor. J. Thoracic Cardiovasc. Surg. 37:679, 1959.

Walker, W. J., Garcia-Gonzalez, E., Hall, R. J., Czarnecki, S. W., Franklin, R. G., Das, S. K., and Cheitlin, M. D.: Interventricular septal defect: analysis of 415 catheterized cases, 90 with serial hemodynamic studies. Circulation *31*:54, 1965.

Wallace, R. B., Rastelli, G. C., Ongley, P. A., Titus, J. H., and McGoon, D. C.: Complete repair of truncus arteriosus defect. J. Thoracic Cardiovasc. Surg. *57*:95, 1969.

Wallace, S., Medellin, H., Dejongh, D., and Gianturco, C.: Systemic heparinization for angiography. Am. J. Roentgenol. *116*:204, 1972.

Wallach, J. B., Lukash, L., and Angrist, A. A.: Frequency of tricuspid stenosis with particular reference to cardiac surgery. Dis. Chest *34*:537, 1958.

Walter, W. H.: Radiographic identification of commonly used pulse generators-1970. J.A.M.A. *215*:1974, 1971.

Wanderman, K. L., Goldstein, M. S., and Faber, J.: Cor pulmonale secondary to severe kyphoscoliosis in Marfan's syndrome. Chest *67*:250, 1975.

Wannamaker, L. W.: Acute rheumatic fever. *In* Heart Disease in Infants, Children and Adolescents, Moss, A. J. and Adams, F. H. (eds.), pp. 801–819. Baltimore, The Williams & Wilkins Co., 1968.

Warden, H. E., Lucas, R. V., Jr., and Varco, R. L.: Right ventricular obstruction resulting from anomalous muscle bundles. J. Thoracic Cardiovasc. Surg. *51*:53, 1966.

Warthen, R. O.: Congenital aneurysm of right anterior sinus of Valsalva (interventricular aneurysm) with spontaneous rupture into the left ventricle. Am. Heart J. *37*:975, 1949.

Waterston, D. J.: Treatment of Fallot's tetralogy in children under one year of age. Rozhl. Chir. *41*:181, 1962.

Watson, D. G.: Aortic valve atresia. J.A.M.A. *179*:14, 1962.

Watson, H.: Natural history of Ebstein's anomaly of tricuspid valve in childhood and adolescence: an international co-operative study of 505 cases. Brit. Heart J. *36*:417, 1974.

Watson, W. L.: Pulmonary arteriovenous aneurysm: a new surgical disease. Surgery *22*:919, 1947.

Webster, J. S., Moberg, C., and Rincon, G.: Natural history of severe proximal coronary artery disease as documented by coronary cineangiography. Am. J. Cardiol. *33*:195, 1974.

Weintraub, A. M. and Zvaifler, N. J.: The occurrence of valvular and myocardial disease in patients with chronic joint deformity: a spectrum. Am. J. Med. *35*:145, 1963.

Weintraub, R. A. and Abrams, H. L.: Mycotic aneurysms. Am. J. Roentgenol. *102*:354, 1968.

Weintraub, R. A., Fabian, C. E., and Adams, D. F.: Ectopic origin of one pulmonary artery from the ascending aorta. Radiology *86*:666, 1966.

Weiss, E.: Calcified plaque of the aorta at the entrance of a patent ductus arteriosus: a point in diagnosis. Am. Heart J. *7*:114, 1931.

Weiss, M. M. and Weiss, M. M., Jr.: The effect of myocardial infarction on the size of the heart. Am. J. Med. Sci. *234*:129, 1957.

Weiss, S., Stead, E. A., Jr., Warren, J. V., and Bailey, O. T.: Scleroderma heart disease with a consideration of certain other visceral manifestations of scleroderma. Arch. Int. Med. *71*:749, 1943.

Weiss, S. and Wilkins, R. W.: The nature of cardiovascular disturbances in nutritional deficiency states (beri-beri). Ann. Int. Med. *11*:104, 1937.

Wellons, H. A., Jr. and Singh, R.: Acute dissecting aortic aneurysm resulting from retrograde brachial arterial catheterization: successful operative intervention. Am. J. Cardiol. *33*:562, 1974.

Westermark, N.: On the roentgen diagnosis of lung embolism. Acta Radiol. *19*:357, 1938.

Wheat, M. W., Jr. and Palmer, R. F.: Drug therapy for dissecting aneurysms. Dis. Chest *54*:372, 1968.

Whitaker, W. and Lodge, T.: The radiological manifestations of pulmonary hypertension in patients with mitral stenosis. J. Fac. Radiol. *5*:182, 1954.

White, P. D.: Heart Disease, ed. 4. New York, The Macmillan Co., 1951.

Whiteleather, J. E. and DeSaussure, R. L.: Experience with a new contrast medium (Hypaque) for cerebral angiography. Radiology *67*:537, 1956.

Wholey, M. H.: Clinical dosimetry during the angiographic examination. Circulation *50*:627, 1974.

Wiederanders, R. E., White, S. M., and Saichek, H. B.: Effect of pulmonary resection on pulmonary artery pressures. Ann. Surg. *160*:889, 1964.

Wigle, E. D., Heimbecker, R. O., and Gunton, R. W.: Idiopathic ventricular septal hypertrophy causing muscular subaortic stenosis. Circulation *26*:325, 1962.

Wilkens, G. D.: Ein Fall von Multiplen Pulmonalis Aneurysm. Beitr. Klin. Tuberk. *38*:1, 1917.

Williams, H. J. and Carey, L. S.: Rubella embryopathy. Am. J. Roentgenol. *97*:92, 1966.

Williams, J. C. P., Barratt-Boyes, B. G., and Lowe, J. B.: Supravalvular aortic stenosis. Circulation *24*:134, 1961.

Williams, R. R., Kent, G. B., Jr., and Edwards, J. E.: Anomalous cardiac blood vessel communicating with the right ventricle. Observations in a case of pulmonary atresia with an intact ventricular septum. Arch. Pathol. *52*:480, 1951.

Wilson, A. C., Simpson, W. L., Richardson, J. P., and Clarebrough, J. K.: Mycotic aneurysms of the aortic root. Aust. N. Z. J. Surg. *42*:113, 1972.

Wilson, J. B., Hood, R. H., Johnson, H. H., Green, A. E., and Bauermeister, M. L.: Primary myocardial fibromas. Radiology *84*:1076, 1965.

Wilson, W.: A review of the causes of rib-notching with a report of an unusual case. Brit. J. Radiol. *33*:765, 1960.

Wilson, W. J., Amplatz, H., and Everhart, F.: Cinefluorographic study of prosthetic cardiac valves. Radiology *88*:779, 1967.

Wilson, W. J., Lee, G. B., and Amplatz, K.: Biplane selective coronary arteriography via femoral approach. Am. J. Roentgenol. *100*:332, 1967.

Windholz, F. and Grayson, C. E.: Roentgen demonstration of calcification in the interventricular septum in cases of heart block. Am. J. Roentgenol. *58*:411, 1947.

Winters, W. L., Jr., Mark, G. E., Jr., and Soloff, L. A.: Left atrial pressure curve in left atrial myxoma. Arch. Int. Med. *107*:384, 1961.

Wittenborg, M. H., Neuhauser, E. B. D., and Sprunt, W. H.: Roentgenographic findings in congenital tricuspid atresia with hypoplasia of the right ventricle. Am. J. Roentgenol. *66*:712, 1951.

Wittenborg, M. H., Tantiwongse, T., and Rosenberg, B. F.: Anomalous course of the left pulmonary artery with respiratory obstruction. Radiology *67*:339, 1956.

Witzleben, C. L.: Idiopathic infantile arterial calcification—A misnomer? Am. J. Cardiol. *26*:305, 1970.

Wolke, K.: Two cases of coarctation (stenosis of the isthmus) of the aorta. Acta Radiol. *18*:319, 1937.

Wolkin, A.: Significance of calcification in ascending portion of aortic arch. Radiology *62*:101, 1954.

Wollenweber, J., Giuliani, E. R., Harrison, C. E., Jr., and Kincaid, O. W.: Pseudotumors of the right heart. Arch. Int. Med. *121*:169, 1968.

Wood, B. P., Young, L. W., and Elbadawi, N. A.: Primary mycotic aneurysm in infancy and childhood. Am. J. Roentgenol. *118*:109, 1973.

Wood, P.: Pulmonary hypertension. Brit. Med. Bull. *8*:348, 1952.

Wood, P.: An appreciation of mitral stenosis. Part II. Investigations and results. Brit. Med. J. *1*:1113, 1954.

Wood, P.: Diseases of the Heart and Circulation, ed. 2., p. 457. Philadelphia, J. B. Lippincott Co., 1956.

Wood, P.: Aortic stenosis. Am. J. Cardiol. *1*:553, 1958.

Woodruff, J. H., Jr.: Calcified heart valves (a comparison of methods for their demonstration). Radiology 79:384, 1962.

Wray, T. M. and Stone, W. J.: Uremic pericarditis: a prospective echocardiographic and clinical study. Clin. Nephrol. 6:295, 1976.

Wright, L. S., Jaffe, R., Lewis, D., and Figley, M. M.: A method for double-contrast stereoscopic study of the internal anatomy of the heart. Radiology 83:1003, 1964.

Wyler, F., Rutishauser, M., Fliegle, C., Buchs, S., and Gradel, E.: Aortic aneurysms as a late complication in the syndrome of supravalvular aortic stenosis, peculiar facies and mental retardation. Am. J. Roentgenol. 119:524, 1973.

Wyman, S. M.: Congenital absence of a pulmonary artery: its demonstration by roentgenography. Radiology 62:321, 1954.

Wyman, S. M.: Dissecting aneurysm of the thoracic aorta: its roentgen recognition. Am. J. Roentgenol. 78:247, 1957.

Wyman, S. M. and Eyler, W. R.: Anomalous pulmonary artery from the aorta associated with intrapulmonary cysts (intralobar sequestration of lung): its roentgenologic recognition and clinical significance. Radiology 59:658, 1962.

Wynn, A.: Gross calcification in the mitral valve. Brit. Heart J. 15:214, 1953.

Yang, S. S., Bentivoglio, L. G., Maranhao, V., and Goldberg, H.: From Cardiac Catheterization Data to Hemodynamic Parameters, F. A. Davis, Co., Philadelphia, 1972.

Yanoff, M. F., Frank, J. H., and Frost, J. W.: Primary mycotic thoracic aorta aneurysm caused by Salmonella choleraesuis. Am. J. Med. 38:145, 1965.

Yater, W. M.: Tumors of the heart and pericardium. Pathology, symptomatology and report of nine cases. Arch. Int. Med. 48:627, 1931.

Yates, J. D., Kirsh, M. M., Sodeman, T. M., Walton, J. A., Jr., and Brymer, J. F.: Coronary ostial stenosis: a complication of aortic valve replacement. Circulation 49:530, 1974.

Youker, J. E.: Prevention of complications during vascular opacification studies. Rad. Clinics N.A. 3(3):453, 1965.

Young, D.: Later results of closure of secundum atrial septal defect in children. Am. J. Cardiol. 31:14, 1973.

Zamalloa, O., De Franceschi, A., and Leachman, R. D.: Clinical and angiographic diagnosis of the "parachute mitral valve." Acta Cardiol. 24:101, 1969.

Zaret, B.L., Pitt, B., and Ross, R. S.: Determination of the site, extent, and significance of regional ventricular dysfunction during acute myocardial infarction. Circulation 45:441, 1972.

Zetterqvist, P.: Atypical coarctation of the aorta with bilateral vertebral-subclavian pathway. A report of the first known case of preligamental aortic arch interruption and its surgical correction. Scand. J. Thoracic Cardiovascular Surg. 1:68, 1967.

Ziady, G. L., Hallidie-Smith, K. A., and Goodwin, J. F.: Conduction disturbances after surgical closure of ventricular septal defect. Brit. Heart J. 34:1199, 1972.

Ziegler, R. F.: Patent ductus arteriosus. In Heart Disease In Infants, Children, and Adolescents. Moss, A. J. and Adams, F. H. (eds.), pp. 338–357. Baltimore, Williams & Wilkins Co., 1968.

Zizmon, J., and Szucs, M. M.: Echinococcus cyst of the heart. Report of a case. Am. J. Roentgenol. 53:15, 1945.

Zoll, P. M., Linenthal, A. J., and Norman, L. R.: Treatment of Stokes-Adams disease by external electric stimulation of the heart. Circulation 9:942, 1954.

Zoll, P. M., Paul, M. H., Linenthal, A. J., Norman, L. R., and Gibson, W.: The effects of external electric currents on the heart. Control of cardiac rhythm and induction and termination of cardiac arrhythmias. Circulation 14:745, 1956.

Zuberbuhler, J. R., and Blank, E.: Hypoplasia of right ventricular myocardium. Am. J. Roentgenol. 110:491, 1970.

Zumbro, G. L., Hinley, L. B., and Tremare, R. L.: Saccular aneurysm of ascending aorta caused by granulomatous aortitis in a child. J. Thoracic Cardiovasc. Surg. 69:397, 1975.

Zvaifler, N. J. and Weintraub, A. M.: Aortitis and aortic insufficiency in chronic rheumatic disorders. A reappraisal. Arthritis and Rheum. 6:241, 1963.

Index

(Page numbers in italic type refer to illustrations.)